From the desk of
Steven R. Garfin, M.D.

AF887248

Instructional Course Lectures

Volume 50 2001

American Academy
of Orthopaedic Surgeons

Instructional Course Lectures

Volume 50 2001
Including index for 1997, 1998, 1999, 2000, and 2001

Edited by
Franklin H. Sim, MD
Professor of Orthopedic Surgery
Department of Orthopedic Surgery
Mayo Clinic
Rochester, Minnesota

American Academy
of Orthopaedic Surgeons
6300 North River Road
Rosemont, IL 60018

American Academy of Orthopaedic Surgeons
Instructional Course Lectures
Volume 50

Board of Directors, 2000

S. Terry Canale, MD, *President*
Richard H. Gelberman, MD
Vernon T. Tolo, MD
William J. Robb III, MD
Andrew J. Weiland, MD
Robert D. D'Ambrosia, MD
James D. Heckman, MD
Joseph P. Iannotti, MD, PhD
Ramon L. Jimenez, MD
Darren L. Johnson, MD
Thomas P. Sculco, MD
John R. Tongue, MD
David A. Halsey, MD
Lowry Jones Jr, MD
Richard B. Welch, MD
Gary E. Friedlaender, MD
William W. Tipton Jr, MD *(ex officio)*

Staff

Vice President, Educational Programs: Mark W. Wieting
Director, Department of Publications: Marilyn L. Fox, PhD
Senior Editor: Lisa Claxton Moore
Manager, Production and Archives: Mary Steermann
Assistant Production Manager: Sophie Tosta
Production Assistants: Kathleen Anderson, Courtney Astle, Karen Danca

Instructional Course Lectures Volume 50
American Academy of Orthopaedic Surgeons

The material presented in *Instructional Course Lectures Volume 50* has been made available by the American Academy of Orthopaedic Surgeons for educational purposes only. This material is not intended to present the only, or necessarily best, methods or procedures for the medical situations discussed, but rather is intended to represent an approach, view, statement, or opinion of the author(s) or producer(s), which may be helpful to others who face similar situations.

Some drugs or medical devices demonstrated in Academy courses or described in Academy print or electronic publications have not been cleared by the Food and Drug Administration (FDA) or have been cleared for specific uses only. The FDA has stated that it is the responsibility of the physician to determine the FDA clearance status of each drug or device he or she wishes to use in clinical practice.

Furthermore, any statements about commercial products are solely the opinion(s) of the author(s) and do not represent an Academy endorsement or evaluation of these products. These statements may not be used in advertising or for any commercial purpose.

All rights reserved. No part of this publication may be reproduced, stored in a retrieval system, or transmitted, in any form, or by any means, electronic, mechanical, photocopying, recording, or otherwise, without prior written permission from the publisher.

Copyright © 2001 by the American Academy of Orthopaedic Surgeons

Contributors

Jeffrey S. Abrams, MD, Associate Medical Director, Princeton Orthopaedic and Rehabilitation Associates, Attending Orthopaedic Surgeon, Princeton Medical Center, Princeton, New Jersey

Alptekin Aksan, MS, Department of Mechanical Engineering, Michigan State University, East Lansing, Michigan

Deborah J. Ammeen, BS, Project Director, Knee Clinical Research, Anderson Orthopaedic Research Institute, Alexandria, Virginia

Kyle Anderson, MD, Senior Staff Team Physician, Detroit Tigers, Department of Orthopaedic Surgery, Henry Ford Health System, Detroit, Michigan

James R. Andrew, MD, Clinical Professor of Surgery, University of Alabama at Birmingham School of Medicine, Medical Director, American Sports Medicine Institute, Alabama Sports Medicine and Orthopaedics Center, Birmingham, Alabama

Christopher C. Annunziata, MD, Fellow, Center for Sports Medicine, University of Pittsburgh, Pittsburgh, Pennsylvania

Michael J. Archibeck, MD, Fellow, Joint Replacement, Department of Orthopaedic Surgery, Rush-Presbyterian-St. Luke's Medical Center, Chicago, Illinois

Steven P. Arnoczky, DVM, Professor and Director, Laboratory for Comparative Orthopaedic Research, Michigan State University, East Lansing, Michigan

David D. Aronsson, MD, Professor, Department of Orthopaedics and Rehabilitation, University of Vermont College of Medicine, Burlington, Vermont

David C. Ayers, MD, Director, Joint Replacement Surgery, Department of Orthopaedic Surgery, Syracuse University New York Upstate Medical University, Syracuse, New York

Kyle F. Baldwin, DPT, Physical Therapy Coordinator, The Bone and Joint Institute at Good Samaritan Hospital, Los Angeles, California

Sue D. Barber-Westin, BS, Director, Clinical Studies, Cincinnati Sports Medicine Research and Education Foundation, Cincinnati, Ohio

Robert L. Barrack, MD, Professor, Orthopaedic Surgery, Department of Orthopaedics and Adult Reconstructive Surgery, Tulane Medical Center, New Orleans, Louisiana

Raman Battish, BS, Department of Orthopaedic Surgery, University of Pennsylvania Hospital, Philadelphia, Pennsylvania

Daniel J. Berry, MD, Associate Professor of Orthopaedics, Mayo Medical School, Consultant in Orthopaedic Surgery, Mayo Clinic, Department of Orthopaedic Surgery, Mayo Foundation, Rochester, Minnesota

Louis U. Bigliani, MD, Chief, The Shoulder Service, Department of Orthopaedic Surgery, College of Physicians and Surgeons, Columbia University, New York, New York

Hugh R.L. Blackley, MB, ChB, FRACS, Consultant Orthopaedic Surgeon, Department of Orthopaedic Surgery, Auckland Hospital, Auckland, New Zealand

Theodore A. Blaine, MD, Fellow, The Shoulder Service, Department of Orthopaedic Surgery, College of Physicians and Surgeons, Columbia University, New York, New York

Robert B. Bourne, MD, FRCSC, A.D. McLachlin Professor, Department of Surgery, University of Western Ontario, London Health Sciences Centre University Campus, London, Ontario, Canada

James P. Bradley, MD, Clinical Associate Professor, Department of Orthopaedics, University of Pittsburgh, Pittsburgh, Pennsylvania

Pieter Buma, PhD, Director of Histomorphology, Department of Orthopaedics, Orthopedic Research Laboratory, University Medical Center Nijmegen, Nijmegen, The Netherlands

John J. Callaghan, MD, Department of Orthopaedics, University of Iowa, Iowa City, Iowa

Henry D. Clarke, MD, Attending Orthopaedic Surgeon, Insall Scott Kelly Institute, Beth Israel Medical Center, New York, New York

William P. Cooney III, MD, Professor of Orthopedic Surgery, Mayo Graduate School of Medicine, Department of Orthopedic Surgery, Mayo Clinic, Rochester, Minnesota

Douglas A. Dennis, MD, Professor, Colorado School of Mines, Clinical Director, Rocky Mountain Musculoskeletal Research Laboratory, Denver, Colorado

Matthew B. Dobbs, MD, Resident Physician, Department of Orthopaedic Surgery, University of Iowa Hospitals and Clinics, Iowa City, Iowa

Lawrence D. Dorr, MD, Director, Bone and Joint Institute, Department of Orthopaedics, Good Samaritan Hospital, Los Angeles, California

Jeffrey R. Dugas, MD, Fellow, Orthopaedic Sports Medicine, American Sports Medicine Institute, Birmingham, Alabama

Michael J. Dunbar, MD, FRCSC, Assistant Professor of Orthopaedics, Clinical Research Scholar, Dalhousie University, Halifax, Nova Scotia, Canada

Clive P. Duncan, MD, FRCSC, Professor and Chairman, Department of Orthopaedics, Faculty of Medicine, University of British Columbia, Vancouver, British Columbia, Canada

Roger C. Dunteman, MD, Fellow, Sports Medicine, Southern California Orthopaedic Institute, Van Nuys, California

Malcolm L. Ecker, MD, Associate Professor of Orthopaedics, Department of Orthopaedics, University of Pennsylvania School of Medicine, Philadelphia, Pennsylvania

Gerard A. Engh, MD, Director, Knee Research, Anderson Orthopaedic Research Institute, Alexandria, Virginia

Diego L. Fernandez, MD, PD, Associate Professor of Orthopaedic Surgery, University of Berne, Department of Orthopaedics, Lindenhof Hospital, Berne, Switzerland

Evan L. Flatow, MD, Lasker Professor of Orthopaedic Surgery, Chief of Shoulder Surgery, Mt. Sinai Medical Center, New York, New York

Michael Q. Freehill, MD, Fellow, The Shoulder Service, Department of Orthopaedic Surgery, College of Physicians and Surgeons, Columbia University, New York, New York

Carol Frey, MD, Assistant Clinical Professor, Department of Orthopaedic Surgery, University of California at Los Angeles, Manhattan Beach, California

Marc J. Friedman, MD, Assistant Clinical Professor of Orthopaedics, University of California at Los Angeles School of Medicine, Southern California Orthopaedic Institute, Van Nuys, California

Reinhold Ganz, MD, Professor and Chairman, Department of Orthopaedic Surgery, University of Berne, Inselspital, Berne, Switzerland

Donald S. Garbuz, MD, MHSc, FRCSC, Clinical Assistant Professor, Department of Orthopaedics, Faculty of Medicine, University of British Columbia, Vancouver, British Columbia, Canada

Jean W.M. Gardeniers, MD, PhD, Department of Orthopaedics, University Medical Centre Nijmegen, Nijmegen, The Netherlands

Steven R. Garfin, MD, Professor and Chairman, Department of Orthopaedics, University of California at San Diego, San Diego, California

Richard H. Gelberman, MD, Reynolds Professor and Chairman, Department of Orthopaedic Surgery, Barnes-Jewish Hospital at Washington University, St. Louis, Missouri

J. Robert Giffin, MD, FRCSC, Clinical and Research Fellow, Center for Sports Medicine, University of Pittsburgh, Pittsburgh, Pennsylvania

Tibor T. Glant, MD, PhD, Professor, Department of Orthopaedics and Biochemistry, Rush-Presbyterian-St. Luke's Medical Center, Chicago, Illinois

Victor M. Goldberg, MD, Professor and Chairman, Department of Orthopaedics, Case Western Reserve University, Cleveland, Ohio

A. Seth Greenwald, DPhil (Oxon), Director, Orthopaedic Research Laboratory, Department of Orthopaedic Research, Mount Sinai Medical Center, Cleveland, Ohio

Allan E. Gross, MD, FRCSC, Professor of Surgery, University of Toronto, Head, Divison of Orthopaedic Surgery, Mount Sinai Hospital, Toronto, Ontario, Canada

Fares S. Haddad, BSc, MCH(Orth), FRCS, Consultant Orthopaedic Surgeon, University College London Hospitals, Department of Orthopaedics, London, United Kingdom

Arlen D. Hanssen, MD, Associate Professor of Orthopaedic Surgery, Mayo Clinic, Mayo Foundation, Rochester, Minnesota

Christopher D. Harner, MD, Professor and Director, Section of Sports Medicine, Department of Orthopaedic Surgery, University of Pittsburgh, Pittsburgh, Pennsylvania

William H. Harris, MD, Alan Gerry Clinical Professor of Orthopaedic Surgery, Harvard Medical School, Orthopaedic Adult Reconstructive Unit, Massachusetts General Hospital, Boston, Massachusetts

Richard J. Hawkins, MD, FRCSC, Orthopaedic Consultant, Steadman Hawkins Clinic, Vail, Colorado

Patrick R.L. Hayes, MD, Chief, Shoulder Service, Department of Orthopedic Surgery, National Navy Medical Center, Bethesda, Maryland

Richard J. Haynes, MD, Chief of Staff, Shriners Hospitals for Children, Houston, Texas

Harry N. Herkowitz, MD, Chairman, Department of Orthopaedic Surgery, William Beaumont Hospital, Royal Oak, Michigan

Richard J. Herzog, MD, FACR, Chief, Division of Teleradiology, Department of Radiology and Imaging, Hospital for Special Surgery, New York, New York

Robert N. Hotchkiss, MD, Chief, Hand Service, Hospital for Special Surgery, New York, New York

David S. Hungerford, MD, Professor of Orthopaedics, Department of Orthopaedics, The Johns Hopkins Medical Institution, Baltimore, Maryland

John N. Insall, MD, Director, Insall-Scott-Kelly Institute for Orthopaedics and Sports Medicine, Chief, Adult Knee Reconstruction, Department of Orthopaedics, Beth Israel Medical Center, New York, New York

Joshua J. Jacobs, MD, Professor, Department of Orthopaedic Surgery, Rush-Presbyterian-St. Luke's Medical Center, Chicago, Illinois

Greg Jaroszynski, MD, FRCSC, Orthopaedic Surgeon, Division of Orthopaedics, Department of Surgery, Joseph Brant Memorial Hospital, Burlington, Ontario, Canada

Miguel A. Jimenez, MD, Resident, Department of Orthopaedic Surgery, Mayo Clinic, Rochester, Minnesota

Jesse B. Jupiter, MD, Director, Orthopaedic Hand Service, Massachusetts General Hospital, Boston, Massachusetts

Spero G. Karas, MD, Assistant Professor, Department of Orthopaedics, University of North Carolina at Chapel Hill, Chapel Hill, North Carolina

Michael A. Kelly, MD, Director, Insall-Scott-Kelly Institute for Orthopaedics and Sports Medicine, Department of Orthopaedic Surgery, Beth Israel Hospital, New York, New York

Graham J.W. King, MD, MSc, FRCS, Associate Professor, Department of Surgery, Hand and Upper Limb Centre, University of Western Ontario, London, Ontario, Canada

Richard D. Komistek, PhD, President and Executive Director, Rocky Mountain Musculoskeletal Research Laboratory, Denver, Colorado

Kenneth A. Krackow, MD, Clinical Director, Department of Orthopaedic Surgery, Kaleida Health/Buffalo General Hospital, Buffalo, New York

Carlos Lavernia, MD, Associate Professor, Orthopaedic Surgery and Biomedical Engineering, Director, Division of Arthritis Surgery, Department of Orthopaedics and Rehabilitation, University of Miami School of Medicine, Miami, Florida

Michael Leunig, MD, Department of Orthopaedic Surgery, University of Berne, Inselspital, Berne, Switzerland

Randall T. Loder, MD, Chief of Staff, Shriner's Hospitals for Children, Minneapolis, Minnesota

Jess H. Lonner, MD, Assistant Professor of Orthopaedic Surgery, Pennsylvania Orthopaedic Institute, University of Pennsylvania School of Medicine, Philadelphia, Pennsylvania

Paul A. Lotke, MD, Professor of Orthopaedic Surgery, Department of Orthopaedic Surgery, University of Pennsylvania Hospital, Philadelphia, Pennsylvania

Kyle Low, MD, Orthopaedic Resident, Department of Orthopaedics, The John Hopkins Medical Institution, Baltimore, Maryland

Bassam A. Masri, MD, FRCSC, Clinical Associate Professor and Head, Division of Reconstructive Orthopaedics, University of British Columbia, Vancouver, British Columbia, Canada

Eric C. McCarty, MD, Assistant Professor and Team Physician, Vanderbilt University, Department of Orthopaedics and Rehabilitation, Vanderbilt University Medical Center, Nashville, Tennessee

Harry A. McKellop, PhD, Director, The J. Vernon Luck Orthopaedic Research Center, Orthopaedic Hospital, University of California at Los Angeles, Los Angeles, California

Dana C. Mears, MD, PhD, Professor and Chief, Division of Orthopaedic Surgery, Albany Medical Center, Albany, New York

Michael A. Mont, MD, Associate Professor of Orthopaedics, Department of Orthopaedics, The John Hopkins Medical Institution, Baltimore, Maryland

Bernard F. Morrey, MD, Professor and Emeritus Chairman, Department of Orthopaedic Surgery, Mayo Clinic, Rochester, Minnesota

Colin F. Moseley, MD, BSc, CM, Chief of Staff, Shriner's Hospitals for Children, Los Angeles, California

Sandeep Munjal, MD, Fellow, Adult Joint Reconstruction, Department of Orthopaedics, Buffalo General Hospital, Buffalo, New York

David W. Murray, MD, FRCS, Professor, Nuffield Orthopaedic Centre, Oxford, England

Charles L. Nelson, MD, Assistant Professor of Orthopaedic Surgery, Department of Orthopaedic Surgery, University of Pennsylvania, Philadelphia, Pennsylvania

Frank R. Noyes, MD, Adjunct Professor, Department of Aerospace Engineering and Engineering Mechanics, University of Cincinnati, Cincinnati, Ohio

Shawn W. O'Driscoll, PhD, MD, FRCS, Professor of Orthopaedic Surgery, Department of Orthopaedic Surgery, Mayo Clinic and Foundation, Rochester, Minnesota

Thomas R. Oxland, PhD, Associate Professor and Director, Division of Orthopaedic Engineering Research, Departments of Orthopaedics and Mechanical Engineering, University of British Columbia, Vancouver, British Columbia, Canada

Douglas E. Padgett, MD, Department of Orthopaedic Surgery, Hospital for Special Surgery, New York, New York

Kostas P. Panagiotopoulos, MD, BSc, Orthopaedic Surgery Resident, Department of Orthopaedic Surgery, Vancouver General Hospital, Vancouver, British Columbia, Canada

Paul M. Pellicci, MD, Department of Orthopaedic Surgery, Hospital for Special Surgery, New York, New York

Glenn B. Pfeffer, MD, Assistant Clinical Professor, Department of Orthopaedics, University of California at San Francisco, San Francisco, California

Matthew J. Phillips, MD, Assistant Clinical Professor of Orthopaedics, Department of Orthopaedic Surgery, State University of New York at Buffalo, Buffalo, New York

Derek Plausinis, MASc, MD, Resident, Orthopaedic Surgery, Department of Orthopaedic Surgery, University of British Columbia, Vancouver, British Columbia, Canada

Wolfgang Rauschning, MD, PhD, Professor of Clinical Anatomy, Academic University Hospital, Uppsala, Sweden

Michael D. Ries, MD, Associate Professor, Department of Orthopaedic Surgery, University of California at San Francisco, San Francisco, California

Graham M. Robbins, MD, Clinical and Research Fellow, Department of Orthopaedics, University of British Columbia, Vancouver, British Columbia, Canada

Kenneth A. Roebuck, PhD, Associate Professor, Department of Immunology, Rush-Presbyterian-St. Luke's Medical Center, Chicago, Illinois

Cecil H. Rorabeck, MD, Professor and Chairman, Division of Orthopaedic Surgery, London Health Science Center, London, Ontario, Canada

Khaled J. Saleh, MD, MSc, FRCSC, Assistant Professor, Department of Orthopaedic Surgery, University of Minnesota, Minneapolis, Minnesota

B. Willem Schreurs, MD, PhD, Department of Orthopaedics, University Medical Centre Nijmegen, Nijmegen, The Netherlands

Richard D. Scott, MD, Associate Clinical Professor, Department of Orthopaedic Surgery, Harvard Medical School, Boston, Massachusetts

Giles R. Scuderi, MD, Associate Chief, Adult Knee Reconstruction, Department of Orthopaedic Surgery, Beth Israel Medical Center, New York, New York

Thomas P. Sculco, MD, Department of Orthopaedic Surgery, Hospital for Special Surgery, New York, New York

Gary S. Shapiro, MD, Department of Orthopaedic Surgery, Hospital for Special Surgery, New York, New York

Alexander Y. Shin, MD, Commander, Medical Corps, United States Navy, Director, Division of Hand and Microvascular Surgery, Department of Orthopaedic Surgery, Naval Medical Center at San Diego, San Diego, California

Klaus A. Siebenrock, MD, Department of Orthopaedic Surgery, University of Berne, Inselspital, Berne, Switzerland

Thomas J.J.H. Slooff, MD, PhD, Professor of Orthopaedics, Department of Orthopaedics, University Medical Centre Nijmegen, Nijmegen, The Netherlands

John W. Sperling, MD, MS, Assistant Professor of Orthopaedic Surgery, Mayo Medical School, Senior Associate Consultant in Orthopaedic Surgery, Mayo Clinic, Rochester, Minnesota

Michael J. Stuart, MD, Assistant Professor and Co-Director of Sports Medicine, Department of Orthopedics, Mayo Clinic, Rochester, Minnesota

Robert M. Szabo, MD, MPH, Professor and Chief, Hand, Microvascular and Upper Extremity Surgery, Department of Orthopaedic Surgery, University of California, Davis Medical Center, Sacramento, California

Robert L. Thornberry, MD, Department of Orthopedic Surgery, Tallahassee Orthopedic Clinic, Tallahassee, Florida

Evangelos Tozakoglou, PhD, Senior Technology Manager, Smith & Nephew Orthopaedics, Memphis, Tennessee

Robert T. Trousdale, MD, Associate Professor of Orthopedic Surgery, Mayo Clinic, Rochester, Minnesota

Thomas E. Trumble, MD, Professor and Chief, Hand and Microvascular Surgery Service, University of Washington, Department of Orthopaedics and Sports Medicine, University of Washington Medical Center, Seattle, Washington

Eeric Truumees, MD, Spine Surgeon, Department of Orthopaedic Surgery, William Beaumont Hospital, Royal Oak, Michigan

John H. Velyvis, MD, Resident and Research Fellow, Division of Orthopaedic Surgery, Albany Medical Center, Albany, New York

Nico Verdonschot, PhD, Director of Implant Biomechanics, Department of Orthopedics, Orthopedic Research Laboratory, University Medical Centre Nijmegen, Nijmegen, The Netherlands

Jon J.P. Warner, MD, Chief, The Harvard Shoulder Service, Associate Professor, Partner's Department of Orthopaedics, Massachusetts General and Brigham and Women's Hospital, Boston, Massachusetts

Russell F. Warren, MD, Surgeon-in-Chief, Hospital for Special Surgery, New York, New York

Daniel Weiland, MD, New York, New York

Stuart L. Weinstein, MD, Ponseti Professor of Orthopaedic Surgery, Department of Orthopaedic Surgery, University of Iowa Hospital and Clinics, Iowa City, Iowa

R. Baxter Willis, MD, Chairman, Department of Orthopaedics, Department of Pediatric Orthopaedic Surgery, Children's Hospital, New Orleans, Louisana

Ian G. Woodgate, FRACS, Department of Orthopaedics, St. Vincent's Hospital, Sydney, New South Wales, Australia

Ken Yamaguchi, MD, Assistant Professor, Chief, Shoulder and Elbow Service, Department of Orthopaedic Surgery, Washington University School of Medicine, St. Louis, Missouri

Foreword

The Instructional Course Lectures have been a rich and very important part of the educational milieu of orthopaedic surgeons for over 50 years. In February 1973, being 3 years into my residency, I was already well aware of their value. All too often, I had been sent scurrying to *The Journal of Bone and Joint Surgery* or the *Instructional Course Lectures* volumes to look up the "right answer" to a question I had asked. Thus, it was with great anticipation that I attended my first annual meeting in Las Vegas. I spent Friday morning listening to Henry Mankin's lecture on vitamin D deficiency, and Bob Jackson's introduction to arthroscopy of the knee. On Saturday morning, I learned about the complications of total hip replacement from Drs. Amstutz, Coventry, Evarts, and Stinchfield. The best lecture of all, however, occurred on Sunday morning, when Drs. Mooney and Sarmiento presented their instructional course on fracture bracing, and we actually had a hands-on demonstration of how to make a functional brace, personally demonstrated by Dr. Sarmiento. I am sure that those courses forever affected the way I practice orthopaedics.

The Instructional Course Lectures were first introduced in 1942. James E.M. Thomson, MD, was the driving force behind this radical departure in orthopaedic education. He tells us, "I was alerted to its usefulness a few years before, when I had had the privilege of taking a 4-hour instructional course on the anatomy of the head at the Annual Meeting of the Academy of O.E.N.T. in Chicago... In those 4 hours, I had a very impressive refresher course on the anatomy of the head. To my surprise, I found there were over 2,000 in attendance at this meeting, and that hundreds of similar courses were in progress most of the day."[1] From that experience, he persuaded the leadership of the AAOS to introduce Instructional Course Lectures at the AAOS Annual Meeting. He had problems: "As with any innovation, this idea had its opponents, as well as proponents. Many were firmly against any deviation from the time-honored, stereotyped, formal scientific discussions and scientific exhibits."[2] Nevertheless, at the annual meeting in 1942, 56 hours of Instructional Courses were presented. The lectures were met with great success and, "the greatest complaint was the inability to hear all the Instructional Courses offered."[3] Because of their popularity, Dr. Thomson was encouraged to publish the lectures, and the first group appeared under the title *Lectures on Peace and War—Orthopaedic Surgery* in 1943.

In his foreword to the 1946 volume, entitled *Regional Orthopaedic Surgery and Fundamental Orthopaedic Problems*, Dr. Thomson indicated that his desire was "...to present orthopaedic problems from a new approach, placing them on a regional and anatomical basis. Therefore, in a presentation of each region, there was a review of the anatomy with particular reference to the importance of the proper surgical approaches and the relation of the soft-tissue and bony structures to possible pathology. Further, that pathology, diagnosis, and treatment of both trauma and disease of each region, was considered."[4]

Volume V, the first volume to actually carry the title *American Academy of Orthopaedic Surgeons Instructional Course Lectures*, was published in 1948. In the foreword to that volume, we find that "as a 'refresher' in orthopaedic surgery, the books should continue to be of particular value to the younger men. No attempt has been made to avoid duplication of subject material. A fresh approach is offered in the selection of a varied faculty."[5]

To this day, the *Instructional Course Lectures* volumes have been a tremendous complement to the scientific articles published in the orthopaedic literature. They are grounded in good science but are embellished and enhanced by the personal experience of the presenter. While allowing the lecturer this freedom of expression always risks the introduction of bias, it also creates the opportunity to season the raw material with experience and expertise. In this way, the scientific information available in the literature is effectively filtered and amplified by the judgment gained by the lecturer through years of clinical experience. It is for this reason that these lectures have had such a profound and long-lasting effect on the education of so many orthopaedic surgeons, both in residency and beyond. The enduring popularity of the Instructional Course Lectures, which are presented from the podium and via surgical demonstration at the Annual Meeting and then are published either in *The Journal of Bone and Joint Surgery* and in these independent volumes, attests to their value as a means of sharing clinical competence and delivering the highest possible quality of care to our patients. Thus, it is with great pride that the Academy presents this 50th volume of *Instructional Course Lectures*, which brings to the 21st century the best available information on the treatment of our patients, presented in the context of clinical experience and judgment by respected leaders in our field.

We pay tribute, and say thanks, to all who have contributed to creating this important foundation of orthopaedic knowledge over the last half century.

James D. Heckman, MD
Past President, American Academy of Orthopaedic Surgeons

---

1. Thomson JEM: Wise or otherwise, in Heck CV (ed): *1933-1983 Fifty Years of Progress In Recognition of the 50th Anniversary of The American Academy of Orthopaedic Surgeons.* Chicago, Illinois, American Academy of Orthopaedic Surgeons, 1983, p 189.
2. Ibid, page 190.
3. Ibid, page 191.
4. Thomson, JEM: *The American Academy of Orthopaedic Surgeons Presents Lectures on Regional Orthopaedic Surgery and Fundamental Orthopaedic Problems.* Selected from the Instructional Courses of the Thirteenth Annual Assembly; January 19-23, 1946, Chicago, Illinois. Ann Arbor, MI, J.W. Edwards, 1947, p v.
5. Blount, WP (ed): *The American Academy of Orthopaedic Surgeons Instructional Course Lectures Volume V.* Ann Arbor, MI, Edwards Brothers, 1948, p v.

Preface

It has been a great privilege to work with the fine staff in the AAOS Publications Department to bring you this 50th volume of the *Instructional Course Lectures* series. It is particularly rewarding because this is the first volume in the new millenium. Since its inception, the *Instructional Course Lectures* series has been one of the major educational tools to help orthopaedic residents amass the knowledge to master their particular specialty. Moreover, it provides the necessary knowledge for the practicing orthopaedic surgeon to stay abreast of new developments.

The 59 chapters in this volume were selected from the more than 180 instructional courses presented at the 2000 AAOS Annual Meeting that was held in Orlando, Florida. These lectures were presented by acknowledged experts in the respective subjects.

The volume presents a spectrum of knowledge of interest to orthopaedic residents, practitioners, and subspecialists that is designed to benefit the clinical care of our patients. The 50th volume is timely in that it provides not only a review of many time-honored techniques, but also presents refinements of existing knowledge and procedures. It also gives insight into the recent explosion of knowledge in new areas of orthopaedics, such as molecular biology and exciting new technology.

I would like to thank the Instructional Course Committee and the many authors who have given of their time and expertise to contribute to this book. It is rather amazing that this high-quality volume can be made available in such a short time frame. This is only possible because of the tremendous expertise in the AAOS Publications Department. Special recognition goes to Marilyn Fox, PhD, Department Director, Lisa Claxton Moore, Senior Editor, who coordinated the solicitation and editing of the manuscripts, Sophie Tosta, Assistant Production Manager, who coordinated and oversaw the production process, and Kathy Anderson, Courtney Astle, and Karen Danca, the editorial and production assistants who provided administrative support. Other members of the Publications Department, Joan Abern, Susan Baim, and David Smith, edited manuscripts and sized figures. In addition, I would like to thank Channon Nation, my secretary, who continues to keep me on task.

I appreciate the opportunity to be involved in the production of such an important and valuable educational resource.

Franklin H. Sim, MD
Rochester, MN

Contents

Section 1 Shoulder and Elbow

	Symposium Thermal Modification of Connective Tissues: Basic Science Considerations and Clinical Implications		
1		3	Steven P. Arnoczky Alptekin Aksan
2	***Symposium*** Arthroscopic Stabilization Plus Thermal Capsulorrhaphy for Anterior Instability With and Without Bankart Lesions: The Role of Rehabilitation and Immobilization ***(with video clip on enclosed CD)***	13	Richard J. Hawkins Spero G. Karas
3	***Symposium*** Diagnosis and Treatment of Shoulder Injuries in the Throwing Athlete: The Role of Thermal-Assisted Capsular Shrinkage	17	James R. Andrews Jeffrey R. Dugas
4	***Symposium*** Thermal Capsulorrhaphy for Instability of the Shoulder: Multidirectional and Posterior Instabilities	23	J. Robert Giffin Christopher C. Annunziata James P. Bradley
5	***Symposium*** Thermal Capsulorrhaphy for Instability of the Shoulder: Concerns and Applications of the Heat Probe	29	Jeffrey S. Abrams
6	***Symposium*** Complications of Thermal Capsulorrhaphy	37	John W. Sperling Kyle Anderson Eric C. McCarty Russell F. Warren
7	Technique of Open Rotator Cuff Repair	43	Theodore A. Blaine Michael Q. Freehill Louis U. Bigliani
8	Mini-Open Rotator Cuff Repair: An Updated Perspective	53	Ken Yamaguchi
9	Management of Massive Irreparable Rotator Cuff Tears: The Role of Tendon Transfer	63	Jon J.P. Warner
10	***Symposium*** Total Shoulder Arthroplasty in the Young Patient ***(with video clip on enclosed CD)***	73	Patrick R.L. Hayes Evan L. Flatow
11	The Unstable Elbow ***(with video clip on enclosed CD)***	89	Shawn W. O'Driscoll Jesse B. Jupiter Graham J.W. King Robert N. Hotchkiss Bernard F. Morrey

Section 2 Hand and Wrist

12 Traumatic and Reconstructive Problems of the Scaphoid — 105 — Jesse B. Jupiter, Alexander Y. Shin, Thomas E. Trumble, Diego L. Fernandez

13 Carpal Instability ***(with video clip on enclosed CD)*** — 123 — Richard H. Gelberman, William P. Cooney III, Robert M. Szabo

Section 3 Spine

14 Radiologic Imaging in Spinal Stenosis — 137 — Richard J. Herzog

15 Spinal Stenosis — 145 — Steven R. Garfin, Wolfgang Rauschning

16 Lumbar Spinal Stenosis: Treatment Options — 153 — Eeric Truumees, Harry N. Herkowitz

Section 4 Hip: Adult Reconstruction—Osteolysis and Osteotomy

17 Bearing Surfaces in Total Hip Replacements: State of the Art and Future Developments — 165 — Harry A. McKellop

18 Cross-Linked Polyethylene: Why the Enthusiasm? — 181 — William H. Harris

19 The Basic Science of Periprosthetic Osteolysis — 185 — Michael J. Archibeck, Joshua J. Jacobs, Kenneth A. Roebuck, Tibor T. Glant

20 Osteolysis of the Femur: Principles of Management — 197 — Michael J. Dunbar, Hugh R.L. Blackley, Robert B. Bourne

Symposium
21 Basis Science of Bone Impaction Grafting — 211 — B. Willem Schreurs, Thomas J.J.H. Slooff, Pieter Buma, Nico Verdonschot

Symposium
22 Acetabular Reconstruction With Bone Impaction Grafting: 20 Years of Experience ***(with video clip on enclosed CD)*** — 221 — B. Willem Schreurs, Jean W.M. Gardeniers, Thomas J.J.H. Slooff

23 Rationale of Periacetabular Osteotomy and Background Work — 229 — Michael Leunig, Klaus A. Siebenrock, Reinhold Ganz

24 Periacetabular Osteotomy: The Bernese Experience — 239 — Klaus A. Siebenrock, Michael Leunig, Reinhold Ganz

25 Trochanteric Slide Osteotomy: Biomechanical Considerations — 247 — Derek Plausinis, Fares S. Haddad, Thomas R. Oxland, Clive P. Duncan

26 Osteotomies Around the Hip: Radiographic Planning and Postoperative Evaluation 253 Fares S. Haddad, Donald S. Garbuz, Clive P. Duncan

Section 5 Hip: Adult Reconstruction—Unstable Total Hip Arthroplasty

27 Unstable Total Hip Arthroplasty: Detailed Overview 265 Daniel J. Berry

28 The Effect of Component Design on Range of Motion to Impingement in Total Hip Arthroplasty ***(with video clip on enclosed CD)*** 275 Robert L. Barrack, Robert L. Thornberry, Michael D. Ries, Carlos Lavernia, Evangelos Tozakoglou

29 The Use of a Constrained Acetabular Component for Recurrent Dislocation 281 Gary S. Shapiro, Daniel Weiland, Thomas P. Sculco, Douglas E. Padgett, Paul M. Pellicci

30 The Unstable Total Hip Arthroplasty: The Role of Postoperative Bracing 289 Kyle F. Baldwin, Lawrence D. Dorr

Section 6 Hip: Adult Reconstruction—Complex Primary Total Hip Arthroplasty

31 Conversion of Hip Arthrodesis to Total Hip Arthroplasty 297 Kostas P. Panagiotopoulos, Graham M. Robbins, Bassam A. Masri, Clive P. Duncan

32 Total Hip Replacement for the Dislocated Hip 307 Greg Jaroszynski, Ian G. Woodgate, Khaled J. Saleh, Allan E. Gross

33 Primary Total Hip Arthroplasty After Infection 317 Graham M. Robbins, Bassam A. Masri, Donald S. Garbuz, Clive P. Duncan

34 Primary Total Hip Arthroplasty After Acetabular Fracture 335 Dana C. Mears, John H. Velyvis

Section 7 Knee: Adult Reconstruction

35 Principles of Revision Total Knee Arthroplasty: Overview 357 Victor M. Goldberg

36 Revision Total Knee Arthroplasty: Planning, Management, Controversies, and Surgical Approaches 359 Henry D. Clarke, Giles R. Scuderi

37 Revision Total Knee Arthroplasty: Planning, Controversies, and Management—Infection 367 Sandeep Munjal, Matthew J. Phillips, Kenneth A. Krackow

38 Periprosthetic Fractures Following Total Knee Arthroplasty 379 Douglas A. Dennis

39 Periprosthetic Osteolysis With Total Knee Arthroplasty 391 Gerard A. Engh, Deborah J. Ammeen

40	Ligament Instability in Total Knee Arthroplasty	399	Michael A. Kelly
41	Patellofemoral Complications Following Total Knee Arthroplasty	403	Michael A. Kelly
42	Infection After Total Knee Arthroplasty	409	Robert T. Trousdale Arlen D. Hanssen
43	Thromboembolic Disease in Total Knee Arthroplasty	415	Miguel A. Jimenez Robert T. Trousdale
44	Maximizing Ultra High Molecular Weight Polyethylene Performance in Total Knee Replacement	421	David C. Ayers
45	Mobile-Bearing Knee Replacement: Concepts and Results	431	John J. Callaghan John N. Insall A. Seth Greenwald Douglas A. Dennis Richard D. Komistek David W. Murray Robert B. Bourne Cecil H. Rorabeck Lawrence D. Dorr
46	Revision Anterior Cruciate Ligament Reconstruction: Report of 11-Year Experience and Results in 114 Consecutive Patients ***(with video clip on enclosed CD)***	451	Frank R. Noyes Sue D. Barber-Westin
47	Evaluation and Treatment of Recurrent Instability After Anterior Cruciate Ligament Reconstruction ***(with video clip on enclosed CD)***	463	Christopher D. Harner J. Robert Giffin Roger C. Dunteman Christopher C. Annunziata Marc J. Friedman

Section 8 Knee: Adult Reconstruction—Osteonecrosis

48	Tibial Osteonecrosis	477	Jess H. Lonner Paul A. Lotke
49	Treatment of Osteonecrosis of the Knee	483	Paul A. Lotke Raman Battish Charles L. Nelson
50	Steroid-Associated Osteonecrosis of the Knee: A Comprehensive Review	489	Kyle Low Michael A. Mont David S. Hungerford
51	Spontaneous Osteonecrosis of the Distal Femur	495	Malcolm L. Ecker
52	Surgical Options for the Middle-Aged Patient With Osteoarthritis of the Knee Joint	499	Arlen D. Hanssen Michael J. Stuart Richard D. Scott Giles R. Scuderi

Section 9 Foot and Ankle

53	Ankle Sprains	515	Carol Frey
54	Plantar Heel Pain	521	Glenn B. Pfeffer

Section 10 Pediatric Orthopaedics

55	Developmental Dysplasia of the Hip: Etiology, Pathogenesis, and Examination and Physical Findings in the Newborn ***(with video clip on enclosed CD)***	**535**	Richard J. Haynes
56	Developmental Dysplasia of the Hip: Assessment and Treatment Before Walking Age	**541**	R. Baxter Willis
57	Developmental Hip Dysplasia and Dislocation: Management of the Older Child	**547**	Colin F. Moseley
58	Slipped Capital Femoral Epiphysis	**555**	Randall T. Loder David D. Aronsson Matthew B. Dobbs Stuart L. Weinstein
59	Natural History and Long-Term Outcomes of Slipped Capital Femoral Epiphysis ***(with video clip on enclosed CD)***	**571**	Matthew B. Dobbs Stuart L. Weinstein

Cumulative Index 1997-2001 **577**

SECTION

1

Shoulder and Elbow

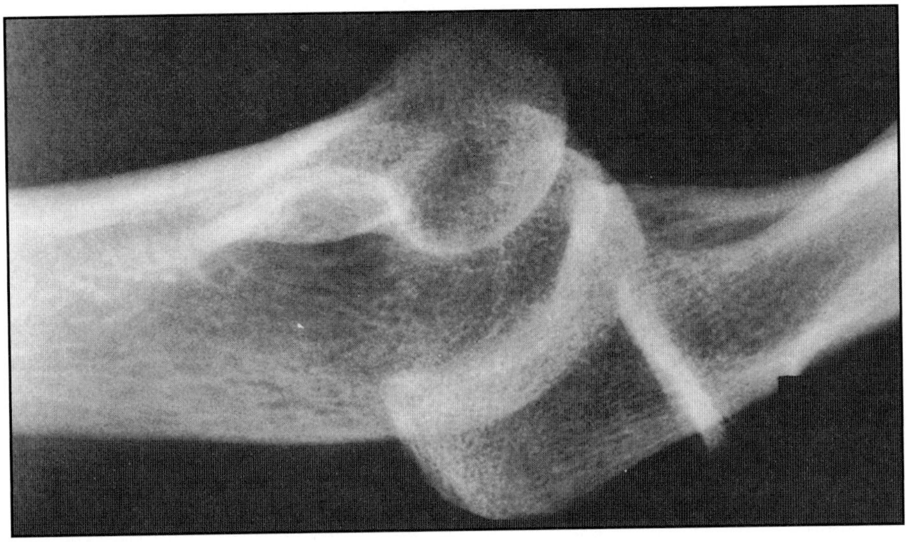

1 ***Symposium***
Thermal Modification of Connective Tissues: Basic Science Considerations and Clinical Implications

2 ***Symposium***
Arthroscopic Stabilization Plus Thermal Capsulorrhaphy for Anterior Instability With and Without Bankart Lesions: The Role of Rehabilitation and Immobilization ***(with video clip on enclosed CD)***

3 ***Symposium***
Diagnosis and Treatment of Shoulder Injuries in the Throwing Athlete: The Role of Thermal-Assisted Capsular Shrinkage

4 ***Symposium***
Thermal Capsulorrhaphy for Instability of the Shoulder: Multidirectional and Posterior Instabilities

5 ***Symposium***
Thermal Capsulorrhaphy for Instability of the Shoulder: Concerns and Applications of the Heat Probe

6 ***Symposium***
Complications of Thermal Capsulorrhaphy

7 Technique of Open Rotator Cuff Repair

8 Mini-Open Rotator Cuff Repair: An Updated Perspective

9 Management of Massive Irreparable Rotator Cuff Tears: The Role of Tendon Transfer

10 ***Symposium***
Total Shoulder Arthroplasty in the Young Patient ***(with video clip on enclosed CD)***

11 The Unstable Elbow ***(with video clip on enclosed CD)***

1

SYMPOSIUM

Thermal Modification of Connective Tissues: Basic Science Considerations and Clinical Implications

Steven P. Arnoczky, DVM
Alptekin Aksan, MS

Introduction

The application of heat as a therapeutic modality has evolved from the use of fire to sterilize wounds and control bleeding to the modern-day use of hyperthermia to treat various forms of cancer.[1] This evolution revolved around a better understanding of the tissue biology associated with the application of thermal energy and an improved ability to control the amount of heat delivered as well as the precision of its application. Although the use of boiling oils, heated metals, and magnified sunlight in medicine has ultimately been replaced by modern electrocautery and laser energy, the major therapeutic uses of these sources of heat in surgery, hemostasis and tissue ablation, remain essentially the same.

The use of thermal energy has recently been proposed as a technique to shrink redundant or lax connective tissues through the well-established mechanism of collagen denaturation.[2-23] Although there have been numerous in vitro[7,10,11,15,16,18,21,22,24-29] and in vivo[5,9,12,13,17,30-32] experimental studies that have investigated the biology and biomechanics of thermally modified tissues, there is still no consensus of opinion as to the optimal therapeutic algorithm (that is, degree of tissue shrinkage required, postoperative regimen), the ultimate mechanism of the reported clinical improvements, or the long-term prognosis of the thermally modified tissues.

This chapter will review the basic science of the thermal modification of connective tissues and examine some of the potential clinical implications associated with its use.

Mechanism of Thermal Shrinkage of Collagen

Ligaments and joint capsules are comprised primarily of type I collagen. The type I collagen molecule is made up of three polypeptide chains that are stabilized in a triple helical arrangement by intramolecular crosslinks.[33] These molecules are, in turn, aggregated into a parallel pattern to form collagen fibrils. This fibrillar arrangement is maintained by intermolecular crosslinks and provides the tissue with its tensile properties. The intramolecular crosslinks are covalent reducible aldehyde bonds that are progressively replaced with irreducible multivalent crosslinks as the tissue ages.[33]

When collagen is heated, the heat-labile intramolecular crosslinks are broken and the protein undergoes a transition from the highly organized crystalline structure to a random, gel-like state (denaturation)[34] (Fig. 1). Collagen "shrinkage" occurs through the cumulative effect of the unwinding of the triple helix (caused by the destruction of the heat-labile intramolecular crosslinks) and the residual tension of the heat-stable intermolecular crosslinks[34,35] (Fig. 2).

While collagen denaturation typically occurs at approximately 65°C,[36] the precise heat-induced behavior of connective tissues and the extent of tissue shrinkage are dependent on several factors including maximum temperature reached and exposure time[35,37] (as discussed in the section on in vitro experimental studies), and the mechanical stress applied to the tissue during heating.[27,38,39] In addition, the thermal properties of a tissue can also vary with species, age,[40] the pH[39] and electrolyte concentration of the surrounding environment,[41] the concentration and orientation of the collagen fibers,[42,43] and the hydration level of the tissue.[44]

Increased collagen content, direction of fiber orientation, and increased tensile load have been shown to increase the

(This chapter has been adapted with permission from Arnoczky SP: Thermal modification of connective tissues: Basic science considerations and clinical implications. J Am Acad Orthop Surg, *in press.)*

One or more of the authors or the departments with which they are affiliated have received something of value from a commercial or other party related directly or indirectly to the subject of this chapter.

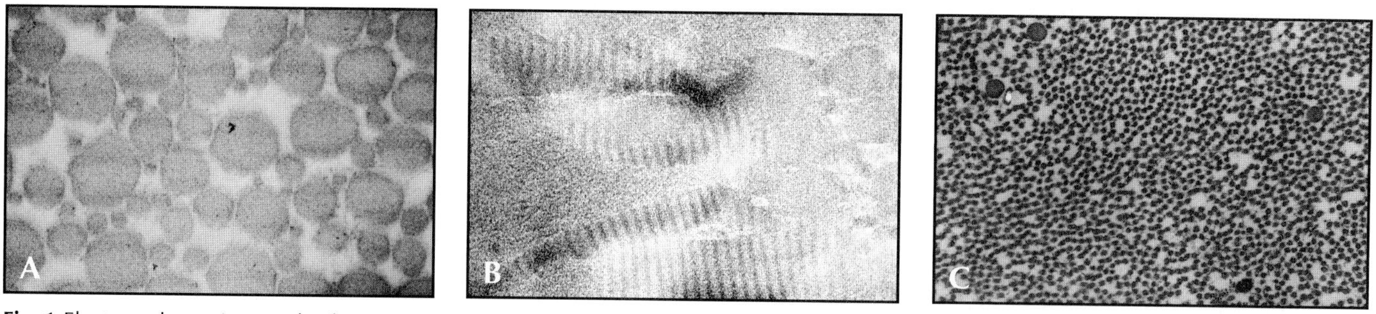

Fig. 1 Electron photomicrograph of a cross section of normal rabbit patellar tendon (**A**) and a rabbit patellar tendon immediately following thermal shrinkage (**B**). Note the random orientation of the collagen fibers (magnification × 34,000). **C**, Electron photomicrograph of a cross section of a rabbit patellar tendon 8 weeks following thermal modification. The tissue is remodeled with a population of small diameter collagen fibers indicative of scar tissue (magnification × 34,000). (Adapted with permission from Arnoczky SP: Thermal modification of connective tissues: Basic science considerations and clinical implications. *J Am Acad Orthop Surg,* in press.)

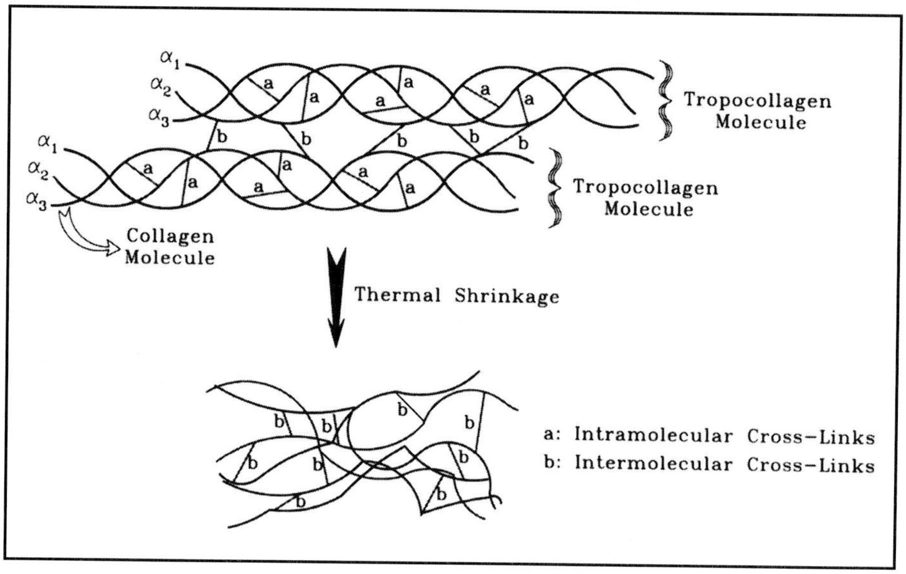

Fig. 2 Schematic showing the molecular mechanism of collagen shrinkage. (Adapted with permission from Arnoczky SP: Thermal modification of connective tissues: Basic science considerations and clinical implications. *J Am Acad Orthop Surg,* in press.)

shrinkage temperature of connective tissue.[42,45] In addition, aging has been shown to increase the shrinkage temperature,[40,42] probably a result of age-related increased ratio of the heat-stable to heat-labile crosslinks.[16] Increased pH of the surrounding medium and dehydration of the tissues are also known to increase the shrinkage temperature.[39,45]

On the macro scale, the effect of heat on dense, regularly-oriented connective tissues (tendons and ligaments) may be summarized as shrinkage along an axis parallel to the dominant direction of fiber orientation accompanied by swelling on the transverse axis. In dense, irregularly-oriented connective tissues (joint capsule), shrinkage still occurs along the long axis of the collagen fibers. However, because the fiber orientation is multidirectional in these tissues the extent and principal axis of shrinkage is less predictable.

In Vitro Studies

Examination and quantification of the thermal response characteristics of collagenous tissues is a difficult task because of the diversity of species and the compositional variance among tissues. During the past four decades, researchers have performed various experiments with tendon, ligament, skin, joint capsule, and corneal tissue specimens harvested from different species (bovine, canine, rat, rabbit, sheep, and human).[10,11,15,25,26,31]

It has been established that when collagenous tissues are exposed to high temperatures (in the range of 65°C to 85°C for most tissue types and species), they undergo rapid denaturation.[34] The outcome of collagen denaturation on the micro scale is tissue shrinkage on the macro scale.[35] At a constant temperature, shrinkage increases with increased heat exposure until it reaches a plateau value beyond which no additional shrinkage is observed. This ultimate value of shrinkage changes with the treatment temperature[35,37] and the mechanical load applied on the tissue during heating.[27,38,39] Heating to excessive temperatures for extended periods of time results in hyalinization, extensive thermal damage, and tissue necrosis.[46]

Hydrothermal heating experiments performed with specimens taken from different regions of cadaver glenohumeral joint capsules point to a correlation between the maximum temperature reached and the amount of tissue shrinkage.[11] Starting with the measurement of 10% shrinkage following 10 minutes of heating at 65°C, a maximum value of 60% shrinkage is reached after 1.5 minutes at 80°C. These results highlight the axiom that the higher the maximum temperature reached during heating, the higher the shrinkage. It is also evident from the same data that the time required to reach the same amount of shrinkage decreases with increasing temperature.

A similar experiment using radiofrequency (RF) heating on specimens harvested from sheep glenohumeral joint capsules yielded to less than 4% shrinkage for temperatures below 65°C and reached a peak value of 14% shrinkage at 80°C.[28]

Discrepancies among these results may have resulted from the interspecies differences in tissue composition and the possible nonthermal effects of the two heating modalities.[20] It is well established in the literature that similar tissues from different species may experience different amounts of shrinkage under identical heating conditions.[25,31] It has also been shown that these differences correlate well with the differences in the physiologic body core temperatures of the species.[47] On the other hand, laser heating causes local dehydration of the tissues due to evaporation of fluids in the target volume, whereas this is not a problem in hydrothermal heating. Additionally, it has been postulated that laser energy enhances healing by stimulating collagen synthesis.[48] Unfortunately, there have been no extensive studies comparing the nonthermal effects of various modalities.

Another important factor in the variety of results reported may be the differences in the application of different heating modalities. In hydrothermal heating, the tissue sample is immersed in a constant temperature bath and the tissue rapidly comes into thermal equilibrium with its surroundings. Therefore, a homogeneous temperature distribution within the tissue could be obtained. On the other hand, in laser or RF heating, the temperature distribution created within the tissue is a function of probe sweep velocity, distance between the target tissue and the probe, and heat penetration depth.[15] These factors combined may easily cause nonhomogeneous heating.[49] Differences between the thermal histories of different regions within the same tissue volume may cause significant changes in ultrastructure and overall behavior, resulting in nonuniform shrinkage.

In the literature, it has been documented that hydrothermal and laser heating caused differences in the collagenous tissue ultrastructure[11] but these differences have not been attributed to any particular reason (nonthermal effects or differences in application). It is also reported in the literature that after heating, if the collagenous tissue is cooled back to room temperature, some collagen molecules regain their triple helical structure (renaturation).[50] This process is accompanied by shrinkage relaxation of the magnitude of 5% to 10% of the shrunken length.[27]

Research done on the effect of mechanical stress on the shrinkage and postheating relaxation characteristics of bovine chordae tendineae yielded interesting results.[27] A fivefold increase in the applied stress caused a decrease in the final plateau value of shrinkage and delayed the renaturation process.[27] The authors suggested that there is a time-temperature-load equivalency in the heat-induced shrinkage behavior of the collagenous tissues. In other words, these parameters are to an extent interchangeable (they have similar effects on the gross tissue behavior) and any change in any of these parameters alters the speed of the shrinkage process. This hypothesis may have very important clinical applications in that the same amount of tissue shrinkage may be obtained at a lower temperature, minimizing the risk of excessive loss of stiffness and thermal damage to the surrounding tissues.

Research performed on cadaver glenohumeral capsular tissues suggests that the stiffness of heated collagenous tissue decreases while viscoelastic properties remain unaltered.[7,11] Stiffness values down to 90% of normal have been measured following aggressive laser heating.[7,11] Similar to the shrinkage response, the decrease in stiffness is also dose-related.[22] The higher the heating (and thus the greater the shrinkage), the greater the loss of stiffness. It has been suggested that the loss of tissue stiffness is of significant concern in that it may make the tissues more vulnerable to postoperative mechanical loading.[8,31]

In Vivo *Studies*

Only a limited number of studies have examined the in vivo effects of thermal modification on connective tissue biology and biomechanics.[9,11,30-32] However, most agree that following thermal modification and subsequent cell death, the modified tissues undergo a repair response characterized by fibroplasia, neovascularization, and fibrovascular scar formation. As demonstrated by studies on sheep[11] and rabbit[9] specimens, tissue begins to undergo a regenerative process as evidenced by hyperplasia and increased fibroblastic activity only 7 days after treatment. Vascularization of the scar region and migration of more fibroblasts to the treated site accompany the long-term healing response of the tissue. After 1 month, newly synthesized collagen molecules and small diameter fibrils are present in the scar area.[9,11]

Subphysiologic loads are known to accelerate healing. On the other hand, it has been observed that when thermally modified tissue is immediately subjected to physiologic loads in the postoperative period, it can elongate to its preoperative length within 4 weeks.[31] Despite the fact that the initial shrinkage values obtained on rabbit patellar tendons with laser treatment in in vivo and in vitro experiments were the same, the in vivo group showed relaxation back to the original length by 4 weeks, and beyond original length by 8 weeks.[31] A recent study has suggested that it may take as long as 12 weeks for thermally modified tissues to regain normal strength.[30] However, another study has shown that during that same period of time the tissue has an increased susceptibility to creep.[32] These findings point to the importance of the need for additional research on the response of thermally modified tissues in the postoperative period and the effects of various rehabilitation regimens (immobilization).

Delivery of Thermal Energy

Basically, two different types of energy systems have been used to thermally modify connective tissues: laser energy and RF energy.[6,51]

Laser Energy

The laser (an acronym for Light Amplification by the Stimulated Emission of Radiation) is an electro-optical device capable of efficiently transmitting energy in the form of an intense beam of light. The radiant energy of the laser beam can be transformed into heat energy through its interaction with tissues. This interaction is dependent on the wavelength of the laser and the properties of the tissue. (Only if light energy is absorbed by the tissues will it be effectively transformed into thermal energy). Holmium:YAG laser light is absorbed by water and because most biologic tissues are composed mainly of water, the tissues are heated.

In addition to the nature of the interaction with the tissue, the extent of the laser thermal effect is also controlled by the power density, spot size, and duration of application. While the total power output of a laser is measured in watts, the power density is measured in watts per square centimeter (watts/cm^2) and is directly correlated with the thermal effect produced in the tissue. The spot size refers to the amount of tissue area upon which the laser light is concentrated and is an important factor in determining power density. Power density can be increased by increasing power output or by decreasing spot size (power density varies as the inverse of the area). Finally, time of laser application, measured in joules (watts/s), can also affect the amount of energy delivered to the tissue and the resultant thermal effect. Pulsing (rapidly alternating the beam off and on) the laser beam allows for a cooling effect between pulses in a fluid medium and can limit heat transfer to adjacent tissues. This helps limit the depth of penetration and tissue damage.

While the holmium:YAG laser was the first system used clinically for the thermal modification of connective tissues, no single therapeutic algorithm has been rigorously tested.[19] Because of the noncontact nature of the holmium:YAG laser probe, there is no specific mechanism for temperature feedback. Thus temperature control, and ultimate thermal effect, are determined by the surgeon through the control of spot size and duration of laser application to a specific area. It has been advocated that the laser be set to a low power setting (10 to 15 watts) and the laser beam defocused (by holding the tip of the probe 2 mm from the surface of the tissue).[51] Once visible tissue shrinkage occurs, the laser beam is then advanced to another area. However, it should be remembered that simply decreasing the spot size (focusing the laser beam by bringing the tip of the probe closer to the tissue) and/or keeping the beam focused too long on the same spot could result in tissue ablation (especially in the relatively thin joint capsule).

Radiofrequency Energy

RF energy is a form of electromagnetic energy. When applied to tissues, rapid oscillation of electromagnetic fields causes movement of charged particles within the tissue and the resultant molecular motion generates heat.[6,51] The electromagnetic energy can be applied between two points on the tip of a probe (bipolar) or between a single electrode tip and a grounding plate (monopolar). In monopolar RF devices the molecular friction created within the tissues adjacent to the RF probe produces heat. Thus, the actual source of heat is the frictional resistance of the tissues rather than the probe itself. In bipolar RF probes the electromagnetic energy follows a much shorter path through the conductive irrigating solution, electrolytes, or tissues between the tips of the probe. In bipolar RF less current is required for a similar effect (compared to monopolar) because the current passes through a much smaller volume of tissue. In addition, the depth of tissue damage (relative to the probe tip) may be less in bipolar applications.

Similar to laser energy, the thermal effect of RF energy in tissues is determined by the level of RF energy (power, impedance), duration of treatment, and nature of the tissues. In addition, electrode type (monopolar or bipolar), size, and shape have an effect.

Some current RF devices are capable of monitoring and/or controlling the temperature at the tip of the probe. While this is thought to provide the highest margin of safety and efficacy, no data (clinical or experimental) has been published to support this claim.[51] Indeed, as with the laser, the extent of thermal modification with RF devices is operator-dependent and relies on the visual observation of the tissue response. Because the tissue response is both time- and heat-dependent, the longer a probe (laser or RF) is left in one place the greater the resulting tissue damage. In addition, the previously mentioned biologic variables of age, tissue thickness, tissue hydration, and tissue quality all affect the thermal response of tissues. Thus, application of a uniform amount of thermal modification with either class of devices appears, at best, subjective.

Although lasers and RF generators differ fundamentally in the way they generate heat within a tissue, both classes of devices are capable of producing temperatures within the critical temperature range (65°C to 75°C) for collagen denaturation and subsequent tissue shrinkage. Although both devices have advantages and disadvantages (price, temperature monitoring, etc) when it comes to cell viability and tissue response, heat is heat. Once critical temperatures are reached, cells will die (45°C)[46,52] and collagen will become denatured (at 65°C)[34,35] no matter what the source of thermal energy. Therefore claims of a better or different type of heat have little bearing on the biologic response of the tissue. Indeed, histologic, ultrastructural, and biomaterial alterations induced by laser and RF energy have been shown to be similar.[6]

Clinical Implications

Although the effect of heat energy on collagen molecules has been well established, the reason for the reported efficacy of this mode of therapy in the treatment of lax or redundant collagenous tissues is less clear. As previously noted, the initial degree of tissue shrinkage (and ultimate tissue damage) is directly related to the amount and rate of thermal energy applied. It has also been shown that the amount of tissue shrinkage is directly related to the loss of tissue stiffness.[7,22,31] Thus, the surgeon is caught in the dilemma of minimizing tissue damage while trying to achieve sufficient tissue shrinkage. Once shrunken (and devitalized) the tissues must be revitalized; during that period of repair they are susceptible to elongation if left unprotected due to the aforementioned compromise in their material properties. Thus, the question remains as to what factor is responsible for the clinical improvement following thermal capsular shrinkage.[3,4,19] Is it the initial connective tissue (capsule and associated structures) shrinkage that appears to tighten the joint and subsequently stabilizes it? Or is it the fibroplasia, capsular thickening, and secondary cicatrix formation that occurs in response to the traumatic insult? Or, could it even be related to the loss of afferent sensory stimulation caused by destruction of sensory receptors?

Maintenance of Initial Capsular Shrinkage

Experimental studies have shown that connective tissues demonstrate a significant loss of stiffness immediately following thermal shrinkage.[7,22,31,32] This loss of stiffness has also been shown to be a significant covariant of shrinkage (more shrinkage results in a greater loss of stiffness). Thus, tightening a lax joint by inducing significant thermal shrinkage in the joint capsule and/or ligaments actually makes these tissues weaker and more compliant, putting them at risk postoperatively. It is also important to note that because most experimental studies have been performed on normal, healthy tissues, the heat response of pathologic tissues is unknown. It is possible that pathologic tissues could respond differently to thermal modification. One study has demonstrated that there is an increased prevalence of reducible crosslinks in joint capsules from pathologic joints irrespective of the age of the patient.[53] This would suggest that collagen from pathologic joints may be more susceptible to thermal modification and could put them at even greater risk in the immediate postoperative period.

If the degree of tissue shrinkage is directly related to the loss of tissue stiffness in the immediate postoperative period, then it is logical to assume that the degree of postoperative tissue repair is directly related to the extent of tissue damage. As previously noted, the application of thermal energy to shrink connective tissue is very subjective and still relies on the visual conformation of the tissue response.[4] With this in mind, it should be remembered that although a temperature of at least 65°C is necessary to shrink connective tissues, a temperature of 45°C is lethal to most cells.[46,52] This would suggest that following thermal application, at minimum, a significant portion of all visibly shrunken tissue has been killed. In addition, it is possible that adjacent, nonshrunken tissue could have been subjected to lethal (> 45°C) temperatures. Thus, the extent of actual tissue injury may not be accurately reflected by the amount of visual shrinkage.

As with all traumatized or devitalized tissues the body will mount an inflammatory response to repair and/or remove and replace the injured tissue.[52] In the case of thermal injury this process is protracted (when compared with traumatic [incisional] injury).[46,52] Numerous experimental studies have documented that thermally modified tissues undergo a repair and remodeling process characterized by fibroplasia (Fig. 3), increased collagen deposition, and a remodeling phase in which the collagen diameter profile changes from a bimodal (large and small diameter) fiber pattern to a unimodal (small diameter) fiber pattern indicative of scar tissue.[9,12,30-32,54] These morphologic changes are associated with a decrease in tensile stiffness and make the tissue susceptible to elongation due to tissue creep.[31,32] Studies have suggested that at least 3 months is required before thermally modified tissue can fully recover its biomechanical properties.[30] Restriction of activity during this time is a recommended consideration for the postoperative regimen.

Thus it appears that the maintenance of initial tissue shrinkage is directly dependent on controlling the postoperative stresses experienced by the tissue and indirectly dependent on the amount of shrinkage induced at the time of surgery.

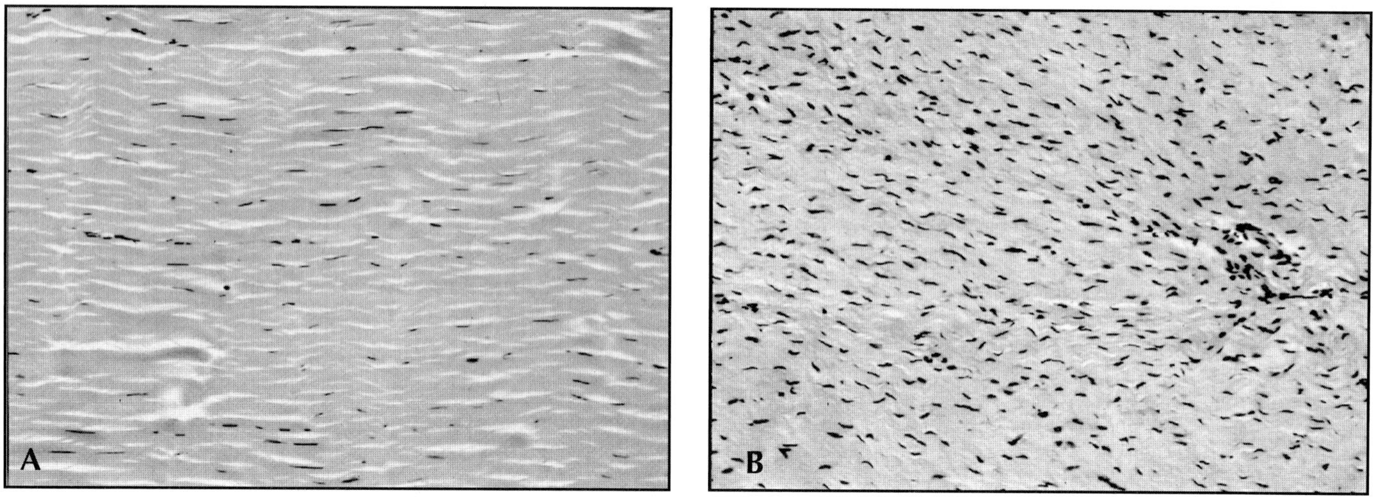

Fig. 3 Photomicrograph of a longitudinal section of a normal rabbit patellar tendon (**A**) and a rabbit patellar tendon 8 weeks following thermal modification (**B**). Note the marked fibroblastic response still present within the tissue at 8 weeks (hematoxylin and eosin, × 100). (Adapted with permission from Arnoczky SP: Thermal modification of connective tissues: Basic science considerations and clinical implications. *J Am Acad Orthop Surg,* in press.)

Posttreatment Capsular Thickening and Cicatrix Formation

Inherent to all wound repair is a period of fibroplasia and collagen deposition which, in most cases, is directly related to the extent of tissue damage (caused either by the initial injury or the subsequent surgery).[52] While extensive fibroplasia and subsequent tissue thickening are an unwelcome sequelae in most surgical procedures, the creation of a hypertrophied joint capsule following thermal modification may actually contribute to the ultimate stability of the joint.

This rationale to shoulder stabilization has historical precedent. Hippocrates treated recurrent shoulder dislocations with a red-hot iron inserted into the axillary region.[55] By creating an eschar in this area it was hoped that the ensuing cicatrix would contract the redundant joint capsule and ultimately stabilize the shoulder.

In the 1950s, in an effort to incite fibroblastic response using minimally invasive techniques, a treatment was developed for the correction of lax ligaments and tendons through the injection of various irritant solutions.[33] The therapy was based on the concept that focal injections of a dextrose solution stimulated the initiation of a generalized inflammatory reaction which, in turn, led to a normal wound healing cascade and the deposition of new collagen, making the thickened structure stronger and stiffer. This treatment was termed prolotherapy (derived from the Latin "to proliferate") and defined as the rehabilitation of an incompetent structure by the generation of new cellular tissue. Hackett[33] described the stabilization of recurrent shoulder dislocations through a series of proliferant injections into the joint capsule. He reported a "beneficial" effect to these patients with a gradual return of joint stability. However, early mobilization of these joints was cautioned because it was believed to possibly result in a disruption of the healing process and a "stretching out" of the tissue. It was concluded that additional research is necessary to clarify the role of immobilization in the healing process and determine the long-term benefits of proliferant injection therapy in treating shoulder instabilities. These same concerns are valid for thermal shrinkage.

In modern-day surgery some open procedures for shoulder stabilization rely on the tightening and reinforcement of the joint capsule to provide stability.[55] It is logical to assume that the exposure and surgical trauma associated with these procedures could also result in postoperative fibroplasia and thickening of the joint capsule, which may contribute to the ultimate stability of the shoulder. Therefore, the inability of arthroscopic shoulder stabilizations to equal the results of open stabilization procedures may be caused, in part, by the decrease in tissue trauma (and attendant fibroplastic response of the joint capsule) associated with this minimally invasive technique. The use of thermal energy to incite an inflammatory cascade in the joint capsule and produce a fibroblastic response may induce the secondary capsular thickening seen in open stabilizations (Fig. 4).

However, attendant to the creation of such a proliferative response is the understanding that excessive fibroplasia (caused by extensive tissue trauma) may also cause problems in the joint (such as arthrofibrosis and adhesive capsulitis) (Fig. 5). Appropriate stresses are required

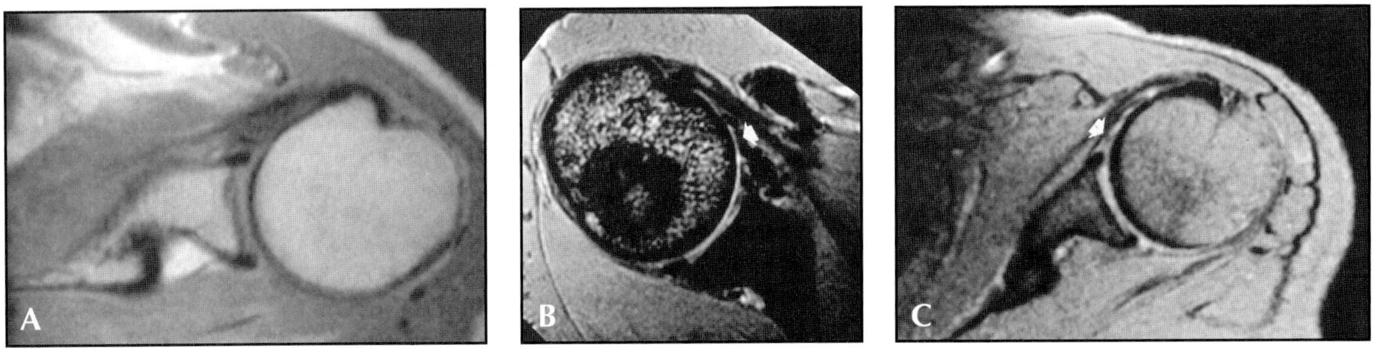

Fig. 4 A, MRI study of a normal shoulder joint. The anterior joint capsule is indistinct. **B**, MRI study of a shoulder 1 year following open stabilization. Note the increased thickness of the anterior joint capsule (*arrow*). **C**, MRI study of a shoulder 1 year following arthroscopic thermal modification of the anterior joint capsule. Note the thickening of the capsule (*arrow*). (Courtesy of Charles Ho, MD, PhD, Menlo Park, CA.)

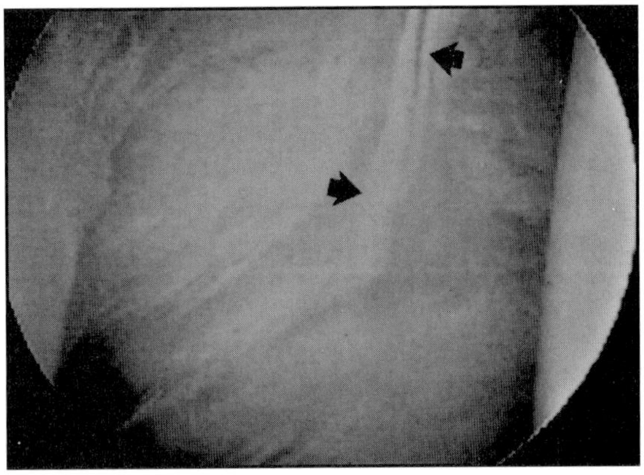

Fig. 5 Arthroscopic view of an anterior capsule of a shoulder joint 1 year following arthroscopic thermal capsular shrinkage. Note the bands of fibrous tissue that have formed secondary to the thermal procedure (*arrows*). It is interesting to note that these bands are oriented at right angles to the normal course of the inferior glenohumeral ligament. (Courtesy of Jonathan Ticker, MD, Massapequa, NY.)

to remodel these healing tissues. This is especially true in the shoulder where various portions of the capsule contribute to joint stability in various arm positions.[56] As with healing in all connective tissues, rehabilitation regimens must be developed to coincide with the various phases of repair in order to permit a functional remodeling of the maturing tissues. The question remains, however, as to the best postoperative protocol with which to adequately modulate scar formation and remodeling following thermal modification.

Loss of Afferent Sensory Stimulation

The joint capsule of the shoulder is a richly innervated structure containing a variety of sensory receptors.[57,58] It seems logical to assume that temperatures that denature and shrink collagen (> 65°C) could also destroy these receptors and alter, if not completely disrupt, the afferent sensory pathway of the shoulder. It has been suggested that in some arthroscopic surgical procedures of the shoulder, destruction (excision) of neural elements may decrease painful stimuli and thus allow more joint movement, strength, and shoulder function.[58] Therefore, thermal modification of the shoulder joint capsule could result in a local or regional anesthesia or kinesthesia of the joint capsule and provide symptomatic relief. This theory has yet to be proven.

It is probable that no one mechanism is totally responsible for the reported clinical improvement in patients following thermal modification of their joint capsule. Indeed, it is entirely possible that initial shrinkage, postoperative capsular thickening, and loss of regional afferent sensory input are mechanisms that may be involved in the ultimate postoperative improvement reported by some clinicians. Careful, long-term follow-up of these patients is needed to provide some insight into what factors most impact on functional outcome following thermal modification of connective tissues.

Summary

Wound healing is a natural and well-orchestrated biologic event. Indeed, the ability of wounds to heal is the foundation on which the practice of surgery is predicated. The successful surgeon maintains a delicate alliance with nature, balancing the magnitude of the surgical insult against the capacity of the tissue for repair. Thermal injury is one of the most traumatic insults a tissue can sustain and the high degree of cell death and matrix alteration associated with thermal burns have been shown to result in a protracted healing time. Thus, the use of thermal energy as a stimulant for tissue shrinkage must be tempered with an appreciation of the biologic events that accompany this phenomenon. Furthermore, it must be realized that the initial degree of capsular shrinkage observed following the application of thermal energy may have little bearing on the long-term biologic and biomechanical status of the joint capsule. Therefore, the desire to see a redundant capsule shrink and become taut at surgery should be weighed very carefully against the level of damage imparted to the tissue to achieve this result. The simple initiation of the healing response may be sufficient to rehabilitate an incompetent structure via the creation of new cellular tissue.[33]

While the ultimate application(s) of thermal modification of connective tissues has yet to be completely defined, its ultimate role may be best suited to that of a low level stimulant for inducing a biologic repair response rather than a highly aggressive mechanism for primary tissue shrinkage.

Acknowledgment

The authors wish to acknowledge the assistance of Charles Ho, MD and Jonathan Ticker, MD in the preparation of this manuscsript.

References

1. Thabit G III: Therapeutic heat: A historical perspective. *Op Tech Sports Med* 1998;6:118-119.
2. Dillingham M: Arthroscopic electrothermal surgery of the knee. *Op Tech Sports Med* 1998; 6:154-156.
3. Fanton GS: Arthroscopic electrothermal surgery of the shoulder. *Op Tech Sports Med* 1998;6:139-146.
4. Fanton GS, Wall MS, Markel MD: Electrothermally-assisted capsule shift (ETAC) procedure for shoulder instability, in *The Science and Applications of ElectroThermal Arthroscopy*. Oratec Interventions, Menlo Park, CA 1998.
5. Hayashi K, Hecht P, Vanderby R, et al: The long-term effect of laser energy on joint capsular tissue. *Trans Orthop Res Soc* 1998;23:1026.
6. Hayashi K, Markel MD: Thermal modification of joint capsule and ligamentous tissues. *Op Tech Sports Med* 1998;6:120-125.
7. Hayashi K, Markel MD, Thabit G III, Bogdanske JJ, Thielke RJ: The effect of nonablative laser energy on joint capsular properties: An in vitro mechanical study using a rabbit model. *Am J Sports Med* 1995;23:482-487.
8. Hayashi K, Massa KL, Thabit G III, et al: Histologic evaluation of the glenohumeral joint capsule after the laser-assisted capsular shift procedure for glenohumeral instability. *Am J Sports Med* 1999;27:162-167.
9. Hayashi K, Nieckarz JA, Thabit G III, Bogdanske JJ, Cooley AJ, Markel MD: Effect of nonablative laser energy on the joint capsule: An in vivo rabbit study using a holmium:YAG laser. *Lasers Surg Med* 1997;20:164-171.
10. Hayashi K, Thabit G III, Bogdanske JJ, Mascio LN, Markel MD: The effect of nonablative laser energy on the ultrastructure of joint capsular collagen. *Arthroscopy* 1996;12:474-481.
11. Hayashi K, Thabit G III, Massa KL, et al: The effect of thermal heating on the length and histologic properties of the glenohumeral joint capsule. *Am J Sports Med* 1997;25:107-112.
12. Hecht P, Hayashi K, Cooley AJ, Fanton GS, Thabit G III, Markel MD: The effect of radiofrequency energy on short term tissue response and heat distribution in joint capsular tissue. *Trans Orthop Res Soc* 1998;23:1039.
13. Hecht P, Hayashi K, Cooley AJ, et al: The thermal effect of monopolar radiofrequency energy on the properties of joint capsule: An in vivo histologic study using a sheep model. *Am J Sports Med* 1998;26:808-814.
14. Lopez MJ, Hayashi K, Fanton GS, Thabit G III, Markel MD: The effect of radiofrequency energy on the ultrastructure of joint capsular collagen. *Arthroscopy* 1998;14:495-501.
15. Naseef GS III, Foster TE, Trauner K, Solhpour S, Anderson RR, Zarins B: The thermal properties of bovine joint capsule: The basic science of laser- and radiofrequency-induced capsular shrinkage. *Am J Sports Med* 1997;25:670-674.
16. Horgan DJ, King NL, Kurth LB, Kuypers R: Collagen crosslinks and their relationship to the thermal properties of calf tendons. *Arch Biochem Biophys* 1990;281:21-26.
17. Pullin JG, Collier MA, Johnson LL, DeBault LE, Walls RC: Holmium:YAG laser-assisted capsular shift in a canine model: Intraarticular pressure and histologic observations. *J Shoulder Elbow Surg* 1997;6:272-285.
18. Selecky MT, Vangsness CT Jr, Liao W-L, Saadat V, Hedman TP: The effects of laser-induced collagen shortening on the biomechanical properties of the inferior glenohumeral ligament complex. *Am J Sports Med* 1999; 27:168-172.
19. Thabit G III: The arthroscopically assisted holmium:YAG laser surgery in the shoulder. *Op Tech Sports Med* 1998;6:131-138.
20. Thabit G III: The arthroscopic monopolar radiofrequency treatment of chronic anterior cruciate ligament instability. *Op Tech Sports Med* 1998;6:157-160.
21. Tibone JE, McMahon PJ, Shrader TA, Sandusky MD, Lee TQ: Glenohumeral joint translation after arthroscopic, nonablative, thermal capsuloplasty with a laser. *Am J Sports Med* 1998;26:495-498.
22. Vangsness CT Jr, Mitchell W III, Nimni M, Erlich M, Saadat V, Schmotzer H: Collagen shortening: An experimental approach with heat. *Clin Orthop* 1997;337:267-271.
23. Brillhart AT: Complications of thermal energy. *Op Tech Sports Med* 1998;6:182-184.
24. Bass LS, Moazami N, Pocsidio J, Oz MC, LoGerfo P, Treat MR: Changes in type I collagen following laser welding. *Lasers Surg Med* 1992;12:500-505.
25. Berend ME, Glisson RR, Seaber AV, Speer KP: Soft tissue shortening with the Ho:YAG laser: Experimental model and structural effects. *Trans Orthop Res Soc* 1996;21:50.
26. Chen SS, Wright NT, Humphrey JD: Heat-induced changes in the mechanics of a collagenous tissue: Isothermal free shrinkage. *J Biomech Eng* 1997;119:372-378.
27. Chen SS, Wright NT, Humphrey JD: Heat-induced changes in the mechanics of a collagenous tissue: Isothermal, isotonic shrinkage. *J Biomech Eng* 1998;120:382-388.
28. Obrzut SL, Hecht P, Hayashi K, Fanton GS, Thabit G III, Markel MD: The effect of radiofrequency energy on the length and temperature properties of the glenohumeral joint capsule. *Arthroscopy* 1998;14:395-400.
29. Spadaro JA, Becker RO: Effects of thermal denaturation on metal binding and ultrastructure in collagen fibrils. *Biochim Biophys Acta* 1972;263:585-592.
30. Sandusky MD, Schulz MM, McMahon PJ, Tibone JE, Lee TQ: The effects of laser on joint capsular tissue: An in vivo rabbit study. *Trans Orthop Res Soc* 1999;24:366.
31. Schaefer SL, Ciarelli MJ, Arnoczky SP, Ross HE: Tissue shrinkage with the holmium:Yttrium aluminum garnet laser: A postoperative assessment of tissue length, stiffness, and structure. *Am J Sports Med* 1997;25:841-848.
32. Wallace AL, Sutherland CA, Marchuk LL, et al: Early in vivo effects of electrothermal shrinkage on viscoelastic properties and cellular responses in a model of ligament laxity. *Trans Orthop Res Soc* 1999;24:309.
33. Hackett GS (ed): *Ligament and Tendon Relaxation (Skeletal Disability) Treated by Prolotherapy (Fibro-Osseous Proliferation)*, ed 3. Springfield, IL, CC Thomas, 1958.
34. Flory PJ, Garrett RR: Phase transitions in collagen and gelatin systems. *J Am Chem Soc* 1958; 80:4836-4845.
35. Allain JC, Le Lous M, Cohen-Solal L, Bazin S, Maroteaux P: Isometric tensions developed during the hydrothermal swelling of rat skin. *Connect Tissue Res* 1980;7:127-133.
36. Fung YC (ed): *Biomechanics: Mechanical Properties of Living Tissues,* ed 2. New York, NY, Springer-Verlag, 1993.
37. Wright NT, Chen SS, Humphrey JD: Time-temperature equivalence of heat-induced changes in cells and proteins. *J Biomech Eng* 1998;120:22-26.
38. Kang T, Resar J, Humphrey JD: Heat-induced changes in the mechanical behavior of passive coronary arteries. *J Biomech Eng* 1995;117: 86-93.

39. Weir CE: Rate of shrinkage of tendon collagen-heat, entropy, and free energy of activation of the shrinkage of untreated tendon: Effect of acid, salt, pickle, and tannage on the activation of tendon collagen. *J Am Leather Chem* 1949;44: 108-138.

40. Le Lous M, Cohen-Solal L, Allain JC, Bonaventure J, Maroteaux P: Age related evolution of stable collagen reticulation in human skin. *Connect Tissue Res* 1985;13:145-155.

41. Privalov PL: Stability of proteins: Proteins which do not present a single cooperative system. *Adv Protein Chem* 1982;35:1-104.

42. Chvapil M, Jensovsky L: The shrinkage temperature of collagen fibres isolated from the tail tendons of rats of various ages and from different places of the same tendon. *Gerontologia* 1963;7:18-29.

43. Le Lous M, Allain JC, Cohen-Solal L, Maroteaux P: Hydrothermal isometric tension curves from different connective tissues: Role of collagen genetic types and noncollagenous components. *Connect Tissue Res* 1983;11: 199-206.

44. Privalov PL: Thermodynamic problems of protein structure. *Annu Rev Biophys Chem* 1989; 18:47-69.

45. Olde Damink LHH, Dijkstra PJ, Van Luyn MJA: Glutaraldehyde as a cross-linking agent for collagen-based biomaterials. *J Mat Sci Mat Med* 1995;6:460-472.

46. Boykin JV Jr, Molnar JA: Burn scar and skin equivalents, in Cohen IK, Diegelmann RF, Lindblad WJ (eds): *Wound Healing: Biochemical and Clinical Aspects.* Philadelphia, PA, WB Saunders, 1992, pp 523-540.

47. Gustavson KH (ed): *The Chemistry and Reactivity of Collagen.* New York, NY, Academic Press, 1956.

48. Reddy GK, Stehno-Bittel L, Enwemeka CS: Laser photostimulation of collagen production in healing rabbit Achilles tendons. *Lasers Surg Med* 1998;22:281-287.

49. Ling FF (ed): *Surface Mechanics.* New York, NY, John Wiley & Sons, 1973.

50. Hormann H, Schlebusch H: Reversible and irreversible denaturation of collagen fibers. *Biochemistry* 1971;10:932-937.

51. Foster TE, Elman M: Arthroscopic delivery systems used for thermally induced shoulder capsulorraphy. *Op Tech Sports Med* 1998;6: 126-130.

52. Peacock EE, Van Winkle W (eds): *Wound Repair,* ed 2. Philadelphia, PA, WB Saunders, 1976.

53. Herbert C, Jayson MI, Bailey AJ: Joint capsule collagen in osteoarthrosis. *Ann Rheum Dis* 1973; 32:510-514.

54. Schunke M, Kruss C, Mecke H, Werner JA: Characteristic features of wound healing in laser-induced incisions. *Adv Otorhinolaryngol* 1995;49:8-14.

55. Matsen FA III, Thomas SC, Rockwood CA Jr, Wirth MA: Glenohumeral Instability, in Rockwood CA Jr, Matsen FA III, Wirth MA, Harryman DT II (eds): *The Shoulder,* ed 2. Philadelphia, PA, WB Saunders, 1998, pp 611-754.

56. O'Brien SJ, Allen AA, Fealy S, Rodeo SA, Arnoczky SP: Developmental anatomy of the shoulder and anatomy of the glenohumeral Joint, in Rockwood CA Jr, Matsen FA III, Wirth MA, Harryman DT II (eds): *The Shoulder*, ed 2. Philadelphia, PA, WB Saunders, 1998, pp 1-33.

57. Hashimoto T, Hamada T, Sasaguri Y, Suzuki K: Immunohistochemical approach for the investigation of nerve distribution in the shoulder joint capsule. *Clin Orthop* 1994;305:273-282.

58. Vangsness CT Jr, Ennis M, Taylor JG, Atkinson R: Neural anatomy of the glenohumeral ligaments, labrum, and subacromial bursa. *Arthroscopy* 1995;11:180-184.

2

SYMPOSIUM

Arthroscopic Stabilization Plus Thermal Capsulorrhaphy for Anterior Instability With and Without Bankart Lesions: The Role of Rehabilitation and Immobilization

Richard J. Hawkins, MD, FRCSC
Spero G. Karas, MD

Introduction

Although open techniques to address anterior shoulder instability have generally provided good results, surgeons have attempted to decrease the morbidity associated with open surgery by using arthroscopically-assisted techniques to address anterior glenohumeral instability. Over the past two decades, arthroscopic treatment of shoulder instability has become increasingly popular. Green and Christensen[1] reported that arthroscopic techniques result in shorter duration of surgery, less blood loss, less narcotic use, and a shorter hospital stay compared with open surgical techniques. However, while some authors have reported excellent results using arthroscopic methods for the management of glenohumeral instability,[2-5] many have not reported success rates equivalent to those of open surgery.[1,6-11] Furthermore, authors have compared their success rates for open versus arthroscopic treatment and have noted inferior outcomes for arthroscopic management of shoulder instability.[8,11]

The failure to address capsular pathology has been indicated as a cause of recurrent instability after arthroscopic Bankart repair.[12-15] Until recently, the difficulty in adequately treating capsular redundancy with arthroscopic methods has contributed to the high failure rate for these procedures. Although the use of heat to treat shoulder instability dates back 2000 years,[16] thermal energy has recently been used to address increased glenohumeral capsular volume associated with instability. Several basic science studies have shown that the application of heat to animal collagen results in significant shrinkage of the collagen network.[17-20] Nonetheless, proper immobilization is necessary to maintain the acute effects of thermal capsular shrinkage. Shaefer and associates[21] reported that rabbit patellar ligaments showed significant shrinkage immediately after thermal treatment with a holmium:YAG laser. However, without an immobilization protocol, these tissues had stretched to their pretreatment length by 4 weeks and beyond their pretreatment lengths at 8 weeks. Schlegel and associates (unpublished data, 1999) noted that rabbit patellar ligaments treated with thermal shrinkage followed by a period of immobilization maintained a contracted morphology.

The rationale for the use of thermal capsulorrhaphy presented here is based on the basic science literature as well as clinical observation. By reducing the capsular laxity associated with anterior instability, thermal shrinkage is likely to improve the outcomes of arthroscopic anterior stabilization. Furthermore, reducing capsular volume with thermal shrinkage might allow the surgeon to accept less than perfect arthroscopic suturing techniques, thus serving as a backup for arthroscopically-assisted anterior instability repairs.

The importance of a meticulous immobilization protocol immediately following thermal capsulorrhaphy for anterior instability cannot be overemphasized. Intraoperative findings and postoperative follow-up seem to indicate that only 25% to 50% of the total contracture from heat capsulorrhaphy take place at the time of heat application. The remaining 50% to 75% occur sometime in the ensuing 6 weeks. A period of immobilization followed by guarded mobilization to allow new fibroblastic growth into the contracted collagen scaffold is required to achieve the desired translational effects while maintaining glenohumeral motion in a functional arc.

Recommended Postoperative Protocol for Anterior Instability

Phase I: Passive Range of Motion (Weeks 1 Through 4)

After arthroscopic anterior reconstruction with thermal capsulorrhaphy is performed, the shoulder is placed in a sling while the patient is in the operating room. Use of the sling continues for 3 weeks; the sling is to be worn at all times during the first postoperative week, with no motion allowed. During week 2, pendulum exercises are permitted. During the third postoperative week, external rotation to neutral or 0° and forward elevation to 90° are performed. Full internal rotation is allowed during week 3. By week 4, passive range of motion is advanced to 30° external rotation and full forward elevation. Pendulum exercises are performed for warm-up prior to each session of passive motion.

Phase II: Active Range of Motion (Week 5)

Active range of motion begins during week 5. Full forward flexion and internal rotation are encouraged. Again, pendulum exercises are performed prior to each active motion session. External rotation is gradually encouraged to progress from 30° at 4 weeks to near full rotation by 12 weeks.

Phase III: Resisted Range of Motion (Weeks 6 Through 12)

During phase III, continued active range of motion is performed. External rotation is advanced to full rotation over the ensuing 6 weeks. Resisted forward flexion, external rotation, and internal rotation are begun. A cord-resisted program of shrugs and rows for strengthening of the periscapular muscle also begins at this time. Eight weeks postoperatively, a weight training program is incorporated into the protocol. However, exercises that introduce stress to the anterior capsule (wide gripped bench press, military press behind the head, and chest flys) are not allowed at this time.

Return to Activities

Patients may return to computer-related jobs after 1 week. Chipping and putting may begin at 8 weeks; however, full golf strokes are not permitted until postoperative week 12. Tennis ground strokes may also begin at 12 weeks; overhead strokes are not permitted for 4 months. Contact sports are allowed after 4 months. Patients are to avoid any stress in the provocative cocking position for at least 4 months.

Outcomes

Between 1994 and 1999, arthroscopically-assisted thermal capsulorrhaphy for anterior instability was performed on 118 patients. The holmium:YAG laser was used for thermal capsulorrhaphy in 70 patients from 1994 to 1997 (unpublished data, 1999). Since 1997, the monopolar radiofrequency (RF) thermal probe has been used for anterior-inferior capsular shrinkage in 88 patients. Concomitant pathology (Bankart or superior labrum anterior posterior lesions) was addressed with arthroscopic suture technique or bioabsorbable tacks. Forty-seven patients were available for follow-up 2 years after the procedure. The overall failure rate for all patients treated with thermal capsulorrhaphy was 6% (3 of 47). The failure rate for laser-treated patients was 3% (1 of 30 patients). Patients treated with RF capsulorrhaphy had a failure rate of 12% (2 of 17 patients). American Shoulder and Elbow Surgeons scores improved from an average of 63 preoperatively to 94 postoperatively. Postoperative satisfaction averaged 9.0 on a 10-point scale. The treatment failed in two patients due to recurrent instability; another failure was caused by postoperative stiffness. There was no incidence of sensory or motor neurapraxia to the axillary nerve; however, one patient required a manipulation under anesthesia for postoperative adhesions.

Summary

The use of thermal energy is an exciting new technology in the treatment of anterior instability with and without Bankart reconstruction. The current approach for treating anterior instability in the absence of a Bankart lesion as discussed here is to perform thermal capsular shrinkage with a monopolar RF heat probe to address laxity in the anterior capsule and the inferior glenohumeral ligaments. If a Bankart lesion is present, repair of the lesion with arthroscopic suture anchors followed by thermal capsulorrhaphy is our treatment of choice. We currently reserve open anterior reconstruction for patients with pathology inappropriate for arthroscopic techniques and in cases where arthroscopic suturing is found to be inadequate intraoperatively. Furthermore, patients who require revision and athletes who engage in contact sports are evaluated on an individual basis to ascertain if arthroscopic techniques are appropriate **(CD-2.1)**.

Nonetheless, basic science research has revealed the importance of a formal period of immobilization followed by guarded mobilization. By using the aforementioned algorithm and postoperative protocol, low recurrence rates have been achieved while at the same time maintaining motion in the functional range. Of course, further follow-up, more patient studies, and peer review publications are required to determine if thermal capsulorrhaphy can replace open procedures as the gold standard for addressing capsular laxity associated with anterior instability.

References

1. Green MR, Christensen KP: Arthroscopic Bankart procedure: Two- to five-year follow-up with clinical correlation to severity of glenoid labral lesion. *Am J Sports Med* 1995;23:276-281.
2. Morgan CD, Bodenstab AB: Arthroscopic Bankart suture repair: Technique and early results. *Arthroscopy* 1987;3:111-122.
3. Arciero RA, Taylor DC, Snyder RJ, Uhorchak JM: Arthroscopic bioabsorbable tack stabilization of initial anterior shoulder dislocations: A preliminary report. *Arthroscopy* 1995;11:410-417.
4. Benedetto KP, Glotzer W: Arthroscopic Bankart procedure by suture technique: Indications, technique, and results. *Arthroscopy* 1992;8:111-115.
5. Wolf EM: Arthroscopic anterior shoulder capsulorrhaphy. *Tech Orthop* 1988;3:67-73.
6. Grana WA, Buckley PD, Yates CK: Arthroscopic Bankart suture repair. *Am J Sports Med* 1993;21:348-353.
7. Walch G, Boileau P, Levigne C, Mandrino A, Neyret P, Donell S: Arthroscopic stabilization for recurrent anterior shoulder dislocation: Results of 59 cases. *Arthroscopy* 1995;11:173-179.

8. Geiger DF, Hurley JA, Tovey JA, Rao JP: Results of arthroscopic versus open Bankart suture repair. *Clin Orthop* 1997;337:111-117.

9. Youssef JA, Carr CF, Walther CE, Murphy JM: Arthroscopic Bankart suture repair for recurrent traumatic unidirectional anterior shoulder dislocations. *Arthroscopy* 1995;11:561-563.

10. Pagnani MJ, Warren RF, Altchek DW, Wickiewicz TL, Anderson AF: Arthroscopic shoulder stabilization using transglenoid sutures: A four-year minimum follow up. *Am J Sports Med* 1996;24:459-467.

11. Guanche CA, Quick DC, Sodergren KM, Buss DD: Arthroscopic versus open reconstruction of the shoulder in patients with isolated Bankart lesions. *Am J Sports Med* 1996;24: 144-148.

12. Mologne TS, McBride MT, Lapoint JM: Assessment of failed arthroscopic anterior labral repairs: Findings at open surgery. *Am J Sports Med* 1997;25:813-817.

13. Speer KP, Deng X, Borrero S, Torzilli PA, Altchek DA, Warren RF: Biomechanical evaluation of a simulated Bankart lesion. *J Bone Joint Surg Am* 1994;76:1819-1826.

14. Speer KP, Warren RF, Pagnani M, Warner JJ: An arthroscopic technique for anterior stabilization of the shoulder with a bioabsorbable tack. *J Bone Joint Surg Am* 1996;78:1801-1807.

15. Warner JJ, Miller MD, Marks P, Fu FH: Arthroscopic Bankart repair with the Suretac device: Part I. Clinical observations. *Arthroscopy* 1995;11:2-13.

16. Adams F (ed): *The Genuine Works of Hippocrates.* New York, NY, William Wood & Co, 1886.

17. Hayashi K, Thabit G III, Bogdanske JJ, Mascio LN, Markel MD: The effect of nonablative laser energy on the ultrastructure of joint capsular collagen. *Arthroscopy* 1996;12:474-481.

18. Hayashi K, Thabit G III, Massa KL, et al: The effect of thermal heating on the length and histologic properties of the glenohumeral joint capsule. *Am J Sports Med* 1997;25:107-112.

19. Hayashi K, Massa KL, Thabit G III, et al: Histologic evaluation of the glenohumeral joint capsule after the laser-assisted capsular shift procedure for glenohumeral instability. *Am J Sports Med* 1999;27:162-167.

20. Hecht P, Hayashi K, Lu Y, et al: Monopolar radiofrequency energy effects on joint capsular tissue: Potential treatment for joint instability: An in vivo mechanical, morphological, and biochemical study using an ovine model. *Am J Sports Med* 1999;27:761-771.

21. Schaefer SL, Ciarelli MJ, Arnoczky SP, Ross HE: Tissue shrinkage with the holmium: yttrium aluminum garnet laser: A postoperative assessment of tissue length, stiffness, and structure. *Am J Sports Med* 1997;25:841-848.

Reference to Video

Hawkins RJ: Arthroscopic Bankart repair with heat probe capsulorrhaphy. *Double and Single Anterior Cannula Techniques.* Vail, CO, Steadman-Hawkins Sports Medicine Foundation, 1999.

3

SYMPOSIUM

Diagnosis and Treatment of Shoulder Injuries in the Throwing Athlete: The Role of Thermal-Assisted Capsular Shrinkage

James R. Andrews, MD
Jeffrey R. Dugas, MD

Introduction

As knowledge about the biomechanical aspects of the throwing motion has increased, so too has understanding of the pathologic conditions associated with throwing. In the majority of throwing athletes at the high school level and beyond, there is increased external rotation as well as decreased internal rotation of the throwing shoulder in abduction when compared with the contralateral shoulder.[1] Thus, the total arc of shoulder motion is not necessarily increased in the throwing shoulder. The increase in external rotation is typically associated with an increase in anterior capsular laxity without frank instability, probably the result of repetitive throwing motion during the course of childhood and adolescent development (Fig. 1). This increase in capsular laxity is normal in the throwing shoulder and should not be considered pathologic.

Any increase in capsular laxity will allow increased translation of the humeral head within the glenoid fossa. The decrease in static stability afforded by the capsule leads to increased reliance on the rotator cuff musculature as a means of providing glenohumeral stability. Unlike the capsule, the dynamic stability provided by the rotator cuff is prone to fatigue, which may lead to abnormal mechanics and increase the potential for injury. This chapter will discuss the typical pathology of the thrower's shoulder, how to confirm the diagnosis, and the treatment of these conditions, specifically, the role of thermal-assisted capsular shrinkage (TACS).

Pathology

Several types of pathology are frequently seen in the throwing shoulder. Labral tears, specifically superior labrum anterior and posterior (SLAP) lesions, and partial-thickness rotator cuff tears associated with internal impingement are among the most common. It is possible, and perhaps even likely, that each of these types of shoulder pathology is related to the increased laxity in the throwing shoulder, which has led to what has been termed overrotation of the humerus in the glenoid, which is considered to be the mechanism of internal impingement.[2] This overrotation can cause a posteriorly directed force by the biceps tendon as it rotates posterior to the center of the humeral head that can potentially result in a peelback phenomenon, as first described by Burkhart and Morgan.[3] In this condition, the superior labrum is peeled away from the glenoid rim (Fig. 2), leading to a type II SLAP lesion, which frequently causes pain. This overrotation can also be

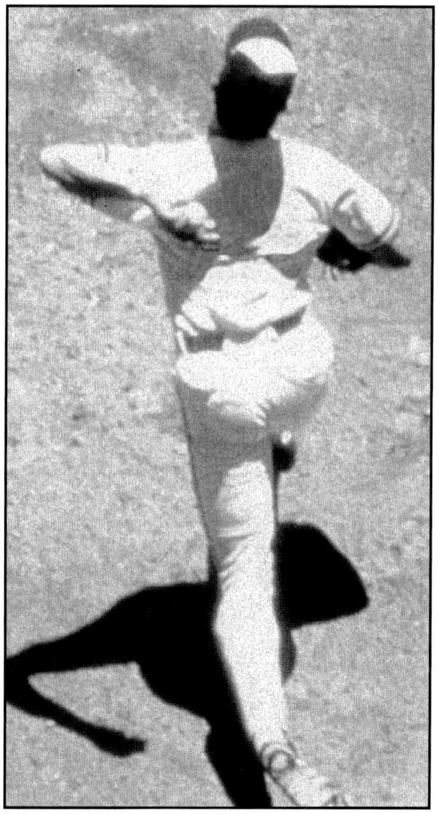

Fig. 1 Note the excessive external rotation of the arm in this professional baseball pitcher. Most throwing athletes demonstrate increased external rotation in abduction.

considered a rotational instability. Obviously, any translational instability can exaggerate this rotational laxity.

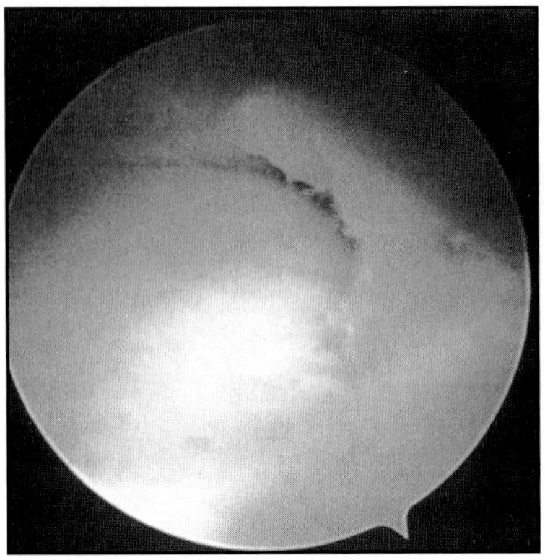

Fig. 2 Arthroscopic view of the left shoulder with the patient in the lateral decubitus position and the arthroscope inserted through a posterior portal. Note the detachment of the superior labrum from the glenoid. This "peelback" of the labrum is likely the result of a posteriorly directed force by the biceps as the arm rotated into maximum external rotation.

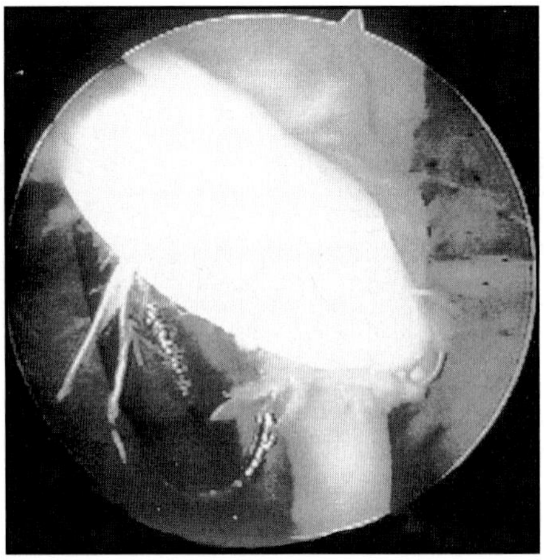

Fig. 3 Arthroscopic view of the partial undersurface tear of the distal aspect of the infraspinatus tendon. The fraying seen here was caused by impingement of the tendon on the posterosuperior glenoid rim. This is the classic internal impingement lesion.

Internal impingement was first described by Walch and associates[2] in 1992. Internal impingement occurs when the posterosuperior glenoid labrum impinges on the posterosuperior rotator cuff fibers with the arm in abduction and maximum external rotation (Fig. 3). Contact between the undersurface of the infraspinatus and the glenoid labrum may lead to abrasion and tearing of the cuff tissue, resulting in a painful shoulder. Typically these are not full-thickness rotator cuff tears, but rather partial-thickness injuries with fraying of the undersurface of the infraspinatus tendon at the level of the glenohumeral joint. This fraying is seen just proximal to the insertion of the tendon rather than at the insertion point. Maximum external rotation of the contralateral shoulder usually does not lead to impingement of the rotator cuff tissue. In a study by Halbrecht and associates,[4] 10 out of 10 throwing shoulders were noted on MRI to have impingement of the infraspinatus tendon in abduction/external rotation. The contralateral shoulders did not demonstrate such impingement.

Labral tears are not uncommon in throwing athletes. SLAP lesions, as first described by Snyder, have been well documented over the past decade.[5-7] It is likely that these lesions in the thrower result from either direct compression of the labrum or from a similar mechanism as the peelback phenomenon, and that labral pathology in the thrower is related to laxity and overrotation as often as it is to primary compression by the humeral head.

Full-thickness rotator cuff tears are distinctly uncommon, but not unheard of, in the thrower. This is probably because insidious progression to full-thickness injury is rarely possible due to the pain and/or decrease in performance that results from a lesser injury, such as a partial-thickness tear. In older, high-level throwers, the partial-thickness tears can penetrate and become full-thickness tears. In the thrower, acute full-thickness rotator cuff tears occur in the presence of direct trauma or dislocation. It is unlikely that the progression from partial-thickness to full-thickness rotator cuff pathology is the direct result of increased laxity in the thrower's shoulder. However, it is possible that such laxity and rotational instability led to the initial insult on the rotator cuff, and that further propagation of the tear occurred with activity.

Diagnosis

In the process of clinical evaluation of the throwing athlete, it is pertinent to obtain an adequate history. Specifically, the throwing history should include most recent activity and changes in level of performance (velocity, control, stamina, pain). Any recent changes in throwing mechanics or schedule should be noted. Any prior history of shoulder or elbow problems or surgery as well as any previous treatment, should be documented.

Physical examination should include visual inspection, palpation, active and passive range of motion tests, manual strength, assessment of neurovascular condition, stability, and other special tests. At our clinic, checking all shoulders for the presence of labral pathology with the active compression test as described by O'Brien and associates[8] is routine, as well as checking for external impingement with the Neer and Hawkins tests.[9,10] A Lachman examination of the shoulder is done with the patient supine and relaxed. The humerus is then abducted and externally rotated as the examiner performs anterior translation of the humeral head. The endfeel, the subjective assessment of the end point of anterior translation, is as important as the amount of translation. In the normal shoulder and the asymptomatic throwing shoulder, the anterior band of the inferior glenohumeral ligament will become the most important static restraint in this position. Normally, with anterior translation of the humeral head, the anterior tissues become taut, leading to a firm end point. In patients with increased laxity, the amount of translation may increase, but the endfeel should not be softened. Careful attention is paid to the overall ligamentous laxity. Toward this end, a sulcus test is performed on both shoulders.

The test for internal impingement is performed by placing the patient supine with the arm abducted and externally rotated. The arm is then forced into maximum external rotation. If this maneuver elicits pain in the posterior aspect of the shoulder in the region of the infraspinatus, the test is positive. Palpation of the posterior aspect of the rotator cuff specifically in the region of the infraspinatus is performed. Any pain in this region should also be noted, because this may be the only outward sign of a partial-thickness rotator cuff tear.

After completeing a thorough history and physical examination, plain radiographs should be obtained. These views include anteroposterior views in internal and external rotation, a Stryker view, and an axillary view. Gadolinium-enhanced MRI is also a valuable diagnostic tool used to confirm the presence of pathology that is suspected on the basis of history and physical examination. MRI will often be able to demonstrate fraying or tearing of the cuff as well as the type and location of labral pathology.

Treatment

Once the diagnosis of a pathologic condition has been made in the throwing athlete, the physician must outline an appropriate treatment plan. It is important to note that one of the most challenging decisions facing clinicians who treat athletes is whether or not surgical treatment is indicated, and when the most appropriate time for surgery might be. The chronic nature of the injury and the amount of disability or decrease in performance that the athlete has or is likely to experience in the future must be carefully weighed against the amount of time required for rehabilitation following surgery in order to return to competition. In many cases, conservative measures, such as prolonged rest, physical therapy, medications, and even injections depending on the nature of the pathology, may be exhausted prior to consideration for surgery.

In treating the throwing athlete who has shoulder pain or decreased performance secondary to shoulder pathology, the choice of surgical procedures must be based on the likelihood of successful return to throwing activities. In the past, shoulder surgery in the throwing athlete may have been a career-ending event. Subacromial impingement is rare in the relatively young throwing athlete population. This may explain the poor results noted with acromioplasty alone, as noted by Kvitne and associates.[11] Payne and associates[12] noted a decrease in the overall results and in the percentage of athletes who returned to competition when increased glenohumeral laxity was present in combination with partial-thickness rotator cuff tears. Many of the patients in this study who had poor results were noted to have insidious rather than acute pain, as well as the frequent presence of labral pathology in those with increased laxity. Similarly, Glasgow and associates[13] noted that débridement of labral lesions in throwing athletes was significantly less successful in throwers with increased glenohumeral laxity when compared to those with stable shoulders. Both of these studies clearly demonstrate the importance of recognizing the presence of increased laxity as a contributor, and possibly even the direct cause of pathology within the throwing shoulder. We believe that in the past, the surgeon's inability to treat acquired laxity in the throwing shoulder without performing a formal open capsular reconstruction has negatively affected outcomes.

Therefore, we began using TACS at our institution in July 1997. Levitz and associates (unpublished data, 2000) recently completed a two-phase retrospective study investigating the treatment with TACS of throwing athletes with shoulder pathology. There were two groups in the first phase of the study. In phase I, group A, the charts of all baseball players (18 Major League, 16 Minor League, 13 college, 2 Korean League, and 2 high school) who underwent shoulder arthroscopy at our institution between January 1, 1995 and December 31, 1996 were reviewed. Fifty-one athletes were identified during that time interval with confirmed partial-thickness undersurface rotator cuff tears at arthroscopy, with follow-up a minimum of 2 years after surgery. Capsular laxity was not addressed in any of these patients. Forty-nine of the 51 patients demonstrated increased glenohumeral laxity on the basis of examination under anesthesia in addition to the internal impingement. One player had subacromial impingement (external impingement), and another did not have increased glenohumeral laxity. Thirteen of the 49 underwent labral repair in addition to rotator cuff débridement. Twenty-seven of the 49 underwent labral débridement in addition to rotator cuff débridement.

In phase I, group B, 30 players who underwent shoulder arthroscopy between July 1997 and December 1997 were identified. Again, each player was noted to have an internal impingement lesion (partial-thickness undersurface rotator cuff tear), with follow-up a minimum of 2 years after surgery. Each of the players in group B underwent TACS in addition to treatment of the rotator cuff pathology.

In phase I, group A (no TACS), 80% of players returned to play. The mean time to return to competition was 7.2 months. At 2 years follow-up, 67% of players were still competing, and 61% were competing at the same or higher level. In phase I, group B (those who had TACS), 93% returned to competition at a mean of 7.4 months. At 2 years follow-up, 93% were still competing, and 86% were competing at the same or higher level.

In the group A patients who underwent only débridement of the partial-thickness rotator cuff tear who had no labral injury requiring repair and did not undergo TACS, 71% were still competing

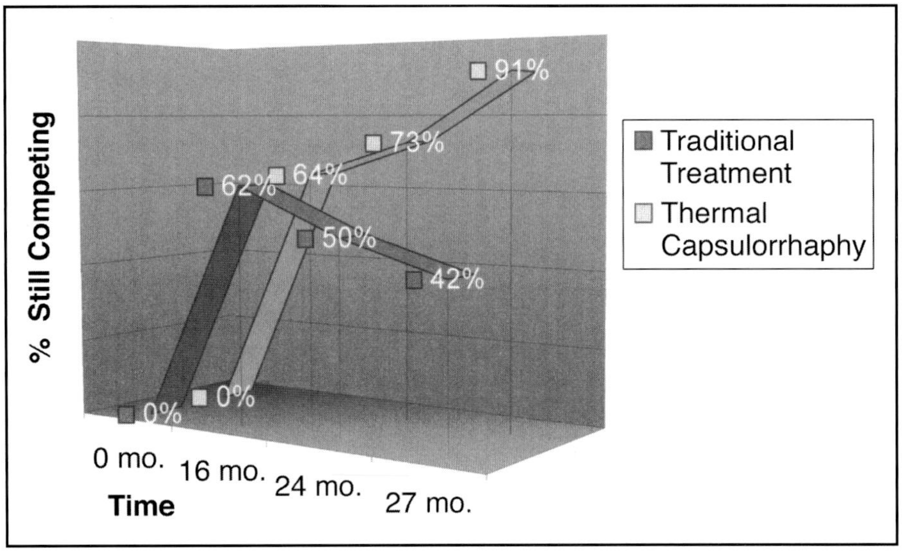

Fig. 4 Internal impingement with SLAP repair. Graphic illustration of the data collected in throwing athletes with and without TACS. Note the improvement in return-to-competition as the interval from surgery increases from 1 to 2 years.

at 2 years postsurgery. In the group B patients who underwent débridement of the partial-thickness rotator cuff tear and TACS who did not have labral injury requiring repair, 100% were still competing at 2 years postsurgery.

In patients who underwent débridement and SLAP repair without TACS, 50% were still competing at 2 years postsurgery. In contrast, 73% of those who underwent débridement and SLAP repair along with TACS were competing at 2 years postsurgery. In reviewing the results in these two groups, the beneficial effect of addressing capsular laxity at the time of arthroscopy is clear.

During the interval between January 1, 1995 and December 31, 1998, a total of 140 TACS procedures were performed, not all involving throwing athletes. No significant complications occurred. One case of axillary neuritis occurred early in the study. The symptoms resolved completely within 6 weeks. Interestingly, improvement in the percentage of athletes who returned to play following TACS was noted as the interval from surgery increased from 1 year to 2 years (Fig. 4). Additionally, it was noted that athletes at the professional level fared better than those performing at the amateur level.

Phase II of the study was then performed to investigate the association of SLAP lesions and capsular laxity. Phase II involved only baseball players at the professional or National Collegiate Athletic Association Division I level. Twenty-three players were identified retrospectively who met the selection criteria and were followed for a minimum of 27 months postsurgery. Of the 12 players who underwent arthroscopic SLAP repair without TACS, 5 of them (42%) were competing at 27 months. Of the 11 players who underwent arthroscopic SLAP repair in addition to TACS, 10 (91%) were competing at 27 months. The mean time to return to play in this group was 11 months.

In a study presented at the 1999 American Orthopaedic Society for Sports Medicine meeting (Traverse City, MI, June 1999) Grana and associates (unpublished data) reported on 19 patients, 14 of whom were throwers with pain as a primary complaint who underwent TACS. These 14 patients had labral pathology (fraying or tear) and 8 of 14 (57%) had internal impingement. At the time of most recent follow-up, 18 of the original 19 had satisfactory results, and all of these patients were asymptomatic. One patient had poor results after a repeat surgery following reinjury. Eight of the 14 throwers returned to throwing (57%).

The results of these studies clearly demonstrate that addressing the capsular laxity at the time of surgery leads to increasing rates of return to play in throwers with increased capsular laxity and intra-articular pathology such as internal impingement and SLAP lesions. No data are available at this time regarding the treatment of throwing athletes with full-thickness rotator cuff tears using open or arthroscopic repair and TACS. Our results do demonstrate that the presence of a SLAP lesion negatively affects the overall results and increases the time necessary to return to competition. As the interval from surgery increases, the overall percentage of players who are able to return to play at the same or higher level tends to increase.

As is the case with nearly any surgical procedure, the postoperative care of the patient is of paramount importance. This is certainly true for the throwing athlete. Since we began using the TACS technique in 1997, our postoperative rehabilitation program has been modified to address the need for physiologic laxity in the thrower without returning to the pathologic laxity that led to surgical treatment in the first place.[14] Currently, we use a standard shoulder sling for the first 2 weeks while the patient is awake, and a shoulder immobilizer for the first 4 weeks while the patient is asleep. During that time, the patient is permitted to remove the sling several times a day to perform range of motion activities with the arm in 0° to 15° of glenohumeral abduction. After the initial 4 weeks, use of the shoulder immobilizer is discontinued, and range of motion is gradually increased so that at 6 weeks after surgery, the patient can abduct the arm to 90° and externally rotate the arm 70° to 80° with the arm abducted. During the 8- to 12-week interval, external rotation in abduction is allowed past 90°, with gradual progression to approximately 115° to 118°. Isometric exercise is allowed for postoperative days 1 through 10. Next, gradual strengthening of the rotator cuff musculature is begun, paying particular attention to the supraspinatus and infraspinatus. An interval throwing program is started when the range of motion is believed to be adequate and soreness has abated, around 4 months. The athlete progresses through the interval throwing program in a stepwise fashion prior to returning to competition. With regard to the initial postoperative period, both shorter (2-week) and longer (6-week) periods of immobilization have been attempted, with less success.

Summary

The treatment of the throwing athlete is complex. Many factors enter into the decision regarding the nature and timing of appropriate intervention. Because of the nature of the mechanical aspects of the throwing motion, increased external rotation (overrotation) is often necessary to throw at a highly competitive level. This increased motion is associated with acquired increased glenohumeral laxity which, by itself, is generally not problematic. However, in the athlete with an overuse-type shoulder injury such as a SLAP lesion or a partial-thickness undersurface tear of the rotator cuff (internal impingement), it is perhaps the increase in glenohumeral laxity that allows such pathology to occur. A careful history and physical examination are important to determine the nature of the injury and the amount of laxity that may be present. Currently, we believe that addressing the capsular laxity arthroscopically at the same time that the intra-articular pathology is addressed is the best form of treatment for these athletes, and affords them the best chance of returning to competition at the same or higher level. Obviously, further follow-up is necessary to determine the long-term results of such treatment.

References

1. King J, Brelsford HJ, Tullos HS: Analysis of the pitching arm of the professional baseball pitcher. *Clin Orthop* 1969;67:116-123.
2. Walch G, Boileau P, Noel E, Donell ST: Impingement of the deep surface of the supraspinatus tendon on the posterosuperior glenoid rim: An arthroscopic study. *J Shoulder Elbow Surg* 1992;1:238-245.
3. Burkhart SS, Morgan CD: The peel-back mechanism: Its role in producing and extending posterior type II SLAP lesions and its effect on SLAP repair rehabilitation. *Arthroscopy* 1998;14:637-640.
4. Halbrecht JL, Tirman P, Atkin D: Internal impingement of the shoulder: Comparison of findings between the throwing and nonthrowing shoulders of college baseball players. *Arthroscopy* 1999;15:253-258.
5. Snyder SJ, Karzel RP, Del Pizzo W, Ferkel RD, Friedman MJ: SLAP lesions of the shoulder. *Arthroscopy* 1990;6:274-279.
6. Andrews JR, Carson WG Jr: Abstract: The arthroscopic treatment of glenoid labrum tears in the throwing athlete. *Orthop Trans* 1984;8:44.
7. Altchek DW, Warren RF, Wickiewicz TL, Oritz G, et al: Arthroscopic labral debridement: A three-year follow-up study. *Am J Sports Med* 1992;20:702-706.
8. O'Brien SJ, Pagnani MJ, Fealy S, McGlynn SR, Wilson JB: The active compression test: A new and effective test for diagnosing labral tears and acromioclavicular joint abnormality. *Am J Sports Med* 1998;26:610-613.
9. Neer CS II, Welsh RP: The shoulder in sports. *Orthop Clin North Am* 1977;8:583–591.
10. Hawkins RJ, Kennedy JC: Impingement syndrome in athletes. *Am J Sports Med* 1980; 8: 151-158.
11. Kvitne RS, Jobe FW, Jobe CM: Shoulder instability in the overhand or throwing athlete. *Clin Sports Med* 1995;14:917-935.
12. Payne LZ, Altchek DW, Craig EV, Warren RF: Arthroscopic treatment of partial rotator cuff tears in young athletes: A preliminary report. *Am J Sports Med* 1997;25:299-305.
13. Glasgow SG, Bruce RA, Yacobucci GN, Torg JS: Arthroscopic resection of glenoid labral tears in the athlete: A review of 29 cases. *Arthroscopy* 1992;8:48-54.
14. Wilk KE: Rehabilitation after shoulder stabilization surgery, in Warren RF, Craig EV, Altchek DW (eds): *The Unstable Shoulder.* Philadelphia, PA, Lippincott-Raven, 1999, pp 367-402.

4

SYMPOSIUM

Thermal Capsulorrhaphy for Instability of the Shoulder: Multidirectional and Posterior Instabilities

J. Robert Giffin, MD, FRCSC
Christopher C. Annunziata, MD
James P. Bradley, MD

Introduction

Arthroscopic stabilization techniques for the treatment of glenohumeral instability continue to improve: incisions are smaller, patient morbidity is lower, and rehabilitation is easier. However, results to date have not matched the success of open procedures, especially in patients with multidirectional or complex patterns of shoulder instability.[1-4] Presumably, the capsular and ligamentous structures, which play a critical role in glenohumeral stability, have not been adequately addressed with arthroscopic stabilization techniques in the past.[2,5]

Recently, radiofrequency (RF) energy has been used to tighten or shrink the glenohumeral ligaments as well as reduce capsular volume.[1,2,6-10] It has become popular to use this energy source alone or in combination with other arthroscopic surgical techniques to treat a variety of shoulder conditions. Several basic science articles have been published on the mechanism of thermal modification of joint capsule and ligamentous tissue.[11-26] The thermal response or shrinkage of the tissue and the effect on its mechanical properties is energy dependent and a function of temperature.

Both laser and RF energy have been shown to cause thermal tissue damage and shortening that is followed by a reparative healing response to regain the tissue's mechanical properties. Although thermal energy has been shown to alter the structure of collagenous tissue, the long-term biomechanical properties of the modified tissue remain unknown. The healing response and the effect of immobilization during this phase in vivo is even less well understood, but early clinical results have been promising in terms of apparent tissue response and symptom resolution.[1,2,7]

Although the technique is currently being widely used throughout the United States, the published literature available regarding patient outcomes is limited. Whether this rapidly evolving technology will have a lasting benefit remains to be determined. Additional prospective outcome studies are necessary to better understand the importance of this new technique in the treatment of glenohumeral instability.[1,2,7]

Shoulder Instability

Shoulder instability spans from occult subluxation to frank dislocation. It commonly affects between 2% and 8% of the population and represents one third of all shoulder-related emergency department visits.[1,27] However, the true incidence of shoulder instability would be grossly underestimated if all activity-related shoulder pain secondary to occult subluxation were also accounted. Glenohumeral instability is primarily a disorder of older adolescents and young adults. Several studies have shown that the recurrence rate of instability is inversely proportional to the age of the patient at the time of the initial injury.[1,28]

Glenohumeral stability is dependent on a variety of well-described anatomic features, including the static restraints of the capsulolabral ligament complex, negative intra-articular pressure, and dynamic compression from a neuromuscularly intact rotator cuff.[5,29-31] Instability can arise from a single traumatic event, recurrent microtrauma, and atraumatic constitutional ligamentous laxity. Furthermore, most instances of unidirectional and multidirectional instability (MDI) are associated with an increase in joint capsule volume. The pathologic feature common to all forms of symptomatic shoulder instability is a varying degree of interstitial damage or plastic deformation of the capsule and/or glenohumeral ligaments.[1,32-34]

Multidirectional Instability

MDI of the shoulder is more common than previously believed in both the athletic and general populations.[32-35] The underlying pathoanatomy is likely to be related to excessive capsuloligamentous laxity, with widening of the rotator interval and a resultant increase in joint capsule volume. The diagnosis of MDI was previously reserved for sedentary individuals with generalized ligamentous laxity, bilateral symptoms, and no history of trauma. However, gymnasts, swimmers, and overhead athletes may have acquired shoulder hyperlaxity secondary to repetitive microtrauma and plastic deformation of the capsule. Furthermore, many of these athletes with MDI have had a superimposed injury and thus may have concomitant Bankart and humeral head lesions.

Patients with MDI may present with pain, overt instability, or vague symptoms in the affected extremity during activities. Provocative motions or activities and associated arm positions that cause symptoms must be elicited carefully because they suggest directions of instability. Patients must be evaluated for evidence of generalized ligamentous laxity, in addition to a thorough examination of the entire shoulder complex. Multiple positive findings may become apparent when the following maneuvers are performed: anterior/posterior load and shift tests, anterior/posterior apprehension and relocation, Fukuda and push-pull tests. It is important to perform the examination with the arm in varying degrees of abduction and rotation to effect different degrees of tension within the capsular ligaments. A sulcus sign of 2 cm is considered pathognomonic for MDI. Finally, examination under anesthesia can provide a more accurate appreciation of the direction and degree of instability in complex cases.

Once the diagnosis of MDI is established, nonsurgical management which includes patient education, activity modification, and a prolonged course of physical therapy is instituted.[36] Emphasis initially is focused on strengthening the rotator cuff, deltoid, and scapular stabilizers, followed by exercises to retrain humeroscapular coordination and proprioception. Exercises are continued for a minimum of 6 months with an expected satisfactory outcome of 90%.[36] If symptoms of pain and functional instability persist following an adequate course of therapy, surgical alternatives should be considered.[3,33,37,38] Surgical treatment must not only address the primary area of pathology but also correct any secondary cartilaginous or bony changes resulting from persistent instability of the shoulder.

Posterior Instability

The diagnosis and treatment of posterior instability of the shoulder continues to present a significant challenge.[39-41] Advances in the understanding and management of the athlete's shoulder have resulted in an increasingly frequent diagnosis of recurrent posterior subluxation. In patients with posterior instability, symptoms are usually present when the arm is used in a position of flexion, adduction, and internal rotation. Traumatic injuries with the arm in this provocative position lead to the onset of symptoms in approximately 50% of patients.[39,41] Repetitive microtrauma from a variety of sporting endeavors (such as football, weight lifting, and overhead sports activities) can also result in symptoms of posterior subluxation. Finally, there is a group of patients with physical characteristics of generalized laxity whose primary complaint is posterior instability.

Pain is the most common symptom in patients with posterior instability. Although variable in location, the pain likely represents edge loading of the humeral head against the glenoid or overuse of the rotator cuff in an attempt to maintain stability. Furthermore, patients will often describe a sensation of clicking or crepitation when the shoulder is placed in certain positions. In approximately 50% of patients with recurrent posterior instability, the instability (positional and muscular) can be demonstrated voluntarily.[39,41] It is important to differentiate between patients who are able to subluxate their shoulders by positioning and muscular activation and those who do so for secondary gain.

Routine physical examination of the shoulder for range of motion and muscle strength is often unremarkable. Although apprehension in the provocative position is an uncommon finding because of patient guarding, it is very helpful in confirming the diagnosis if posterior translation reproduces the patient's symptoms. Posterior glenohumeral joint tenderness can usually be appreciated as well. Stress testing should also be performed in the anterior and inferior directions to assess the shoulder for MDI.

Nonsurgical management is the mainstay of treatment for patients with atraumatic posterior instability.[36,39] Treatment is directed toward decreasing the patient's pain with rest, anti-inflammatory medications, and avoidance of provocative arm positions and activities. Physical therapy exercises consisting of scapular stabilization and rotator cuff strengthening (especially of the external rotators) will improve the dynamic stabilization of the joint. Voluntary dislocators are best treated with extensive rehabilitation. Patients with traumatic posterior dislocations generally respond better to conservative treatment than do those with anterior dislocations.[36] However, patients with large reverse Bankart lesions or marked instability are less likely to respond to exercise therapy alone. Surgery should be considered in those patients for whom an extensive rehabilitation program has failed.[39,42,43]

Goals of Surgery

Successful treatment of shoulder instability is dependent on accurate recognition of the pattern of the instability and complete assessment of the extent of soft-tissue injury. Surgical stabilization of the glenohumeral joint is an option in those patients for whom an extensive rehabilitation program has failed because of continued pain and/or instability. Persons who have symptoms during desired activities or who are unable to participate in their sports may also elect surgical treatment. Although open procedures have been the treatment of choice for many years, there remains considerable room for improvement in the treatment of shoulder instability. For newer techniques to gain acceptance, the treatment must adequately address the pathology, be relatively easy to perform, and remain cost-effective.

Surgical Technique

Arthroscopic thermal capsulorrhaphy of the shoulder does not require any special setup and typically can be performed through standard anterior, posterior, and posterior accessory arthroscopy portals. Either the beach chair or lateral decubitus position can be used based on the preference of the surgeon. Following an examination under anesthesia, a diagnostic arthroscopy is then performed. Any associated labral lesions (such as superior labrum anterior and posterior [SLAP], Bankart) found at the time of arthroscopy must be concomitantly stabilized.

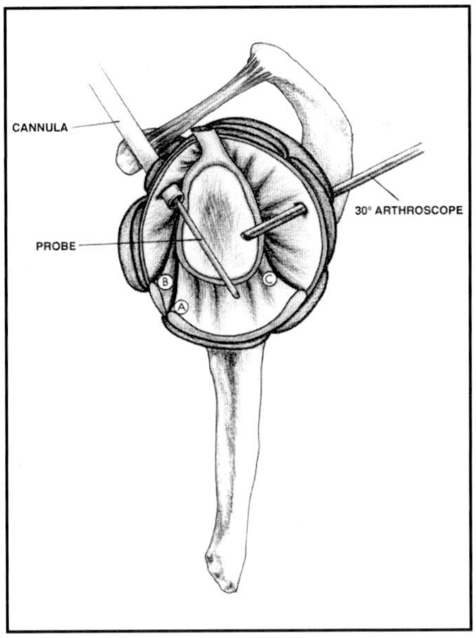

Fig. 1 Thermal capsulorrhaphy for primarily anterior instability is performed with the probe entering anteriorly. The sequence of treatment progresses from the anterior recess of the axillary pouch in an anterosuperior direction. The anterior band of inferior glenohumeral ligament complex (**A**), middle glenohumeral ligament (**B**), and posterior band of inferior glenohumeral ligament complex (**C**) are shown. (© Cyndi Slagel)

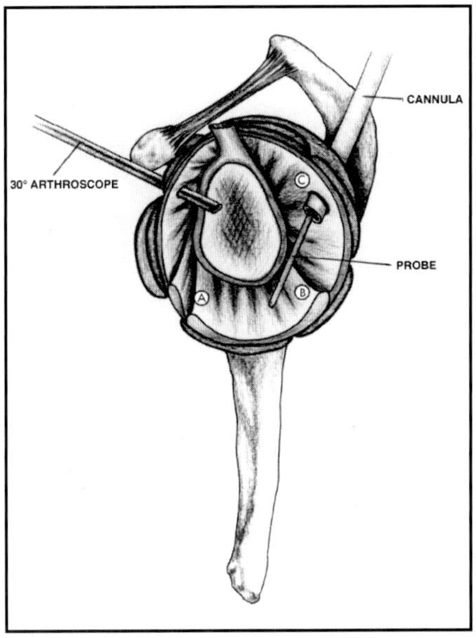

Fig. 2 Posterior instability can be performed with the portal setup reversed and treatment progressing from the posterior recess of the axillary pouch in a posterosuperior direction. The anterior band of inferior glonohumeral ligament complex (**A**), posterior band of inferior glenohumeral ligament complex (**B**), and posterior capsule (**C**) are shown. (© Cyndi Slagel)

Capsular Response

RF energy heats the capsule via a probe that is in contact with the tissue. The capsular response to the thermal energy is dependent on both temperature and time. Thus, the speed with which the probe is moved across the tissue will affect the amount of shrinkage obtained. Caution must be taken not to leave the probe in one position while activated. Maintenance of the temperature in the therapeutic range must be monitored while the surgeon visually inspects for the capsular response. Areas of the capsule with higher collagen density, that is, the middle and inferior glenohumeral ligaments, will respond more dramatically. The least responsive area is the posterior superior capsule, which is relatively thin.

Treatment Sequence

In order to optimize arthroscopic visualization while performing the procedure, the surgeon should treat the areas of the capsule in a specific sequence depending on the instability pattern of the shoulder. Thermal capsulorrhaphy can be accomplished in patients with primarily anterior instability by having the probe enter anteriorly while viewing from the posterior portal. The surgeon should begin in the anterior portion of the auxiliary recess, moving toward the anterior capsular structures from an inferior to superior direction (Fig. 1). Posterior pathology can be addressed in the reverse sequence and portal setup (Fig. 2).

For patients with MDI, the posterior and inferior portions of the capsule need to be addressed in addition to the anterior capsuloligamentous structures. If necessary, an accessory posterior portal can be safely established approximately 1.0 to 1.5 cm below the standard posterior portal (GS DeFelice, MD, RJ Williams, MD, RF Warren, MD, Vancouver, British Columbia, unpublised data, 1999) (Fig. 3). The probe is then introduced parallel to the arthroscope, providing excellent access to the patulous central axillary pouch and posterior band of the inferior glenohumeral ligament. Extreme care must be exercised while using the probe in this area because of the close proximity of the axillary nerve to the capsule.[44] Furthermore, the arm should not be abducted beyond 30° intraoperatively in order to avoid pulling the axillary nerve closer to the inferior capsule.

Postoperative Care

A period of postoperative immobilization in a sling is critical to a successful outcome following thermal capsulorrhaphy. The sling is removed only for personal hygiene, and passive range of motion exercises are delayed for 2 weeks for anterior instability and 4 weeks for posterior instability. Motion is then reintroduced progressively over the next several weeks under the guidance of a physical

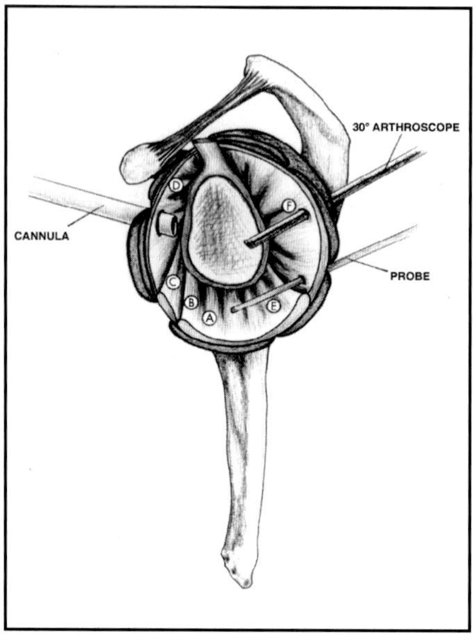

Fig. 3 Multidirectional instability is performed through a combination of portals in the sequence shown. The rotator interval (**D**) must also be addressed. An accessory posterior portal can be safely established for improved access of the inferior capsule. Care must be taken in this region because of the proximity of the axillary nerve. The ancillary pouch (**A**), anterior band of inferior glenohumeral ligament complex (**B**), middle glenohumeral ligament (**C**), posterior band of inferior glenohumeral ligament complex (**E**), and posterior capsule (**F**) are shown. (© Cyndi Slagel)

therapist. Patients with MDI require 6 weeks of immobilization; stiffness following the procedure has not been a problem clinically. Strengthening is begun with isometric rotator cuff exercises and is advanced to active strengthening as motion is allowed.

Animal studies[12,14,17,18] have suggested that thermal capsulorrhaphy creates a shortened scaffold upon which new fibroblasts invade and lay down collagen. This process may take 4 to 6 weeks to begin and perhaps several months to mature. Theoretically, any activities or exercises that potentially would stretch out the shrunken capsule before it is reinforced with a new collagen layer should be avoided during rehabilitation.

Early Clinical Results

One of the greatest difficulties in evaluating this new surgical technique is that patient selection criteria have not been clearly established.[2] The problem is due in part to the complex nature of shoulder instability and recognition of its various patterns. A variety of types of shoulder pathology appear similar clinically, yet respond to treatment very differently. Furthermore, the amount of motion and translation for one person may be abnormal and produce symptoms in another, thus making the examination of the contralateral shoulder extremely important.

A multicenter prospective study (JP Bradley, MD, DF D'Alessandro, MD, PM Connor, MD, unpublished data, 1999) of thermal capsulorrhaphy for multidirectional, posterior, and anterior instabilities of the shoulder is currently underway. To date, 120 patients have been enrolled in the study since the study was initiated in April 1997. Inclusion criteria for subject participation were mild to moderate instability (1+ to 2+) in one or more planes and no prior surgery for stabilization.[45] Any associated SLAP or Bankart lesions were concomitantly stabilized at the time of thermal capsulorrhaphy.

The average patient age was 22.3 years (range, 15 to 40 years), and a preliminary report of the first 60 shoulders in 58 patients has a minimum follow-up of 6 months, with an average follow-up of 12 months (range, 6 to 28 months). Of these first 58 patients, 32 were female and 26 were male. The dominant shoulder was involved in 65% of the patients and the nondominant shoulder in 35%. Seventy-six percent of the patients participated in athletics, 57% at the college or high school level and 2% professionally; the rest were involved in recreational sports. A nonsurgical course of exercise and strengthening prior to surgery was unsuccessful in all patients.

Patient self-evaluation forms, including a visual analog pain scale, shoulder performance questionnaire, visual analog satisfaction scale, and American Shoulder and Elbow Surgeons (ASES) assessment score were completed preoperatively, 3 and 6 months postoperatively, and at 6-month intervals thereafter. All patients underwent the same surgical technique using a monopolar device to heat the tissue to 65° to 67° in areas of the capsule determined by the etiology of the instability and its shrinkage response.

The overall group average preoperative ASES score was 47 and the average postoperative score was 86 of 100 points. Patient satisfaction averaged 8.2 on a visual scale of 1 to 10 and overall rating was graded as excellent in 23 patients (38%), satisfactory in 23 patients (38%), and unsatisfactory in 14 patients (23%). The 58 patients were separated into clinical subgroups based on their instability pattern: 12 with dislocations (20%), 13 with subluxations (22%), and 33 (2 bilateral) with MDI (58%).

In four of the patients, symptomatic subluxations were primarily in the posterior direction. Patient satisfaction for this small group following treatment was graded as excellent in two patients (50%) and satisfactory in two patients (50%).

The group of patients with MDI comprised 26 females and 7 males. Associated findings and procedures performed at arthroscopy included one Bankart and three SLAP repairs. The average preoperative ASES score was 43 and the average postoperative score was 87. Overall patient satisfaction was graded as excellent in 13 shoulders (37%), satisfactory in 12 shoulders (34%), and unsatisfactory in 10 shoulders (29%). Four of these patients had symptoms of recurrent instability: three were successfully treated with revision open inferior capsular shifts, and one was deferred because of lack of adequate capsular tissue to ensure a successful open repair. The other complication to date was a reactive synovitis to a bioabsorbable fixation device used for a SLAP repair.

Because of a high failure rate in the patients with MDI, changes were made in the length of postoperative immobilization (from 2 to 6 weeks) and rehabilitation protocols. These modifications appear to have improved the outcome for the second group of 60 patients enrolled in the study.

Other Reported Results

We are unaware of any current study that has been published in a peer-reviewed journal reporting patient outcome following thermal capsulorrhaphy. However, a limited number of reports in non–peer-reviewed articles and unpublished reports exist from which to draw conclusions.

Fanton[7] reported on 54 patients treated with thermal capsulorrhaphy who had a minimum follow-up of 2 years. Two thirds of the patients were treated with thermal capsulorrhaphy alone and the remainder required supplemental fixation of the capsule to the glenoid rim. He reported a success rate exceeding 90%, with only six patients having fair or poor results. One of the six was a patient with MDI who had recurring posterior instability symptoms and was treated with open repair. There were two complications: one patient developed an adhesive capsulitis that required prolonged physical therapy, and another developed a temporary sensory axillary neuritis that resolved at 4 weeks.

Savoie and Field[9] reported on 30 patients treated with thermal capsulorrhaphy and arthroscopic suture plication of the rotator interval. All patients were reexamined 22 to 28 months postoperatively using the UCLA, Rowe, and Neer-Foster rating scales. Patient satisfaction was graded satisfactory in 28 patients (93%) and unsatisfactory in 2 patients (7%). Both patients with unsatisfactory results had a recurrence of instability and were subsequently treated with open capsular repairs. Two other patients reported episodic shoulder irritation during participation in sports, which responded to anti-inflammatory medication.

Thabit[10] reported on the short-term follow-up of 41 shoulders treated with laser-assisted capsulorrhaphy for MDI and unidirectional instability. Anterior instability was present in 27 shoulders, MDI in 12, and posterior instability in 2. The average age of the patients was 27.5 years and follow-up ranged from 2 to 12 months. The Rowe instability scale was used to evaluate both subjective and objective results and the average postoperative score was 88.2 of 100 points. All competitive athletes returned to their preinjury level of sports participation and there was a strong positive inverse outcome with age.

Hawkins reported the results of 40 patients (including five professional football players) treated with thermal capsulorrhaphy who had a minimum 1 year follow-up (RJ Hawkins, MD, unpublished data, 2000). Of the 27 patients with anterior instability, 8 had an associated arthroscopic Bankart repair; their average postoperative ASES score was 88 of 100 points and patient satisfaction score was 9.3 (on a scale of 1 to 10). The other 19 patients were treated with capsulorrhaphy alone and their average ASES and satisfaction scores were 83 and 9.3, respectively. The 8 MDI patients in the series fared well, with an average ASES score of 89 and satisfaction score of 8.0, compared with the posterior instability patients, who reported scores of 83 and 6.0. One patient in each of the treatment groups had recurrent instability.

In 28 high-level baseball players treated with thermal capsulorrhaphy who had a minimum follow-up of 16 months (JR Andrews, MD, unpublished data, 2000), the mean rehabilitation time was 6.3 months before the athletes returned to play. Of the 80% who returned to competition, 79% were competing at the same or higher level.

Summary

Early results of thermal capsulorrhaphy appear to be favorable and the procedure seems safe when used appropriately to enhance shoulder stability, either in isolation or combination with other arthroscopic procedures. Basic science research has shown that the capsular response to thermal energy and its effect on the mechanical properties of the tissue is dependent on both time and temperature. Additional work is needed to better understand the tissue's healing response and the time required to restore its mechanical properties. Although short-term results are encouraging, longer-term follow-up and studies cited in peer-reviewed publications are needed.

References

1. Fanton GS, Wall MS: Thermally-assisted arthroscopic stabilization of the shoulder joint, in Warren RF, Craig EV, Altchek DW (eds): *The Unstable Shoulder*. Philadelphia, PA, Lippincott-Raven, 1999, pp 329-343.
2. Anderson K, McCarty EC, Warren RF: Thermal capsulorrhaphy: Where are we today? *Sports Med Arthrosc Rev* 1999;7:117-127.
3. Altchek DW, Warren RF, Skyhar MJ, Ortiz G: T-plasty modification of the Bankart procedure for multidirectional instability of the anterior and inferior types. *J Bone Joint Surg Am* 1991;73: 105-112.
4. Rowe CR, Patel D, Southmayd WW: The Bankart procedure: A long-term end-result study. *J Bone Joint Surg Am* 1978;60:1-16.
5. Speer KP, Deng X, Borrero S, Torzilli PA, Altchek DA, Warren RF: Biomechanical evaluation of a simulated Bankart lesion. *J Bone Joint Surg Am* 1994;76:1819-1826.
6. Ellenbecker TS, Mattalino AJ: Glenohumeral joint range of motion and rotator cuff strength following arthroscopic anterior stabilization with thermal capsulorraphy. *J Orthop Sports Phys Ther* 1999;29:160-167.
7. Fanton GS: Arthroscopic electrothermal surgery of the shoulder. *Op Tech Sports Med* 1998;6:139-146.
8. Hayashi K, Markel MD: Thermal modification of joint capsule and ligamentous tissue. *Op Tech Sports Med* 1998;6:120-125.
9. Savoie FH III, Field LD: Thermal versus suture treatment of symptomatic capsular laxity. *Clin Sports Med* 2000;19:63-75.

10. Thabit G III: The arthroscopically assisted holmium:YAG laser surgery in the shoulder. *Op Tech Sports Med* 1998;6:131-138.

11. Abelow SP: Use of lasers in orthopedic surgery: Current concepts. *Orthopedics* 1993;16:551-556.

12. Hayashi K, Markel MD, Thabit G III, Bogdanske JJ, Thielke RJ: The effect of nonablative laser energy on joint capsular properties: An in vitro mechanical study using a rabbit model. *Am J Sports Med* 1995;23:482-487.

13. Hayashi K, Massa KL, Thabit G III, et al: Histologic evaluation of the glenohumeral joint capsule after the laser-assisted capsular shift procedure for glenohumeral instability. *Am J Sports Med* 1999;27:162-167.

14. Hayashi K, Nieckarz JA, Thabit G III, Bogdanske JJ, Cooley AJ, Markel MD: Effect of nonablative laser energy on the joint capsule: An in vivo rabbit study using a holmium:YAG laser. *Lasers Surg Med* 1997;20:164-171.

15. Hayashi K, Thabit G III, Bogdanske JJ, Mascio LN, Markel MD: The effect of nonablative laser energy on the ultrastructure of joint capsular collagen. *Arthroscopy* 1996;12:474-481.

16. Hayashi K, Thabit G III, Massa KL, et al: The effect of thermal heating on the length and histologic properties of the glenohumeral joint capsule. *Am J Sports Med* 1997;25:107-112.

17. Hayashi K, Thabit G III, Vailas AC, Bogdanske JJ, Cooley AJ, Markel MD: The effect of nonablative laser energy on joint capsular properties: An in vitro histologic and biochemical study using a rabbit model. *Am J Sports Med* 1996;24:640-646.

18. Hecht P, Hayashi K, Cooley AJ, et al: The thermal effect of monopolar radiofrequency energy on the properties of joint capsule: An in vivo histologic study using a sheep model. *Am J Sports Med* 1998;26:808-814.

19. Lopez MJ, Hayashi K, Fanton GS, Thabit G III, Markel MD: The effect of radiofrequency energy on the ultrastructure of joint capsular collagen. *Arthroscopy* 1998;14:495-501.

20. Naseef GS III, Foster TE, Trauner K, Solhpour S, Anderson RR, Zarins B: The thermal properties of bovine joint capsule: The basic science of laser- and radiofrequency-induced capsular shrinkage. *Am J Sports Med* 1997;25:670-674.

21. Obrzut SL, Hecht P, Hayashi K, Fanton GS, Thabit G III, Markel MD: The effect of radiofrequency energy on the length and temperature properties of the glenohumeral joint capsule. *Arthroscopy* 1998;14:395-400.

22. Schaefer SL, Ciarelli MJ, Arnoczky SP, Ross HE: Tissue shrinkage with the holmium:yttrium aluminum garnet laser: A postoperative assessment of tissue length, stiffness, and structure. *Am J Sports Med* 1997;25:841-848.

23. Sherk HH: The use of lasers in orthopaedic procedures. *J Bone Joint Surg Am* 1993;75:768-776.

24. Tibone JE, McMahon PJ, Shrader TA, Sandusky MD, Lee TQ: Glenohumeral joint translation after arthroscopic, nonablative, thermal capsuloplasty with a laser. *Am J Sports Med* 1998;26:495-498.

25. Vangsness CT Jr, Mitchell W III, Nimni M, Erlich M, Saadat V, Schmotzer H: Collagen shortening: An experimental approach with heat. *Clin Orthop* 1997;337:267-271.

26. Wall MS, Deng XH, Torzilli PA, Doty SB, O'Brien SJ, Warren RF: Thermal modification of collagen. *J Shoulder Elbow Surg* 1999;8:339-344.

27. Hovelius L: Anterior dislocation of the shoulder in teen-agers and young adults: Five-year prognosis. *J Bone Joint Surg Am* 1987;69:393-399.

28. Henry JH, Genung JA: Natural history of glenohumeral dislocation: Revisited. *Am J Sports Med* 1982;10:135-137.

29. Bowen MK, Warren RF: Ligamentous control of shoulder stability based on selective cutting and static translation experiments. *Clin Sports Med* 1991;10:757-782.

30. O'Brien SJ, Neves MC, Arnoczky SP, et al: The anatomy and histology of the inferior glenohumeral ligament complex of the shoulder. *Am J Sports Med* 1990;18:449-456.

31. Warner JJ, Deng XH, Warren RF, Torzilli PA: Static capsuloligamentous restraints to superior-inferior translation of the glenohumeral joint. *Am J Sports Med* 1992;20:675-685.

32. Pollock RG, Bigliani LU: Glenohumeral instability: Evaluation and treatment. *J Am Acad Orthop Surg* 1993;1:24-32.

33. Neer CS II, Foster CR: Inferior capsular shift for involuntary inferior and multidirectional instability of the shoulder: A preliminary report. *J Bone Joint Surg Am* 1980;62:897-908.

34. Schenk TJ, Brems JJ: Multidirectional instability of the shoulder: Pathophysiology, diagnosis, and management. *J Am Acad Orthop Surg* 1998;6:65-72.

35. Cordasco FA, Bigliani LU: Multidirectional shoulder instability: Open surgical treatment, in Warren RF, Craig EV, Altchek DW (eds): *The Unstable Shoulder*. Philadelphia, PA, Lippincott-Raven, 1999, pp 249-261.

36. Burkhead WZ Jr, Rockwood CA Jr: Treatment of instability of the shoulder with an exercise program. *J Bone Joint Surg Am* 1992;74:890-896.

37. Cooper RA, Brems JJ: The inferior capsular-shift procedure for multidirectional instability of the shoulder. *J Bone Joint Surg Am* 1992;74:1516-1521.

38. Pagnani MJ, Warren RF: Multidirectional instability: Medial T-plasty and selective capsular repairs. *Sport Med Arthrosc Rev* 1993;1:249-258.

39. Bowen MK, Warren RF: Recurrent posterior subluxation: Open surgical treatment, in Warren RF, Craig EV, Altchek DW (eds): *The Unstable Shoulder*. Philadelphia, PA, Lippincott-Raven, 1999, pp 237-247.

40. Boyd HB, Sisk TD: Recurrent posterior dislocation of the shoulder. *J Bone Joint Surg Am* 1972;54:779-786.

41. Fronek J, Warren RF, Bowen M: Posterior subluxation of the glenohumeral joint. *J Bone Joint Surg Am* 1989;71:205-216.

42. Bigliani LU, Pollock RG, McIlveen SJ, Endrizzi DP, Flatow EL: Shift of the posteroinferior aspect of the capsule for recurrent posterior glenohumeral instability. *J Bone Joint Surg Am* 1995;77:1011-1020.

43. Wirth MA, Groh GI, Rockwood CA Jr: Capsulorrhaphy through an anterior approach for the treatment of atraumatic posterior glenohumeral instability with multidirectional laxity of the shoulder. *J Bone Joint Surg Am* 1998;80:1570-1578.

44. Eakin CL, Dvirnak P, Miller CM, Hawkins RJ: The relationship of the axillary nerve to arthroscopically placed capsulolabral sutures: An anatomic study. *Am J Sports Med* 1998;26:505-509.

45. Richards RR: A standardized method for the assessment of shoulder function. *J Shoulder Elbow Surg* 1994;3:347-352.

5

SYMPOSIUM

Thermal Capsulorrhaphy for Instability of the Shoulder: Concerns and Applications of the Heat Probe

Jeffrey S. Abrams, MD

Introduction

The use of thermal energy during open surgery has become routine. Its application in coagulation and the cutting of tissue is safe and has been associated with few complications. Recently, a more subtle form of thermal energy has been used to modify tissue. The application of thermal energy through laser or radiofrequency techniques can alter collagen within the glenohumeral capsule, resulting in contracture.[1,2] As minimally invasive surgery is being performed more often, the heat probe is now being used in the treatment of shoulder instability. As with many new exciting orthopaedic procedures, there is the potential for failure and complications. Therefore, surgeons need to be familiar with the concerns, limitations, and potential complications associated with the use of thermal energy in order to safely use this technique.

The treatment of shoulder instability continues to evolve. Success rates have been considered high with the elimination of recurrent events. As surgeons attempted to maximize range of motion following surgical reconstruction, the stabilization rate has decreased.[3] The goal was to enable overhead athletes to return to their desired sport, as well as reduce the potential for arthritis from an overconstrained joint.[4-6] Returning a shoulder to near normal range of motion, without the risk of subluxation or dislocation, is a fundamental challenge.

Shoulder stabilization has traditionally been performed during open surgery, and more recently, arthroscopically. The use of the arthroscope has eliminated the detachment or division of the surrounding rotator cuff, in turn reducing morbidity, pain, and risk of detachment. An articular approach is applied to the damaged structures. Early reports of successfully reducing recurrence of traumatic anterior instability using arthroscopy have not equaled the success of open techniques. Although labral reattachment can be achieved with suture anchors, the deficiency has been identified as persistent capsular laxity.[7] Use of the heat probe may be one way to reduce capsular laxity and improve the arthroscopic results.

Shoulder instability can occur from multiple minor traumatic events that result in stretching rather than detachment or tears of ligaments. Certain individuals may have a genetic predisposition that is compounded by repetitive overuse activities. Treatment is directed at reducing capsule volume. Sutures have been used to plicate the capsule and transfer thickened portions of the capsule ligaments to a more desirable location during both open and arthroscopic surgery.[8] Use of the heat probe may be an alternative or an additional way to restore capsule tension and increase thickness of deficient tissues in shoulders with multidirectional and posterior instability.

Superior labral tears and internal impingement have been discovered arthroscopically in the throwing shoulder of the overhead athlete.[9] During maximum flexion, external rotation, and extension, the articular surface of the rotator cuff comes in contact with the posterosuperior glenoid. Stretching of the capsule during early acceleration may accentuate the posterior contact forces, creating tears along the articular side of the rotator cuff and the posterosuperior labrum.[10,11] This pain syndrome is worsened by capsule stretching, which allows for increased external rotation. Although gross instability is not seen, it is believed that microinstability exists, allowing the physiologic contact forces to become pathologic.[10] Andrews and Dugas (chapter 3) have presented early results using the heat probe to alter the capsule, creating minimal reduction in external rotation and allowing patients to return to pain-free throwing.

Discussion of Complications

The advantages of using the heat probe should be weighed against the possibility of failure and potential for complications. One issue is the difficulty in understanding and appreciating proper capsule tension arthroscopically. The learning curve for a procedure is often related to technique. Visualizing pathologic capsule laxity is a challenging process that takes time and experience. Surgeons who have had little experience in arthroscopic surgery have become interested in the heat probe because of the "look and touch" technical ease. Many have chosen to avoid the technical challenges of sutures and knot-tying and may not have developed the visual acuity needed for quantifying capsule tension.

Failure and complications attributed to the newness of the technique have been identified as the popularity of the heat probe increases. These complications include inconsistent tissue shrinkage; capsule ablation; overconstrained shoulder; and neurologic complications.

The prudent surgeon will understand these limitations and be prepared for an alternative plan. Augmenting procedures, or the so-called belt and suspenders approach, may allow technical experience to be gained while reducing risk factors for failure. The risk of neurologic injury can be reduced if the surgeon is armed with a familiarity with shoulder anatomy and an understanding of capsular volume. Thermal shrinkage will play a role in the future of arthroscopic management of shoulder instability, as complications and failure risks are reduced. However, inexperience and overuse may jeopardize the popularity of the heat probe.

Inconsistent Tissue Shrinkage

Tissue shrinkage may be directly affected by the manner of heat application, collagen temperature, and individualized collagen characteristics. Those surgeons who have attempted thermal capsule shrinkage have been faced with a variable visual response at the time of heat application. Choice of temperature probe, surgical technique, and condition of the collagen comprising the joint capsule may play a role.

The history of thermal shrinkage began with laser-assisted capsular shifts.[12,13] The instrumentation was expensive, space-consuming, and brought unique risks to the personnel that required eye protection. Nevertheless, successful capsular reduction was able to be achieved. Radiofrequency energy application has piqued increased interest because of its reduced cost, smaller size, and avoidance of laser exposure concerns. Both techniques produce heat that can reach the capsule tissue and cause alterations in molecular structure, allowing shrinkage. Currently, monopolar (Oratec Interventions, Menlo Park, CA) and bipolar (Arthrocare, Arthrocare Corporation, Sunnyvale CA; Mitek, Johnson & Johnson, Norwood, MA) probes are available. The difference in design determines depth of penetration, which may play a role in applications. The bipolar devices can produce elevated heat transfer along the surface. The heat returns through the probe, making these devices more applicable to tissue ablation as in preparation of an acromioplasty. The monopolar device dissipates heat as it travels to the grounding pad. An elevated temperature is present throughout the entire thickness of the capsule, which may have a greater role in shrinkage.

The optimal temperature for collagen shrinkage is approximately 65°C. Naseef and associates[14] have shown that temperature and length of exposure to heat are important factors. Although higher temperatures allow for greater degrees of collagen shrinkage, the mechanical strength of tissue may be diminished.[15] However, a reduction in tissue temperature would be expected to lead to a reduced initial response. Arthroscopy is performed in a saline environment, which may play a role in modifying the temperature. Reducing fluid flow and warming the saline are ways to modify the cooling effect. Despite the creation of a desired probe delivery temperature, not all tissue types react in a uniform manner. Repetitive use of the probe may only exacerbate this scenario, and possibly increase the risk of additional complications.

Certain individuals are born with collagen that allows for increased flexibility and translation of the glenohumeral joint.[16] Variations in collagen quality and content can be found; therefore, it is not surprising that a variable response can follow capsular shrinkage. This may be noted during application of the heat probe, or possibly postoperatively during the remodeling and healing phases. Many patients with global laxity need significant reduction in capsular volume. As tissue shrinkage exceeds 15%, mechanical deterioration and loss of capsule stiffness may be seen. These conditions may be inadequate for joint stabilization. The temptation to create further capsule shrinkage places the mechanical strength of the capsule at risk. Nonthermal techniques to reduce capsule volume can exceed 15% reduction in capsule length without this concern.

Certain individual shoulders may have variable responses within the same shoulder. It is not clear if this is caused by changes in thickness, capsular content, or those due to injury. Portions of the capsule may have a dramatic visual effect during capsular shrinkage, while visual effects in other regions are less impressive or even absent.

The collagen content may be different based on patient age and history of prior surgery. Capsular response to heat would appear to be less dramatic in older athletes. The composition of the capsule may be similar to skin and demonstrate less contractile properties when exposed to the thermal treatment. In patients with prior history of stabilization surgery, the effect of heat on many shoulders will be minimal. It could be surmised that the content of the capsule changes with age and with prior surgery, altering its responsiveness to thermal capsulorrhaphy.

The surgeon should be prepared for the possibility of inconsistent tissue shrinkage before surgery. Options include arthroscopic capsule sutures or conversion to open surgical correction. Expectation of a delayed response to thermally modified tissue may lead to mutual disappointment of the surgeon and the patient.

Surgeons performing arthroscopy who are comfortable with placing sutures, advancing capsular ligaments, and reducing capsular volume can proceed. The patient can expect results that have been shown to be acceptable in the literature.[17,18] The length of surgery may have been increased, but the goal of leaving the operating room with satisfaction will have been achieved. Surgeons need to be prepared to use additional measures to complete the surgery if thermal response is inadequate.

Capsule Ablation

Capsular shrinkage requires denaturation of the collagen within the joint capsule. The heat-labile crosslinks of the triple helix molecule are disrupted, allowing for shrinkage and collagen fibril swelling.[19] Capsule ablation occurs when heat destroys the collagen infrastructure, resulting in amorphous gelatinous tissue. The healing and remodeling process requires viable cells to produce new collagen that is superimposed on the shrunken lattice. In this instance, the remodeling process is aborted. There is a vulnerable period whereby the structural strength is compromised and tissue stiffness is reduced.[20] Aggressive stretching can result in increased laxity and probable failure. In cases of tissue ablation, the remodeling phase is either aborted or significantly delayed, and capsule strength is not restored. Currently, it has been recommended to protect shoulders from stretching for a minimum of 6 weeks, with some shoulders requiring 12 weeks to remodel.[21]

The presetting of radiofrequency power can determine the temperature of a heat probe. It has been shown that 65°C is the desired temperature to create the thermal effect and allow proper depth of penetration. Higher settings may provide temperatures that can produce more shrinkage, but risk tissue stiffness deficits. Factors including water temperature and flow may play a role in the tissue temperature at the time of the procedure. Surgeons often reduce the flow to allow elevated temperatures to be exposed to the capsule. Discoloration of the tissue and visible tissue contracture are the visual cues of capsular shrinkage. The tissue temperature at the time of exposure and whether excessive heat is producing irreversible changes within the capsule are not always apparent. Capsule ablation is relatively uncommon, with anecdotal cases being presented. Surgeons experienced in arthroscopic thermal shrinkage have not reported this problem in their practice; however, this lack of examples may represent the inexperience of some surgeons, who may be overzealous in their application of heat.

The monopolar probe (Oratec) is a device that can preprogram the energy and temperature as well as measure the tissue temperature at the tip of the probe. This probe can deliver to a tissue depth of 4.7 mm. The bipolar devices currently in use (Arthrocare, Mitek) deliver energy through the conductive solution between the probe tips and has reduced penetration of 1 mm. Initiating full-thickness capsular alteration is the goal of capsular shrinkage, making the Oratec device more applicable, but possibly at a greater risk of injury to the capsule.

Arthroscopic stabilization procedures have had success rates below those of open surgery during their developmental phase. However, revision surgery following arthroscopic stabilization techniques has been relatively easy. Scar tissue is rarely a problem and is usually easier to remove or release than after open surgery. Tissue mobility can be restored and repair can generally be performed using the available capsule after failure or with subsequent traumas. In instances of capsule ablation, this is rarely the case. Reports of absent capsule, thin, friable capsule, and other deficiencies are being reported. Salvage techniques to stabilize the joint via extra-articular structures need to be supplemented. These techniques were largely abandoned because results were less than optimal. In addition, loss of capsular tissue may not provide successful stabilization even with tendinous augmentation. The potential success of surgical revision diminishes after capsule ablation. These procedures are generally performed on high-demand athletes and further injury is not an unexpected outcome.

Overconstrained Shoulder

Shoulder stiffness following surgery may result from the formation of adhesions. The heat probe induces a biologic reaction, which in certain individuals may be variable. In some shoulders, the response to the heat probe may be intensified. Immobilization has been shown to be an important aspect during the period when the shoulder is structurally deficient. Schlegel and associates have reported on immobilization of thermally treated rabbit tendon (unpublished data, Anaheim, CA, 1999). Denaturation can significantly weaken the capsule, allowing it to be vulnerable to stretch with physiologic stresses. Subluxating shoulders treated with capsular shrinkage have been reported to progress to a dislocation when the capsular strength has not been restored. Immobilization is important during the early vulnerable phase, but can also initiate overconstraint, as certain shoulders do not regain their proper flexibility afterward.

Currently, Schlegel and Hawkins (personal communication, 1999) have shown success rates to be improved with immobilization. They have advised that shoulders be frequently reevaluated postoperatively to determine when to allow mobility and when to initiate rehabilitation. Individual tissue responses will make a cookbook approach impossible. Patients who are at greater risk for stiffness, such as redheads, blonds, and those with the propensity for keloid formation, need close scrutiny. It is unclear what makes their potential response different from others. Reexamination at 2-week intervals is currently advised.

Loss of rotation is not always associated with the area of the shoulder that was treated with the probe. Reports of isolated regions undergoing thermal capsulorrhaphy can result in global shoulder contracture. An intensified fibroblast response may simulate global capsulitis, leading to adhesions. As a result, physicians are often faced with an unhappy patient with the classic frozen shoulder postoperatively. Imagine how the patient must feel when their original complaint was shoulder pain, with full range of motion. The diagnosis of microinstability was explained followed by thermal shrinkage, and this prolonged complication developed postoperatively. Careful patient selection, frequent monitoring during the postoperative period, and good communication of limits of early motion are currently recommended.

Neurologic Complications

A main concern with the use of the heat probe is damage to neurologic structures such as peripheral nerves adjacent to the capsule or the proprioceptive afferent capsular nerves. Neurologic injury may be reversible, partial, or complete. The complication of a complete axillary nerve palsy is devastating, and return to normal function is impossible.

A number of sensory nerve injuries occur following thermal shrinkage, commonly in the axillary nerve distribution along the deltoid. These injuries may produce pain and dysesthesia and are considered incomplete injuries. The time for healing of this complication is often 6 weeks, but may be longer depending on the extent of the injury. The axillary nerve has always been cause for concern for shoulder surgeons. It passes anteroinferiorly along the inferior capsule and exits posteriorly below the teres minor. The axillary nerve's proximity to the capsule has been measured in cadavers.[22] With the arm in traction, abduction, and capsular pouch inflation, the references may be distorted. The axillary nerve passes along the anteroinferior capsule near the glenoid at approximately the 5 o'clock position (right shoulder). It travels midcapsule at the 6 o'clock position, and continues to deviate to the humeral shaft as it passes posteriorly. Concentration of heat on the capsule at areas closest to the nerve may place this structure at greatest risk. Shoulders with loose damaged capsules or patients with multidirectional instability have not been used as cadaveric specimens, making conclusions uncertain as to a safe distance.

Experts have suggested that heat probe directional movement and possible avoidance of certain capsular regions should be considered to avoid neurologic complications. Unfortunately, the inferior pouch adjacent to the axillary nerve is often a desirable area for thermal treatment. Some dexterity is needed to reach certain areas of the capsule. The surgeon needs to use multiple portals to address the capsule on either side of the humeral head. By modifying the tip of the probe, certain areas may be contacted without significant pressure. Pressing on the capsule may increase the temperature penetration, placing peripheral structures at risk. A preferred technique would be to place the probe adjacent to the labral capsule junction, achieve visual contraction, and gently move the probe laterally. Again, the capsule should not be pressed, but rather its surface dusted. As the capsule contracts, it elevates to the probe rather than the probe pressing down on the capsule. So that advanced denaturation or heat penetration to peripheral structures are avoided, the probe should not be concentrated in any given area.

The capsular structures are altered as a result of exposure to heat. Vessels along the capsule surface are visibly altered. There are afferent nerves within the capsule that are affected by elevated temperature. The role of the pacinian corpuscles is to provide joint position and sensory feedback. Permanent injury to these nerves may theoretically alter the patient's perception of pain and position. Charcot shoulder joints seen in syringomyelia, diabetes, tabes dorsalis, or leprosy can lead to early signs of degeneration. It is not known whether this condition can occur with thermally overtreated capsules.

Certain pain syndromes in the shoulder may benefit from selective denervation. Microinstability has been identified as the cause of pain, even though increased translation cannot be demonstrated. Successful use of the heat probe may be due to alteration in the capsular nerves, and not necessarily restoration of capsular integrity. Reduction of humeral head translation is generally associated with some change in range of movement. Certain painful throwing syndromes have been improved with minimal loss of motion. The question remains: Is this improvement because of a reduction in excessive external rotation, reduction in humeral head translation, reduction of internal impingement, or a capsular modification anteriorly? In patients with microinstability, it may be a combination of several of these factors.

Current Applications

Despite several uncertainties, the heat probe has been shown to be useful in certain settings. With time this list may become longer or shorter depending on long-term clinical outcomes. When surgeons combine surgical techniques, the success rate may be improved. On the other hand, it is more difficult to report on success of a particular instrument or technique because the reason for success is not always clear. Arthroscopic procedures have been criticized due to reduced fixation of damaged structures when compared with open techniques. Augmentation of repairs can improve success rates. Lack of compliance by patients, therapists, and overly enthusiastic surgeons may also be alleviated somewhat by this approach. Sutures, combined with the heat probe, allow for internal fixation stability. The parallels to fracture fixation suggest an internal support maintains tissue position while the biologic repair phase completes itself. This reduces the risk of stretching during the fibroblastic phase, when rehabilitation is started. As with fracture fixation, the biologic repair process is necessary for success.

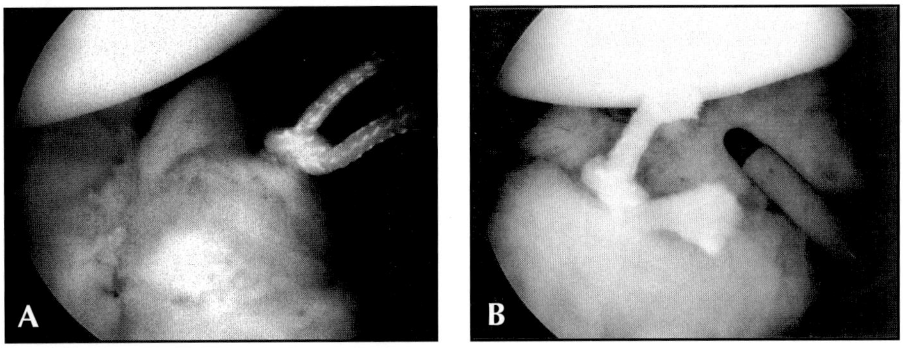

Fig. 1 Heat probe application in anterior stabilization. Suture anchors are used to repair the labrum. Increased capsule tension is created with the heat probe. **A**, Anterior labrum repaired with suture anchors. **B**, Capsule tensioned along midsubstance of the ligament.

Traumatic Anterior Instability

A common articular finding following traumatic anterior dislocation is a Bankart labral detachment. The anterior band of the inferior glenohumeral ligament loses its normal function in the provocative position. Several authors have demonstrated the associated capsule elongation, in vitro, associated with labral detachments.[23,24] One reason for arthroscopic failure is believed to be the lack of restoration of capsule tension, despite successful reattachment of the labrum.[7] Early on, arthroscopic repairs of the Bankart lesion emphasized labral reattachment. Tensioning lateral to the glenoid repair that occurs via closure of the arthrotomy site was not emphasized. Plastic deformation of the ligament reduces its ability to reduce translation. The heat probe can play a role in reversing ligament changes lateral to the glenoid (Fig. 1).

A detached labrum needs to be repaired using techniques other than thermal. The highest success rates have been reported with use of suture anchors on the articular margin of the glenoid.[25] At the completion of the labral repair, capsule tension should be evaluated. If the capsule is attached to the humeral head laterally and the glenoid medially, but does not control humeral head translation (out of traction), then further tensioning is needed. Use of the heat probe to address the inferior glenohumeral and middle glenohumeral ligaments may produce the desired midligament changes. Care should be taken to avoid damage to the sutures near the glenoid. Absorbable sutures along the superior margin of the middle glenohumeral ligament will give additional superior support to the inferior pouch.

Recurrent Posterior Subluxation

Recurrent posterior subluxation can develop as a result of a single traumatic event, multiple smaller traumatic events, or as a predominant symptom of multidirectional instability. The arthroscope may help to directly address multiple areas within the joint, reducing posterior and posteroinferior translation. Shoulders that have involuntary posterior subluxation and that subluxate during elevation with a palpable reduction have the best chance for success. Patients with willful subluxation that can be demonstrated with the arm at the side by selective muscle contraction have the poorest surgical results.

Labral detachments occur but are less common than those associated with anterior instability. In patients in whom a reverse Bankart exists, suture anchor repair of the detached labrum is important. The heat probe can then be placed in the inferior pouch while viewing from an anterior portal (Fig. 2). The inferior ligament and the posterior capsule are treated. Sutures are placed augmenting the posterosuperior band of the inferior glenohumeral ligament, and posterior capsule recess is reduced. The scope is then placed in the posterior-viewing portal while the remaining aspects of the inferior ligament are treated.

The rotator capsular interval lies between the middle and superior glenohumeral ligaments. Sutures parallel to the glenoid reduce inferior translation of the humeral head in the adducted shoulder. Augmentation here may be helpful to further stabilize the shoulder that has increased inferior translation and posterior findings.[26] Although not all shoulders with posterior instability have multidirectional instability, it seems likely that many would require additional fixation.

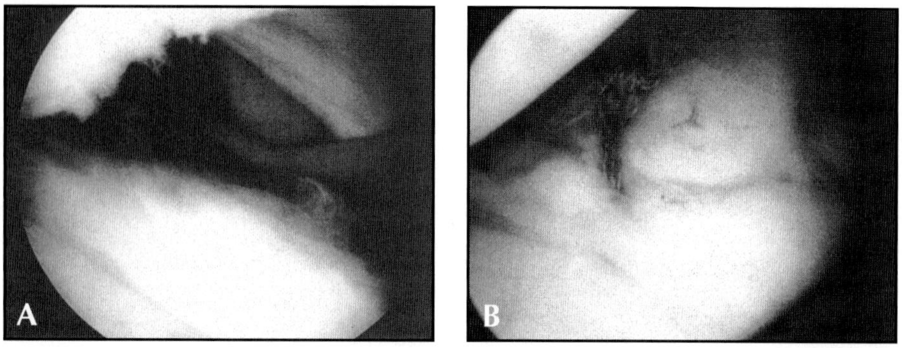

Fig. 2 Recurrent posterior subluxation requires capsular shrinkage of the inferior pouch and posterior sulcus. Suture reinforcement will augment the posterior band of the inferior glenohumeral ligament and close the capsule to the labrum. **A**, Posterior capsule probed to reduce pouch. **B**, Suture supports posterosuperior band of inferior glenohumeral ligament and posterior capsule.

Internal Impingement

Experienced overhead throwers and racquet enthusiasts develop several adaptations in shoulder function during their careers. Increases in external rotation and reduction of internal rotation may be seen compared to their nondominant extremity. Several shoulders with abnormal articular side changes along the supraspinatus have been identified with the arthroscope. With the arm in the throwing or cocked position, this part of the rotator cuff can be seen to contact the posterosuperior glenoid rim or labrum. The term internal impingement as popularized by Jobe[10] and Walch and associates[11] is when this contact has become pathologic and damage can be identified in the contacting structures.

During the acceleration phase of throwing, many pitchers can demonstrate an excessive degree of external rotation. By thrusting the torso forward, the arm extension is increased, creating the potential for greater contact of the rotator cuff and greater tuberosity along the glenoid rim. Internal impingement is usually treated by rest and rehabilitation. Resistant cases may undergo arthroscopic débridement and rehabilitation. Andrews and Dugas (chapter 3) have presented early results of shoulders with thermal treatment to the anteroinferior capsule. A minor reduction in external rotation can eliminate or reduce the contact of the articular side of the cuff with the labrum (Fig. 3). The rotator cuff symptoms are temporarily or permanently alleviated and the structure is allowed to heal.

Although internal impingement has been classified as microinstability, the most common symptom is pain, not apprehension. Does heat along the capsule interfere with the sensory message or is there a mechanical improvement? Successful results are reported with return to near full motion, suggesting minimal alteration in the joint capsular length. There has been good success returning to sport, especially in the absence of a superior labral anterior and posterior (SLAP) lesion. A period of rest, capsular alteration, and possibly a reduction of internal impingement abrasion forces may all contribute to this success. Superior labral repair is completed using nonthermal techniques and further modifies the glenohumeral relationship.

Multidirectional Instability

Patients with excessive inferior translation and who have excessive glenohumeral translation in both the anterior and posterior direction are classified as having multidirectional instability. Since Neer and Foster's[8] original description, the inferior capsular shift has become the most popular surgical approach. Surgical correction includes reduction of the inferior pouch and furthers tensioning to the most symptomatic direction, either anterior or posterior.

The abducted shoulder relies on the inferior glenohumeral ligament to reduce inferior translation, similar to a hammock between two trees. In the adducted shoulder, this structure is lax and the superior structures play a greater role.[26] Open surgery requires the detachment and reattachment of the thick inferior capsule to create a shift. This allows for indirect tensioning of the hidden capsule. Arthroscopic surgery allows for superior advancement of the posterior and anterior bands of the inferior hammock, reducing volume but not placing this ligament in a new location.

Use of the heat probe can further address the pouch laterally adjacent to the humeral head. Capsular plication can reinforce the superior bands of the inferior capsule ligaments or other areas of deficiency. Rotator capsular interval closure is an important aspect of this treatment (Fig. 4). Preventing inferior migration of the humeral head while the arm is supported at the side is critical to the success.

Concerns remain regarding the genetic predisposition of these individuals. Multidirectional instability is a difficult entity to reverse. An improvement in stability, followed by rehabilitation, allows the patient to return to most desired activities. The long-term prognosis remains guarded, however.

Results

The early results of thermal capsulorrhaphy should be viewed with caution. Complications and catastrophes are anecdotally mentioned, and the incidence is difficult to identify with cur-

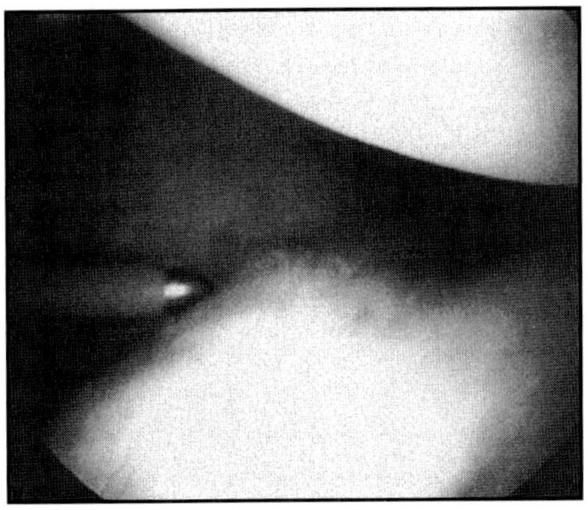

Fig. 3 Overhead throwers may develop anterior microinstability accentuating internal impingement. Anterior capsular shrinkage may reduce external rotation, limiting posterior contact forces. The inferior and middle glenohumeral ligament are treated.

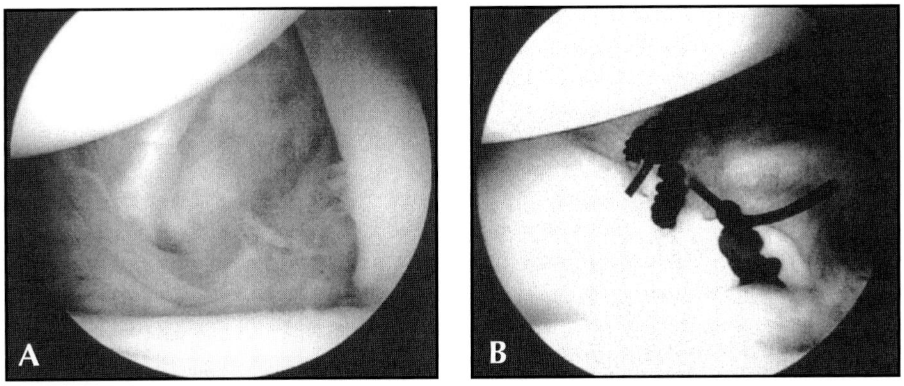

Fig. 4 Rotator capsular interval closure is shown. The superior band of the middle glenohumeral ligament is closed to the superior glenohumeral ligament. This method is used when it is desirable to reduce inferior translation, as in posteroinferior multidirectional instability, or further reduce anterior translation. **A**, Open rotator capsular interval. **B**, Advancement of the middle glenohumeral ligament, closing the interval.

rent use, although use of the heat probe is increasing. The enthusiasm may be the result of the technical ease of procedure. Surgeons who have not performed arthroscopic stabilization have attempted thermal capsulorrhaphy. Inappropriate applications may create dissatisfaction in the public's eye, with the additional stigma of surgical complications.

I have used the heat probe as an adjunct to arthroscopic shoulder stabilization. The learning curve of identifying capsule laxity, increased glenohumeral translation, and what the capsule should look like at the end of the procedure took years to appreciate. There are other arthroscopic techniques to achieve reduction in capsule volume and increased selective capsule tension and to repair capsular tears or detachments. The probe can be selectively used to treat midsubstance capsular ligaments when laxity is appreciated.

Approximately 20% of anterior shoulder repairs have required additional capsule tension at the end of the suture anchor repair. In 30 shoulders, the current success rate of 94% has been achieved with the combined techniques. The capsule must be intact at both attachment points prior to considering this technique.[25]

Posterior subluxation cases are routinely done with a heat probe and sutures. After reviewing 25 cases, repair was successful in 92% (unpublished data). This success may be related to multiple approaches including addressing inferior glenohumeral ligament, posterior capsule, and rotator interval. Immobilization of 4 weeks in an Ultrasling (DonJoy, Carlsbad, CA) is important. Postoperative external rotation to 30° was permitted, but flexion, cross chest movement, and internal rotation were limited.

Overhead throwers and tennis players with pain syndrome are usually improved with nonsurgical techniques. Early results would suggest that more than 90% of patients resume overhead sports activities. It is not clear whether the longevity of the repair will hold up after return to the offending activity. Stiffness was noted in one patient, but a satisfactory range of motion was eventually achieved. Repair of damaged tissue, that is, SLAP repair, is still emphasized and clearly plays a role in joint stabilization.

Multidirectional instability among athletes, particularly gymnasts and swimmers, is common. Many do respond to a conservative approach. Use of the heat probe and sutures has improved symptoms in 80% of the 20 patients studied (unpublished data). Some teenagers have not returned to swimming despite restoration of the range of motion and stability. Other social issues may come into play that affect their decisions at this age. When asked, however, most will acknowledge an improvement in their shoulders.

Future Plans

The use of thermal energy for treatment of shoulder instability is still a relatively new option. Animal models are being used to identify tissue response. Mechanical strength of tissue is altered early during this procedure. In certain studies, it is restored by 12 weeks. It is unclear whether the human shoulder capsule will require the same amount of recovery time. There are many reports of early return to athletics, with some athletes returning prior to the completion of the healing period. Histologic studies would suggest that hyalinization and restoration of capsule stiffness and strength may be deficient during recovery. Additional studies will be necessary to identify long-term results.

Technical complications can be difficult, if not impossible, to correct. There has been little instruction on the application of the heat probe. Understanding safe zones in which to work may reduce injury to extra-articular structures. Techniques allowing portions of capsule tissue to remain viable may allow a resource for new tissue to overgrow the altered capsule. Techniques that will reduce complications and correct certain pathologies need to be developed.

Disruption of capsular structures, including pacinian corpuscles, may reduce pain, and possibly alter proprioception. Overzealous use of the probe may alter these structures and potentially destroy the capsule. One of the more promising aspects of arthroscopic treatment of instability is the desirable visualization and tissue mobility in patients revisited due to reinjury or surgical failure. Capsule ablation may prove a nightmare and distinguish itself as a unique complication of this technique.

Summary

The use of the heat probe, in my experience, is another instrument to address shoulder instability; however, it will probably not replace suture repairs. Sutures may be used to (1) reattach soft tissue to bone, (2) repair capsule tears lateral to the glenoid, (3) close intervals including the rotator capsular interval, and (4) provide internal fixation to thermally treated tissue. Surgeons need to be able to perform suture repairs to plicate tissues that do not have significant response during the heat application. Most capsular volume reduction procedures require some form of capsular inflammation to stimulate a healing process. The heat probe can be used in a manner similar to the rasp. Sutures will provide internal fixation during the long reparative and remodeling phases.

Greater knowledge is necessary regarding techniques, postoperative management, limitation of the procedures, and long-term outcomes. Improvements in application will hopefully reduce complications. Abuse of the heat probe by the inexperienced places its popularity in jeopardy. Following the experts' advice, remaining current in the literature, and improving techniques at laboratory courses will offer the best results to patients.

References

1. Hayashi K, Thabit G III, Bogdanske JJ, Mascio LN, Markel MD: The effect of nonablative laser energy on the ultrastructure of joint capsular collagen. *Arthroscopy* 1996;12:474-481.
2. Vangsness CT Jr, Mitchell W III, Nimni M, Erlich M, Saadat V, Schmotzer H: Collagen shortening: An experimental approach with heat. *Clin Orthop* 1997;337:267-271.
3. Ungersbock A, Michel M, Hertel R: Factors influencing the results of a modified Bankart procedure. *J Shoulder Elbow Surg* 1995;4: 365-369.
4. Jobe FW, Giangarra CE, Kvitne RS, Glousman RE: Anterior capsulolabral reconstruction of the shoulder in athletes in overhand sports. *Am J Sports Med* 1991;19:428-434.
5. Bigliani LU, Kurzweil PR, Schwartzbach CC, Wolfe IN, Flatow EL: Inferior capsular shift procedure for anterior-inferior shoulder instability in athletes. *Am J Sports Med* 1994;22: 578-584.
6. Hawkins RJ, Angelo RL: Glenohumeral osteoarthrosis: A late complication of the Putti-Platt repair. *J Bone Joint Surg Am* 1990;72: 1193-1197.
7. Abrams JS: Arthroscopic shoulder stabilization for recurrent subluxation and dislocation. *J Shoulder Elbow Surg* 1993;2:25.
8. Neer CS II, Foster CR: Inferior capsular shift for involuntary inferior and multi-directional instability of the shoulder: A preliminary report. *J Bone Joint Surg Am* 1980;62:897-908.
9. Abrams JS: Special shoulder problems in the throwing athletes: Pathology, diagnosis, and nonoperative management. *Clin Sports Med* 1991;10:839-861.
10. Jobe CM: Posterior superior glenoid impingement: Expanded spectrum. *Arthroscopy* 1995; 11:530-536.
11. Walch G, Boileau P, Noel E, Donell ST: Impingement of the deep surface of the supraspinatus tendon on the posterosuperior glenoid rim: An arthroscopic study. *J Shoulder Elbow Surg* 1992;1:238-245.
12. Abelow SP: Laser capsulorrhaphy for multidirectional instability of the shoulder. *Op Tech Sports Med* 1997;5:244-248.
13. Hayashi K, Markel MD, Thabit G III, Bogdanske JJ, Thielke RJ: The effect of nonablative laser energy on joint capsule properties: An in vitro mechanical study using a rabbit model. *Am J Sports Med* 1995;23:482-487.
14. Naseef GS III, Foster TE, Trauner K, Solhpour S, Anderson RR, Zarins B: The thermal properties of bovine joint capsule: The basic science of laser- and radiofrequency-induced capsular shrinkage. *Am J Sports Med* 1997;25:670-674.
15. Wall MS, Deng XH, Torzilli PA, Doty SB, O'Brien SJ, Warren RF: Thermal modification of collagen. *J Shoulder Elbow Surg* 1999;8: 339-344.
16. Belle RM, Hawkins RJ: Collagen typing and production in multidirectional instability of the shoulder. *Orthop Trans* 1991;15:188.
17. Snyder SJ, Strafford BB: Arthroscopic management of instability of the shoulder. *Orthopedics* 1993;16:993-1002.
18. Cole BJ, L'Insalata J, Irrgang J, Warner JJP: Comparison of arthroscopic and open anterior shoulder stabilization: A two to six year follow-up study. *J Bone Joint Surg Am* 2000; 82:1108-1114.
19. Allain JC, Le Lous M, Cohen-Solal, Bazin S, Maroteaux P: Isometric tensions developed during the hydrothermal swelling of rat skin. *Connect Tissue Res* 1980;7:127-133.
20. Schaefer SL, Ciarelli MJ, Arnoczky SP, Ross HE: Tissue shrinkage with the holmium:yttrium aluminum garnet laser: A postoperative assessment of tissue length, stiffness, and structure. *Am J Sports Med* 1997;25:841-848.
21. Hecht P, Hayashi K, Lu Y, et al: Monopolar radiofrequency energy effects on joint capsular tissue: Potential treatment for joint instability: An in vivo mechanical, morphological, and biochemical study using an ovine model. *Am J Sports Med* 1999;27:761-771.
22. Eakin CL, Dvirnak P, Miller CM, Hawkins RJ: The relationship of the axillary nerve to arthroscopically placed capsulolabral sutures: An anatomic study. *Am J Sports Med* 1998;26: 505-509.
23. Bigliani LU, Pollock RG, Soslowsky LJ, Flatow EL, Pawluk RJ, Mow VC: Tensile properties of the inferior glenohumeral ligament. *J Orthop Res* 1992;10:187-197.
24. Speer KP, Deng X, Borrero S, Torzilli PA, Altchek DA, Warren RF: Biomechanical evaluation of a simulated Bankart lesion. *J Bone Joint Surg Am* 1994;76:1819-1826.
25. Abrams JS: Shoulder stabilization and evolving trends in arthroscopic repair. *Sports Med Arthrosc Rev* 1999;7:104-116.
26. Warner JJ, Deng XH, Warren RF, Torzilli PA: Static capsuloligamentous restraints to superior-inferior translation of the glenohumeral joint. *Am J Sports Med* 1992;20:675-685.

6

SYMPOSIUM

Complications of Thermal Capsulorrhaphy

John W. Sperling, MD, MS
Kyle Anderson, MD
Eric C. McCarty, MD
Russell F. Warren, MD

Introduction

The treatment of glenohumeral instability with thermal energy continues to gain increasing attention since the first clinical series was reported in 1994 (G Thabit, MD, Squaw Valley, CA, unpublished data, 1994). The appeal of smaller incisions, decreased morbidity, and lack of retained instrumentation are some of the factors driving this trend. Along with the multiple benefits of an arthroscopic procedure as compared with an open procedure, thermal shrinkage also has its own particular complications—proven and theoretical. While there have been publications supporting the underlying basic science of thermal shrinkage, there have been few peer-reviewed publications discussing clinical trials. In addition, the clinical criteria and indications for its use are not well defined. Therefore, when examining potential complications of this procedure, the inherent risks of any arthroscopic shoulder instability surgery as well as those risks specific to this procedure should be examined. This chapter will discuss potential complications of capsular shrinkage and strategies to minimize or avoid these problems.

One or more of the authors or the departments with which they are affiliated have received something of value from a commercial or other party related directly or indirectly to the subject of this chapter.

Literature Review

Currently, there are few reported studies that specifically examine the complications and rate of failure of thermal capsular shrinkage. In 1999, Fanton and Wall[1] reported the results of 34 patients who were evaluated for a minimum of 1 year following radiofrequency (RF) thermal capsulorrhaphy. The patients had no associated labral or rotator cuff pathology. The average Bankart score improved from 24 to 93 (on a scale of 0 to 100). There was one patient with an axillary neuritis, involving the sensory portion of the nerve, that resolved 3 weeks following surgery. One patient developed adhesive capsulitis. Another patient had recurrence of instability that required revision open stabilization. At the time of revision, 9 months following the primary procedure, biopsy of the treated capsule revealed increased fibroblasts, dense collagenation, and increased vascularity along the synovial surface of the capsule.

Bradley presented the results of 60 patients who underwent thermal shrinkage with a 6-month minimum follow-up (average 12 months) (JP Bradley, MD, Orlando, FL, unpublished data, 2000). There were 12 shoulders with a history of a dislocation, 13 shoulders with a history of subluxation, and 35 shoulders with a history of multidirectional instability (MDI).

Among the 12 patients with a history of dislocation, there were 7 Bankart lesions and 2 superior labrum anterior and posterior (SLAP) lesions. At follow-up, there were seven excellent, three satisfactory, and two unsatisfactory results. Of the 13 patients with a history of subluxation, there were 3 SLAP lesions and 1 Bankart lesion. There were three excellent, eight satisfactory, and two unsatisfactory results. Of the 35 shoulders with MDI, there were 3 SLAP lesions and 1 Bankart lesion. There were 13 excellent, 12 satisfactory, and 10 unsatisfactory results. Among those patients with MDI, there was recurrent instability in four patients: one patient underwent a diagnostic scope with a deferred open shift and three patients underwent capsular shifts without recurrent instability after the shift. The author notes that a separate rehabilitation protocol for patients with MDI was designed after the first 60 patients and this modification has subsequently improved the outcome of MDI patients.

Additional surgery was performed on six shoulders overall. In one shoulder, arthroscopic release following thermal shrinkage with a SLAP repair was performed. In five shoulders with recurrent instability, the following additional surgical procedures were performed:

Table 1
Risk for failure of thermal capsulorrhaphy

Proposed Risk Factor	Group I (n=91)	Group II (n=15)
Prior surgery (frequency %)	6 (6.5%)	7 (46%)*
Multiple dislocations	10 (11%)	8 (53%)*
Contact sports	10 (11%)	6 (40%)
Multidirectional instability	4 (4.4%)	3 (20%)
Concurrent procedures	49 (54%)	9 (60%)

*$P = < .05$

diagnostic scope (one), anterior capsule labral reconstruction (one), and capsular shift (three). Additionally, there were two instances of axillary neuritis that resolved within 6 weeks.

Andrews reported on the results of 122 patients who underwent monopolar thermal shrinkage between July 1997 and October 1998 (JR Andrews, MD, Orlando, FL, unpublished data, 2000). There was one instance of a transient axillary neuritis that had completely resolved by 3 months from the time of surgery. Of the 122 patients, 26 throwing athletes with internal impingement were evaluated for a minimum of 9 months and completed a subsequent sports season. These 26 patients were compared with a group of 56 throwers who underwent surgery for internal impingement prior to the use of thermal shrinkage. Of those treated with thermal shrinkage, 79% returned to compete at the same or a higher level versus 61% who were treated prior to the use of thermal shrinkage.

Savoie and Field[2] studied the results of 30 patients with MDI who underwent RF thermal shrinkage from January 1997 to July 1997 using a monopolar temperature specific probe. The comparison group consisted of 26 patients with MDI who underwent an arthroscopic capsular shift from 1990 to 1993 with a transglenoid suture technique and 32 patients who underwent laser capsular shrinkage from 1995 to 1996. Twenty-eight of the 30 patients treated with RF capsular shrinkage had satisfactory results at a minimum follow-up of 22 months. There was recurrent instability in two patients. One patient underwent revision open capsular shift at another institution. According to the authors, the capsule appeared normal at surgery. The other patient underwent arthroscopic posterior capsule plication.

There was recurrent instability in one patient in the laser-treated group, with an average follow-up of 27 months. This patient underwent revision surgery without mention of the quality of the capsular tissue. Among those treated with suture fixation, there was recurrent instability in three patients. All three patients underwent revision surgery.

Jensen reported on a series of 15 patients in whom thermal capsulorrhaphy failed (KL Jensen, MD, Orlando, FL, unpublished data, 2000). Review of the patients' records revealed that prior to thermal shrinkage, four patients had no clinical evidence of glenohumeral instability, six had MDI, and five had traumatic instability in the setting of underlying asymptomatic MDI. At the time of revision surgery, the capsule was thin and friable in five patients and appeared normal in three patients. It was noted that thermal shrinkage may not have been the best treatment for these patients, and that successful management of a patient with a failed thermal shrinkage depends on the accurate determination of the initial injury and underlying diagnosis. In addition, near-complete absence of capsular tissue in several patients who have undergone revision surgery following a failed thermal shrinkage has been noted.

Recurrent Instability

The cause of recurrent instability following capsular shrinkage can be attributed to certain factors before, during, and after surgery.

Preoperative Factors

Failure to obtain an accurate history, perform a thorough physical examination, and obtain proper imaging studies can result in misdiagnosis and lead to failure of treatment. Accurately determining the direction (anterior, posterior, inferior, bidirectional, multidirectional) and magnitude of instability is critical.

In regard to proper patient selection, few clinical studies have identified which patients are at an increased risk for failure of thermal capsulorrhaphy. Therefore, the results of 106 patients who underwent thermal capsulorrhaphy at the Hospital for Special Surgery were reviewed (K Anderson, MD, Orlando, FL, unpublished data, 2000). From this group, 15 patients were identified to have failed capsular shrinkage. Failures were defined as re-dislocation, re-operation, or a L'Insalata shoulder rating score of less than 70 (range: 17 to 100).[3] The investigators proposed several potential risk factors for failure based on clinical observation and failure patterns in previous studies of instability (Table 1). Importantly, the risk factors were chosen prior to data analysis. The frequency of the risk factors was then compared between the failure group (n=15) and the nonfailure group (n=91).

Prior Surgery Reports on revision shoulder stabilization have indicated that prior surgery represents a risk factor for failure.[4,5] Therefore, previous surgery on the affected shoulder was chosen as a potential risk factor for failure of thermal shrinkage. In addition, it is believed that scar tissue may have more limited

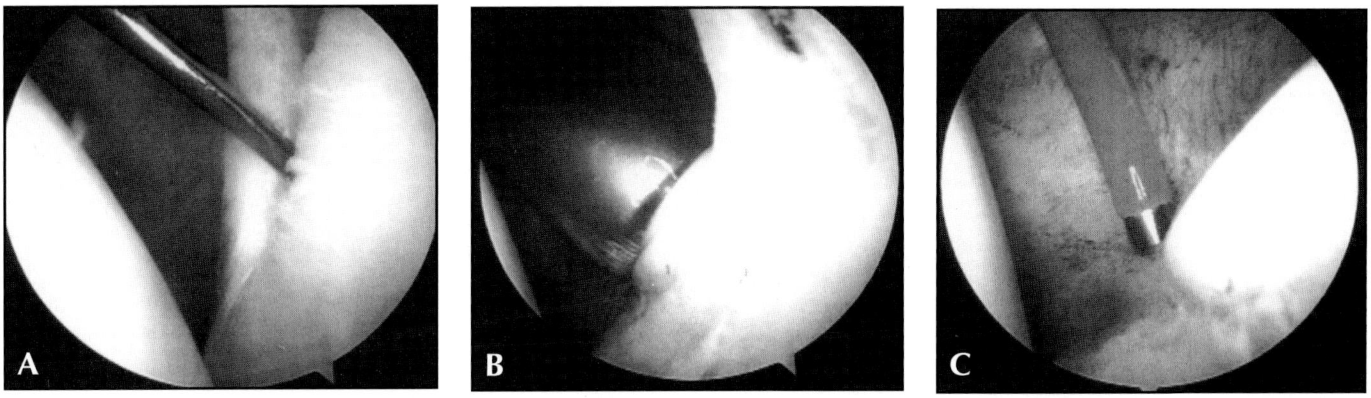

Fig. 1 Arthroscopic view of a Bankart lesion (**A**), capsular laxity treated with Suretac fixation (**B**), and capsular shrinkage (**C**).

capacity for shrinkage. Early arthroscopic observations suggested a less dramatic response when scar tissue was treated with the thermal probe as compared with native capsular tissue. Presumably scar tissue, which is less organized than native capsular tissue, would have less capacity to shorten and maintain this new length.

A history of prior surgery on the affected shoulder was significantly more common among the patients in whom thermal shrinkage failed compared with those patients with a successful outcome. Of the 13 patients that presented after having had prior surgery, thermal capsulorrhaphy failed in 7 patients.

Multiple Preoperative Dislocations A history of multiple dislocations prior to treatment was seen more often in the failure group as compared with the nonfailure group. Patients with multiple preoperative dislocations have been shown to be at higher risk for failure with other arthroscopic stabilization procedures.[6,7] In this setting, multiple preoperative dislocations may indicate a higher degree of instability and capsular stretch that is beyond the limits of thermal capsulorrhaphy.

Contact Sports Participation Forty percent of the failure group participated in contact sports compared with less than 11% of the nonfailure group. This difference was not statistically significant; however, the numbers were too limited to exclude contact sports participation as a risk factor for failure. Contact sports participation has been suggested as a risk factor for failure in previous reports on arthroscopic stabilization procedures.[8] In a recent study, new trauma was a cause of failure in 17 of 49 patients who had undergone stabilization procedures.[4] The potential of a new traumatic event occurring while participating in contact sports is of particular concern when the biomechanical properties of the healed capsular tissue remain unknown. Additional research is needed before the advisability of return to contact sports after thermal capsulorrhaphy can be determined.

Multidirectional Instability In our study of failures, there appeared to be a larger percentage of patients with MDI among those in whom thermal shrinkage had failed compared with the nonfailure group. However, the numbers available were insufficient to statistically prove or exclude MDI as a significant risk factor. Some inconsistencies in the literature regarding the success of treatment of MDI with thermal shrinkage may be the result of a lack of uniformity in the diagnostic criteria for MDI. The primary direction of instability may be important in the outcome of these patients. Dramatic improvements have been noted in some patients with MDI. However, the surgeon should exercise caution when using thermal capsulorrhaphy alone in the treatment of patients with MDI.

Concurrent Procedures Patients undergoing a concurrent arthroscopic procedure (labral or biceps anchor repair) at the time of thermal shrinkage were not at an increased risk of failure. In fact, other studies have shown that the addition of thermal capsulorrhaphy to labral repair improved the rate of return to competitive activity at the same or higher level (JR Andrews, MD, Orlando, FL, unpublished data, 2000). The role of thermal capsulorrhaphy as an adjunct to other arthroscopic procedures may prove to be the most effective use of this technology (Fig. 1).

Intraoperative Factors

Proper instrumentation and adequate visualization must be obtained to optimize the results of thermal shrinkage. This includes proper patient positioning, satisfactory anesthesia, adequate fluid flow, and excellent hemostasis. In order for the physician to have optimum visualization, a particular sequence of thermal treatment is performed. The preferred technique for anterior instability involves placing the probe through

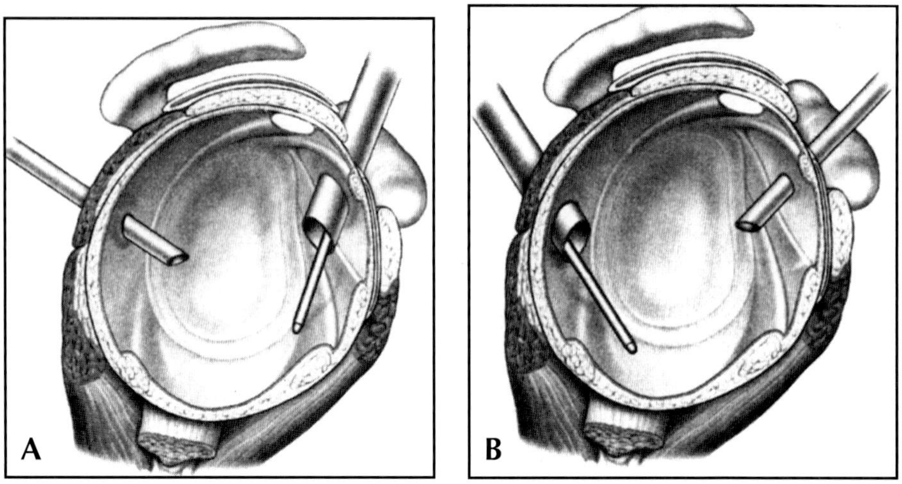

Fig. 2 A, Treatment of anterior instability. The probe is placed through the anterior portal with the scope viewing from the posterior portal. **B**, Treatment of posterior instability. The reverse portal set-up and shrinkage sequence are shown. (Reproduced with permission from Anderson KA, McCarty EC, Warren RF: Thermal capsulorrhaphy: Where are we today? *Sports Med Arthrosc Rev* 1999;7:117-127.)

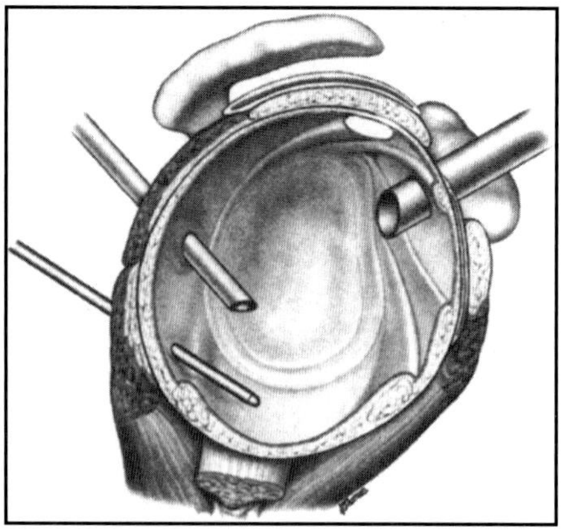

Fig. 3 Placement of an accessory posteroinferior portal can improve access to the inferior capsule. (Reproduced with permission from Anderson KA, McCarty EC, Warren RF: Thermal capsulorrhaphy: Where are we today? *Sports Med Arthrosc Rev* 1999;7:117-127.)

the anterior portal with the scope viewing from the posterior portal (Fig. 2, *A*). The probe is then advanced from the posterior axillary pouch toward the anterior capsular structures. Posterior thermal treatment is performed with the reverse portal set-up and shrinkage sequence (Fig. 2, *B*). MDI is addressed initially with the probe in the anterior portal. Following shrinkage of the anterior capsular structures, the probe is switched to the posterior portal with the arthroscope placed in the anterior portal. An accessory posteroinferior portal may be helpful to properly visualize the inferior capsule (Fig. 3). The temperature and duration of probe exposure must be carefully monitored during shrinkage in the axillary pouch.

Management of the rotator interval may not be adequately addressed with capsular shrinkage. Rotator interval insufficiency has been noted to be a component of inferior and posterior instability, and MDI.[9-11] There are no specific guidelines to determine when the rotator interval should be tightened. In the report by Savoie and Field,[2] thermal shrinkage was combined with tightening of the rotator interval in all cases. We have chosen thermal treatment of the rotator interval in cases of posterior instability or MDI.

Postoperative Factors

Failure to comply with immobilization or a therapy program after surgery may also be a cause for failure. An experimental study by Schaefer and associates[12] suggests that tissues may stretch out if exposed too early to physiologic loads. Wall and associates[13] have demonstrated that shrinkage increases with added energy; however, mechanical properties decline. Perhaps the amount of shrinkage necessary in some patients, while achievable, is at too great a cost in tissue strength.

Motion Restriction

Restricted motion has been reported following capsular shrinkage with both RF and laser devices.[14,15] Fanton[15] reported that one patient developed adhesive capsulitis following RF shrinkage requiring prolonged physical therapy. Thabit[14] suggested performing manipulation of the shoulder under anesthesia 3 to 5 months following surgery if motion has not recovered.

Current shrinkage techniques depend on direct visual response of the capsular tissue to gauge the amount of capsular shrinkage indicated. Moreover, there are no definitive guidelines to determine when adequate capsular contraction has occurred. Excessive capsular contraction with restricted motion may occur.

Following shrinkage, range of motion is restricted in patients with unidirectional instability for 4 weeks and in patients with MDI for 5 to 6 weeks.

Nerve Injury

Transient injury to the axillary nerve has recently been reported (JR Andrews, MD, and JP Bradley, MD, Orlando, FL, unpublished data, 2000). Because of the close proximity of the axillary nerve to the inferior aspect of the capsule, tightening between the 5 o'clock and 7 o'clock positions in patients with a thin capsule is not recommended.[1] In addition, in patients with "very hypermobile" MDI, the temperature and power setting should be lowered and gradually increased until the necessary capsular response is observed.[1] It was also noted that the arm should not be abducted more than 30° to avoid pulling the axillary nerve closer to the inferior capsule.[1]

Potential nerve injury from capsular shrinkage raises an important technical concern: depth of thermal penetration. The depth of thermal penetration is a function of the quality of the target tissue, the time of exposure, the probe settings, the type of probe, and the method of application.[16] In a recent study, the temperature along the axillary nerve during RF-induced thermal capsular shrinkage was investigated (EC McCarty, MD, Orlando, FL, unpublished data, 2000). Thermometer probes were used to measure the temperature at various points along the axillary nerve in 16 specimens during capsular shrinkage with an RF probe (65°). The shoulders were tested in 0°, 45°, and 90° of abduction. At 0° of abduction, temperature increases above 50° along the teres minor branch of the axillary nerve were evident in 4 of 6 specimens at 0° of abduction, 4 of 5 specimens at 45° of abduction, and 3 of 4 specimens at 90° of abduction. Temperature within the axillary nerve proper was elevated only at 90° of abduction.

Failure to understand the neurovascular anatomy of the shoulder may also lead to injury during creation of the portal. Inattention to proper traction may lead to brachial plexus strains. To avoid injury to the cervical or brachial plexus, care also must be directed toward correct neck and head positioning.

Summary

As the popularity of thermal capsular shrinkage continues to increase, analysis of complications and failures will continue to provide helpful information in guiding patient selection and decreasing morbidity. Patients who are undergoing revision surgery or who have a history of multiple preoperative dislocations appear to be at higher risk for failure with thermal shrinkage surgery. Caution should be exercised for patients who participate in contact or collision sports, as well as those with MDI. Further study may determine whether thermal shrinkage is most appropriate for microinstability or used as an adjunct to other stabilization procedures.

References

1. Fanton GS, Wall MS: Thermally-assisted arthroscopic stabilization of the shoulder joint, in Warren RF, Craig EV, Altchek DW (eds): *The Unstable Shoulder*. Philadelphia, PA, Lippincott-Raven, 1999, pp 329-343.
2. Savoie FH III, Field LD: Thermal versus suture treatment of symptomatic capsular laxity. *Clin Sports Med* 2000;19:63-75.
3. L'Insalata JC, Warren RF, Cohen SB, Altchek DW, Peterson MG: A self-administered questionnaire for assessment of symptoms and function of the shoulder. *J Bone Joint Surg Am* 1997;79:738-748.
4. Levine WN, Arroyo JS, Pollock RG, Flatow EL, Bigliani LU: Open revision stabilization surgery for recurrent anterior glenohumeral instability. *Am J Sports Med* 2000;28:156-160.
5. Zabinski SJ, Callaway GH, Cohen S, Warren RF: Revision shoulder stabilization: 2- to 10-year results. *J Shoulder Elbow Surg* 1999;8:58-65.
6. Roberts SN, Taylor DE, Brown JN, Hayes MG, Saies A: Open and arthroscopic techniques for the treatment of traumatic anterior shoulder instability in Australian rules football players. *J Shoulder Elbow Surg* 1999;8:403-409.
7. Koss S, Richmond JC, Woodward JS Jr: Two- to five-year followup of arthroscopic Bankart reconstruction using a suture anchor technique. *Am J Sports Med* 1997;25:809-812.
8. O'Neill DB: Arthroscopic Bankart repair of anterior detachments of the glenoid labrum: A prospective study. *J Bone Joint Surg Am* 1999;81:1357-1366.
9. Schwartz E, Warren RF, O'Brien SJ, Fronek J: Posterior shoulder instability. *Orthop Clin North Am* 1987;18:409-419.
10. Nobuhara K, Ikeda H: Rotator interval lesion. *Clin Orthop* 1987;223:44-50.
11. Harryman DT II, Sidles JA, Harris SL, Matsen FA III: The role of the rotator interval capsule in passive motion and stability of the shoulder. *J Bone Joint Surg Am* 1992;74:53-66.
12. Schaefer SL, Ciarelli MJ, Arnoczky SP, Ross HE: Tissue shrinkage with the holmium:yttrium aluminum garnet laser: A postoperative assessment of tissue length, stiffness, and structure. *Am J Sports Med* 1997;25:841-848.
13. Wall MS, Deng XH, Torzilli PA, Doty SB, O'Brien SJ, Warren RF: Thermal modification of collagen. *J Shoulder Elbow Surg* 1999; 8:339-344.
14. Thabit G III: The arthroscopically assisted holmium:YAG laser surgery in the shoulder. *Op Tech Sports Med* 1998;6:131-138.
15. Fanton GS: Arthroscopic electrothermal surgery of the shoulder. *Op Tech Sports Med* 1998;6:139-146.
16. Foster TE, Elman M: Arthroscopic delivery systems used for thermally induced shoulder capsulorraphy. *Operative Techniques in Sports Medicine* 1998;6:126-130.

7

Technique of Open Rotator Cuff Repair

Theodore A. Blaine, MD
Michael Q. Freehill, MD
Louis U. Bigliani, MD

Introduction

Rotator cuff repair is a common surgical procedure first described by Codman in 1911.[1,2] Since his initial series reporting 67% satisfactory results, several other authors have made modifications to open rotator cuff repair techniques. McLaughlin[3-5] described the pathogenesis of rotator cuff tears and emphasized surgical principles in achieving a tension-free repair. Further modifications in technique, including the use of anterior acromioplasty, cuff mobilization, and transosseous sutures were later proposed by Neer. With current surgical techniques, good to excellent results in both functional improvement (70% to 95%) and pain relief (85% to 100%) have recently been reported.[6-20]

However, the repair of large and massive tears remains a technical challenge. There is a higher incidence of postoperative failure that is related to a number of factors. The quality of remaining tissue may be poor,[8] and significant tendon retraction, bursal scarring, and adhesions to adjacent structures often accompany massive tears.[3,8,21-27] In many instances, the evolution of mobilization techniques has allowed for reconstruction of these large defects. In addition, local tendon transposition, tendon transfers, and tissue grafting with autograft, allograft, and synthetic material have all been described as potential options in repairing or augmenting the cuff repair.[3,8,21,24,25,28-32] Overall, satisfactory results have been attained more often in studies using mobilization or transposition of existing rotator cuff tissue.[5,8] This chapter will describe the technical aspects and considerations for open repair of large and massive rotator cuff tears.

Preoperative Evaluation

Patients with large or massive rotator cuff tears frequently complain of pain. Symptoms are often chronic in nature with a nocturnal component interrupting normal sleep. The use of narcotic analgesics is common in these patients. Physical examination may reveal significant weakness in forward elevation and external rotation, accompanied by atrophy of the spinati muscles. Patients will present with a wide discrepancy between active and passive range of motion. Patients with large tears have a positive lag sign, which indicates weakness of external rotation. A positive drop sign—inability to maintain neutral rotation with the arm at the side—usually indicates a tear of the infraspinatus and teres minor. Often patients with massive tears cannot actively elevate the arm above 90° of elevation. Patients with painless weakness require an expanded differential diagnosis. It is important that neurologic lesions, including cervical radiculopathy, brachial neuritis, suprascapular neuropathy, or syringomyelia, be considered in the diagnosis. A majority of patients will have signs and symptoms of subacromial impingement as this is often a contributing factor to full-thickness rotator cuff tears.

Routine radiographic evaluation should include supraspinatus outlet, axillary, and anteroposterior views in neutral, internal, and external rotation (Fig. 1). This evaluation allows determination of acromial morphology, the presence of an acromial spur, and an estimation of the acromiohumeral interval.[31] Patients with large or massive tears have a decreased acromiohumeral distance. In our series of massive tears, the average acromiohumeral interval was 7.1 mm. Early signs of cuff tear arthropathy must be considered in patients with superior migration of the humeral head, superior glenoid wear, and erosion into the acromioclavicular joint.[34]

Additional imaging studies may be necessary in the patient who has not responded to nonsurgical treatment. Arthrography, ultrasonography, and MRI can confirm the presence of a large or massive tear. MRI is the preferred modality because information regarding tear size, tear location, and tissue quality can be more clearly elucidated[35] (Fig. 2). It is important to perform MRI studies in the scapular plane to evaluate the infraspinatus attachment as more proximal cuts to determine muscle atrophy. Axillary images are needed to evaluate the subscapularis tendon and subluxation, dislocation, or rupture of the long head of the biceps.

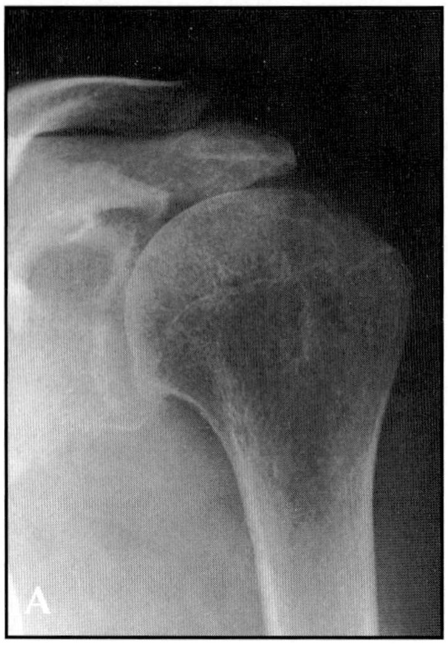

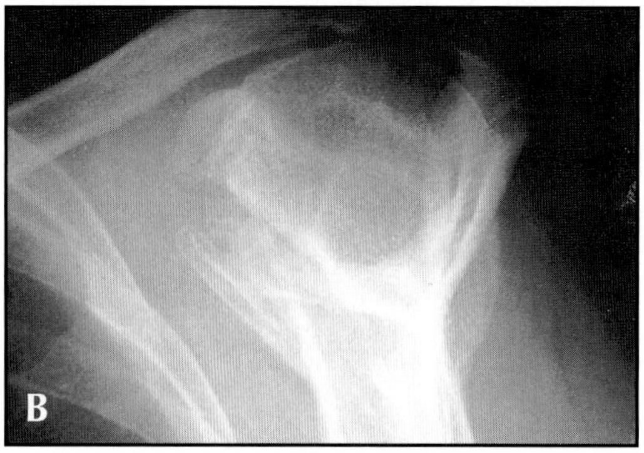

Fig. 1 **A,** Anteroposterior and **B,** lateral radiographs of a patient with a massive rotator cuff tear. There is proximal humeral migration and a decreased acromiohumeral interval.

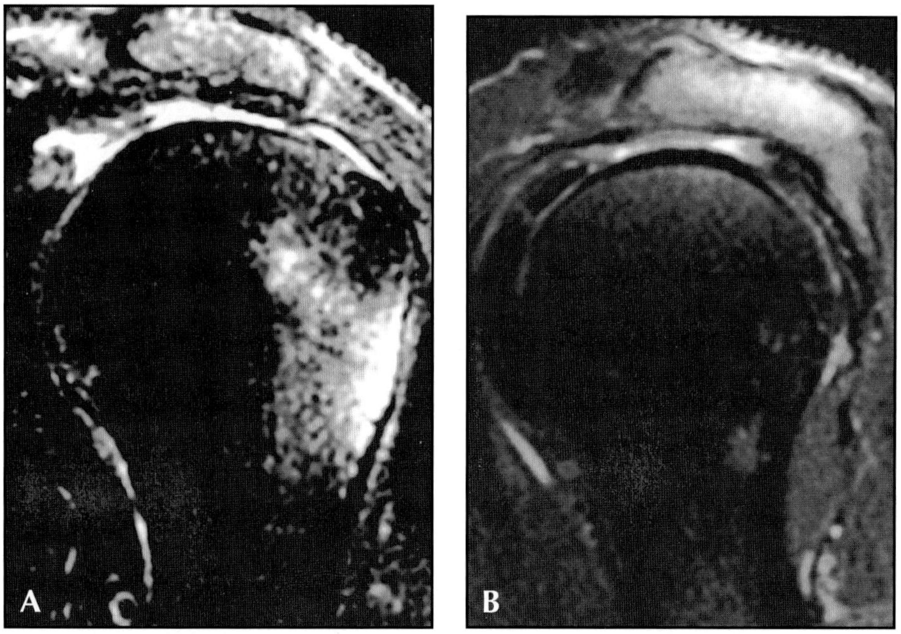

Fig. 2 **A,** Coronal oblique and **B,** sagittal oblique MRI studies in a patient with a massive rotator cuff tear.

Surgical Technique

Excellent results have been reported with the use of arthroscopic or combined approaches (mini-open) in the treatment of small and medium tears.[36-38] Large and massive tears, however, are managed more appropriately with open techniques. The technique of open repair has four distinct facets: the surgical approach, the decompression, the mobilization and repair, and the postoperative rehabilitation program. At our institution we have attained excellent intraoperative anesthesia and postoperative pain relief with interscalene regional anesthesia, which lasts between 8 and 9 hours.[39] This method has increased patient satisfaction and decreased postoperative pain, thus decreasing narcotic usage.

Approach

The patient is placed on the operating table in a supine position. An interscalene regional block is performed by the anesthesia team, and the patient is then placed in a modified beach chair position with the torso angled approximately 60° from the horizontal plane. The head is placed in a beach chair adapter or McConnell headrest with the neck in neutral position, which allows access to the superior and posterior aspects of the shoulder. The arm is draped free to permit full rotation, elevation, and rotation. Osseous landmarks are identified prior to incision. Antibiotics (first-generation cephalosporin or vancomycin for penicillin-allergic patients) are administered before skin incision is performed. The approach is initiated on the anterosuperior aspect of the shoulder with a 10- to 12-cm incision within Langer's lines. This approach promotes improved cosmesis with diminished potential for hypertrophic scar formation. The incision extends from the lateral aspect of the anterior acromion toward the lateral tip of the coracoid. This extensile incision allows for access to the acromioclavicular joint, the superior aspect of the subscapularis, and the posterior rotator cuff. The subcutaneous layer is divided, and needle-tip electrocautery is used to expose the superficial deltoid fascial layer. It is imperative to keep the fascial layer intact while creating full-thickness subcutaneous flaps. This allows for anatomic reconstruction of the deltoid split after cuff repair. Mobilization of the flaps is performed to allow exposure of the acromioclavicular joint, the anterolateral acromion, and the lateral deltoid in preparation for the deltoid split.

Kessel and Watson[40] initially described a transacromial or acromial-splitting approach for exposure of the rotator cuff. More recently, this approach has been advocated as an option in the management of massive tears involving the posterior cuff.[41] Satisfactory results were reported in 70% of the patients despite a 24% fibrous union rate. Complete detachment of the deltoid origin and modifications have been described as a method of obtaining unimpeded access to the rotator cuff.[42] Theoretically, these techniques can increase the possibility of deltoid origin disruption or symptomatic nonunion and should be avoided.[41,43,44] With modifications that consist of osseous detachment of the deltoid muscle, good results have been reported in 89%, and there are no complications related to deltoid function.[45] We prefer an approach that involves a deltoid split performed with electrocautery beginning 5 mm anterior to the acromioclavicular joint and extending past the anterolateral acromion. A strong, healthy cuff of tissue remains, allowing for excellent tissue reapproximation and preservation of the deltoid origin. The deltoid split is extended slightly posterior within a raphe of the middle deltoid for a distance of 3 to 4 cm past the tip of the lateral acromion, which safely avoids the axillary nerve (Fig. 3). The split is centered over the greater tuberosity to allow for improved visualization of the posterior cuff with internal rotation. Stay suture placement at the distal end of the split is performed to prevent propagation that may injure the axillary nerve. The superficial lateral bursal tissue is excised to improve visualization. The lateral aspect of the coracoacromial ligament is identified. The ligament should be removed in a subperiosteal fashion with electrocautery from the undersurface of the acromion and acromioclavicular joint and tagged so that it can be repaired back to the acromion in a more medial position after cuff repair (Fig. 4). This may aid in maintaining the "buffering" function of the coracoacromial arch and prevent anterosuperior humeral head subluxation in patients who have compromised rotator cuff function.[46,47] Exposure of the ligament and acromion can be facilitated by placing a wide, flat retractor (Darrach) inferior to the acromion, allowing the humeral head to be levered inferiorly. The entire rotator cuff can be visualized with simple maneuvering of the humerus in flexion, extension, and rotation.

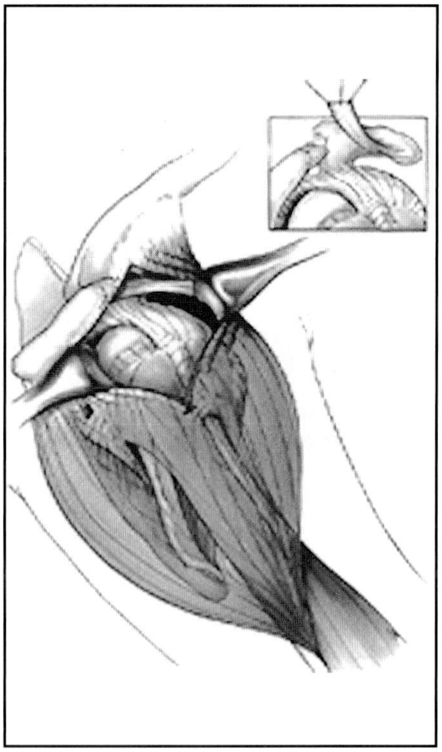

Fig. 3 Deltoid split for a distance of 3 to 4 cm. The coracoacromial ligament is preserved. (Reproduced with permission from Bigliani LU: Rotator cuff repair, in Bigliani LU, Flatow EL, Pollock RA, Post MP (eds): *The Shoulder: Operative Technique*. Baltimore, MD, Williams & Wilkins, 1998, pp 133-135.)

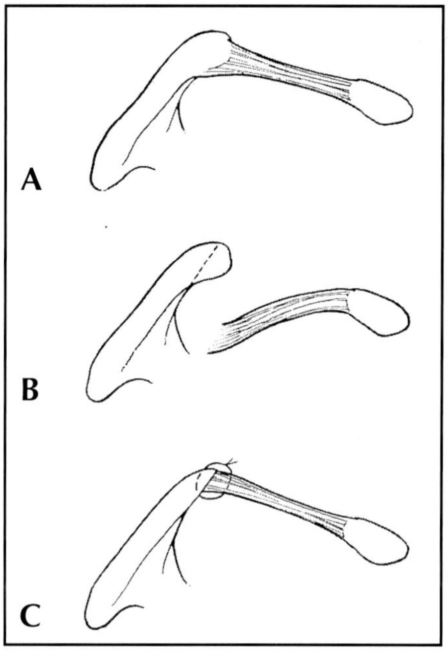

Fig. 4 Repair of the coracoacromial ligament. (Reproduced with permission from Bigliani LU: Rotator cuff repair, in Bigliani LU, Flatow EL, Pollock RA, Post MP (eds): *The Shoulder: Operative Technique*. Baltimore, MD, Williams & Wilkins, 1998, pp 133-135.)

Decompression

The etiology of subacromial impingement can involve three elements: the anterolateral coracoacromial ligament, the anteroinferior acromion, and the acromioclavicular joint.[17,18] A decompression usually includes a coracoacromial ligament release as well as an anterior acromioplasty. If the acromioclavicular joint is symptomatic, then a modified or complete acromioclavicular joint arthroplasty is indicated. Meticulous elevation of the deltoid origin is performed to expose the anterior aspect of the acromion, and adherent cuff and bursal tissue is cleared from the inferior aspect of the acromion. Prior to performing the acromioplasty, the thickness of the acromion and the presence of a spur should be assessed. A thin, sharp, beveled osteotome is then used to perform the acromioplasty, keeping the bevel directed superiorly to avoid excessive bone removal or fracture (Fig. 5). The osteotomized region should consist of the full acromial width, leaving a smooth contour on the anteroinferior acromion. A double-action rongeur, rasp, or burr can also be used when performing a modified acromioplasty. A complete acromioclavicular arthroplasty or distal clavicle resection is reserved for patients who

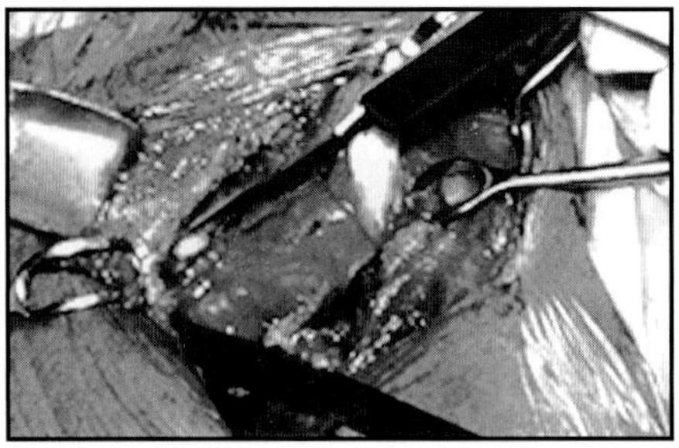

Fig. 5 A conservative acromioplasty is performed with a sharp, beveled osteotome. Prior to performing the procedure, the acromion is palpated to assess its thickness.

exhibit associated tenderness and pain with cross-body adduction during clinical examination. The resection should allow for preservation of the superior acromioclavicular ligaments, thereby maintaining anterior-posterior stability of the joint. If patients do not have tenderness but have inferior osteophytes extending inferiorly from the acromioclavicular joint, then a modified acromioclavicular arthroplasty where just the undersurface of the joint is resected should be performed.

Also, lateral or radical acromioplasty should be avoided because these procedures are often deforming in nature.[48] Radical acromionectomy weakens the deltoid by removing the fulcrum provided by the acromion. As a result, the middle deltoid can become permanently contracted. Subsequently, these patients frequently present with associated functional deficits and diminished range of motion.[49] In addition, these aggressive techniques have demonstrated an increased incidence of postoperative complications, including sinus tract formation and deltoid origin disruption.[50,51] Moreover, revision surgery becomes technically demanding with a greater opportunity for an unsatisfactory outcome.[52-56]

Bursal Resection

The subacromial bursa is bordered superiorly by the acromion and coracoacromial ligament, medially by the coracoid process, laterally by the deltoid muscle, and inferiorly by the rotator cuff tendons and the greater tuberosity.[57] The role of bursal resection in rotator cuff surgery is controversial. Many surgeons believe that the bursa is important in the healing process that leads to repair of a degenerated rotator cuff tendon.[58-60] Others routinely resect the subacromial bursa, primarily to obtain better exposure to the rotator cuff.[61] Recent studies have identified an increase in inflammatory mediators, afferent nerve endings and their products in inflamed subacromial bursa.[62-66] Often with full-thickness rotator cuff tears the bursa is thickened, inflamed, or fibrotic; therefore, resection of the bursa can reduce the pain and inflammation produced by this reactive bursal membrane. For bursal resection, the superficial inflamed and fibrotic tissue overlying the rotator cuff is grasped with a straight Adson clamp and extensive resection is performed using Mayo or Metzenbaum scissors. The distal end of the bursa may be a considerable distance from the edge of the acromion. Care should be taken to avoid resection of the rotator cuff tendons, which often are tightly adhered to the fibrotic bursal tissue. The thick fibrotic bursa will lead to the edge of rotator cuff tendon that can be differentiated by identifying the capsule on the deep articular side of the cuff.

Assessment of Tear

After subacromial decompression and bursal resection, the size of the tendon defect is determined by several parameters. The width of the tear at its insertion to the greater tuberosity can be measured as well as its greatest diameter in any direction. Small tears are less than 1 cm in width; medium tears are 1 to 3 cm; large tears 3 to 5 cm, and massive tears greater than 5 cm in width.[67] The tear can also be characterized by the number of tendons involved. Large and massive tears typically involve two or more tendons. This technique of classification, however, may be unreliable because of confluence of the tendons at their insertion into the greater tuberosity.[68]

The presence of associated pathology should also be noted. In a review of 200 shoulder arthroscopies for patients with full-thickness tears, 60.5% had associated intra-articular pathology, including 15% biceps tendon lesions. However, only three of these (1.5%) were considered major lesions that required surgical intervention.[69] A low incidence of biceps tendon pathology in association with rotator cuff tears was noted, with only 33 subluxations or dislocations at a tertiary referral center over a 9-year period. If a biceps tear is present, a subscapularis tear should be suspected. Some authors have argued that the biceps tendon has a humeral head depressing function and should be preserved in patients with massive rotator cuff tears.[70] These recommendations have been questioned by a more recent study examining biceps activity using electromyography, where biceps activity remained low (1.6%-4.4% maximum muscle contraction), even in the setting of a rotator cuff tear.[71] We recommend biceps tenodesis in conjunction with rotator cuff repair if greater than 50% of the biceps tendon is involved or significant dislocation is present. We do not advocate biceps transection, posterior transposition, tenodesis of the distal part, or using the proximal part as a substitute for a deficient rotator cuff. On rare occasions the biceps can be sutured in situ into the cuff repair to achieve continuity.

Cuff Mobilization

The first step in cuff mobilization is to identify the leading edge of the torn rotator cuff tendons anteriorly, superiorly, and posteriorly. It is helpful to tag the edges of the tendons with nonabsorbable sutures. The Gerber retractor may be used for better visualization during cuff mobilization. The rotator

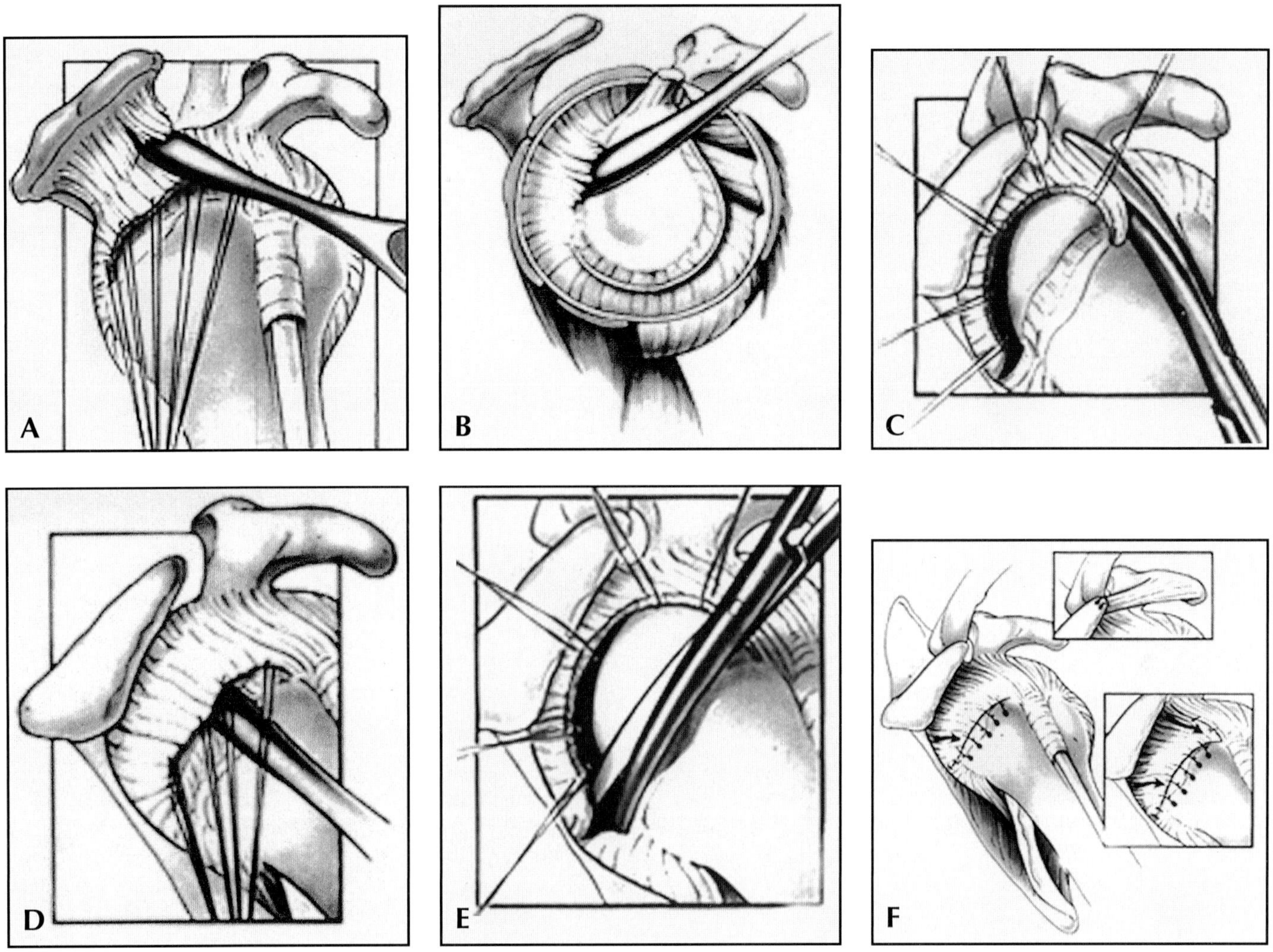

Fig. 6 Cuff mobilization. **A**, The adherent rotator cuff is elevated from the undersurface of the acromion. **B**, The rotator cuff is released from the glenoid rim with an elevator. **C**, Interval slide. The rotator interval and coracohumeral ligament are incised to the coracoid base. **D** and **E**, The tendon is mobilized posteriorly using blunt and sharp dissection. **F**, The rotator cuff is mobilized to the tuberosity. Simple transosseous sutures secure a tension-free repair. (Reproduced with permission from Bigliani LU: Rotator cuff repair, in Bigliani LU, Flatow EL, Pollock RA, Post MP (eds): *The Shoulder: Operative Technique*. Baltimore, MD, Williams & Wilkins, 1998, pp 133-135.)

cuff is released from any subacromial adhesions by sweeping a periosteal elevator in the subacromial space (Fig. 6, *A*). Sharp dissection may be performed when needed with Mayo scissors, and dissection is continued around anteriorly over the subscapularis tendon and beneath the coracoid. Often the leading edge of the torn rotator cuff is stuck up under the acromion or more laterally under the origin of the deltoid muscle as it leaves the acromion. The edge of tendon is closely adherent and gives an impression that there is no rotator cuff tissue. However, soft tissue can be palpated and with sharp dissection the leading edge of tendon can be liberated and then mobilized. Posterolateral adhesions between the rotator cuff and deltoid in the lateral gutter should also be addressed.[72]

Dissection is then performed on the articular side of the remaining rotator cuff tendons to free any attachments to the glenoid rim (Fig. 6, *B*). This is accomplished with a combination of both blunt and sharp dissection. Blunt dissection should be performed initially and if sharp dissection is required, great care should be taken with posterior dissection to avoid injury to the suprascapular nerve.[73] In a previous study on dissection of the suprascapular nerve in 90 cadavers, the suprascapular nerve was on average between 2.5 and 3 cm medial to the glenoid rim.[74] Therefore, a relative safe zone for dissection in the posterosuperior aspect of the glenoid is within 2 cm of the glenoid rim. A Gerber retractor may be used during posterior cuff mobilization to improve visualization. This retractor increases the acromiohumeral distance by depressing the humeral head.

Often, the coracohumeral ligament and the anteromedial portion of the supraspinatus tendon is retracted and scarred down to the base of the coracoid. In this case, an interval slide—a complete longitudinal release of the rotator interval and coracohumeral ligament to the superior aspect of the coracoid—may be performed (Fig. 6, *C*). In an anatomic study of the coracohumeral ligament and its insertions present in 55 cadavers, 14 (25%) inserted into the supraspinatus tendon, and 16 (29%) had a secondary slip of insertion to the subscapularis tendon in addition to the usual insertion in the rotator interval.[75] We have found that release of the coracohumeral ligament from its origin at the base of the coracoid allows an additional excursion of the supraspinatus tendon of 1 to 1.5 cm. This technique has also obviated the need for subscapularis transfer in most cases. The coracohumeral ligament is released at its origin from the coracoid process using Mayo scissors and electrocautery. Dissection should not be performed medial to the coracoid because of the risk of injury to the musculocutaneous nerve and axillary vessels.

Often, there is differential retraction of the rotator cuff tendons.[76] If the supraspinatus is retracted more medially than the subscapularis, dividing the rotator interval can free the supraspinatus from its contracture to the subscapularis, allowing advancement to its insertion at the tuberosity. Differential retraction can also occur posteriorly between the supraspinatus and infraspinatus tendons. A similar interval release can be performed between these tendons to allow supraspinatus advancement. This can also be performed by both sharp and blunt dissection (Fig. 6, *D* and *E*). We prefer spreading gently with scissors rather than cutting with a knife when visualization is less than optimal. An alternative technique of supraspinatus advancement has previously been described by Debyre and others which involves elevating the muscle from its scapular origin.[25,26] This technique should be avoided as it will significantly weaken the muscle and tendon.

Subscapularis tendon transfer has also been advocated in cases of massive tears.[24] We have performed transfer of the upper one third of the tendon in severe cases but have been dissatisfied with the results. In 1994, Burkhart and associates[77] demonstrated that this transfer may lead to superior migration of the humeral head by destabilizing force couples. We prefer partial repair over transfer of the subscapularis tendon, as even partial transfer of an intact subscapularis may further destabilize the shoulder and adversely affect active motion.

The mobility of the remaining cuff tendons must be assessed following release. To achieve satisfactory repair, the tendons should extend past the anatomic neck of the humerus with the arm in a functional position. In the beach chair position, the arm is in relative extension, which puts great stress across the rotator cuff. Placing the arm in the functional position of approximately 10° to 15° of forward flexion, abduction, and internal rotation will facilitate repair. If interval slides have been performed as described, tendons should be repaired first to the tuberosity, followed by interval closure with nonabsorbable sutures.

Preparation of Tendon and Bone

Once the tendon has been mobilized adequately and traction sutures placed in the tendon ends, attention is turned to performing a tension-free tendon to bone repair. Débridement of the tendon edges to healthy bleeding tissue has been proposed by several authors.[78] More recent studies using laser Doppler flowmetry in patients with rotator cuff tears have demonstrated that the tendon edges are well vascularized.[79] Furthermore, Uhthoff and associates[80] have demonstrated healthy granulation tissue present over the tendon edges indicating a neovascular response. We believe that maximum tendon length should be maintained and therefore do not recommend routine débridement of the tendon edges.

Once the rotator cuff tendons have been successfully mobilized to reach the greater tuberosity of the humerus, the bone must be prepared for tendon insertion. We do not recommend making a bony trough because this will increase the distance of tendon excursion and may create a sharp edge of bone over which the tendon has to pass. It is important to have bleeding bone adjacent to the anatomic neck of the humerus to promote healing from tendon to bone. However, recent studies have demonstrated that the healing of rotator cuff tendons to cortical bone is comparable to healing in a cancellous bony trough.[81] Therefore, we perform only minimal débridement of the cortical bone on the superficial aspect of the greater tuberosity using a scalpel blade, rongeur, or burr. The tendon should be advanced to the proximal aspect of the greater tuberosity past the anatomic neck.

Sutures and Suture Anchors

McLaughlin[4] emphasized in his early work that the primary concern in rotator cuff repair is to obtain tension-free apposition of tendon to bone. Because the humeral head is spherical, there is obligatory rotation with movement; and preliminary data reveal that stress and strain occur in oblique directions and not in a straight line. Therefore, despite the importance placed on the concept of suture and suture anchor pullout strength, it is important to emphasize that minimal tissue tension in all directions is critical to successful rotator cuff repair. Great care should be taken to ensure that excessive stress is not placed on the repair until adequate healing has occurred.

Multiple studies have been performed to determine the strength of transosseous versus suture anchors in rotator cuff repair. A transosseous suture technique is preferred, unless the bone stock is insufficient to provide a reasonable bone tunnel. Studies have shown that suture pullout strength is increased by placing the transosseous sutures in the hard bone distal to the tuberosity and by using a wide bridge of bone.[82] A 1- to 1.5-cm bridge is preferred between the medial and lateral drill holes with the lateral hole exiting in the hard cortical bone distal to the tip of the tuberosity. Holes are connected and enlarged using a small curette to allow passage of nonabsorbable sutures with a medium-sized Mayo needle. Simple sutures are used, because the mechanical strength of mattress sutures have been demonstrated to be inferior.[83] Other investigators have also recommended augmenting the insertion site with a plastic or metal button.[82,84,85] Suture fixation with transosseous bone tunnels has been found to be adequate in most cases.

Once the bone tunnels are made, 0 to #1 braided nylon sutures are passed through the holes. A larger caliber of suture is not necessary, as failure is typically noted at the knot of the suture or at the bony insertion.[83] Larger sutures may also promote excess scar formation or direct impingement of the knot underneath the acromion. Sutures are then passed through the tendon, grasping at least 1 cm of tissue. Because of the concern that Mason Allen sutures do not slide or allow slack and may lead to suture breakage, we typically use simple sutures for repair. However, in compromised tendon tissue, a modified Mason Allen stitch may be used for better grasping power.[86] The Mason-Allen stitch is a locking stitch where the transverse suture limb is placed perpendicular to the tendon fibers in the tendon edge. The vertical limb of the suture then loops behind the transverse limb, allowing the suture to grasp both the tendon and the transverse suture limb for improved holding power. Although any locking suture configuration may be used to improve grasping power in the compromised tendon (such as the Krackow or Bunnell stitch), the Mason-Allen stitch has been found to be the simplest and most effective when it is required. The arm is then held in 10° to 15° of flexion and 10° of abduction with slight internal rotation while the sutures are tied. The anterior and posterior tendon to bone stitches are tied first and then the middle sutures. It is important to tie the knots on top of the tendon to create superior compression. The knot can also be advanced distally over the tuberosity to avoid impingement. The longitudinal component of the tear may then be closed side to side, followed by the lateral portion of the rotator interval (Fig. 6, *E*).

Multiple studies have examined the pullout strength of suture anchors and compared them to the transosseous technique. One study has demonstrated improved anchor strength over transosseous sutures, although the transosseous technique for this study used only an 8 mm bony bridge and horizontal mattress sutures, which have been shown to be inadequate in other studies.[87] A second study comparing four different suture anchors with the transosseous technique found comparable results in all techniques, with the exception of one anchor that was found to be inferior.[88] The transosseous technique is preferred because it is both less expensive and does not pose the risk of hardware migration that suture anchors present.[89] We are not opposed to the use of suture anchors, however, especially as newer bioabsorbable anchors that do not have the risks of retained hardware become available.

Deficient Rotator Cuff

Many procedures have also been proposed to augment a deficient rotator cuff. Although rotator cuff débridement alone for "irreparable tears"[90] caused by the disastrous complication of anterosuperior humeral head migration is not advised,[91] the routine use of allografts or synthetic grafts in this setting is not advocated.[29,30] Instead, partial repair of the rotator cuff has been used successfully. Burkhart and associates[22] initially described this technique in 14 patients with "irreparable" rotator cuff tears, with the goal of restoring force couples and converting the defect to a "functional cuff tear." Complete coverage of the defect was not essential, and average residual defect size measured 2.9 cm^2. With this technique, forward elevation improved from 59.6° preoperatively to 150.4° postoperatively, and only one patient had a poor result according to the UCLA score. We have had success using a modification of this partial repair technique, leaving the posterolateral aspect of the head uncovered.

If a partial repair is not adequate, transfer of either the latissimus dorsi or teres major in cases of posterior cuff deficiency or pectoralis major transfer in the absence of a subscapularis tendon has been performed.[32] With the tendon mobilization techniques described here as well as partial repair proposed by Burkhart, we have seldom had to use tendon transfer procedures.

As mentioned previously, in large to massive tears, the coracoacromial ligament is reattached in a more medial position to provide improved anterosuperior stability.[46,47] Firm reattachment is performed with 0 or No. 1 nonabsorbable sutures with transosseous sutures placed through the acromion.

Deltoid Reattachment and Closure

Deltoid reattachment is a critical component of rotator cuff repair. In a study of 31 patients undergoing surgical treatment for failed rotator cuff repair, poor results were associated with previous lateral acromionectomy or deltoid detachment.[52] In another study, there was a 48% incidence of prior deltoid detachment or lateral acromionectomy in those patients

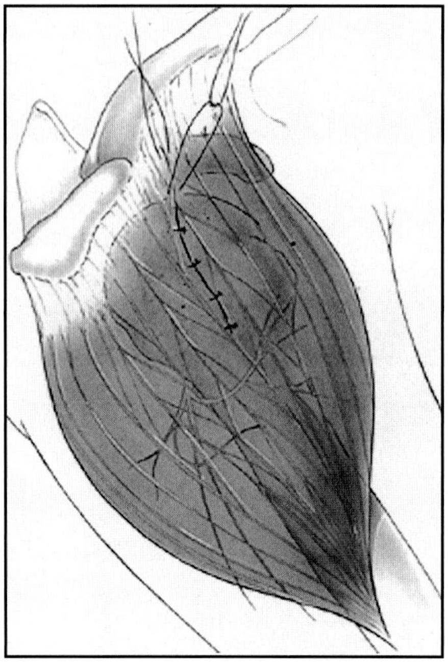

Fig. 7 Meticulous deltoid repair to the cuff of tissue at the anterior acromial edge using nonabsorbable sutures is shown.

presenting for a second rotator cuff repair.[55] For deltoid reapproximation, we repair the longitudinal deltoid split with nonabsorbable sutures in a simple fashion. The anterior portion of the deltoid fascia is then reapproximated to the cuff or soft tissue origin on the acromion with 0 or No. 1 nonabsorbable sutures (Fig. 7). Drill holes through bone are used only if the deltoid tissue is adequate to hold the sutures. Absorbable sutures are then placed in the subcutaneous tissue, followed by a running subcuticular monocryl stitch for the skin closure.

Rehabilitation

The rehabilitation begins with passive-assisted range of motion exercises on the first postoperative day. Patients with large or massive tears undergo a modified Neer phase I protocol for 6 weeks that includes pendulum exercises, passive-assisted forward elevation to 140°, and passive-assisted external rotation (while supine) to 30°. Pulley exercises are avoided for the first 6 weeks in order to protect the cuff repair. Strengthening with isometric exercises is also initiated at 6 weeks, accompanied by active-assisted range of motion. Use of weights is avoided for at least 3 months in the rehabilitation period to avoid re-tear of the cuff. Early use of weights has been reported to cause cuff failure.[19,43] However, resistance exercises with light weights (1 to 3 lb) can be initiated at 12 weeks, progressing to dynamic strengthening exercises at 6 to 8 months. Patients should be aware that full return of strength may take as long as 12 to 18 months.[8]

Results

With these techniques, long-term results for repair of large and massive rotator cuff tears have been excellent. In a 7-year average follow-up study of 61 patients who underwent repair of massive rotator cuff tears, 85% excellent or satisfactory results were achieved by Neer's criteria.[8] Ninety-two percent of patients had adequate pain relief and the ability to raise the arm above the horizontal position. Only two re-tears occurred, and these were secondary to significant trauma. In a more recent study at the New York Orthopaedic Hospital of 231 shoulder massive rotator cuff tears there were 90% satisfactory results with primary rotator cuff repair. Function was improved postoperatively, with average active forward elevation 160°, external rotation 55°, and internal rotation to T-9. This represented an average improvement of 46° elevation, 22° external rotation, and internal rotation of two vertebral levels. External rotation power was improved from an average of 3.1 to 4.7. Satisfactory results were slightly less (76.5%) in patients with four-tendon involvement. These results support the role of open primary rotator cuff repair for patients with large to massive rotator cuff tears.

Summary

With current surgical techniques, open rotator cuff repair can provide significant functional improvement and pain relief in the majority of patients. Important principles include performing anterior acromioplasty, bursal resection, rotator cuff mobilization, tension-free repair to the greater tuberosity with nonabsorbable sutures, and meticulous deltoid repair. In massive rotator cuff tears, the coracoacromial ligament should be repaired to prevent anterosuperior instability, and partial repair of the rotator cuff is recommended over performing transfer procedures. Postoperative rehabilitation requires the patient to avoid active exercises for 6 weeks and weights for 3 months. With these techniques, 85% to 90% satisfactory results can be expected.

References

1. Codman EA: Complete rupture of the supraspinatus tendon: Operative treatment with report of two successful cases. *Boston Med Surg J* 1911;164:708-710.
2. Codman EA (ed): *The Shoulder: Rupture of the Supraspinatus Tendon and Other Lesions In or About the Subacromial Bursa.* Boston, MA, Thomas Todd, 1934.
3. McLaughlin HL: Lesions of the musculotendinous cuff of the shoulder: I. The exposure and treatment of tears with retraction. *J Bone Joint Surg Am* 1944;26:31-51.
4. McLaughlin HL: Repair of major cuff ruptures. *Surg Clin North Am* 1963;43:1535-1540.
5. McLaughlin HL, Asherman EG: Lesions of the musculotendinous cuff of the shoulder: IV. Some observations based upon the results of surgical repair. *J Bone Joint Surg Am* 1951;33:76-86.
6. Cofield RH: Rotator cuff disease of the shoulder. *J Bone Joint Surg Am* 1985;67:974-979.
7. Ellman H, Hanker G, Bayer M: Repair of the rotator cuff: End-result study of factors influencing reconstruction. *J Bone Joint Surg Am* 1986;68:1136-1144.
8. Bigliani LU, Cordasco FA, McIlveen SJ, et al: Operative treatment of massive cuff tears: Long term results. *J Shoulder Elbow Surg* 1992;1:120-130.
9. Rokito AS, Cuomo F, Gallagher MA, Zuckerman JD: Long-term functional outcome of repair of large and massive chronic tears of the rotator cuff. *J Bone Joint Surg Am* 1999;81:991-997.

10. Gupta R, Leggin BG, Iannotti JP: Results of surgical repair of full-thickness tears of the rotator cuff. *Orthop Clin North Am* 1997;28: 241-248.

11. Iannotti JP, Bernot MP, Kuhlman JR; Kelley MJ; Williams GR: Postoperative assessment of shoulder function: A prospective study of full-thickness rotator cuff tears. *J Shoulder Elbow Surg* 1996;5:449-457.

12. Iannotti JP: Full-thickness rotator cuff tears: Factors affecting surgical outcome. *J Am Acad Orthop Surg* 1994;2:87-95.

13. Worland RL, Arredondo J, Angles F, Lopez-Jimenez F: Repair of massive rotator cuff tears in patients older than 70 years. *J Shoulder Elbow Surg* 1999;8:26-30.

14. Adamson GJ, Tibone JE: Ten-year assessment of primary rotator cuff repairs. *J Shoulder Elbow Surg* 1993;2:57-63.

15. Bassett RW, Cofield RH: Acute tears of the rotator cuff: The timing of surgical repair. *Clin Orthop* 1983;175:18-24.

16. Misamore GW, Ziegler DW, Rushton JL II: Repair of the rotator cuff: A comparison of results in two populations of patients. *J Bone Joint Surg Am* 1995;77:1335-1339.

17. Neer CS II: Impingement lesions. *Clin Orthop* 1983;173:70-77.

18. Neer CS II, Flatow EL, Lech O: Tears of the rotator cuff: Long-term results of anterior acromioplasty and repair. *Orthop Trans* 1988;12:673-674.

19. Packer NP, Calvert PT, Bayley JI, Kessel L: Operative treatment of chronic ruptures of the rotator cuff of the shoulder. *J Bone Joint Surg Br* 1983;65:171-175.

20. Pollock RG, Black AD, Self EB, Flatow EL, Bigliani LU: Abstract: Surgical management of rotator cuff disease. *J Shoulder Elbow Surg* 1996;5:S37.

21. Bateman JE: The diagnosis and treatment of ruptures of the rotator cuff. *Surg Clin North Am* 1963;43:1523-1530.

22. Burkhart SS, Nottage WM, Ogilvie-Harris DJ, Kohn HS, Pachelli A: Partial repair of irreparable rotator cuff tears. *Arthroscopy* 1994;10: 363-370.

23. Bush LF: The torn shoulder capsule. *J Bone Joint Surg Am* 1975;57:256-259.

24. Cofield RH: Subscapular muscle transoposition for repair of chronic rotator cuff tears. *Surg Gynecol Obstet* 1982;154:667-672.

25. Debyre J, Patte D, Elmelik E: Repair of ruptures of the rotator cuff of the shoulder: With a note on advancement of the supraspinatus muscle. *J Bone Joint Surg Br* 1965;47:36-42.

26. Ha'eri GB, Wiley AM: Advancement of the surpraspinatus muscle in the repair of ruptures of the rotator cuff. *J Bone Joint Surg Am* 1981;63:232-238.

27. Neviaser JS: Ruptures of the rotator cuff of the shoulder: New concepts in the diagnosis and operative treatment of chronic ruptures. *Arch Surg* 1971;102:483-485.

28. Neviaser RJ, Neviaser TJ: Transfer of subscapularis and teres minor for massive defects of the rotator cuff, in Bayley I, Kessel L (eds): *Shoulder Surgery*. Berlin, Germany, Springer-Verlag, 1982, pp 60-63.

29. Neviaser JS, Neviaser RJ, Neviaser TJ: The repair of chronic massive ruptures of the rotator cuff of the shoulder by use of a freeze-dried rotator cuff. *J Bone Joint Surg Am* 1978;60: 681-684.

30. Ozaki J, Fujimoto S, Masuhara K, Tamai S, Yoshimoto S: Reconstruction of chronic massive rotator cuff tears with synthetic materials. *Clin Orthop* 1986;202:173-183.

31. Karas SE, Giachello TL: Subscapularis transfer for reconstruction of massive tears of the rotator cuff. *J Bone Joint Surg Am* 1996;78:239-245.

32. Gerber C, Vinh TS, Hertel R, Hess CW: Latissimus dorsi transfer for the treatment of massive tears of the rotator cuff: A preliminary report. *Clin Orthop* 1988;232:51-61.

33. Weiner DS, Macnab I: Superior migration of the humeral head: A radiological aid in the diagnosis of the rotator cuff. *J Bone Joint Surg Br* 1970;52:524-527.

34. Neer CS II, Craig EV, Fukuda H: Cuff-tear arthropathy. *J Bone Joint Surg Am* 1983;65: 1232-1244.

35. Tirman PF, Steinbach LS, Belzer JP, Bost FW: A practical approach to imaging of the shoulder with emphasis on MR imaging. *Orthop Clin North Am* 1997;28:483-515.

36. Gartsman GM, Hammerman SM: Full-thickness tears: Arthroscopic repair. *Orthop Clin North Am* 1997;28:83-98.

37. Weber SC: Abstract: All arthroscopic versus mini-open repair in the management of complete tears of the rotator cuff. *Arthroscopy* 1997; 13:398.

38. Pollock RG, Flatow EL: The rotator cuff: Full-thickness tears: Mini-open repair. *Orthop Clin North Am* 1997;28:169-177.

39. Brown AR, Weiss R, Greenberg C, Flatow EL, Bigliani LU: Interscalene block for shoulder arthroscopy: Comparison with general anesthesia. *Arthroscopy* 1993;9:295-300.

40. Kessel L, Watson M: The painful arc syndrome: Clinical classification as a guide to management. *J Bone Joint Surg Br* 1977;59:166-172.

41. Paulos LE, Meislin RJ, Drawbert J: The acrominon- splitting approach for large and massive rotator cuff tears. *Am J Sports Med* 1994;22:306-312.

42. Cubbins WR, Callahan JJ, Scuderi CS: The reduction of old or irreducible dislocations of the shoulder joint. *Surg Gynecol Obstet* 1934;58:129-135.

43. Neviaser RJ, Neviaser TJ: Reoperation for failed rotator cuff repair: Analysis of fifty cases. *J Shoulder Elbow Surg* 1992;1:283-286.

44. Sher SJ, Iannotti JP, Warner JJ, Groff Y, Williams GR: Surgical treatment of postoperative deltoid origin disruption. *Clin Orthop* 1997;343:93-98.

45. Habernek H, Weinstabl R, Schabus R, Schmid L: A new approach to the subacromial space: Technique and 2-year results in 28 rotator-cuff repair cases. *Acta Orthop Scand* 1993;64:92-94.

46. Flatow EL, Weinstein DM, Duralde XA, Compito CA, Pollock RG, Bigliani LU: Abstract: Coracoacromial ligament preservation in rotator cuff surgery. *J Shoulder Elbow Surg* 1994;3:S73.

47. Flatow EL, Connor PM, Levine WN, Arroyo JS, Pollock RG, Bigliani LU: Abstract: Coracoacromial arch reconstruction for antero-superior subluxation after failed rotator cuff surgery: A preliminary report. *J Shoulder Elbow Surg* 1997;6:228.

48. Neer CS II, Marberry TA: On the disadvantages of radical acromionectomy. *J Bone Joint Surg Am* 1981;63:416-419.

49. Bigliani LU, Steinmann S, Flatow EL, et al: Complications, in Iannotti JP (ed): *Rotator Cuff Disorders: Evaluation and Treatment*. Park Ridge, IL, American Academy of Orthopaedic Surgeons, 1991, pp 63-74.

50. Hammond G: Complete acromionectomy in the treatment of chronic tendinitis of the shoulder: A follow-up of ninety operations on eighty-seven patients. *J Bone Joint Surg Am* 1971;53:173-180.

51. Groh GI, Simoni M, Rolla P, Rockwood CA: Loss of the deltoid after shoulder operations: An operative disaster. *J Shoulder Elbow Surg* 1994;3:243-253.

52. Bigliani LU, Cordasco FA, McIlveen SJ, Musso ES: Operative treatment of failed repairs of the rotator cuff. *J Bone Joint Surg Am* 1992;74: 1505-1515.

53. Wolfgang GL: Surgical repair of tears of the rotator cuff of the shoulder: Factors influencing the result. *J Bone Joint Surg Am* 1974;56: 14-26.

54. Cordasco FA, Bigliani LU: The treatment of failed rotator cuff repairs. *Instr Course Lect* 1998; 47:77-86.

55. DeOrio JK, Cofield RH: Results of a second attempt at surgical repair of a failed initial rotator-cuff repair. *J Bone Joint Surg Am* 1984;66:563-567.

56. Neviaser RJ: Evaluation and management of failed rotator cuff repairs. *Orthop Clin North Am* 1997;28:215-224.

57. Strizak AM, Danzig L, Jackson DW, Resnick D, Staple T: Subacromial bursography: An anatomical and clinical study. *J Bone Joint Surg Am* 1982;64:196-201.

58. Rahme H, Nordgren H, Hamberg H, Westerberg CE: The subacromial bursa and the impingement syndrome: A clinical and histological study of 30 cases. *Acta Orthop Scand* 1993;64:485-488.

59. Ishii H, Brunet JA, Welsh RP, Uhthoff HK: 'Bursal reactions' in rotator cuff tearing, the impingement syndrome, and calcifying tendinitis. *J Shoulder Elbow Surg* 1997;6:131-136.

60. Uhthoff HK, Sarkar K: Surgical repair of rotator cuff ruptures: The importance of the subacromial bursa. *J Bone Joint Surg Br* 1991;73:399-401.

61. Gerber C: Massive rotator cuff tears, in Iannotti JP, Williams GR Jr (eds): *Disorders of the Shoulder: Diagnosis and Management*. Philadelphia, PA, Lippincott-Williams & Wilkins, 1999, pp 57-92.

62. Soifer TB, Levy H, Soifer FM, Kleinbart F, Vigorita V, Bryk E: Neurohistology of the subacromial space. *Arthroscopy* 1996;12:182-186.

63. Gotoh M, Hamada K, Yamakawa H, Inoue A, Fukuda H: Increased substance P in subacromial bursa and shoulder pain in rotator cuff diseases. *J Orthop Res* 1998;16:618-621.

64. Gotoh M, Hamada K, Yamakawa H, et al: Increased interleukin-1 beta production in the synovium of glenohumeral joints with anterior instability. *J Orthop Res* 1999;17:392-397.

65. Rodeo SA, Hannafin JA, Tom J, Warren RF, Wickiewicz TL: Immunolocalization of cytokines and their receptors in adhesive capsulitis of the shoulder. *J Orthop Res* 1997,15:427-436.

66. Stone D, Green C, Rao U, et al: Cytokine-induced tendinitis: A preliminary study in rabbits. *J Orthop Res* 1999;17:168-177.

67. Post M, Silver R, Singh M: Rotator cuff tear: Diagnosis and treatment. *Clin Orthop* 1983;173: 78-91.

68. Clark JM, Harryman DT II: Tendons, ligaments, and capsule of the rotator cuff: Gross and microscopic anatomy. *J Bone Joint Surg Am* 1992;74:713-725.

69. Gartsman GM, Taverna E: The incidence of glenohueral joint abnormalities associated with full-thickness, reparable rotator cuff tears. *Arthroscopy*. 1997;13:450-455.

70. Kumar VP, Satka K, Balasubralmaniam P: The role of the long head of biceps brachii in the stabilization of the head of the humerus. *Clin Orthop* 1989;244:172-175.

71. Yamaguchi K, Riew KD, Galatz LM, Syme JA, Neviaser RJ: Biceps activity during shoulder motion: An electromyographic analysis. *Clin Orthop* 1997;336:122-129.

72. Cordasco FA, Bigliani LU: The rotator cuff: Large and massive tears: Technique of open repair. *Orthop Clin North Am* 1997;28:179-193.

73. Warner JP, Krushell RJ, Masquelet A, Gerber C: Anatomy and relationships of the suprascapular nerve: Anatomical constraints to mobilization of the supraspinatus and infraspinatus muscles in the management of massive rotator-cuff tears. *J Bone Joint Surg Am* 1992;74:36-45.

74. Bigliani LU, Dalsey RM, McCann PD, April EW: An anatomical study of the suprascapular nerve. *Arthroscopy* 1990;6:301-305.

75. Neer CS II, Satterlee CC, Dalsey RM, Flatow EL: The anatomy and potential effects of contracture of the coracohumeral ligament. *Clin Orthop* 1992;280:182-185.

76. Codd TP, Flatow EL: Anterior acromioplasty, tendon mobilization, and direct repair of massive rotator cuff tears, in Burkhead WZ Jr (ed): *Rotator Cuff Disorders*. Baltimore, MD, Williams & Wilkins, 1996, pp 323-334.

77. Burkart SS, Nottage WM, Ogilvie-Harris DJ, Kohn HS, Pachelli A: Partial repair of irreparable rotator cuff tears. *Arthroscopy* 1994;10: 363-370.

78. Rathbun JB, Macnab I: The microvascular pattern of the rotator cuff. *J Bone Joint Surg Br* 1970;52:540-553.

79. Swiontkowski MF, Iannotti JP, Boulas HJ, Esterhai JL: Intraoperative assessment of rotator cuff vascularity using Laser Doppler Flowmetry, in Post M, Morrey BF, Hawkins RJ (eds): *Surgery of the Shoulder*. St. Louis, MO, Mosby-Year Book, 1990; pp 208-212.

80. Uhthoff HK, Sarkar K, Lohr J: Repair in rotator cuff tendons, in Post M, Morrey BF, Hawkins RJ (eds): *Surgery of the Shoulder*. St. Louis, MO, Mosby-Year Book, 1990, pp 216-219.

81. St Pierre P, Olson EJ, Elliott JJ, O'Hair KC, McKinney LA, Ryan J: Tendon-healing to cortical bone compared with healing to a cancellous trough: A biomechanical and histological evaluation in goats. *J Bone Joint Surg Am* 1995;77:1858-1866.

82. Caldwell GL, Warner JP, Miller MD, Boardman D, Towers J, Debski R: Strength of fixation with transosseous sutures in rotator cuff repair. *J Bone Joint Surg Am* 1997;79: 1064-1068.

83. Burkhart SS, Fischer SP, Nottage WM, et al: Tissue fixation security in transosseous rotator cuff repairs: A mechanical comparison of simple versus mattress sutures. *Arthroscopy* 1996; 12:704-708.

84. Burkhart SS, Johnson TC, Wirth MA, Athanasiou KA: Cyclic loading of transosseous rotator cuff repairs: Tension overload as a possible cause of failure. *Arthroscopy* 1997;13: 172-176.

85. Sward L, Hughes JS, Amis A, Wallace WA: The strength of surgical repairs of the rotator cuff: A biomechanical study on cadavers. *J Bone Joint Surg Br* 1992;74:585-588.

86. Gerber C, Schneeberger AG, Beck M, Schlegel U: Mechanical strength of repairs of the rotator cuff. *J Bone Joint Surg* Br 1994;76:371-380.

87. Reed SC, Glossop N, Ogilvie-Harris DJ: Full-thickness rotator cuff tears: A biomechanical comparison of suture versus bone anchor techniques. *Am J Sports Med* 1996;24:46-48.

88. Craft DV, Moseley JB, Cawley PW, Noble PC: Fixation strength of rotator cuff repairs with suture anchors and the transosseous suture technique. *J Shoulder Elbow Surg* 1996;5:32-40.

89. Zuckerman JD, Matsen FA III: Complications about the glenohumeral joint related to the use of screws and staples. *J Bone Joint Surg Am* 1984;66:175-180.

90. Rockwood CA Jr, Williams GR Jr, Burkhead WZ Jr: Debridement of degenerative, irreparable lesions of the rotator cuff. *J Bone Joint Surg Am* 1995;77:857-866.

91. Wiley AM: Superior humeral dislocation: A complication following decompression and debridement for rotator cuff tears. *Clin Orthop* 1991;263:135-141.

8

Mini-Open Rotator Cuff Repair: An Updated Perspective

Ken Yamaguchi, MD

Introduction

Once regarded as a "cutting edge" procedure performed only by a select few arthroscopists, the mini-open or arthroscopically assisted rotator cuff repair has quickly become a popular procedure and for many the standard of care for rotator cuff repair.[1-8] In just 5 to 10 years, the mini-open repair has gained acceptance comparable to formal open repair and ironically now lies as a "sensible" middle ground between the traditional formal open repair and the unproven, newer complete arthroscopic rotator cuff repair techniques.[9,10] From several standpoints, the mini-open or arthroscopically assisted approach to rotator cuff repair combines many of the advantages of the former open repair and complete arthroscopic repair while avoiding many of the disadvantages. As complete arthroscopic rotator cuff repair becomes a more viable option, mini-open repair represents an excellent transitional procedure in which a surgeon can become experienced in many of the arthroscopic-specific techniques such as release, tendon mobilization, suture and suture anchor placement necessary in order to perform complete arthroscopic repairs. This chapter will review some of the relevant history regarding the mini-open repair, the relationship to the formal open and arthroscopic repair alternatives, specifics of surgical technique, and the overall results reported with mini-open repair. Additionally, a rationale for the use of the mini-open repair technique for rotator cuff tears of all sizes and as a transition procedure toward complete arthroscopic repair, if desirable, will be described.

Table 1
Fundamentals of rotator cuff repair

Glenohumeral inspection
Anterior-inferior acromioplasty
Release of the coracoacromial ligament
Complete release/mobilization of any fixed contracted tendons around the following structures:
Glenoid labrum
Superficial bursa
Coracoid base (coracohumeral ligament)
Rotator interval
Posterior interval (scapular spine)
Tendon grasping suture placement
Secure bone fixation
Minimize deltoid surgical insult/meticulous repair
Early restoration of passive motion and surgeon-directed rehabilitation

Historical Considerations

The advent of shoulder arthroscopy has had an important impact on the evolution of rotator cuff treatment. Since the initial description of arthroscopic subacromial decompression by Ellman and Kay[11] only a short time ago, there has been a significant trend toward more minimally invasive surgery to accomplish the same results seen previously with the formal open repair. It is important, however, to review formal open repairs as the gold standard or benchmark when reviewing results with arthroscopic treatment. Many of the fundamental principles required in the successful outcome from formal open repair (Table 1) are applicable to achieving good outcome from the mini-open or complete arthroscopic repairs.

The surgical experience with formal open repair of the rotator cuff as presented in the peer-reviewed literature has been extensive.[12-26] Codman[27,28] reported on his experience with rotator cuff repair first described as early as 1911 in which he noted 20 of 31 patients with successful results after repair of full-thickness tears. In 1972, Neer[29] reported results on rotator cuff repair employing routine anterior acromioplasty. He reported 19 of 20 satisfactory results and highlighted four important principles for open rotator cuff surgery: (1) anterior-inferior acromioplasty or reshaping rather than acromionectomy; (2) meticulous repair of the deltoid origin and avoidance of those procedures that may place this area at risk for injury; (3) releasing, mobilizing, and repairing the torn rotator cuff tendons; (4) early restoration of passive motion through surgeon-directed and individualized rehabilitation. These principles have been generally accepted and have led to relatively uniform open treatment of full-thickness rotator cuff tears. Not surprisingly, many subsequent large series of rotator cuff repairs have shown similarly good results. In a series of 100 consecutive rotator cuff repairs with a mean follow-up of 4.2 years, Hawkins and and associates[18] showed that 86% had no or slight pain and average postoperative improvement in abduction of 44°. In a later series of 245 shoulders, Neer and associates[22] reported a 92% excellent or satisfactory rating. Multiple later series have shown similar results for either small or massive repairs.[12-17,20,21,24-26] A common denominator for the articles referred to above has been the adherence to strict surgical principles of deltoid preservation, anterior-inferior acromioplasty, cuff mobilization, and then repair.

Despite a track record of a high percentage of good or excellent results, the formal open repair was associated with some disadvantages. The open repair required some form of anterior deltoid takedown combined with a lateral deltoid split; if associated with a long, difficult procedure, open repair could also be associated with some traction injury. Although the surgical injury imparted to the deltoid has generally been reported to repair and heal in a predictable fashion, experienced shoulder surgeons report a 0.5% incidence of deltoid avulsion.[19,30-32] The incidence reported by less experienced shoulder surgeons may be substantially higher. Loss of the integrity of the anterior deltoid origin is a serious and devastating complication for which there are no satisfying surgical alternatives.[30,32-33] In the context of a rotator cuff tear, results following loss of anterior deltoid function were almost uniformly poor.

Fortunately, deltoid-related complications from formal open approaches appear to be rare. However, a formal open approach has two additional disadvantages related to surgical insult to the deltoid during the rotator cuff repair. The deltoid takedown and repair usually requires a period of protection in order to avoid any inadvertent avulsion. This may preclude accelerated rehabilitation in terms of active-assisted or active motion in smaller rotator cuff tears. Additionally, although not formally qualified, the open repair appears to be associated with more perioperative pain than mini-open or complete arthroscopic alternatives.[1,6,8,34-36] The increased pain may be related to the transdeltoid approach required for formal open repair. This pain can hinder early rehabilitation and early motion as well. Finally, formal open repair, while highly successful over the long term, has been associated with significant recovery times.[24,25] It is generally considered to require 18 months for full recovery to take place. These recovery times appear to be longer than those required for mini-open or complete arthroscopic approaches and again may be related to surgical insult to the deltoid.

In order to avoid anterior deltoid detachment, Levy and associates,[3] in a preliminary report, and then Paulos and Kody[6] in a long-term follow-up study first described the arthroscopically enhanced "mini approach" to rotator cuff repair in 1994. The authors described a technique performed in the lateral decubitus position in which an arthroscopic decompression was first performed followed by an open rotator cuff repair through a lateral deltoid split. As the anterior-inferior acromioplasty had been performed in an arthroscopic fashion, an anterior deltoid detachment was no longer necessary. The rotator cuff repair technique at this point was essentially the same as a complete open repair. All releases were performed in an open fashion and then a combination of transosseous sutures and suture anchors used to secure bone-tendon fixation. Paulos and Kody reported 88% good and excellent results at average follow-up of 48 months.[6] In their opinion, the technique resulted in less perioperative morbidity and, because the deltoid muscle was not detached, more safe initiation of rehabilitation exercises. Conceptionally, the strategy of arthroscopic decompression and then lateral deltoid split has been appealing and several subsequent studies have shown comparable good and excellent results.

Although the results reported thus far have been encouraging, mini-open repair generally is not advised for all rotator cuff tears.[7] For those who rely on open rotator cuff releases and mobilization, the small lateral approach is generally insufficient for repairs of large or massive size tears. For this reason, small, easily mobilized tears are the best indication for the originally described mini-open repair[4,7,9,10] However, with increasing experience in arthroscopic mobilization and tagging of rotator cuff tears, large or massive tears are becoming more easily amenable to repair through mini-open lateral deltoid-splitting approaches.

Strategy and Indications for Surgery

In general, there have been two strategies for surgical technique when using the mini-open repair. The more established method has been arthroscopic decompression followed by a standard open repair through a lateral deltoid split. This technique was initially described by Paulos and Kody.[6] An alternative strategy uses more extensive arthroscopic assistance. In this case, an arthroscopic decompression is performed as in the previous scenario, but in addition an extensive rotator cuff mobilization is performed during the arthroscopic portion procedure. Afterward, arthroscopic tagging sutures or stay sutures are placed and perhaps preparation of the greater tuberosity, débridement of the rotator cuff tendon, and placement of suture anchors are all done arthroscopically. The small lateral deltoid split is then performed in order to place tendon gripping sutures on the previously mobilized

Table 2
Comparison of mini-open surgical techniques

	Inspection	Decompression	Releases	Placement of Tagging Sutures	Tendon Gripping Stitches	Bone-Tendon Fixation
Arthroscopically-assisted open repair	Arthroscopic	Arthroscopic	Open	Open	Open	Open
Mini-open assisted arthroscopic repair	Arthroscopic	Arthroscopic	Arthroscopic	Arthroscopic	Open	Open

cuff and then to fixate the cuff to bone using the surgeon's preferred method, whether it be suture anchors or transosseous sutures.

The two strategies of mini-open repair are fundamentally different in the manner in which arthroscopic assistance is used (Table 2). In the more established method, arthroscopic surgery is used simply to perform a decompression and plays a small role in the actual performance of the rotator cuff repair. This method can be referred to by the traditional designation of an arthroscopically assisted open repair technique. In the second strategy, the decompression and rotator cuff repair are primarily performed arthroscopically and a small portal-extension approach is performed simply to obtain secure tendon to bone fixation of a previously mobilized cuff. This surgical strategy can be referred to as a mini-open assisted arthroscopic rotator cuff repair. In the first case, the emphasis is on open repair techniques; in the second, the emphasis is on arthroscopic repair. Because a lateral open deltoid-splitting approach is used in both strategies, the term mini-open repair can be applicable to both. However, the surgical techniques are distinctly different and associated with different advantages and disadvantages (Table 3).

Table 3
Comparison of rotator cuff repair techniques

	Formal Open	Arthroscopically Assisted Open Repair	Mini-Open Assisted Arthroscopic Repair	Complete Arthroscopic Repair
Glenohumeral evaluation	No	Yes	Yes	Yes
Limited mobilization	Yes	Yes	Yes	Yes
Extensive mobilization	Yes	No	Yes	Yes
Limited deltoid surgical insult	No	No/Yes	Yes	Yes
Tendon-gripping stitches (Mason-Allen)	Yes	Yes	Yes	No
Transosseous sutures	Yes	Yes	Yes	No
Suture anchors	Yes	Yes	Yes	Yes
Early passive motion	Yes	Yes	Yes	Yes
Early active assisted motion	No/Yes	Yes	Yes	Yes
Early active motion (small tears)	No	Yes	Yes	Yes

For the more established arthroscopically assisted open repair technique, less arthroscopic experience or expertise is required. For those surgeons with less experience in performing shoulder arthroscopy, the technique is less technically demanding and more readily performed. However, this technique is directly limited by the size of the lateral deltoid split. When using a smaller approach for larger or massive rotator cuff tears that are chronic in nature, performing all necessary surgical releases can be difficult, if not impossible, through a limited transdeltoid opening. If a large or massive rotator cuff repair is attempted in this fashion, the surgeon is essentially "squeezing" a large operation through a small opening. Although a formal anterior deltoid takedown is not performed in a classic mini-open approach, attempting to repair a large tear can still lead to significant deltoid injury from surgical traction. This may help explain why some surgeons have reported increased episodes of frozen shoulder and even deltoid injury following mini-open repair.

In contrast, a mini-open assisted arthroscopic repair should not be limited by the size of the lateral deltoid split. All rotator cuff preparation is done in an arthroscopic fashion including débridement of cuff edges, extensive releases, cuff mobilization, tuberosity preparation, and even suture anchor placement if desired. Because the rotator cuff has been previously mobilized and tagged, the tendon edges can be delivered directly to the small opening for placement of tendon gripping sutures and then fixation to bone. Because a majority of the surgery has been performed arthroscopically, the

Table 4
Progression toward minimally invasive rotator cuff repair

Formal open repair
↓
Arthroscopically assisted open repair (Arthroscopic decompression followed by lateral open repair)
↓
Mini-open assisted arthroscopic repair (Arthroscopic decompression, arthroscopic rotator cuff preparation followed by mini-open exposure for bone-tendon fixation)
↓
Complete arthroscopic repair

time requirement and exposure for the deltoid splitting portion should be reduced and deltoid injury minimized.

The technique, however, is associated with some significant disadvantages. A large amount of arthroscopic experience around the shoulder is probably a prerequisite for most surgeons in order to obtain expertise in performing all the necessary surgical releases and suture placement. The technique also relies heavily on uncompromising visualization of the rotator cuff and surrounding structures. Without this, the surgeon can be easily misled during rotator cuff preparation. However, as technically demanding as the arthroscopic portion of this procedure can be, it is still significantly easier from a technical standpoint than complete arthroscopic repair (Table 4). Additionally, in comparison to complete arthroscopic repair, more secure bone to tendon fixation is probably possible, because tendon-gripping Mason-Allen sutures and bone augmentation can be used.[37,38]

Surgical Technique

Basic Setup

Open and arthroscopic shoulder surgery at my institution is performed with the patient under interscalene block regional anesthesia and supplemental laryngeal masked general anesthesia (LMA). The interscalene block regional anesthesia has been a reliable and safe method for obtaining intraoperative and postoperative pain relief.[39] The intraoperative pain relief obtained with the block significantly reduces the general anesthetic requirements for the LMA. Laryngeal mask anesthesia is performed in addition to the interscalene block to obtain a more reliable, responsive control of systolic blood pressure, which is essential for the more complex arthroscopic techniques. The patient is placed in a semisitting, upright beach chair position with the back elevated to approximately 70° to 80°. A shoulder arthroscopic positioning device is often helpful. In my institution, a universal locking head and arm holder is used. Once the patient is positioned on the table with the medial aspect of the scapula in line with the lateral aspect of the table, 20 mL of 0.25% bupivacaine hydrochloride containing epinephrine is injected into the subacromial space. Early injection of the bupivacaine hydrochloride with epinephrine prior to prepping and draping of the patient allows for enhanced vascular constriction from the epinephrine. This step can significantly decrease surgical bleeding and improve visualization. Once the shoulder is prepped and draped, all bony landmarks are carefully outlined with a marking pen to help facilitate accurate portal placement.

Accurate portal placement is especially important when instituting advanced arthroscopic techniques about the shoulder. The posterior portal is generally drawn approximately 1 to 2 cm inferior to the posterior edge of the acromion and 2 cm medial to the posterior lateral corner. This portal is generally drawn slightly more superior than the usual posterior portal for arthroscopy in order to obtain a better line of sight to the subacromial bursa for arthroscopic repair. The anterior portal is positioned just lateral to the palpable coracoid tip. The lateral portal is generally placed 1 cm posterior and 3 cm inferior to the anterior lateral corner of the acromion. The exact placement of this portal is determined by needle localization during arthroscopy.

The arthroscope is first placed in the glenohumeral joint through the posterior portal. A standard glenohumeral inspection is performed. Of particular importance, the biceps tendon should be visualized carefully. Often the pathology in the biceps tendon is in the intertubercular groove portion and not readily seen on initial inspection of the intra-articular portion. A hook should be used to pull the tendon into the joint and ensure there are no structural difficulties with the tendon laterally. In those situations in which there is structural pathology to the tendon; such as a partial tear, atrophy, or chronic enlargement, either biceps tenodesis or tenotomy is preferred as the treatment of choice.[40] In those situations in which the tendon either looks normal or inflamed, surgical treatment for the biceps is not recommended. Next, the rotator cuff tear should be visualized and the tear location and size qualified. This will give an idea as to where the appropriate lateral portal placement should be. Finally, the subscapularis should be carefully visualized and its integrity verified.

Rotator cuff mobilization starts with an intra-articular release. This should be performed with the arthroscope in the posterior portal and a hook multipolar cautery device in the anterior portal. Normally a pouch is present superior to the glenoid labrum between the undersurface of the rotator cuff and the superior or posterior-superior portion of the lateral glenoid neck. A hook probe should be placed in this location to determine if the rotator cuff is scarred to the superior labrum. The release is performed by taking the hook cautery and sharply releasing adhesions between the undersurface of the cuff and the superior glenoid labrum starting from anterior and progressing toward posterior (Fig. 1). The multipolar cautery is oriented away from the suprascapular nerve, which is medial. A circumferential release around the posterior, anterior-superior and posterior-superior labrum can be accomplished all the way to the posterior portal. This release is probably the most important to obtain mobilization of the cuff. In addition, it is probably more readily performed arthroscopically than open, where access to the posterior glenoid and posterior-superior rim is difficult secondary to obstruction by the humeral head. Once this intra-articular release has been performed, the arthroscope is then withdrawn and attention placed to the subacromial space.

An arm holder is used in order to apply inline traction on the humerus. The arm is adducted, forward flexed, and slightly internally rotated. This opens up the subacromial space for good visualization. The arthroscope is then redirected into the subacromial space from posterior. Upon entrance into the subacromial bursa, a needle is used to localize the appropriate location for the lateral portal. The lateral portal location should allow a parallel orientation of the burr to the undersurface of the acromion, and it should also be centered over the middle of the rotator cuff tear. In general, this portal is located 1 cm posterior to the anterior-lateral corner of the acromion and 3 cm interior. The portal is made in the direction of Langer's skin lines in a horizontal fashion.

A subacromial bursectomy is then performed, initially starting out with the full radius resector and usually followed by a multipolar electrocautery device. Care should be taken to visualize the cuff first to make sure that bursa, and not rotator cuff, is being débrided. The anteriormost portions of the bursa are débrided first and the débridement also includes the undersurface of the acromion, which is excavated of soft tissues from the anterior-inferior edge and posteriorly. The arthroscope is then generally switched to the lateral portal and the cautery device placed posterior (Fig. 2). The cautery device is then swept from lateral toward medial and then from anterior toward posterior, again excavating bursa off of the rotator cuff all the way medial to the base of the acromion. Generally, a complete removal of bursa from the underlying rotator cuff can be achieved in this fashion. Because the arthroscope is placed laterally, visualization can be obtained all the way around the teres minor posteriorly and inferiorly. Excellent visualization of the subacromial space and the undersurface of the acromion should be obtained in this fashion. At this time, the scope is replaced into the posterior portal and a burr placed into the anterior portal and an anterior-inferior acromioplasty performed. The degree of acromioplasty performed and whether or not a coracoacromial ligament release is also added depends on the reparability[41] of the cuff tear and the size

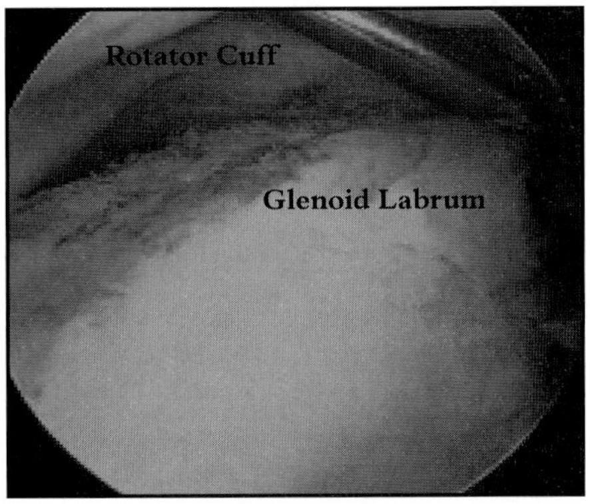

Fig. 1 Release of superior glenoid adhesions.

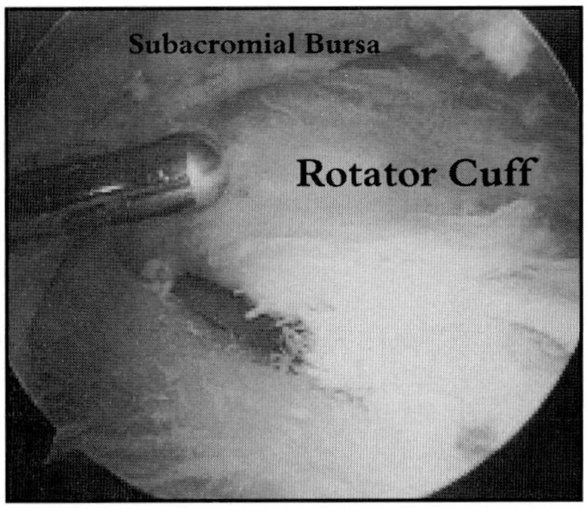

Fig. 2 Release of the superficial surface of the rotator cuff.

of the anterior-inferior spur if present. These are precautions to avoid anterior-superior instability.[33] At this point, the mini-open approach through a lateral deltoid split can be performed if the surgeon is not experienced with the more technically difficult arthroscopic procedures.

It should be noted that throughout the subacromial procedure, careful attention should be applied to blood pressure control. As a general rule, systolic blood pressure should not exceed 120 mm Hg. The pump pressure is generally placed at 40 mm Hg, but it can be raised to 60 mm Hg (as necessary to control bleeding). Elevated pump pressures, however, are associated with more rapid soft-tissue distention and edema, conditions that will eventually obscure visualization. Following decompression, an uncompromising visualization of the rotator cuff should be achieved (Fig. 3). The rotator cuff tear should be seen from its most anterior aspect all the way to its most posterior aspect. This is a prerequisite to performing further rotator cuff preparation arthroscopically.

At this point, an arthroscopic shaver is placed into the lateral portal and débridement performed of the greater tuberosity for later rotator cuff repair. The tuberosity is slightly decorticated and extraneous soft tissue removed. A formal bone

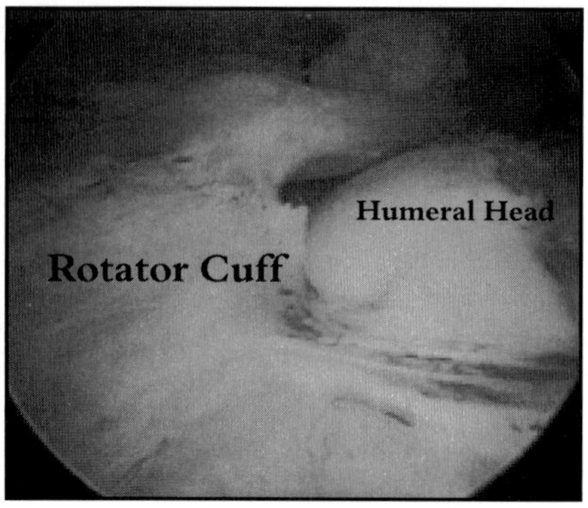

Fig. 3 Arthroscopic visualization of the rotator cuff.

trough is not performed and is contraindicated if a suture anchor is used. Next, the shaver is used to débride any of the torn cuff edge that appears to be nonviable or attenuated. Care should be taken here to do only a limited débridement.

At this point, stay suture placement is initiated. Several different alternative devices are available to achieve this. The Caspari suture punch (Linvatec, Largo, FL) is delivered through the lateral portal (Fig. 4). A place in the midportion of the rotator cuff tear is selected and the suture punch is used to grasp this location. The suture punch is then used to access the mobility of the rotator cuff tendon. For the majority of cases, a release of the rotator cuff from the superior glenoid labrum as well as a superficial bursa generally results in a significant mobilization of the rotator cuff tissue. In rare cases, when assessing the cuff with the suture punch, further releases may be necessary. If the releases are necessary, the suture punch is withdrawn and the arthroscope is placed to the lateral portal. A cautery device is then placed into the anterior portal and this is brought down into the base of the coracoid. At this point, a coracohumeral ligament release is performed right down to the base of the coracoid on the superficial surface. It should be noted that the base of the coracoid has already been débrided on the articular side during the circumferential glenoid release. The sharp débridement can be taken from the base of the coracoid all the way out laterally to the bicipital groove as a rotator interval release as necessary, although this option is rarely needed. Finally, if this release is not sufficient, a posterior interval release can be performed arthroscopically. The scope remains in the lateral portal and the electrocautery device is then switched back to the posterior portal. The base of the acromion and scapular spine can be visualized quite readily from the lateral portal and the cautery device is delivered to this location. The rotator cuff is then mobilized from the scapular spine and base of the acromion in a sharp fashion. Once these releases are performed, mobility of the cuff is reassessed by grasping the tissue with a Caspari suture punch.

After all of these releases are performed, it is a rare case in which the rotator cuff will not be reducible to the greater tuberosity. At this point, multiple shuttle-relay devices (Linvatec, Largo, FL) are delivered by the Caspari suture punch into the anterior, middle, and posterior portions of the rotator cuff tear. In general, these stay sutures are separated by 1 cm and the number required depends on the transverse dimension of the rotator cuff tear. Use of a shuttle-relay device, or alternatively, a No. 1 prolene doubled onto itself allows the surgeon to use these sutures both to control the rotator cuff into a reduced location and also to later pass either transosseous sutures or suture anchors into the cuff for bone fixation.

At this point the mini-open approach is initiated. The horizontal lateral incision is enlarged to a length of 3 to 4 cm (Fig. 5). The subcutaneous tissue is then undermined to expose underlying deltoid fascia. The deltoid is then split inline, with fibers incorporating the arthroscopic puncture site. This split is generally taken up to the acromion and distally about 3 to 4 cm. As the cuff has been previously mobilized and stay sutures already placed, a surprisingly small deltoid split is necessary at this time. Further bursectomy can be performed around the split site to improve visualization, but this is generally not necessary secondary to the extensive bursectomy previously performed with the electrocautery device. Rotating the arm allows different portions of the cuff to be visualized through the deltoid split.

Bone-tendon fixation is then performed at this time. If the tear is small and easily mobilized, then simple stitches placed through suture anchors, which are embedded in the superior lateral aspect of the greater tuberosity, are preferred. For large tears under some tension, Mason-Allen stitches in the cuff, once again placed through suture anchors in the superior lateral location on the greater tuberosity, are preferred.[37,42] Alternatively, transosseous fixation can be used; however, many studies have documented that suture anchors placed in the superior-lateral portion of the greater tuberosity to be at a strength equal to or greater than that of transosseous sutures.[42-44]

Results

The reported outcome from mini-open or arthroscopically assisted rotator cuff repair performed through a lateral deltoid-splitting approach has been generally good and comparable to long-term results seen in multiple open rotator cuff repair series.[1,3-8,41] First reported in 1990 as a preliminary report of 1-year follow-up on 25 patients treated with an arthroscopic subacromial decompression and then lateral deltoid-splitting open repair, Levy and associates[3] reported that 80% of the patients had good or excellent results according to the UCLA shoulder rating. Flynn and associates[45] reported a satisfactory outcome from mini-open repair performed in 10 recreational athletes who participated in overhead and nonthrowing sports. Accelerated rehabilitation appeared to be present as all

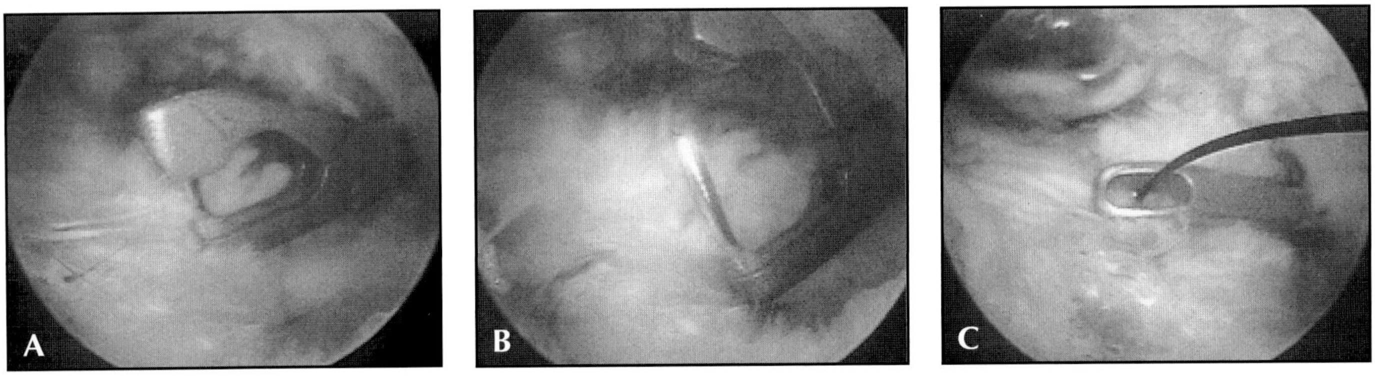

Fig. 4 The Caspari suture punch (Linvatec, Largo, FL) is helpful to insert stay sutures into the rotator cuff. **A** and **B**, This suture punch can be inserted from the lateral portal. **C**, A monofilament suture or a shuttle relay device is then inserted into the rotator cuff to pull traction into the lateral deltoid split.

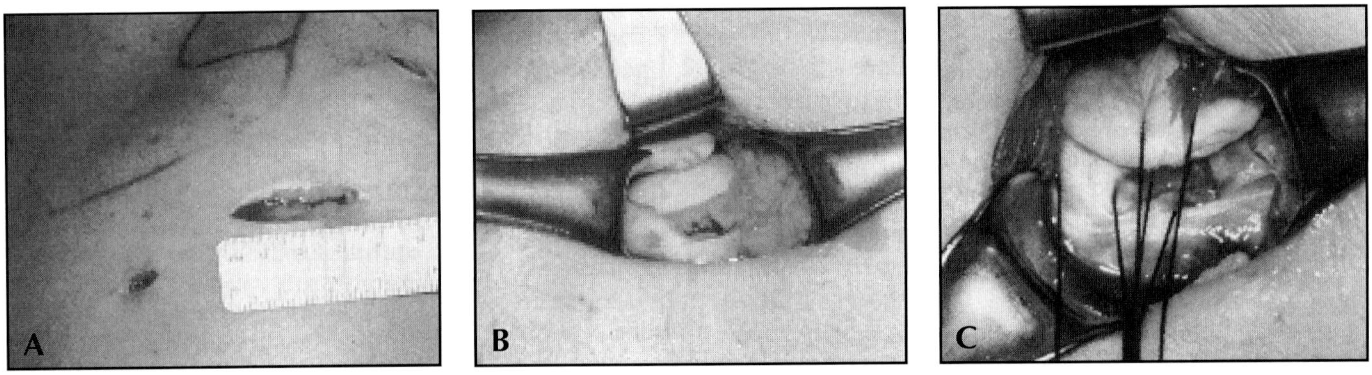

Fig. 5 The mini-open approach. **A**, The anterior-lateral portal is extended. This portal usually measures between 3 and 4 cm in length. Skin incisions within Langer's lines are preferred. **B**, Once subcutaneous dissection is performed, a deltoid split is made in line with the previous portal wound to expose the tear. **C**, Stay sutures are then placed. If arthroscopic preparation has been performed, the previously placed stay sutures can then be brought out through the portal to pull the rotator cuff into view. (Reproduced with permission from Bigliani LU: Rotator cuff repair, in Post M, Bigliani LU, Flatow EL, Pollack RG (eds): *The Shoulder: Operative Technique*. Baltimore, MD, Williams & Wilkins, 1998, pp 133-165.)

these patients returned to their sports within 9 months.

Paulos and Kody[6] presented the first long-term results in 18 patients with an average follow-up of 46 months. In this series, 88% had excellent or good results with the only two poor results seen in patients with pending worker's compensation cases. Pain and function were significantly improved. In another long-term study, Liu and Baker[4] reviewed 44 patients with full-thickness tears treated with an arthroscopically assisted approach. The average follow-up was 4.2 years and 84% of the patients had an excellent or good result. With this surgical technique, the authors correlated outcome to size of tear and showed less satisfactory results in large and massive tears. The authors also showed the procedure to be associated with a shortened hospital stay and more rapid rehabilitation, presumably from less soft-tissue damage. Blevins and associates[2] also reported on results of a large series of patients in which large rotator cuff tears were repaired in addition to the smaller or easily accessible tears. In this study, 83% of the patients achieved a good or excellent rating based on the Hospital for Special Surgery shoulder score. The authors concluded that the procedure was effective for larger rotator cuff tears, but it was more technically demanding. Warner and associates[7] reported on an average 4-year follow-up of 24 patients who were specifically selected for arthroscopically assisted rotator cuff repair. In this focused series, 17 patients underwent a transosseous arthroscopically assisted rotator cuff repair when intraoperative selection criteria showed an avulsion-type tear configuration with good tendon quality and absence of subscapularis tendon involvement. Using specific selection criteria, the authors showed that the arthroscopically assisted repair can achieve excellent results. Average American Shoulder and Elbow Surgeons Function Index of 96 out of 100 was achieved, along with an 89 out of 100 activity of daily living score.

Two studies have sought to compare open and arthroscopically assisted rotator cuff repairs. Baker and Liu[1] compared open and arthroscopically assisted rotator cuff repairs in 37 patients. The open group had 80% good or excellent results compared with 85% for the arthroscopically assisted repair group. Of the patients who had an open repair, 88% were satisfied in comparison to 92% for the arthroscopically assisted repair group. The shoulder strength and functional outcome did not differ significantly between the two groups; however, the arthroscopically assisted repair group had shorter hospital stays and returned to their previous activity an average of 1 month earlier.

Weber and Schaefer[8] also compared mini-open and formal open repair in a retrospective series. The authors studied 69 patients who had open repair and 60 patients in a mini-open group with a minimum 2-year follow-up. The mini-open repair group was seen to require significantly less parenteral narcotics and had shorter hospital stays. The final outcome, however, was not significantly different between the two groups. The authors concluded that the primary advantage of a mini-open technique was to offer a significant decrease in perioperative morbidity without compromising long-term results.

Summary

The mini-open rotator cuff or arthroscopically assisted surgical procedure for repair of the rotator cuff has become a popular procedure with proven clinical results. The development of this procedure has followed a natural progression toward more minimally invasive means to accomplish rotator cuff repair. For many, it represents a middle ground between the traditional formal open repair and the newer complete arthroscopic rotator cuff repairs. As arthroscopic rotator cuff repair becomes more refined and accepted,[35,36,45-48] the mini-open repair can also represent an excellent transitional technique to someday accomplish the more technically difficult complete arthroscopic repair. Whether used as the definitive rotator cuff repair procedure or as a transitional procedure toward arthroscopic repair, the mini-open repair can be thought of as two different types of procedures, an arthroscopically assisted open repair in which the actual repair is performed in a primarily open fashion, or as a mini-open assisted arthroscopic repair in which most of the repair is performed arthroscopically and an open exposure provided just for bone-tendon fixation. With either strategy, the mini-open repair represents an excellent technique for treating full-thickness rotator cuff tears and offers many of the advantages of either formal or complete arthroscopic repair while minimizing many of the disadvantages.

References

1. Baker CL, Liu SH: Comparison of open and arthroscopically assisted rotator cuff repairs. *Am J Sports Med* 1995;23:99-104.
2. Blevins FT, Warren RF, Cavo C, et al: Arthroscopic assisted rotator cuff repair: Results using a mini-open deltoid splitting approach. *Arthroscopy* 1996;12:50-59.
3. Levy HJ, Uribe JW, Delaney LG: Arthroscopic assisted rotator cuff repair: Preliminary results. *Arthroscopy* 1990;6:55-60.
4. Liu SH, Baker CL: Arthroscopically assisted rotator cuff repair: Correlation of functional results with integrity of the cuff. *Arthroscopy* 1994;10:54-60.
5. Liu SH: Arthroscopically-assisted rotator-cuff repair. *J Bone Joint Surg Br* 1994;76:592-595.
6. Paulos LE, Kody MH: Arthroscopically enhanced "mini approach" to rotator cuff repair. *Am J Sports Med* 1994;22:19-25.
7. Warner JJ, Goitz RJ, Irrgang JJ, Groff YJ: Arthroscopic-assisted rotator cuff repair: Patient selection and treatment outcome. *J Shoulder Elbow Surg* 1997;6:463-472.
8. Weber SC, Schaefer R: Abstract: "Mini-open" versus traditional open repair in the management of small and moderate size tears of the rotator cuff. *Arthroscopy* 1993;9:365-366.
9. Pollock RG, Flatow EL: The rotator cuff: Full-thickness tears: Mini-open repair. *Orthop Clin North Am* 1997;28:169-77.
10. Yamaguchi K, Flatow EL: Arthroscopic evaluation and treatment of the rotator cuff. *Orthop Clin North Am* 1995;26:643-659.
11. Ellman H, Kay SP: Arthroscopic subacromial decompression for chronic impingement: Two-to five-year results. *J Bone Joint Surg Br* 1991;73:395-398.
12. Adamson GJ, Tibone JE: Ten-year assessment of primary rotator cuff repairs. *J Shoulder Elbow Surg* 1993;2:57-63.
13. Bigliani L, Cordasco F, McIlveen S, et al: Operative treatment of massive rotator cuff tears: Long-term results. *J Shoulder Elbow Surg* 1992;1:120-130.
14. Gazielly DF, Gleyze P, Montagnon C: Functional and anatomical results after rotator cuff repair. *Clin Orthop* 1994;304:43-53.
15. Grana WA, Teague B, King M, Reeves RB: An analysis of rotator cuff repair. *Am J Sports Med* 1994;22:585-588.
16. Gupta R, Leggin BG, Iannotti JP: Results of surgical repair of full-thickness tears of the rotator cuff. *Orthop Clin North Am* 1997;28:241-248.
17. Hattrup SJ: Rotator cuff repair: Relevance of patient age. *J Shoulder Elbow Surg* 1995; 4:95-100.
18. Hawkins RJ, Misamore GW, Hobeika PE: Surgery for full-thickness rotator-cuff tears. *J Bone Joint Surg Am* 1985;67:1349-1355.
19. Karas EH, Iannotti JP: Failed repair of the rotator cuff: Evaluation and treatment of complications. *Instr Course Lect* 1998;47:87-95.
20. Kronberg M, Wahlstrom P, Brostrom L-A: Shoulder function after surgical repair of rotator cuff tears. *J Shoulder Elbow Surg* 1997;6:125-130.
21. Kirschenbaum D, Coyle MP Jr, Leddy JP, Katsaros P, Tan F Jr, Cody RP: Shoulder strength with rotator cuff tears: Pre- and postoperative analysis. *Clin Orthop* 1993;288:174-178.
22. Neer CS II, Flatow EL, Lech O: Tears of the rotator cuff: Long term results of anterior acromioplasty and repair. *Orthop Trans* 1988;12:673-674.
23. Neer CS II (ed): *Shoulder Reconstruction*. Philadelphia, PA, WB Saunders, 1990, pp 41-142.
24. Rokito AS, Cuomo F, Gallagher MA, Zuckerman JD: Long-term functional outcome of repair of large and massive chronic tears of the rotator cuff. *J Bone Joint Surg Am* 1999;81:991-997.
25. Rokito AS, Zuckerman JD, Gallagher MA, Cuomo F: Strength after surgical repair of the rotator cuff. *J Shoulder Elbow Surg* 1996;5:12-17.
26. Romeo AA, Hang DW, Bach BR Jr, Shott S: Repair of full thickness rotator cuff tears: Gender, age, and other factors affecting outcome. *Clin Orthop* 1999;367:243-255.
27. Codman EA (ed): *The Shoulder: Rupture of the Supraspinatus Tendon and Other Lesions In or*

About the Subacromial Bursa. Boston, MA, Thomas Todd, 1934.

28. Codman EA: Complete rupture of the supraspinatus tendon: Operative treatment with report of two successful cases. *Boston Med Surg J* 1911;164:708-710.
29. Neer CS II: Anterior acromioplasty for the chronic impingement syndrome in the shoulder: A preliminary report. *J Bone Joint Surg Am* 1972;54:41-50.
30. Mansat P, Cofield RH, Kersten TE, Rowland CM: Complications of rotator cuff repair. *Orthop Clin North Am* 1997;28:205-213.
31. Mormino MA, Gross RM, McCarthy JA: Captured shoulder: A complication of rotator cuff surgery. *Arthroscopy* 1996;12:457-461.
32. Yamaguchi K: Complications of rotator cuff repair. *Tech Orthop* 1997;12:33-41.
33. Wiley AM: Superior humeral dislocation: A complication following decompression and débridement for rotator cuff tears. *Clin Orthop* 1991;263:135-141.
34. Gartsman GM: Arthroscopic management of rotator cuff disease. *J Am Acad Orthop Surg* 1998;6:259-266.
35. Gartsman GM, Brinker MR, Khan M: Early effectiveness of arthroscopic repair for full-thickness tears of the rotator cuff: An outcome analysis. *J Bone Joint Surg Am* 1998;80:33-40.
36. Gartsman GM, Hammerman SM: Full-thickness tears: Arthroscopic repair. *Orthop Clin North Am* 1997;28:83-98.
37. Gerber C, Schneeberger AG, Beck M, Schlegel U: Mechanical strength of repairs of the rotator cuff. *J Bone Joint Surg Br* 1994;76:371-380.
38. Gerber C, Schneeberger AG, Perren SM, Nyffeler RW: Experimental rotator cuff repair: A preliminary study. *J Bone Joint Surg Am* 1999;81:1281-1290.
39. Brown AR, Weiss R, Greenberg C, Flatow EL, Bigliani LU: Interscalene block for shoulder arthroscopy: Comparison with general anesthesia. *Arthroscopy* 1993;9:295-300.
40. Sethi N, Wright R, Yamaguchi K: Disorders of the long head of the biceps tendon. *J Shoulder Elbow Surg* 1999;8:644-654.
41. Gartsman GM: Arthroscopic assessment of rotator cuff tear reparability. *Arthroscopy* 1996;12:546-549.
42. Burkhart SS, Diaz Pagan JL, Wirth MA, Athanasiou KA: Cyclic loading of anchor-based rotator cuff repairs: Confirmation of the tension overload phenomenon and comparison of suture anchor fixation with transosseous fixation. *Arthroscopy* 1997;13:720-724.
43. Reed SC, Glossop N, Ogilvie-Harris DJ: Full-thickness rotator cuff tears: A biomechanical comparison of suture versus bone anchor techniques. *Am J Sports Med* 1996;24:46-48.
44. Barber FA, Cawley P, Prudich JF: Suture anchor failure strength: An in vivo study. *Arthroscopy* 1993;9:647-652.
45. Flynn L, Flood S, Clifford S, et al: Arthroscopically assisted rotator cuff repair with the Mitek anchor. *Am J Arthroscopy* 1991;1:15-18.
46. Snyder SJ: Technique of arthroscopic rotator cuff repair using implantable 4-mm Revo suture anchors, suture Shuttle Relays, and no. 2 nonabsorbable mattress sutures. *Orthop Clin North Am* 1997;28:267-275.
47. Stollsteimer GT, Savoie FH III: Arthroscopic rotator cuff repair: Current indications, limitations, techniques, and results. *Instr Course Lect* 1998;47:59-65.
48. Tauro JC: Arthroscopic rotator cuff repair: Analysis of technique and results at 2- and 3-year follow-up. *Arthroscopy* 1998;14:45-51.

9

Management of Massive Irreparable Rotator Cuff Tears: The Role of Tendon Transfer

Jon J.P. Warner, MD

The Problem

Most rotator cuff tears can be repaired by conventional methods. Even in the case of massive tears, repair or reconstruction is usually feasible and the outcome is usually good.[1,2] While there is no universal agreement on the definition, in North America Cofield's[3] definition of a massive tear as one with a diameter of 5 cm or greater is used. Furthermore, there appear to be two distinct patterns of tears, each with a different epidemiology, mechanism of injury, associated disability, and prognosis.[4] The more common, posterosuperior configuration involves the supraspinatus and the infraspinatus, and the less common, anterosuperior configuration involves the subscapularis and the supraspinatus.

Massive posterosuperior rotator cuff tears are not common. Even in clinical practices limited to the treatment of shoulder problems, less than one third of all rotator cuff tears are massive. Neer[5] reported that, of 340 rotator cuff tears operated on over a 13-year period, 145 were massive. Bigliani and associates[2] described 61 massive rotator cuff tears requiring surgery over a 6-year period. Ellman and associates[6] reported that 9 of 54 rotator cuff repairs involved a massive tear. Harryman and associates[7] reported that 28 of 105 surgically-treated tears were massive. Of 407 rotator cuff tears that I repaired surgically over a period of 6 years, 146 were massive posterosuperior lesions (unpublished data).

Massive anterosuperior rotator cuff tears are even less common. A recent European study included 88 combined subscapularis and supraspinatus tendon tears from seven centers; 24 such tears were reported in a series of 301 tears that were repaired over a 5-year period.[4] Of 105 tears reported on by Harryman and associates,[7] 22 involved the subscapularis as well as the supraspinatus. Of the 407 rotator cuff tears that I repaired surgically during a period of 6 years, 19 were combined supraspinatus and subscapularis tears (unpublished data).

Although most tears that involve two or more tendons can be repaired with good results, in some patients the size of the defect and the quality of the tendon tissue preclude secure repair to bone.[7-9] As these tears are, by definition, massive, not all can be repaired. An irreparable tear is one in which the quality of the tendon tissue is so poor that direct tendon-to-bone repair is not possible. In such cases, alternative surgical techniques are considered. Both open and arthroscopic débridement have been suggested; however, while some authors have thought that this provides good pain relief and function, strength is not restored.[10-12] Furthermore, the durability of this pain relief has been questioned.[13] In general, this technique is best suited for elderly patients whose predominant symptom is pain. Tendon allografts and synthetic fabrics have also been used in such patients but without reproducible results.[14,15]

Both local tendon transposition and distant tendon transfer have been proposed to manage irreparable rotator cuff tears in patients who have both pain and weakness. The former has included use of a portion of the subscapularis and the teres minor to cover a large superior defect of the rotator cuff.[16-18] While some surgeons have reported success with these methods, the results have not been reproducible by others. In Europe, anterior deltoid transposition has also been suggested for the reconstruction of irreparable tears of the cuff;[19-21] however, this technique has not gained favor in North America.

Historically, extrinsic tendon transfer about the shoulder has been proposed for the management of paralysis.[22-25] Transfer of the trapezius tendon was once recommended for the management of massive rotator cuff tears;[26] however, the results of this technique were not reproducible. Several authors[27,28] have suggested that the teres major may be a reasonable substitute for an infraspinatus muscle with an irreparable lesion; however, clinically it has been found that this tendon is too short and bulky for transfer.[9] In 1988, Gerber and associates[9] documented the anatomic potential and clinical effectiveness of latissimus dorsi tendon transfer for the management of the functional deficit associated with a massive irreparable posterosuperior rotator cuff tear. Gerber's[29] long-term follow-up study of this series, reported in 1992, added to the enthusiasm for this method. Others[30,31] have reported similarly successful outcomes with this approach. This is currently the favored method for the reconstruction of irreparable massive posterosuperior rotator cuff tears.

The principal problem with management of irreparable anterosuperior tears is the subscapularis component of the tear. This is the most important muscle-tendon unit for both function and stability of the glenohumeral joint.[32-36] Although subscapularis rupture has been well recognized as a complication of anterior dislocation, it has only recently been appreciated that disruption of this structure without instability can lead to severe pain and weakness.[33,34,37-40] While Gerber and associates[33,34] highlighted the physical findings that allow the detection of subscapularis rupture and the technical steps necessary for repair, little has been written about the management of an irreparable subscapularis tendon tear. Recent anecdotal experience and one published report[32] have suggested that transfer of the pectoralis major may be a method for the management of chronic irreparable subscapularis deficiency. No other type of tendon transfer has proved useful in this situation.

Preoperative Considerations

All considerations with regard to treatment must be placed in the context of the individual patient's disability and expectations for pain relief and functional recovery. Concomitant medical problems must also be considered, as they have a bearing on the patient's potential for recovery and for postoperative compliance with therapy.

Pathoanatomy and Pathomechanics

The functional contribution of a muscle to the rotation of a joint is determined by multiplying its physiologic cross-sectional area by its leverage. Physiologic cross-sectional area is an expression of a muscle's force potential.[41] The leverage of a muscle is determined by drawing a perpendicular line from the muscle's line of action to the center of rotation of the joint.[42] If this analysis is applied to the rotator cuff muscles, it is clear that the supraspinatus makes a small (14%) contribution to the overall moment arm for abduction of the shoulder,[41,42] whereas the infraspinatus and teres minor contribute 32% and the subscapularis contributes 52%.[41] Thus, the anterior and posterior components of the rotator cuff are of primary importance in determining the rotation of this joint.

The excursion of the rotator cuff tendons is also relatively small (range, 0.5 to 4.0 cm) during scapular abduction. In comparison, the deltoid muscle has an excursion of 6.5 cm during abduction.[35] The rotator cuff muscles are thus critical stabilizers of the humeral head, providing a fixed fulcrum for rotation powered by the deltoid during abduction.[35] Disruption of the supraspinatus in combination with either the infraspinatus or the subscapularis can result in loss of the fulcrum for the rotation that is necessary for full abduction.[36,43-45]

The role of the long head of the biceps remains a matter of some debate. While some authors[46-48] have provided evidence for its action as a humeral head depressor, others[49,50] have suggested that it does not play an important biomechanical role in the setting of a massive rotator cuff tear.

Clinical[10,12] and experimental[36,37] work has demonstrated that, in some patients who have a massive rotator cuff tear, shoulder function remains good. In these patients, the tear involves the entire supraspinatus and, while it may extend into the subscapularis or the infraspinatus, it does not disrupt these tendons inferior to the equator of the humeral head. Thus, the remaining anterior and posterior aspects of the rotator cuff can exert sufficient force to maintain a fixed fulcrum for rotation of the humeral head in the glenoid. Extension of the tear inferior to the equator results in biomechanical decompensation with loss of containment of the humeral head.[9,29,36,37] Paradoxically, some patients with a smaller rotator cuff tear may have very poor function while others with a larger tear may maintain good function. The fact that tear size does not always correlate with function is reflected in the literature in terms of the disparity among treatment outcomes.[2,3,10,12] Several surgeons have suggested that this disparity between tear size and function can be explained by the degree of atrophy and fatty degeneration of the muscles of the rotator cuff[34,51] (Fig. 1).

Another important factor that must be considered is the integrity of the coracoacromial arch. This structure may act as a stabilizer against unchecked anterosuperior movement of the humeral head in the setting of a tendon tear involving the supraspinatus and at least one other tendon.[52,53] Thus, it is now commonly recommended that the arch be preserved in the surgical management of such patients.

Because massive rotator cuff tears are found in a heterogeneous population of patients, it remains difficult to select the optimal form of treatment. The determination that a rotator cuff tear is irreparable can be made prior to surgery. Currently, it is possible to identify individuals who have poor quality tissue and a large tear that preclude successful primary tendon repair. Factors that predict these findings include profound weakness of external rotation, superior displacement of the humeral head, and MRI imaging showing not only atrophy but also fatty replacement of the muscles of the rotator cuff. An anteroposterior radiograph that shows an acromiohumeral interval of less than 5 mm usually means that the tear involves at least two tendons of the rotator cuff. Hersche and Gerber[54] demonstrated that the duration of the tendon tear is associated with the stiffness of the muscle-tendon unit at the time of surgery. I have found that the degree of fatty replacement of the muscle seen on a preoperative MRI study predicts the quality and stiffness of the tendon tissue as well. Therefore, primary repair or local reconstruction of the torn rotator cuff tendon is not recommended for patients with this combination of findings.

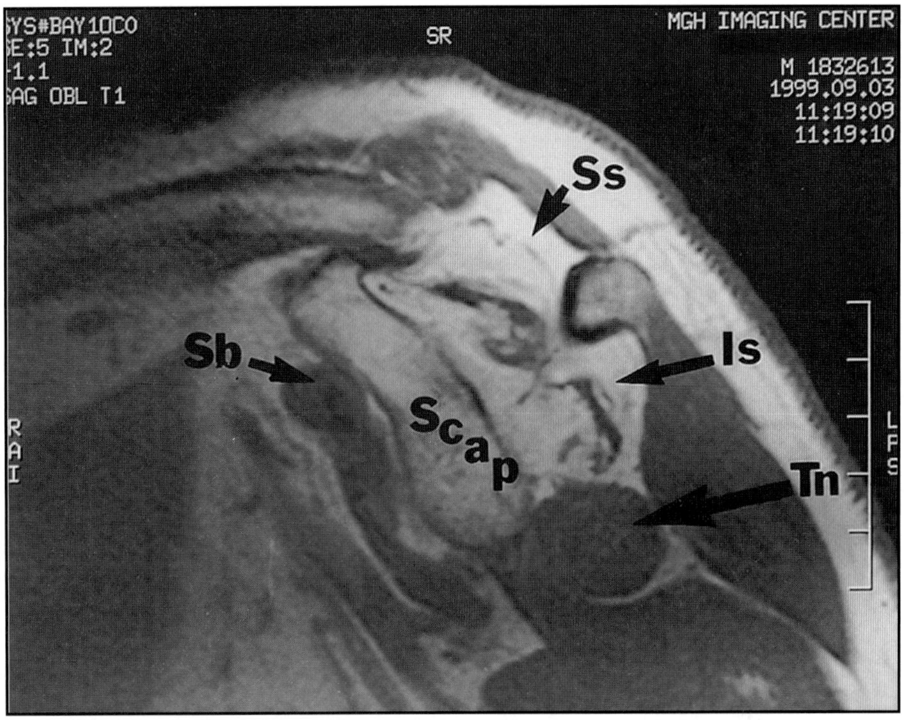

Fig. 1 Oblique sagittal plane MRI study of a left shoulder with a chronic massive tear involving the supraspinatus (Ss) and the infraspinatus (Is). These muscles are atrophic and have a signal characterized as fat. The teres minor (Tn) and the subscapularis (Sb) are not torn and do not demonstrate fatty replacement. Scap = scapula.

Indications for Tendon Transfer

The clinical experience of several authors provides some guidelines for the appropriate selection of patients for tendon transfer for the reconstruction of an irreparable tear.[9,29-31] In general, it is appropriate to consider tendon transfer for patients who have a painful rotator cuff tear that is associated with poor function and in whom there is a low probability that primary reconstruction will be successful.

For patients who have had failure of a prior tendon repair, the indications for tendon transfer are less clear; a number of factors may mitigate against successful improvement of function in this situation.[29,30] These factors include disruption of the coracoacromial arch, deltoid deficiency, stiffness, and nerve injury. In addition, with an irreparable tear of the supraspinatus and infraspinatus, disruption of the subscapularis is a relative contraindication for latissimus dorsi tendon transfer.[9] This is due to disruption of the anterior component of the anteroposterior force couple of the rotator cuff.

The Mechanical Basis of Tendon Transfer for Reconstruction of the Rotator Cuff

The anatomic and biomechanical basis of muscle transfer has been previously published.[55] The relative length of a muscle and its line of action relative to the center of rotation of the joint determine its usefulness as a transfer to restore motion. The rotator cuff muscles have a relatively short amplitude compared with extrinsic shoulder muscles such as the deltoid, pectoralis major, and latissimus dorsi. For the most part, the important function of the rotator cuff that needs to be restored is its action as an external and internal rotator of the humeral head. Thus, the function of the infraspinatus or subscapularis is of primary concern. The subscapularis has an amplitude of 7.3 cm and is the strongest of the rotator cuff muscles.[55] It acts as a powerful internal rotator, but it also maintains the stability of the humeral head by pulling it both downward and posteriorly during abduction of the arm. It acts in synergy with the infraspinatus both to abduct the shoulder and to provide centering of the humeral head in the glenoid.

Comparison of the orientation of the subscapularis with that of other muscles about the shoulder reveals that there are no tendons available for optimal restoration of function if the subscapularis cannot be repaired. Use of the trapezius and the pectoralis major has been proposed.[32] Clinical experience with the trapezius has not been reported in the peer-reviewed literature, to my knowledge, but its line of action seems unfavorable as a substitute for subscapularis function. The pectoralis major has a favorable amplitude (14.4 cm for the clavicular head and 18.8 cm for the sternal head), but its line of action is anterior to the normal orientation of the subscapularis as it originates from the chest wall and thus it cannot pull the humeral head backward.[32,55] Several surgeons have suggested that this line of action can be improved if the pectoralis major is transferred underneath the conjoined tendon and to the lesser tuberosity; however, I am aware of no published reports of this technique.

Transfer of the trapezius[26] or the lateral head of the deltoid[19,21] has been proposed for use in the management of supraspinatus tendon insufficiency; however, neither technique has been shown to

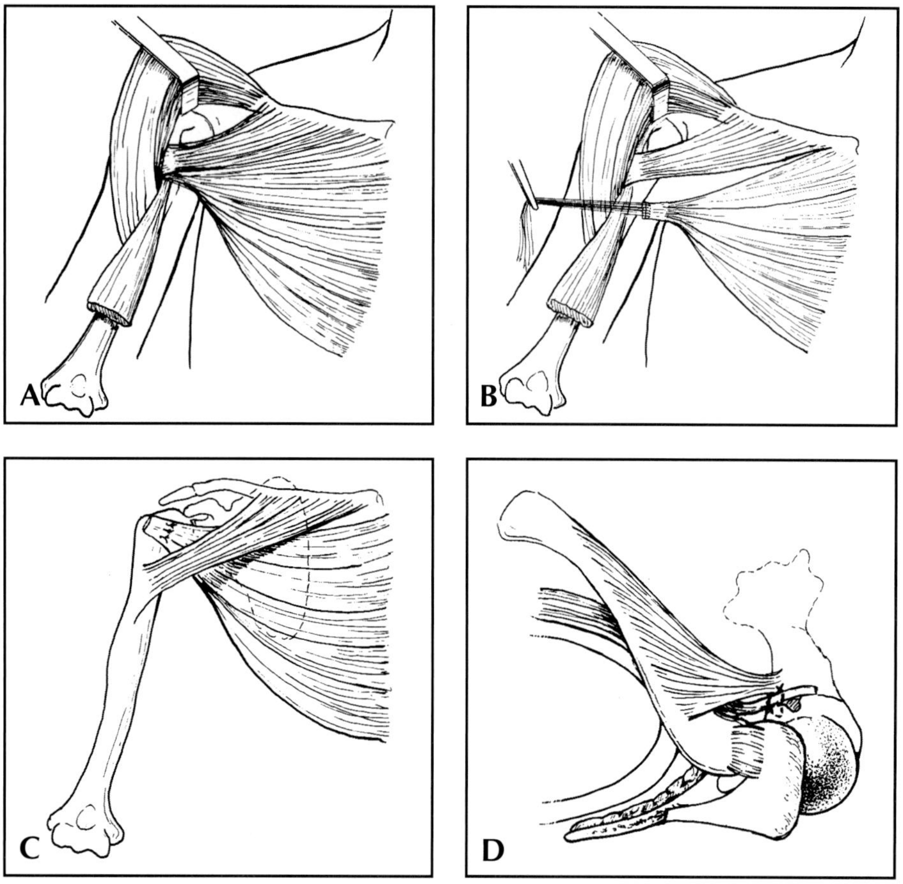

Fig. 2 Drawings showing the surgical technique for the pectoralis major tendon transfer. **A**, The superior and inferior borders of the pectoralis major are exposed. **B**, The sternal portion is dissected, with preservation of the clavicular portion. **C**, The sternal portion is transferred underneath the clavicular portion and is repaired into the lesser tuberosity. **D**, The sternal head of the pectoralis passes underneath the clavicular head, which acts as a pulley, keeping the line of pull of the sternal head closer to the line of the subscapularis tendon.

be effective when there is an irreparable infraspinatus or subscapularis tear.

Disruption of the infraspinatus is always associated with a supraspinatus tear. The combination, which is irreparable, is very disabling for some patients because they lose not only abduction but also external rotation, which prevents movement of the hand to the mouth or to the top of the head. The two muscles that have been proposed as best suited to restore external rotation and abduction are the teres major and the latissimus dorsi. The maximum potential amplitude of the infraspinatus is 8.6 cm, that of the latissimus dorsi is 34 cm, and that of the teres major is 15 cm. Each of these muscles has sufficient strength to be effective as a transferred muscle. While the teres major appears to qualify as a good substitute on the basis of its line of action, it has a rather bulky short tendon, and experimental study has demonstrated that it may not reach superior to the posterior portion of the greater tuberosity when it is transferred underneath the acromion.[28] The latissimus dorsi has been shown to have sufficient excursion to be transferred over the humeral head; however, this muscle crosses both the scapulothoracic and the glenohumeral articulation, and its function is completely different from that of the muscle for which it is acting as a substitute. It normally functions as a powerful adductor and extends the humerus.

My personal preference is to use a modified pectoralis major transfer for reconstruction of an irreparable subscapularis tendon tear and to use a latissimus dorsi transfer for reconstruction of an irreparable infraspinatus tear.

Split Pectoralis Major Transfer for Reconstruction of an Irreparable Subscapularis Tear

The technical steps for the mobilization and repair of the subscapularis were described by Gerber and associates.[9] It is important to attempt to mobilize the subscapularis tendon because even a partial repair may be of some advantage. It is sometimes possible to repair the inferior portion of the tendon while the superior one half remains irreparable. The pectoralis major can then be used to augment the function of the deficient portion.

Wirth and Rockwood[32] described use of the superior portion of the pectoralis major for reconstruction. With their technique, this portion is released from the humerus and transferred lateral to the bicipital groove with the arm in internal rotation. My approach modifies this technique for several reasons. First, the sternal portion of the pectoralis is identified and used for the transfer because this component has sufficient strength and amplitude to act effectively as a transfer. Second, transfer of this component of the pectoralis underneath the remaining clavicular portion of the tendon brings its line of action closer to that of the subscapularis muscle (Fig. 2).

Surgical Technique An extended deltopectoral approach is used. The deltopectoral groove is identified, and the dissection proceeds through this interval to the level of the clavipectoral fascia. The interval underneath the conjoined tendon is developed by both blunt and sharp dissection. There is usually a thin layer of tissue overlying the humeral head; this is not the subscapularis but rather scar tissue in continuity with the subscapularis tendon that has retracted medially deep to the conjoined tendon. This layer is detached along the lesser tuberosity from superior to inferior. Often, a few remaining muscle fibers of the subscapularis attached inferiorly to the lesser tuberosity are visible. A humeral head retractor is then inserted into the joint to displace the humeral head posteriorly, improving exposure for mobilization of the scarred subscapularis tendon. A long, thin retractor is then placed underneath the conjoined tendon, and the axillary nerve and the circumflex vessels are identified. The circumflex vessels are mobilized and then controlled with suture ligature, and the axillary nerve is mobilized and a vessel loupe is placed underneath it. Dissection then frees the inferior scar of the subscapularis while protecting the axillary nerve. Sutures are placed through the scarred edge of the subscapularis so that it can be manipulated to allow for release of adhesions. Sharp dissection releases the contracted subscapularis from the labrum, and the muscle is then mobilized from its fossa. Finally, the scarred coracohumeral ligament is released from the base of the coracoid process. When there is fatty replacement of the muscle, the muscle-tendon unit feels stiff. Usually, the entire subscapularis tendon cannot be repaired to the lesser tuberosity, but in some cases its inferior portion can be reattached to the lesser tuberosity with use of a transosseous repair technique.[4,34]

The pectoralis major is then exposed, and the dissection is continued medially on its superficial surface. Knowledge of the anatomy of the tendon insertion is important for harvesting the sternal head of the muscle. The sternal portion originates from the inferior part of the sternum and the fifth and sixth ribs. Its tendon courses superiorly underneath that of the clavicular head, so that it twists 180° and inserts superiorly on the humerus. The interval between the two heads and the orientation of the tendon usually can be clearly identified (Fig. 3). This interval is then developed bluntly just medial to the muscle-tendon junction, and a large clamp is placed underneath the sternal portion of the muscle. The clamp is replaced with a Penrose drain. The dissection then proceeds distally, with separation of the two components of the tendon and detachment of the sternal portion from the humerus. Nonabsorbable No. 2 braided sutures are placed in the tendon end. The muscle split between the two heads is extended about 3 to 4 cm medially in order to facilitate transfer of the sternal head underneath the clavicular head. After decortication of the area of the lesser tuberosity and the bicipital groove, the tendon is repaired to bone with use of either bone anchors or a transosseous repair technique. This is done with the arm in neutral rotation and the pectoralis pulled superiorly to the top of the lesser tuberosity. The incision is then closed in layers, and the arm is placed in a shoulder immobilizer.

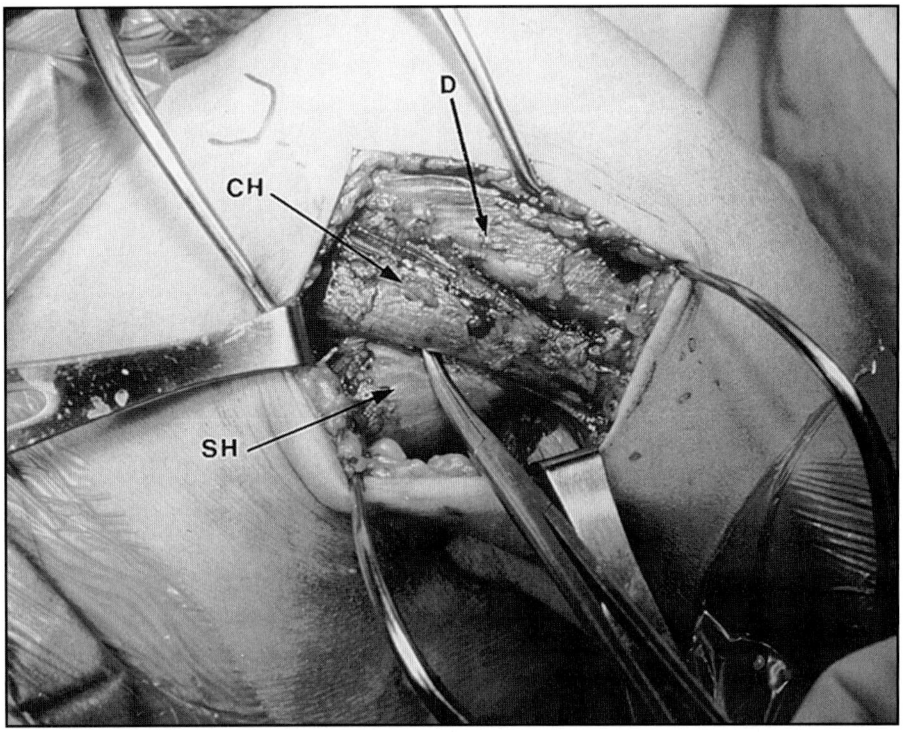

Fig. 3 Photograph showing the interval between the sternal head (SH) and the clavicular head (CH) of the pectoralis major. The sternal head passes posterior to the clavicular head as it approaches its insertion on the humerus. D = deltoid.

Postoperative care consists of immobilization in a sling for 4 weeks, during which time passive flexion is performed below the horizontal and passive external rotation is limited to about 30°. After 4 weeks, active assisted motion is commenced. Strengthening exercises are delayed for 4 months.

Results Experience with transfer of the pectoralis major for the reconstruction of irreparable subscapularis tears is limited. Wirth and Rockwood[32] reported on 13 patients with an irreparable subscapularis tendon tear who had had failure of a capsular repair for the treatment of instability. Seven of these patients had transfer of the pectoralis major only, five had transfer of both the pectoralis major and the pectoralis minor, and one had transfer of the pectoralis minor only. Ten patients had a satisfactory outcome, and three had failure of the

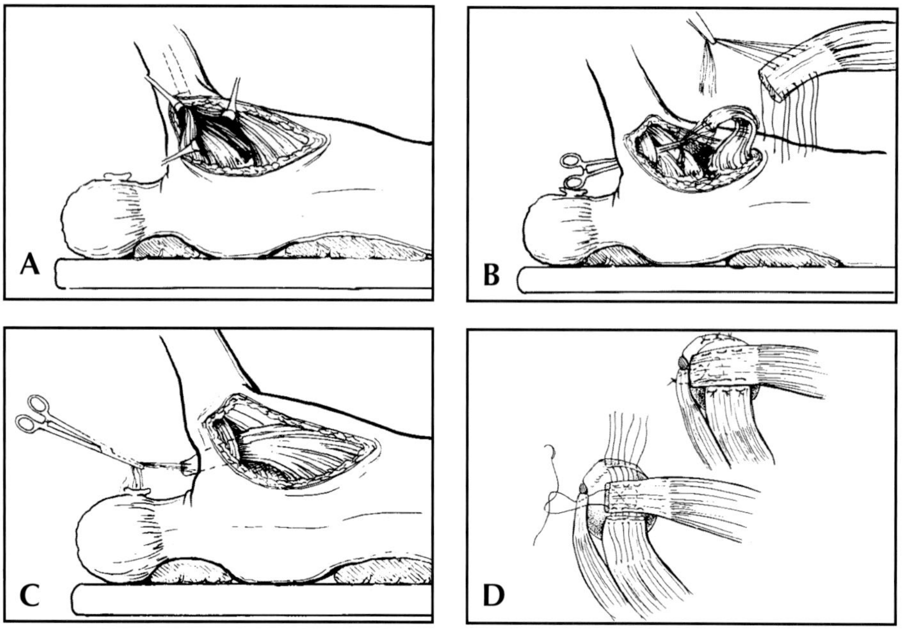

Fig. 4 Drawings showing the surgical technique for the latissimus dorsi tendon transfer. **A,** The patient is placed in the lateral decubitus position, and an accessory posterior incision is made in order to identify and harvest the latissimus dorsi tendon. **B,** The tendon is detached from the humerus and then dissected retrograde to the neurovascular pedicle. The tendon is freed from its fascial connections to the chest wall. Sutures are then placed in the tendon prior to its transfer underneath the acromion. **C,** The tendon is transferred underneath the deltoid and the acromion. **D,** With the shoulder abducted and in external rotation, the tendon is secured to the remnant of the rotator cuff tendons medially, to the greater tuberosity laterally, and to the subscapularis anteriorly.

procedure. All of the patients with a satisfactory outcome had resolution of the instability as well as a marked reduction in pain. Two patients had restoration of a normal lift-off test.[32] (This test measures the ability to lift the internally rotated arm off of the lower back, and it indicates normal terminal internal rotation performed by the subscapularis.)

My experience with split pectoralis major transfer has included 10 patients over the past 4 years. In five patients, the procedure was done after failure of prior rotator cuff surgery; in three, it was done after failure of surgery for the treatment of instability; and in two, it was done in the setting of instability after hemiarthroplasty. All patients had pain and the perception of instability when the arm was placed either overhead or behind the plane of the body. The results were graded according to pain relief, improved function, and resolution of instability. All patients thought that the shoulder was stable and indicated that the pain had decreased, although only six reported minimal or no pain. Functional gains were more limited, with only two patients indicating marked improvement and the ability to participate in sports such as golf and tennis. Three patients thought that they had much improvement, but they still had limited overhead use of the arm, and five had minimal functional improvement despite relief of pain and of the sense of apprehension. No patient had a normal lift-off test.

Latissimus Dorsi Transfer for Reconstruction of an Irreparable Posterosuperior Rotator Cuff Tear

The technique for transfer of the latissimus dorsi tendon to reconstruct posterosuperior rotator cuff tears has been described in detail previously.[4,9,29] Over the 8 years of my experience, it has been modified technically as described below.

Surgical Technique The patient is placed in the lateral decubitus position and is stabilized on a long beanbag, which is contoured to support the torso (Fig. 4, *A*). The entire arm and hemithorax are prepared with use of sterile technique and are draped. An anterosuperior incision is made in order to expose the rotator cuff tear. This incision begins on top of the shoulder, over the lateral one third of the acromion, and continues anteriorly about 1 cm lateral to the coracoid process. In all cases, an attempt is made to preserve the coracoacromial arch. This is done by splitting the deltoid from the lateral aspect of the acromion and elevating it subperiosteally off of the anterior aspect. The interval between the deltoid and the coracoacromial ligament is identified, so that the latter is not detached from the acromion. The lateral deltoid split also allows easier access to the posterior aspect of the rotator cuff, improving exposure for transfer of the tendon. The edges of the rotator cuff are then identified, and steps to mobilize the retracted tendon edges are performed. These steps include release of the coracohumeral ligament, extra-articular lysis of adhesions that may be tethering the tendons, and intra-articular release in the plane between the labrum and the tendon surface. This will increase tendon excursion only modestly, usually less than a centimeter. Braided nonabsorbable No. 2 sutures are then placed through the tendon edges.

The greater tuberosity is then prepared by abrading its surface and placing holes from the edge of the tuberosity to the lateral cortex of the humerus. Loops of braided No. 2 suture are placed through these holes so that sutures from the transferred tendon can be passed subsequently.

In order to harvest the latissimus dorsi tendon, a separate posterior incision is

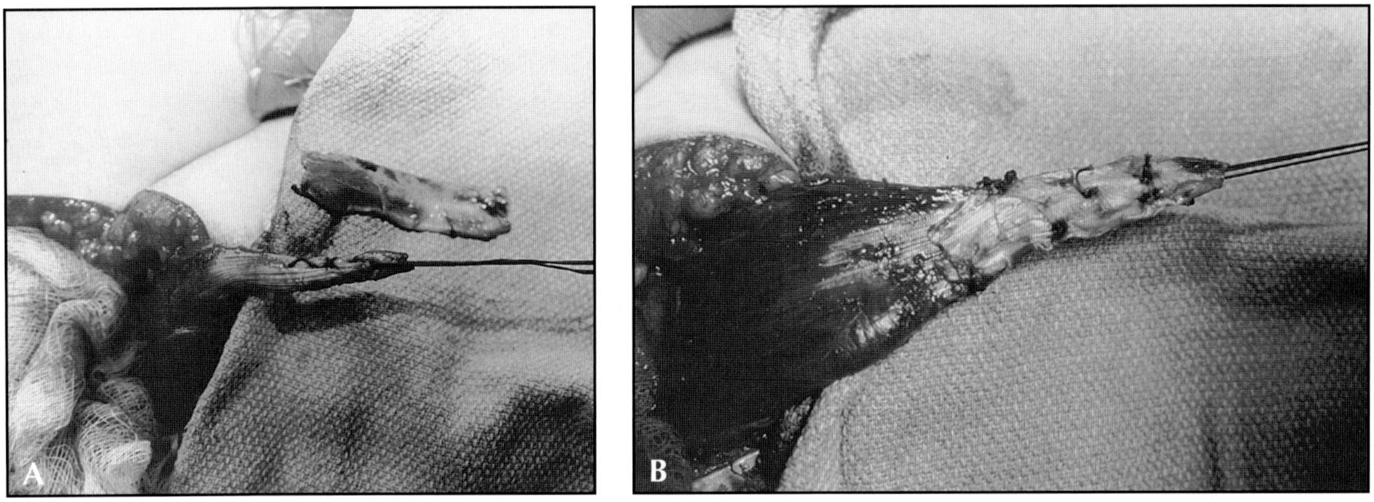

Fig. 5 A, The latissimus dorsi tendon is often small and thin. The fascia lata autograft that will be used to augment the tendon is shown in the background of the photograph. **B,** Photograph showing the latissimus dorsi tendon after the fascia lata autograft has been sewn over it to reinforce it prior to transfer.

made over the muscle belly and curved superiorly over the posterior aspect of the deltoid at the level of the joint line. The posterior aspect of the deltoid, the long head of the triceps, the teres major, and the latissimus dorsi muscles are identified. The latissimus dorsi is then dissected free from the teres major and the fascia of the chest wall. There are often substantial connections between the latissimus dorsi and the teres major, so dissection is easier if it begins at the level of the muscle and continues toward its insertion. The arm is positioned in flexion and internal rotation, which makes access to the tendon insertion easier. Long retractors are used to expose the tendon insertion while an assistant holds the arm in this position. Once the tendon has been detached from its insertion on the humerus, several No. 2 braided sutures are placed through the end of the tendon in order to maintain tension on it as it is dissected in a retrograde fashion (Fig. 4, *B*). The tendon is freed from fascial extensions to the chest wall, and the neurovascular pedicle is isolated and protected. The muscle-tendon unit has been sufficiently mobilized for transfer when the tendon end can reach superior to the posterior aspect of the acromion. Braided nonabsorbable No. 2 sutures are then placed through the tendon's lateral edge to be used to repair the tendon to the greater tuberosity once it has been transferred underneath the acromion.

The interval underneath the deltoid and the acromion is developed by both blunt and sharp dissection, and the tendon is then transferred with use of a curved clamp (Fig. 4, *C*). The arm is positioned in 45° of abduction in the scapular plane and 30° of external rotation and is held in that position with use of a special articulated arm-holder (McConnell Shoulder Holder; McConnell, Greenville, TX) until the transferred tendon is sutured in place. Use of the arm-holder seems to work better than having an assistant hold the arm, as it allows better exposure of the shoulder because of its thin profile. It also maintains the arm in a consistent position, whereas an assistant might become fatigued and allow the arm position to move during the tendon transfer and repair. At this stage, a lamina spreader placed between the greater tuberosity and the acromion may help with exposure for suturing of the tendon. The tendon is held in position over the greater tuberosity while it is sutured along its medial edge to the remaining cuff tendons and then to the subscapularis as well (Fig. 4, *D*). Finally, the sutures in the lateral edge of the tendon are transferred through the greater tuberosity with use of the loops of the previously placed suture.

Because the latissimus tendon is thin and I have noted late rupture of the graft in 20% to 30% of cases, the tendon is now routinely augmented with autogenous fascia lata (Fig. 5, *A*). A 2 × 4-cm strip of iliotibial band is harvested from the ipsilateral thigh and sewn over the tendon in order to reinforce it (Fig. 5, *B*).

Postoperative care is very important following this transfer. For the first 6 weeks, the patient continually wears an abduction brace that maintains the arm in 45° of abduction and 30° of external rotation in order to allow the tendon to heal without tension. Throughout this period, a therapist performs passive motion with the arm in abduction and external rotation, but internal rotation and adduction are not permitted. This motion ensures that the tendon graft does not adhere to the surrounding soft tissue and that the glenohumeral joint does not become stiff. After 6 weeks, the brace is removed and the patient is encouraged to perform activities of daily living.

The patient is then taught to initiate and maintain active contraction of the latissimus dorsi during flexion and external rotation of the arm. This is not the normal phase of activity for this musculotendinous unit, so a concerted effort must be made to retrain the muscle. This is achieved in two ways. With the first method, the arm is positioned in the midrange of abduction and the patient is asked to adduct the shoulder toward the midline, which causes the latissimus dorsi to contract. As the latissimus dorsi contracts, the arm is guided into flexion and the patient is coached to maintain this contraction in order to facilitate flexion. Gradually, the patient acquires the ability to maintain contraction of the latissimus dorsi. Similarly, the patient is asked to maintain contraction as the arm is moved into external rotation.

The second method for retraining the latissimus dorsi is with use of biofeedback. A small biofeedback unit with cutaneous electrode pads is applied over the muscle belly of the latissimus dorsi. This unit provides audible feedback (a higher pitch indicates more muscle activity) and visual feedback (red to green indicates more muscle activity). The patient tries to maintain contraction of the latissimus dorsi during flexion and external rotation and is gradually able to do so through biofeedback. Overall, it may take between 6 and 12 months for complete training of the transferred muscle.

Results Gerber and associates[9] originally reported good-to-excellent short-term results in four patients who were followed for more than 1 year after a latissimus dorsi transfer. Gerber[29] subsequently evaluated 16 patients who had been followed for an average of 33 months after such a transfer. He reported an excellent subjective result in eight patients, a good result in five, a fair result in two, and a poor result in one. The average improvement in flexion was 53°. Aoki and associates[31] reported on 12 shoulders at an average of 36 months after a latissimus dorsi transfer. The subjective improvement was rated as excellent in four shoulders, good in four, fair in one, and poor in three. The average improvement in flexion was 36°. Miniaci and MacLeod[30] reported on 17 patients who had undergone a latissimus dorsi transfer for revision of a failed rotator cuff repair. At an average of 51 months postoperatively, 14 of the 17 patients had marked relief of pain and increased function. My experience has been more varied. Of 407 rotator cuff repairs performed by my colleagues and myself over 6 years, 22 were latissimus dorsi tendon transfers (unpublished data). Of these 22 transfers, 6 were done to reconstruct an irreparable rotator cuff tear that had not been treated with prior surgery and 16 were performed after failure of a prior repair of a rotator cuff tear. When the results were analyzed according to these two groups, the outcomes were quite different. Of the 16 patients who had had a revision, only 8 reported a satisfactory outcome, and the average gain in flexion was 44°. Negative prognostic factors included a prior deltoid injury, associated stiffness, and poor tendon quality of the remaining rotator cuff. In contrast, a satisfactory outcome was achieved in five of the six patients who had had the latissimus dorsi transfer as a primary procedure, and the average gain in flexion was 60°. Late rupture of the transferred tendon was thought to have occurred in about 20% to 30% of the patients on the basis of the inability of the examiner to palpate contraction of the muscle and on the basis of a decrease in shoulder function. While others have not reported this problem, to my knowledge, I believe that it was due to the relatively small size of the latissimus tendon and the good early results in some patients, which led to increased activity before adequate healing was obtained. This has led me to augment these tendon transfers with autogenous iliotibial band. In the past year, four such procedures have been performed, and none have led to a late rupture at the time of this writing.

Summary

The inability to repair a rotator cuff tear is not uncommon, and in practices devoted to the management of shoulder injuries up to 30% of rotator cuff tears may be irreparable. The anterior and posterior components of the rotator cuff are the most important deficient areas. In the case of an irreparable subscapularis tendon tear, pain relief and stability appear to be reliably achieved by a split pectoralis major transfer; however, functional improvement is less certain because the biomechanics associated with this tendon transfer do not appear to be optimal. In the case of an irreparable posterosuperior rotator cuff tear, a latissimus dorsi tendon transfer reliably restores flexion and relieves pain; however, its use after failure of prior rotator cuff surgery makes the outcome less predictable. Both anterior and posterior reconstructions with tendon transfer require precise surgical technique and patient compliance with postoperative rehabilitation.

References

1. Rokito AS, Cuomo F, Gallagher MA, Zuckerman JD: Long-term functional outcome of repair of large and massive chronic tears of the rotator cuff. *J Bone Joint Surg Am* 1999;81:991–997.
2. Bigliani LU, Cordasco FA, McIlveen SJ, Musso ES: Operative repairs of massive rotator cuff tears: Long-term results. *J Shoulder Elbow Surg* 1992;1:120–130.
3. Cofield RH: Rotator cuff disease of the shoulder. *J Bone Joint Surg Am* 1985;67:974–979.
4. Warner JJP, Gerber C: Treatment of massive rotator cuff tears: Posterior-superior and anterior-superior, in Iannotti JP (ed): *The Rotator Cuff: Current Concepts and Complex Problems*. Rosemont, IL, American Academy of Orthopaedic Surgeons, 1998, pp 59–94.
5. Neer CS II (ed): *Shoulder Reconstruction*. Philadelphia, PA, WB Saunders, 1990, pp 41–142.
6. Ellman H, Hanker G, Bayer M: Repair of the rotator cuff: End result study of factors influencing reconstruction. *J Bone Joint Surg Am* 1986;68:1136–1144.

7. Harryman DT II, Mack LA, Wang KY, Jackins SE, Richardson ML, Matsen FA III: Repairs of the rotator cuff: Correlation of functional results with integrity of the cuff. *J Bone Joint Surg Am* 1991;73:982–989.
8. Gazielly DF, Gleyze P, Montagnon C: Functional and anatomical results after rotator cuff repair. *Clin Orthop* 1994;304:43–53.
9. Gerber C, Vinh TS, Hertel R, Hess CW: Latissimus dorsi transfer for the treatment of massive tears of the rotator cuff: A preliminary report. *Clin Orthop* 1988;232:51–61.
10. Rockwood CA Jr, Williams GR Jr, Burkhead WZ Jr: Debridement of degenerative, irreparable lesions of the rotator cuff. *J Bone Joint Surg Am* 1995;77:857–866.
11. Apoil A, Dautry P, Moinet P, Koechlin P: The syndrome "rupture of the cap of the rotations of the scapula:" A propos of 70 cases. *Rev Chir Orthop Reparatrice Appar Mot* 1977:63(suppl 2): 145–149.
12. Burkhart SS: Arthroscopic debridement and decompression for selected rotator cuff tears. Clinical results, pathomechanics, and patient selection based on biomechanical parameters. *Orthop Clin North Am* 1993;24:111–123.
13. Melillo AS, Savoie FH III, Field LD: Massive rotator cuff tears: Debridement versus repair. *Orthop Clin North Am* 1997;28:117–124.
14. Neviaser JS, Neviaser RJ, Neviaser TJ: The repair of chronic massive ruptures of the rotator cuff of the shoulder by use of freeze-dried rotator cuff. *J Bone Joint Surg Am* 1978;60:681–684.
15. Ozaki J, Fujimoto S, Masuhara K, Tamai S, Yoshimoto S: Reconstruction of chronic massive rotator cuff tears with synthetic materials. *Clin Orthop* 1986;202:173–183.
16. Cofield RH: Subscapular muscle transposition for repair of chronic rotator cuff tears. *Surg Gynecol Obstet* 1982;154:667–672.
17. Debeyre J, Patte D, Elmelik E: Repairs of ruptures of the rotator cuff of the shoulder: With a note on advancement of the supraspinatus muscle. *J Bone Joint Surg Br* 1965;47:36–42.
18. Neviaser RJ, Neviaser TJ: Transfer of subscapularis and teres minor for massive defects of the rotator cuff, in Bayley I, Kessel L (eds): *Shoulder Surgery*. Berlin, Germany, Springer-Verlag, 1982, pp 60–63.
19. Apoil A, Augereau B: Deltoid flap repair of large losses of substance of the shoulder rotator cuff. *Chirurgie* 1985;111:287–290.
20. Dierickx C, Vanhoof H: Massive rotator cuff tears treated by a deltoid muscular inlay flap. *Acta Orthop Belg* 1994:60:94–100.
21. Gazielly DF: Deltoid muscular flap transfer for massive defects of the rotator cuff, in Burkhead WZ Jr (ed): *Rotator Cuff Disorders*. Baltimore, MD, Williams & Wilkins, 1996, pp 356–367.
22. L'Episcopo JB: Tendon transplantation in obstetrical paralysis. *Am J Surg* 1934; 25:122–125.
23. Covey DC, Riordan DC, Milstead ME, Albright JA: Modification of the L'Episcopo procedure for brachial plexus birth palsies. *J Bone Joint Surg Br* 1992;74:897–901.
24. Hoffer MM, Wickenden R, Roper B: Brachial plexus birth palsies: Results of tendon transfers to the rotator cuff. *J Bone Joint Surg Am* 1978;60:691–695.
25. Phipps GJ, Hoffer MM: Latissimus dorsi and teres major transfer to rotator cuff for Erb's palsy. *J Shoulder Elbow Surg* 1995;4:124–129.
26. Mikasa M: Trapezius transfer for global tear of the rotator cuff, in Bateman JE, Welsh RP (eds): *Surgery of the Shoulder*. Philadelphia, PA, BC Decker, 1984, pp 196–199.
27. Combes JM, Mansat M: Lambeau de muscle grand rond dans les ruptures massives de la coiffe des rotateurs: Etude experimentale, in Bonnel F, Blotman F, Mansat M (eds*): L'epaule: L'epaule Degenerative, l'epaule Traumatique, l'epaule du Sportif*. Paris, France, Springer, 1993, pp 318–330.
28. Wang AA, Strauch RJ, Flatow EL, Bigliani LU, Rosenwasser MP: The teres major muscle: An anatomic study of its use as a tendon transfer *J Shoulder Elbow Surg* 1999; 8:334–338.
29. Gerber C: Latissimus dorsi transfer for the treatment of irreparable tears of the rotator cuff. *Clin Orthop* 1992;275:152–160.
30. Miniaci A, MacLeod M: Transfer of the latissimus dorsi muscle after failed repair of a massive tear of the rotator cuff: A two to five-year review. *J Bone Joint Surg Am* 1999:81:1120–1127.
31. Aoki M, Okamura K, Fukushima S, Takahashi T, Ogino T: Transfer of latissimus dorsi for irreparable rotator-cuff tears. *J Bone Joint Surg Br* 1996;78:761–766.
32. Wirth MA, Rockwood CA Jr: Operative treatment of irreparable rupture of the subscapularis. *J Bone Joint Surg Am* 1997:79:722–731.
33. Gerber C, Krushell RJ: Isolated rupture of the tendon of the subscapularis muscle: Clinical features in 16 cases. *J Bone Joint Surg Br* 1991;73:389–394.
34. Gerber C, Hersche O, Farron A: Isolated rupture of the subscapularis tendon. *J Bone Joint Surg Am* 1996;78:1015–1023.
35. McMahon PJ, Debski RE, Thompson WO, Warner JJ, Fu FH, Woo SL: Shoulder muscle forces and tendon excursions during glenohumeral abduction in the scapular plane. *J Shoulder Elbow Surg* 1995;4:199–208.
36. Thompson WO, Debski RE, Boardman ND III, at al: A biomechanical analysis of rotator cuff deficiency in a cadaveric model. *Am J Sports Med* 1996;24:286–292.
37. Burkhart SS: Reconciling the paradox of rotator cuff repair versus debridement: A unified biomechanical rationale for the treatment of rotator cuff tears. *Arthroscopy* 1994;10:4–19.
38. DePalma AF, Cooke AJ, Prabhakar M: The role of the subscapularis in recurrent anterior dislocations of the shoulder. *Clin Orthop* 1967;54:35–49.
39. Neviaser RJ, Neviaser TJ, Neviaser JS: Concurrent rupture of the rotator cuff and anterior dislocation of the shoulder in the older patient. *J Bone Joint Surg Am* 1988;70:1308–1311.
40. Turkel SJ, Panio MW, Marshall JL, Girgis FG: Stabilizing mechanisms preventing anterior dislocation of the glenohumeral joint. *J Bone Joint Surg Am* 1981;63:1208–1217.
41. Keating JF, Waterworth P, Shaw-Dunn J, Crossan J: The relative strengths of the rotator cuff muscles: A cadaver study. *J Bone Joint Surg Br* 1993;75:137–140.
42. Bassett RW, Browne AO, Morrey BF, An KN: Glenohumeral muscle force and moment mechanics in a position of shoulder instability. *J Biomech* 1990;23:405–415.
43. Bernageau J: Roentgenographic assessment of the rotator cuff. *Clin Orthop* 1990;254:87–91.
44. LeClerq R: Diagnostic de la rupture du sous-epineoux. *Rev Rheum* 1950;10:510–515.
45. Weiner DS, Macnab I: Superior migration of the humeral head: A radiological aid in the diagnosis of tears of the rotator cuff. *J Bone Joint Surg Br* 1970;52:524–527.
46. Itoi E, Kuechle DK, Newman SR, Morrey BF, An KN: Stabilising function of the biceps in stable and unstable shoulders. *J Bone Joint Surg Br* 1993;75:546–550.
47. Kumar VP, Satku K, Balasubramaniam P: The role of the long head of biceps brachii in the stabilization of the head of the humerus. *Clin Orthop* 1989:244:172–175.
48. Warner JJ, McMahon PJ: The role of the long head of the biceps brachii in superior stability of the glenohumeral joint. *J Bone Joint Surg Am* 1995;77:366–372.
49. Yamaguchi K, Riew KD, Galatz LM, Syme JA, Neviaser RJ: Biceps activity during shoulder motion: An electromyographic analysis. *Clin Orthop* 1997;336:122–129.
50. Walch G, Boileau P, Noel E, Liotard JP, Dejour H: Surgical treatment of painful shoulders caused by lesions of the rotator cuff and biceps, treatment as a function of lesions: Reflections on the Neer's concept. *Rev Rhum Mal Osteoartic* 1991;58:247–257.
51. Goutallier D, Postel JM, Bernageau J, Lavau L, Voisin MC: Fatty muscle degeneration in cuff ruptures: Pre- and postoperative evaluation by CT scan. *Clin Orthop* 1994;304:78–83.
52. Arntz CT, Matsen FA III, Jackins S: Surgical management of complex irreparable rotator cuff deficiency. *J Arthroplasty* 1991;6:363–370.
53. Flatow EL, Raimondo RA, Kelkar R, et al: Abstract: Active and passive restraints against superior humeral translation: The contribution of the rotator cuff, the biceps tendon and the coracoacromial arch. *Orthop Trans* 1996:20:121.
54. Hersche O, Gerber C: Passive tension in the supraspinatus musculotendinous unit after long-standing rupture of its tendon: A preliminary report. *J Shoulder Elbow Surg* 1998;7:393–396.
55. Gerber C, Hersche O: Tendon transfers for the treatment of irreparable rotator cuff defects. *Orthop Clin North Am* 1997;28:195–203.

10
SYMPOSIUM

Total Shoulder Arthroplasty in the Young Patient

Patrick R.L. Hayes, MD
Evan L. Flatow, MD

Introduction

Neer ushered in the era of modern shoulder arthroplasty in 1953, reporting on his first anatomic humeral head prosthesis.[1] In 1955 he described using his redesigned vitallium, anatomic humeral head prosthesis (the Neer I) in patients with four-part fractures, fracture-dislocations, and osteonecrosis (ON).[2,3] He then expanded the indications for humeral head replacement to include degenerative glenohumeral arthritis.[4] In the 1970s several authors reported on the implantation of a polyethylene glenoid component with which the humeral prosthesis articulated.[4-7] The Neer II prostheses was designed to articulate with any of Neer's glenoid components.[4] Since then, many other shoulder prostheses have been developed. To date the most reliable long-term results in shoulder arthroplasty with respect to pain relief, restoration of function, and longevity of the prosthesis appear to occur with unconstrained prostheses of anatomic design.[4,8-19]

As success with shoulder arthroplasty has grown and orthopaedists have become more familiar and adept with the technique, the indications for shoulder arthroplasty have expanded. In young patients with severe proximal humerus fractures; ON; posttraumatic, inflammatory, and degenerative arthritides; humeral replacement and total shoulder arthroplasty remain viable options.[20-23] It is critical, however, to remember the limits of the technique, to remain clear on the indications and contraindications, and to accurately educate patients on the risks, benefits, alternatives, and expected outcomes of shoulder arthroplasty in the young patient.

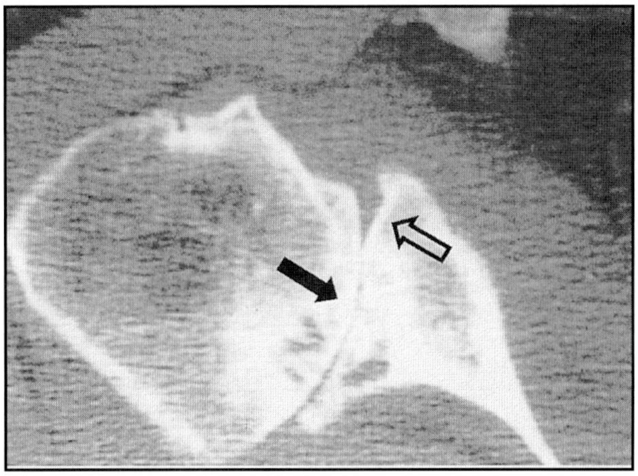

Fig. 1 CT scan showing eccentric posterior glenoid wear in this patient with OA. Version is easily seen on CT. The hollow arrow shows native glenoid contour; the solid arrow shows posterior eroded contour.

Alternatives

Shoulder arthroplasty remains the optimal procedure for pain relief and restoration of function in most shoulders with severe articular disease.[20-23] In more moderate cases the pathology may not warrant such definitive intervention, and in some settings prosthetic replacement is contraindicated. It is important to be familiar with conservative and other surgical options in treating glenohumeral pathology.[24]

Etiology of the arthritis plays an important part in a patient's natural history and prognosis after arthroplasty. The shoulder joint is an uncommon site of primary osteoarthritis (OA). Radiographic signs of OA in the shoulder include large inferior osteophytes, sclerosis, subchondral cysts, and posterior erosion of the glenoid (Fig. 1). An OA presentation in young patients often is the result of trauma[24] or of prior instability repairs. Humeral trauma or surgery that alters shoulder biomechanics and results in humeral roughness or eccentric loading of the glenoid eventually can progress to glenoid degeneration.[22,23,25] Radiographic findings do not necessarily correlate with symptoms.

In rheumatoid arthritis (RA), the glenohumeral joint is commonly involved

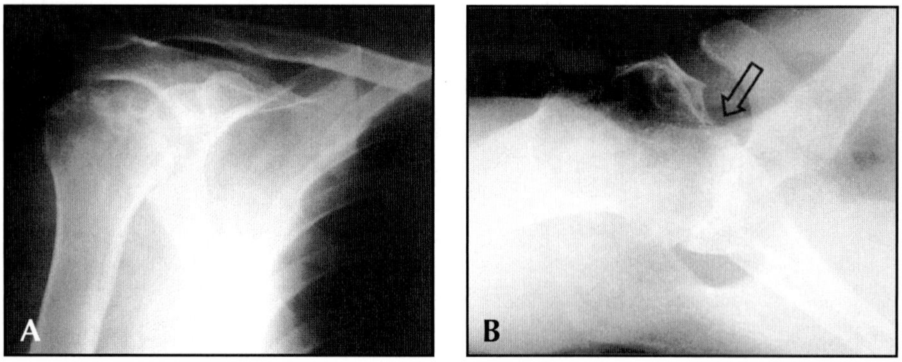

Fig. 2 Radiographs from a patient with glenohumeral RA. **A,** AP view. Note the subchondral erosions, relative osteopenia, and absence of osteophytes. **B,** Axillary view. Note central glenoid erosion, relative osteopenia, periarticular erosions, and lack of osteophytes. The arrow points to anterior periarticular erosion.

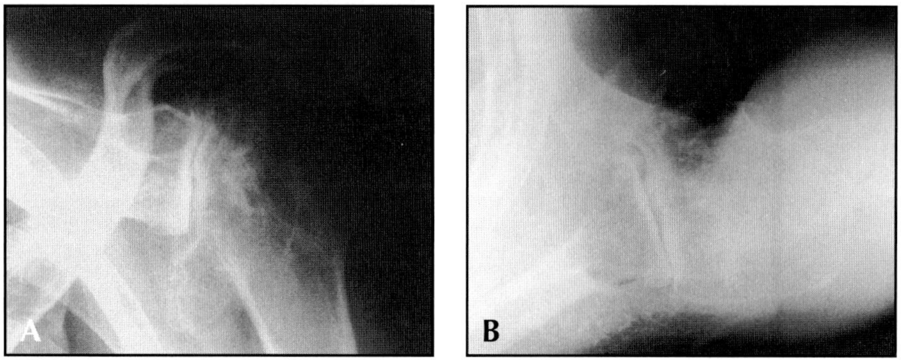

Fig. 3 Radiograph from a patient with Cruess stage V idiopathic ON. **A,** AP view. Note joint space narrowing, huge inferior humeral osteophyte, and humeral head collapse. The dotted line marks the native cortex and underscores the size of the humeral osteophyte. **B,** Axillary view. Flattened humeral head caused like changes on the glenoid.

and is usually part of a polyarthropathy[26] (Fig. 2). Symptomatic RA of the shoulder typically occurs in women between 35 and 55 years of age who have positive rheumatoid factor.[24] Loss of motion, fatigue, and muscle weakness occur. Rotator cuff tears occur in approximately 25% of these patients.[24]

ON can occur in patients with trauma, steroid use, alcoholism, sickle-cell disease, hemophilia, a history of decompression sickness, lipid storage diseases, or lupus erythematosus.[23,27,28] Often the cause is unknown. Disease progression was staged by Cruess as follows: preradiographic stage (I), humeral head involvement (II), subchondral humeral head fracture (crescent sign, III), humeral head collapse (IV), and glenoid involvement (V) (Fig. 3). The later stages of ON are typically more symptomatic, are more likely to progress, and most often require prosthetic replacement.[27]

Degenerative glenohumeral arthritis can occur after stabilization surgery for instability.[29,30] This arthritis may result from postsurgical, iatrogenic subluxations; persistent multidirectional instability; inadequate or inappropriate surgery; or as a complication of hardware, and it is often multifactorial in nature[30] (Fig. 4). In Bigliani and associates' series,[29] symptomatic arthritis came to prosthetic replacement an average of 16 years after the initial stabilization procedure.

Nonsurgical Treatment

Patient education about natural history and prognosis can ensure that the patients understand what to expect and how they can influence their disease process. Understanding what is in store allows them to make realistic job and recreational choices, participate in strength and motion preserving exercises, and avoid detrimental activities.

Physical therapy can especially benefit patients who are stiff and weak prior to the onset of end-stage arthritis. Motion and strength can be restored or at least maintained. End-stage arthritis with stiffness secondary to joint incongruity actually may be exacerbated with aggressive stretching exercises. Preferential strengthening of muscles that specifically resist instability may be beneficial in patients with a component of instability.[31] Cold therapy is useful in reducing inflammation and calming down shoulders after stretching and strengthening. Heat can help alleviate chronic pain and facilitate gaining joint motion. Ultrasound works to increase tissue temperature and blood flow to a depth of 5 cm.[24,32] Occupational therapy can provide strategies and assistive devices to patients with glenohumeral arthritis who struggle with daily functional limitations.

Local anesthetic injections can be valuable in determining the pain generators about a painful shoulder.[33-35] Steroid injections can efficaciously alleviate symptoms in the shoulder with RA, although the value of steroid injections is less clear in OA.[24,36,37] Nonsteroidal anti-inflammatory drugs (NSAIDs) also can be very effective in treating inflammatory glenohumeral arthritis. In OA it is not clear that NSAIDs are any better than acetaminophen.[38]

Surgical Alternatives

Arthroscopic débridement for degenerative arthritis of the knee has been used with reasonable success in the appropriate setting.[39] The indications for débridement of degenerative arthritis of the glenohumeral joint are not as clear. Often degenerative lesions of the glenohumeral joint are found incidentally during diagnostic arthroscopy.[40,41]

Results of arthroscopic débridement appear to depend on the extent of the degenerative changes found.[42] One series looked at arthroscopic débridement of OA of the shoulder in 54 patients with 3 years' follow-up. If mild changes were present, two thirds did well; if severe changes were seen, only one third were doing well at follow-up. Those who had débridement of degenerative labral tears did well.

Abrasion arthroplasty has been suggested in the shoulder, but its benefit remains to be proven.[24,43] In ON, abrasion of small lesions on the humeral head with removal of loose bodies may be helpful.[44] In a study by Weinstein and associates,[45] 27 patients were followed for an average of 30 months after arthroscopic débridement of degenerative arthritis of the shoulder. Loose bodies were removed, degenerative labral tissue and cartilage were débrided, and subacromial bursectomy was performed. Patients experienced significant gains in function and pain relief, with 78% satisfactory results. The authors concluded that arthroscopic débridement is a useful procedure in patients with mild glenohumeral OA. The addition of bursectomy in this series may have increased the success compared with results seen in other series.[24]

The efficacy of subacromial decompression (SAD) in the presence of glenohumeral arthritis has been established by two other series. Simpson and Kelley[46] performed SAD, bursectomy, and glenohumeral débridement in 24 patients with RA and advanced glenohumeral involvement. Nineteen of 22 patients at 30-months follow-up had good pain relief and significantly improved range of motion. Ellowitz and associates[47] looked at 21 patients who had OA with grade IV chondral changes in the glenohumeral joint. They performed SAD and reported uniformly good results. Given these results, Skedros and associates[24] could not recommend glenohumeral débridement as an isolated procedure in glenohumeral arthritis, and urged consideration of SAD and bursectomy as part of the débridement.

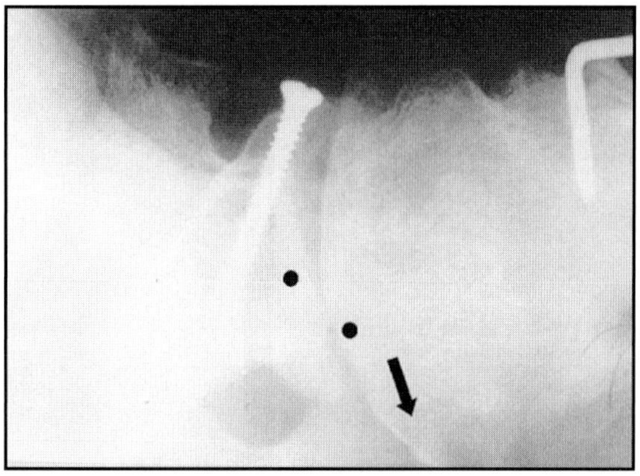

Fig. 4 Axillary view from a 32-year-old patient with painful arthritis of the glenohumeral joint following multiple procedures for instability, including a coracoid transfer and a Putti-Platt procedure, performed approximately 10 years earlier. Dots show the center of the glenoid and the humerus. The arrow underscores the fixed posterior subluxation that contributed to the arthrosis.

Capsular release has a role in the stiff, painful shoulder with mild arthritic changes. Hawkins and Angelo[48] reported arthritis in 10 patients who had previously undergone Putti-Platt capsulorrhaphies for anterior instability. Four patients were taken to surgery, all received open capsular releases to restore external rotation, and two received humeral head replacements. Ogilvie-Harris and Wiley[42] arthroscopically débrided 14 frozen shoulders with associated OA. If more than 20° of motion were lost, an arthroscopic capsular release was performed. Brems[30] reviewed arthritis of dislocation and found a large number of patients who developed arthritis in the setting of instability had had previous reconstructive procedures. Common factors contributing to the development of arthritis included failure to diagnose direction or degree of instability, inadequate or nonanatomic surgical reconstruction, prominent hardware, surgery on the wrong side of the joint, and inappropriate use of arthroscopic techniques. Brems[30] advocated soft-tissue rebalancing and prosthetic replacement in these patients if the cartilage surfaces were destroyed. Ideally, humeral head replacement without glenoid resurfacing could be performed if the surgery was performed before severe glenoid involvement.

Surgical synovectomy can give good local pain relief and improve motion in inflammatory arthropathies about the shoulder.[24] The synovectomy can be performed arthroscopically.[49] Done early in the disease process, it can slow disease progression. The procedure may have to be repeated in tenacious inflammatory arthropathies. The best overall symptomatic relief is obtained when the shoulder is the most symptomatic of the joints involved. It was found on 6-year follow-up of open shoulder synovectomies, that 75% of late stage RA patients were satisfied, 70% had improvements in swelling and motion, and 50% had lasting reduction in pain.[24]

Addressing comorbidities in mild or moderate arthritis can give significant relief and buy time before glenohumeral replacement, if the comorbidities are the dominant pain generators. Diagnostic injections can help identify portions of pain from symptomatic acromiocalvicular joints or subacromial bursae. According to Pollock,[50] cuff repair and humeral head replacement is the treatment of choice in severely painful shoulders with RA that have rotator cuff tears. If the cuff appears

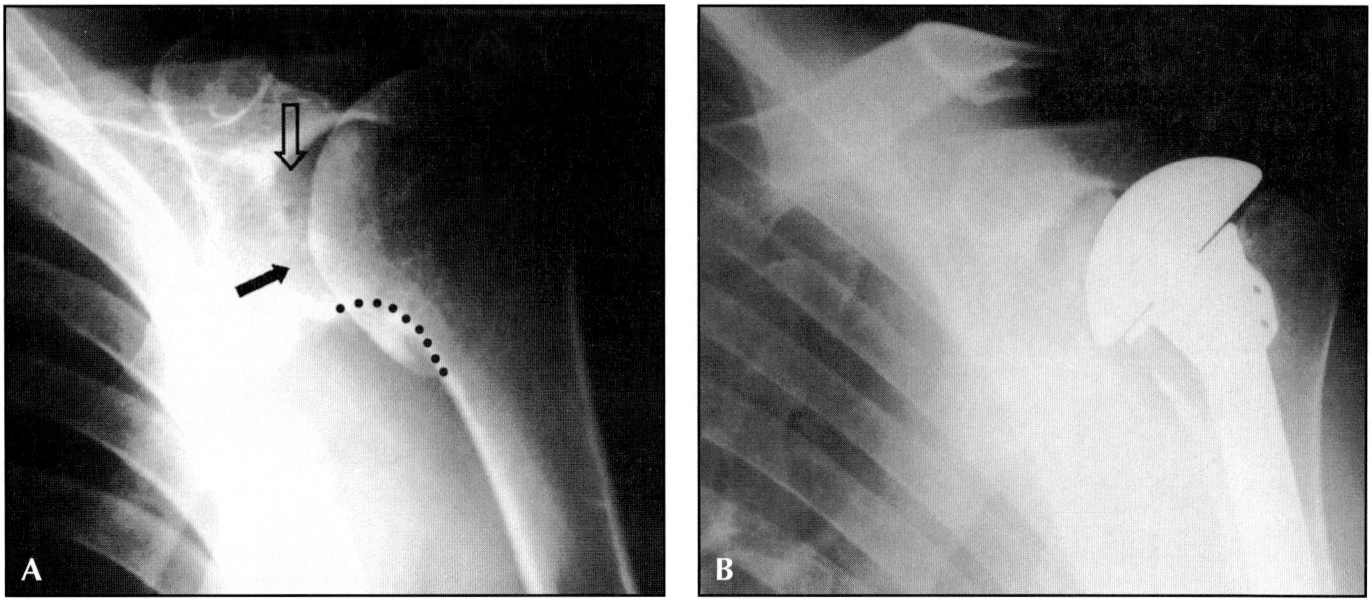

Fig. 5 Radiograph from a 35-year-old patient with painful glenohumeral arthritis and stiffness after multiple instability reconstructions performed during his late teens and early 20s. **A**, Dotted line outlines native cortex and shows size of inferior osteophyte. The solid arrow points to change in contour of humeral head from flattening; the hollow arrow points to nonmetallic anchor hole from prior repair for instability. **B**, AP view of hemiarthroplasty with biologic resurfacing of glenoid with reflected capsule.

to be dysfunctional and unable to center the glenoid even after repair, the glenoid should not be replaced.[51,52] Skedros and associates[24] recommended cuff repair without replacement in symptomatic tears if the arthritis is minor.

Benjamin and associates[53,54] described periarticular osteotomies for symptomatic treatment of glenohumeral arthritis. This is rarely done in the United States. The theory is that the osteotomies reduce subchondral venous congestion and bring new blood flow to the area with healing. The procedure has not been reported by other surgeons in peer reviewed journals.[24]

Osteotomies through the humerus have been described to correct abnormal glenohumeral biomechanics and reduce instability.[55] Theoretically this may prevent development of arthritis from fixed or recurrent instability. As pointed out by Brems,[30] most arthritis in the setting of instability usually occurs as the result of an unbalanced joint after previous surgery attempting to address the instability.[30] Glenoid osteotomies have been suggested to reduce increased glenoid retroversion and posterior instability.[56,57] In a patient with marked glenoid retroversion and instability, a scapular neck osteotomy may correct the abnormal biomechanics and avoid posterior glenoid wear. True glenoid hypoplasia is uncommon, and only a small percentage of these patients develop degenerative arthritis. If this arthritis occurs, most patients can be managed with a program of physical therapy.[58] If bone stock is inadequate, glenoid replacement should not be performed.

Most surgeons are reluctant to offer prosthetic replacement to young, active, high-demand patients, for fear of loosening and eventual failure. Alternative techniques have been developed which débride, resect, reshape, or fuse the articular surfaces. Humeral head resection results in significant loss of strength and motion because the fulcrum for the shoulder is lost.[23] In the era of arthroplasty, fusion is reserved for salvage efforts. Indications may include combined deltoid and rotator cuff dysfunction, irreparable rotator cuff tears with painful cuff tear arthropathy, paralytic disorders in infancy, joint destroying infections, failed arthroplasty, recurrent dislocations uncontrolled by other procedures, painful arthritis in patients who require power but not motion, and resections after tumors.[59] Fusion significantly limits the ability to place the hand in space and often transfers the stresses and pain to the periscapular muscles.

Interposition arthroplasty has been reported on both sides of the joint. The techniques described include reducing in size, then resurfacing the humeral head with a biologic membrane, and smoothing or flattening the glenoid and covering it with biologic tissue as well. The main indication appears to be in the young patient with end-stage RA who has an intact rotator cuff and is capable of following the postoperative regimen. Loss of cuff integrity and large destructive cysts in the humeral head are contraindica-

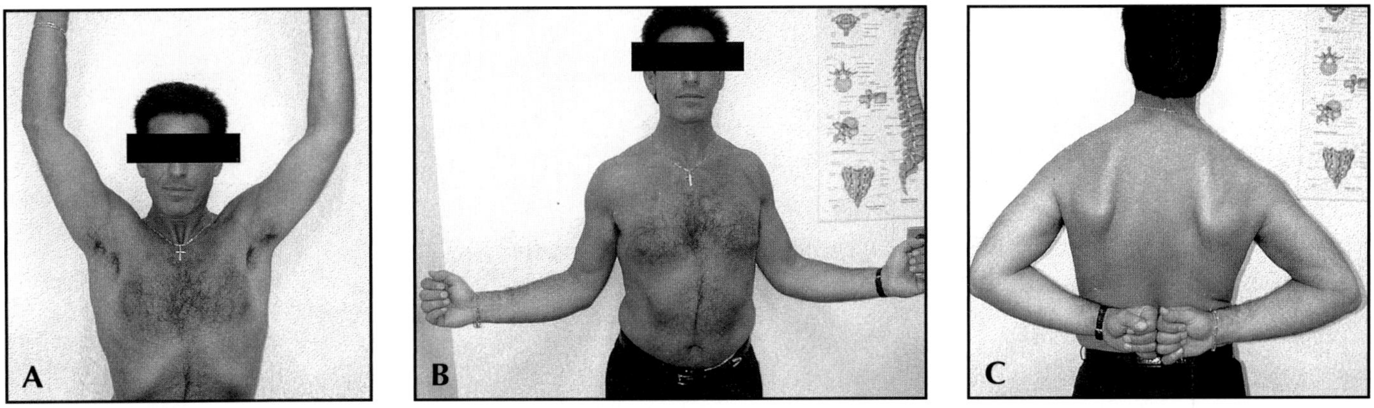

Fig. 6 Photographs of a patient who had infectious arthritis 1 year after left humeral head replacement with fascial arthroplasty. **A**, Maximum forward flexion compared with the normal side. **B**, Maximum external rotation. **C**, Maximum internal rotation. The patient is able to play golf and lift light weights.

tions. Burkhead and Hutton[60] reported on early results of biologic resurfacing of the glenoid with humeral head replacement in the young patient with glenohumeral arthritis. Excellent results were obtained in five of six patients at a minimum of 2 years' follow-up, with excellent pain relief and significant gains in motion (Figs. 5 and 6).

Indications and Contraindications

Shoulder arthroplasty is performed in many young patients with painful conditions of the glenohumeral joint, whose symptoms are refractory to conservative measures and less definitive procedures. The most common diagnoses in the young shoulder arthroplasty patient include trauma, posttraumatic arthritis, arthritis after reconstruction of instability, inflammatory arthritis, and ON of the humeral head.

Humeral head replacement (HHR) is offered to patients with severe pain and dysfunction of the shoulder resulting from destruction of the humeral head. HHRs work best in patients with functioning deltoid and rotator cuff muscles and a balanced soft-tissue envelope that centers the humeral head on the glenoid.[50-52] Soft tissues may have to be balanced or repaired, and the glenoid may have to be smoothed at surgery to achieve this.[23] In Levine and associates' series,[61] HHRs were most successful in the patients with OA who had concentric glenoid wear. Poorer results, with less forward elevation and external rotation, were seen in patients with increased posterior wear and were attributed to a less stable fulcrum for the humeral head. Rodosky and Bigliani[62] believed that patients with OA and eccentric glenoid wear do better with glenoid resurfacing. This belief is a relative indication to be weighed against the relative contraindication of resurfacing a glenoid in a young person.

HHR may be offered in the setting of prior infection (Fig. 7). The infection must have been quiescent for over 12 months, with laboratory tests and cultures negative for signs of active infection. Smith and Matsen[63] recommend a noncemented HHR. The glenoid is not replaced, and the patient is warned the humeral component will have to be removed if the infection recurs.

Nerve or muscle damage causing muscle imbalance and subluxation of the glenohumeral joint is another contraindication to glenoid replacement. Severe rotator cuff dysfunction can allow superior migration of the humerus and eccentric loading of the glenoid component, which increases the risk of early glenoid loosening,[64] the so-called "rocking horse" glenoid. Deltoid dysfunction could cause fixed inferior subluxation or dislocation of the humeral prosthesis.

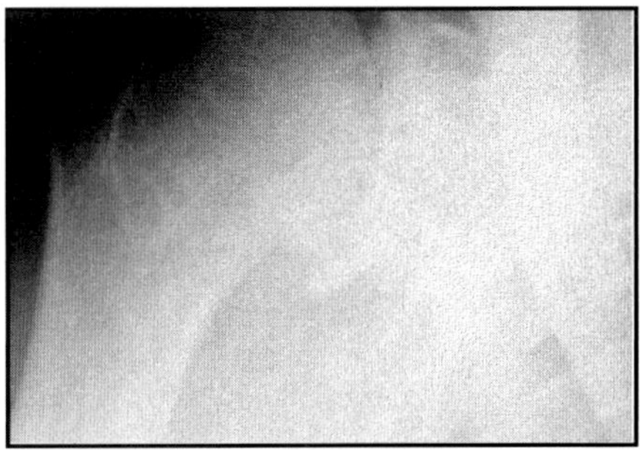

Fig. 7 AP view of postinfectious arthritis in a patient with prior hematogenous *Staphylococcus* infection. Note the erosive appearance and absence of osteophytes.

Caution is warranted in neuropathic arthropathy of the shoulder.[65] Central lesions such as syringomyelia and metabolic processes such as diabetes and chronic alcoholism can cause neuropathic arthropathy. The same lack of sensation that led to the joint destruction can loosen any prosthesis that is inserted. The neuropathy may progress and cause loss of rotator cuff or deltoid function. Arthroplasty is not recommended.

Glenoid replacement generally is avoided in the young, active patient for fear of loosening. In a series of patients

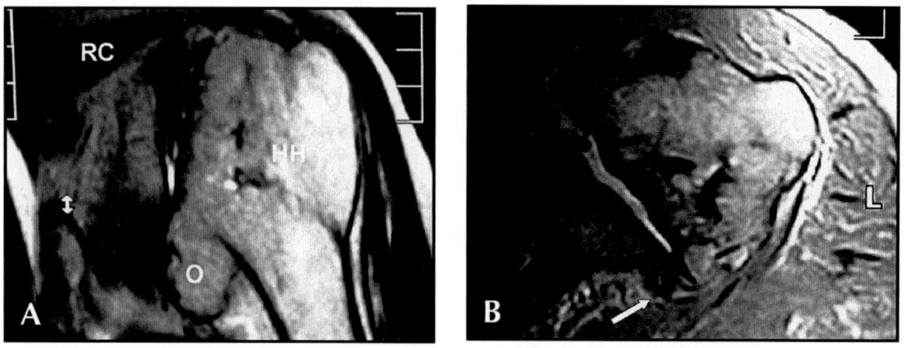

Fig. 8 A, Sagittal oblique MRI study of the patient in Figure 3. RC = rotator cuff, HH = humeral head, O = osteophyte. Cuff looks intact but thinned. **B,** Axial MRI study. Note how clear version is on this image. The arrow points to a posterior osteophyte that overhangs the posterior glenoid, which made dislocation of the glenohumeral joint impossible without extensive releases.

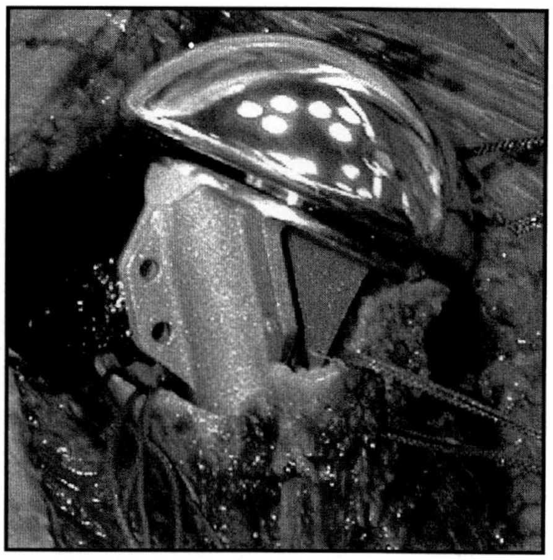

Fig. 9 HHR in a four-part fracture. Sutures are used to reattach tuberosities. Cement is always used to afford rotational stability. The stem may need to be cemented superior to the shaft fracture to obtain appropriate tension in myofascial sleeve.

younger than 50 years of age,[66] complete radiolucent lines around the glenoid were seen in 59% of 34 total shoulder arthroplasties (TSAs) at a mean follow-up of 12.3 years. Torchia and associates[19] reported the presence of radiolucent lines at the bone-cement interface of glenoid components in 84% of their patients followed an average of 12 years. By radiographic signs, 44% were definitely loose, and looseness was associated with pain. Biologic resurfacing should be considered if glenoid involvement is present in the young patient (Fig. 5). Revising a loose glenoid is technically demanding and may not be possible because of bone loss (2 of 9 in a small series).[67] Recurrent loosening after revision can occur (two of seven). Given these data, we recommend attempting humeral replacement and biologic resurfacing in the young, active patient with destruction on both sides of the joint (Fig. 6).

If the nonreplaced glenoid becomes symptomatic, resurfacing the glenoid can be undertaken as a later procedure with reasonable success. Sperling and Cofield[25] reported on 22 revisions of painful humeral replacements to TSAs. Revisions were performed an average of 4.4 years after their humeral replacements. Most patients had marked pain relief and increased motion after revision. This further reinforces a staged approach in the young patient, performing HHR and possibly biologic resurfacing, then addressing the glenoid later if it becomes symptomatic.

Glenoid resurfacing is avoided in patients with nonfunctioning deltoids or rotator cuffs,[23,50,51] a history of infection, inadequate bone stock to support a glenoid, very tight shoulders despite releases, and patients who cannot comply with the postoperative restrictions.

Preoperative Planning

Preoperative imaging studies are critical in planning for TSA. Standard plain films obtained include a true anteroposterior (AP) view in slight external rotation and a good quality axillary view. The AP will show superior migration suspicious for rotator cuff dysfunction. This view will also show joint space narrowing and humeral and glenoid osteophytes (Fig. 3, *A*). The axillary delineates the version of the glenoid and any rim erosions present (Fig. 3, *B*). If bony anatomy or glenoid involvement remains in question, a CT scan or MRI study can provide additional information about the glenoid (Figs. 1 and 8). MRI will show the condition of the rotator cuff. Electromyograms and nerve conduction studies may be necessary to evaluate or document preoperatively the patient's neural status.

In fracture cases, the goals of the procedure include preserving vascularity of the fracture fragments, getting the fracture to heal, and restoring appropriate tension in the soft-tissue envelope to restore function of the deltoid and rotator cuff postoperatively.[23,68,69] With significant comminution or bone loss, radiographs of the opposite, normal humerus with radiographic markers to correct for magnification may be helpful in planning where to seat the cemented humeral prosthesis. Traction radiographs or a CT scan can help define the fracture lines and the size and orientation of the fragments. Bone graft can be obtained from the discarded humeral head if this is available. Heavy suture or wire may be used to repair tuberosity fragments to each other and to the humeral stem (Fig. 9).

In tumor cases imaging studies including MRI and bone scintigraphy can delineate the extent of the tumor including skip lesions. Bulk allografts and custom prostheses may be needed; these must be planned for preoperatively.

Technique

Meticulous handling of the soft tissues is critical to successful TSA. The patient is met in the holding area before receiving anesthesia, and the surgical site and plan are confirmed. Usually, regional anesthesia is administered with interscalene block without general anesthesia. The patient is placed in the beach chair position over the edge of the table so that the extremity to be operated on can be adducted and extended in a vertical position without hitting the side of the table. Two folded towels are placed under the medial border of the scapula to support the glenoid. A headrest is used, and the head is taped in place.

The patient is prepped and draped. Bony landmarks, old scars, and the proposed incision are drawn on the skin. A medium-sized antimicrobial incise drape is placed over the surgical site, enveloping the shoulder.

The skin incision is made through dermis from superiomedial to the coracoid, crossing the coracoid, down toward the anterior aspect of the deltoid insertion on the upper arm. Needle tip electrocaudery is used to divide fat down to the fascia, which is left on the muscles. Medial and lateral skin flaps are raised to allow palpation of the anterior clavicle, the coracoid, and the insertion of the deltoid. A fatty triangle will open up at the superior edge of the deltopectoral interval. Near its insertion the deltoid will curve away from the pertoralis, opening up the interval. **(CD-10.1)**

The cephalic vein is identified and preferentially taken medially to avoid trauma to the vein during preparation of the humerus. The vein is unroofed, and any branches are cauterized or ligated. Branches reliably occur superiorly in the fat triangle near the coracoid, periodically along the lateral and deep aspects of the vein, and along the superior border of the pectoralis, right next to the deltoid tendon insertion.

Sweeping a finger in the interval further develops the deltopectoral interval. Any adhesions should be divided with electrocautery. The clavipectoral fascia is divided lateral to the strap muscle fibers lateral to the conjoined tendon. If the deltoid is still adherent, it is freed from underlying tissue as well. Bursa is resected for exposure. The axillary nerve can be located by sweeping a finger under the strap muscles, over the front of the subscapularis. The tug test[70] will reliably help identify the course of the axillary nerve in index procedures without scarring from previous trauma. The spaces under the acromion and deltoid must be fully developed. Retractors are placed under the deltoid and the strap muscles. For additional exposure, the anterior free edge of the coracoacromial ligament can be resected. The superior centimeter of the pectoralis can be divided as well. This usually is not repaired.

At this point, different surgical techniques are used to handle a variety of clinical situations. In fracture cases, technique depends on the fracture configuration. In old fractures, great care must be taken to incise scar, meticulously developing the planes described above. The axillary nerve must carefully be identified and freed from scar. The patient is not paralyzed, and electrocautery is used for the dissection. Nerve stimulation from the cautery warns the surgeon of the nerve's proximity.

With acute three- and four-part fractures,[68,69,71-73] the soft-tissue attachments to the tuberosities are preserved. The biceps is followed into the glenoid, and the rotator interval is opened. The tuberosity fragments are mobilized, preserving their cuff attachments, and the humeral head is removed. Sutures placed through the bone-tendon junction of each tuberosity piece can assist the surgeon in mobilizing these fragments from each other and enveloping adhesions. Any cartilage remaining on the tuberosities is removed. The humeral shaft is prepared for a cemented humeral stem. Version for the humeral component is selected, using the forearm as a goniometer. Less version may be selected for locked posterior dislocations. Drill holes and suture or wires are placed in the shaft before cementing the stem. Cement must be used in fracture cases to afford rotational stability because the proximal fins of the prosthesis do not engage the distal humeral shaft. The humerus is cemented above the fractured shaft the appropriate amount to restore height and soft-tissue tension (Fig. 9). If little comminution is present, the bony fragments can assist in assessing this length. Preoperative measurements and intraoperative soft-tissue tension must also be considered. The tuberosity fragments are repaired to the shaft and to the stem with wire or heavy suture. Cancellous bone may have to be removed from the tuberosities to allow them to fit around the cemented humeral stem.

In surgical neck fractures that go on to nonunions,[72] the inferior part of the humeral head often undergoes significant erosion. Prosthetic hemiarthroplasty can simultaneously bridge the nonunion and replace the eroded humeral head. An attempt can be made to approach the humeral head osteotomy through the rotator interval to preserve subscapularis insertion and blood supply to the proximal fragment. The subscapularis and capsule may have to be taken down in the usual fashion if this soft-tissue sparing approach is not successful or if releases are needed to regain motion. The subscapularis insertion can be taken with bone to facilitate healing. The prosthesis skewers the proximal humerus if there is adequate bone, preserving a ring of metaphysis proximally. Otherwise a horseshoe of metaphyseal bone is fashioned to fit around the proximal stem. The humeral prosthesis is cemented in the shaft in the correct position, with the appropriate amount of tension in the deltoid to

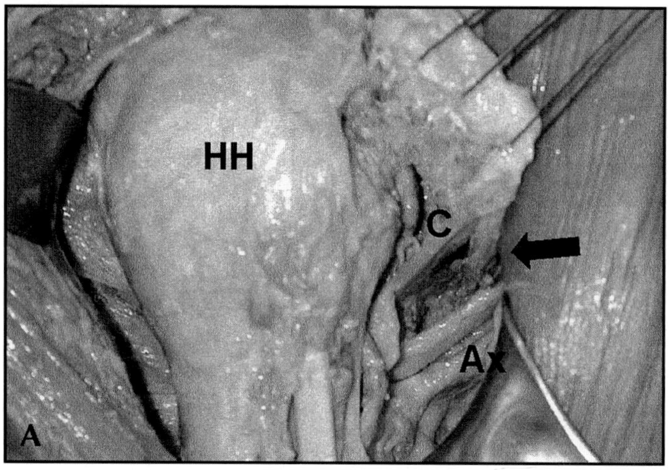

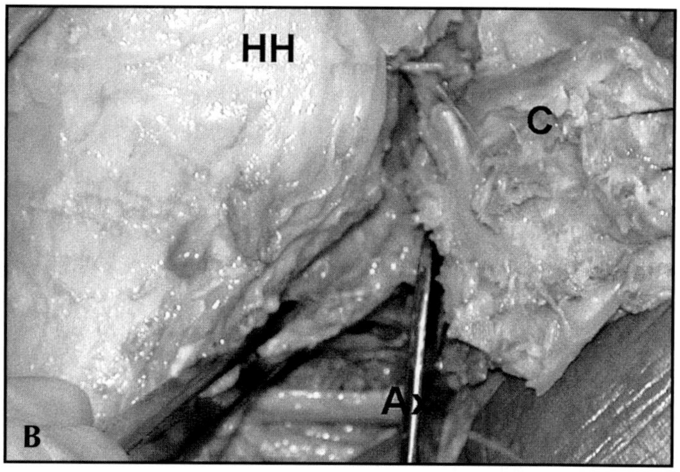

Fig. 10 A, Exposure in a cadaver after subscapularis release, just before dividing the capsule off the posterior aspect of the subscapularis. The anterior labrum can be left to deepen the socket in hemiarthroplasties. The capsule can be harvested off the subscapularis and reflected over the freshened glenoid surface for biologic resurfacing. In TSA, the anterior capsule and labrum are excised. HH = humeral head, C = capsule, Ax = axillary nerve. The arrow points to the subscapularis muscle anterior to the capsule. **B,** Cadaveric dissection showing standard anterior capsulectomy to release medial tethering effect on the subscapularis.

restore function. The nonunion site is bone grafted and can be reinforced with wire or heavy suture.

For chronic malunions of the proximal humerus, the different fragments may have collapsed on each other and coalesced into an amorphous ball. To replace the humeral head, the tuberosity fragments may have to be osteotomized off the shaft and each other. Reconstruction proceeds as in a three- or four-part fracture after the tuberosity fragments have been mobilized. Length may be considerably more difficult to judge than in the acute setting.

In inflammatory and degenerative arthritis, the circumflex vessels are ligated routinely. The subscapularis and capsule are divided together a centimeter medial and parallel to the biceps. If loss of external rotation is present preoperatively, completely freeing the subscapularis usually restores much of this motion. In cases of severe internal rotation contracture, z-lengthening of the subscapularis with a laterally based flap of capsule has been described.[23] For moderate contractures, the tendon of the subscapularis can be taken down adjacent to the bicipital groove and repaired to the humeral osteotomy site. This effectively lengthens the subscapularis, especially at its inferior aspect. We have rarely found these measures to be necessary, and in our hands the subscapularis is routinely repaired to its anatomic insertion at the end of the surgical procedure.

The capsule is stripped off the humerus past the 6 o'clock position. Medial to the biceps, inferior to the subscapularis, the soft tissue on the inframedial neck of the humerus is dissected subperiosteally. It is critical during dissection in this area to know at all times exactly where the nerve lies and to protect it. The subscapularis is freed from soft-tissue attachments in the rotator interval, at the inferiomedial base of the coracoid, and along its inferior border. The rotator interval tissue overlying the biceps as it enters the glenohumeral joint is released, effectively releasing the coracohumeral ligament.

The humeral head is dislocated, the glenoid is inspected, and a decision is made regarding the glenoid. If the glenoid is mildly involved and a biologic resurfacing is appropriate (given the patient's age and degree of glenoid involvement), the anterior capsular flap can be used to resurface it. The capsule must be harvested off the undersurface of the subscapularis to create a medially based flap. Care is taken to preserve length of the capsular flap so that it can reach the posterior and superior edges of the glenoid. The glenoid is reamed to a bleeding surface. The capsular flap is then sewn to the glenoid peripherally through the labrum and anchored centrally with suture anchors (Fig. 10).

If the glenoid is to be replaced, we proceed with our standard TSA technique. The capsule is excised from the posterior surface of the subscapularis to remove its medially tethering effect on the tendon. By pulling on the traction sutures placed along its cut edge, excursion of the subscapularis is tested. If more excursion is needed, the superior, rolled edge of the subscapularis is "recessed" with an oblique cut. This step can give an additional 7 to 10 mm excursion, in our experience. In stiff shoulders it is important to release the anterior edge of the supraspinatus from the superior base of the coracoid.

In intact proximal humerii, the canal of the humerus is found with a small, sharp hand reamer. The humerus is reamed by hand until cortical contact is obtained for noncemented humerii. If cement is used, the stem 1 to 2 mm under the diameter that was reamed is selected. The humeral cutting guide is placed on the final reamer and prongs that insert in the guide show the surgeon where 20° and 40° of retroversion fall in relation to the forearm. The forearm is used as a goniometer to select version for the cut. Metal fingers on the guide can help assess where the cut will be in relation to the cuff. The cut is made and the head fragment is used to assist in selection of prosthetic head size. The trial broach is inserted. Prostheses with a thin proximal body preserve proximal bone stock, and humeral fracture during broach insertion is less of a problem. The lateral fin of the prosthesis should fall on average 12 mm behind the biceps groove. The proximal plate of the prosthesis can be recessed into cancellous bone by using a special reamer. A trial head with variable offset is placed on the broach. Using the prosthetic head as a template, osteophytes are removed around the proximal humerus to make the bone even with the prosthesis. If the glenoid is replaced, the head must have the same radius of curvature as the glenoid component. If only the humerus is replaced, the head that is selected should match the size and the curvature of the head removed and the native glenoid.

If the glenoid is to be replaced, the trial head is removed and a Fukuda retractor is placed behind the posterior glenoid. The broach in the humerus partially protects the humerus from crushing during retraction, although some injury to the anterior metaphysis can still occur. A two-pronged retractor is placed medially on the anterior glenoid neck to hold back the subscapularis and strap muscles. Protecting the axillary nerve from damage, the inferior capsule is resected near the glenoid to facilitate further exposure. Overhanging soft tissue and labrum are resected, and any remaining cartilage on the glenoid is scraped away. These tissues are preserved in hemiarthroplasty to deepen the articulating socket for the HHR.

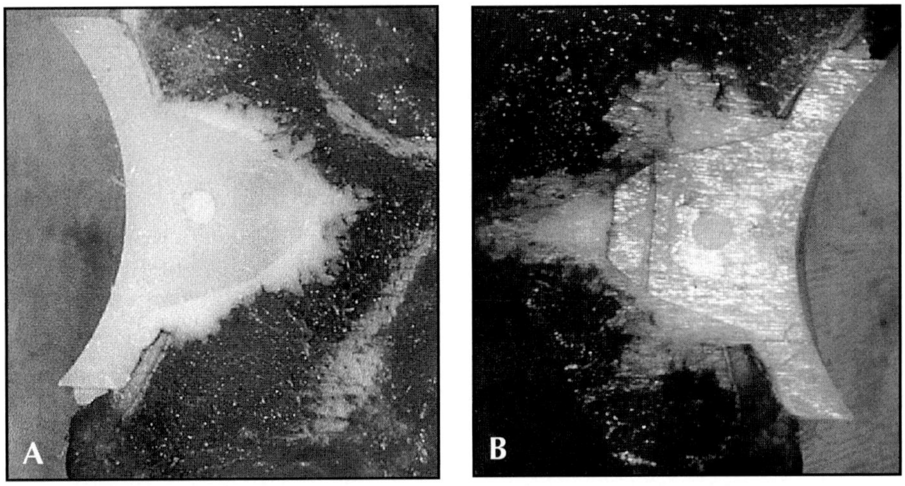

Fig. 11 Cadaveric specimen. **A,** Cut in coronal plane after cementing the glenoid with standard finger packing technique. **B,** Cut in coronal plane after cementing the glenoid with third-generation technique: serial pressurization of "wet" cement with special pressurization tools and sponges.

In OA, erosions occur posteriorly or centrally (Fig. 1). In arthritis following instability procedures, erosions occur opposite the side of the capsular reefing, if the capsule was overtightened (Fig. 4). If there is rim erosion on one side of the glenoid, a burr may be used to even the surface, prior to reaming. Care must be taken not to remove so much bone that the prosthesis cannot be inserted or supported. The glenoid size is selected from trials, choosing the biggest size that allows no overhang of the glenoid component. Reamers are used to smooth the glenoid surface. Straight reamers are preferred because these are easier to control, but adequate glenoid exposure is essential. For cemented glenoids, keel or peg fixation have been used. We prefer peg fixation in small glenoids. Prosthetic designs with anterior and posterior pegs can force the surgeon to place peg holes in thin areas, causing fracture or perforation of the rim.

Trial reduction of the glenoid is performed to ensure the glenoid fits well, there is no rocking of the prosthesis against the glenoid, there is good rim coverage circumferentially, and there is no soft-tissue interposition. Third-generation cement technique is used while cementing the glenoid. The cancellous bone in the vault is prepared with pulsatile lavage, with thrombin-soaked gel foam, and finally with peroxide-soaked sponges. The cement is injected in the holes using a Tumey syringe. The cement is injected and pressurized a total of four times in rapid succession using special cement pressurizing instruments, then the prosthesis is inserted. These techniques have been shown to increase depth of penetration of cement into the bony glenoid in cadaver studies by 50% (Fig. 11). The glenoid prosthesis is held in place until the cement cures.

The proximal humerus is again exposed, and the broach is removed. The humeral canal is prepared for cementing similarly to the glenoid. A cement restrictor is placed 1 to 2 cm distal to the length of the stem. Sutures are placed through the proximal humerus prior to cementing to repair the subscapularis to bone. The humeral stem is cemented in place without excessive pressurization to avoid cement extrusion in the humerus. Care is taken to orient the stem in the appropriate position, and it is held securely in place until the cement cures. The humerus can also be inserted without cement. There is some controversy over which technique is best in the young patient.

Final trial reduction is performed. Care is taken to select a head size that allows 50% translation of the humeral head posteriorly and allows the hand to reach the opposite axilla. The top of the HHR should be superior to the greater tuberosity to avoid impingement. The neck of the proximal humerus is again inspected, and final contouring of the metaphysis is performed to create a smooth contour from neck to prosthetic head. The subscapularis is repaired anatomically with sutures through bone. Drains may be placed if needed. The deltopectoral interval is loosely approximated, and the superficial layers are closed meticulously.

Postoperative Course

Any drains are removed the first or second postoperative day. The arm is placed in a Velpeau dressing with a pillow under the elbow to protect the subscapularis repair while the interscalene block remains in effect. Starting the day after surgery, the patient is switched to a sling and is seen by a therapist twice a day. Neer Phase I exercises are begun postoperative day 1, including pendulum exercises, passive external rotation with a stick to 45°, and passive forward flexion to 140°, using a door pulley. These limits may need to be modified if the subscapularis is tight after repair or the tissue quality is poor. The patient is allowed to remove the sling for sponge bathing and exercises and is discharged from the hospital usually after 2 days. At 2 weeks additional assisted motion in all planes and isometrics are added except for resisted internal rotation and passive external rotation past 45°. At 6 weeks assisted motion in all planes is allowed and light resistive exercises are added in all planes. At 12 weeks more resistance and terminal stretching are added.

Results

Results in general from TSA are excellent. In Torchia and associates' series,[19] 113 TSA patients operated on between 1975 and 1981 were reviewed. Survivorship at 10 and 15 years was 93% and 87%, respectively. At a mean of 12.2 years' follow-up, relief of moderate or severe pain was achieved in 83%. Significant gains in motion were achieved, although gains in elevation were related to the condition of the rotator cuff.

Results in TSA can be markedly influenced by the underlying pathology. In OA early outcome data show substantial and statistically significant improvement in pain, motion, function, and general health by 6 months after surgery, and these remain stable, at least, with short-term follow-up.[17] Long-term follow-up studies are currently sparse in the literature for OA. In 1996 Wirth and Rockwood[74] surveyed the literature and found only four series with an average of more than 4 years' follow-up that included patients with OA.[74] OA in the young patient is rare, and arthritis of the glenohumeral joint in the young patient is usually secondary to trauma, prior instability repairs, ON, or inflammatory arthropathy.

Hemiarthroplasty for fractures has had less successful results. Zyto and associates[75] reviewed 27 hemiarthroplasty patients for fractures at an average of 39 months' follow-up. Most of their patients were older (median age 71 years). The median Constant score was 51 for three-part and 46 for four-part fractures. Median flexion was 70°, and 9 of the 27 patients still had moderate or severe pain. Movin and associates[76] looked at 29 patients, average age 71 years, at an average of 3 years after surgery. They also found significant persistent disability with pain, limited motion, and difficulty with activities of daily living. Goldman and associates[77] reported similar results in their series of 26 patients, average age 67 years, at 30 months' follow-up. Seventy-three percent of their population reported no or only slight pain. They concluded hemiarthroplasty was reliable for pain relief but much less predictable in restoring function, in three- and four-part proximal humerus fractures.

Bigliani[73] reviewed the literature with respect to hemiarthroplasty for proximal humerus fractures. Seventy-seven percent of 355 patients had excellent or satisfactory results. Achieving a relatively painless shoulder is reliable, with most studies reporting greater than 90% satisfactory pain relief. Return of active motion and function was more variable. Bigliani[73] reported expected forward flexion after hemiarthroplasty for proximal humerus fractures ranged from 90° to 120°. Factors cited as contributing to compromised motion and function included age, gender, motivation, fracture type, and timing of surgery. Adherence to technical details including restoration of humeral length and version, reconstruction and healing of the tuberosities, and soft-tissue tensioning are important. An extended supervised rehabilitation is also necessary in maximizing a patient's functional result. In 1994, Compito and associates[78] reported that unsatisfactory results in this type of patient were associated with tuberosity detachment, prosthetic loosening, inadequate or noncompliant rehabilitation, preoperative nerve injury, humeral malposition, dislocation, deep infection, and ectopic bone formation.

Arthritis following instability repairs is the most common cause of arthritis in patients younger than 40 years according to Brems.[30] In Samilson and Prieto's[79] series of 74 patients without prior surgery, older patients at first dislocation were at higher risk for developing arthritis. No correlation was found between the number of dislocations, the severity of initial trauma, and the presence of a Hill-Sachs lesion or a glenoid rim fracture and the development of arthritis. In surgical patients, the main risk factor for development of arthritis after instability repair is creation of an unbalanced joint, causing subluxation in the opposite direction and rim loading. Other surgical factors include failure to diagnose direction or degree of instability, inadequate or nonanatomic surgical reconstruction, prominent hardware, surgery on the wrong side of the joint, and inappropriate use of arthroscopic techniques. Arthroplasty after instability repair occurred an average of 16 years after the index procedure in Bigliani and associates' series.[29] Brems[30] reported that the average age of his patients was 38. He argued against fusion or chielectomy in these patients and for shoulder arthroplasty despite their young age, advocating glenoid replacement as well if the cartilage was destroyed. Releasing contractures and balancing the soft tissues, with particular attention to version of the components is critical. No long-term data after arthroplasty on this particular group are available.

In ON, the results of arthroplasty are often obscured by reporting results in mixed series with more common diagnoses. In 1998 Hattrup[80] gleaned 64 cases of shoulder arthroplasy for ON of the humeral head from the literature. Generally excellent results for pain relief and range of motion can be expected. Rutherford and Cofield[81] reported on 17 shoulders with 2 to 6.5 years' follow-up after shoulder arthroplasty for ON. Eleven had hemiarthroplasties and 6 had TSAs. Active abduction averaged 161° in the hemiarthroplasties and 150° in the total shoulder replacements. Differences between steroid-induced and posttraumatic ON have been reported by several authors. Tanner and Cofield[82] noted that reconstruction in the posttraumatic shoulder can be complicated by scarring, stiffness, cuff damage, nerve injury, and bony deformity. In nontraumatic causes of ON, scarring and stiffness are not present until the last stages of the disease. Hattrup[80] concluded pain relief and motion are generally excellent in ON. Results are superior in steroid-induced ON compared to posttraumatic ON.

Generally good and excellent results for shoulder arthroplasty can be expected in the patient with RA. Neer and associates[8] in a mixed series reported results in 43 patients with RA who received TSAs with a minimum of 2 years' follow-up. Twenty-eight were excellent, 12 were satisfactory, and 3 were unsatisfactory. Fourteen had rotator cuff tears that were repaired at surgery. All patients had excellent pain relief. The three failures were unable to actively elevate the arm past 90°. Cofield[13] reported on 29 arthroplasty patients with RA in a larger series of mixed diagnoses. The rotator cuff was normal in 5 and thinned in 17 patients. Pain relief was generally good or excellent. Postoperative abduction and external rotation averaged 103° and 35°, respectively. Stewert and Kelly[83] looked at 37 TSAs in patients with RA at 7 to 13 years' follow-up. Seventy-eight percent were pain free or had only slight discomfort. Abduction and external rotation postoperatively averaged 75° and 38°, respectively. In most series TSA is highly successful for pain relief in patients with RA. Significant gains in motion and function can also be obtained, even though postoperative elevation on average is 90°.[84]

Younger patients with arthroplasty may not fare as well as the older patient. Sperling and associates[66] reviewed 74 Neer hemiarthroplasties and 34 Neer TSAs in patients younger than 50 years of age with a mean of 12.3 years' follow-up. Both techniques resulted in significant long-term pain relief and significant gains in active abduction and external rotation with no statistically significant difference between the two groups. Results were graded according to a modified system of Neer and of Cofield. Thirty-five of 74 hemiarthroplasties and 17 of 34 TSAs had an unsatisfactory result according to the rating system. Caution was emphasized in offering shoulder arthroplasty to patients younger than age 50 years.[66]

Complications

TSA yields good or excellent results in over 90% of patients in midrange follow-up (< 10 years).[85] Despite these excellent results, Cofield and Edgerton[14] put the overall rate of complications in shoulder arthroplasty at 14% in their review. Complications can be related to one or more of the following: patient selection, underlying diagnoses (patient factors), surgical technique, rehabilitation, and natural history of the underlying diagnoses and shoulder arthroplasty.

Strict adherence to appropriate indications for TSA and hemiarthroplasty will limit a surgeon's postoperative complications. Replacing the glenoid in a rotator cuff deficient shoulder or performing arthroplasty in an unreliable patient with unrealistic expectations dooms the patient and the surgeon to increased complications.

Results from various diagnoses differ and were discussed above. OA most reliably fares well after TSA. RA has less reliable pain relief and restoration of function.[84] Arthroplasty for fracture[78] and for posttraumatic ON[80] typically gives the patient significant motion and pain relief but can fail to provide full active motion or function as discussed previously.

Cuomo and Checroun[85] reported instability occurs after shoulder arthroplasty in 0 to 22% of patients. Post and Pollock[23] put it at 1% to 2%. Appropriate version of the glenoid and humeral components are critical. Total combined retroversion of the glenoid and humeral components should average 35° to 45°. The largest glenoid that the bony glenoid can circumferentially support should be inserted. With a fixed radius of curvature, this will increase the wall height of the glenoid circumferentially, increasing stability.[85,86]

Anterior instability can be caused by excessive anteversion of either component, loss of subscapularis or anterior deltoid function, and excessive posterior capsular tightness.[85] Subscapularis rupture can lead to anterior instability postoperatively. Poor tendon repair, inadequate mobilization, poor tissue quality, oversized components, and inappropriate therapy can put the subscapularis at risk. Circumferential release of the subscapularis and, occasionally, lengthening are required to restore functional external rotation without placing excessive stress on the subscapularis repair.

Posterior instability typically is caused by excessive overall retroversion. Preoperative studies are obtained to assess glenoid version and posterior wear. The anterior high side can be smoothed with a burr and the glenoid reamed to lessen the glenoid retroversion.[23,87] Rarely bone grafting may be used to correct posterior deficiency[88] but severe bone loss will prevent glenoid resurfacing. Humeral retroversion can be decreased, but not too much, to avoid anterior instability. Intraoperative rotator cuff and capsular detachment can occur during the humeral osteotomy and contribute to instability. This cut should be made under direct vision. Newer humeral cutting guides are available in some systems. If these structures are detached they should be repaired to bone intraoperatively.

Placing the HHR too low in the humerus effectively lengthens the deltoid and leads to inferior instability.[23,85] The top of the head should rise about 5 mm above the tuberosity to avoid postoperative impingement. In cases with proximal bone loss the prosthesis may have to be cemented superior to the shaft fracture. Inferior instability can also be caused by axillary nerve palsy. Superior instability results from cuff dysfunction and overpull of the deltoid. Small rotator cuff tears should be repaired at the time of surgery. If the rotator cuff is likely not to center the head in the glenoid, the glenoid should not be replaced.[64] After releases and placement of components, the HHR should subluxate 50% on the glenoid, and the subscapularis should come to the humerus easily. Ideally the shoulder should externally rotate to 40° without excess tension on the subscapularis after repair. Treating the deltoid and rotator cuff with care, repairing the subscapularis securely, and taking care with soft-tissue balancing and version are critical in avoiding postoperative instability.

Postoperative rotator cuff tears occur from 1% to 13% of TSAs.[85] Degenerative changes in the cuff can progress years after arthroplasty. Progressive superior migration of the head may occur[23] as the deltoid overpowers the dysfunctional rotator cuff. Pain and dysfunction may result. Reoperation to repair a rotator cuff tear is best accomplished in acute traumatic tears with a sudden loss of function.

Nerve injury after shoulder arthroplasty rarely is reported.[23,85] Most represent traction neurapraxias and can be treated expectantly.[89] Lynch and associates[89] reported on 18 neurologic deficits after arthroplasty; 11 good and 5 fair recoveries were reported at 1 year. Traction on the brachial plexus in adduction, exernal rotation, and extension was postulated as the mechanism of injury. Careful attention to protecting the nerves and supporting the elbow during humeral preparation to take tension off the plexus is recommended. Nerves can be damaged by extruded cement. Care must be taken to avoid cortical perforations. Blunt-tipped humeral reamers are available to minimize these perforations. Excessive cement pressurization in fragile, osteoporotic bone can cause fractures and cement extrusion. Nerves can be damaged by crush or stretch from retractors. Care must be taken in placing and holding retractors to avoid crushing or stretching nerves. Serial electromyogram/nerve conduction studies can document nerve recovery. Failure of a dense, isolated peripheral nerve palsy to show improvement after 3 months may be reason to explore the nerve.

Infection is reported to occur in from 0.3% to 0.5%.[14,23] It is higher in immunocompromised patients and in patients who have had previous surgeries on the shoulder. Remote sites of potential bacteremia (teeth, bladder) need to be evaluated and treated preoperatively to minimize postoperative risk of infection. Routine preoperative antibiotics are given. Postoperative prophylactic antibiotics are given as recommended by the American Heart Association before dental, urologic and other procedures likely to cause transient bacteremia.[16] Any signs of infection postoperatively must be evaluated aggressively.

Intraoperative fractures are uncommon but do occur, especially in fragile osteoporotic or rheumatoid bone.[23] Humeral fractures during dislocation can be avoided by complete soft-tissue releases and gentle dislocation with adduction and external rotation. In endstage ON or a locked posterior dislocation, the humeral head can hang up on the posterior glenoid rim and make dislocation particularly difficult (Fig. 8, *B*). Translating the head away from the glenoid to disengage the humeral head from the posterior rim before external rotation

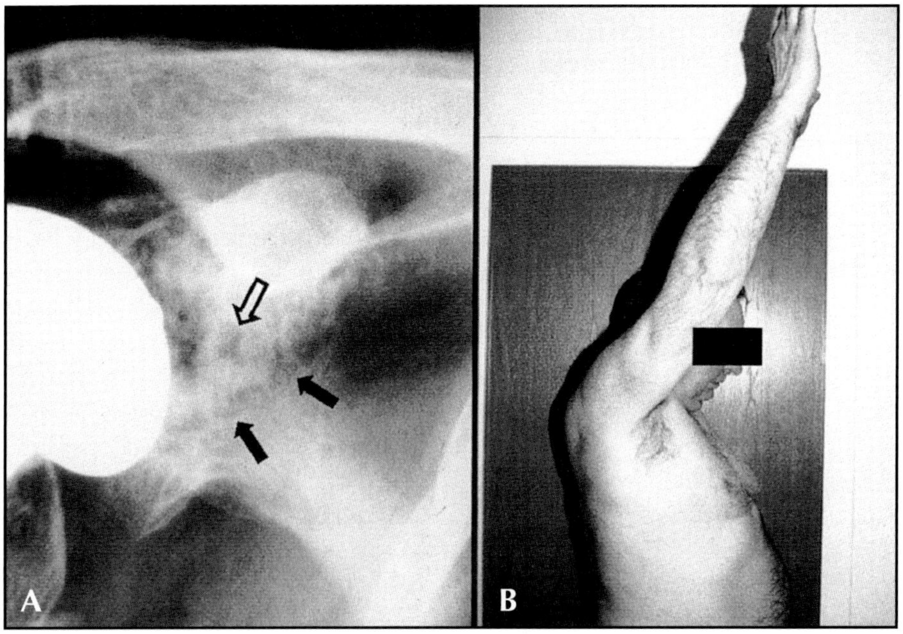

Fig. 12 Nineteen-year follow-up with evidence on left of glenoid loosening. **A,** Solid arrows point out wide radiolucent line at the bone-cement interface. The hollow arrow points to the prosthesis-cement interface. **B,** Patient has good function. He does not desire revision for current level of symptoms.

can ease dislocation.[85] Humeral fractures also can occur during broach or prosthesis insertion if the lateral fin contacts cortical bone, and the proximal body of the component is a large wedge. Thinner proximal body humeral components are available. Removing cortical bone behind the lateral fin with a thin rongeur before seating the broach is recommended.[85] In very weak bone it is recommended to avoid excessive pressurization, which can fracture the humerus.

On the glenoid side eccentric drilling can cause perforation of cortical bone on the scapular neck. It can be difficult determining the center of the glenoid. In OA, osteophytes typically occur posteriorly and inferiorly, which can lead the surgeon to placing the center hole too low and too posterior. Preoperative imaging studies and palpating the scapular neck intraoperatively can help the surgeon orient on the glenoid. A provisional shallow centering hole can be placed for reaming. This hole can be deepened after reaming, once the surgeon is satisfied the centering hole is appropriate. Perforations should be bone grafted or dammed prior to cementing. Glenoid fractures can occur during broaching or placement of a keeled prosthesis if the glenoid is small and the slot is narrow or not properly excavated. We use a pegged glenoid in small bony glenoids and use a keeled component in larger glenoids.

Humeral prostheses can be fixed with cement or press fit. Several authors assert uncemented humerii do as well as cemented stems. Advocates cite bone preservation and ease of surgery as reasons for using uncemented techniques. In the series by Sperling and associates[66] looking at shoulder arthroplasties in patients younger than age 50 years with an average follow-up of 12.3 years, radiolucent lines were present around the humeral prosthesis in 24% of the hemiarthroplasties and 53% of the TSAs. If humeral loosening occurred, which was rare before 10 years, it occurred in uncemented humerii.[66] Torchia and associates[19] reported humeral components shifted position in 49% of their press-fit components and in none of the cemented stems. Humeral component loosening was not associated with pain. It is unclear whether noncemented techniques result in bone preservation during later humeral revisions in the young patient, as asserted by proponents of this technique.

Glenoid loosening is the main problem with long-term survivorship in TSA, particularly in the young patient. A radiolucent line around the glenoid component was seen in 59% of the TSAs in Sperling and Cofield's series.[25] Erosion of the glenoid was present in 68% of the hemiarthroplasties. Torchia and associates[19] reported definite glenoid loosening was present in 44% of their patients, and glenoid loosening was associated with pain. In our experience, however, the ache associated with loosening is often not enough, in the patient's opinion, to warrant a revision surgery (Fig. 12).

Survivorship analysis for shoulder arthroplasty was conducted by Sperling and associates[66] in patients younger than age 50 years. Estimated survival of the hemiarthroplasties was 92% at 5 years, 83% at 10 years, and 73% at 15 years. Risk of revision was higher for hemiarthroplasties performed after trauma than for RA. Estimated survival for TSA was 97% at 5 and at 10 years, and 84% at 15 years. The risk of revision for TSA increased if a rotator cuff tear was present at the time of the surgery.[66]

Complications in shoulder arthroplasty may be minimized by appropriate patient selection; a thorough understanding of the anatomy, biomechanics, and underlying complications of particular disease states; meticulous attention to soft-tissue balancing, bony preparation, and component placement; and adherence to an appropriate, surgeon-directed rehabilitation program.

Discussion

In the young patient with glenohumeral arthritis, shoulder arthroplasty can generally result in excellent pain relief and significant gains in active motion. Care must be taken to exhaust measures short of arthroplasty in the young, active patient with a long life expectancy, given the finite survivorship of prosthetic components in patients younger than 50 years of age.

Careful preoperative studies help select and plan the appropriate procedure. History, physical examination, radiographic studies, and diagnostic injections can isolate the pain generators about the shoulder, including or excluding the acromioclavicular joint, subacromial bursa, glenohumeral joint, and sites outside the shoulder such as the cervical spine.

Nonsurgical means must be fully used to restore comfort and function, including activity modification; stretching and strengthening; ice, heat, and other physical modalities; pharmaceutical agents; and judicious use of steroid injections. Smaller procedures, such as débridement arthroscopy, subacromial decompression, distal clavicle resection, rotator cuff repair, and capsular releases may play a role, depending on the clinical setting.

Knowing the condition of the rotator cuff, deltoid, and neurovascular status about the shoulder is vital in planning shoulder arthroplasty. If any doubt exists, appropriate preoperative studies such as MRI or electromyography are ordered. We avoid glenoid replacement in the young patient, favoring biologic resurfacing in moderately involved glenoids. Glenoids are not replaced in patients with previous infections, nonfunctioning deltoids or rotator cuffs, tight shoulders despite releases, or in patients in whom it is known that there will be noncompliance with postoperative restrictions.

Results of shoulder arthroplasty are significantly influenced by the underlying pathogenesis, degree of arthrosis, and any concomitant comorbidities (like rotator cuff tears). Patients with OA typically fare very well with pain relief and restoration of function, although pure OA requiring shoulder arthroplasty in patients younger than age 40 years is very rare. Arthoplasty after fractures reliably relieves pain and results in significant gains of motion, but restoration of function and full active motion is less predictable. In ON, results are typically excellent in steroid-induced and other nontraumatic causes of ON. Prosthetic replacement of traumatic ON can be technically more difficult and results are not as good as in the atraumatic setting. In RA longevity of prostheses is statistically better than in the posttraumatic setting. Pain relief is excellent but restoration of function depends to a large degree on the condition of the rotator cuff.

Shoulder arthroplasty has a unique set of foibles in the young patient. Subtle nuances in pathogenesis (such as arthritis of dislocation) and unique clinical considerations (such as return to the work force and patient longevity) are seen that are not encountered in the older patient. Prosthetic survivorship is much more an issue in the young. Limitations of current techniques influence surgical decisions (such as whether to replace the glenoid or offer biologic resurfacing). Understanding the unique pathogenesis, surgical alternatives, technical considerations, and clinical results with arthroplasty in the young patient can help the shoulder surgeon choose wisely in offering surgical solutions to his young patients with glenohumeral arthritis.

References

1. Neer CS, Brown TH Jr, McLaughlin HL: Fracture of the neck of the humerus with dislocation of the head fragment. *Am J Surg* 1953;85:252-258.
2. Neer CS II: Articular replacement for the humeral head. *J Bone Joint Surg Am* 1955;37:215-228.
3. Neer CS II: Indications for replacement of the proximal humeral articulation. *Am J Surg* 1955;89:901-907.
4. Neer CS II: Replacement arthroplasty for glenohumeral osteoarthritis. *J Bone Joint Surg Am* 1974;56:1-13.
5. Post M, Jablon M, Miller H, Singh M: Constrained total shoulder joint replacement: A critical review. *Clin Orthop* 1979;144:135-150.
6. Hughes M, Neer CS II: Glenohumeral joint replacement and postoperative rehabilitation. *Phys Ther* 1975;55:850-858.
7. Paradis DK, Ferlic DC: Shoulder arthroplasty in rheumatoid arthritis. *Phys Ther* 1975;55:157-159.
8. Neer CS II, Watson KC, Stanton FJ: Recent experience in total shoulder replacement. *J Bone Joint Surg Am* 1982;64:319-337.
9. Neer CS II, Kirby RM: Revision of humeral head and total shoulder arthroplasties. *Clin Orthop* 1982;170:189-195.
10. Neer CS II: Unconstrained shoulder arthroplasty. *Instr Course Lect* 1985;34:278-286.
11. Figgie HE III, Inglis AE, Goldberg VM, Ranawat CS, Figgie MP, Wile JM: An analysis of factors affecting the long-term results of total shoulder arthroplasty in inflammatory arthritis. *J Arthroplasty* 1988;3:123-130.
12. Post M, Jablon M: Constrained total shoulder arthroplasty: Long-term follow-up observations. *Clin Orthop* 1983;173:109-116.
13. Cofield RH: Total shoulder arthroplasty with the Neer prosthesis. *J Bone Joint Surg Am* 1984;66:899-906.
14. Cofield RH, Edgerton BC: Total shoulder arthroplasty: Complications and revision surgery. *Instr Course Lect* 1990;39:449-462.
15. Fenlin JM Jr, Ramsey ML, Allardyce TJ, Frieman BG: Modular total shoulder replacement: Design rationale, indications, and results. *Clin Orthop* 1994;307:37-46.
16. Wirth MA, Rockwood CA Jr: Complications of shoulder arthroplasty. *Clin Orthop* 1994;307:47-69.
17. Matsen FA III: Early effectiveness of shoulder arthroplasty for patients who have primary glenohumeral degenerative joint disease. *J Bone Joint Surg Am* 1996;78:260-264.
18. Cofield RH: Uncemented total shoulder arthroplasty: A review. *Clin Orthop* 1994;307:86-93.
19. Torchia ME, Cofield RH, Settergren CR: Total shoulder arthroplasty with the Neer prosthesis: Long-term results. *J Shoulder Elbow Surg* 1997;6:495-505.
20. Neer CS II (ed): *Shoulder Reconstruction*. Philadelphia, PA, WB Saunders, 1990.
21. Friedman RJ (ed): Total shoulder arthroplasty. *Orthop Clin North Am* 1998;29.
22. Matsen FA III, Rockwood CA Jr, Wirth MA, Lippitt SB: Glenohumeral arthritis and its management, in Rockwood CA Jr, Matsen FA III, Wirth MA, Harryman DT II (eds): *The Shoulder*, ed 2. Philadelphia, PA, WB Saunders, 1998, vol 2, pp 840-964.
23. Post M, Pollock RG: Operative treatment of degenerative and arthritic diseases of the glenohumeral joint, in Post M, Flatow EL, Bigliani

LU, Pollock RG (eds): *The Shoulder: Operative Technique.* Baltimore, MD, Williams & Wilkins, 1998, pp 73-131.

24. Skedros JG, O'Rourke PJ, Zimmerman JM, Burkhead WZ Jr: Alternatives to replacement arthroplasty for glenohumeral arthritis, in Iannotti JP, Williams GR Jr (eds): *Disorders of the Shoulder: Diagnosis and Management.* Philadelphia, PA, Lippincott-Williams & Wilkins, 1999, pp 485-499.
25. Sperling JW, Cofield RH: Revision total shoulder arthroplasty for the treatment of glenoid arthrosis. *J Bone Joint Surg Am* 1998;80:860-867.
26. Barrett WP, Thornhill TS, Thomas WH, Gebhart EM, Sledge CB: Nonconstrained total shoulder arthroplasty in patients with polyarticular rheumatoid arthritis. *J Arthroplasty* 1989;4:91-96.
27. Hattrup SJ, Cofield RH: Osteonecrosis of the humeral head: Relationship of disease stage, extent, and cause to natural history. *J Shoulder Elbow Surg* 1999;8:559-564.
28. Cruess RL: Experience with steroid-induced avascular necrosis of the shoulder and etiologic considerations regarding osteonecrosis of the hip. *Clin Orthop* 1978;130:86-93.
29. Bigliani LU, Weinstein DM, Glasgow MT, Pollock RG, Flatow EL: Glenohumeral arthroplasty for arthritis after instability surgery. *J Shoulder Elbow Surg* 1995;4:87-94.
30. Brems JJ: Arthritis of dislocation. *Orthop Clin North Am* 1998;29:453-466.
31. Hurley JA, Anderson TE, Dear W, Andrish JT, Bergfeld JA, Weiker GG: Posterior shoulder instability: Surgical versus conservative results with evaluation of glenoid version. *Am J Sports Med* 1992;20:396-400.
32. Lehmann JF, Warren CG, Scham SM: Therapeutic heat and cold. *Clin Orthop* 1974;99:207-245.
33. Neer CS II: Impingement lesions. *Clin Orthop* 1983;173:70-77.
34. Rowe CR: Injection technique for the shoulder and elbow. *Orthop Clin North Am* 1988;19:773-777.
35. Kerlan RK, Glousman RE: Injections and techniques in athletic medicine. *Clin Sports Med* 1989;8:541-560.
36. Hollingworth GR, Ellis RM, Hattersley TS: Comparison of injection techniques for shoulder pain: Results of a double blind, randomised study. *Br Med J* 1983;287:1339-1341.
37. Blair B, Rokito AS, Cuomo F, Jarolem K, Zuckerman JD: Efficacy of injections of corticosteroids for subacromial impingement syndrome. *J Bone Joint Surg Am* 1996;78: 1685-1689.
38. Dieppe P: Drug treatment of osteoarthritis. *J Bone Joint Surg Br* 1993;75:673-674.
39. Jackson RW: Arthroscopic surgery. *J Bone Joint Surg Am* 1983;65:416-420.
40. Ellman H, Harris E, Kay SP: Early degenerative joint disease simulating impingement syndrome: Arthroscopic findings. *Arthroscopy* 1992;8:482-487.
41. Ellman H: Shoulder arthroscopy: Current indications and techniques. *Orthopedics* 1988;11:45-51.
42. Ogilvie-Harris DJ, Wiley AM: Arthroscopic surgery of the shoulder: A general appraisal. *J Bone Joint Surg Br* 1986;68:201-207.
43. Johnson LL: Arthroscopic abrasion arthroplasty historical and pathologic perspective: Present status. *Arthroscopy* 1986;2:54-69.
44. Hayes JM: Arthroscopic treatment of steroid-induced osteonecrosis of the humeral head. *Arthroscopy* 1989;5:218-221.
45. Weinstein DM, Bucchieri JS, Pollock RG, Flatow EL, Bigliani LU: Abstract: Arthroscopic debridement of the shoulder for osteoarthritis. *Arthroscopy* 1993;9:366.
46. Simpson NS, Kelly IG: Extra-glenohumeral joint shoulder surgery in rheumatoid arthritis: The role of bursectomy, acromioplasty, and distal clavicle excision. *J Shoulder Elbow Surg* 1994;3:66-69.
47. Ellowitz AS, Rosas R, Rodosky MW, Buss DD: Abstract: The benefit of arthroscopic subacromial decompression for impingement in patients found to have unsuspected glenohumeral osteoarthritis. *64th Annual Meeting Proceedings.* Rosemont, IL American Academy of Orthopaedic Surgeons, 1997, p 206.
48. Hawkins RJ, Angelo RL: Glenohumeral osteoarthrosis: A late complication of the Putti-Platt repair. *J Bone Joint Surg Am* 1990;72:1193-1197.
49. Caspari: Shoulder arthroscopy: A review of the current state of the art. *Contemp Orthop* 1982;4:523-530.
50. Pollock RG: Prosthetic replacement in rotator cuff-deficient shoulders. *J Shoulder Elbow Surg* 1992;1:173-186.
51. Flatow EL: Prosthetic replacement in the rotator cuff deficient shoulder in, Vastamäki M, Jalovaara P (eds): *Surgery of the Shoulder.* Amsterdam, The Netherlands, Elsevier, 1995, pp 335-345.
52. Codd TP, Pollock RG, Flatow EL: Prosthetic replacement in the rotator cuff-deficient shoulder. *Tech Orthop* 1993;8:174-183.
53. Benjamin A: Double osteotomy of the shoulder. *Scand J Rheumatol* 1974;3:65.
54. Benjamin A, Hirschowitz D, Arden GP: The treatment of arthritis of the shoulder joint by double osteotomy. *Int Orthop* 1979;3:211-216.
55. Kronberg M, Brostrom LA: Rotation osteotomy of the proximal humerus to stabilise the shoulder: Five years' experience. *J Bone Joint Surg Br* 1995;77:924-927.
56. Hawkins RH: Glenoid osteotomy for recurrent posterior subluxation of the shoulder: Assessment by computed axial tomography. *J Shoulder Elbow Surg* 1996;5:393-400.
57. Johnston GH, Hawkins RJ, Haddad R, Fowler PJ: A complication of posterior glenoid osteotomy for recurrent posterior shoulder instability. *Clin Orthop* 1984;187:147-149.
58. Wirth MA, Lyons FR, Rockwood CA Jr: Hypoplasia of the glenoid: A review of sixteen patients. *J Bone Joint Surg Am* 1993;75:1175-1184.
59. Gonzalez-Diaz R, Rodriguez-Merchan EC, Gilbert MS: The role of shoulder fusion in the era of arthroplasty. *Int Orthop* 1997;21:204-209.
60. Burkhead WZ Jr, Hutton KS: Biologic resurfacing of the glenoid with hemiarthroplasty of the shoulder. *J Shoulder Elbow Surg* 1995;4:263-270.
61. Levine WN, Djurasovic M, Glasson JM, Pollock RG, Flatow EL, Bigliani LU: Hemiarthroplasty for glenohumeral osteoarthritis: Results correlated to degree of glenoid wear. *J Shoulder Elbow Surg* 1997;6:449-454.
62. Rodosky MW, Bigliani LU: Indications for glenoid resurfacing in shoulder arthroplasty. *J Shoulder Elbow Surg* 1996;5:231-248.
63. Smith KL, Matsen FA III: Total shoulder arthroplasty versus hemiarthroplasty: Current trends. *Orthop Clin North Am* 1998;29:491-506.
64. Franklin JL, Barrett WP, Jackins SE, Matsen FA III: Glenoid loosening in total shoulder arthroplasty: Association with rotator cuff deficiency. *J Arthroplasty* 1988;3:39-46.
65. Hatzis N, Kaar TK, Wirth MA, Toro F, Rockwood CA Jr: Neuropathic arthropathy of the shoulder. *J Bone Joint Surg Am* 1998;80:1314-1319.
66. Sperling JW, Cofield RH, Rowland CM: Neer hemiarthroplasty and Neer total shoulder arthroplasty in patients fifty years old or less: Long-term results. *J Bone Joint Surg Am* 1998;80:464-473.
67. Hawkins RJ, Greis PE, Bonutti PM: Treatment of symptomatic glenoid loosening following unconstrained shoulder arthroplasty. *Orthopedics* 1999;22:229-234.
68. Fischer RA, Nicholson GP, McIlveen SJ, McCann PD, Flatow EL, Bigliani LU: Primary humeral head replacement for severely displaced proximal humerus fractures. *Orthop Trans* 1993;16:779.
69. Levine WN, Connor PM, Yamaguchi K, et al: Humeral head replacement for proximal humeral fractures. *Orthopedics* 1998;21:68-73.
70. Flatow EL, Bigliani LU: Tips of the trade: Locating and protecting the axillary nerve in shoulder surgery: The tug test. *Orthop Rev* 1992;21:503-505.
71. Connor PM, Flatow EL: Complications of internal fixation of proximal humeral fractures. *Instr Course Lect* 1997;46:25-37.
72. Duralde XA, Flatow EL, Pollock RG, Nicholson GP, Self EB, Bigliani LU: Operative treatment of nonunions of the surgical neck of the humerus. *J Shoulder Elbow Surg* 1996;5:169-180.

73. Bigliani LU: Proximal humerus fractures, in Post M, Flatow EL, Bigliani LU, Pollock RG (eds): *The Shoulder: Operative Technique.* Baltimore, MD, Williams & Wilkins, 1998, pp 43-71.

74. Wirth MA, Rockwood CA Jr: Complications of total shoulder-replacement arthroplasty. *J Bone Joint Surg Am* 1996;78:603-616.

75. Zyto K, Wallace WA, Frostick SP, Preston BJ: Outcome after hemiarthroplasty for three- and four-part fractures of the proximal humerus. *J Shoulder Elbow Surg* 1998;7:85-89.

76. Movin T, Sjoden GO, Ahrengart L: Poor function after shoulder replacement in fracture patients: A retrospective evaluation of 29 patients followed for 2-12 years. *Acta Orthop Scand* 1998;69:392-396.

77. Goldman RT, Koval KJ, Cuomo F, Gallagher MA, Zuckerman JD: Functional outcome after humeral head replacement for acute three- and four-part proximal humeral fractures. *J Shoulder Elbow Surg* 1995;4:81-86.

78. Compito CA, Self EB, Bigliani LU: Arthroplasty and acute shoulder trauma: Reasons for success and failure. *Clin Orthop* 1994;307:27-36.

79. Samilson RL, Prieto V: Dislocation arthropathy of the shoulder. *J Bone Joint Surg Am* 1983;65:456-460.

80. Hattrup SJ: Indications, technique, and results of shoulder arthroplasty in osteonecrosis. *Orthop Clin North Am* 1998;29:445-451.

81. Rutherford CS, Cofield RH: Osteonecrosis of the shoulder. *Orthop Trans* 1987;11:239.

82. Tanner MW, Cofield RH: Prosthetic arthroplasty for fractures and fracture-dislocations of the proximal humerus. *Clin Orthop* 1983;179:116-128.

83. Stewart MP, Kelly IG: Total shoulder replacement in rheumatoid disease: 7- to 13-year follow-up of 37 joints. *J Bone Joint Surg Br* 1997;79:68-72.

84. Waldman BJ, Figgie MP: Indications, technique, and results of total shoulder arthroplasty in rheumatoid arthritis. *Orthop Clin North Am* 1998;29:435-444.

85. Cuomo F, Checroun A: Avoiding pitfalls and complications in total shoulder arthroplasty. *Orthop Clin North Am* 1998;29:507-518.

86. Iannotti JP, Williams GR: Total shoulder arthroplasty: Factors influencing prosthetic design. *Orthop Clin North Am* 1998;29:377-391.

87. Ibarra C, Dines DM, McLaughlin JA: Glenoid replacement in total shoulder arthroplasty. *Orthop Clin North Am* 1998;29:403-413.

88. Neer CS II, Morrison DS: Glenoid bone-grafting in total shoulder arthroplasty. *J Bone Joint Surg Am* 1988;70:1154-1162.

89. Lynch NM, Cofield RH, Silbert PL, Hermann RC: Neurologic complications after total shoulder arthroplasty. *J Shoulder Elbow Surg* 1996;5:53-61.

Reference to Video

Flatow E, Yassamin H: Intraoperative video. New York, NY, Mt. Sinai Hospital, 2000.

11

The Unstable Elbow

Shawn W. O'Driscoll, PhD, MD, FRCS
Jesse B. Jupiter, MD
Graham J. W. King, MD, MSc, FRCS
Robert N. Hotchkiss, MD
Bernard F. Morrey, MD

Biomechanics of Elbow Dislocation

Pathoanatomy

The pathoanatomy of an elbow dislocation can be thought of as a disruption of the circle of soft tissue or bone, or both, that begins on the lateral side of the elbow and progresses to the medial side in three stages (Fig. 1, *A*). In stage 1, the lateral collateral ligament is partially or completely disrupted (the ulnar part is disrupted). This disruption results in posterolateral rotatory subluxation of the elbow, which can reduce spontaneously (Fig. 1, *B*). Stage 2 involves additional disruption anteriorly and posteriorly. There is an incomplete posterolateral dislocation of the elbow in which the concave medial edge of the ulna rests on the trochlea. On a lateral radiograph of the elbow, the coronoid process appears to be perched on the trochlea. This dislocation can be reduced with use of minimal force or by the patient manipulating his or her own elbow. Stage 3 is subdivided into three parts. In stage 3A, all of the soft tissues around and including the posterior part of the medial collateral ligament are disrupted, leaving only the important anterior band (the anterior medial collateral ligament) intact. This permits posterior dislocation by a posterolateral rotatory mechanism. The elbow pivots on the intact anterior band of the medial collateral ligament. Reduction is accomplished by gentle manipulation of the elbow beginning with supination and valgus stress, temporarily recreating the deformity, followed by application of traction, varus stress, and pronation simultaneously. The intact anterior medial collateral ligament provides stability if the forearm is kept in pronation to prevent posterolateral rotatory subluxation during valgus stress-testing. Stage 3A instability is most commonly seen in the presence of fractures of the radial head and coronoid process. In stage 3B, the entire medial collateral complex is disrupted. Varus, valgus, and rotatory instability are all present following reduction. In stage 3C, the instability is so severe that the elbow can dislocate even when it is immobilized in a cast in 90° of flexion. This degree of instability occurs because the entire distal aspect of the humerus has been stripped of soft tissues. Usually, reduction can be maintained only by flexing the elbow beyond 90° to 110°. The flexor-pronator and common extensor muscle origins are important secondary stabilizers of the elbow. These pathoanatomic stages all correlate with clinical degrees of elbow instability. Most commonly, elbow dislocations involve disruption of both the medial and the lateral collateral ligament and, therefore, are at least stage 2.[1-3]

Thus, dislocation is the final stage of three sequential stages of elbow instability resulting from posterolateral ulnohumeral rotatory subluxation, with soft-tissue disruption that progresses from the lateral to the medial side. This finding has been confirmed in a study of cadaveric elbows.[4] Twelve of 13 elbows could be dislocated posteriorly with the anterior medial collateral ligament intact. In each stage, the pathoanatomy correlated with the pattern and degree of instability.

This circle of disruption is referred to as the Horii circle and is analogous to the Mayfield spiral of soft tissue or osseous disruption, or both, in carpal instability (Fig. 1, *A*). As disruption progresses from the lateral to the medial side, it may pass through the soft tissues or bone, or both. Therefore, an elbow dislocation is most commonly associated with a torn capsule, but the capsule may be intact if the coronoid process is fractured. Because energy is dissipated with a fracture before the elbow dislocates, the anterior bundle of the medial collateral ligament is often intact when the radial head and coronoid process are both fractured.

This parallel between the pathoanatomy and the degree of displacement explains the spectrum of instability,

One or more of the authors or the departments with which they are affiliated have received something of value from a commercial or other party related directly or indirectly to the subject of this chapter.

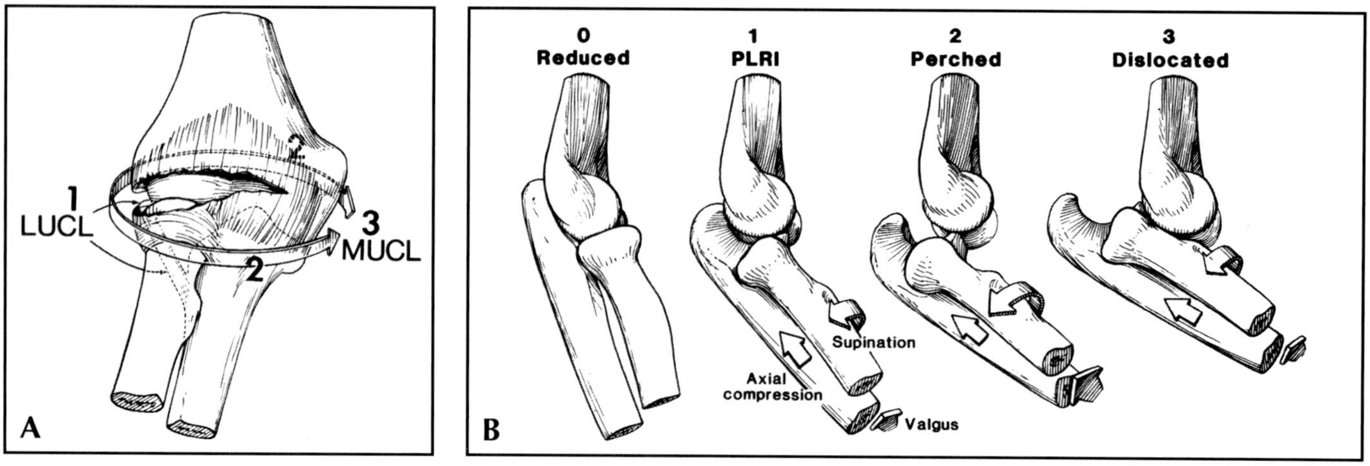

Fig. 1 A, Drawing of the Horii circle of soft-issue injury. The injury progresses from the lateral to the medial side in three stages. In stage 1, the ulnar part of the lateral collateral ligament, the lateral ulnar collateral ligament (LUCL), is disrupted. In stage 2, the other lateral ligamentous structures and the anterior and posterior aspects of the capsule are disrupted. In stage 3, the medial ulnar collateral ligament (MUCL) is either partially disrupted, involving the posterior medial ulnar collateral ligament only (stage 3A), or completely disrupted (stage 3B). The common extensor and flexor origins are often disrupted as well. **B,** Drawings showing the spectrum of elbow instability, from subluxation to dislocation. The three stages correspond with the pathoanatomic stages of capsuloligamentous disruption in **A**. The arrows indicate the forces and moments responsible for displacements. PLRI = posterolateral rotatory instability. (Reproduced with permission from the Mayo Foundation, Rochester, MN.)

ranging from posterolateral rotatory instability to posterior dislocation with or without disruption of the anterior medial collateral ligament. Such a posterolateral rotatory mechanism for dislocation would be compatible with those suggested in the 1960s by Osborne and Cotterill[5] and by Roberts.[6]

Constraints to Elbow Instability

The elbow has both static and dynamic constraints, which are analogous to the defenses of a fortress (Fig. 2). The three primary static constraints to elbow instability are the ulnohumeral articulation, the medial collateral ligament, and the lateral collateral ligament, especially the ulnar part of the lateral collateral ligament (also referred to as the lateral ulnar collateral ligament). The secondary constraints include the radial head, the common flexor and extensor origins, and the capsule. The dynamic stabilizers include the muscles that cross the elbow joint and produce compressive forces at the articulation. The anconeus, triceps, and brachialis are the most important muscles in this regard. Originating near the lateral epicondyle and inserting broadly on the ulna in a fan shape, the anconeus seems designed to serve its major function as a dynamic stabilizer, preventing posterolateral rotational displacement of the elbow. A word of caution: the nerve to the anconeus, which enters the muscle proximally, is divided with the traditional olecranon osteotomy for distal humeral fractures.

An elbow with its three primary constraints intact will be stable. If the coronoid process is fractured or lost, the radial head becomes a critical stabilizer. The radial head must not be removed when a dislocated elbow is associated with a fractured coronoid process unless the coronoid process and the ligaments can be securely fixed. The management of injuries to these structures is discussed in the ensuing sections.

Classification of Elbow Instability

Elbow instability can be classified into different types according to five criteria: (1) the articulation or articulations involved (the elbow or the radial head); (2) the direction of displacement (valgus, varus, anterior, or posterolateral rotatory); (3) the degree of displacement (subluxation or dislocation); (4) the timing (acute, chronic, or recurrent); and (5) the presence or absence of associated fractures.[7]

As described in detail in the section on pathoanatomy, elbow instability can be considered a spectrum consisting of three stages (Fig. 1, *B*). In stage 1, the elbow subluxates in a posterolateral direction and the patient has a positive lateral pivot-shift test (Fig. 3). In stage 2, the elbow dislocates incompletely so that the coronoid process is perched on the trochlea. In stage 3, the elbow dislocates fully so that the coronoid process rests behind the humerus. Stage 3 is subclassified into three categories. In stage 3A, the anterior band of the medial collateral ligament is intact and the elbow is stable to valgus stress following reduction. In stage 3B, the elbow dislocates fully and the anterior band of the medial collateral ligament is disrupted so that the elbow is unstable in varus, valgus, and posterolateral rotation.

Some flexion (30° to 45°) is usually required to prevent subluxation. In stage 3C, the entire distal aspect of the humerus is stripped of soft tissues, rendering the elbow unstable even in a cast. Reduction can be maintained usually only by flexing the elbow more than 90°. Each stage has specific clinical, radiographic, and pathologic features that are predictable and have implications for treatment. The pathologic characteristics can be predicted from the degree of instability.

Evaluation of Acute Dislocations and Fracture-Dislocations

Acute Elbow Dislocations

Dislocated elbows must be evaluated for functional stability after reduction of the dislocation. Following reduction, instability is assessed by gently moving the elbow through a range of motion. If the elbow appears to subluxate or dislocate, a splint is applied and anteroposterior and lateral radiographs are made. If no subluxation is seen on radiographs, the patient is discharged with the arm in the splint or a sling. The patient should be reevaluated in 5 to 7 days. If the elbow subluxates or dislocates in extension or is noncongruent on the radiographs made at the follow-up visit, the forearm should be pronated and the stability of the elbow should be reassessed. If stability is restored, a hinged brace or cast-brace is applied with the forearm in full pronation. An extension block of 30° is sometimes necessary. If the elbow requires an extension block of more than 30° to 45°, surgical repair should be considered. Extension blocks should be gradually eased so that by 3 weeks the brace allows full motion. At each follow-up examination, the elbow should be reevaluated in exactly the same manner.

Instability may need to be assessed with the patient under general anesthesia, as this is sometimes the only way to adequately examine the joint for stability. This examination is easiest to

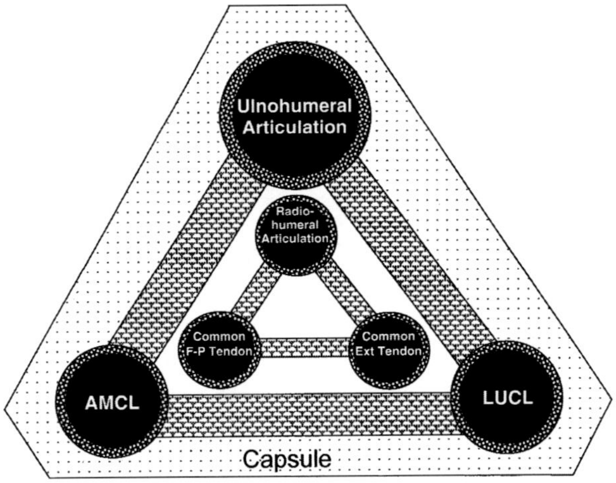

Fig. 2 Drawing showing the static and dynamic constraints to instability, which can be considered analogous to the defenses of a fortress. The three primary static constraints to elbow instability are the ulnohumeral articulation, the anterior medial collateral ligament (AMCL), and the lateral collateral ligament, especially the ulnar part of the lateral collateral ligament, which is also referred to as the lateral ulnar collateral ligament (LUCL). The secondary constraints include the radial head, the common flexor and extensor tendon origins, and the capsule. Dynamic stabilizers include the muscles that cross the elbow joint and produce compressive forces at the articulation. F-P = flexor-pronator. (Reproduced with permission from the Mayo Foundation, Rochester, MN.)

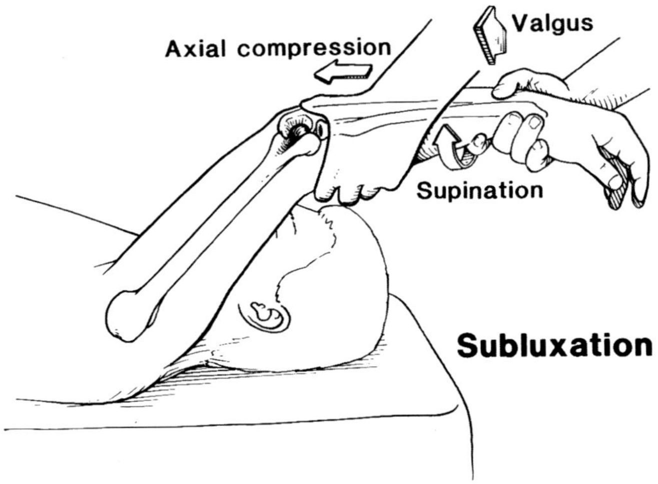

Fig. 3 Drawing showing the lateral pivot-shift test for posterolateral rotatory instability of the elbow, which is performed with the patient's arm overhead. A supination-valgus moment is applied during flexion, causing the elbow to subluxate maximally at about 40° of flexion. Additional flexion causes reduction (with a palpable, visible clunk, if successful). This test creates apprehension in the patient, who notes the sensation that the elbow is about to dislocate. (Reproduced with permission from the Mayo Foundation, Rochester, MN.)

perform and the findings are easiest to interpret with the arm in the overhead position. The arm then resembles a leg, and the elbow resembles a knee. To most surgeons, this is extremely helpful. The elbow is examined for valgus, varus, and posterolateral rotatory instability. Valgus stress-testing is performed with the forearm fully pronated so that posterolateral rotatory instability is not mistaken for valgus instability.[8] This happens because the ulna and the radius rotate as a unit away from the humerus in response to valgus stress when the lateral collateral ligament is disrupted. Forced pronation prevents posterolateral rotatory instability because the intact medial soft tissues are used as a hinge or fulcrum, just as the periosteum is used for this purpose during the reduction of a supracondylar fracture in a child. Varus stress-testing is easiest to perform with the shoulder fully internally rotated. Both valgus and varus stress-testing are performed with the elbow in full extension and then in about 30° of flexion. Flexion unlocks the olecranon from the olecranon fossa. Posterolateral rotatory instability is diagnosed with use of the lateral pivot-shift maneuver of the elbow. If there is severe soft-tissue disruption, this test can have a false-negative result. With severe soft-tissue disruption, the elbow can sometimes remain dislocated even when it is flexed past 90°. If suspected, this problem can be avoided by the examiner using his or her thumb to prevent the elbow from fully dislocating (or limiting the degree of subluxation during the pivot-shift test).

Lateral Pivot-Shift Maneuver

Currently, the most common method of performing this test is with the patient placed supine on the examining table with the affected extremity overhead[9] (Fig. 3). The elbow is supinated, and a mild to moderate forced valgus stress is applied while the elbow is flexed past approximately 40°. This maneuver results in apprehension or frank subluxation of the radius and the ulna in a rotatory fashion from the humerus. A visible, palpable clunk or an actual pivot shift may be elicited by this maneuver. If instability is not elicited, the test is still positive if there is apprehension, and the diagnosis can be made on this basis. The posterolateral rotatory drawer test involves placing the elbow in approximately 40° of flexion and applying an anterior-posterior force on the ulna and the radius to subluxate the forearm away from the humerus on the lateral side (pivoting on the intact medial ligaments).

Stress radiographs are made in the anteroposterior plane with application of valgus and varus stress and the arm overhead as described above. With the shoulder in 90° of abduction and full external rotation, stress radiographs are also made with the arm in supination and pronation to detect posterolateral rotatory instability and to determine if the medial side opens up with pronation (indicating disruption of the medial soft tissues).

Evaluation and Management of Acute Fracture-Dislocations

The evaluation of a patient who has sustained a fracture-dislocation is very structured, and it is also essential. Stress radiographs should be made, with use of an image intensifier, in the anteroposterior plane with valgus stress and then with varus stress. When valgus stress-testing is performed, the forearm must be held fully pronated with moderated force to prevent posterolateral rotatory subluxation and false-positive valgus instability. With the shoulder in 90° of abduction and full external rotation, lateral stress radiographs are also made with the forearm in supination and pronation to detect posterolateral rotatory instability and to determine if the medial side opens up with pronation (indicating disruption of the medial soft tissues).

The Terrible-Triad Injury

The elbow is one of the most stable articulations in the skeletal system, and when one or more parts of its articular supporting architecture is disrupted in the presence of a dislocation the risk of recurrent instability or arthrosis is substantial.[10-12] The fundamental goal in the management of fracture-dislocation of the elbow (a so-called complex dislocation) is the restoration of the osseous-articular restraints, thereby converting the injury to a so-called simple dislocation, which has been demonstrated in a number of studies to have a generally favorable long-term prognosis.[11,12] Most of the principles of managing complex instability of the elbow can be derived from an understanding of the pathomechanics and treatment of the terrible-triad injury. Hotchkiss[13] used the phrase "terrible triad" for the combination of an elbow dislocation and fractures of the radial head and coronoid process. It received this name because of the major disability that so often results from this injury.[13] The terrible triad often affects young active individuals, and the complications include persistent instability, nonunion, malunion, and osseous proximal radioulnar synostosis. In approaching the management of the terrible-triad injury, the individual injuries to the coronoid process, radial head, and collateral ligaments must be considered.

Fractures of the Coronoid Process

Regan and Morrey[14] classified fractures of the coronoid process into three types. Type I is a small fleck of bone, type II involves 50% of the height of the coronoid process or less, and type III involves more than 50% of the height of the coronoid process. Type I fractures have been incorrectly referred to as avulsion fractures, but Cage and associates[15] showed, in a cadaver study, that they are not, as nothing attaches to the tip of the coronoid process. They represent shear fractures, similar to a Bankart lesion of the shoulder, and they occur during subluxation or dislocation of the elbow.[8] Regan and Morrey[14] found that the prevalence of instability rises, and the prognosis deteriorates, according to the amount of the coronoid process that is fractured.

When the coronoid process is fractured, with or without concomitant fracture of the olecranon, restoration of the intrinsic stability of the elbow depends to a large degree on reestablishment of the anatomic dimensions of the trochlear notch. Fracture of the coronoid process at its base compromises stability in two ways. First, the anterior buttress, which serves to resist the normal posteriorly directed forces occurring with elbow flexion, and second, the anterior band of the medial collateral ligament, the insertion of which is attached to the coronoid fracture fragment, are rendered incompetent.[14-18]

Beredjiklian and associates, in a biomechanical study performed on cadaver, confirmed the role of the coronoid process as a primary stabilizer of the elbow and its critical role in the presence of a radial head fracture and ligament injury (P Beredjiklian, MD, et al, Minneapolis, MN, unpublished data, 1989). O'Driscoll and associates demonstrated, in a cadaveric model simulating the terrible-triad injury, that the coronoid process is a primary stabilizer of the elbow (S O'Driscoll, MD, et al, New Orleans, LA, unpublished data, 1998). Persistent instability was progressively more likely as the amount of coronoid resection increased, even with the radial head present. However, with even a small deficiency in the coronoid process, the radial head became a critically important secondary stabilizer.

The surgical exposures of the coronoid process depend on the associated lesions. A universal posterior skin incision, just lateral to the tip of the olecranon, permits deep access to both the medial and the lateral side of the elbow and provides the versatility needed to treat these injuries. In general, small (type I and many type II) fractures found in association with radial head fractures and dislocated elbows can be approached from the lateral side, as described in the literature.[19] An exception is a medial coronoid fragment (often part of a comminuted type II or type III coronoid fracture), which is more appropriately approached medially. The fractured radial head is retracted gently to permit access to the coronoid process. The medial approach is facilitated when the injury includes avulsion of the origin of the flexor-pronator muscle mass. Elevation of the ulnar origin of the flexor-pronator muscle group allows visualization of the coronoid process. When it is part of a complex proximal ulnar fracture, the coronoid process can occasionally be reduced, and the reduction can be held by exposure through the olecranon fracture itself.[20]

Internal fixation of smaller (type I or type II) fragments may present not only technical problems but also problems that may jeopardize the tenuous blood supply to the coronoid process. We prefer to use the technique in which two braided sutures are passed over the top of the small coronoid fragment, pulled out through drill-holes in the ulna, and tied over the bone[21] (Fig. 4). If the capsule is attached to the fragment, the sutures should be passed through the capsule as well. Reattachment of a fractured coronoid fragment provides important stability through the capsular attachments, just as a volar plate advancement arthroplasty does for an unstable fracture-dislocation of the proximal interphalangeal joint.

Larger (type III and some type II) fractures of the coronoid process require anatomic reduction and stable internal fixation. The best techniques are not yet known, as experience with treating these injuries is limited. However, it is likely that screw fixation and the use of a buttress plate are necessary for most such fractures. This is particularly true for medial coronoid fractures.

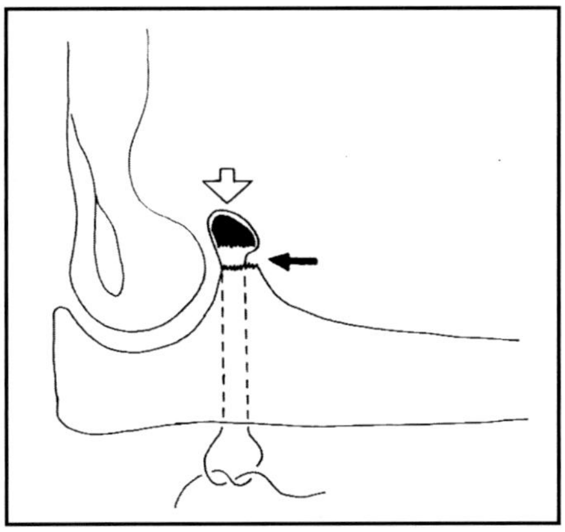

Fig. 4 Drawing showing internal fixation of smaller coronoid fragments (type I or II) with two braided sutures that are passed through the ulna and over the top of the small coronoid fragment and then tied over the bone.[24] If the capsule is attached to the fragment, the sutures should be passed through the capsule as well.

In some instances, the coronoid may not be amenable to fixation because of the size or comminution of the fracture or because of a delay between the injury and the treatment. When the coronoid fracture is associated with a complex fracture of the radial head, a portion of the radial head can be shaped and secured with one or two interfragmentary screws. Alternative sources of osteochondral bone include tricortical iliac crest bone graft, an allograft coronoid, and the proximal tip of the olecranon. If iliac crest bone graft is used, the capsule should be interposed between the graft and the trochlea to prevent direct contact and cartilage erosion.

Results and Complications

To our knowledge, the results of treatment of the terrible-triad injury have not been reported in a single series, but anecdotal experience justifies the name. In a series reviewed by Jupiter (unpublished data) of 56 patients who had a fracture-dislocation that was treated in Boston, 13 patients had a posterior dislocation of the elbow associated with a fracture of the radial head and coronoid process. Ten of the 13 elbows remained unstable following surgical treatment, with early arthrosis seen in all, and only 4 of the 13 patients had a satisfactory outcome. All but one had a type II coronoid fracture, and one had a type III fracture. It is of note that none of the type II lesions had stable internal fixation. It is also noteworthy that 90% of the patients who had removal of the fractured radial head had an unsatisfactory outcome, whereas only one third of the patients in whom the radial head was fixed had an unsatisfactory result.

These data support the concept that the terrible triad is a grave and complex injury and suggest that lesions of both the coronoid process and the radial head need to be stabilized or reconstructed whenever possible.

Fractures of the Radial Head

Fractures of the radial head are commonly associated with dislocation of the elbow and with isolated disruption of the medial collateral ligament, lateral collateral ligament, or interosseous membrane, or all three.[22-24] Fractures of the coronoid process, olecranon, and capitellum are also frequently associated with radial head fractures and may further impair elbow stability.[25,26] The presence of these concomitant injuries has important implications with regard to the management of a radial head fracture.

Anatomy and Biomechanics

The radial head has a concave dish that articulates with the capitellum. The posteromedial two thirds of the radial head articulates with the lesser sigmoid notch of the ulna, whereas the anterolateral one third of the radial head has no articulation. Therefore, internal fixation devices can be placed anterolaterally on the radial head without impingement against the ulna during rotation of the forearm.[27]

The radiocapitellar articulation accounts for as much as 60% of the load transfer across the elbow, and resisted isometric flexion can generate forces up to four times body weight.[28,29] Depressed fractures of the radial head decrease the surface area available for load transfer and decrease elbow stability by virtue of a loss of congruity of the articulating disk of the radial head with the capitellum. The radial head is an important valgus stabilizer of the elbow, particularly in the setting of an incompetent medial collateral ligament, which typically is disrupted in most fracture-dislocations.[2,4,22,24,25,30-36]

Classification

Mason[37] classified radial head fractures into three types. Type I indicates an undisplaced fracture; type II, a fracture with displaced wedge fragments; and type III, a comminuted fracture. Johnson[38] added a fourth type, a radial head fracture associated with an elbow dislocation. More recently, a management-based classification system was developed.[19] Type I indicates a fracture that is undisplaced or minimally displaced (less than 2 mm); type II, a fracture that is displaced but amenable to internal fixation; and type III, a fracture that is not amenable to internal fixation with use of current techniques. The latter classification is preferable because of its implications with regard to treatment.

Imaging

Anteroposterior, lateral, and oblique radiographs of the elbow usually provide sufficient information for the diagnosis and treatment of radial head fractures. Tomography or CT can be useful for evaluating selected fractures that are difficult to classify and can be helpful for preoperative planning. Posteroanterior radiographs of both wrists should be made for patients who have associated wrist pain and for those who have a comminuted fracture of the radial head because such patients have been found to have a higher prevalence of interosseous ligament injury.[22]

Treatment

A concomitant dislocation of the elbow should be reduced, and the radial head fracture should then be managed on its own merits. Decision making is influenced by patient-related factors (age, bone quality, and activity level) and fracture-related factors (fracture size, displacement, and location). For example, an older patient with osteoporosis and a comminuted radial head fracture is a poor candidate for internal fixation, with radial head arthroplasty being the preferred option in the setting of an associated elbow dislocation.

Undisplaced or minimally displaced radial head fractures (Hotchkiss type I) are occasionally seen with elbow dislocations, but displaced radial head fractures are more common when the elbow has been dislocated. As already mentioned, elbow dislocations with a radial head fracture also are typically associated with a coronoid fracture. When the elbow is dislocated and more than one third of the radial head is fractured and displaced greater than 2 mm (Hotchkiss type II), open reduction and internal fixation of the radial head fracture should be attempted when it is technically possible[19,39-41] (Fig. 5).

The management of displaced radial head fractures that are not amenable to internal fixation with use of current techniques (Hotchkiss type III) is controversial. Fragment excision, delayed excision of the radial head, and replacement of the radial head have all been considered. Acute excision of the radial head without replacement is contraindicated when there is concomitant disruption of the medial collateral ligament or the interosseous membrane.[24,31,32] Displaced fractures that block the rotation of the forearm and are too small, comminuted, or osteoporotic for stable internal fixation should be managed with fragment excision. The two prerequisites for fragment excision are evidence that the fragments to be excised do not articulate with the lesser sigmoid notch of the ulna and involvement of less than one third of the radial head. Delayed excision of the radial head can be used for an isolated, comminuted, displaced fracture that involves more than one third of the radial head and does not block forearm rotation, but it is not an option in a patient who has had a fracture-dislocation.[42-44] Arthroplasty of the radial head is indicated for displaced, comminuted radial head fractures when stable internal fixation is not possible and the fracture involves more than one third of the radial head.[45-52]

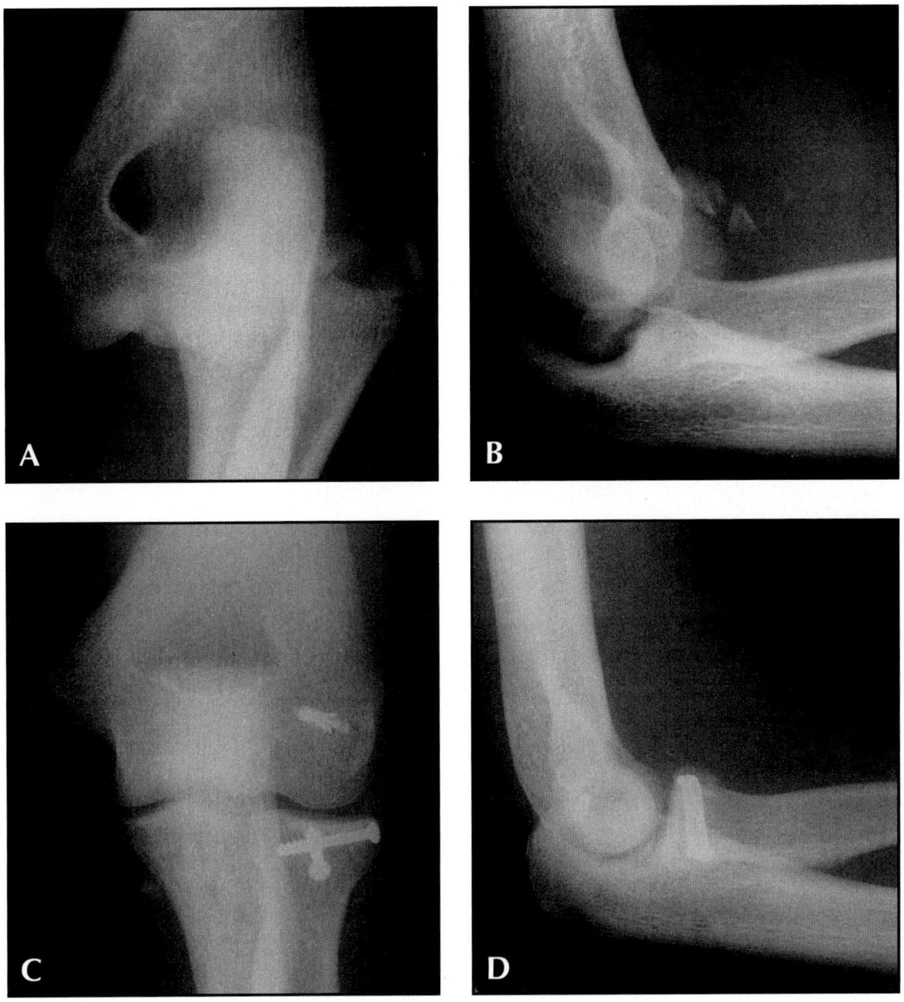

Fig. 5 Radiographs of the elbow of a 24-year-old man who fell off a mountain bike. **A** and **B,** Anteroposterior and lateral radiographs showing dislocation of the elbow with a type II radial head fracture, according to the classification system of Hotchkiss,[13] and a type II coronoid fracture, according to the system of Regan and Morrey.[14] **C** and **D,** Anteroposterior and lateral radiographs demonstrating an anatomic reduction after open reduction and internal fixation of the radial head and repair of the coronoid process with sutures. Early postoperative elbow motion was permitted, and a good result was achieved.

Surgical Techniques

The patient is placed in the supine position on the operating table with a tourniquet in place. Prophylactic antibiotic therapy is administered, and general or regional anesthesia is initiated. As in the case of a coronoid fracture, a posterior elbow incision is used. This approach decreases the risk of a cutaneous nerve injury compared with that associated with a separate medial incision.[53,54] Disruption of the lateral collateral ligament complex and the common extensor muscles from the lateral epicondyle is commonly noted in patients with an elbow dislocation. This approach also simplifies the surgical exposure of the radial head.[2] The interval between the anconeus and the extensor carpi ulnaris (the Kocher interval) is identified and developed. The lateral collateral ligament is incised at the midportion of the radial head, with the surgeon staying anterior to the lateral ulnar collateral ligament.[44,55] The annular ligament often must be divided to improve exposure. **(CD-11.1)**

Internal fixation is performed with use of 1.5-, 2.0-, or 2.7-mm screws and plates or 3.0-mm cannulated screws, depending on the size of the fragment. If plate fixation is used, the plate should be placed on the nonarticular portion of the radial head, which is the lateral part of the radial head when the arm is in neutral rotation.[56] Screws should be countersunk to avoid impingement with the lesser sigmoid notch. Threaded Kirschner wires may be useful for small fragments not amenable to screw fixation. Smooth Kirschner wires should be avoided because of their tendency to migrate during the postoperative period.

A radial head with a fracture that is not amenable to fixation should be replaced with a metallic radial head when there is a medial collateral or interosseous ligament injury.[24,31,32,45] Silicone implants have been used in the past; however, they have a high rate of failure due to fracture and fragmentation.[24,31,32,45,52] The fragmentation of silicone often produces synovitis. Clinical series of patients managed with metallic implants have shown good results.[47,48] Most metallic radial head implants have a monoblock design that makes implantation difficult because a wide surgical exposure is necessary. Recently, modular metallic radial head prostheses have become available. These prostheses have wider sizing options, and they may be easier to implant. A word of caution: the coronoid fragment should not be removed when the radial head is excised.

Following fragment excision, open reduction and internal fixation, or radial head replacement, the lateral collateral ligament complex and the common extensor muscle origins should be carefully repaired back to the lateral epicondyle with use of heavy sutures through drill-holes or suture anchors.[55] The fascial interval between the anconeus and the extensor carpi radialis also should be closed to augment lateral stability of the elbow.[57] The elbow should be carefully evaluated for stability, and concomitant injuries (for example, those involving the medial collateral ligament or the coronoid process) should be repaired when appropriate.

Postoperative Management

Indomethacin (75 mm daily) has been recommended for patients with complex elbow dislocations, to control postoperative pain and to potentially reduce the prevalence of heterotopic ossification.[56,58,59] This medication should be avoided by patients with a history of peptic ulcer disease or a known allergy. An early range of motion within a safe arc should be initiated, depending on associated fractures and ligamentous injuries. An extension-splinting program[60] is initiated as soon as stability improves, and the splint is worn at night for 12 weeks.

Complications

Osteonecrosis might be expected following open reduction and internal fixation of most radial head fractures, as the fragments typically have a precarious blood supply or no blood supply. Fortunately, the fragments usually heal and late collapse is uncommon. Nonunion is usually associated with osteonecrosis and seems to be more common in patients with a fracture involving the radial neck. Malunion is usually a consequence of inadequate fracture fixation or collapse due to osteonecrosis. Osteoarthritis is seen as a consequence of articular cartilage injury from the initial dislocation, late instability, or articular incongruity. Stiffness is a common sequela of a radial head fracture and may be due to capsular contracture or heterotopic ossification. Late axial or valgus instability is uncommon unless the radial head has been excised.

Hinged External Fixation for Unstable Elbows

It is not possible (or wise) to restore stability surgically after all dislocations or fracture-dislocations. In other cases, the constraints may have been repaired, but not securely, and need protection.

Indications

As with most surgical devices and methods, the two most important factors of success are how and when to apply them. This is especially true of hinged fixators about the elbow because of the difficulty and the time that application of the device adds to the procedure and to postoperative care. However, failure to use the device when indicated may result in a stiff and dislocated elbow, the worst of all worlds for a patient with a traumatized elbow.

The three primary indications are: (1) persistent instability in association with an acute fracture-dislocation despite attempted ligament repair and fracture fixation or radial head replacement, or both; (2) gross acute instability in a patient who is not a candidate for surgery; and (3) delayed treatment (approximately 4 weeks or more after the time of injury) of a dislocated and stiff elbow. A relative indication is the need to protect the stability and the fracture reduction during rehabilitation following surgical treatment of an unstable elbow.

The severity of a dislocation is seldom assessed, but it should be evaluated when hinged fixation is considered for the treatment of instability. Gross instability is not a condition that is easily recognized, but there are a few distinguishing features. In most cases, the patient has one or more of the following features: (1) a high-energy injury—that is, an injury sustained in a fall from a considerable height or in a motor-vehicle accident; (2) previous failed attempts at reduction or surgical repair of the dislocation; (3) multidirectional instability on examination after attempted or achieved reduction; and (4) a concomitant fracture of the radial head or the coronoid process, or both (the terrible triad of the elbow). None of these features alone creates a grossly unstable elbow, but if any one is present the others should be looked for.

Hinged fixation is used most commonly as a secondary device to protect surgically repaired or healing structures while permitting and assisting proper kinematic motion. Even if they are not repaired, the medial ligaments usually heal with mechanical integrity if they are protected. Conversely, the lateral ligaments should be repaired or reconstructed, as detailed in other sections.

There are a few situations in which application of the devices alone may be both adequate and optimal. In patients who have polytrauma, time may not permit full anatomic restoration of all structures. In this setting, protecting the elbow in a reduced position before definitive care will assist in the subsequent treatment.

Surgical Technique

At the present time, three very different hinged external fixators for the elbow are commercially available. They each have their own advantages and disadvantages. With two of the devices, the use of a temporary axis pin is crucial to replicate the kinematic axis of the elbow. In earlier reports and designs, the axis pin was left in place in the distal part of the humerus for the duration of use.[59] However, because pin-tract infection at the site of the axis pin led to joint infections, a temporary axis pin is now used with all of the devices. The long-term use of a pin through the axis of rotation at the distal aspect of the humerus is no longer recommended.

In most cases, repair of the fractures and ligaments obviates the need for a fixator. To determine if a fixator is needed, the stability of the joint should be gently tested before application of the fixator, while the ligament sutures are held under tension. If the elbow is stable and the fractures require minimal protection, no fixator is needed.

When the hinged fixator is applied after fixation of the fractures, care must be taken not to disrupt the ligament repair and the delicate fracture fixation. Repair of the coronoid process, so crucial to long-term success yet often quite vulnerable to loading during application of the hinge, must be protected during placement of the device. It is often better to position the sutures for ligament repair without securing them with knots, in anticipation of fixator placement. Because of unfamiliarity with the device or the complexity of fixator application, the repaired ligaments and fractures could be subjected to failure loads, defeating the purpose of the repair efforts. If the sutures for ligament repairs are tied in place after the fixator is applied, tension in the repairs is achieved with confidence that there is no eccentric displacement of the repair.

Technical Tips

The proper technical application of these devices cannot be overemphasized. The most crucial and usually the first step of hinged fixator application is replication of the recognized axis of rotation. If the axis is not replicated or if pin placement in the humerus or ulna impedes motion, the use of the device is entirely compromised and provides little, if any, value. Because the axis of elbow motion is within the distal aspect of the humerus, the frame is attached to the humerus first. A temporary joint-axis pin is placed, and the frame is built from this temporary axis pin. Once the fixator is properly attached to the humerus, the ulna may be reduced and attached to the fixator.

In most cases in which surgery is performed on a grossly unstable elbow, both the medial and the lateral aspect of the distal part of the humerus are exposed and visible. This permits visualization of the instant center of rotation on both sides. The temporary axis pin should penetrate both central points of rotation, ensuring proper function of the hinge. If the distal part of the humerus is not directly visible, the pin and axis must be visualized with fluoroscopic imaging. There are many methods for placement of the axis pin across the distal aspect of the humerus, and these are usually detailed in the instructional materials provided for each particular device. Anterior cruciate ligament drill guides or variations of them may help.

On the medial side, injury to the ulnar nerve is avoided by exposing the nerve anchor or transposing it, or both. The center of rotation from the medial view is slightly distal and anterior to the medial epicondyle. From the lateral view, the center of rotation is in the center of the capitellum. If there is concern about the location on visual inspection, fluoroscopic images should be made. Both the anteroposterior and lateral views are needed to properly ascertain the pin location. As one gains experience, the localization and placement becomes less time-consuming and challenging.

After the axis pin is properly placed in the distal part of the humerus, pin fixation of the frame to the humerus must be done. Adjustment of pin fixation may be necessary if plates on the distal part of the humerus or the proximal part of the ulna interfere with the normal pin position.

Secure fixation of the frame to the distal part of the humerus may require more than just two pins (one medial and one lateral) in the supracondylar region of the humerus. In such cases, an extension can be added onto the frame, with half-pins placed in the humerus more proximally. When pins are placed more proximally in the humerus, the radial nerve should be protected from injury. The half-pins should also be placed to avoid impaling muscle or tendon, because this will impede movement. Placement of pins in the ulna is usually simpler.

Half-pins attached to the fixator should be placed so that there is no skin under tension. The skin tension against the pins should be inspected in all positions of flexion and extension. Skin under tension should be released. Redness, pain, and drainage are avoided by meticulous pin-site care. If skin tension is noted later, it should be released. Antibiotics may be needed if there is erythema and increased pain.

Loss of reduction and mechanical failure can occur. Frequent clinical examination and radiographs to confirm maintenance of the reduction are mandatory. The clamps, nuts, bolts, and frames should be inspected frequently for any loosening during the first few weeks. As rehabilitation activity becomes more vigorous, there is also more stress on the components, which can lead to loosening of the pins

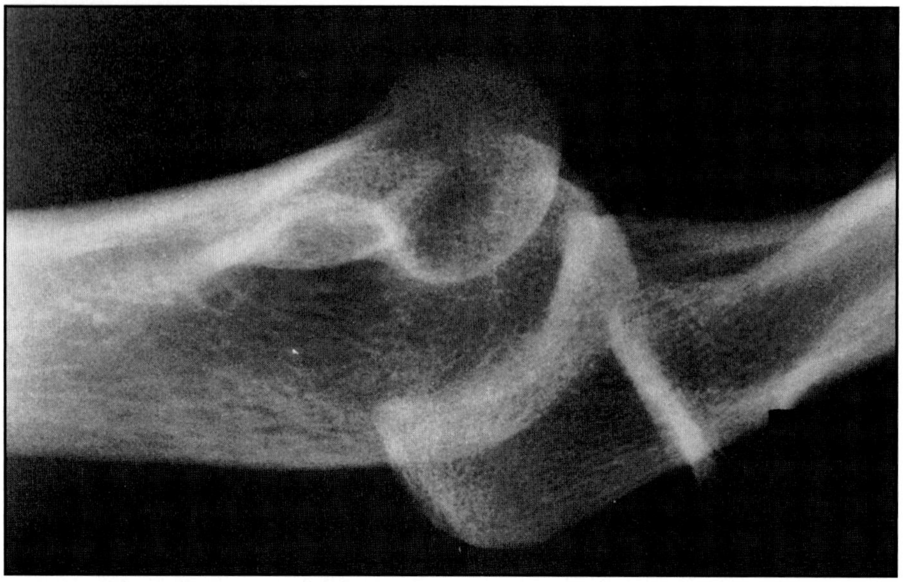

Fig. 6 Lateral radiograph of an elbow with recurrent posterolateral rotatory instability, showing the radial head to be aligned posterior to the capitellum. The ulnohumeral relationship does not appear to be grossly abnormal but, in fact, reveals subtle subluxation.

in the bone or component failure, or both. The components should be routinely inspected for signs of fatigue.

Recurrent Elbow Instability

Lateral collateral ligament insufficiency is most commonly seen after elbow dislocation, particularly in young patients. It is the essential lesion leading to elbow instability.[35] While most studies have indicated that both the medial and the lateral collateral ligament complex are acutely disrupted with an elbow dislocation, the residual insufficiency most commonly involves the lateral collateral ligament complex for reasons that have not yet been elucidated. This insufficiency gives rise to recurrent posterolateral rotatory instability.[4]

History

In the vast majority of patients, dislocation with or without fracture accounts for the injury.[61] Sometimes the problem is quite obvious, as the patient is able to demonstrate the instability; however, it may be more subtle. Sometimes the patient has noticed only pain and discomfort and is not aware of instability. Additional symptoms include painful catching, slippage, or clicking with flexion and extension. A feeling of slippage of the joint in and out of place may be reported by the patient. The elbow position most typically associated with symptoms is approximately 40° of flexion with the forearm in supination. The subluxation reduces in pronation. The patient may have noted that specific activity such as pushing on the armrests when rising from a chair reproduces the symptoms of instability.

The physical examination includes the lateral pivot-shift maneuver, the posterolateral rotatory drawer test, and the apprehension test. In some instances, varus stress-testing may suggest a lateral collateral ligament insufficiency. Rising from a chair while pushing on the armrests has been suggested by Morrey and Regan[61] to be particularly helpful, either to demonstrate the instability or as an apprehension-eliciting maneuver.

Radiographs

Classically, the elbow appears normal on anteroposterior radiographs or there is slight widening of the radiohumeral joint. On lateral radiographs, the radial head may appear to be situated posterior to the capitellum (Fig. 6). Special studies, MRI, and CT have not been necessary or useful in our experience.

Arthroscopy

In some instances, when the presentation does not suggest the injury or the findings on the physical examination are not convincing, or when there is a possiblity of an intra-articular lesion, arthroscopic examination of the elbow may be helpful. Arthroscopy will reveal the laxity of the radiohumeral joint and thus confirm the lesion.

Management

In our experience, the ligament does not become stable over time, except possibly when a patient is seen in the very early stages. By definition, this is a recurrent problem, and it needs a surgical reconstruction or the patient must live with the problem. The latter is rarely acceptable to the patient, as symptoms interfere with daily activity.

Surgical Technique

The patient is placed supine on the operating table, and the arm is brought across the chest. A 10-cm incision is made at the Kocher interval, roughly equidistant proximal and distal to the epicondyle. The dissection proceeds through the Kocher interval, with separation of the anconeus from the extensor carpi ulnaris and identification of the lateral collateral ligament complex, the supracondylar ridge, and the crest of the supinator. The anconeus is further reflected from the margin of the supinator crest and from the lateral face of the proximal part of the ulna. The tubercle of the supinator ridge is palpated. The lateral epicondyle is exposed along with 2 cm of the proximal supracondylar ridge anteriorly and posteriorly. **(CD-11.2)**

The insertion site for the tendon graft is then prepared by creating two

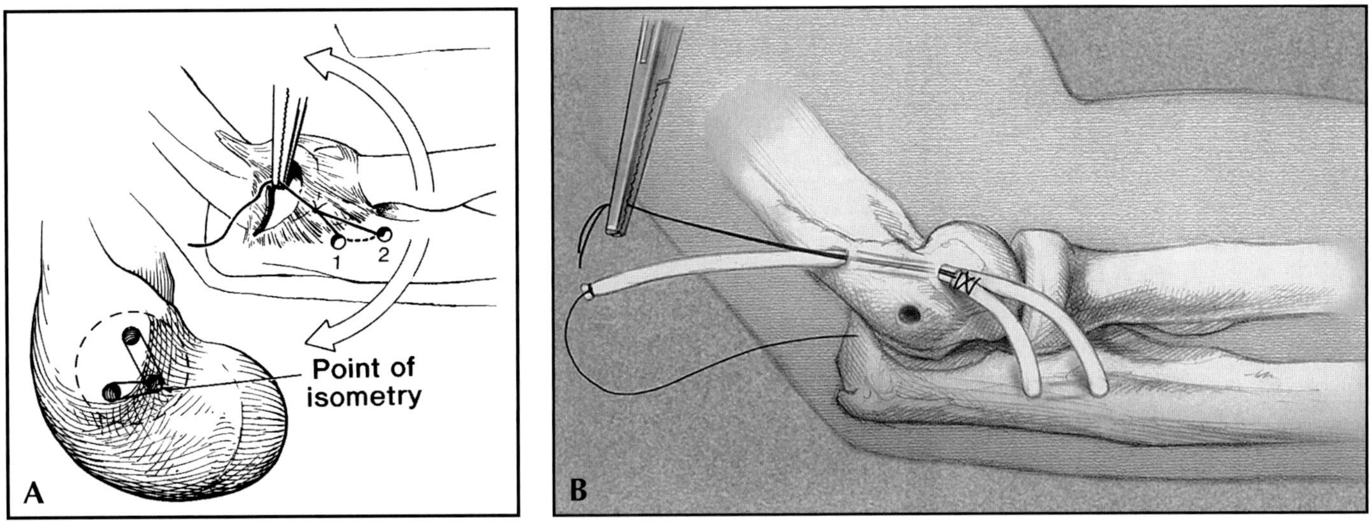

Fig. 7 A, Drawing showing a suture being passed through the osseous tunnels in the ulna distal to the tubercle of the supinator crest. The isometric point is determined by the point at which there is no laxity or increased tension on the suture through the arc of elbow flexion. **B,** Drawing showing a tendon (palmaris longus) graft placed through holes in the ulna and brought into the isometric origin near the lateral epicondyle, out through an exit tunnel proximally, and back into the bone for fixation. (Reproduced with permission from the Mayo Foundation, Rochester, MN.)

drill-holes in the ulna: one near the tubercle on the supinator crest (which is felt by stressing the elbow in varus or supination) and the other, 1.25 cm proximally at the base of the annular ligament (Fig. 7, *A*). A suture is passed through these two holes and tied to itself. It is then pulled toward the lateral epicondyle and grasped with a hemostat at the estimated isometric center of the rotation of the elbow. The isometric ligament origin is then determined by flexion and extension of the elbow to see if the suture moves. No movement occurs when the suture and hemostat are on the isometric point. The isometric point is more anterior than is usually thought to be the case. It is important to remember that instability occurs in extension so the graft must be taut in extension. A Y-shaped tunnel is placed in the lateral epicondyle, with the isometric spot widened in order to accept a three-ply graft. Currently, one of us (BFM) prefers to use the plantaris tendon if a substantial palmaris longus is not present. A 16-cm graft allows a reliable three-ply passage across the joint (Fig. 7, *B*). There are a number of options for fixing the graft into the humerus. One or both limbs of the graft pass into the isometric origin. We prefer to place a stitch in the first two limbs of the graft after the graft is passed through the tunnel in the ulna. Both this stitch (the yoke stitch) and the graft are then passed through one of the tunnels in the humerus. The free end of the graft just reaches the tunnel, ensuring a two-ply passage as the free end of the tendon graft is brought through the holes in the epicondylar region and back down distally across the joint. This end is usually passed back into the ulnar tunnel if sufficient length is present. If not, it is sutured to itself distally near the ulnar tunnel. Once this has been done, the forearm is placed in 40° of flexion and full pronation while axial tension is placed on the yoke stitch, which is then tied. This applies additional tension to the reconstruction.

Rehabilitation

The elbow is placed in 70° to 80° of flexion with the forearm in full pronation. The arm is held in this position for 10 to 14 days, and then the patient is permitted protected motion in a hinged brace for 2 to 6 weeks, with flexion allowed as tolerated. After 6 weeks, the patient may remove the hinged splint for sedentary activities, but otherwise the splint is worn for most activities. At the end of an additional 6 weeks, the use of the splint is discontinued, but conscious protection is recommended for a total of 12 weeks after surgery. Supination is gradually allowed and encouraged, but excessive force is avoided. After 12 weeks, activity is gradually resumed, with 100% activity allowed at 6 months.

Results

Although we are currently reassessing our clinical experience, to date it has been suggested that, if there is no degenerative arthritis and if the radial head is intact, approximately 90% of patients have a satisfactory outcome with no subsequent recurrent subluxation.[62-64] If the radial head is excised or if there is degenerative arthritis of the ulnohumeral joint, the satisfactory result decreases to between 67% and 75%. Delayed laxity, redislocation,

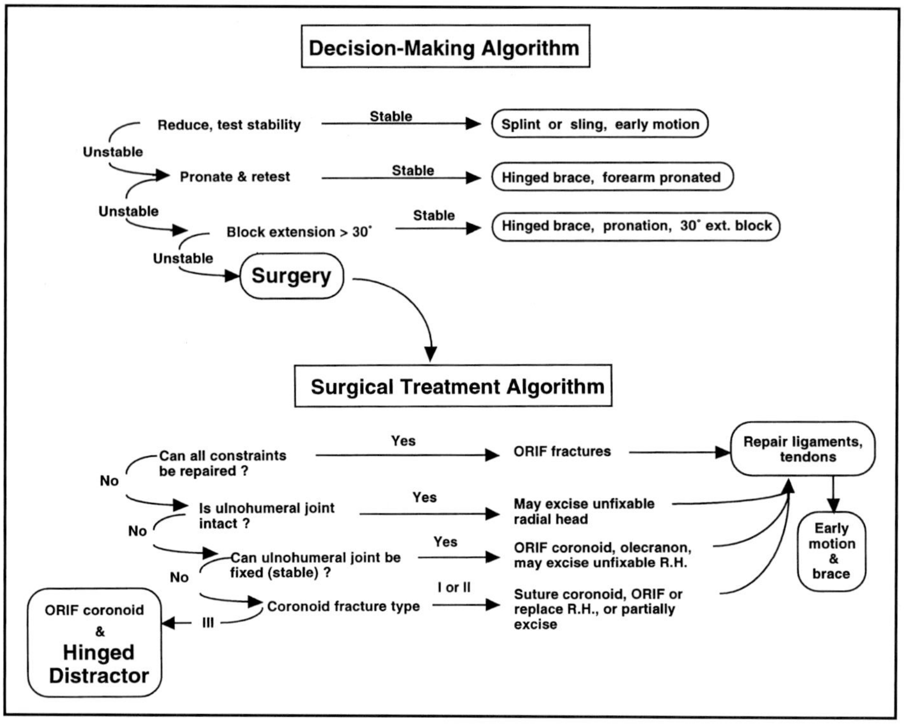

Fig. 8 Chart showing the decision-making algorithm for acute dislocations and fracture-dislocations. The term stable implies functional stability, meaning that the elbow does not apparently subluxate in the functional arc of motion and appears reduced on plain radiographs. ORIF = open reduction and internal fixation; RH = radial head. (Reproduced with permission from the Mayo Foundation, Rochester, MN.)

and reinjury have been observed, usually in association with substantial stress. We accept a mild (10°) flexion contracture, because the most vulnerable position of instability is in full extension.

Summary of Treatment Principles

Reduction of Acute Dislocations and Management After Reduction

The initial treatment of an elbow dislocation without associated fractures is a closed reduction. The reduction should be done with the forearm in supination to clear the coronoid process under the trochlea, thereby minimizing additional trauma to the medial soft tissues that have not yet been disrupted. Essentially, the deformity is recreated in order to make the reduction possible and easy. A simple principle to follow in managing a patient after reduction is to place the elbow in a splint for a brief period (3 to 5 days) and then to start allowing movement unless the elbow tends to subluxate or dislocate. One must be vigilant. Subluxation or dislocation must be detected by careful examination throughout the comfortable range of motion and by radiographic examination, with anteroposterior and lateral radiographs made initially after the reduction and every five to seven days for the first three weeks. If subluxation or dislocation is detected clinically or radiographically at any time, a change of treatment is required.

The so-called stage or degree of instability dictates the treatment. If the elbow feels stable in all positions of forearm rotation, a hinged brace is not necessary. Such stability is usual. When the elbow is stable to valgus stress only with the forearm in pronation (that is, a stage 3A dislocation), the injury is treated immediately in a cast-brace that allows unlimited flexion and extension and holds the forearm in full pronation. A summary of these treatment principles is depicted in Figure 8.

Management of Acute Fracture-Dislocations

The presence of fractures usually changes the management, and almost always these fractures should be treated surgically. In general, the approach to the unstable elbow is to fix the bones internally and then repair the ligaments (particularly on the lateral side) so that early motion can be commenced.

The coronoid process is an important part of the force-bearing surface of the elbow and is important for stability. Type I and type II fractures (those involving 50% of the height of the coronoid process or less) should be fixed if the joint is subluxated or dislocated. Type III fractures (those involving more than 50% of the coronoid process) cause instability and should be fixed. Type III fracture-dislocations have traditionally been associated with a poor prognosis.

Fractures of the radial head associated with an elbow dislocation or subluxation are best managed by internal fixation when technically possible. When the radial head is comminuted and has to be excised, prosthetic replacement is indicated if the elbow is unstable and cannot be rendered stable by ligament reconstruction alone.

Repair of an Acute Ligament Injury

Repair of an acute ligament injury is indicated in all fracture-dislocations requiring internal fixation of the radial head or the coronoid process, or both, and following reduction of a dislocation if gross instability does not allow early protected motion in a cast-brace without subluxation. In such cases, the ligament or ligaments may have been avulsed and can be repaired directly to bone with heavy sutures. In some cases, passing a heavy absorbable suture through the same course as that for a late ligament reconstruction and fixing it to the normal ligament attachments on the epicondyle and the ulna augments the repair.

References

1. Josefsson PO, Gentz CF, Johnell O, Wendeberg B: Surgical versus nonsurgical treatment of ligamentous injuries following dislocations of the elbow joint. *Clin Orthop* 1987;214:165-169.
2. Josefsson PO, Gentz CF, Johnell O, Wendeberg B: Surgical versus non-surgical treatment of ligamentous injuries following dislocation of the elbow joint: A prospective randomized study. *J Bone Joint Surg Am* 1987;69:605-608.
3. Josefsson PO, Johnell O, Wendeberg B: Ligamentous injuries in dislocations of the elbow joint. *Clin Orthop* 1987;221:221-225.
4. O'Driscoll SW, Morrey BF, Korinek S, An KN: Elbow subluxation and dislocation: A spectrum of instability. *Clin Orthop* 1992;280:186-197.
5. Osborne G, Cotterill P: Recurrent dislocation of the elbow. *J Bone Joint Surg Br* 1966;48: 340-346.
6. Roberts PH: Dislocation of the elbow. *Br J Surg* 1969;56:806-815.
7. O'Driscoll SW: Classification and spectrum of elbow instability: Recurrent instability, in Morrey BF (ed): *The Elbow and Its Disorders*, ed 2. Philadelphia, PA, WB Saunders, 1993, pp 453-463.
8. O'Driscoll SW: Elbow instability. *Hand Clin* 1994;10;405-415.
9. O'Driscoll SW, Bell DF, Morrey BF: Posterolateral rotatory instability of the elbow. *J Bone Joint Surg Am* 1991;73:440-446.
10. Broberg MA, Morrey BF: Results of treatment of fracture-dislocations of the elbow. *Clin Orthop* 1987;216:109-119.
11. Josefsson PO, Gentz CF, Johnell O, Wendeberg B: Dislocations of the elbow and intraarticular fractures. *Clin Orthop* 1989;246;126-130.
12. Ring D, Jupiter JB: Fracture-dislocation of the elbow. *J Bone Joint Surg Am* 1998;80:566-580.
13. Hotchkiss RN: Fractures and dislocations of the elbow, in Rockwood CA Jr, Green DP, Bucholz RW, Heckman JD (eds): *Fractures in Adults*, ed 4. Philadelphia, PA, Lippincott-Raven, 1996, pp 929-1024.
14. Regan W, Morrey BF: Fractures of the coronoid process of the ulna. *J Bone Joint Surg Am* 1989;71:1348-1354.
15. Cage DJ, Abrams RA, Callahan JJ, Botte MJ: Soft tissue attachments of the ulnar coronoid process: An anatomic study with radiographic correlation. *Clin Orthop* 1995;320:154-158.
16. An KN, Hui FC, Morrey BF, Linscheid RL, Chao EY: Muscles across the elbow joint: A biomechanical analysis. *J Biomech* 1981;14: 659-669.
17. Meeder PJ, Holz U: Replacement-plasty of the coronoid process in unstable elbow joint dislocations with avulsion fracture of the coronoid process and radius head crush fracture. *Aktuelle Traumat* 1985;15:89-90.
18. Stankovi P, Zuhlke V, Persitzky V: Isolated fractures of the coronoid processus of the ulna. *Unfallheilkunde* 1976;79:395-398.
19. Hotchkiss RN: Displaced fractures of the radial head: Internal fixation or excision? *J Am Acad Orthop Surgeons* 1997;5:1-10.
20. McWhorter GL: Fracture of both the coronoid and the olecranon processes of the ulna: Indications for operation and treatment. *J Bone Joint Surg* 1972:767-777.
21. O'Driscoll SW: Olecranon and coronoid fractures, in Norris TR (ed): *Orthopaedic Knowledge Update: Shoulder and Elbow*. Rosemont, IL, American Academy of Orthopaedic Surgeons, 1997, 405-413.
22. Davidson PA, Moseley JB Jr, Tullos HS: Radial head fracture: A potentially complex injury. *Clin Orthop* 1993;297:224-230.
23. Morrey BF (ed): *The Elbow and Its Disorders*, ed 2. Philadelphia, PA, WB Saunders, 1993.
24. Sellman DC, Seitz WH Jr, Postak PD, Greenwald AS: Reconstructive strategies for radioulnar dissociation: A biomechanical study. *J Orthop Trauma* 1995;9:516-522.
25. King GJW, Morrey BF, An KN: Stabilizers of the elbow. *J Shoulder Elbow Surg* 1993;2: 165-174.
26. Regan W, Morrey BF: Classification and treatment of coronoid process fractures. *Orthopedics* 1992;15:845-848.
27. Smith GR, Hotchkiss RN: Radial head and neck fractures: Anatomic guidelines for proper placement of internal fixation. *J Shoulder Elbow Surg* 1996;5:113-117.
28. Amis AA, Dowson D, Wright V: Elbow joint force predictions for some strenuous isometric actions. *J Biomech* 1980;13:765-775.
29. Halls AA, Travill A: Transmission of pressures across the elbow joint. *Anat Rec* 1964;150: 243-247.
30. Frankle MA, Koval KJ, Sanders RW, Zuckerman JD: Radial head fractures associated with elbow dislocations treated by immediate stabilization and early motion. *J Shoulder Elbow Surg* 1999;8:355-360.
31. Hotchkiss RN, Weiland AJ: Valgus stability of the elbow. *J Orthop Res* 1987;5:372-377.
32. King GJ, Zarzour ZD, Rath DA, Dunning CE, Patterson SD, Johnson JA: Metallic radial head arthroplasty improves valgus stability of the elbow. *Clin Orthop* 1999:368;114-125.
33. Mehlhoff TL, Noble PC, Bennett JB, Tullos HS: Simple dislocation of the elbow in the adult: Results after closed treatment. *J Bone Joint Surg Am* 1988;70:244-249.
34. Morrey BF, Chao EY, Hui FC: Biomechanical study of the elbow following excision of the radial head. *J Bone Joint Surg Am* 1979;61:63-68.
35. Morrey BF, Tanaka S, An K-N: Valgus stability of the elbow: A definition of primary and secondary constraints. *Clin Orthop* 1991;265: 187-195.
36. Pribyl CR, Kester MA, Cook SD, Edmunds JO, Brunet ME: The effect of the radial head and prosthetic radial head replacement on resisting valgus stress at the elbow. *Orthopedics* 1986;9:723-726.
37. Mason ML: Some observations on fractures of the head of the radius with a review of one hundred cases. *Br J Surg* 1954;42:123-132.
38. Johnson G: A follow-up of one hundred cases of fracture of the head of the radius with a review of the literature. *Ulster Med J* 1952;31:51-56.
39. Esser RD, Davis S, Taavao T: Fractures of the radial head treated by internal fixation: Late results in 26 cases. *J Orthop Trauma* 1995;9: 318-323.
40. Geel CW, Palmer AK, Ruedi T, Leutenegger AF: Internal fixation of proximal radial head fractures. *J Orthop Trauma* 1990;4:270-274.
41. King GJ, Evans DC, Kellam JF: Open reduction and internal fixation of radial head fractures. *J Orthop Trauma* 1991;5:21-28.
42. Goldberg I, Peylan J, Yosipovitch Z: Late results of excision of the radial head for an isolated closed fracture. *J Bone Joint Surg Am* 1986;68:675-679.
43. Janssen RP, Vegter J: Resection of the radial head after Mason type-III fractures of the elbow: Follow-up at 16 to 30 years. *J Bone Joint Surg Br* 1998;80:231-233.

44. Miki D, Vukadinovi SM: Late results in fractures of the radial head treated by excision. *Clin Orthop* 1983;181:220-228.

45. Carn RM, Medige J, Curtain D, Koenig A: Silicone rubber replacement of the severely fractured radial head. *Clin Orthop* 1986;209: 259-269.

46. Gupta GG, Lucas G, Hahn DL: Biomechanical and computer analysis of radial head prostheses. *J Shoulder Elbow Surg* 1997;6:37-48.

47. Harrington IJ, Tountas AA: Replacement of the radial head in the treatment of unstable elbow fractures. *Injury* 1981;12:405-412.

48. Knight DJ, Rymaszewski LA, Amis AA, Miller JH: Primary replacement of the fractured radial head with a metal prosthesis. *J Bone Joint Surg Br* 1993;75:572-576.

49. Morrey BF, Askew L, Chao EY: Silastic prosthetic replacement for the radial head. *J Bone Joint Surg Am* 1981;63:454-458.

50. Stoffelen DV, Holdsworth BJ: Excision or Silastic replacement for comminuted radial head fractures: A long-term follow-up. *Acta Orthop Belg* 1994;60:402-407.

51. Swanson AB, Jaeger SH, La Rochelle D: Comminuted fractures of the radial head: The role of silicone-implant replacement arthroplasty. *J Bone Joint Surg Am* 1981;63:1039-1049.

52. Vanderwilde RS, Morrey BF, Melberg MW, Vinh TN: Inflammatory arthritis after failure of silicone rubber replacement of the radial head. *J Bone Joint Surg Br* 1994;76:78-81.

53. Dowdy PA, Bain GI, King GJW, Patterson SD: The midline posterior elbow incision: An anatomical appraisal. *J Bone Joint Surg Br* 1995;77:696-699.

54. Patterson SD, King GJ, Bain GI: Abstract: A posterior global approach to the elbow. *J Bone Joint Surg Br* 1995;77(suppl 3):316.

55. Morrey BF, An K-N: Articular and ligamentous contributions to the stability of the elbow joint. *Am J Sports Med* 1983;11:315-319.

56. Segstro R, Morley-Forster PK, Lu G: Indomethacin as a postoperative analgesic for total hip arthroplasty. *Can J Anaesth* 1991;38: 578-581.

57. Cohen MS, Hastings H II: Rotatory instability of the elbow: The anatomy and role of the lateral stabilizers. *J Bone Joint Surg Am* 1997;79: 225-233.

58. Kjaersgaard-Andersen P, Ritter MA: Prevention of formation of heterotopic bone after total hip arthroplasty. *J Bone Joint Surg Am* 1991;73:942-947.

59. Knelles D, Barthel T, Karrer A, Kraus U, Eulert J, Kolbl O: Prevention of heterotopic ossification after total hip replacement: A prospective, randomised study using acetylsalicylic acid, indomethacin and fractional or single-dose irradiation. *J Bone Joint Surg Br* 1997;79:596-602.

60. Morrey B, Regan W: Post-traumatic stiffness: Distraction arthroplasty, in Morrey BF (ed): *The Elbow and Its Disorders*, ed 2. Philadelphia, WB Saunders, 1993, pp 472-491.

61. Morrey B, Regan W: Physical examination of the elbow, in Morrey B (ed): *The Elbow and Its Disorders*, ed 3. New York, NY, WB Saunders, 2000.

62. Nestor BJ, O'Driscoll SW, Morrey BF: Ligamentous reconstruction for posterolateral rotatory instability of the elbow. *J Bone Joint Surg Am* 1992;74:1235-1241.

63. Hamilton CD, Glousman RE, Jobe FW, Brault J, Pink M, Perry J: Dynamic stability of the elbow: Electromyographic analysis of the flexor pronator group and the extensor group in pitchers with valgus instability. *J Shoulder Elbow Surg* 1996;5:347-354.

64. Linscheid RL, O'Driscoll SW: Elbow dislocations, in Morrey BF (ed): *The Elbow and Its Disorders*, ed 2. Philadelphia, PA, WB Saunders Company, 1993, pp 441-452.

References to Video

Morrey BF: Distal humerus fractures: Surgical exposure. *Elbow Cadaveric Surgical Demonstration.* Rosemont, IL, American Academy of Orthopaedic Surgeons, Summer Institute, 1999.

Morrey BF: Lateral instability. *Elbow Cadaveric Surgical Demonstration.* Rosemont, IL, American Academy of Orthopaedic Surgeons, Summer Institute, 1999.

SECTION

2

Hand and Wrist

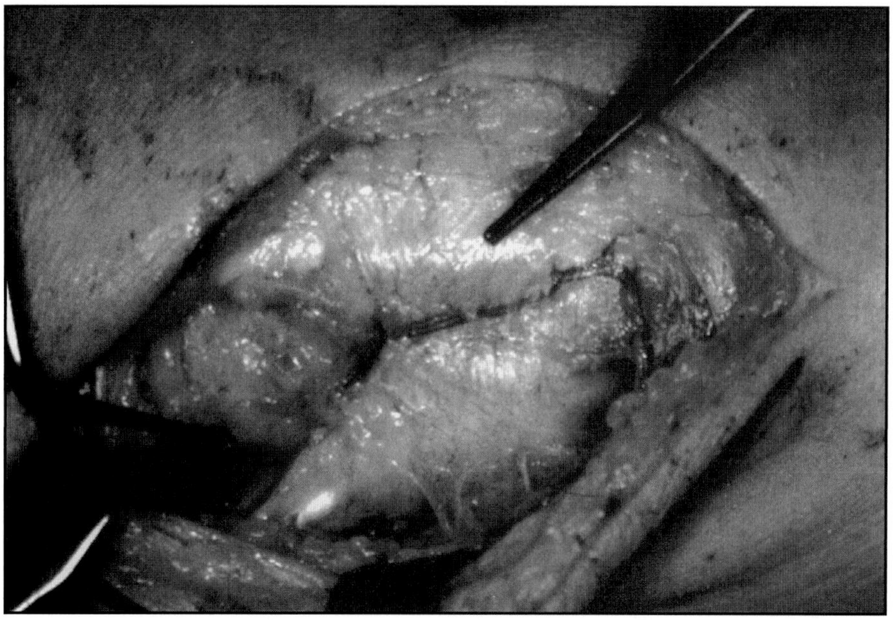

12 Traumatic and Reconstructive Problems of the Scaphoid

13 Carpal Instability ***(with video clip on enclosed CD)***

12

Traumatic and Reconstructive Problems of the Scaphoid

Jesse B. Jupiter, MD
Alexander Y. Shin, MD
Thomas E. Trumble, MD
Diego L. Fernandez, MD, PhD

Introduction

The treatment of traumatic and reconstructive problems of the carpal scaphoid can be fraught with difficulty. Scaphoid fractures more commonly occur in young, active adults, many of whom are uniquely dependent on the integrity of upper limb function for work or sport.[1-10] It is remarkable that, despite the enormity of publications on the subject, the management of scaphoid fractures still is based to a large extent on anecdote and tradition.

The past decade has witnessed substantial technical improvements in the diagnostic and surgical treatment of the scaphoid fracture and associated complications.[11] MRI has enabled presence of an occult fracture to be determined on the day of injury; it also has enabled preoperative assessment of the vascular status of the proximal pole.[12-16] Refinements in internal fixation techniques, especially those involving minimally invasive screw fixation with fluoroscopic or arthroscopic control, have permitted the reduction of prolonged cast immobilization and diminished the overall cost.[17-23] Standardized techniques of vascularized pedicled bone grafting have dramatically improved the salvage of avascular proximal pole fractures or nonunions, ultimately reducing the need for functionally unpredictable reconstructive wrist procedures.[24-33]

Functional Anatomy

The bony anatomy of the carpus was first clearly identified by Andreas Vesalius in 1548.[34] He numbered the carpal bones from radial to ulnar, starting in the proximal row followed by those in the distal row. In 1653, Michael Lyser, a Flemish anatomist, coined the term "cotyloides" derived from the Greek term *kotyloeides*, which means cup-shaped, to describe the scaphoid. In the 1700s, Alexander Monroe used the term "scaphoideum" from the Greek word *scaphon*, meaning boat-shaped, while Albinus of Leiden used the Latin word, *navicular* (also meaning boat-shaped) to describe this carpal bone.[35,36] At present, the International Federation of Societies for Surgery of the Hand recognizes the term scaphoid and its equivalent to describe this carpal bone.[37]

Osteogenesis of the scaphoid arises from the fusion of two chondrified elements called centralia. The radiale and ulnare distal centralia fuse at approximately 9 weeks gestation. Failure of fusion results in an os centrale, which is present in approximately 1.5% of the population.[38]

The scaphoid is the largest bone in the proximal carpal row, playing an integral role in the stability of the carpus. Articular facets encompass nearly 80% of the scaphoid surface area. The lateroproximal facet is a convex surface articulating with the scaphoid fossa of the radius. The lunar shaped medial facet forms the articulation with the lunate. The distal medial facet is concave and faces the lateral aspect of the head of the capitate. Last, the distal facet is convex and divided by a sagittal smooth ridge forming articular facets for the trapezoid and trapezium.

The rounded prominence on the volar radial aspect is termed the scaphoid tuberosity or distal pole. This locus provides the zone of attachment for the radioscaphocapitate and scaphotrapezial-trapezoid ligaments in addition to acting as a pivot point for the flexor carpi radialis. The dorsal surface of the scaphoid has a nonarticular region called the scaphoid ridge into which nearly 80% of the vascular elements enter the bone.[39,40] In addition, the dorsal scaphoid provides a site of attachment for the dorsal scaphotriquetral ligament.

The vascular supply of the scaphoid has been described by a number of investigators.[29,39-41] Taleisnik and Kelly[41] suggested that most of the vascular supply arises from three branches of the radial artery, with the laterovolar vessel providing the main contribution to the intraosseous circulation. Studies by Gelberman and Menon[39] demonstrated two major vessels providing blood supply to the scaphoid. The proximal pole and 70% to 80% of the scaphoid receive their blood supply from vessels entering the dorsal ridge, while the tuberosity and distal 20%

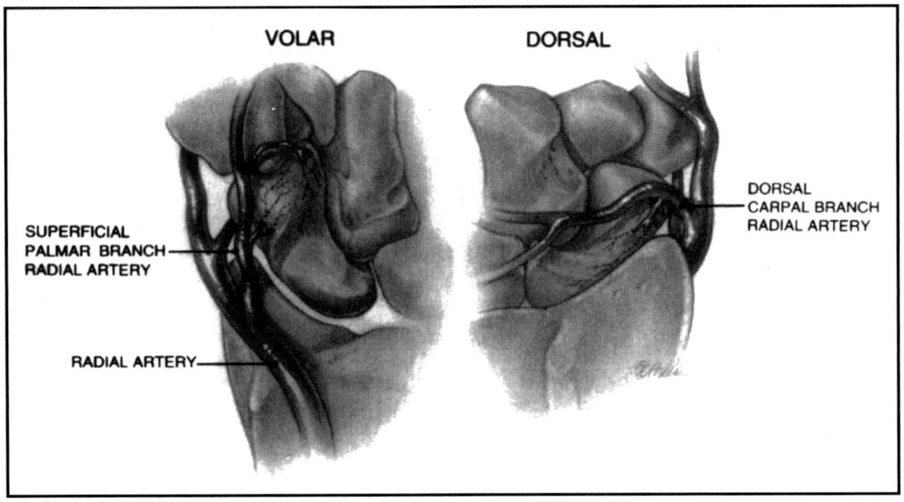

Fig. 1 The vascular supply to the scaphoid. Two main pedicles include a dorsal and volar artery; both are branches of the radial artery. (Reproduced with permission from Amadio PC, Taleisnik J: Fractures of the carpal bones, in Green DP (ed): *Operative Hand Surgery*, ed 4. Philadelphia, PA, Churchill Livingstone, 1999.)

to 30% of the scaphoid are supplied from the volar vessels (Fig. 1).

Given that the majority of vascular elements enter at or distal to the waist of the scaphoid, it has long been thought that a volar surgical approach is safer than the dorsal approach. In reality, however, no approach completely avoids jeopardizing the vascular supply.

Fracture Assessment and Scaphoid Imaging

Scaphoid fractures account for almost two thirds of all carpal fractures. Therefore, a high degree of suspicion should follow after a hyperextension injury to the wrist.[42] In general, axial load on the thenar eminence, with the wrist extended beyond 90°, may result in a scaphoid fracture. There truly may be no such injury as a sprained wrist, adding to the difficulty in determining the true incidence of scaphoid fractures. The classic clinical signs include pain with pronation against resistance;[43] tenderness in the anatomic snuff box;[2] and scaphoid tuberosity tenderness.[44] The axial compression test[45] associated with wrist swelling has been shown to be the most accurate indicator of a scaphoid fracture, even in the presence of normal radiographs.[46]

The standardized radiographs should include anteroposterior (AP) and lateral views of the wrist as well as special scaphoid views including a posteroanterior view, with the wrist in ulnar deviation, pronated obliquely at 45° and ulnarly elevated obliquely at 45°.

Upward of 2% to 3% of acute fractures will not be seen on the initial radiographs and can be termed occult fractures.[47] Conversely, normal bone markings (dorsal lip of the radius or the dorsal ridge or tuberosity of the scaphoid) may render fracture exclusion difficult. Comparative views of the uninjured wrist may be helpful in these instances.[48]

When faced with clinical findings consistent with a scaphoid fracture but having normal-appearing radiographs, the classic teaching has been to immobilize the hand and wrist and repeat radiographs at 10 days, and even at 3 weeks if tenderness persists. At that point, 99-Tc nuclear bone scans, trispiral tomography, or CT scans are indicated. It must be kept in mind that nuclear bone scans are not totally specific, with up to a 15% false-positive rate.[48,49] CT scans should be performed in the true longitudinal axis of the scaphoid.[50,51] Sagittal plane images are obtained by placing the patient prone in the scanner, with the hand placed over the head in full pronation and neutral flexion. The plane of the scaphoid is similar to that defined by the axis of the thumb metacarpal fully abducted to the plane of the hand. For coronal images, the forearm is supinated to neutral. Thin (1 mm) cuts are obtained, and reconstructed three-dimensional (3-D) images ordinarily will not be required.[52] Since the advent of MRI, an immediate and accurate diagnosis is now feasible and treatment can be initiated, avoiding traditional time delays[12-15] (Fig. 2).

Fracture Classification

A number of classification systems have been adapted for scaphoid fractures and are well represented in the literature. However, it is important to recognize that studies using CT,[51,52] dry cadaver bones, or methylmethacrylate models of the scaphoid[53] have demonstrated how difficult it is to accurately characterize the plane of the fracture using standard radiographs.

Russe[54] in 1960 classified the fractures by the direction of the fracture line to the long axis of the scaphoid. Three patterns were identified, including a horizontal oblique plane, and transverse and vertical oblique directions (Fig. 3). The vertical oblique patterns were considered more likely to have problems with healing as a result of presumed shearing forces across the fracture.

McLaughlin and Parkes[55] in 1969 provided a prognostic classification as well as treatment recommendations based on the fracture pattern. Type A defined incomplete fractures treated with a splint; type B, nondisplaced but with a hemiarthrosis, treated with cast immobilization or internal fixation in selected

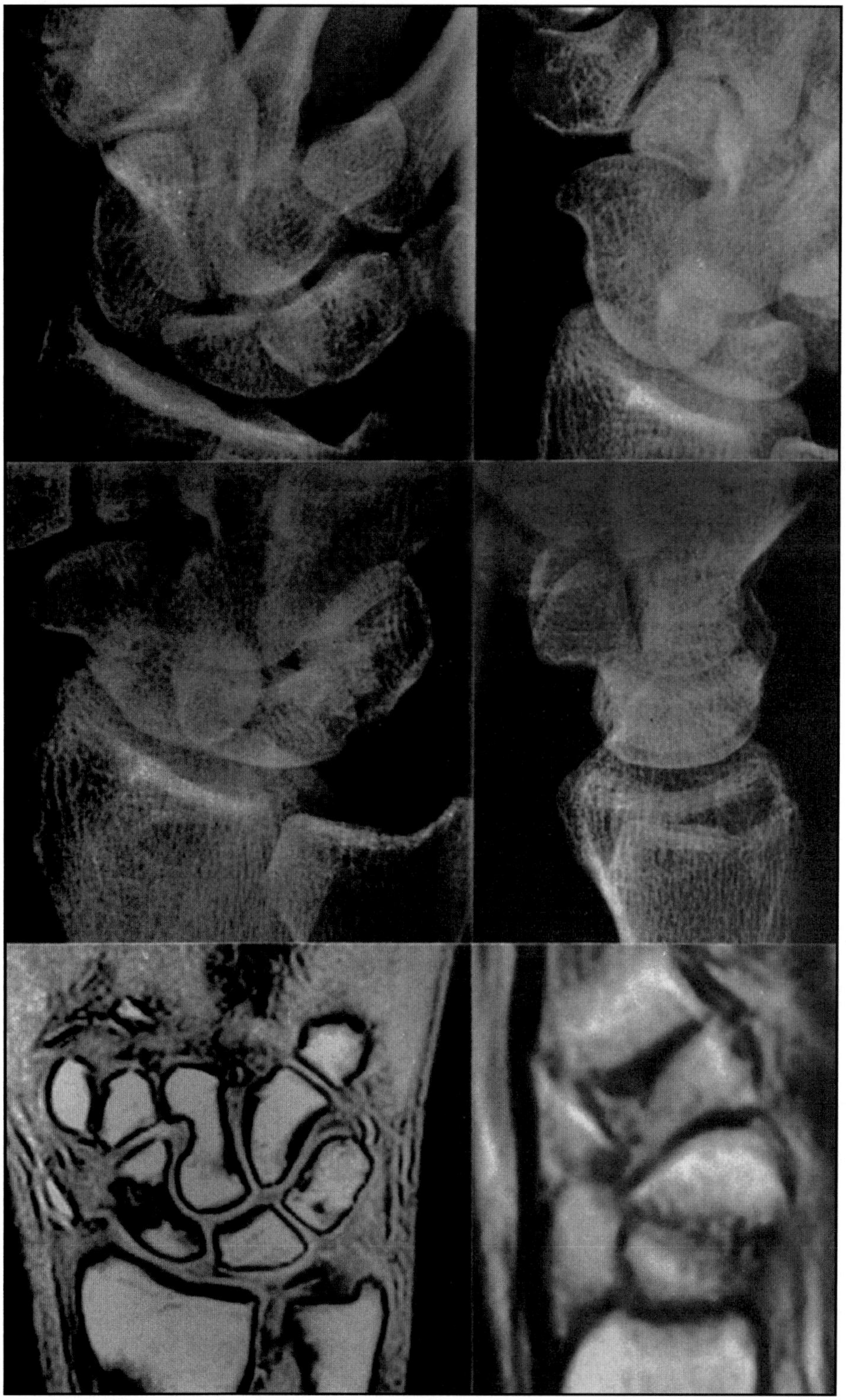

Fig. 2 *Top* and *middle* panels show an occult scaphoid fracture not visible on conventional scaphoid views that was confirmed with MRI *(bottom)* performed on the day of injury.

cases; and type C, displaced fractures requiring surgical intervention.

Herbert and Fisher[56] in 1984 classified the scaphoid fractures into stable

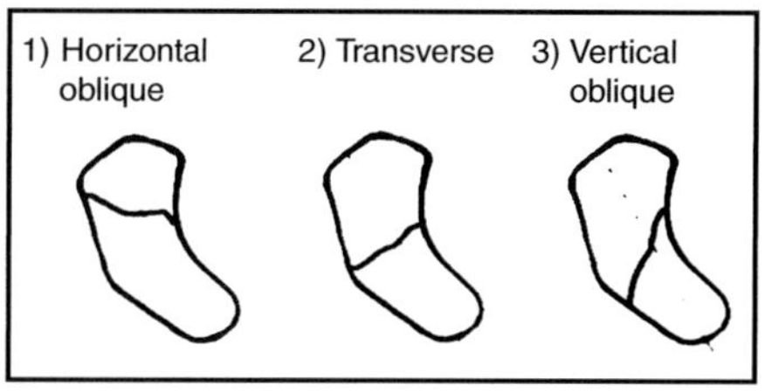

Fig. 3 Russe's scaphoid fracture classification. (Reproduced with permission from Taleisnik J (ed): *The Wrist.* New York, NY, Churchill Livingstone, 1985.)

versus unstable patterns, adding subgroups defined by location, comminution, and associated perilunate injury (Fig. 4). They considered any fracture that crosses both cortices to be unstable. Their concern as to defining instability as a major risk factor with regard to healing has been well supported by numerous studies in the literature.[2,56,57]

Additional radiographic parameters of fracture instability include displacement at the fracture site greater than 1 mm; an intrascaphoid angle greater than 60° and a capitolunate angle greater than 15°.[2]

In light of the recognized difficulties of accurately defining fracture classifications of the scaphoid from routine radiographic views, one of us (DLF) has grouped the fractures, irrespective of the direction of the fracture line or its location, into two main groups: stable and unstable. Stable fractures include the occult, incomplete, and complete nondisplaced fracture. The unstable fractures are grouped prognostically and according to the complexity of their surgical treatment into completely displaced, comminuted, dislocated, or combined fractures. The management recommendations for each group are provided in the form of a diagnostic and treatment algorithm (Figs. 5 and 6 and Tables 1 through 3).

Nonsurgical Treatment

Nonsurgical treatment of most scaphoid fractures remains the standard in most

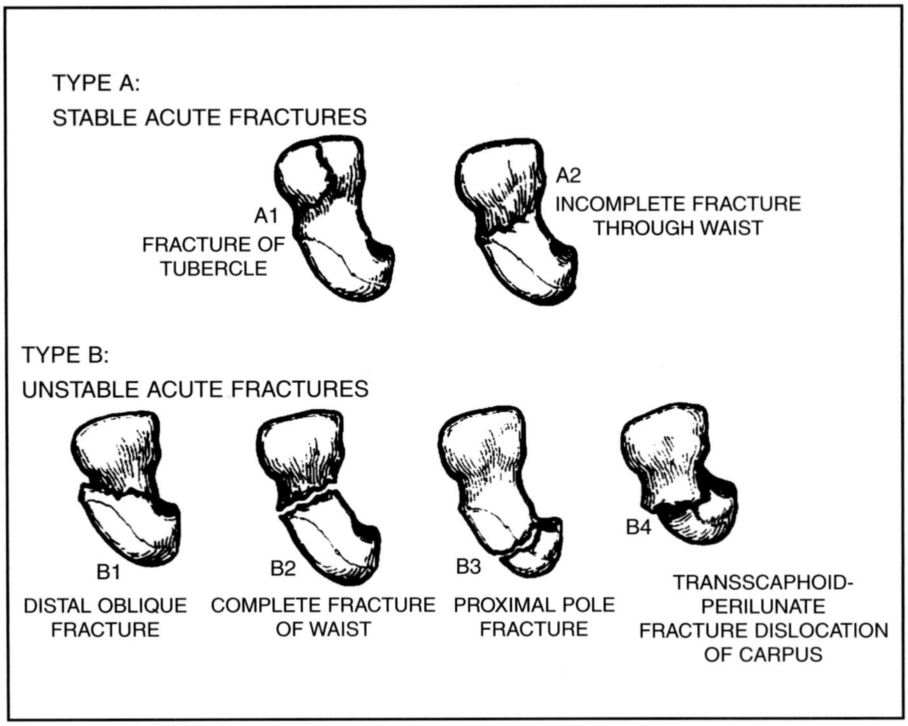

Fig. 4 Herbert scaphoid fracture classification. (Reproduced with permission from Herbert TJ (ed): *The Fractured Scaphoid.* St Louis, MO, Quality Medical Publishing, 1990, p 52.)

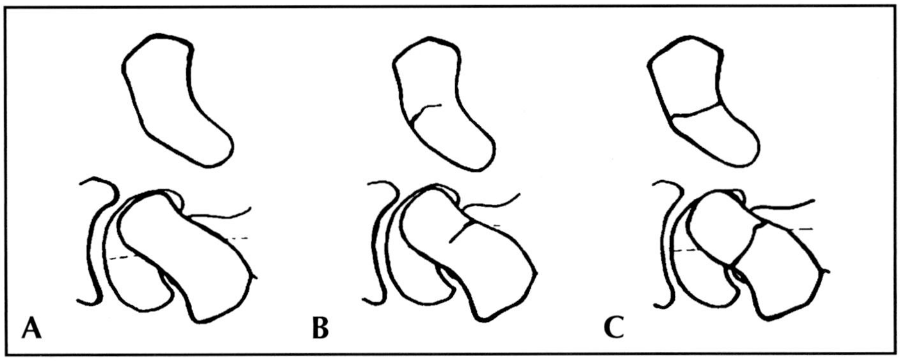

Fig. 5 Fractures of the scaphoid: stable fracture patterns. **A**, Occult. **B**, Incomplete. **C**, Complete nondisplaced.

Table 1
How to confirm healing of scaphoid fractures

Absence of tenderness
Disappearance of fracture line in various planes (scaphoid views)
Presence of regular sclerosis at fracture site
Bridging bony trabeculae in trispiral tomograms or CT scans
If any doubt (delayed union):
A low signal intensity on a magnetic resonance T1-weighted image combined with a high signal intensity on a T2-weighted image is an indicator of fracture, and on follow-up provides information as to progression of healing
The signal intensity resumes the iso-level in both fracture fragments on T1- and T2-weighted images when union is complete
No sign of implant loosening

centers, yet a number of questions remain, not the least of which includes the indications for cast immobilization. Additional questions include the type of immobilization, the position of the hand and wrist in the cast, the duration of cast immobilization, determination of fracture union, and when to allow return to sport.[59]

The clear indications for cast treatment include a fracture of the distal pole that does not involve a large segment of the articular surface, as well as fractures at the waist that are nondisplaced or impacted and in an anatomically acceptable position (Table 4). Perhaps the best definition of acceptability was developed by Amadio and associates,[60] who defined intrascaphoid angles based on sagittal CT images. An acceptable position would include those fractures with a lateral intrascaphoid angle less than 35° (normal 24° ± 5°) and an AP intrascaphoid angle greater than 35° (normal 40° ± 5°) (Fig 7). In addition, any gap at the fracture site should be less than 1 mm.

The data in the literature are in conflict regarding whether or not cast immobilization should extend above the elbow. Gellman and associates,[3] in a prospective study of 51 patients treated with either above or below elbow thumb spica casts for undisplaced fractures, evaluated patients at an average of 12 months after treatment. Those fractures treated with an above-elbow cast healed at an average of 9.5 weeks compared to 12.7 weeks for those treated with below elbow immobilization. No nonunions and two delayed unions were observed among the above elbow group compared with two nonunions and six delayed unions in the below elbow group. In an additional study, Kim and associates[61] suggested that noncompliance was also a factor in outcome, perhaps minimized by more extensive immobilization.

By contrast, in a prospective randomized study of 100 patients by Alho

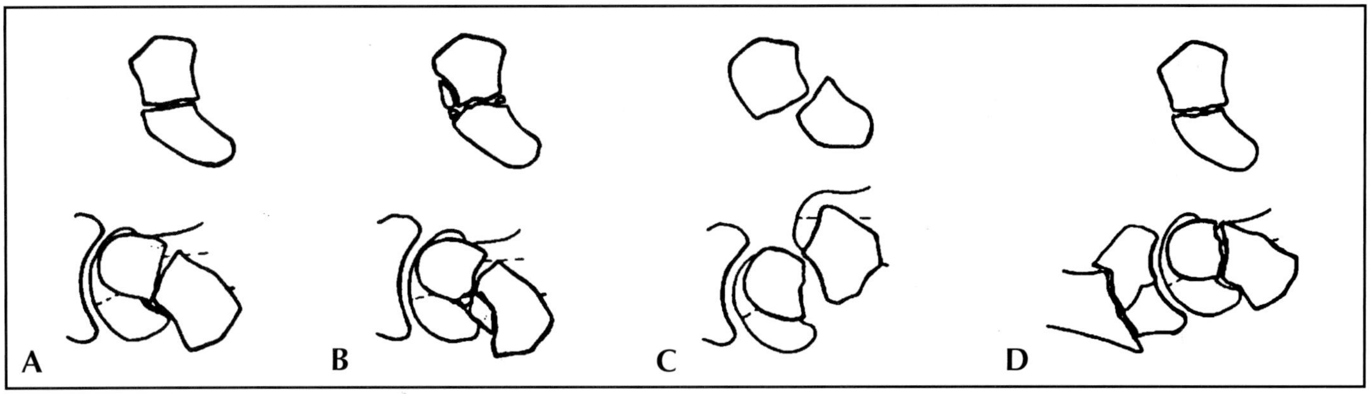

Fig. 6 Fractures of the scaphoid: unstable fracture patterns. **A**, Complete displaced. **B**, Comminuted. **C**, Dislocated. **D**, Combined.

and Kankaanpaau,[62] no difference was demonstrated between patients treated with an above or below elbow cast. Falkenberg,[63] in a biomechanical study, found no motion at a simulated scaphoid fracture with forearm rotation. Based upon these data, a stable, nondisplaced fracture in a reliable patient can be treated effectively with a below-thumb spica cast, whereas the issue of noncompliance would favor above elbow immobilization.

The issue of optimal wrist position has also been the source of biomechanical and clinical investigation. Experimental studies have suggested that palmar flexion and radial deviation of the wrist will help to reduce a gap at the scaphoid fracture site but will lead to collapse at the fracture site.[2,42,64] Ulnar deviation of the wrist, while more effective in reducing the fracture, will tend to cause distraction. As a result of these conflicting observations, we favor immobilization of the wrist in a neutral position.

The duration of cast immobilization is based on a number of factors. In general, patients should be evaluated on a monthly basis with repeat radiographs and cast changes as needed. When standard radiographs show definite signs of fracture healing for two consecutive examinations, the cast is discontinued and a long opponens splint is applied for an additional month. Nondisplaced or impacted fractures located at the distal waist should heal within 2 to 3 months, the midwaist 3 to 4 months, and the proximal third 4 to 5 months.[8,65]

Table 2
Management of stable fractures of the scaphoid

Occult	Incomplete	Complete Nondisplaced
If initial radiographs negative, splint for 10 days	Splint for 3 weeks and confirm healing with trispiral tomograms or CT scans	Try conservative treatment: 4 weeks long arm thumb spica 8 weeks short thumb spica
If tenderness persists, radiographs at 10 days, repeat 3 weeks	If doubt, use MRI	Or
Or		Percutaneous screw fixation and functional after-treatment if patient unwilling or unable to tolerate long periods of immobilization due to economic, social, or medical reasons (Herbert)
Immediate MRI to confirm nature of injury and treat accordingly		

A clear determination of union may not always be accurately obtained from standard radiographs or clinical examination.[1] Dias and associates[57] submitted a series of radiographs to a panel of experts and found poor agreement at 3 months after injury with regard to fracture union. The most accurate depiction of the status of fracture healing will be obtained with a CT scan, with sagittal cuts obtained in line with the longitudinal axis of the scaphoid.[51] Other factors that have been identified to be associated with fracture union include the absence of tenderness, disappearance of the fracture line in standard radiographs, sclerosis at the fracture line, and iso-level appearance of T1- and T2-weighted MRI studies.

The literature would support a favorable outcome from cast immobilization of stable fractures. Baumeister and Greinemann[66] observed union in 136 of 138 patients retrieved for follow-up; Alho and Kankaanpaau[62] found union in 90 of 100 patients; Cooney and associates[2] in 100% of patients; and Khan and al Harby[5] found that 35 of 45 united in a prospective study.

The final issue surrounding cast immobilization centers about when an

Table 3
Management of unstable scaphoid fractures

Compete Displaced	Comminuted	Dislocated	Combined
Reducible fracture: Limited open or percutaneous fixation with fluoroscopic and/or arthroscopic control Irreducible fracture: Open reduction and internal fixation Volar approach for distal and waist fractures Dorsal approach for proximal third fractures	Same as for displaced Depending on extent of comminution bone grafting should be considered Bone graft source: Distal radius Iliac crest	Transscaphoperilunate dislocation; naviculo-capitate syndrome (Fenton): Scaphoid screw fixation from volar or dorsal approach depending on fracture location and direction of displacement Choice of surgical approach: Palmar: Median nerve decompression Palmarly displaced lunate and/or proximal scaphoid pole Repair of palmar capsule Scaphoid reconstruction easier Dorsal: Better view of midcarpal joint and lunotriquetral junction Combined: Complete exposure-global assessment useful for old dislocation, simplifies bone and ligament reconstruction	Fracture of the scaphoid and distal radius: Conservative treatment feasible if both fractures reducible and stable after closed reduction. Otherwise, surgical treatment of both fractures. Radius Percutaneous pins External fixation Bone graft Plate fixation Combined methods depending on fracture type Scaphoid Screw fixation as in isolated complete fractures Warning: Ligamentotaxis alone is contraindicated because it distracts the scaphoid fracture

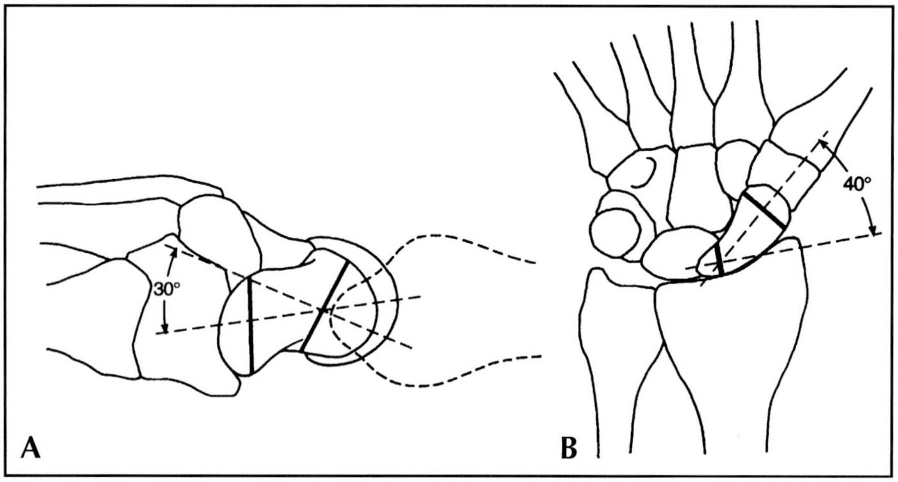

Fig. 7 The lateral and anterior interscaphoid angles are measured by drawing lines perpendicular to the diameter of the proximal and distal poles. Patients with a lateral interscaphoid angle of greater than 30° (**A**) or an anterior interscaphoid angle of less than 40° (**B**) reflect angulation and rotation of the scaphoid. (Reproduced with permission from Trumble TE: Principles of hand surgery and therapy, in *Fractures and Dislocations of the Carpus.* Philadelphia, PA, WB Saunders, 2000.)

athlete can safely return to sports. As a general rule, recreational athletes should be held out from sports until assurance of fracture union. Scholarship or professional athletes can be permitted to participate using a custom cast.[67]

Surgical Management

The decision making for acute fractures of the scaphoid is best based on a combination of factors including the complexity of the fracture, the technical abilities of the surgeon, and the patient's needs and functional expectations. Certainly, irreducible, unstable fractures; comminuted fractures; and fractures associated with perilunate dislocations or fractures of the distal radius require surgical exposure to guarantee restoration of anatomic articular congruency as well as to provide ligament repair when indicated.[68] In addition, comminuted fractures often require autogenous bone grafting to help correct deformity and accelerate healing.

For stable fractures or those with minimal displacement, there may be indications for surgical treatment, especially for individuals who find the potential of prolonged cast immobilization less attractive. In addition, the unpredictability of healing for any scaphoid fracture[69] has also stimulated interest by some toward percutaneous screw fixation for all scaphoid fractures.[18,42,70] Barton,[48] noting the inability to predict outcome solely from the initial radiographic presentation, stated that "all these classifications fail, in that some with a 'poor' prognosis will unite and some with a 'good' prognosis will not. As far as I know, there is no reliable way of predicting the outcome in undisplaced fractures." We have made similar observations, occasionally witnessing an adequately treated stable waist fracture develop into a nondisplaced cystic nonunion (Fig. 8), in contrast to a slightly displaced proximal pole fracture that healed with cast immobilization (Fig. 9).

With the advent of percutaneous techniques of screw fixation with fluoroscopic or arthroscopic control,[22,23] a number of series have reported favorable outcomes. Wozasek and Moser[23] achieved an 89% union rate in a series of 130 patients, 30% with stable fractures and 70% with unstable patterns. Inoue and Shionoya[70] reported a 100% union rate in a series of 40 patients using percutaneously placed Herbert screws. When these authors compared this group with 39 patients treated with cast immobilization, they observed a shorter time to union and an earlier return to work in the surgically treated group. A similar union rate of 100% was reported by Haddad and Goddard.[18]

The advent of cannulated screw systems has substantially facilitated percutaneous screw fixation of the scaphoid. Using image intensification, a more

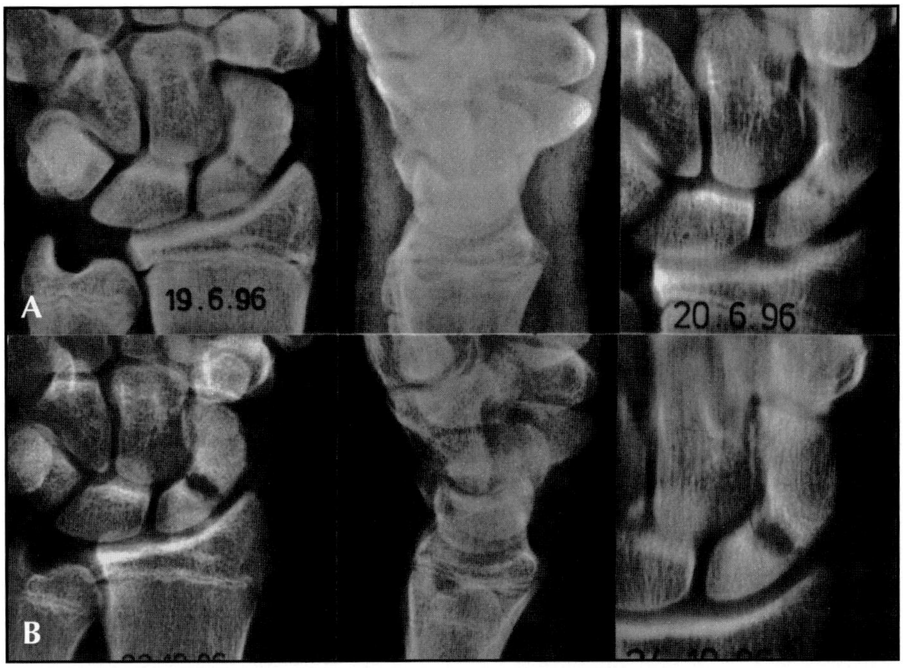

Fig. 8 A, Radiographs and AP tomograms of a nondisplaced "stable" fracture of the scaphoid in a 15-year-old patient. **B,** Following cast immobilization for 12 weeks, radiographs 4 months postinjury showed cystic changes and ultimately a nonunion.

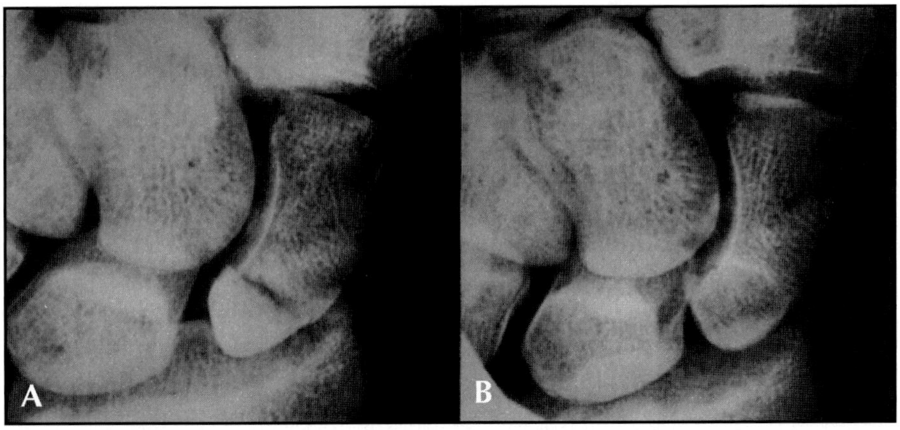

Fig. 9 A, Displaced unstable fracture associated with avascular changes in the proximal pole. **B,** Uneventful healing and normal bone density after 3 months of immobilization in a below-elbow cast.

Table 4
Indications for cast treatment of acute scaphoid fractures

Translation less than 1.0 mm
No evidence of angulation or collapse on lateral radiographs; lateral intrascaphoid angle < 30°
No evidence of collapse on anteroposterior radiographs; anteroposterior scaphoid angle > 40°
Minimal comminution
Fracture located in waist or tubercle
No evidence of carpal instability
Isolated injury

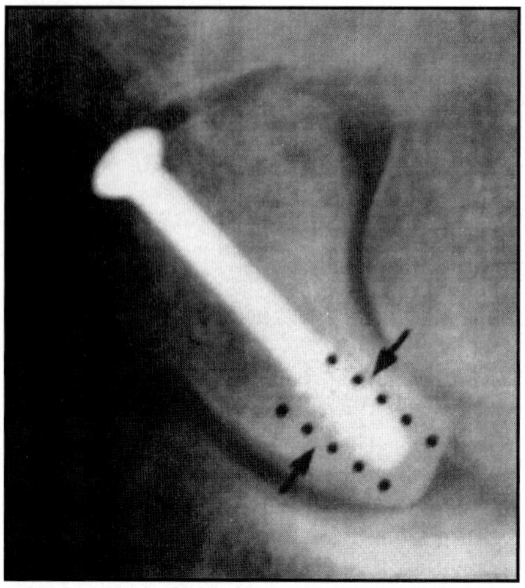

Fig. 10 Central placement of a screw enhances the stability of internal fixation of a scaphoid fracture or nonunion. The development of cannulated screws has enhanced the ability to achieve this stability. (Reproduced with permission from Trumble TE, Clark T, Kreder HJ: Nonunion of the scaphoid: Treatment with cannulated screws compared with treatment with Herbert screws. *J Bone Joint Surg Am* 1994;78:1929-1937.)

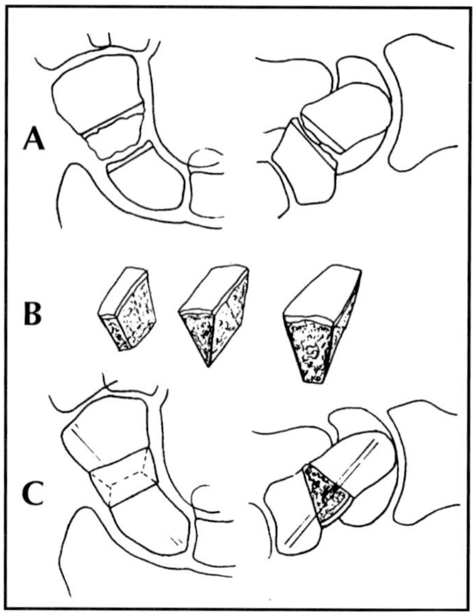

Fig. 11 Preoperative planning for the interpositional bone graft technique. **A,** Resection of the sclerotic borders of the nonunion. **B,** Iliac crest corticocancellous graft with rectangular, triangular, and trapezoidal cross-section, dependent on the size and shape of the defect. **C,** The anticipated final result connecting the "humpback deformity" and lunate rotation and showing ideal screw positioning in the anteroposterior and sagittal planes.

Table 5
Potential pitfalls of screw fixation

Distal entrance site not prepared by excision of the foot process of the trapezium
Failure to correct "humpback" deformity
Small proximal pole fracture
Failure to place threads of the tip of the screw across the fracture site
Screw not centrally placed

accurate placement of the cannulated guide wire and subsequent screw is facilitated (Fig. 10). Trumble and associates,[71] in a retrospective study of 34 patients in whom a nonunion of the scaphoid was treated with a bone graft and one of two types of screws, observed that the time to union was significantly shorter when the screw had been placed in the central third of the scaphoid ($P < 0.05$). In addition, 17 of the 18 patients with a cannulated screw had a central placement compared with 7 of the 16 patients with a noncannulated screw ($P < 0.01$) (Table 5).

An additional advantage of a percutaneous screw placement is the avoidance of injury to the volar carpal ligaments, which can lead to carpal instability after open reduction through a palmar approach.[72] Garcia-Elias and assoicates,[73] comparing patients treated for nonunion with a volar approach and those with a dorsal approach found similar union rates, but the palmar approach caused a significant increase in the scapholunate angle ($P < 0.05$) and consequently augmented carpal collapse.

Scaphoid Nonunion and Malunion

It has become clear from the data in a number of publications[4,59,74-78] that ununited fractures of the scaphoid associated with displacement or angulation as well as malunited fractures will have a higher likelihood of associated osteoarthritis and impaired wrist function. In one study by Jiranek and associates,[79] upward of 50% of patients treated for a scaphoid nonunion with a conventional inlay bone graft were found to have united with deformity. Although there was no significant subjective difference between those patients whose scaphoid healed anatomically compared to those with deformity, there was a significant difference in the functional results between these two groups. Tsuyuguchi and associates[80] also found a statistically significant correlation between improved wrist function and improved carpal alignment following anterior wedge-shaped grafting for an established scaphoid nonunion.

Two of the most important factors affecting the success in gaining union are the time elapsed between the initial fracture and the treatment of the nonunion,[81] and the presence of osteonecrosis of the proximal fragment.[82] These parameters, as well as the presence of periscaphoid arthritic changes, must be carefully evaluated as they represent major impediments to gaining union with conventional bone grafting techniques.

In general terms, the categories of reconstruction of an ununited scaphoid can be divided into: (1) an established nonunion without secondary degenerative changes within the wrist in which sound union of the scaphoid is the major goal; (2) a scaphoid nonunion with early degenerative changes in which establishing union of the scaphoid has to be combined with an additional procedure such as a radial styloidectomy;[83] and (3) a scaphoid nonunion with advanced degenerative wrist arthritis for which only a salvage procedure (that is, resection arthroplasty,

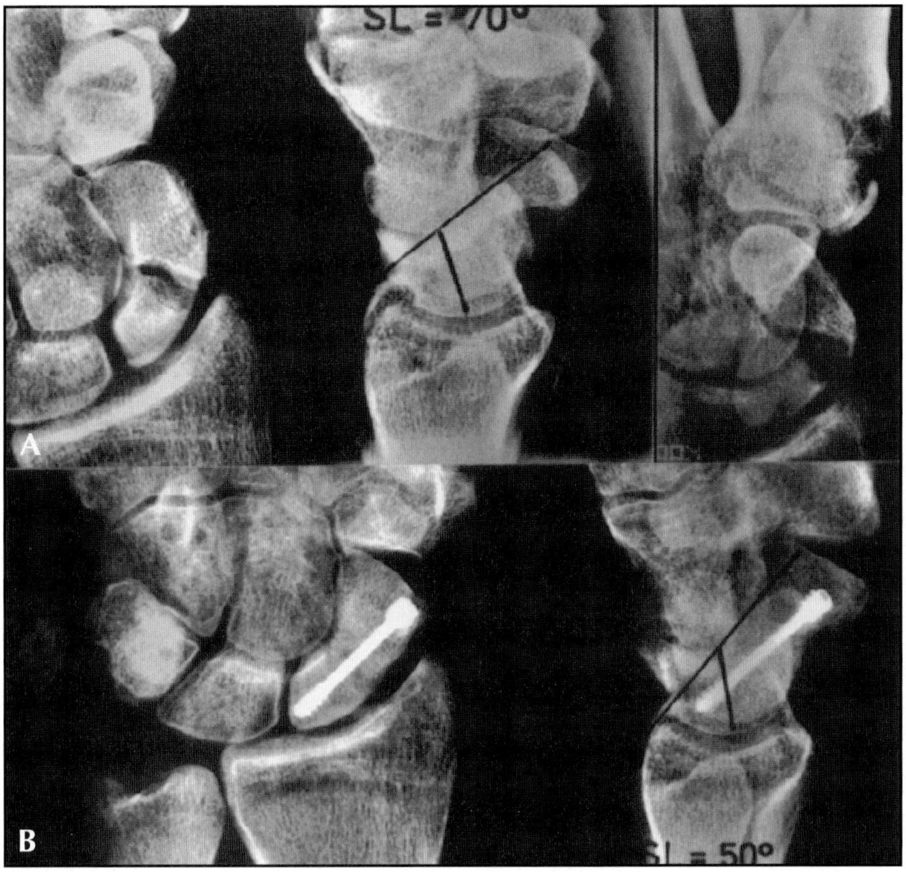

Fig. 12 An unstable scaphoid nonunion with a scapholunate angle of 70°. **A,** Following interpositional anterior wedge grafting, solid union and correct carpal alignment were obtained (scapholunate angle of 50°). **B,** Scaphoid views 5 years after surgery reveal maintenance of the carpal architecture and no evidence of degenerative changes.

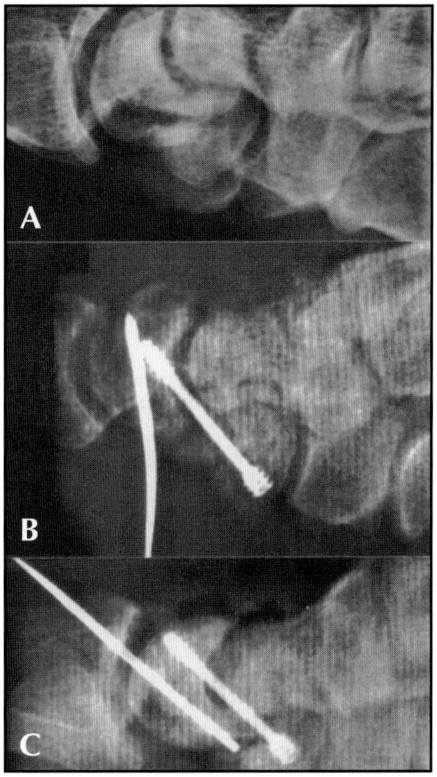

Fig. 13 If a dorsal intercalary segmental instability malalignment of the lunate cannot be reduced (**A**), the corrected lunate rotation is held with a K-wire driven through the palmar pole (**B**). The lunate is obliquely pinned to the radius and the K-wire retrieved through the dorsal skin (**C**). The wire is left in place for 8 weeks.

partial or total wrist fusion) should be considered.

For the first category, the surgical considerations are based on the concept of stability, the location of the nonunion, and the presence or absence of osteonecrosis. Stable, ununited scaphoid fractures in an anatomically acceptable position still profit from conventional inlay bone grafting.[2,6,34,54,82,84-89]

The surgical management of the unstable, angulated, or displaced nonunions located at the scaphoid waist or distal third along with intact blood supply to the proximal pole is based on gaining a more anatomic intrascaphoid angle and scaphoid length. This is best accomplished with an anteriorly placed interpositional graft along with stable internal fixation.[56,71,85,90-93]

Anterior Interpositional Wedge Graft Technique

Deformity associated with an established nonunion or malunion is complex. Based on the position of the distal fragment, the deformity includes: (1) flexion (humpback); (2) ulnar deviation (radial angulation); (3) pronation (rotatory malalignment); (4) shortening; and (5) on occasion, translation with articular displacement.[51,52,94,95] The restoration of the length and alignment through distraction of the nonunion restores the scaphoid's role as the radial column of the carpus, which corrects the initial carpal collapse and associated dorsal lunate rotation.[90,91]

Preoperative Planning

To correct the angular deformity and restore more normal length, the amount of resection of sclerotic bone at the site of the nonunion and the size of the required bone graft are calculated preoperatively by carefully tracing the radiographic findings in the AP and lateral views of the injured and contralateral wrists. This will also permit preoperative assessment of carpal height (collapse) and the scapholunate and lunocapitate angles. When instability exists at the nonunion site, the nonunion gap will open in maximal ulnar

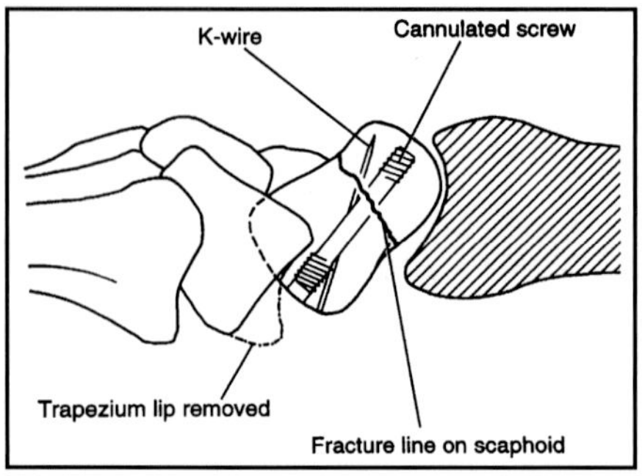

Fig. 14 By removal of the nonarticular volar foot process of the trapezium, a screw can be more successfully inserted along the longitudinal access of the scaphoid and more centrally placed into the proximal pole. (Reproduced with permission from Trumble TE: Principles of hand surgery and therapy, in *Fractures and Dislocations of the Carpus*. Philadelphia, PA, WB Saunders, 2000.)

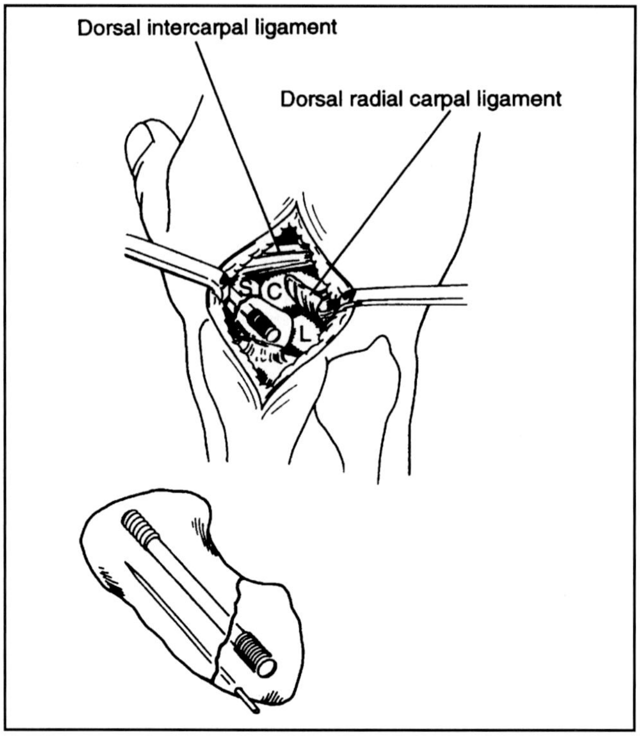

Fig. 15 The dorsal approach to a proximal pole fracture or nonunion will limit the risk of fracture displacement and facilitate central screw placement. It is important not to damage the scapholunate ligament when performing the internal fixation. (Reproduced with permission from Trumble TE: Principles of hand surgery and therapy, in *Fractures and Dislocations of the Carpus*. Philadelphia, PA, WB Saunders, 2000.)

deviation of the wrist and radiographs of both wrists taken in this position will be very useful in determining the amount of interpositional bone graft that will be required (Fig. 11). The size and form of the graft may be calculated in millimeters. Even more exact calculations can be made using CT or especially 3-D CT imaging.[51,52,94]

Surgical Technique

Nonunions located at the waist of distal third of the scaphoid are exposed through the palmar approach attributed to Russe.[54] The incision begins in the distal forearm and extends distally into the thenar eminence, with a radially-directed 2 cm oblique limb taking care that the angle of the incision lies within the transverse skin crease of the wrist to avoid a subsequent hypertrophic scar. The anterior capsule is incised in line with the skin from the distal radius to the scaphotrapezial joint, taking care to expose the most palmar-radial corner of the scaphoid, limiting the risk of injury to its vascular supply. The capsular flaps that contain the stout radioscaphocapitate ligament are held on both sides with stay sutures to facilitate anatomic closure at the end of the procedure. Sclerotic or irregular borders at the site of the nonunion are then resected with a small oscillating saw to enhance the surface contact between the graft and the scaphoid fragments. Cystic defects within the scaphoid are curetted and filled with small autogenous cancellous bone graft chips. The flexion deformity and shortening of the scaphoid are corrected by distraction of the nonunion site on the palmar and radial aspect using a small spreader clamp or, alternatively, by hyperextending the wrist over a rolled towel. The dorsal rotation of the lunate is simultaneously corrected by pushing the palmar pole toward the radius either with a fine bone spike or by using a Kirschner wire (K-wire) inserted through the palmar pole of the lunate. A small corticocancellous bone graft, obtained from the iliac crest and shaped according to the preoperative plan and intraoperative dimensions of the defect, is next inserted with the cortical aspect of the graft oriented on the palmar surface (Fig. 12).

In the event that neutral rotation of the lunate cannot be achieved, a smooth K-wire is inserted through the palmar pole into the lunate fossa of the radius and brought out percutaneously through the dorsal aspect of the forearm (Fig. 13).

We prefer stable fixation of the reconstructed scaphoid using a screw placed from the distal fragment into the proximal scaphoid. As noted, central screw placement into the proximal fragment is critical to ensure stability as well as enhance union. When directing a screw from distal to proximal, the extra-articular foot process of the trapezium needs to be removed to gain access to the entry location that will facilitate central placement of the screw. If not removed, the screw will be directed too dorsal in the proximal fragment (Fig. 14). In addition, if the flexion deformity is not adequately corrected, the likelihood is that the screw will be too

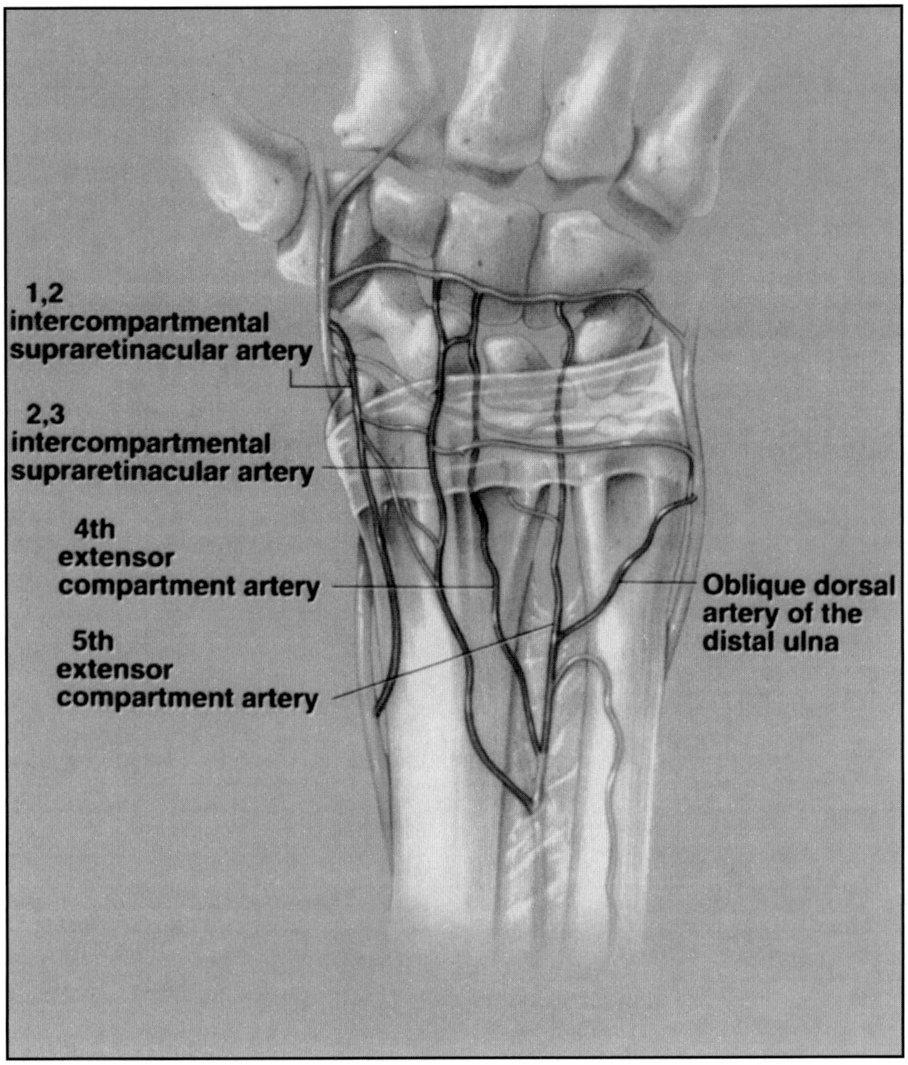

Fig. 16 The longitudinal vessels of the dorsal distal radius comprise two intercompartmental supraretinacular vessels (1,2 and 2,3 ICSRA) and two compartmental arteries (fourth and fifth extensor compartment arteries). (Reproduced with permisson of the Mayo Foundation, Rochester, MN.)

palmar. When realignment renders the reconstruction unstable, a K-wire in addition to a screw will add to the stability of the internal fixation and enhance healing.[95]

More proximally located nonunions with well vascularized bony fragments are best managed through a dorsal surgical approach combining autogenous cancellous bone graft and a screw placed from proximal to distal (Fig. 15).

With stable fixation of the scaphoid, wrist immobilization can be discontinued 2 weeks after the procedure except in those cases in which K-wire fixation of the lunate into the radius was required. In the latter cases, immobilization is needed for 8 weeks. Once immobilization is discontinued, the patient is encouraged to use the hand and wrist for activities of daily living. A removable thermoplastic wrist brace or splint is also routinely provided. Heavy manual work and strenuous sports activities are not permitted until a minimum of 12 weeks after surgery provided union is confirmed on radiographs.

Vascularized Pedicled Bone Graft

Ununited scaphoid fractures characterized by impaired vascularity or frank osteonecrosis as well as those having failed conventional bone grafting represent far more difficult management problems.[6,27,43,48,80,81,96-100] The development of vascularized pedicled distal radius bone grafts has offered a relatively straightforward surgical procedure performed through a single incision for the bone graft harvest, inserting the graft into the site of nonunion, and for the placement of internal fixation. The results of this technique have proven successful in a number of published reports.[25,27-29,31,33,93,101]

Vascular Anatomy

The blood supply to the distal dorsal radius is relatively constant and provided by a series of longitudinal vessels that demonstrate consistent spatial relationships to surrounding anatomic structures. The radial ulnar and anterior and posterior interosseous arteries contribute nutrient vessels to the distal radius and ulna. The vessels directly supplying nutrient branches to the dorsal radius and ulna are best described by their relationship to the extensor compartments of the wrist and extensor retinaculum. They are considered intercompartmental when located between compartments and compartmental when lying within an extensor compartment.

There are two consistent intercompartmental vessels that lie superficial to the extensor retinaculum and are further described as supraretinacular. These two vessels, the 1,2 and 2,3 intercompartmental supraretinacular arteries (1,2 and 2,3 ICSRA) are located on the retinaculum between their numbered compartments (Fig. 16). The retinaculum under these vessels is adherent to an underlying bony tubercle separating the compartments, allowing nutrient vessels to penetrate the distal radius.

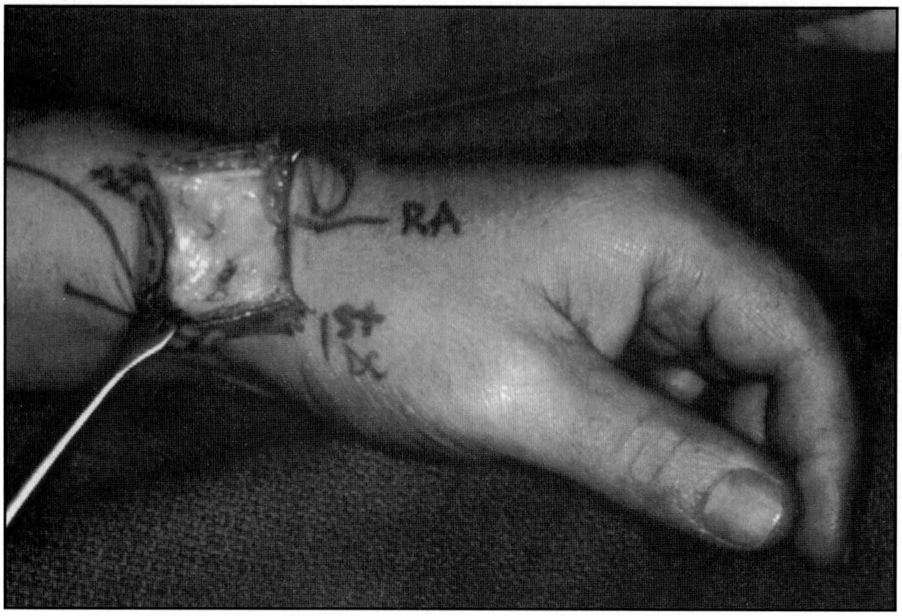

Fig. 17 A curvilinear incision over the dorsal radial aspect of the radiocarpal joint provides a single incision for exposure of the graft site and carpus.

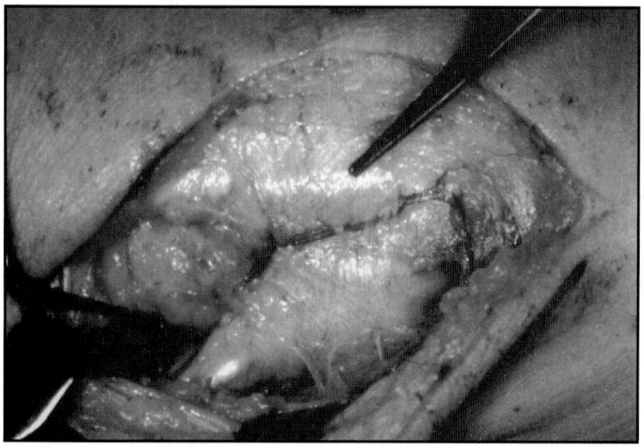

Fig. 18 With blunt dissection of the subcutaneous tissues, the 1,2 intercompartmental supraretinacular vessels are easily identified. (Reproduced with permission of the Mayo Foundation, Rochester, MN.)

The 1,2 ICSRA originates from the radial artery approximately 5 cm proximal to the radiocarpal joint and courses beneath the brachioradialis muscle to lie on the dorsal surface of the extensor retinaculum. Distally, it enters the anatomic snuffbox to anastomose to the radial artery and/or the radiocarpal arch. It is accompanied by venae comitantes and is the smallest of the four vessels. The distal origin is the ascending irrigating branch previously described by Zaidemberg and associates.[33] Its superficial location makes its dissection straightforward. Its pedicle has a short arc of rotation, and its nutrient artery branches to bone are small in number and caliber, but it is ideally located for grafts to the scaphoid.

The 2,3 ICSRA originates proximally from the anterior interosseous artery or the posterior division of the anterior interosseous artery. It lies superficial to the extensor retinaculum directly on Lister's tubercle and anastomoses with the dorsal intercarpal arch, the dorsal radiocarpal arch, or the fourth extensor compartmental artery. Its nutrient artery branches penetrate deep into cancellous bone. Like the 1,2 ICSRA, the 2,3 ICSRA is easily harvested and used as a vascularized pedicled bone graft. The arc of rotation is much greater and can reach the entire proximal row.

Pedicled bone grafts based on the 1,2 ICSRA are useful for most scaphoid nonunions. The harvest of this bone graft utilizes a dorsal surgical approach for both the graft and exposure of the scaphoid. The extremity is elevated for exsanguination without using an Esmarch bandage and a tourniquet inflated. A gentle curvilnear dorsal radial incision is used to expose the scaphoid and bone graft donor site (Fig. 17). Branches of the superficial radial nerve are identified and protected, the subcutaneous tissues are gently retracted, and the 1,2 ICSRA and venae comitantes will be seen on the surface of the retinaculum between the first and second extensor tendon compartments (Fig. 18). The vessels are dissected toward their distal anastomosis with the radial artery (toward the anatomic snuff box). The first and second dorsal extensor compartments are opened at the level of the bone graft site to create a cuff or retinaculum containing the vessels and their nutrient arteries to bone. The graft is centered approximately 1.5 cm proximal to the radiocarpal joint to include the nutrient vessels. Before elevation of the bone graft, a transverse dorsal-radial capsulotomy is made to expose the scaphoid nonunion site (Fig. 19).

With proximal pole fracture nonunions, a dorsal inlay graft is most appropriate. Curettes are used to remove any fibrous tissue from the nonunion site. Osteotomes or high-speed burrs are used to prepare a slot that spans the fracture site to receive the bone graft. If the proximal pole fragment is too small to create a slot, the graft is shaped to lie within the concavity of the proximal pole. After preparation of the nonunion site, the graft is elevated. Graft elevation begins with ligation of the 1,2 ICSRA and accompanying veins proximal to the graft. The vessels are mobilized distal to the graft to separate them from the radius and joint capsule, but leaving them applied to the graft itself. Osteotomes create the radial, ulnar, and proximal osteotomies of the graft. The distal osteotomy is performed in two stages, moving the pedicle radial then ulnarward to prevent injury to the pedicle. The graft is then gently levered out to create a distally based pedicle (Fig. 20).

Once elevated, the tourniquet is deflated, and the bone graft is observed for pulsatile bleeding. After satisfactory vascularity of the graft is determined, the graft is resized as needed, transposed beneath the radial wrist extensors, and press fit into the prepared slot in the nonunion site (Fig. 21). Supplemental internal fixation with K-wires or scaphoid screws may be safely placed without jeopardy to the pedicle. The wrist capsule and extensor retinaculum are reapproximated with nonabsorbable sutures. A bulky above-elbow plaster thumb spica splint is applied.

In the event that scaphoid foreshortening and angular deformity require a interpositional bone graft, a vascularized wedge graft may be placed through a dorsoradial approach. In this case, the scaphoid is prepared prior to graft elevation. When used as a wedge graft, the vessels are placed palmarly to allow a palmar cortical strut for stability. A graft sufficiently large to fill the internal scaphoid defect is harvested as previously described. The graft is carefully trimmed to match the dimensions of the defect, such that it will be used as a volar cortical strut. The graft is then inserted into the defect with the vascular pedicle placed palmarly and secured with K-wires or compression screw fixation, and the wound is closed as previously described.

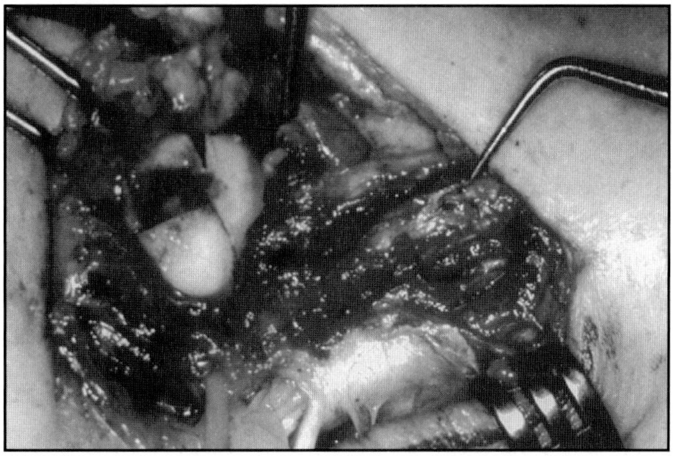

Fig. 19 An arthrotomy of the radiocarpal capsule enables exposure of the proximal scaphoid, which is prepared to receive the graft.

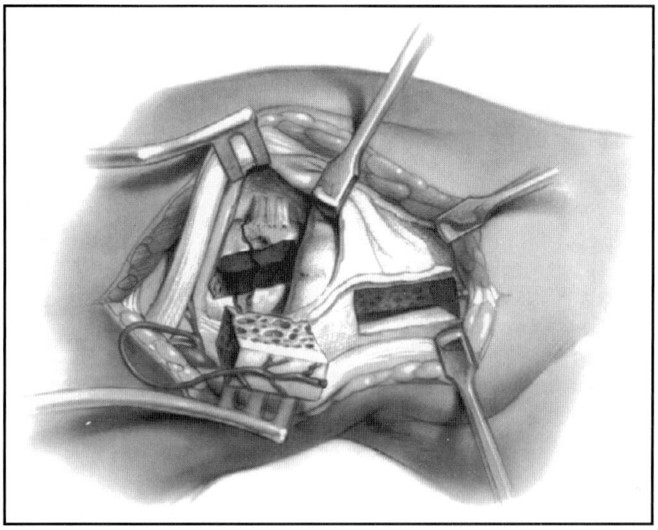

Fig. 20 As depicted in the schematic, after proximal ligation of the 1,2 intercompartmental supraretinacular vessels and creation of the bone graft with osteotomes, the graft is gently mobilized to be contoured to fit snugly into the scaphoid. (Reproduced with permission of the Mayo Foundation, Rochester, MN.)

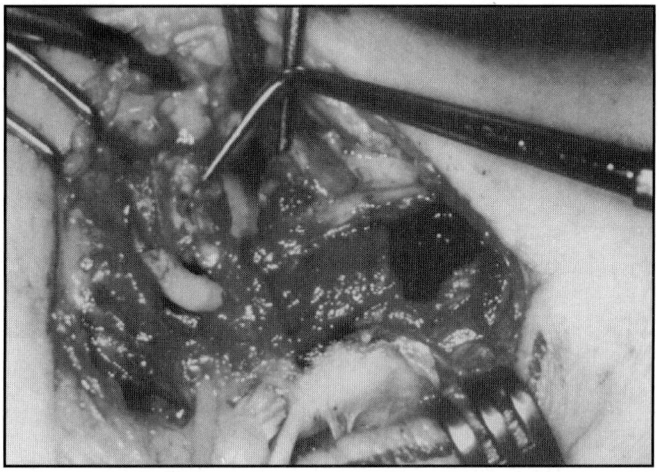

Fig. 21 With the graft impacted into the scaphoid defect (probe), additional fixation with K-wires or a screw may be placed at this time.

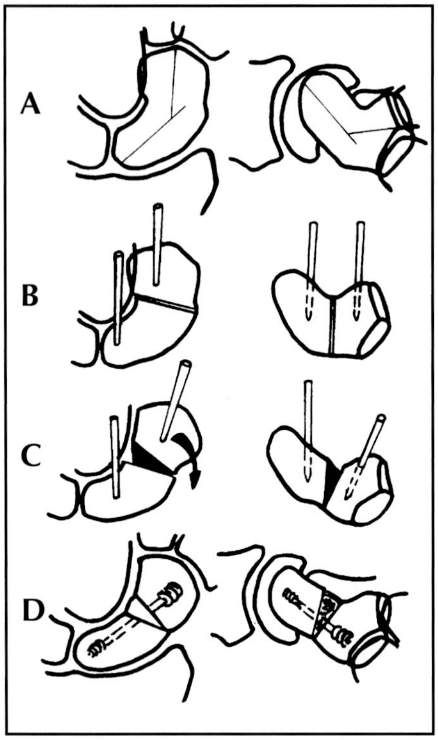

Fig. 22 The surgical technique for reconstruction of a malunited scaphoid fracture is demonstrated in this schematic. **A,** The anteroposterior and lateral interscaphoid angles have been measured on tracings of the scaphoid radiographs. **B,** A transverse osteotomy is made at the original fracture site. The parallel placed K-wires in both fragments are to be used as "joy-sticks" during angular and rotational correction. **C,** Correction of the deformity consists of extension, supination (arrow), and radial deviation of the distal fragment. **D,** Internal fixation with a screw after insertion of the palmar and ulnarly based trapezoidal bone graft.

Corrective Osteotomy for Malunion

A number of studies have suggested that deformity of the scaphoid, even in the face of union, may lead to pain as well as a loss of active wrist extension.[4,59,76,95,102] Altered wrist kinematics, articular incongruity, and a dorsal intercalary segment instability pattern all represent potential causes for long-term problems, including arthritis, and correction of deformity should be considered in symptomatic patients.[103]

The classic deformity found with a symptomatic malunion of the scaphoid includes shortening flexion in the sagittal plane and ulnar deviation of the distal fragment in the frontal plane. A rotational malalignment with pronation of the distal fragment in the horizontal plane is also present.[48,85,104] For preoperative assessment in addition to the comparative radiographs used for treatment of nonunions, trispiral tomography or 3-D reconstructed CT scans are used to evaluate the intrascaphoid angles.[59]

Surgical Technique

The scaphoid is exposed through a palmar approach and two 0.045-in K-wires are introduced parallel to one another on each side of the planned osteotomy site and are used as joy sticks to manipulate the scaphoid fragments into the corrected position after completion of the osteotomy. They also serve to confirm intraoperatively the accuracy of correction of the angles subtended by the K-wires (extension and derotation) (Fig. 22, *A*). The osteotomy is performed transversely at the old fracture site with a small oscillating saw, taking particular care not to damage the point of entry of the dorsal ridge vessels. The wrist is extended over a rolled towel, opening up the palmar gap for the required amount of correction. Restoration of full wrist extension follows correction of the flexion and pronation deformity of the distal fragment of the scaphoid. The reduction can be assessed intraoperatively by observing the new positions of the K-wires in both the sagittal and horizontal planes (Fig. 22, *B*). Ulnar deviation is corrected by opening the osteotomy on the ulnar side with a small spreader clamp. A corticocancellous wedge graft shaped to fit the defect is obtained from the iliac crest or distal radius and inserted into the osteotomy gap while an assistant maintains the corrected position by holding the K-wires in the corrected position. Temporary placement of a K-wire across the two fragments and bone graft performed under fluoroscopic control is helpful before placement of a screw for definitive fixation (Fig. 22, *C*). The redundant edges of the bone graft are smoothed off with a burr, and the wrist capsule, including the strong radiocarpal oblique ligaments, is closed with nonabsorbable interrupted sutures.

Postoperatively, a long opponens thumb splint is applied for 10 to 14 days. Following suture removal, the wrist is immobilized in a thumb spica cast for 3 weeks followed by a removable wrist splint. At 8 weeks after surgery, scaphoid views as well as CT scans are used to assess union. Comparative radiographs with the contralateral wrist that permit measurement of the scapholunate angle will be a useful indicator of residual dorsal carpal instability[80,85] (Fig. 23).

Wrist Arthritis Following Scaphoid Nonunion

Scaphoid Nonunion Advanced Collapse

The patterns of arthritis associated with a scaphoid nonunion were initially identified by Watson and associates.[105,106] This condition is similar to that associated with chronic scapholunate ligament incompetence, in that the wrist has lost the structural support of the scaphoid, which normally maintains the anatomic orientation of the scaphoid and distal radius as well as the capitate within the center of rotation of the wrist.

Four stages of arthritis exist and include: stage I, characterized by osteophyte formation of the radial styloid without substantial narrowing of the radius-scaphoid articulation; stage II reflecting progression of arthritis to now involve the radioscaphoid joint; stage III now involving the capitolunate articulation; and stage IV in which arthritis has involved all but the lunate-radius articulation (Fig. 24).

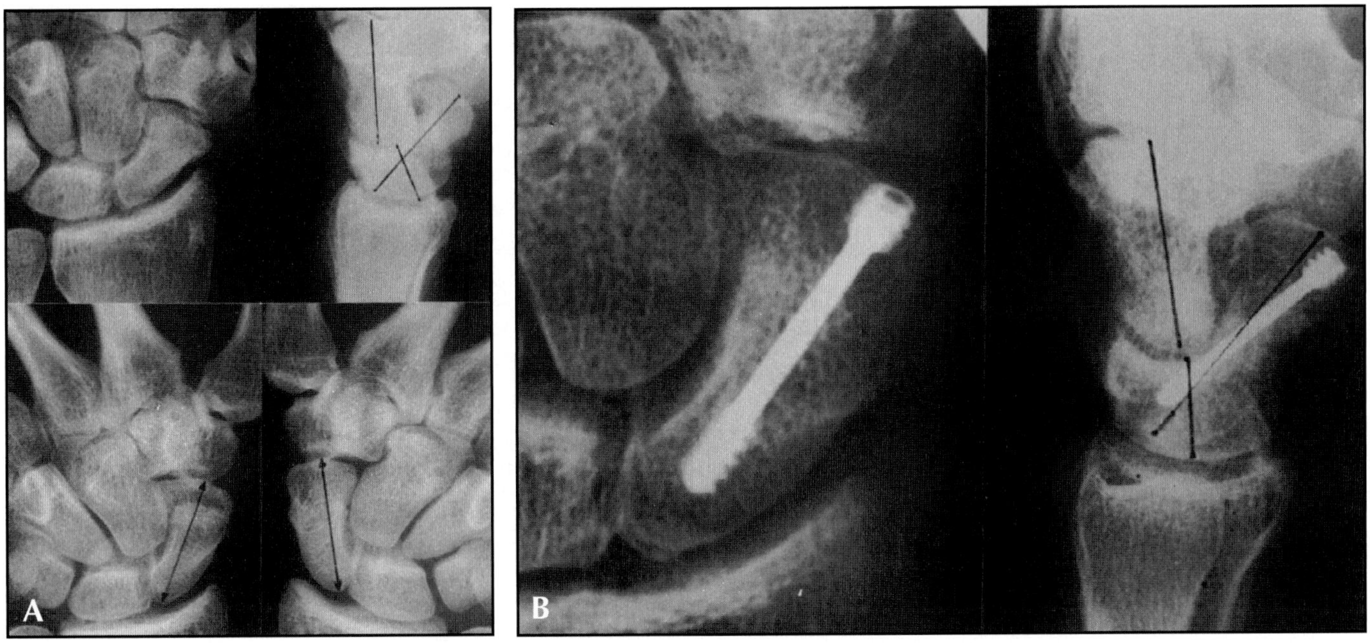

Fig. 23 A symptomatic malunited scaphoid fracture was corrected with osteotomy and realignment. **A,** The malunion of the scaphoid was located in the distal third associated with a dorsal intercalary segmental instability carpal malalignment. The scapholunate angle was 68° (*top*). The preoperative estimation of scaphoid length in the ulnarly deviated AP views of both wrists (*bottom*). **B,** Late follow-up radiographs show anatomic restoration of the scaphoid following the osteotomy. The scapholunate angle was reduced to 40°.

The management of the stage I wrist depends on whether or not criteria exist to warrant an attempt at gaining union. If so, combined with a radial styloidectomy, the outcome will be favorable. Alternatively, if the proximal pole of the scaphoid has demonstrated significant collapse or has other poor prognostic factors for predicting success with an attempt to gain union, a soft-tissue arthroplasty can be performed through a dorsoradial approach.[98] This results in a permanent pseudarthrosis at the fracture site.

The surgical technique most used for patients with stage II arthritis include proximal row carpectomy and a four-bone intercarpal arthrodesis involving the capitate, lunate, triquetrum, and hamate in conjunction with scaphoid excision.[105-109]

In one retrospective study involving 24 patients, Tomaino and associates[108] observed that patients treated with a proximal row carpectomy, when compared with a group who had a four-bone fusion, required a shorter period of immobilization and had improved range of wrist motion. By the same token, follow-up radiographs demonstrated the development of progressive arthrosis between the capitate and radius in the patients treated with proximal row carpectomy.

When intercarpal arthritis has progressed to stage III, involving the capitate-lunate articulation, decision making focuses on either an attempt to retain some wrist motion with a four-bone intercarpal fusion or performing a total wrist arthrodesis. The latter is to be considered as well for patients with stage IV involvement.

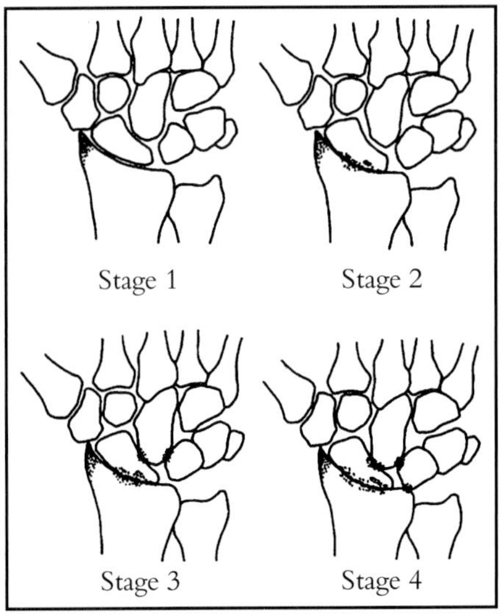

Fig. 24 Scapholunate advanced collapse pattern arthritis presents in four stages: Stage 1: Osteophyte formation or beaking of the radial styloid without significant narrowing of the radioscaphoid articulations. Stage 2: In this stage the arthritis has progressed to involve the radioscaphoid articulation. Stage 3: In this stage the arthritis has progressed to involve the capitate-lunate articulation. Stage 4: In this stage the arthritis has progressed to pancarpal involvement.

Summary

The management of acute scaphoid fractures should be oriented on the concept of fracture stability, ease of reduction, associated ligamentous injury, and risk of impaired blood supply, rather than the direction of the fracture line or location of the fracture within the scaphoid. The lack of predictability of successful fracture union and prognostic discrepancies of historic and contemporary classifications may be related to subtle differences of the internal vascular architecture of each scaphoid. Because the possibility of impaired vascularity is greater with fractures located in the proximal third, stable internal fixation is indicated to provide mechanical stability and fracture surface contact to enhance revascularization. Improved healing rates in a shorter time and earlier rehabilitation with percutaneous techniques of internal fixation have produced a clear shift from classic conservative treatment to internal skeletal fixation.

Although the rates of union of well-vascularized nonunions have not been dramatically improved with the use of internal fixation as compared with inlay bone grafting, the restoration of scaphoid anatomy and prevention of malunion and associated carpal collapse with interpositional bone grafting techniques will reduce the risk of osteoarthritis.

References

1. Barton NJ: Apparent and partial non-union of the scaphoid. *J Hand Surg Br* 1996;21:496-500.
2. Cooney WP, Dobyns JH, Linscheid RL: Fractures of the scaphoid: A rational approach to management. *Clin Orthop* 1980;149:90-97.
3. Gellman H, Caputo RJ, Carter V, Aboulafia A, McKay M: Comparison of short and long thumb-spica casts for non-displaced fractures of the carpal scaphoid. *J Bone Joint Surg Am* 1989;71:354-357.
4. Herbert TJ (ed): *The Fractured Scaphoid*. St. Louis, MO, Quality Medical Publishing, 1990.
5. Khan FA, al Harby S: Fresh scaphoid fractures (analysis of 45 cases). *Afr J Med Sci* 1995;24:201-206.
6. Kleinert JM, Zenni EJ Jr: Nonunion of the scaphoid: Review of literature and current treatment. *Orthop Rev* 1984;13:125-141.
7. Langhoff O, Andersen JL: Consequences of late immobilization of scaphoid fractures. *J Hand Surg Br* 1988;13:77-79.
8. Leslie IJ, Dickson RA: The fractured carpal scaphoid: Natural history and factors influencing outcome. *J Bone Joint Surg Br* 1981;63: 225-230.
9. Morgan DA, Walters JW: A prospective study of 100 consecutive carpal scaphoid fractures. *Aust N Z J Surg* 1984;54:233-241.
10. Stewart MJ: Fractures of the carpal navicular (scaphoid): A report of 436 cases. *J Bone Joint Surg Am* 1954;36:998-1006.
11. Munk B, Frokjaer J, Larsen CF, Johannsen HG, Rasmussen LL, Edal A, Rasmussen LD: Diagnosis of scaphoid fractures: A prospective multicenter study of 1,052 patients with 160 fractures. *Acta Orthop Scand* 1995;66:359-360.
12. Breitenseher MJ, Metz VM, Gilula LA, et al: Radiographically occult scaphoid fractures: Value of MR imaging in detection. *Radiology* 1997;203:245-250.
13. Gaebler C, Kukla C, Breitenseher M, Trattnig S, Mittlboeck M, Vecsei V: Magnetic resonance imaging of occult scaphoid fractures. *J Trauma* 1996;41:73-76.
14. Hunter JC, Escobedo EM, Wilson AJ, Hanel DP, Zink-Brody GC, Mann FA: MR imaging of clinically suspected scaphoid fractures. *Am J Roentgenol* 1997;168:1287-1293.
15. Imaeda T, Nakamura R, Miura T, Makino N: Magnetic resonance imaging in scaphoid fractures. *J Hand Surg Br* 1992;17:20-27.
16. Trumble TE: Avascular necrosis after scaphoid fracture: A correlation of magnetic resonance imaging and histology. *J Hand Surg Am* 1990;15:557-564.
17. Filan SL, Herbert TJ: Herbert screw fixation of scaphoid fractures. *J Bone Joint Surg Br* 1996;78:519-529.
18. Haddad FS, Goddard NJ: Acute percutaneous scaphoid fixation: A pilot study. *J Bone Joint Surg Br* 1998;80:95-99.
19. Maudsley RH, Chen SC: Screw fixation in the management of the fractured carpal scaphoid. *J Bone Joint Surg Br* 1972;54:432-441.
20. McLaughlin HL: Fracture of the carpal navicular (scaphoid) bone: Some observations based on treatment by open reduction and internal fixation. *J Bone Joint Surg Am* 1954;36:765-774.
21. Rettig AC, Kollias SC: Internal fixation of acute stable scaphoid fractures in the athlete. *Am J Sports Med* 1996;24:182-186.
22. Whipple TL: Acute scaphoid fracture fixation, in Vastamaki M, Vilkki S, Raatikainen T, Viljakka T (eds): *Current Trends in Hand Surgery*. Amsterdam, The Netherlands, Elsevier Science, 1995, pp 75-77.
23. Wozasek GE, Moser KD: Percutaneous screw fixation for fractures of the scaphoid. *J Bone Joint Surg Br* 1991;73:138-142.
24. Barth A: Histologische untersuchungen über knochenimplantationen. *Beitr Anat Pathol* 1895;17:65-142.
25. Bishop AT: Vascularized pedicle grafts from the dorsal distal radius: Design and application for carpal pathology. *Curr Prac Hand Surg* 1997:307-313.
26. Dell PC, Burchardt H, Glowczewskie FP Jr: A roentgenographic, biomechanical, and histological evaluation of vascularized and non-vascularized segmental fibular canine autografts. *J Bone Joint Surg Am* 1985;67:105-112.
27. Guimberteau JC, Panconi B: Recalcitrant non-union of the scaphoid treated with a vascularized bone graft based on the ulnar artery. *J Bone Joint Surg Am* 1990;72:88-97.
28. Kawai H, Yamamoto K: Pronator quadratus pedicled bone graft for old scaphoid fractures. *J Bone Joint Surg Br* 1988;70:829-831.
29. Kuhlmann JN, Mimoun M, Boabighi A, Baux S: Vascularized bone graft pedicled on the volar carpal artery for non-union of the scaphoid. *J Hand Surg Br* 1987;12:203-210.
30. Shaffer JW, Field GA, Wilber RG, Goldberg VM: Experimental vascularized bone grafts: Histopathologic correlations with postoperative bone scan: The risk of false-positive results. *J Orthop Res* 1987;5:311-319.
31. Shin AY, Sheetz KK, Bishop AJ, Berger RA: Vascularized pedicled bone graft from the distal radius. *Arch Am Acad Orthop Surg* 1999; 2:94-106.
32. Weiland AJ, Hotchkiss RN: Vascularized bone grafts, in Green DP, Hotchkiss RN (eds): *Operative Hand Surgery*, ed 3. New York, NY, Churchill Livingstone, 1993, pp 1179-1199.
33. Zaidemberg C, Siebert JW, Angrigiani C: A new vascularized bone graft for scaphoid nonunion. *J Hand Surg Am* 1991;16:474-478.
34. Vesalius A: *De Humani Corporis Fabrica*. Basileae, Libri 7, Oporini, Plate 16, 1543.
35. Johnson RP: The evolution of carpal nomenclature: A short review. *J Hand Surg Am* 1990;15:834-838.
36. McMurrich JP: The nomenclature of the carpal bones. *Anat Rec* 1914;8:173-182.
37. *Terminology for Hand Surgery. Publication of the International Federation of Societies for Surgery of the Hand (IRSSH)*. Brentwood, England, Westbury Press, 1990.
38. Ebri B, Ros R, Monzon A: Contribucion al estudio de los huesos accesorios de la Mano. *Rev Mano* 1982;24:65-76.
39. Gelberman RH, Menon J: The vascularity of the scaphoid bone. *J Hand Surg Am* 1980;5: 508-513.
40. Gelberman H, Panagis JS, Taleisnik J, Baumgaertner M: The arterial anatomy of the human carpus: The extraosseous vascularity. *J Hand Surg Am* 1983;8:367-375.
41. Taleisnik J, Kelly PJ: The extraosseous and intraosseous blood supply of the scaphoid bone. *J Bone Joint Surg Am* 1966;48:1125-1137.
42. Weber ER: Biomechanical implications of scaphoid waist fractures. *Clin Orthop* 1980;149:83-89.
43. Verdan C, Narakas A: Fractures and pseudarthrosis of the scaphoid. *Surg Clin North Am* 1968;48:1083-1095.
44. Freeland P: Scaphoid tubercle tenderness: A better indicator of scaphoid fractures? *Arch Emerg Med* 1989;6:46-50.
45. Chen SC: The scaphoid compression test. *J Hand Surg Br* 1989;14:323-325.

46. Grover R: Clinical assessment of scaphoid injuries and the detection of fractures. *J Hand Surg Br* 1996;21:341-343.

47. Jacobsen S, Hassani G, Hansen D, Christensen O: Suspected scaphoid fractures: Can we avoid overkill? *Acta Orthop Belg* 1995;61:74-78.

48. Barton NJ: Twenty questions about scaphoid fractures. *J Hand Surg Br* 1992;17:289-310.

49. Murphy DG, Eisenhauer MA, Powe J, Pavlofsky W: Can a day 4 bone scan accurately determine the presence or absence of scaphoid fracture? *Ann Emerg Med* 1995;26:434-438.

50. Bain GI, Bennett JD, Richards RS, Slethaug GP, Roth JH: Longitudinal computed tomography of the scaphoid: A new technique. *Skeletal Radiol* 1995;24:271-273.

51. Sanders WE: Evaluation of the humpback scaphoid by computed tomography in the longitudinal axial plane of the scaphoid. *J Hand Surg Am* 1988;13:182-187.

52. Nakamura R, Imaeda T, Horii E, Miura T, Hayakawa N: Analysis of scaphoid fracture displacement by three-dimensional computed tomography. *J Hand Surg Am* 1991;16:485-492.

53. Compson JP: The anatomy of acute scaphoid fractures: A three-dimensional analysis of patterns. *J Bone Joint Surg Br* 1998;80:218-224.

54. Russe O: Fracture of the carpal navicular: Diagnosis, non operative treatment, and operative treatment. *J Bone Joint Surg Am* 1960;42:759-768.

55. McLaughlin HL, Parkes JC II: Fracture of the carpal navicular (scaphoid) bone: Gradations in therapy based upon pathology. *J Trauma* 1969;9:311-319.

56. Herbert TJ, Fisher WE: Management of the fractured scaphoid using a new bone screw. *J Bone Joint Surg Br* 1984;66:114-123.

57. Dias JJ, Taylor M, Thompson J, Brenkel IJ, Gregg PJ: Radiographic signs of union of scaphoid fractures: An analysis of inter-observer agreement and reproducibility. *J Bone Joint Surg Br* 1998;70:299-301.

58. Clay NR, Dias JJ, Costigan PS, Gregg PJ, Barton NJ: Need the thumb be immobilised in scaphoid fractures? A randomised prospective trial. *J Bone Joint Surg Br* 1991;73:828-832.

59. Kaneshiro SA, Failla JM, Tashman S: Scaphoid fracture displacement with forearm rotation in a short-arm thumb spica cast. *J Hand Surg Am* 1999;24:984-991.

60. Amadio PC, Berquist TH, Smith DK, Ilstrup DM, Cooney WP III, Linscheid RL: Scaphoid malunion. *J Hand Surg Am* 1989;14:679-687.

61. Kim WC, Shaffer JW, Idzikowski C: Failure of treatment of ununited fractures of the carpal scaphoid: The role of non-compliance. *J Bone Joint Surg Am* 1983;65:985-991.

62. Alho A, Kankaanpaau U: Management of fractured scaphoid bone: A prospective study of 100 fractures. *Acta Orthop Scand* 1975;46: 737-743.

63. Falkenberg P: An experimental study of instability during supination and pronation of the fractured scaphoid. *J Hand Surg Br* 1985;10:211-213.

64. Weber ER, Chao EY: An experimental approach to the mechanism of scaphoid waist fractures. *J Hand Surg Am* 1978;3:142-148.

65. Böhler L, Trojan E, Jahna H: Behandlungsergebnisse von 734 frischen einfachen Brüchen des Kahnbeinkorpers der hand. *Wiederhestel Traumatol* 1954;2:86-111.

66. Baumeister HH, Greinemann H: Conservative treatment of scaphoid bone fracture of the wrist. *Unfallchirurg* 1989;92:175-179.

67. Riester JN, Baker BE, Mosher JF, Lowe D: A review of scaphoid fracture healing in competitive athletes. *Am J Sports Med* 1985;13:159-161.

68. Szabo RM, Manske D: Displaced fractures of the scaphoid. *Clin Orthop* 1988;230:30-38.

69. Desai VV, Davis TR, Barton NJ: The prognostic value and reproducibility of the radiological features of the fractured scaphoid. *J Hand Surg Br* 1999;24:586-590.

70. Inoue G, Shionoya K: Herbert screw fixation by limited access for acute fractures of the scaphoid. *J Bone Joint Surg Br* 1997;79:418-421.

71. Trumble TE, Clarke T, Kreder HJ: Non-union of the scaphoid: Treatment with cannulated screws compared with treatment with Herbert screws. *J Bone Joint Surg Am* 1996;78: 1829-1837.

72. Rettig ME, Raskin KB: Retrograde compression screw fixation of acute proximal pole scaphoid fractures. *J Hand Surg Am* 1999;24: 1206-1210.

73. Garcia-Elias M, Vall A, Salo JM, Lluch AL: Carpal alignment after different surgical approaches to the scaphoid: A comparative study. *J Hand Surg Am* 1988;13:604-612.

74. Lindstrom G, Nystrom A: Natural history of scaphoid non-union with special reference to "asymptomatic" cases. *J Hand Surg Br* 1992;17:697-700.

75. Mack GR, Bosse MJ, Gelberman RH, Yu E: The natural history of scaphoid non-union. *J Bone Joint Surg Am* 1984;66:504-509.

76. Nakamura R, Imaeda T, Tsuge S, Watanabe K: Scaphoid non-union with D.I.S.I. deformity: A survey of clinical cases with special reference to ligamentous injury. *J Hand Surg Am* 1991;16:156-161.

77. Ruby LK, Stinson J, Belsky MR: The natural history of scaphoid non-union: A review of fifty-five cases. *J Bone Joint Surg Am* 1985;67:428-432.

78. Steiger R, Sennwald G: Late results of operated scaphoid pseudarthroses. *Handchir Mikrochir Plast Chir* 1990;22:152-155.

79. Jiranek WA, Ruby LK, Millender LB, Bankoff MS, Newberg AH: Long-term results after Russe bone-grafting: The effect of malunion of the scaphoid. *J Bone Joint Surg Am* 1992;74:1217-1228.

80. Tsuyuguchi Y, Murase T, Hidaka N, Ohno H, Kawai H: Anterior wedge-shaped bone graft for old scaphoid fractures or non-unions: An analysis of relevant carpal alignment. *J Hand Surg Br* 1995;20:194-200.

81. Schuind F, Haentjens P, Van Innis F, Vander Maren C, Garcia-Elias M, Sennwald G: Prognostic factors in the treatment of carpal scaphoid nonunions. *J Hand Surg Am* 1999;24:761-776.

82. Green DP: The effect of avascular necrosis on Russe bone grafting for scaphoid nonunion. *J Hand Surg Am* 1985;10:597-605.

83. Mazet R Jr, Hohl M: Radial styloidectomy and styloidectomy plus bone graft in the treatment of old ununited carpal scaphoid fractures. *Ann Surg* 1960;152:296-302.

84. Andrews J, Miller G, Haddad R: Treatment of scaphoid nonunion by volar inlay distal radius bone graft. *J Hand Surg Br* 1985;10:214-216.

85. Fernandez DL: Anterior bone grafting and conventional lag screw fixation to treat scaphoid nonunions. *J Hand Surg Am* 1990;15:140-147.

86. Schneider LH, Aulicino P: Nonunion of the carpal scaphoid: The Russe procedure. *J Trauma* 1982;22:315-319.

87. Stark HH, Rickard TA, Zemel NP, Ashworth CR: Treatment of ununited fractures of the scaphoid by iliac bone grafts and Kirschner-wire fixation. *J Bone Joint Surg Am* 1988;70: 982-991.

88. Trumble TE, Gilbert M, Murray LW, Smith J, Rafijah G, McCallister WV: Displaced scaphoid fractures treated with open reduction and internal fixation with a cannulated screw. *J Bone Joint Surg Am* 2000;82:633-641.

89. Warren-Smith CD, Barton NJ: Non-union of the scaphoid: Russe graft vs. Herbert screw. *J Hand Surg Br* 1988;13:83-86.

90. Cooney WP, Linscheid RL, Dobyns JH, Wood MB: Scaphoid nonunion: Role of anterior interpositional bone grafts. *J Hand Surg Am* 1988;13:635-650.

91. Fernandez DL: A technique for anterior wedge-shaped grafts for scaphoid nonunions with carpal instability. *J Hand Surg Am* 1984;9:733-737.

92. Manske PR, McCarthy JA, Strecker WB: Use of the Herbert bone screw for scaphoid nonunions. *Orthopedics* 1988;11:1653-1661.

93. Trumble T (ed): Fractures and dislocations of the carpus, in *Principles of Hand Surgery and Therapy*. Philadelphia, PA, WB Saunders, 2001.

94. Belsole RJ, Hilbelink DR, Llewellyn JA, Dale M, Greene TL, Rayhack JM: Computed analyses of the pathomechanics of scaphoid waist nonunions. *J Hand Surg Am* 1991;16:899-906.

95. Lynch NM, Linscheid RL: Corrective osteotomy for scaphoid malunion: Technique and long-term follow-up evaluation. *J Hand Surg Am* 1997;22:35-43.

96. Adams BD, Blair WF, Reagan DS, Grundberg AB: Technical factors related to Herbert screw fixation. *J Hand Surg Am* 1988;13:893-899.

97. Alnot JY, Bellan N, Oberlin C, De Cheveigne C: Fractures and nonunions of the proximal pole of the carpal scaphoid bone: Internal fixation by a proximal to distal screw. *Ann Chir Main* 1988;7:101-108.

98. Boeckstyns ME, Kjaer L, Busch P, Holst-Nielsen F: Soft tissue interposition arthroplasty for scaphoid nonunion. *J Hand Surg Am* 1985;10:109-114.

99. Roy-Camille R: Fractures et pseudarthrosis du scaphoide moge. Utilsation d'un Greffo pedicule. *Actual de Chir Orthop R Poincare* 1965;4:197-214.

100. Shah J, Jones WA: Factors affecting the outcome in 50 cases of scaphoid nonunion treated with Herbert screw fixation. *J Hand Surg Br* 1998;23:680-685.

101. Chacha PB: Vascularised pedicular bone grafts. *Int Orthop* 1984;8:117-138.

102. Birchard D, Pichora D: Experimental corrective scaphoid osteotomy for scaphoid malunion with abnormal wrist mechanics. *J Hand Surg Am* 1990;15:863-868.

103. Burgess RC: The effect of a simulated scaphoid malunion on wrist motion. *J Hand Surg Am* 1987;12:774-776.

104. Fernandez DL, Martin CJ, Gonzalez del Pino J: Scaphoid malunion: The significance of rotational malalignment. *J Hand Surg Br* 1998;23:771-775.

105. Watson HK, Ballet FL: The SLAC wrist: Scapholunate advanced collapse pattern of degenerative arthritis. *J Hand Surg Am* 1984;9: 358-365.

106. Watson HK, Weinzweig J, Zeppieri J: The natural progression of scaphoid instability. *Hand Clin* 1997;13:39-49.

107. Ashmead D IV, Watson HK, Damon C, Herber S, Paly W: Scapholunate advanced collapse wrist salvage. *J Hand Surg Am* 1994;19:741-750.

108. Tomaino MM, Miller RJ, Cole I, Burton RI. Scapholunate advanced collapse wrist: Proximal row carpectomy or limited wrist arthrodesis with scaphoid excision? *J Hand Surg Am* 1994; 19:134-142.

109. Viegas SF: Limited arthrodesis for scaphoid nonunion. *J Hand Surg Am* 1994;19:127-133.

13

Carpal Instability

Richard H. Gelberman, MD
William P. Cooney III, MD
Robert M. Szabo, MD, MPH

Anatomy

The intracapsular ligaments of the wrist are divided into intrinsic and extrinsic components.[1-9] The two most important intrinsic (interosseous) ligaments, the scapholunate and lunotriquetral ligaments, are divided into dorsal, proximal, and palmar regions (Fig. 1). The thickest and strongest region of the scapholunate ligament is located dorsally, and that of the lunotriquetral ligament is located palmarly.[1,10]

There are three strong palmar extrinsic radiocarpal ligaments: the radioscaphocapitate, long radiolunate, and short radiolunate ligaments.[2] The radioscaphocapitate ligament, which extends from the radial styloid process through a groove in the waist of the scaphoid to the palmar aspect of the capitate, acts as a fulcrum around which the scaphoid rotates (Fig. 2). The long radiolunate ligament, which lies parallel to the radioscaphocapitate ligament, extends from the palmar rim of the distal part of the radius to the radial margin of the palmar horn of the lunate. The long radiolunate ligament and the palmar region of the lunotriquetral interosseous ligament, thought to be in continuity in earlier studies, were previously labeled the radiotriquetral ligament.[7] Located between the radioscaphocapitate and long radiolunate ligaments, at the level of the midcarpal joint, is an area of capsular weakness known as the space of Poirier. The short radiolunate ligament, which is contiguous with palmar fibers of the triangular fibrocartilage complex, originates from the palmar margin of the distal part of the radius and inserts into the proximal part of the palmar surface of the lunate. The radioscapholunate ligament (the ligament of Testut), previously thought to be an important stabilizer of the scaphoid, is now considered to be a neurovascular pedicle derived from the anterior interosseous and radial arteries and from the anterior interosseous nerve.[3] The ulnolunate and the ulnotriquetral ligaments arise from the

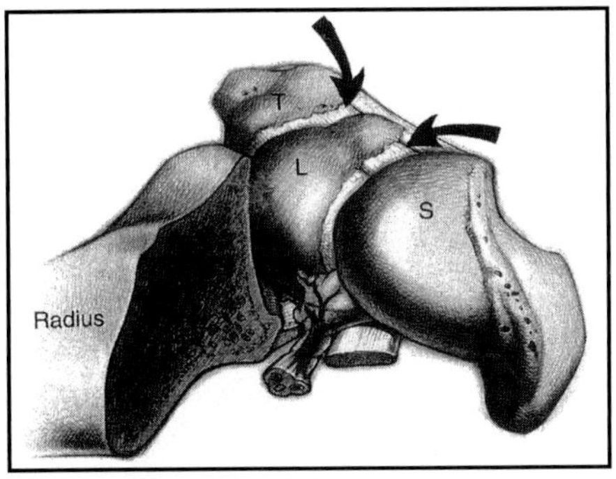

Fig. 1 Illustration demonstrating the scapholunate and lunotriquetral interosseous ligaments (*arrows*). S = scaphoid, L = lunate, T = triquetrum. (Adapted with permission from Berger RA: The gross and histologic anatomy of the scapholunate interosseous ligament. *J Hand Surg Am* 1996;21:172.)

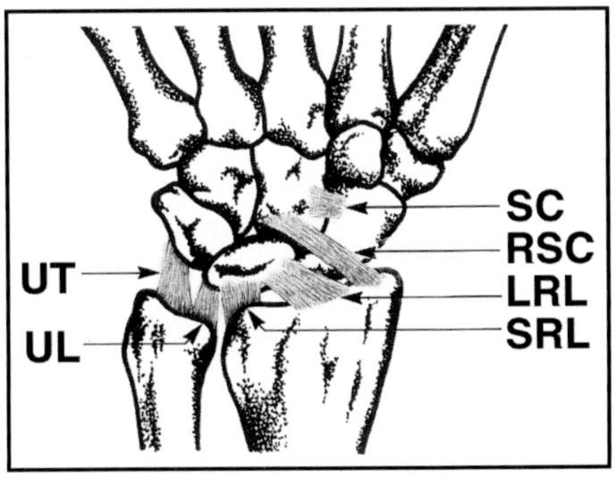

Fig. 2 Illustration demonstrating the palmar wrist ligaments. UT = ulnotriquetral, UL = ulnolunate, SC = scaphocapitate, RSC = radioscaphocapitate, LRL = long radiolunate, SRL = short radiolunate. The space between the long radiolunate and short radiolunate ligaments is where the ligament of Testut (or the radioscapholunate ligament), now known to be a neurovascular pedicle, enters the radiocarpal joint.

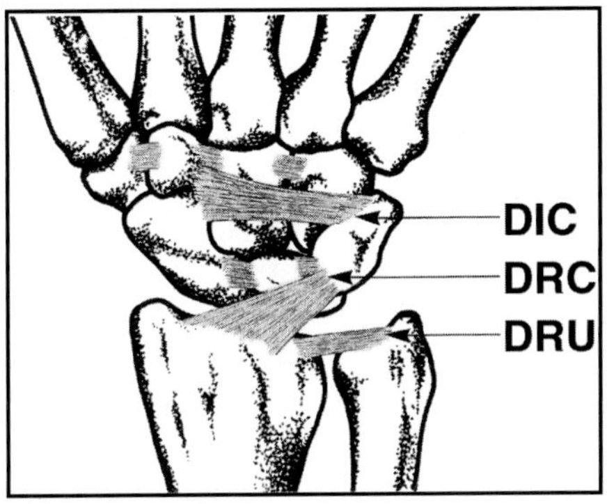

Fig. 3 Illustration demonstrating the dorsal wrist ligaments. DIC = dorsal intercarpal, DRC = dorsal radiocarpal, DRU = dorsal radioulnar.

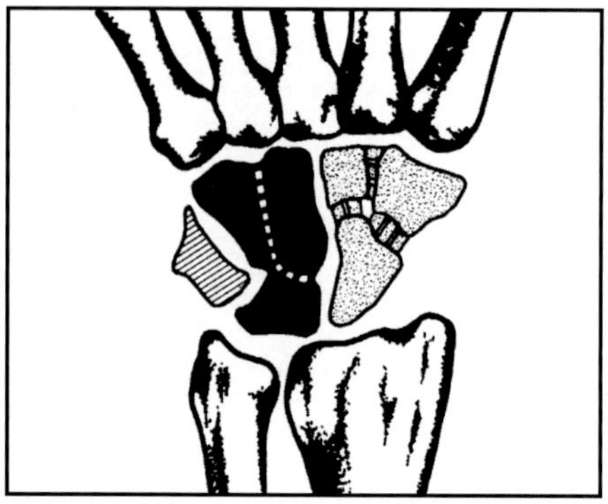

Fig. 4 Illustration demonstrating Navarro's columnar carpus.[12] The lateral column comprises the scaphoid, trapezium, and trapezoid; the central column comprises the lunate, capitate, and hamate; and the medial column comprises the triquetrum and pisiform. (Adapted with permission from Lichtman DM, Schneider JR, Swafford AR, Mack GR: Ulnar midcarpal instability: Clinical and laboratory analysis. *J Hand Surg Am* 1981;6:515-523.)

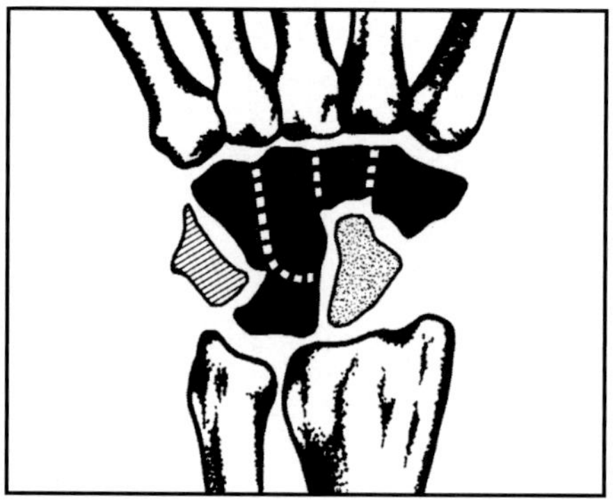

Fig. 5 Illustration demonstrating Taleisnik's modification of the columnar carpus.[8] The trapezium and trapezoid are included in the central column, and the pisiform is eliminated from the medial column. (Adapted with permission from Lichtman DM, Schneider JR, Swafford AR, Mack GR: Ulnar midcarpal instability: Clinical and laboratory analysis. *J Hand Surg Am* 1981;6:515-523.)

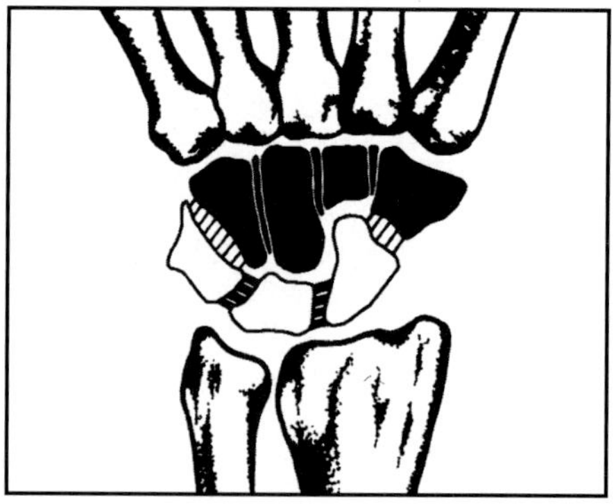

Fig. 6 Illustration demonstrating the oval ring concept of Lichtman and associates.[14] (Adapted with permission from Lichtman DM, Schneider JR, Swafford AR, Mack GR: Ulnar midcarpal instability: Clinical and laboratory analysis. *J Hand Surg Am* 1981;6:515-523.).

volar edge of the triangular fibrocartilage and insert into the lunate and the triquetrum, respectively. The dorsal radiocarpal ligament originates from the dorsal margin of the distal part of the radius and extends ulnarly and distally to attach to the lunate, the lunotriquetral interosseous ligament, and the dorsal tubercle of the triquetrum[11] (Fig. 3). The dorsal intercarpal ligament originates from the triquetrum and extends radially to insert into the lunate, the dorsal groove of the scaphoid, and the trapezium.

Kinematics

There are two prevailing theories, the columnar and oval ring concepts, that have been used to characterize carpal kinematics. The columnar carpus concept, introduced by Navarro in 1921, describes the carpus as a series of three longitudinal columns (the central [flexion-extension], lateral [mobile], and medial [rotational] columns)[12] (Fig. 4). Taleisnik modified Navarro's theory, adding the trapezium and trapezoid to the central column and eliminating the pisiform from the medial column[8] (Fig. 5). The scaphoid is considered to be the stabilizing link for the midcarpal joint, and the triquetrum is thought to be the pivot point for carpal rotation.[8,9] Flexion and extension occur through the central column, and radial and ulnar deviation occur by rotation of the scaphoid laterally and the triquetrum medially. With the proximal row independence and oval ring concepts, Linscheid[13] and Lichtman and associates[14] characterized the carpus as a ring that allows reciprocal motion during radial and ulnar deviation and flexion and extension of the wrist (Fig. 6). Central to this concept is the observation that radial and ulnar deviation and flexion and extension occur reciprocally between the radiocarpal and midcarpal joints (that is, movement by one row is in the opposite direction from that by the other). An interruption of the proximal carpal row at any point in the ring results in carpal instability.

Terminology

The carpus is considered clinically unstable if it exhibits symptomatic malalignment, is not able to bear loads, and does not have normal kinematics during any portion of its arc of motion.[15] Static instability refers to carpal malalignment that can be detected on standard posteroanterior and lateral radiographs.[16] Dynamic instability refers to carpal malalignment that is reproduced with physical examination maneuvers and when stress radiographs are made. With dynamic instability, there is no evidence of carpal bone malalignment on plain radiographs. The terms dorsal intercalated instability and volar intercalated instability refer to the appearance of the lunate, the intercalated segment, on the lateral radiograph.[17] In dorsal intercalated instability, the lunate is angulated dorsally in the sagittal plane and the capitate is displaced dorsal to the radiometacarpal axis (radiolunate angle, more than 10°) (Fig. 7). In volar intercalated instability, the lunate angulates palmarly (radiolunate angle, 10° in a palmar direction), which causes the capitate to become displaced palmar to the radiometacarpal axis.

Other terms have been introduced to clarify various patterns of carpal instability. Carpal instability dissociative connotes an injury to one of the major intrinsic carpal ligaments, such as that seen in scapholunate dissociation and perilunate dislocation. Carpal instability nondissociative indicates an injury to a major extrinsic ligament, such as occurs in dorsal carpal subluxation, midcarpal instability, volar carpal subluxation, or capitate-lunate instability. Carpal instability adaptive refers to carpal instability resulting from an external cause, such as that seen at the radiocarpal or midcarpal joint following severe malunion of the distal part of the radius.

Mechanisms of Injury

In an experimental study, Mayfield and associates[18,19] determined that the mechanism of injury for most carpal dislocations is a fall on the outstretched hand causing wrist extension, ulnar deviation, and intercarpal supination. Sequential ligamentous injury, called progressive perilunar instability, was noted to be initiated on the radial aspect of the wrist and to extend across the perilunate ligaments to the ulnar aspect of the wrist. Four stages of progressive perilunar instability were defined, including scapholunate dissociation caused by injury to the scapholunate interosseous and palmar radioscaphocapitate ligaments (stage I), dislocation of the capitolunate joint through the space of Poirier (stage II), separation of the triquetrum from the lunate with associated injury to the lunotriquetral and ulnotriquetral ligaments (stage III), and palmar lunate dislocation due to injury to the dorsal radiocarpal ligament (stage IV). Transradial styloid, transscaphoid, and transcapitate fractures are associated with perilunate injuries that progress from lateral to medial, ultimately involving the lunotriquetral ligament, the volar ulnocarpal ligaments, and the ulnar styloid process.[20]

Radiographic and Other Diagnostic Studies

Six radiographs are made for wrists with suspected carpal instability. These include posteroanterior, lateral, radial and ulnar deviation, and flexion and extension views.[21] An additional posteroanterior radiograph of the wrist with a clenched and loaded fist is made to rule out scapholunate instability. The alignment of the proximal and distal carpal rows is measured with Gilula's method. The midcarpal joint is visualized as an acetabulum or cup where the capitate and hamate articulate with the proximal carpal row. Interruption of the normal carpal arc of either the proximal or the distal carpal row indicates an instability pattern.

The use of radionuclide bone scans as screening tools is indicated for the localization of the cause of obscure wrist pain such as that caused by a chondral fracture.[22] While a positive bone scan provides information on the location of a wrist abnormality, it is rarely diagnostic. A negative bone scan, which suggests that a serious injury has not occurred, does not rule out carpal instability, especially in the early stages when reactive bone changes have not yet taken place. Overall, bone scanning is not as helpful as other studies in the evaluation of wrists with suspected carpal instability.

Arthrography of the wrist, performed alone or with videofluoroscopy, is a useful study in the evaluation of a wrist with carpal instability.[23] While wrist dynamics are best assessed with fluoroscopy, arthrography remains the standard study for the carpal ligaments and the triangular fibrocartilage complex.[24] Midcarpal, radiocarpal, and distal radioulnar arthrography (triple-phase injection) provides valuable definitive data on the integrity of the intrinsic intercarpal ligaments. Contrast material injected into the midcarpal joint does not extend into the radiocarpal joint unless there is either an acute or a degenerative intrinsic ligament tear (Fig. 8). For injuries of the triangular fibrocartilage complex, selective injection of the distal radioulnar joint is carried out. However, in some cases, both the radiocarpal and the distal radioulnar joint must be inspected to show a communicating defect. While false-positive and false-negative arthrograms have been reported, arthrography is of considerable value as a primary study for intrinsic carpal ligament injury.

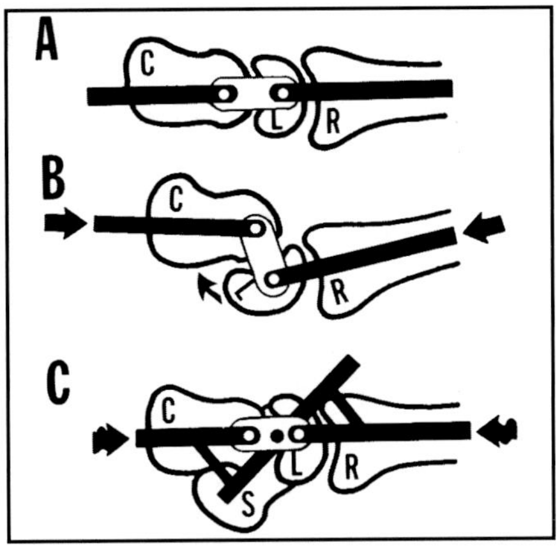

Fig. 7 **A,** The wrist has been described as a link joint, noting that instability occurs in compression because of the intercalated segment (the proximal carpal row represented by the lunate [L]) (**B**). **C,** The scaphoid (S) links the radius to the distal carpal row and provides stability against compression forces during wrist flexion and extension. C = capitate, R = radius. (Reproduced with permission from Green DP: Carpal dislocation and instabilities, in Green DP (ed): *Operative Hand Surgery*, ed 3. New York, NY, Churchill Livingstone, 1993, p 863.)

Tomography of the wrist (polytomography or CT), which is useful for evaluating the alignment of the carpal bones, is most helpful for assessing the fractures and fracture-dislocations that are frequently associated with carpal instability.[25] Complex motion polytomography is of special value for obtaining biplanar images of the carpus. Computed axial topography,[26] which provides useful cross-sectional images, is particularly helpful if three-dimensional reconstruction is performed. In the evaluation of wrist injuries, tomography is generally limited to cases in which a carpal fracture is suspected.

MRI, used frequently for the evaluation of wrist pain, is less helpful than other studies for the assessment of a wrist with carpal instability.[27,28] MRI is

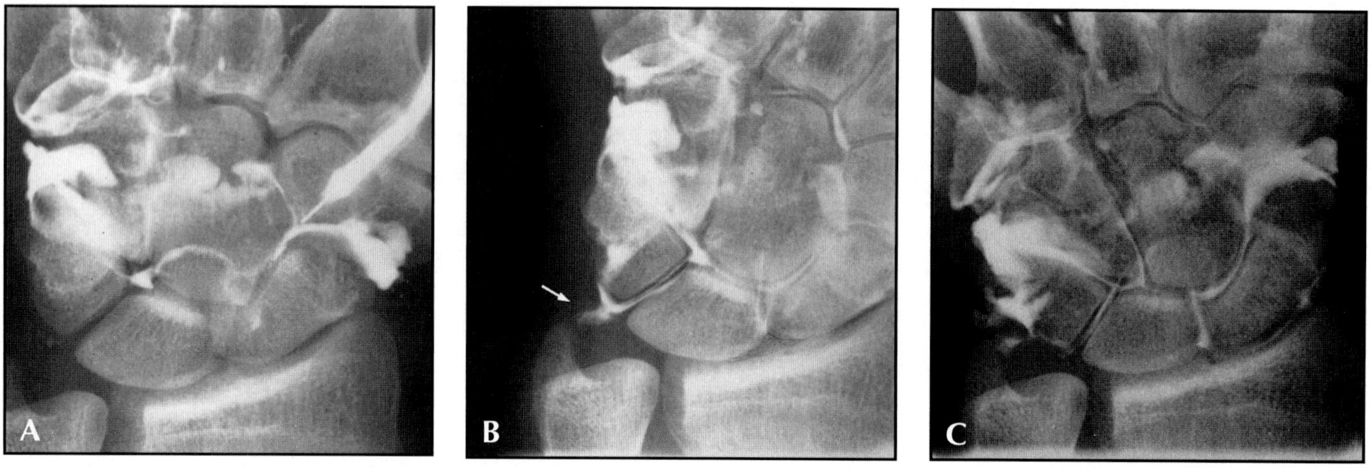

Fig. 8 Midcarpal arthrograms diagnostic for a lunotriquetral ligament tear. **A**, Contrast material is injected into the midcarpal joint. **B**, Contrast material is noted to extend across the lunotriquetral joint *(arrow)*. **C**, Contrast material fills the scapholunate interval but does not cross at this location into the radiocarpal joint.

most useful for evaluating suspected cases of osteonecrosis of bone and tumors of bone or soft tissue. While it can be helpful for visualizing the triangular fibrocartilage complex, it is not particularly useful for the evaluation of carpal ligament injuries unless gadolinium enhancement is performed.[28,29] The consistency with which both the radiocarpal and the interosseous ligaments are demonstrated, however, is not sufficient for this to be a primary method of evaluation.

Arthroscopy has replaced arthrography in many centers as the definitive diagnostic study for wrists with suspected carpal instability.[30,31] Recent reports have indicated that arthroscopic evaluation of the wrist is more accurate and specific than arthrography in detecting the site and extent of ligament injury.[21,32] Diagnostic wrist arthroscopy includes an examination of both the radiocarpal and the midcarpal joint. In the radiocarpal joint, triangulation probing of the scapholunate interosseous ligament, the lunotriquetral interosseous ligament, and the triangular fibrocartilage complex is carried out. The volar carpal ligaments are assessed in a radial-to-ulnar direction to determine whether extrinsic ligament injury has occurred. Midcarpal arthroscopy, with use of a triangulation probe, is performed routinely. The space between the scaphoid and lunate bones is assessed for evidence of ligamentous laxity. A diagnosis of partial or complete carpal ligament injury is established on the basis of the ease of separation of the scaphoid from the lunate and of the lunate from the triquetrum. If the probe can be rotated within the joint, a tear of the scapholunate or lunotriquetral interosseous ligament is suggested. If either the probe or the arthroscope can be passed from the midcarpal to the radiocarpal joint, rotatory subluxation of the scaphoid (a complete scapholunate ligament tear with extrinsic ligament laxity) is confirmed. Within the radiocarpal joint, a triangulation probe assists in the assessment of the size, location, and extent of tears of the triangular fibrocartilage complex. Associated osseous injuries (fractures of the proximal pole of the scaphoid or dorsal triquetral chip fractures) can be visualized also. Wrist arthrography and arthroscopy may be carried out in sequence within the operating room. Comprehensive intraoperative assessment currently includes fluoroscopy of the wrist with the patient under anesthesia in the operating room, followed by wrist arthrography and then by wrist arthroscopy, if indicated. Dynamic fluoroscopic imaging studies and arthroscopy are particularly useful when performed sequentially in the operating room to confirm the presence of a ligamentous injury and to plan the appropriate surgical approach. **(CD-13.1)**

Acute Static Scapholunate Dissociation

Acute static scapholunate dissociation, which may occur as an isolated entity or as a late sequela of a perilunate dislocation, results from injury to the scapholunate interosseous and palmar radioscaphoid ligaments.[33] Depending on the extent of ligamentous injury, there is either diffuse tenderness of the carpus or point tenderness over the scapholunate interval. Radiographs reveal all five key features of rotatory subluxation of the scaphoid (Figs. 9 and 10). Although ligamentous repair within 3 weeks after the injury is preferred,[34,35] delayed repair can be carried out as long as 4 to 6 months from the time of the injury. Several factors govern the feasibility of delayed ligamentous repair (repair later

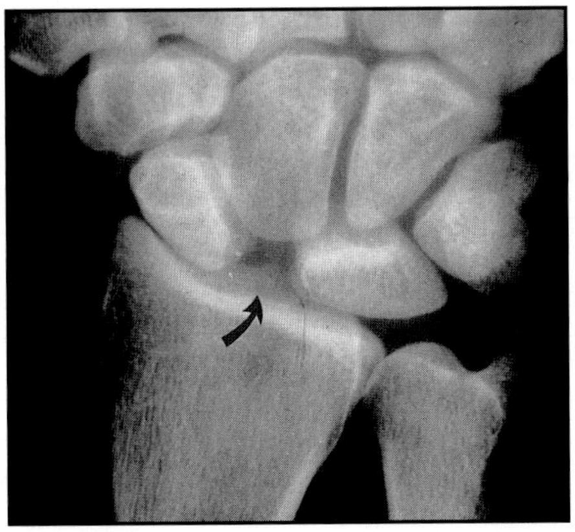

Fig. 9 Posteroanterior radiograph of a wrist with acute static scapholunate dislocation. The scaphoid is flexed (foreshortened), there is a scaphoid ring sign, the distance between the proximal aspect of the ring and the proximal pole of the scaphoid is less than 7 mm, and there is a gap between the scaphoid and the lunate of greater than 3 mm (*arrow*). In addition, the lunate and the triquetrum are dorsiflexed (the lunate is quadrilateral in shape, and the triquetrum is displaced distally on the hamate), while the scaphoid is flexed (the ring sign), which indicates an interruption in the proximal carpal row at the scapholunate interval.

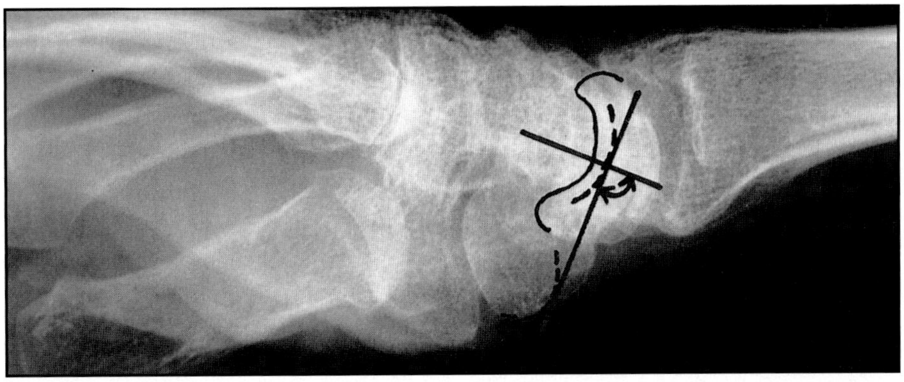

Fig. 10 Lateral radiograph of a wrist with acute static scapholunate dissociation. The scapholunate angle is increased as measured with the tangential measurement method. The longitudinal axis of the scaphoid is demonstrated by creating a line that connects the proximal surfaces of the two poles of the scaphoid. The angle is 90°.

than 3 weeks after the time of the injury); these factors include the identification of a substantial, reparable scapholunate interosseous ligament and the isolation of a palmar flexed scaphoid that can be reduced without the necessity for extensive circumferential dissection. The extent to which the scaphoid becomes fixed in palmar flexion is dependent on the magnitude of the initial capsular injury, with scarring and capsular contracture increasing over time.

Neither closed reduction alone nor closed reduction and percutaneous pin fixation is uniformly successful in maintaining carpal alignment and in achieving satisfactory long-term outcomes in wrists with acute scapholunate instability. The preferred method of treatment is open reduction of the carpus through a dorsal approach, pinning of the scaphoid to the lunate and to the capitate with two 0.045-in (0.114-cm) Kirschner wires,[36-39] and direct repair of the scapholunate ligament. Ligament repair is carried out either with direct suture for ligaments torn in their midsubstance or with pull-out sutures or suture anchors for ligaments avulsed from bone. The wrist is immobilized in neutral position in an above-the-elbow thumb-spica cast for 8 weeks,[34] following which time the pins are removed and active motion is initiated.

Chronic Scapholunate Dissociation

For wrists in which the scapholunate interosseous ligament cannot be repaired primarily, attempts to reconstruct the dorsal and palmar ligaments of the scaphoid with any combination of late ligamentous repair, tendon-grafting, and capsulodesis, while feasible,[40] have not provided consistent pain relief and have not maintained the alignment of the carpus over the long term.[36,41,42] Either scaphotrapeziotrapezoid or scaphocapitate intercarpal arthrodesis is effective surgical management. Each has been shown to produce similar reductions in the global range of motion of the wrist and comparable effects on relative intercarpal motion.[43] While some experimental studies have shown that these intercarpal arthrodeses cause increased loads across the radioscaphoid joint,[44,45] increased shear stresses on the lunate, and increased tension on the surrounding ligaments,[43] others have indicated that the long-term functional results are satisfactory.[45-50] Most authors have recommended that radial styloidectomy be carried out at the time of scaphotrapeziotrapezoid and scaphocapitate arthrodeses to avoid radial styloid-scaphoid impingement. Following both of these limited intercarpal arthrodeses, residual flexion and extension of the wrist is 50% to 60% of that on the contralateral side and residual radial and ulnar deviation is 60% to 70% of that on the contralateral side.[47,48,51-53] The most common complications are nonunion, which is seen in as many as 30% of patients, and radioscaphoid impingement.[54-56]

Acute Perilunate Dislocation

With acute perilunate dislocation, the typical findings on physical examination are swelling, pain, and deformity of the wrist and the typical finding on radiographic examination is gross disturbance of the intercarpal relationships (Fig. 11, *A*). With dorsal perilunate dislocation, lateral radiographs demonstrate that the longitudinal axis of the capitate is displaced dorsal to the longitudinal axis of the radius (Fig. 11, *B*). With

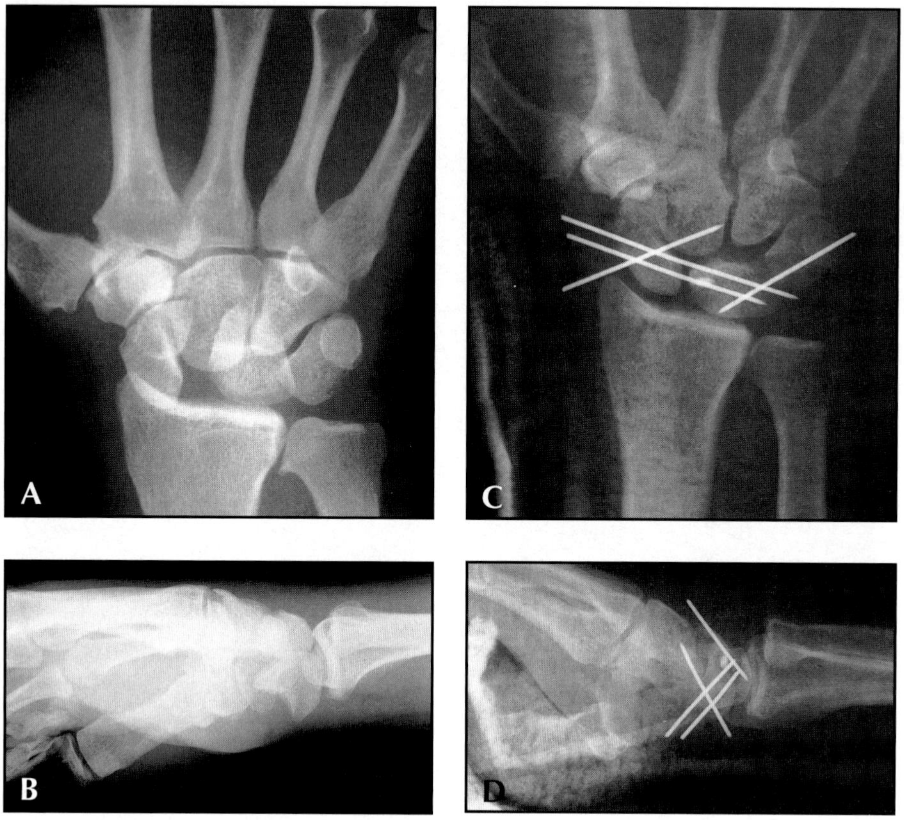

Fig. 11 Radiographs of a wrist with acute stage III dorsal perilunate dislocation according to the system of Mayfield and associates.[18,19] **A**, Preoperative posteroanterior radiograph demonstrating overlap of the carpal bones (normally only the trapezium and the trapezoid, and the triquetrum and the pisiform, overlap on the posteroanterior radiograph), a triangular shape to the lunate, and a scapholunate gap of 7 mm. **B**, Preoperative lateral radiograph demonstrating that while the lunate is palmar flexed it rests in the lunate fossa of the radius. The scaphoid and the capitate are displaced dorsal to the longitudinal axis of the radius. **C**, Postoperative posteroanterior radiograph demonstrating reduction of the scaphoid with fixation of the scaphoid to the lunate with two 0.045-in (0.114-cm) Kirschner wires. A third Kirschner wire secures the scaphoid to the capitate. The scapholunate interosseous ligament was reattached to the lunate with a suture anchor. The lunotriquetral joint was reduced, and the triquetrum was secured to the lunate with a 0.045-in Kirschner wire. The lunotriquetral ligament was repaired by direct suture. **D**, Postoperative lateral radiograph demonstrating that the capitate and the lunate are colinear with the radius and that the capitate is concentric with the articular surface of the lunate.

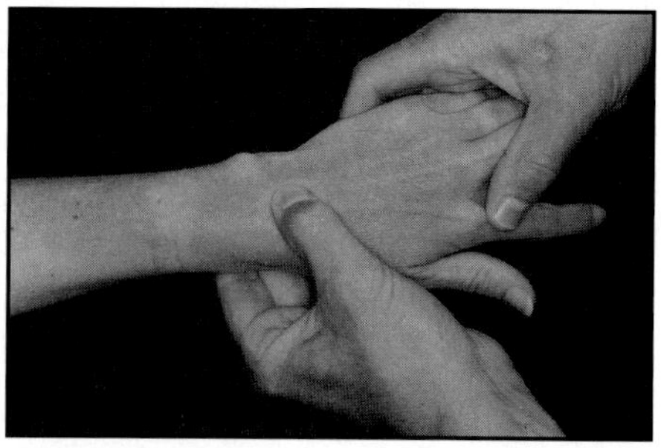

Fig. 12 Photograph demonstrating how point tenderness over the scapholunate interval is elicited in wrists with dynamic scapholunate instability.

lunate dislocation, the longitudinal axis of the capitate is colinear with the axis of the radius and the lunate is displaced palmarly.[17] Distortion of the concentric arcs of the proximal and distal rows indicates that the injury has extended to the ulnar side of the carpus. If initial radiographs are confusing, it is helpful to make distraction radiographs with 10 to 15 lb (4.5 to 6.8 kg) of fingertrap traction. Radiographs of the contralateral wrist in neutral alignment are made, and measurements are made from reference points on the lunate and scaphoid.

Previous investigators have noted that there is a low likelihood of achieving long-term success with closed reduction of an acute perilunate dislocation, with or without percutaneous pin fixation.[57] Currently, the treatment of choice is immediate closed reduction followed by open ligamentous repair through a dorsal approach. Closed reduction is carried out in the emergency room with traction (10 lb [4.5 kg] for 10 min) applied to the hand with fingertraps. The fingertraps are then removed, and manual longitudinal traction is applied. As the wrist is extended, the lunate is stabilized by the examiner's thumb. With traction maintained, the wrist is gradually palmar flexed and the capitate is reduced into the concavity of the lunate.[58] The patient is then taken to the operating room, and regional or general anesthesia is administered. A longitudinal dorsal incision is made from the base of the index and long metacarpals, over Lister's tubercle to the distal aspect of the forearm. Dissection of the carpus is carried out beneath the infratendinous retinaculum of the fourth dorsal compartment. The scapholunate and lunotriquetral interosseous ligaments are inspected. After reduction of the scapholunate joint, three to four 0.045-in (0.114-cm) Kirschner wires are inserted, extending from the scaphoid to the lunate, from the scaphoid to the capitate, and on occasion from the radius to the lunate. If the lunotriquetral ligament is torn, the lunotriquetral joint is reduced and pinned with an additional 0.045-in Kirschner wire (Fig. 11, *C* and *D*). The scapholunate and lunotriquetral interosseous ligaments are repaired with direct suture with 4.0 braided Dacron

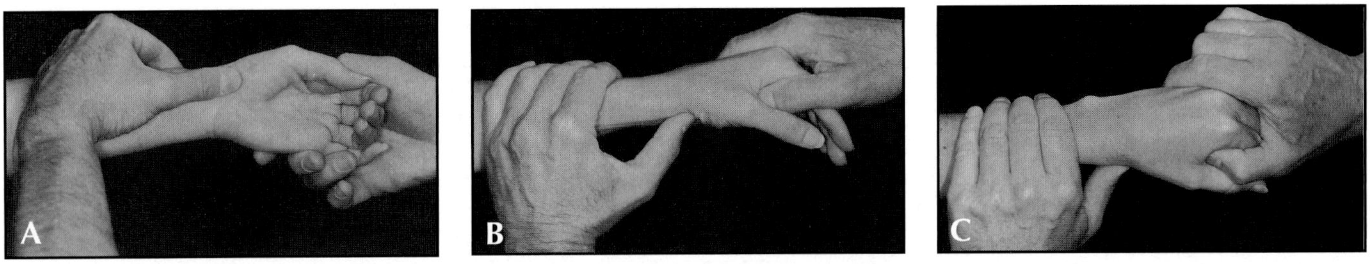

Fig. 13 Photographs demonstrating the scaphoid shift maneuver. Volar (**A**) and lateral (**B**) views showing how the maneuver is performed by applying pressure over the scaphoid while the wrist is held in ulnar deviation. **C**, As the wrist is brought from ulnar to radial deviation, the scaphoid's proximal pole returns to its position in the scaphoid fossa of the radius. The patient notes wrist pain with the maneuver, and both the patient and the examiner note a clunking sensation.

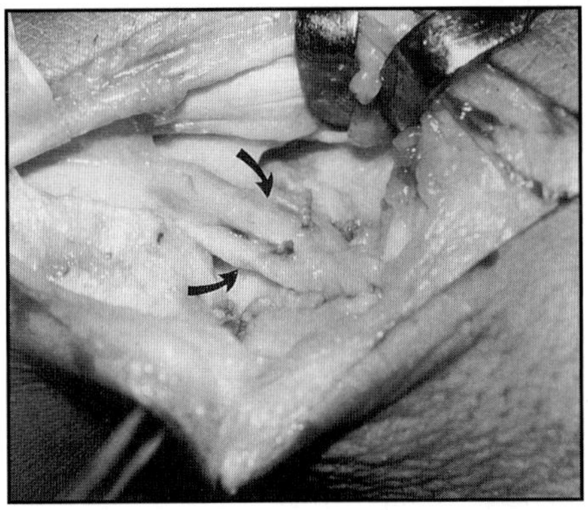

Fig. 14 Dorsal capsulodesis is performed by creating a transversely directed trough in the distal portion of the scaphoid. A 1-cm wide dorsal radius-based capsular flap, aligned with the longitudinal axis of the thumb metacarpal *(arrows)*, is attached to the scaphoid with suture anchors.

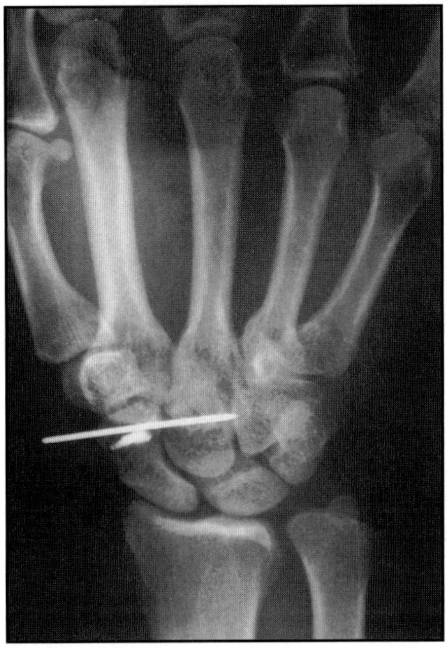

Fig. 15 Radiograph showing dorsal capsulodesis. One or two 0.045-in (0.114-cm) Kirschner wires, inserted through the scaphoid's distal pole, provide stabilization to the capitate. The wrist is immobilized postoperatively in 20° of extension and ulnar deviation for 6 weeks.

or with suture anchors. Currently, a palmar incision is made in addition, particularly if there is a palmar lunate (stage IV) dislocation that cannot be reduced closed or if there are findings indicative of acute carpal tunnel syndrome.[18,19]

Postoperatively, the wrist is immobilized in an above-the-elbow plaster-reinforced compression dressing for 14 days. A below-the-elbow thumb-spica cast is then applied and is maintained for an additional 6 weeks. Eight weeks postoperatively, the cast is removed, the pins are removed, and active motion is initiated.[59] In a recent multicenter study of perilunate dislocations and fracture-dislocations, the authors noted that both open injury and a delay in treatment had adverse effects on outcomes and that postoperative arthritis was common (seen in as many as 56% of cases).[20,57,60]

Transscaphoid Perilunate Dislocation

Initial evaluation and treatment is similar to that carried out for perilunate dislocation.[20,57,59,60] Internal fixation of the scaphoid is performed with insertion of a compression screw through a dorsal incision. Injury to the dorsolateral branches of the radial artery, which enter the scaphoid through the dorsal ridge, can be avoided by direct visualization and protection of the dorsolateral vascular leash. An additional Kirschner wire may be placed in the scaphoid to provide rotational stability. Immobilization in a thumb-spica cast is maintained until there are clinical and radiographic signs of scaphoid union as evidenced by the absence of tenderness in the anatomic snuffbox on physical examination and the appearance of trabeculae extending across the fracture site on plain radiographs.

Scaphoid Dislocation

Palmar radial displacement of the proximal pole of the scaphoid from the scaphoid fossa of the distal part of the radius is diagnostic of a scaphoid rather than a perilunate dislocation. The interposition of capsular or ligamentous tissue may prevent closed reduction. Treatment, which is similar to that recommended for acute scapholunate dissociation, consists of open reduction of the scapholunate joint, insertion of two 0.045-in (0.114-cm) Kirschner wires extending from the scaphoid to the lunate and from the scaphoid to the capitate, and direct repair of the scapholunate interosseous

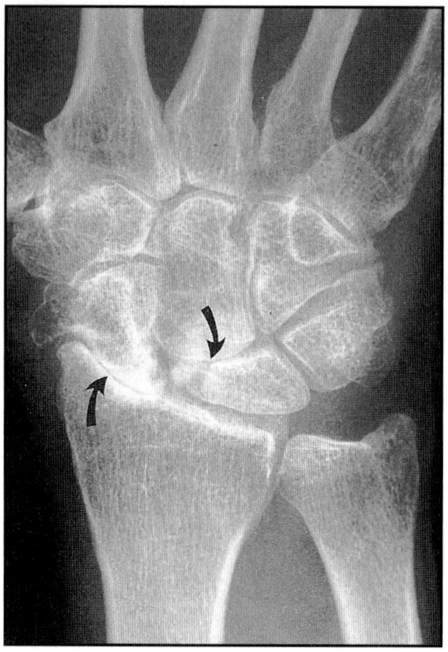

Fig. 16 Posteroanterior radiograph of the wrist, demonstrating stage III scapholunate advanced collapse. There is severe narrowing of the radioscaphoid joint space, from the tip of the styloid process of the radius to the lateral edge of the scaphoid fossa, and narrowing of the capitolunate joint space *(arrows)*. The radiolunate joint is preserved.

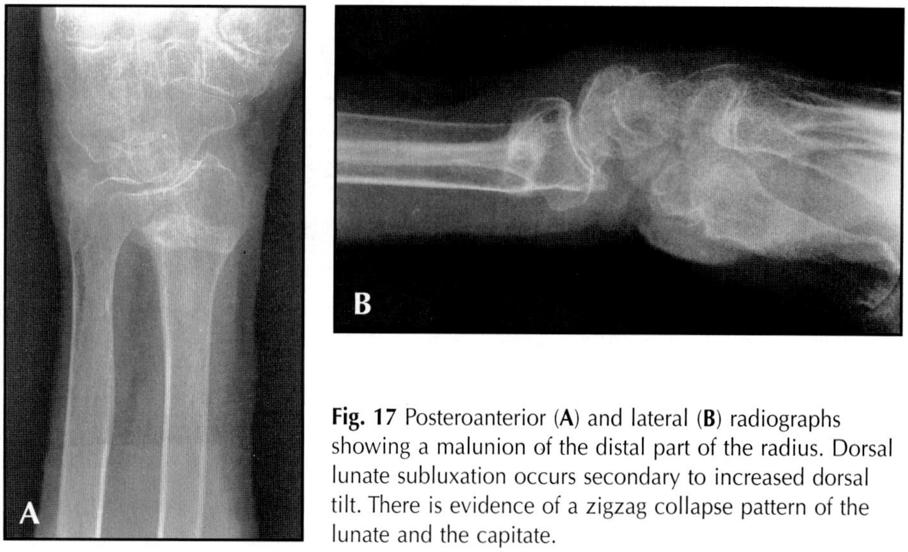

Fig. 17 Posteroanterior (**A**) and lateral (**B**) radiographs showing a malunion of the distal part of the radius. Dorsal lunate subluxation occurs secondary to increased dorsal tilt. There is evidence of a zigzag collapse pattern of the lunate and the capitate.

ligament. Immobilization in a below-the-elbow thumb-spica cast is maintained for 8 weeks, after which time active motion is initiated.

Dynamic Scapholunate Instability

Initially described by Taleisnik[61] in 1980, dynamic scapholunate instability is the most common cause of wrist pain and instability in adolescents and young adults.[62] Although a precise anatomic cause has not been determined, it is likely that attenuation of the palmar radioscaphoid and the scapholunate interosseous ligaments is the basis for this instability pattern.[8,61,63-66] While radiographic findings are frequently normal,[60,63,67] consistent findings on physical examination confirm the diagnosis. There is point tenderness over the scapholunate interval (Fig. 12), and provocative tests reproduce symptoms of instability. The scaphoid shift maneuver, performed as described by Watson and associates,[68] is the most useful clinical test. To perform this maneuver, pressure is applied to the palmar tubercle of the scaphoid by the examiner's thumb with the wrist in ulnar deviation (Fig. 13, *A* and *B*). In wrists with instability, the scaphoid is displaced dorsally over the lip of the radius. As the wrist is brought from ulnar to radial deviation, the scaphoid's proximal pole returns to its position in the scaphoid fossa of the radius (Fig. 13, *C*). As the scaphoid reduces, a clunking sensation and wrist pain are noted. Although 110 (11%) of 1000 randomly examined wrists were found to have unilateral, asymptomatic increased mobility of the scaphoid on the scaphoid shift test,[69] patients with dynamic instability are distinguished by their symptoms of instability and pain with this maneuver. The unaffected wrist is examined, and an assessment for generalized ligamentous laxity is carried out. Additional studies, such as three-portal wrist arthrography and wrist arthroscopy, have not been found to be helpful in confirming the diagnosis.[62]

In a recent study, 19 patients (20 wrists) with dynamic instability were treated nonsurgically with splinting of the wrist, oral administration of nonsteroidal anti-inflammatory medication, and modification of activities.[62] No patient in that study, however, had a substantial reduction in symptoms, even after 12 weeks and longer durations of nonsurgical treatment.

For wrists with persistent incapacitating pain and instability after a trial of nonsurgical care, dorsal capsulodesis, as described by Blatt[63,70] and as modified by Wintman and associates,[62] is the treatment of choice (Figs. 14 and 15). Results, reported in three recent studies, have been consistent with regard to the effectiveness of this procedure in eliminating symptoms of instability and pain in more than 90% of patients and in the achievement of high levels of satisfaction as reported on questionnaires.[36,62,63] Patients reported that substantial improvements occurred in activities such as brushing teeth, opening automobile doors, shoveling, sweeping, throwing, and using a screwdriver.[62] Although dorsal capsulodesis has been shown to cause a mean loss of wrist flexion of 15°, this procedure appears to provide superior outcomes when compared with the alternative methods that

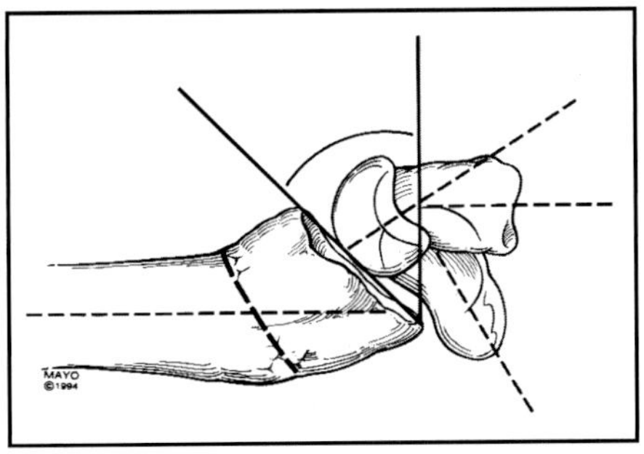

Fig. 18 Schematic of a wrist with midcarpal instability demonstrating flexion of the lunocapitate joint. The dotted oblique line through the distal part of the radius is the site of the proposed corrective osteotomy. (Reproduced with permission from the Mayo Foundation, Rochester, MN.)

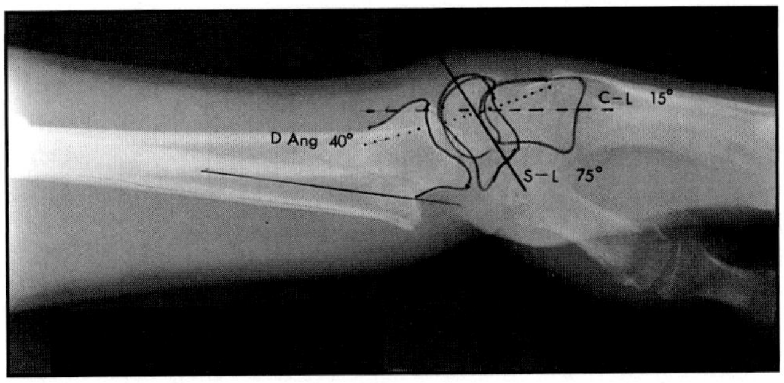

Fig. 19 Radiograph showing a malunion of the distal part of the radius with 40° of dorsiflexion of the distal part of the radius, a scapholunate angle of 75°, and a lunocapitate angle of 15°.

have been used for the treatment of dynamic instability, such as triscaphoid arthrodesis, which causes a far greater loss of wrist motion in all planes.[36]

Dorsal Wrist Ganglia and Dynamic Carpal Instability

Dorsal wrist ganglia, which most often originate from the scapholunate interosseous ligament in the young adults, have been shown to be associated with symptoms and signs of dynamic scapholunate instability. In a recent study[71] of 18 patients (19 wrists) with a dorsal wrist ganglion and dynamic scapholunate instability, treatment consisted of excision of the ganglion to the level of the scapholunate interosseous ligament and postoperative immobilization of the wrist in 20° of extension for 2 weeks. On follow-up evaluation, two patients had continued wrist pain and one had a recurrent ganglion. All but one patient in this series, including two who had signs of generalized ligamentous laxity, had a stable nontender wrist on follow-up physical examination at 1 year. It appears that postoperative dorsal capsular scarring following ganglion excision and 2 weeks of wrist immobilization stabilizes the scaphoid sufficiently to alleviate symptoms and signs of dynamic scapholunate instability.

Scapholunate Advanced Collapse

The most common form of wrist arthritis, scapholunate advanced collapse, evolves in a predictable sequence.[72] Injury to the scapholunate interosseous and palmar radioscaphoid ligaments has been shown to lead to a progressive shift of the pressure centroid of the scaphoid,[73] which is noted to result in a change in the regions of peak intra-articular contact between the scaphoid and the distal part of the radius. Three distinct time-related degenerative changes occur in scapholunate advanced collapse; these consist of joint-space narrowing between the tip of the styloid process of the radius and the distal outer aspect of the scaphoid in stage I, degenerative changes along the entire articular surface between the radius and the scaphoid in stage II, and narrowing of the capitolunate joint space in stage III (Fig. 16). The observation that the radiolunate joint is spared consistently in wrists with scapholunate advanced collapse has served as the anatomic basis for several of the most widely used treatment methods over the past two decades.

Initial treatment consists of oral administration of nonsteroidal anti-inflammatory medication, application of a wrist splint, and modification of activities. For wrists with stage I scapholunate advanced collapse that are resistant to nonsurgical measures, surgical treatment designed to stabilize the carpus so that compressive and shear forces are transmitted through the normal radioscapholunate articulation is recommended. As ligament reconstruction has not proved to be consistently effective in maintaining correction of the excessively flexed scaphoid, intercarpal arthrodesis has become the surgical procedure of choice. Either scaphotrapeziotrapezoid or scaphocapitate arthrodesis achieves the goal of maintaining the scaphoid in an alignment that is 50° to 55° to the longitudinal axis of the radius when the wrist is in neutral position, and each is effective in reducing pain and slowing the progression of degenerative arthritis. Radial styloidectomy, performed simultaneously and consisting of removal of 7 mm of the radial styloid process dorsally and 4 mm palmarly, consistently minimizes symptoms due to abutment and eliminates pain due to arthritis at the distal aspect of the radioscaphoid joint.

For wrists with degenerative arthritis involving the entire radioscaphoid joint (stage II) or the radioscaphoid and capitolunate joints (stage III), a motion-preserving reconstructive procedure, either capitate-lunate-hamate-triquetrum (four-corner) arthrodesis with scaphoid excision or proximal row carpectomy, is recommended.

Studies by Imbriglia and associates[74] and by Neviaser[75] on proximal row carpectomy have indicated that, while high levels of wrist motion and grip strength are maintained, there is persistent pain, a failure to return to strenuous work, and a recommendation for

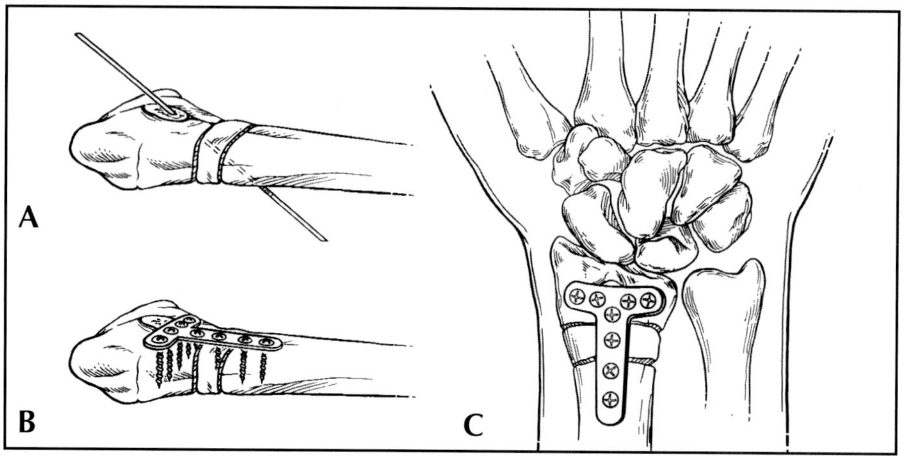

Fig. 20 Schematic of a corrective osteotomy, showing interposition of bone graft from the iliac crest to restore the length and tilt of the distal part of the radius. **A,** The graft is shown in place with temporary Kirschner wire fixation. **B,** A lateral view of T-plate fixation with the interposition graft. **C,** A posteroanterior view of the graft and T-plate in place.

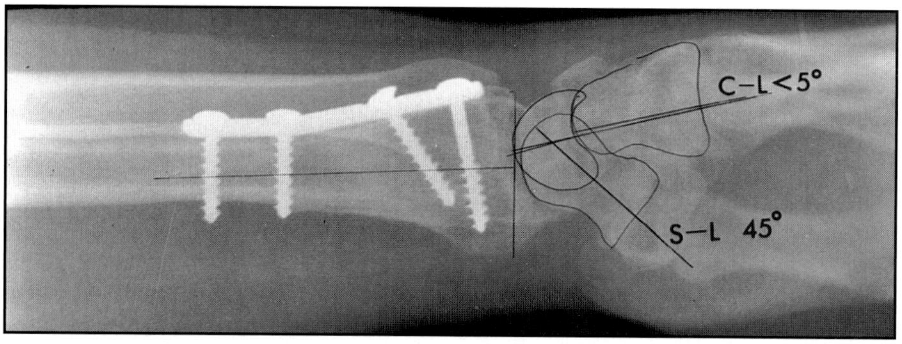

Fig. 21 Postoperative lateral radiograph showing the scapholunate angle corrected to 45° and the lunocapitate angle corrected to less than 5° after corrective osteotomy for the treatment of malunion of the distal part of the radius.

conversion to arthrodesis in as many as 15% of patients. Although carefully performed four-corner arthrodesis with scaphoid excision provides levels of patient satisfaction and grip strength that are similar to those seen with proximal row carpectomy, values for the range of motion of the wrist are 15° to 20° lower.[72,76] Attempts to limit the arthrodesis to the capitolunate joint in order to achieve a higher postoperative range of motion of the wrist have been unsuccessful because of high rates of nonunion.[77]

Recent studies have confirmed that proximal row carpectomy maintains an arc of wrist flexion and extension that is approximately 20° greater than the motion arc that is achieved with four-corner arthrodesis. Although grip-strength values and overall patient-satisfaction scores have been similar, specific complications have been noted with each procedure. Proximal row carpectomy appears to be particularly unpredictable in laborers and in wrists with stage III scapholunate advanced collapse. Four-corner arthrodesis has been associated with failure rates of as high as 30%,[78] and isolated capitolunate arthrodesis has been associated with a nonunion rate of 50% (four of eight).[79] Studies have indicated that either scaphotrapeziotrapezoid or scaphocapitate arthrodesis with radial styloidectomy is indicated for stage I scapholunate advanced collapse.[51,72] For stage II, either four-corner arthrodesis with scaphoid excision or proximal row carpectomy is an effective reconstructive procedure. There is general consensus that either limited wrist arthrodesis with scaphoid excision or proximal row carpectomy with fascial interposition is the procedure of choice for stage III scapholunate advanced collapse.[78-81]

Adaptive Instability

Dorsiflexion malunion after fracture of the distal part of the radius is the most common cause of adaptive carpal instability.[82,83] The osseous deformity leads to malalignment of the bones of the proximal carpal row, loss of wrist flexion, and radiocarpal or midcarpal instability. Biomechanical studies have shown that there is a shift of load from the radius to the ulna (from 20% to 67% of the total load) when dorsal angulation is increased beyond 15° of dorsal tilt (a 26° loss of normal palmar tilt).[84,85] Fernandez[86] observed that symptoms occurred most frequently when dorsal angulation of the distal part of the radius was greater than 20°, and other authors have recommended that 15° to 30° of dorsal angulation be considered an indication for distal radial osteotomy.

Adaptive instability of the carpus may occur at either the radiocarpal or the midcarpal joint.[87,88] With radiocarpal instability, dorsal radiocarpal subluxation occurs as the lunate contact area translates dorsally along the inclined plane of the distal part of the radius (Fig. 17). For the hand to become realigned with the forearm, flexion takes place at the radiolunate joint. With midcarpal instability, the angular relationship between the articular surface of the radius and the longitudinal axis of the lunate remains unchanged. For the hand to become realigned with the forearm, palmar flexion occurs at the lunocapitate level (Figs. 18 and 19). Instability occurs gradually, after the fracture has united, as the midcarpal joint is stressed during loading of the wrist. With both types of instability, a zigzag collapse deformity of the carpus results. While the condition is initially dynamic, both radiocarpal and midcarpal instability may become static over time.[89] Adaptive carpal instability results in a change of the moment arm of the flexor and extensor tendons, an alteration in carpal kinematics,[85] and a loss of power transmission across the wrist. With radial shortening and progressively increasing positive ulnar variance, the proximal row of carpal bones abuts the distal end of the ulna, either limiting rotation of the radius or causing palmar or dorsal displacement of the carpus.

Patients with adaptive carpal instability most frequently present with wrist pain, which is often delayed in onset for several weeks to months after fracture-healing, and loss of wrist motion and grip strength. Additional sequelae may include median neuropathy at the wrist and tendon rupture.[82,83]

The preferred treatment for radial dorsiflexion malunion in young patients (those younger than 50 years of age) who have greater than 5 mm of shortening consists of surgical restoration of both radial length and palmar tilt. Recent modifications in preoperative planning and surgical technique have improved the outcome of dorsal opening-wedge osteotomy, which is the procedure of choice[86,90] (Figs. 20 and 21). Postoperatively, the adaptive instability pattern corrects spontaneously in most cases and forearm rotation is restored. For wrists in which the adaptive instability pattern has become static, either ligament reconstruction or intercarpal arthrodesis is recommended.

References

1. Berger RA, Blair WF, Crowninshield RD, Flatt AE: The scapholunate ligament. *J Hand Surg Am* 1982;7:87-91.
2. Berger RA, Landsmeer JM: The palmar radiocarpal ligaments: A study of adult and fetal human wrist joints. *J Hand Surg Am* 1990; 15:847-854.
3. Berger RA, Kauer JM, Landsmeer JM: Radioscapholunate ligament: A gross anatomic and histologic study of fetal and adult wrists. *J Hand Surg Am* 1991; 16: 350-355.
4. Berger RA: The anatomy and basic biomechanics of the wrist joint. *J Hand Ther* 1996;9:84-93.
5. Berger RA: The gross and histologic anatomy of the scapholunate interosseous ligament. *J Hand Surg Am* 1996;21:170-178.
6. Berger RA: The ligaments of the wrist: A current overview of anatomy with considerations of their potential functions. *Hand Clin* 1997;13:63-82.
7. Mayfield JK, Johnson RP, Kilcoyne RF: The ligaments of the human wrist and their functional significance. *Anat Rec* 1976;186:417-428.
8. Taleisnik J: The ligaments of the wrist. *J Hand Surg Am* 1976;1:110-118.
9. Taleisnik, J: Wrist: Anatomy, function, and injury. *Instr Course Lect* 1978;27:61-87.
10. Ritt MJ, Bishop AT, Berger RA, Linscheid RL, Berglund LJ, An KN: Lunotriquetral ligament properties: A comparison of three anatomic subregions. *J Hand Surg Am* 1998;23:425-431.
11. Viegas SF, Yamaguchi S, Boyd NL, Patterson RM: The dorsal ligaments of the wrist: Anatomy, mechanical properties, and function. *J Hand Surg Am* 1999;24:456-468.
12. Navarro A: Luxaciones del carpo. *Anal Fac Med Montevideo* 1921;6:113-141.
13. Linscheid RL: Kinematic considerations of the wrist. *Clin Orthop* 1986;202:27-39.
14. Lichtman DM, Schneider JR, Swafford AR, Mack GR: Ulnar midcarpal instability: Clinical and laboratory analysis. *J Hand Surg Am* 1981;6:515-523.
15. The Anatomy and Biomechanics Committee of the International Federation of Societies for Surgery of the Hand: Definition of carpal instability. *J Hand Surg Am* 1999;24:866-867.
16. Larsen CF, Amadio PC, Gilula LA, Hodge JC: Analysis of carpal instability: Description of the scheme. *J Hand Surg Am* 1995;20:757-764.
17. Linscheid RL, Dobyns JH, Beabout JW, Bryan RS: Traumatic instability of the wrist: Diagnosis, classification, and pathomechanics. *J Bone Joint Surg Am* 1972;54:1612-1632.
18. Mayfield JK, Johnson RP, Kilcoyne RK: Carpal dislocations: Pathomechanics and progressive perilunar instability. *J Hand Surg Am* 1980;5:226-241.
19. Mayfield JK: Patterns of injury to carpal ligaments: A spectrum. *Clin Orthop* 1984; 187:36-42.
20. Herzberg G, Comtet JJ, Linscheid RL, Amadio PC, Cooney WP, Stalder J: Perilunate dislocations and fracture-dislocations: A multicenter study. *J Hand Surg Am* 1993;18:768-779.
21. Cooney WP III, Linscheid RL, Dobyns JH: Carpal instability: Ligament repair and reconstruction, in Neviaser RJ (ed): *Controversies in Hand Surgery*. New York, NY, Churchill Livingstone, 1990, pp 125-145.
22. Maurer AH: Nuclear medicine in evaluation of the hand and wrist. *Hand Clin* 1991;7:183-200.
23. Braunstein EM, Louis DS, Greene TL, Hankin FM: Fluoroscopic and arthrographic evaluation of carpal instability. *AJR Am J Roentgenol* 1985;144:1259-1262.
24. Levinsohn EM, Rosen ID, Palmer AK: Wrist arthrography: Value of the three-compartment injection method. *Radiology* 1991; 179:231-239.
25. Berquist TH (ed): *Imaging of Orthopaedic Trauma and Surgery*. Philadelphia, PA, WB Saunders, 1986.
26. Sanders WE: Evaluation of the humpback scaphoid by computed tomography in the longitudinal axial plane of the scaphoid. *J Hand Surg Am* 1988;13:182-187.
27. Berger RA, Linscheid RL, Berquist TH: Magnetic resonance imaging of the anterior radiocarpal ligaments. *J Hand Surg Am* 1994;19:295-303.
28. Gabl M, Lener M, Pechlaner S, Judmaier W: The role of dynamic magnetic resonance imaging in the detection of lesions of the ulnocarpal complex. *J Hand Surg Br* 1996; 21:311-314.
29. Pederzini L, Luchetti R, Soragni O, et al: Evaluation of the triangular fibrocartilage complex tears by arthroscopy, arthrography, and magnetic resonance imaging. *Arthroscopy* 1992;8:191-197.
30. Whipple TL, Cooney WP III, Osterman AL, Viegas SF: Wrist arthroscopy. *Instr Course Lect* 1995;44:139-145.
31. Savoie FH III, Grondel RJ: Arthroscopy for carpal instability. *Orthop Clin North Am* 1995;26:731-738.
32. Weiss AP, Akelman E: Diagnostic imaging and arthroscopy for chronic wrist pain. *Orthop Clin North Am* 1995;26:759-767.
33. Mayfield JK: Mechanism of carpal injuries. *Clin Orthop* 1980;149:45-54.
34. Taleisnik J: Scapholunate dissociation, in Strickland JW, Steichen JB (eds): *Difficult Problems in Hand Surgery*. St. Louis, MO, CV Mosby, 1982, pp 341-348.
35. Cooney WP III, Linscheid RL, Dobyns JH: Fractures and dislocations of the wrist in, Rockwood CA Jr, Green DP, Bucholz RW (eds): *Fractures in Adults*, ed 3. Philadelphia, PA, JB Lippincott, 1991, pp 563-678.
36. Lavernia CJ, Cohen MS, Taleisnik J: Treatment of scapholunate dissociation by ligamentous repair and capsulodesis. *J Hand Surg Am* 1992;17:354-359.
37. Cohn I: Dislocations of the semilunar carpal bone. *Ann Surg* 1921;73:621-628.
38. Conyers DJ: Scapholunate interosseous reconstruction and imbrication of palmar ligaments. *J Hand Surg Am* 1990;15:690-700.

39. Fisk GR: Malalignment of the scaphoid after lunate dislocation. *Ann Chir Main* 1984;3:353-356.

40. Dagum AB, Hurst LC, Finzel KC: Scapholunate dissociation: An experimental kinematic study of two types of indirect soft tissue repairs. *J Hand Surg Am* 1997;22: 714-719.

41. Glickel SZ, Millender LH: Ligamentous reconstruction for chronic intercarpal instability. *J Hand Surg Am* 1984;9:514-527.

42. Wyrick JD, Youse BD, Kiefhaber TR: Scapholunate ligament repair and capsulodesis for the treatment of static scapholunate dissociation. *J Hand Surg Br* 1998;23:776-80.

43. Garcia-Elias M, Cooney WP, An KN, Linscheid RL, Chao EY: Wrist kinematics after limited intercarpal arthrodesis. *J Hand Surg Am* 1989;14:791-799.

44. Viegas SF, Patterson RM, Peterson PD, et al: Evaluation of the biomechanical efficacy of limited intercarpal fusions for the treatment of scapho-lunate dissociation. *J Hand Surg Am* 1990;15:120-128.

45. Kleinman WB, Carroll C IV: Scapho-trapezio-trapezoid arthrodesis for treatment of chronic static and dynamic scapho-lunate instability: A 10-year perspective on pitfalls and complications. *J Hand Surg Am* 1990;15:408-414.

46. Watson HK, Belniak R, Garcia-Elias M: Treatment of scapholunate dissociation: Preferred treatment. STT fusion vs other methods. *Orthopedics* 1991;14:365-370.

47. Minami A, Kato H, Iwasaki N, Minami M: Limited wrist fusions: Comparison of results 22 and 89 months after surgery. *J Hand Surg Am* 1999;24:133-137.

48. Mih AD: Limited wrist fusion. *Hand Clin* 1997;13:615-25.

49. Eckenrode JF, Louis DS, Greene TL: Scaphoid-trapezium-trapezoid fusion in the treatment of chronic scapholunate instability. *J Hand Surg Am* 1986;11:497-502.

50. Kleinman WB: Long-term study of chronic scapho-lunate instability treated by scapho-trapezio-trapezoid arthrodesis. *J Hand Surg Am* 1989;14:429-445.

51. Watson HK, Hempton RF: Limited wrist arthrodeses: The triscaphoid joint. *J Hand Surg Am* 1980;5:320-327.

52. Gellman H, Kauffman D, Lenihan M, Botte MJ, Sarmiento A: An in vitro analysis of wrist motion: The effect of limited intercarpal arthrodesis and the contributions of the radiocarpal and midcarpal joints. *J Hand Surg Am* 1988;13:378-383.

53. Douglas DP, Peimer CA, Koniuch MP: Motion of the wrist after simulated limited intercarpal arthrodeses: An experimental study. *J Bone Joint Surg Am* 1987;69:1413-1418.

54. McAuliffe JA, Dell PC, Jaffe R: Complications of intercarpal arthrodesis. *J Hand Surg Am* 1993;18:1121-1128.

55. Frykman EB, Af Ekenstam F, Wadin K: Triscaphoid arthrodesis and its complications. *J Hand Surg Am* 1988;13:844-849.

56. Ishida O, Tsai TM: Complications and results of scapho-trapezio-trapezoid arthrodesis. *Clin Orthop* 1993;287:125-130.

57. Adkison JW, Chapman MW: Treatment of acute lunate and perilunate dislocations. *Clin Orthop* 1982;164:199-207.

58. Green DP, O'Brien ET: Classification and management of carpal dislocations. *Clin Orthop* 1980;149:55-72.

59. Szabo RM, Newland CC: Open reduction and ligamentous repair for acute lunate and perilunate dislocations, in Gelberman RH (ed): *The Wrist*. New York, NY, Raven Press, 1994, pp 167-182.

60. Campbell RD Jr, Thompson TC, Lance EM, Adler JB: Indications for open reduction of lunate and perilunate dislocations of the carpal bones. *J Bone Joint Surg Am* 1965;47:915-937.

61. Taleisnik J: Post-traumatic carpal instability. *Clin Orthop* 1980;149:73-82.

62. Wintman BI, Gelberman RH, Katz JN: Dynamic scapholunate instability: Results of operative treatment with dorsal capsulodesis. *J Hand Surg Am* 1995;20:971-979.

63. Blatt G: Capsulodesis in reconstructive hand surgery: Dorsal capsulodesis for the unstable scaphoid and volar capsulodesis following excision of the distal ulna. *Hand Clin* 1987; 3:81-102.

64. Kleinman WB: Management of chronic rotary subluxation of the scaphoid by scapho-trapezio-trapezoid arthrodesis: Rationale for the technique, postoperative changes in biomechanics, and results. *Hand Clin* 1987;3: 113-133.

65. Taleisnik J: Carpal instability. *J Bone Joint Surg Am* 1988;70:1262-1268.

66. Watson HK, Black DM: Instabilities of the wrist. *Hand Clin* 1987;3:103-111.

67. Moneim MS: The tangential posteroanterior radiograph to demonstrate scapholunate dissociation. *J Bone Joint Surg Am* 1981;63: 1324-1326.

68. Watson HK, Ashmead D IV, Makhlouf MV: Examination of the scaphoid. *J Hand Surg Am* 1988;13:657-660.

69. Watson H, Ottoni L, Pitts EC, Handal AG: Rotary subluxation of the scaphoid: A spectrum of instability. *J Hand Surg Br* 1993;18:62-64.

70. Blatt G: Dorsal capsulodesis for rotary subluxation of the scaphoid, in Gelberman RH (ed): *The Wrist*. New York, NY, Raven Press, 1994, pp 147-165.

71. Hwang JJ, Goldfarb CA, Gelberman RH, Boyer MI: The effect of dorsal carpal ganglion excision on the scaphoid shift test. *J Hand Surg Br* 1999;24:106-108.

72. Watson HK, Ballet FL: The SLAC wrist: Scapholunate advanced collapse pattern of degenerative arthritis. *J Hand Surg Am* 1984;9:358-365.

73. Viegas SF, Tencer AF, Cantrell J, et al: Load transfer characteristics of the wrist: Part II. Perilunate instability. *J Hand Surg Am* 1987;12:978-985.

74. Imbriglia JE, Broudy AS, Hagberg WC, McKernan D: Proximal row carpectomy: Clinical evaluation. *J Hand Surg Am* 1990;15:426-430.

75. Neviaser RJ: On resection of the proximal carpal row. *Clin Orthop* 1986;202:12-15.

76. Ashmead D IV, Watson HK, Damon C, Herber S, Paly W: Scapholunate advanced collapse wrist salvage. *J Hand Surg Am* 1994;19:741-750.

77. Kirschenbaum D, Schneider LH, Kirkpatrick WH, Adams DC, Cody RP: Scaphoid excision and capitolunate arthrodesis for radioscaphoid arthritis. *J Hand Surg Am* 1993;18:780-785.

78. Wyrick JD, Stern PJ, Kiefhaber TR: Motion-preserving procedures in the treatment of scapholunate advanced collapse wrist: Proximal row carpectomy versus four-corner arthrodesis. *J Hand Surg Am* 1995;20:965-970.

79. Tomaino MM, Miller RJ, Cole I, Burton RI: Scapholunate advanced collapse wrist: Proximal row carpectomy or limited wrist arthrodesis with scaphoid excision? *J Hand Surg Am* 1994;19:134-142.

80. Krakauer JD, Bishop AT, Cooney WP: Surgical treatment of scapholunate advanced collapse. *J Hand Surg Am* 1994;19:751-759.

81. Salomon GD, Eaton RG: Proximal row carpectomy with partial capitate resection. *J Hand Surg Am* 1996;21:2-8.

82. Cooney WP: External fixation of distal radial fractures. *Clin Orthop* 1983;180:44-49.

83. Taleisnik J, Watson HK: Midcarpal instability caused by malunited fractures of the distal radius. *J Hand Surg Am* 1984;9:350-357.

84. Short WH, Palmer AK, Werner FW, Murphy DJ: A biomechanical study of distal radial fractures. *J Hand Surg Am* 1987;12:529-534.

85. Pogue DJ, Viegas SF, Patterson RM, et al: Effects of distal radius fracture malunion on wrist joint mechanics. *J Hand Surg Am* 1990; 15:721-727.

86. Fernandez DL: Correction of post-traumatic wrist deformity in adults by osteotomy, bone-grafting, and internal fixation. *J Bone Joint Surg Am* 1982;64:1164-1178.

87. Amadio PC, Botte MJ: Treatment of malunion of the distal radius. *Hand Clin* 1987;3:541-561.

88. Ireland DCR: Radiocarpal instability and radiocarpal dislocations, in Cooney WP, Linscheid RL, Dobyns JH (eds): *The Wrist: Diagnosis and Operative Treatment*. St. Louis, MO, Mosby-Year Book, 1998, pp 569-587.

89. Cooney WP III, Linscheid RL, Dobyns JH: Carpal instability: Treatment of ligament injuries of the wrist. *Instr Course Lect* 1992; 41:33-44.

90. Jupiter JB, Ruder J, Roth DA: Computer-generated bone models in the planning of osteotomy of multidirectional distal radius malunions. *J Hand Surg Am* 1992;17:406-415.

Reference to Video

Weiss AP: Arthroscopic wrist anatomy. *Diagnostic Wrist Arthroscopy*. Rosemont, IL, American Academy of Orthopaedic Surgeons, Annual Meeting, 1998.

SECTION

3

Spine

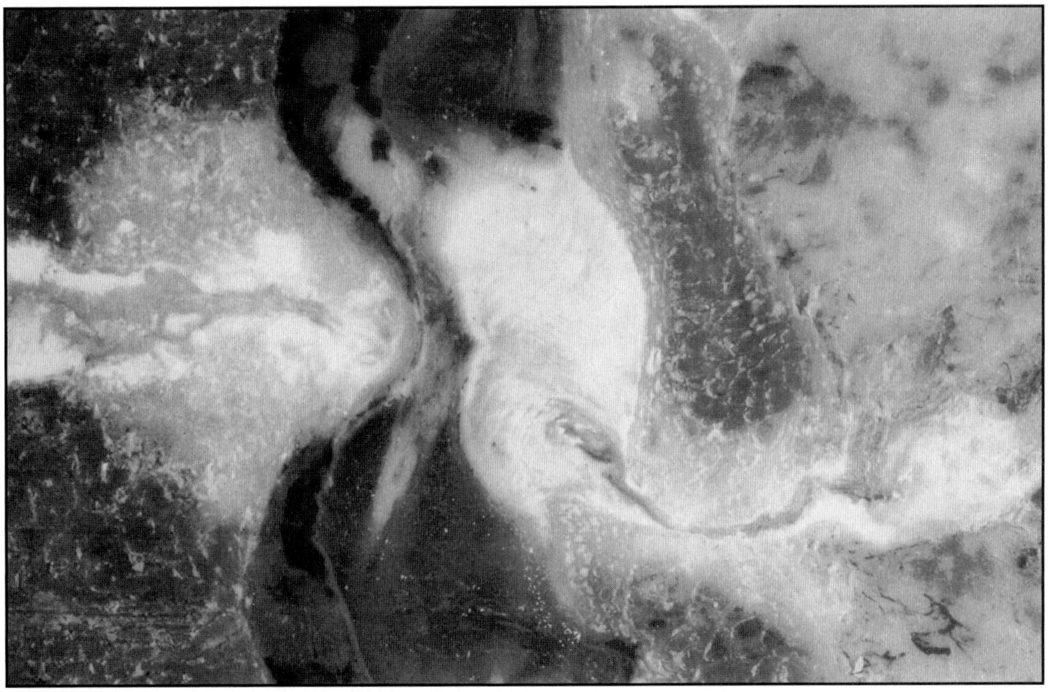

14 Radiologic Imaging in Spinal Stenosis

15 Spinal Stenosis

16 Lumbar Spinal Stenosis: Treatment Options

14

Radiologic Imaging in Spinal Stenosis

Richard J. Herzog, MD

Introduction

Lumbar spinal stenosis has been defined as any type of narrowing of the central spinal canal, nerve root canals (lateral recess), or the neural foramina.[1] The narrowing may be due to osseous or soft-tissue elements. When stenosis causes intractable pain, weakness, or functional disability, it may be necessary to order a diagnostic imaging test to assess the nature and extent of the pathoanatomic changes of the spine to select the optimal form of therapy. Radiologic imaging studies provide a snapshot in time of the degenerative process affecting many patients with stenotic symptoms. These studies provide morphologic information, the significance of which can be determined only by precise correlation to the patient's clinical condition. The radiologic studies currently used for the evaluation of patients with stenotic symptoms include plain films, myelography, CT, CT-myelography, and MRI. The value of these tests depends on their sensitivity, specificity, precision, reliability, accuracy, risk, cost, and availability.

Prior to 1970, plain film radiography was the primary radiologic study available to evaluate patients with symptoms of spinal stenosis. Plain films only provide direct information on the morphology and alignment of the osseous components of the spinal motion segments. Any pathologic process that causes osseous destruction, degeneration, or remodeling can be detected on plain films if a sufficient amount of bone is affected. Plain film findings that may be associated with symptomatic spinal stenosis include end plate proliferation and remodeling, facet arthrosis, malalignment in the sagittal or coronal plane, a developmentally small spinal canal, postoperative or posttraumatic spinal deformity, and any pathologic condition that may cause enlargement of the osseous structures, for example, Paget's disease.

Plain Radiographs

To determine the value of plain radiographs in the workup of patients with symptoms of spinal stenosis, it is necessary to know the spectrum of findings detected on plain films obtained on asymptomatic patients. Frymoyer and associates[2] evaluated the plain films of 292 patients, including 96 with no history of back pain, 134 with a history of previous or current moderate back pain, and

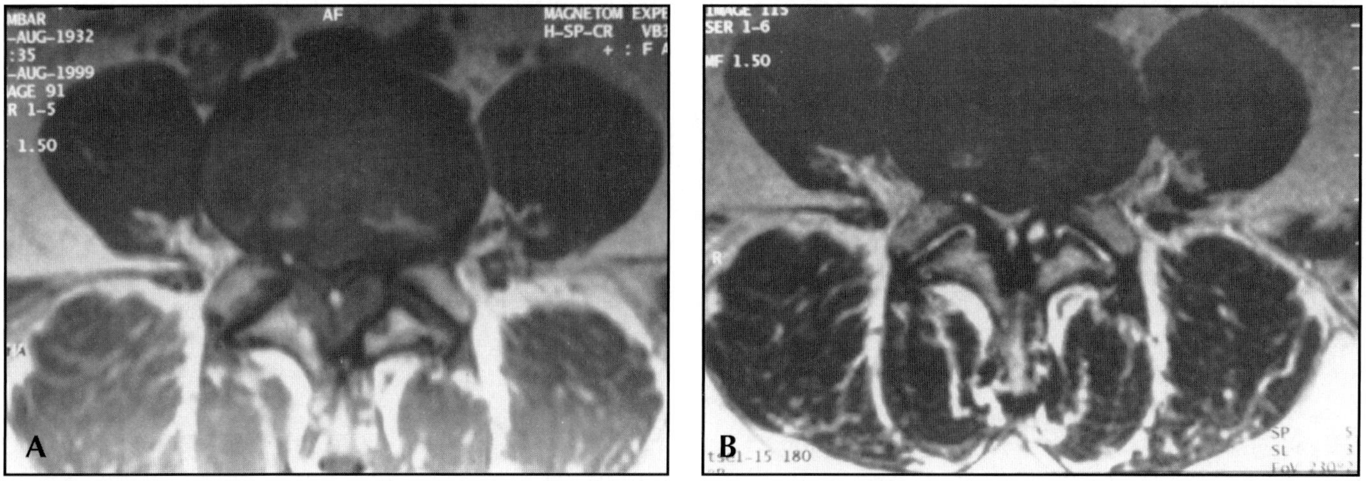

Fig. 1 At the L4-5 level, on the T1-weighted (**A**) and T2-weighted (**B**) axial images, there is severe compression of the thecal sac by a posterior midline disk protrusion and hypertrophied ligamenta flava. The left ligamentum flavum contains a small synovial cyst.

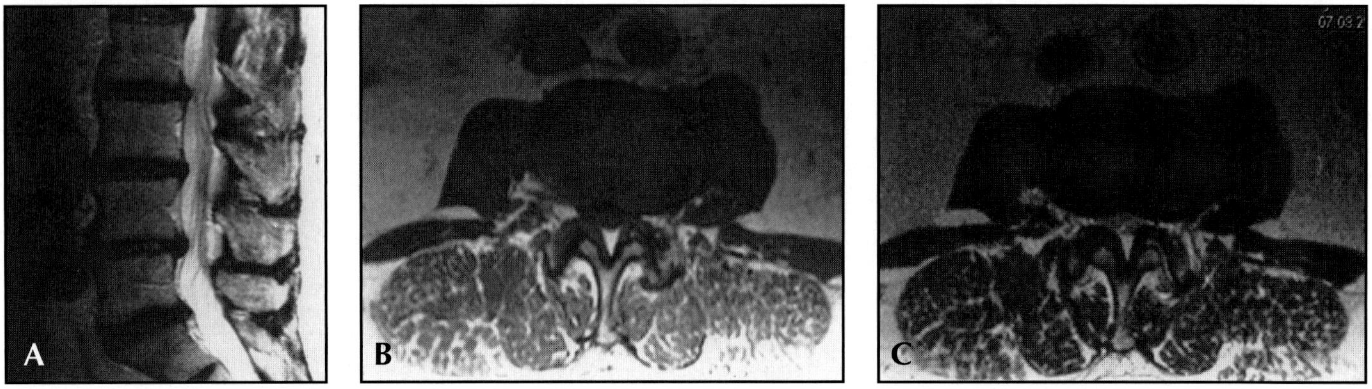

Fig. 2 In a patient with neurogenic claudication, the midline T2-weighted sagittal image (**A**) depicts multisegmental degenerative changes along with a posterior midline disk protrusion at the L4-5 level. Axial images orthogonal to the disk space are obtained to assess the degree of thecal sac deformation. On the T1-weighted (**B**) and T2-weighted (**C**) axial images at the L2-3 level, mild/moderate right and moderate/severe left facet arthrosis along with posterior bulge of the disk results in severe constriction of the thecal sac. Only a minimal amount of cerebrospinal fluid surrounds the cauda equina.

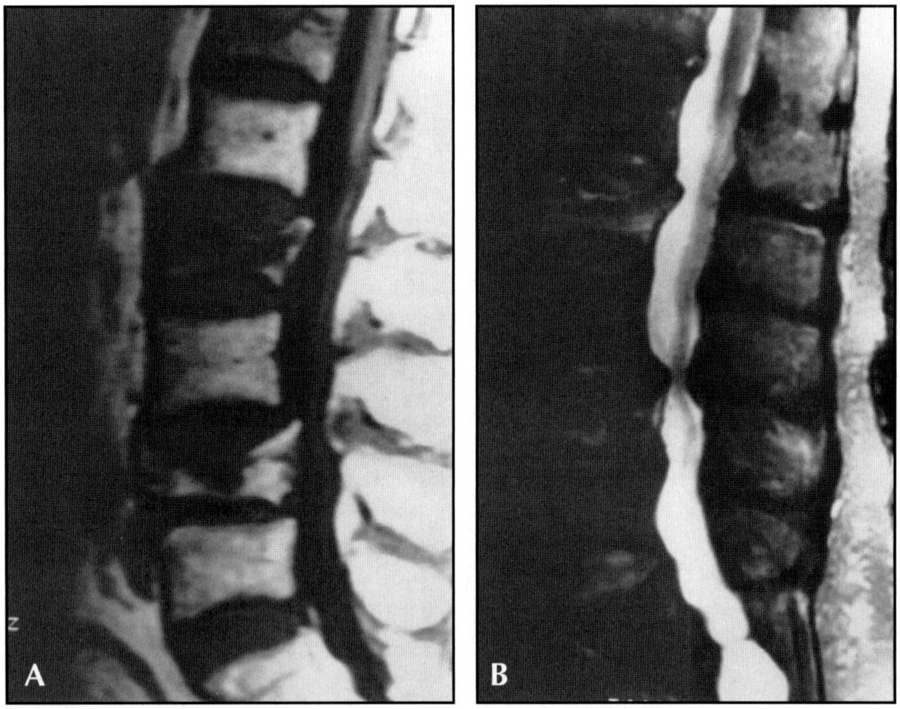

Fig. 3 In an elderly patient with a history of a fall and who is currently experiencing neurogenic claudication, the T1-weighted (**A**) and T2-weighted fat saturated (**B**) sagittal images depict severe central canal stenosis at the L1-2 and L3-4 levels due to osteopenic compression fractures. There are changes of Kummel's disease in the L2 vertebral body.

62 with a history of prior or current severe back pain. In the three groups, the frequency of transitional vertebrae, Schmorl's nodes, disk vacuum phenomenon, claw spurs, and disk-space narrowing at the L3-4 and L5-S1 disk levels were similar. Traction spurs and disk-space narrowing at the L4-5 level had a positive correlation to severe low back pain. Witt and associates[3] compared the plain film findings in patients with and without back pain. There was no difference in the prevalence of disk degeneration or spondylosis when comparing the 238 patients with low back pain and sciatica to 68 asymptomatic patients. The prevalence of disk degeneration and spondylosis increased with age in the two groups. Torgerson and Dotter[4] evaluated 217 asymptomatic patients between the ages of 40 and 70 years, and 387 symptomatic patients with back pain in the same age range. They found a higher incidence of spondylolysis and spondylolisthesis in the symptomatic patients

Plain films provide a global depiction of the severity of degenerative spinal disease, but they are extremely limited in determining the precise location of neural entrapment. When interpreting plain films, each spinal motion segment should be scrutinized for the presence of disk degeneration, facet arthrosis, and central canal or neural foraminal stenosis. Spinal alignment in the sagittal and coronal planes must be assessed as well as any rotatory deformity. The routine plain film evaluation of the lumbar spine includes an erect anteroposterior (AP) view, a lateral view that includes the spine from the thoracolumbar junction to the upper sacrum, and a cone-downed lateral view of the lumbosacral junction. Flexion and extension and lateral bending views may be warranted in the initial assessment of a patient if dynamic instability is clinically suspected, or if there is evidence of malalignment on the routine radiographs. Erect films are needed for the assessment of spinal balance. In patients with scoliosis, specific supine stress views may be obtained to determine the structural versus the functional component of the deformity. After the initial examination of the spine, repeat plain films should be limited to the assessment of new symptoms or evaluation of the stability of spinal alignment.

Computed Tomography and Magnetic Resonance Imaging

With the development and implementation of radiologic cross-sectional imaging studies, for example, MRI and CT with multiplanar reformations (CT/MPR), it became possible to directly evaluate all the osseous components of each spinal motion segment in the three anatomic planes of the body, as well as to assess the soft-tissue structures. With CT, it also is possible to create a three-dimensional model of the spine that may facilitate the comprehension of complex anatomic relationships. With CT's excellent delineation of osseous structures, it is the optimal modality to characterize the nature and degree of osseous stenosis, whether related to the vertebral end plates or facet joint. The advantage of MRI is its ability to depict the soft-tissue structures that may precipitate stenotic symptoms, for example, thickened ligamenta flava, hypertrophied facet capsules, prominent epidural fat, and herniated disk material (Fig. 1). MRI provides direct information concerning nerve root entrapment and the degree of thecal sac deformation. Another advantage of MRI compared with CT is the greater length of the spine that can be evaluated on a standard MRI examination.

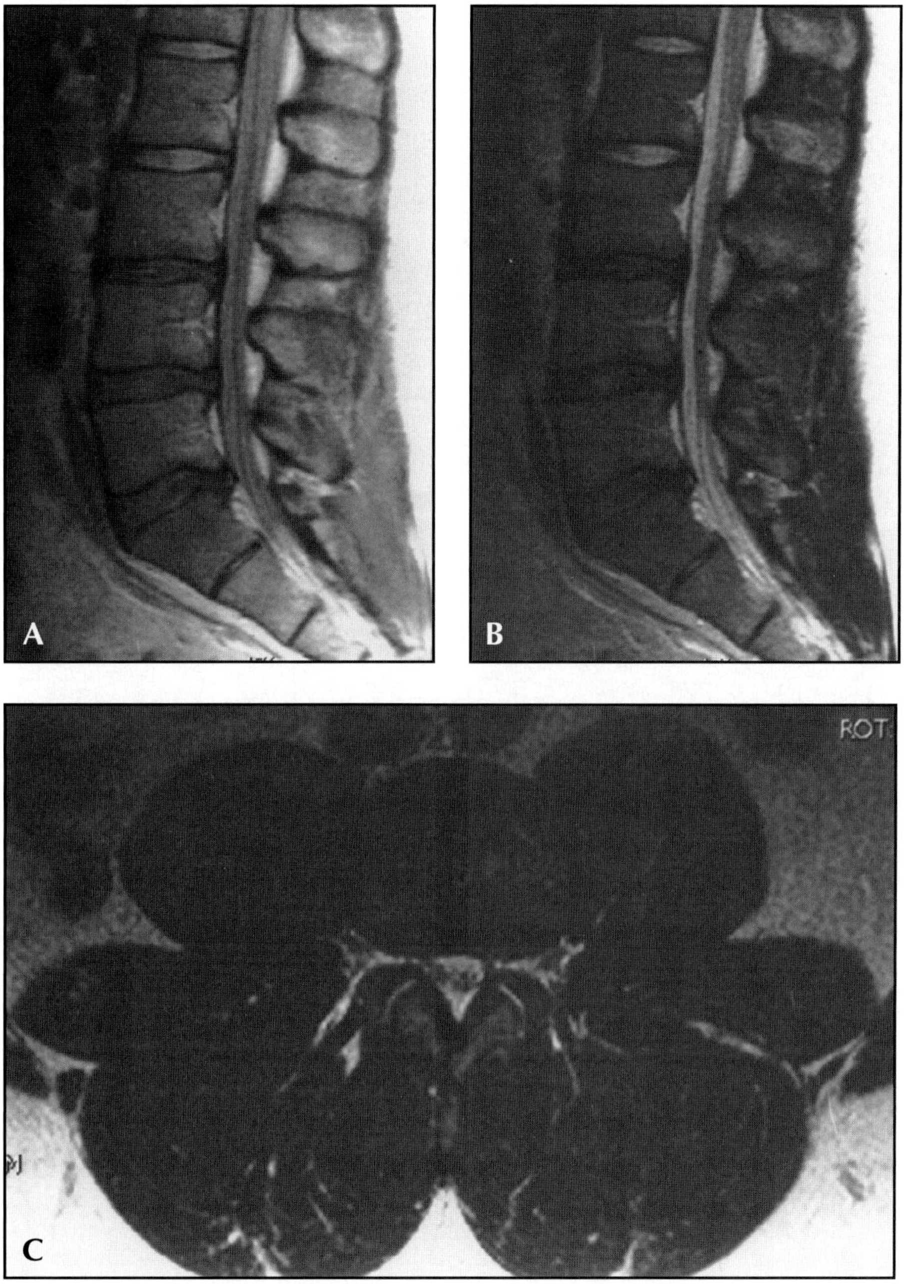

Fig. 4 On the proton-density-weighted (**A**) and T2-weighted (**B**) sagittal images there is mild/moderate developmental stenosis of the lumbar central spinal canal from L3 to L5, along with changes of disk degeneration at the L3-5 and L5-S1 levels. On the T2-weighted axial image (**C**) at the L3-4 level, there is developmental central canal stenosis and mild thecal sac deformation.

To achieve the maximum amount of information on a CT or MRI study it is necessary to perform the optimal imaging examination. A routine CT examination of the lumbar spine includes sequential axial 3 mm-thick sections from the pedicle of L3 through the L5-S1 disk level. Thin axial sections are needed for optimal spatial resolution and to create the computer-generated sagittal reformations that should be obtained for every patient. Coronal reformations

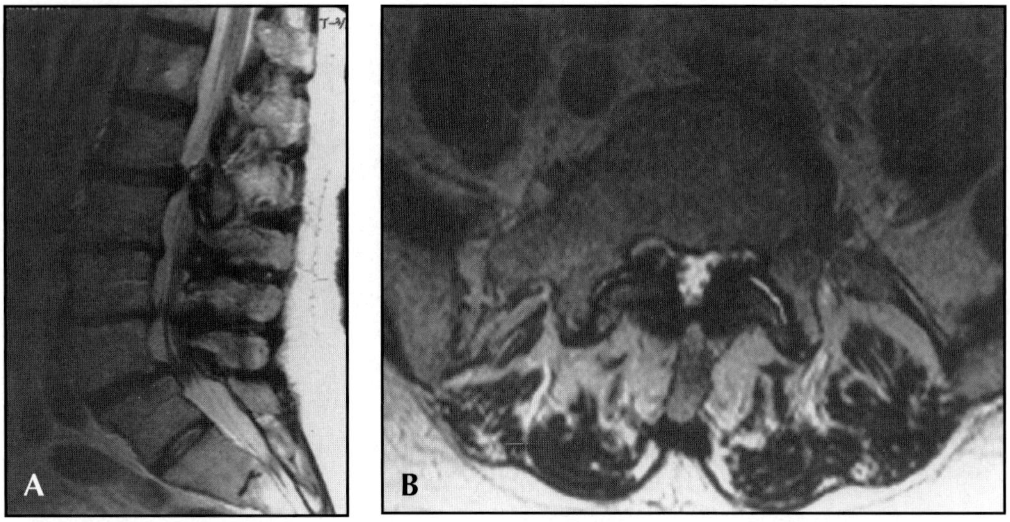

Fig. 5 In a patient with back and leg pain, on the T2-weighted sagittal image (**A**), there is multisegmental central canal stenosis along with a degenerative anterolisthesis at the L4-5 level. On the T2-weighted axial image (**B**), at the L4-5 level, moderate/severe facet arthrosis is causing moderate central canal stenosis along with stenosis of the subarticular lateral recesses and entrapment of the L5 nerve roots.

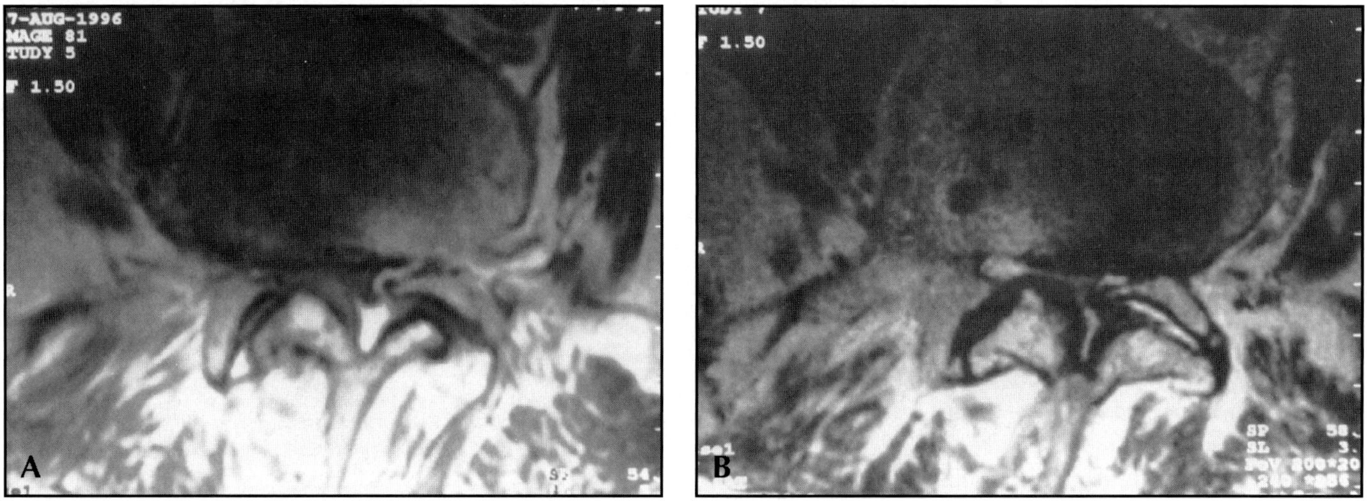

Fig. 6 At the L4-5 level, on the T1-weighted (**A**) and T2-weighted (**B**) axial images, there is severe central canal stenosis predominantly due to facet arthrosis and hypertrophy of the right ligamentum flavum. Facet tropism is present with the right facet joint oriented more sagittally than the left. Only the more sagittally oriented right facet joint is anteriorly subluxated.

are needed to assess spinal alignment in patients with scoliosis or in patients with a segmental lateral listhesis. All CT images should be evaluated in both soft-tissue and bone windows.

When possible, MRI examinations of the lumbar spine should be performed on a high field strength MRI system (1.0 to 1.5 Tesla) to achieve rapid high-resolution imaging. Low field strength (0.1 to 0.3 Tesla) MRI systems are indicated for obese patients or patients with claustrophobia who can not undergo an examination in a high field strength system. Almost all open MRI scanners are low field strength systems. The routine MRI examination of the lumbar spine performed on a patient with back or leg pain will include: a T1 or proton-density-weighted sagittal sequence and a fast spin-echo T2-weighted sagittal sequence (typically fat saturated), using a section thickness of 4 mm and an interslice gap of 0.5 mm; a T1 or proton-density-weighted axial sequence with a section thickness of 4 mm and an interslice gap of 0.5 mm; and a fast spin echo T2-weighted axial sequence with a section thickness of 3 to 4 mm and an interslice gap of 0.5 mm. At least one axial sequence should have contiguous sections from the pedicle of L2 or L3 through the L5-S1 disk level and not merely angled sections through the disk spaces.

Disk degeneration may induce segmental instability and secondary hypertrophy and hyperplasia of the connective tissue elements. The degenerative tissue may encroach into the central spinal canal,

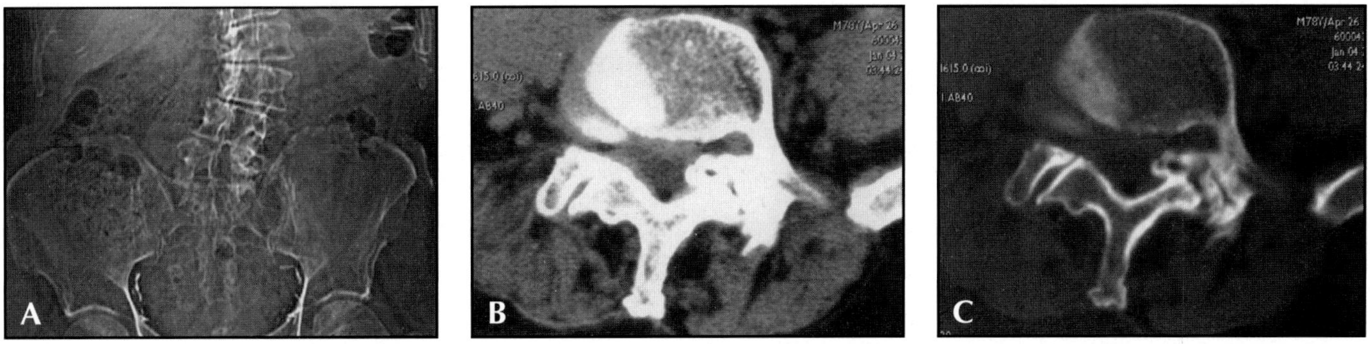

Fig. 7 On a patient with a mild/moderate lumbar rotatory levoscoliosis and a left lateral listhesis at the L3-4 level (**A**), CT demonstrates asymmetrical facet arthrosis and moderate/severe central canal stenosis at the L3-4 level depicted on the axial images photographed for soft-tissue (**B**) and bone (**C**) resolution.

the subarticular lateral recess, or the neural foramina and impinge, entrap, or compress the neural structures. The central canal narrowing may involve the bony canal alone or the dural sac, or both.[1] The degenerative changes most often associated with central canal stenosis include posterior bulging of the disk, osteophytes projecting off the vertebral body end plates, hypertrophy and bony proliferation of the facet joints, and hypertrophy of the ligamenta flava and anterior facet capsules.[5,6] The goal of both MRI and CT/MPR in the evaluation of patients presenting with back pain, radiculopathy, or intermittent claudication is not just to demonstrate the presence of stenosis, but to define that spinal components are causing the stenosis (Fig. 2).

Degenerative spinal disease is a continuous subclinical process which may not evoke symptoms. Abnormalities are frequently detected on CT and MRI studies performed on asymptomatic individuals.[7] The spondylotic changes do not represent false positive findings, but true pathologic changes of spinal structures that are not evoking symptoms. In addition to degenerative osseous changes that may lead to stenosis of the central spinal canal, other osseous abnormalities that may cause stenosis include posttraumatic deformities (Fig. 3), overgrowth of a spinal fusion, Paget's disease, fluorosis and vertebral hemangiomas. Intraspinal masses, for example, synovial cysts and epidural lipomatosis, may also precipitate symptoms of neurogenic claudication.

In order to obtain a true AP diameter of the lumbar central spinal canal, axial images orthogonal to the long axis of the spinal canal or midline sagittal images must be obtained. With the excellent spatial resolution of osseous structures, CT/MPR is the best examination to ascertain precise osseous spinal measurements. The classification of spinal stenosis as congenital, developmental, and acquired is helpful when evaluating a small spinal canal.[8,9] Congenital stenosis is a result of disturbed fetal development and may occur as one element of a congenital malformation of the lumbar spine. Developmental stenosis is a growth disturbance of the posterior elements, involving the pedicles, lamina, or articular processes, resulting in decreased volume of the spinal canal. In the lumbar spine, a true midline osseous sagittal diameter measuring less than 12 mm is considered relative stenosis, and a diameter of less than 10 mm is considered absolute stenosis.[10] This diameter is measured from the middle of the posterior surface of the vertebral body to the point of junction of its spinous process and laminae. With developmental stenosis, the reserve capacity of the spinal canal is reduced, thus predisposing the neural elements to impingement or compression by any material encroaching into the central canal (Fig. 4). Developmental central canal stenosis may be associated with developmental narrowing of the neural foramina. Acquired stenosis is the narrowing of the central spinal canal, the subarticular lateral recess, or the neural foramina by degenerative changes of the discovertebral joint, facet joints, and ligamenta flava. Acquired stenosis may be superimposed on developmental stenosis. Central and neural foraminal stenosis frequently coexist in the same patient.

Spinal degeneration may be associated with altered spinal alignment, scoliosis, or spondylolisthesis. Spondylolisthesis is defined as a slip of the spine, and depending on the relationship of the vertebral bodies at the involved motion segment, the displacement will be an anterolisthesis, a retrolisthesis, or a lateral listhesis. Degenerative spondylolisthesis is an important cause of central canal stenosis and most frequently involves the L4-5 disk level (Fig. 5). Disk degeneration along with degenerative changes of sagittally-oriented facet joints predispose the motion segment to an anterolisthesis, which rarely progresses beyond a grade I slip because there is an

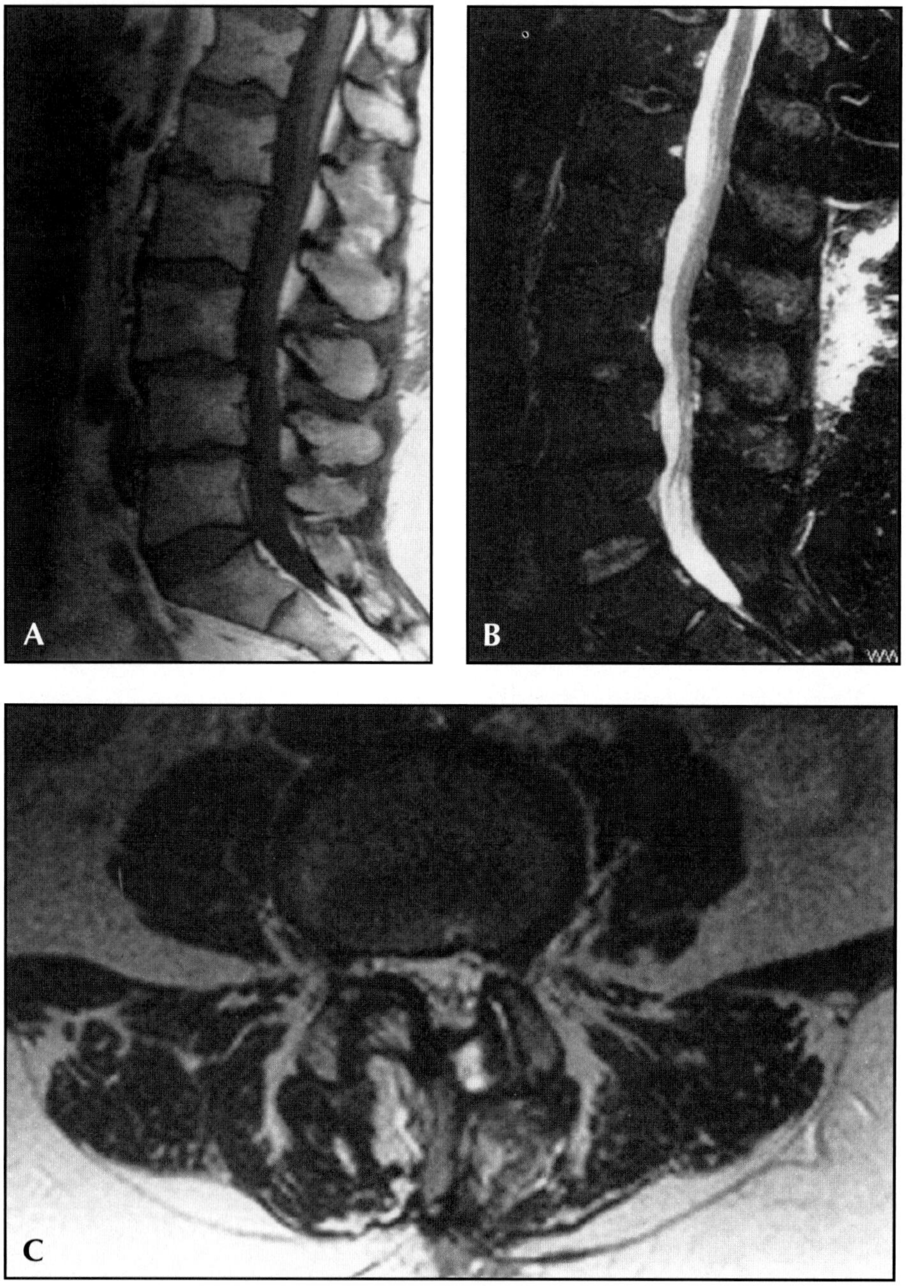

Fig. 8 In a patient who developed a new anterolisthesis at the L3-4 level and new right leg radicular symptoms after an L3-4 left laminectomy, on the T1-weighted (**A**) and T2-weighted (**B**) sagittal images, there is a grade I anterolisthesis at the L3-4 level along with changes of multisegmental disk degeneration. On the T2-weighted axial image (**C**) anterior subluxation of the right inferior articular process of L3 results in compression of the right L4 axillary pouch. A left laminectomy defect is present.

intact neural arch. The combination of osseous ridges projecting off the anteromedial margin of the facet joints, hypertrophy of the ligamenta flava, posterior bulge of the disk, and an anterolisthesis may result in severe central canal and subarticular lateral recess stenosis. If there is asymmetry in the orientation of the facet joints (facet tropism), the anterolisthesis may have a rotatory component and asymmetrical stenosis of the subarticular lateral recesses (Fig. 6). Asymmetrical central canal stenosis is also seen in adult patients with scoliosis and a degenerative lateral listhesis (Fig. 7). In postoperative patients who develop new radicular symptoms, MRI is excellent for detecting nerve root entrapment resulting from spinal instability (Fig. 8).

Myelography

Myelography provides opacification of the thecal sac and a means to assess its dimensions in both the supine and erect positions, including stress views with flexion and extension. Many clinicians prefer myelography and CT-myelography for the assessment of patients with stenosis. Erect myelography provides the opportunity to assess the size of the thecal sac in various stressful positions that may provoke the patient's symptoms. Although erect myelography provides a more provocative stress examination than a supine MRI, CT, or myelographic study, its is still unclear whether the information provided on an erect myelogram is unique in predicting patient outcome or needed in selecting the optimal mode of therapy. Some studies have shown no relationship between preoperative myelograms and postoperative outcome; however, Herno and associates[11] reported that the severity of myelographic findings was significantly related to the outcome of patients who underwent surgery for spinal stenosis. Seventy-six percent of patients with a complete or subtotal block on nonfunctional myelography (not erect or stressed) had a good or excellent outcome after spinal surgery.

Because there is potential morbidity with myelography, the question arises whether the same information can be achieved with CT or MRI. Wildermuth and associates[12] recently reported on the comparison of supine and erect MRI (with the patient seated in flexion or extension) to supine and erect myelography in a group of 30 patients, most of whom were being evaluated for stenotic symptoms. They demonstrated a high (r = 0.81 to 0.97) correlation between MRIs and myelographic measurements. They demonstrated only a small positional difference in dural sac diameters from the supine to the erect position, and they concluded that the additional information gained on the erect MRI study when compared to that obtained on the standard supine MRI examination is limited.

Neural foraminal stenosis should always be considered as a possible etiology for radicular symptoms. Considering that all neural foramina in the spinal column have a vertical and horizontal dimension as well as a length, the foramen is truly a three-dimensional structure, that is, a canal. Pathologic changes of any structure that borders the neural foramen may impinge or compress the exiting nerve root or dorsal root ganglion. The most common etiology of neural foraminal stenosis are osteophytes projecting off the vertebral end plates[5,13] (Fig. 9).

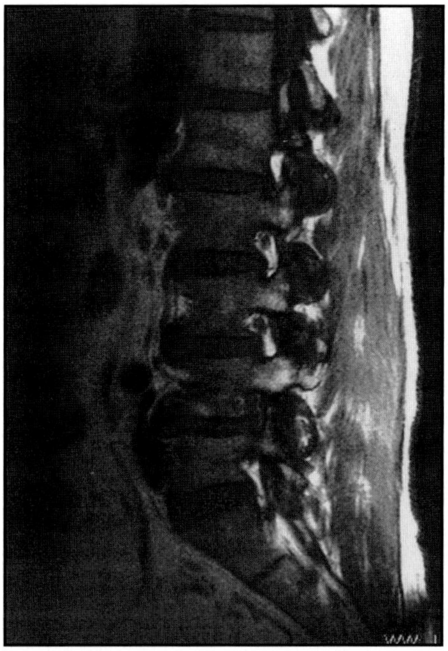

Fig. 9 Bulging of the disk and end plate proliferation results in mild neural foraminal stenosis at the L2-3 and L3-4 levels and moderate stenosis at the L4-5 level. There is impingement of the left L4 nerve root in the neural foramen on the T1-weighted sagittal image.

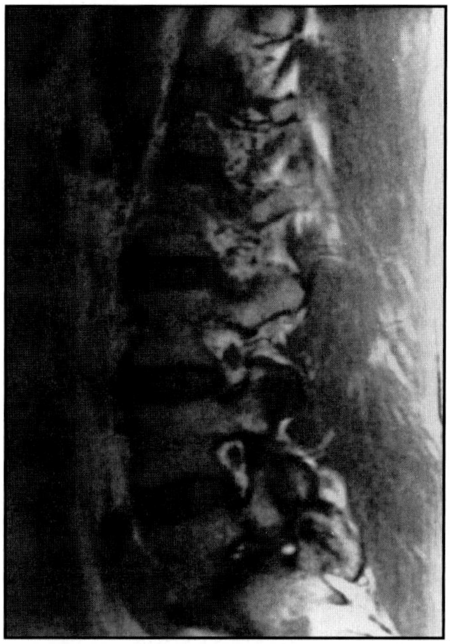

Fig. 10 In a patient with a grade II isthmic spondylolisthesis at the L5-S1 disk level, there is severe cephalocaudal stenosis of the neural foramen and compression of the L5 nerve root between the base of the L5 pars interarticularis and the superior end plate of S1 on the proton density-weighted sagittal image.

Degenerative changes of the superior articular process may lead to decreased volume of the posterosuperior compartment of the neural foramen, potentially causing neural compression. Decreased disk height results in cephalocaudal stenosis of the neural foramen, which may be amplified with an anterolisthesis (Fig. 10). Sagittal imaging is mandatory with both MRI and CT to evaluate the neural foramina for the presence of stenosis. Extraforaminal (far-out) stenosis[14] may occur at the L5-S1 disk level because of the apposition of the base of the transverse process of L5 to the adjacent sacral ala.

Evaluation and Diagnosis

While plain films, CT, MRI, and myelography are currently used to evaluate patients with stenotic symptoms, there are few controlled studies documenting the relative value of these tests for the evaluation of these patients. Amundsen and associates[15] reported on 100 patients with symptomatic lumbar spinal stenosis who were evaluated with plain films, myelography, and CT. As emphasized by the authors, this cohort group was a selected group of patients who were hospitalized for sciatica, but workup determined that lumbar stenosis and not a disk herniation, neoplasm, or inflammatory process was the cause of their symptoms. The radiologic studies were used to determine the type and degree of stenosis. As stated by the authors, the criteria for diagnosing central and lateral (lateral recess and neural foramina) stenosis are difficult to define. Stenosis was determined by evaluating the shape of the spinal canal, the appearance of the facet joints, and the measured dimensions of pedicle length, interpedicular width, and sagittal diameter of the thecal sac.

The diagnosis of stenosis was based on the combination of visual impression by the radiologists and direct measurements, which makes the results of this study difficult to validate by other investigators. In their cohort group, 95% had back pain in addition to sciatica. Lateral stenosis was demonstrated in 51 patients and central canal stenosis in 49. A degenerative spondylolisthesis was present in 12 patients. There was no difference in the symptoms of patients with lateral and central stenosis. Claudication was present in both groups and at all degrees of stenosis. There was no significant correlation between the severity of pain and the degree of stenosis. The radiologic changes were more extensive than expected by the clinical findings, and multilevel changes were detected in patients with lateral and central canal stenosis. The number of the clinically symptomatic nerve roots could not be predicted from the radiologic findings. The authors concluded that clinical and radiologic assessment together are necessary to determine the diagnosis of symptomatic lumbar spinal stenosis. They also stated that perhaps the determination of the cross-sectional area of the spinal canal may provide useful information in the evaluation of patients with stenosis. While CT is the best method to measure the cross-sectional area of the osseous central canal, MRI is optimal to measure the cross-sectional area of the thecal sac.

Herno and associates[16] reported on the lack of correlation between CT findings and patients' symptoms after laminectomy for lumbar spinal stenosis. The structural changes identified on the postoperative CT study did not correlate significantly with the patients' pain patterns, walking capacity, or subjective disability. Herno and associates[17] also recently reported on a long-term (10-year) postoperative follow-up study of patients with lumbar spinal stenosis. MRI was used for the evaluation of these patients, and the authors found no significant difference in patient symptoms whether or not they had stenosis diagnosed on the MRI study. They did find that evidence of disk degeneration had a significant effect on patient walking capacity. The poor correlation of MRI to patient symptoms may have been affected by the lack of quantitative measurements used in the study to characterize the degree of stenosis.

An important question, which to date has not been resolved, is which study, myelography, CT, CT-myelography, or MRI, should be ordered when additional information is needed in the evaluation of a patient with spinal stenotic symptoms. Considering the rapid evolution of MRI and CT technology, a study on their effectiveness may be difficult to complete and still provide relevant information on the appropriate application of these diagnostic tests. The recent Cochrane review reported that there is no scientific evidence on the effectiveness of any form of surgical decompression or fusion for degenerative lumbar spondylosis compared with natural history, placebo, or conservative management.[18] Perhaps using the optimal imaging study in the assessment of these patients may improve surgical management and patient outcome.

References

1. Arnoldi CC, et al: Lumbar spinal stenosis and nerve root entrapment syndromes: Definition and classification. *Clin Orthop* 1976;115:4-5.
2. Frymoyer JW, Newberg A, Pope MA, Wilder DG, Clements J, MacPherson B: Spine radiographs in patients with low-back pain: An epidemiological study in men. *J Bone Joint Surg Am* 1984;66:1048-1053.
3. Witt I, Vestergaard A, Rosenklint A: A comparative analysis of x-ray findings of the lumbar spine in patients with and without lumbar pain. *Spine* 1984;9:299-300.
4. Torgerson WR, Dotter WE: Comparative roentgenographic study of the asymptomatic and symptomatic lumbar spine. *J Bone Joint Surg Am* 1976;58:850-853.
5. Rauschning W: Normal and pathologic anatomy of the lumbar root canals. *Spine* 1987;12:1008-1019.
6. Schneck CD: The anatomy of lumbar spondylosis. *Clin Orthop* 1985;193:20-37.
7. Boden SD, David DO, Dina TS, Patronas NJ, Wiesel SW: Abnormal magnetic-resonance scans of the lumbar spine asymptomatic subjects. *J Bone Joint Surg Am* 1990;72:403-408.
8. Verbiest H: Fallacies of the present definition, nomenclature, and classification of the stenosis of the lumbar vertebral canal. *Spine* 1976;1: 217-225.
9. Verbiest H: Words, images, knowledge, and reality: Some reflections from the neurosurgical perspective. *Acta Neurochirugica* 1983;69:163-193.
10. Verbiest H: Results of surgical treatment of idiopathic development stenosis of the lumbar vertebral canal. *J Bone Joint Surg Br* 1977;59:181-188.
11. Herno A, Airaksinen O, Saari T, Miettinen H: The predictive value of preoperative myelography in lumbar spinal stenosis. *Spine* 1994;19:1335-1338.
12. Wildermuth S, Zanetti M, Duewell S, et al: Lumbar spine: Quant itative and qualitative assessment of positional (upright flexion and extension) MR imaging and myelography. *Radiology* 1998;207:391-398.
13. Bohatirchuk F: The aging vertebral column (macro- and historadiographical study). *Br J Radiol* 1955;28:389-404.
14. Wiltse L: Far-out syndrome, in Rothman LG, Glenn WVJ (eds): *Multiplanar CT of the Spine.* Baltimore, MD, University Park Press, 1985, pp 384-393.
15. Amundsen T: Lumbar spinal stenosis: Clinical and radiologic features. *Spine* 1995;20: 1178-1186.
16. Herno A, Airaksinen O, Saari T: Computed tomography after laminectomy for lumbar stenosis. *Spine* 1994;19:1975-1978.
17. Herno A, Partanen K, Talaslahti T, et al: Long-term clinical and magnetic resonance imaging follow-up assessment of patients with lumbar spinal stenosis after laminectomy. *Spine* 1999;24:1533-1537.
18. Gibson JNA, Grant IC, Waddell G: The Cochrane review of surgery for lumbar disc prolapse and degenerative lumbar spondylosis. *Spine* 1999;24:1820-1832.

15

Spinal Stenosis

Steven R. Garfin, MD
Wolfgang Rauschning, MD, PhD

Introduction

Spinal stenosis by definition is a narrowing of the spinal canal, which is a common finding in an aging or degenerative spine.[1,2] Clinically, it describes a condition, usually found in older individuals, of leg pain, leg weakness, and difficulty ambulating, that may or may not be associated with a neurologic deficit. Although the imaging and pathoanatomic findings are fairly ubiquitous (and might be universal if everyone lived long enough), symptoms do not occur in all people despite similar radiographic findings.

The stenosis can occur centrally across the cauda equina, or more laterally.[3-5] The degenerative changes include disk bulging, thickening and overriding of laminae and ligamentum flavum, and arthritic changes with hypertrophy of the facets and facet capsules (Figs. 1 through 7). The stenosis may be associated with degenerative spondylolisthesis, frequently at the L4-5 segmental level.

Laterally, the nerve roots may be compressed within three areas around the facet joints. This lateral compression can occur subarticularly, in the foramen, or extraforaminally. It may involve the dorsal root ganglion (DRG).[6]

Congenital stenosis occurs in individuals with small pedicles, such as in achondroplastic dwarfs. It also may occur in normal-sized individuals with large vertebral bodies; short, round pedicles; and protruding disks. This stenosis frequently becomes symptomatic in the 30- to 45-year age range.

Acquired stenosis occurs over time. It can be associated with normal degenerative changes, or with posttraumatically or iatrogenically induced pars defects. The latter can occur during surgery when the pars and/or facet joints are removed, or thinned, excessively.

The symptoms of stenosis may be related to local changes involving one root as a result of a hypertrophic facet, degenerative disk, or facet cyst (ganglion). The latter usually occurs at the L4-5 level. There can be segmental changes, which often clinically involve one motion segment. This usually is L4-5 and often is associated with degenerative spondylolisthesis at that level. Frequently, however, the symptoms are related to generalized, multilevel involvement.

With our current level of knowledge, normal, age-related disk degeneration is difficult to separate from pathologic changes leading to symptoms.[7-10] The degenerative process usually begins at age 20 years in men and age 30 years in women. By age 50 years, 95% of the population have imaging and/or pathologic changes that demonstrate degenerative changes.[11] The degenerative cascade, as described by Kirkaldy-Willis and associates,[3] occurs relatively concurrently in the disk and the facet joints. The disk changes proceed from small tears to circumferential or radial tears. In young individuals this may lead to herniated disks. The early changes of degeneration are followed by decreased disk height, possible instability, and osteophyte formation, all of which can lead to compromise of the space available for the cauda equina or nerve roots. At the same time, facet degeneration

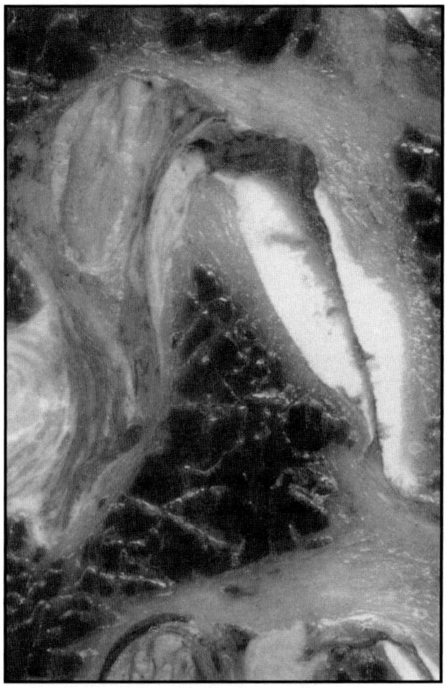

Fig. 1 Sagittal high-power photograph of the L4-5 facet joint and foramen in a spine that had been positioned in extension. Extension induces a posterior translation of L4 on L5. The tip of the inferior articular process contacts the pars interarticularis of L5 which also contacts, from inferiorly, the superior articular process of S1. The joint capsules also elongate. The ligamentum flavum and a joint capsule attach broadly to the anterior surface of the superior articular process, which is pushed into the subpedicular notch and compresses and flattens the dorsal root ganglion posteriorly.

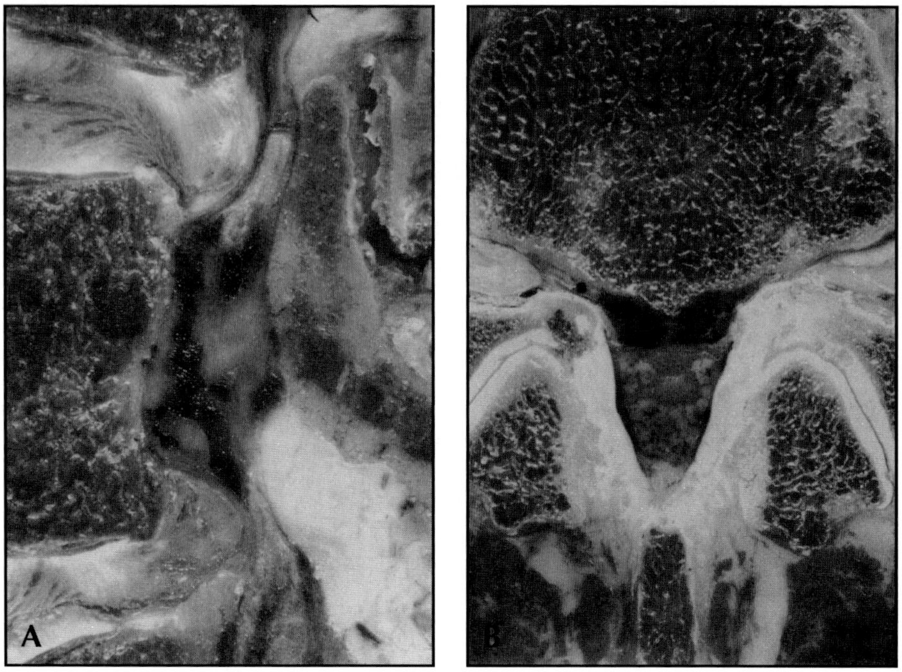

Fig. 2 A, Sagittal section, and **B,** Cross section showing pronounced disk degenerations L4-5 and L5-S1. The intact torso had been frozen in axial rotation. At L4-5 the root traversing the lateral recess is severely compressed. Anteriorly there is a motion-induced (functional) retrolisthesis of L4 on L5 that also causes the disk to move posteriorly. Posteriorly the lateral portion of the lamina and the most medial portion of the superior articular process of L5 have moved anteriorly. Note the gaping (vacuum phenomenon) in the joint. At L5-S1, disk material pushes the outermost anulus posteriorly and has caused detachment of periosteum from the vertebral body (contained disk herniation). At the lower insertion of the anulus a spondylophyte projects posteriorly, compressing the S1 root against the infolding ligamentum flavum.

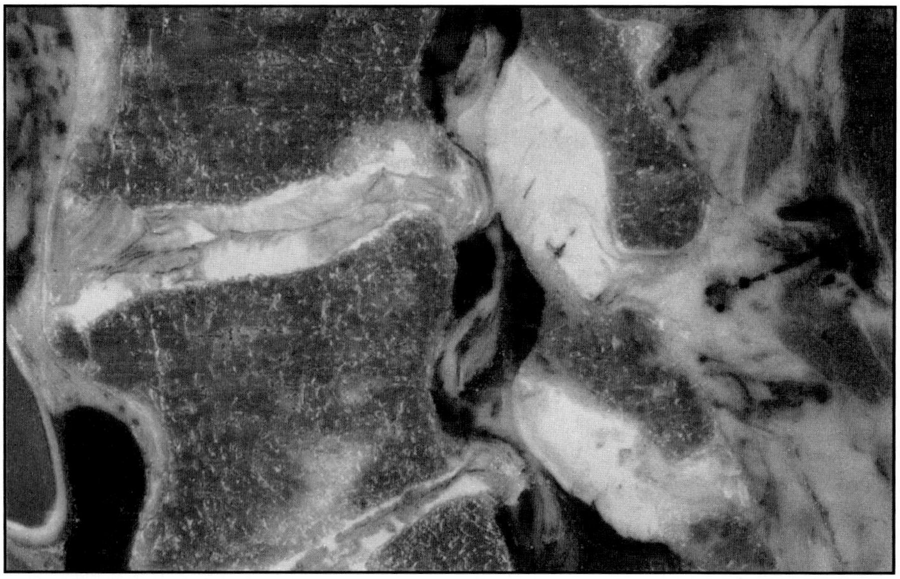

Fig. 3 Sagittal section through a moderately degenerated lower lumbar spine of a 77-year-old man who had a history of intermittent claudication. This section is carried through the lateral recesses of L4-5 and L5-S1. The L4-5 disk is grossly disrupted and protrudes both anteriorly (underneath the anterior longitudinal ligament) and posteriorly into the lateral recess, abutting the markedly thickened and infolding ligamentum flavum, thereby completely blocking the epidural veins, which are engorged both above and below this obstruction level. The L5-S1 disk is completely resorbed with total loss of disk height. Focal end-plate sclerosis and erosions of the end plates are obvious. A (probably still contained) disk herniation tracks inferiorly and reaches the ligamentum flavum, again obstructing the epidural veins at this level.

occurs, including synovial reactions followed by cartilage erosion, osteophyte formation, perhaps some "slippage," and associated bone and capsular thickening. In general, disk degeneration precedes visible facet changes, although in 20% of individuals, facet degeneration can be found without disk degeneration.[12]

The primary biochemical constituents of a disk include collagen, proteoglycans, and water.[13,14] Collagen provides connectivity and stability. Type I collagen is found primarily in the anulus and type II in the nucleus.[14,15] The absolute amount of collagen increases with age. This particularly reflects an increase in type I collagen. Proteoglycans help retain water within their intertwined structures, thereby providing an ability to enhance swelling pressure and turgor.[16-20] Over time there is a loss of water content, from 90% in children decreasing to 70% in adults. There also is an associated decrease in proteoglycans, with increased link proteins and increased proteolysis.

Facet joint arthritis occurs in a process similar to that found in other major joints. Cartilage degeneration is followed by increased, or altered, bone contact stresses with localized sclerosis and adjacent osteoporosis as weight bearing across the joint is redistributed. These abnormal forces can lead to osteophyte formation, further joint deterioration, and associated facet capsule buckling. As the joint narrows, instability, including progressive anterior subluxation, can occur with an alteration of the configuration of the joint, particularly in those that start with a more sagittal orientation.[21]

If there is increased lordosis across the degenerative section with more weight bearing posteriorly, hypertrophy of the laminae and spinous processes can occur. This hypertrophy, coupled with disk protrusion and osteophytes, can lead to circumferential bony as well as ligamentous and disk related stenosis.

Instability across a motion segment can occur by translation (anterolisthesis or retrolisthesis) or rotation. Retrolisthesis occurs when facets allow the segment to settle posteriorly; this usually occurs at L5-S1. Anterolisthesis usually is associated with facet erosion or alignment alteration, particularly when there is a preexisting sagittal configuration of the joint;[21-23] this usually occurs at L4-5 and to a lesser extent at L3-4. Rotational changes are often associated with degenerative scoliosis. These changes also occur with some facet laxity; they may create narrowing across the neuroforamen and impingement of the nerve by the joint, particularly when there is associated disk settling and facet and capsular hypertrophy.

The changes seen in spinal stenosis are also seen in normal disk degeneration. These changes include progressive loss of disk height, posterior disk bulging, gradual increase of lordosis, degenerative changes in the facet joint, osteophyte formation, and, occasionally, degenerative spondylolisthesis. The unanswered question, therefore, is why some people have back and/or leg pain related to these processes and the majority do not.

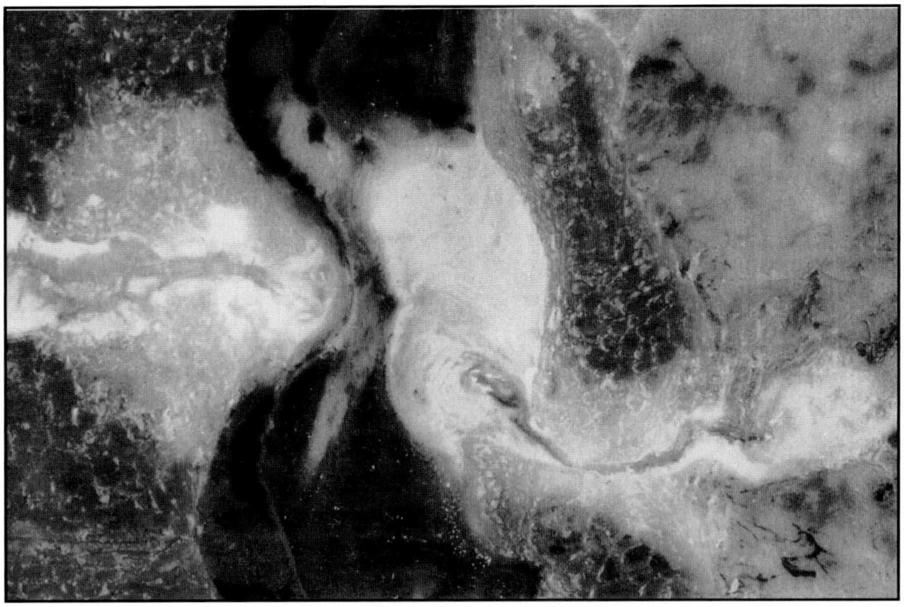

Fig. 4 Close-up view of the midlumbar spinal canal in a severely degenerated and stenotic specimen from an elderly male adult who had a history of prolonged low back pain with radicular symptoms. The intervertebral disk is completely reabsorbed. Posterior to the vertebra, the ventral internal veins are engorged. At the posterior aspect of the disk a beak-shaped spondylotic ridge projects into the spinal canal. The bone of this projecting osteophyte has a light color (sclerotic); note that the outermost anulus fibrosus (darker color) is still present. Posteriorly the loss of segmental height leads to an approximation of the spinous processes and laminae (kissing spines). The interlaminar ligamentum flavum is probably only thickened by retraction due to the redundance; it mushrooms into the spinal canal and compresses the traversing intrathecal root against the hard spondylophytic beak.

Pain usually occurs with a combination of compression and inflammation. Compression alone usually does not lead to pain. The pain from a herniated disk, which tends to be an excruciating, lancinating pain, is often different than the more diffuse, difficult to describe leg pains related to spinal stenosis. This difference may be related to the asymmetric, rapid compression related to a sudden onset of disk herniation and associated chemical irritation (inflammation), as opposed to the more gradual, global, circumferential type of compression associated with spinal stenosis. The latter occurs slowly and gives the neural elements time to adjust to their altered state and environment.

Compression, however, is important in the clinical symptoms related to spinal stenosis.[24,25] The degree, as well as the duration, of compression is important.[26] Schonstrom and associates[27] have demonstrated that many patients develop symptoms when the amount of cauda equina compression compromises over two thirds of the space available for the cauda equina. This compression leads to an increase in the pressure within the cauda equina to 100 mm Hg. When the narrowing is to 63% of normal, the intrathecal pressure raises to 50 mm Hg. The same pressures have been shown to have significant effects.[24,28-33] At a pressure of 50 mm Hg there is decreased capillary flow, decreased electrophysiologic conduction, and increased edema formation within and along the nerve roots. Pressures greater than this lead to

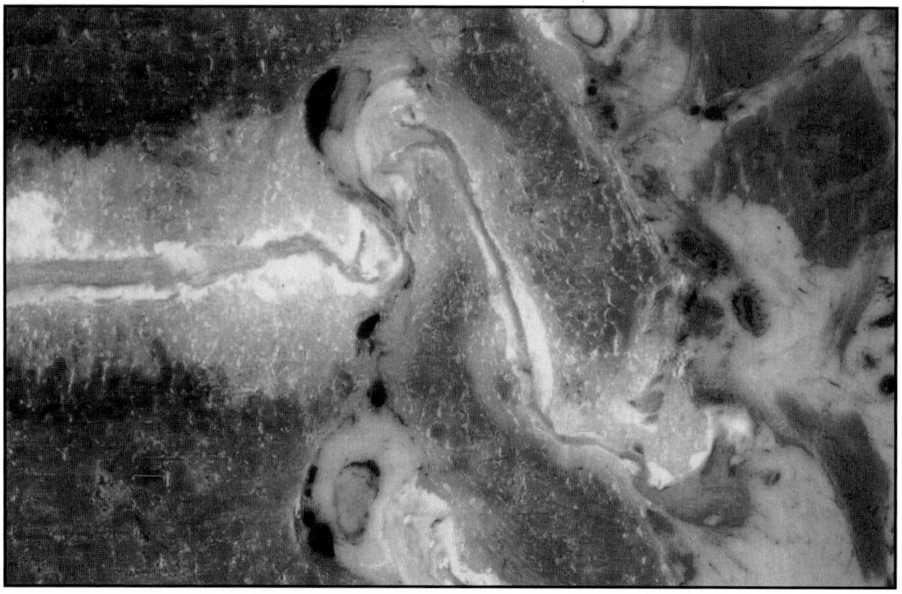

Fig. 5 Sagittal section through the L4-5 neuroforamen illustrates the five components that contribute to the extremely severe stenosis of the foramina in this specimen. The almost complete loss of intervertebral disk height causes the pedicle of L4 to "fall down" on or compress the root like a guillotine, thereby also kinking it (up-down stenosis). The second component is a front-back stenosis that is caused by the slight retrolisthesis of L4 on L5 induced by the obliquity of the facet joint in the sagittal plane. The mass effect is caused by the superior articular process of L5 intruding into the neuroforamen from below; the outermost anulus fibrosus is partially ossified and extruded, obliterating the lower portion of the foramen; and the ligamentum flavum is redundant and thickened.

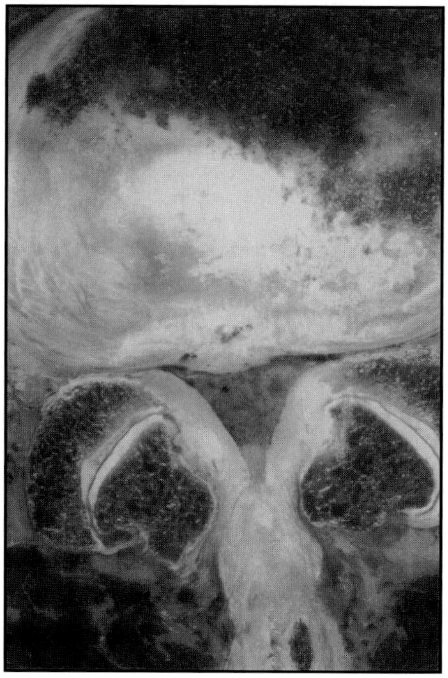

Fig. 6 Severe degenerative spinal stenosis at the L4-5 level in a 70-year-old patient with a history of intermittent claudication and occasional radicular leg pain. The central and lateral stenosis is most pronounced at this motion segment level and is almost exclusively caused by soft tissues. Anteriorly, the circumferentially ballooning disk narrows the thecal sac anteriorly and also completely obliterated the retrodiscal portion of the root canals (neuroforamina). The facet joints, especially the superior articular processes are moderately hypertophied. The thecal sac is severely compressed posterolaterally by the thick ligamentum flavum and assumes a triangular slit-shaped configuration.

arteriolar compromise and more dramatic electrophysiologic and pathophysiologic changes.

Although not measuring pain per se, findings in animal models are consistent with cadaveric and, more significantly, human anatomic cross-sectional area studies in individuals with symptoms of spinal stenosis. Delamarter and associates[34] also demonstrated the clinical significance of 50% to 75% canal compromise in terms of loss of cauda equina function and ability to functionally improve if the decompression is relieved. Other authors have shown that the magnitude and duration of compression affect the sensory components of spinal nerve roots and the cauda equina more than motor function or motor root conduction.[26,35-37] Pressures above systolic, maintained for over 2 hours, can lead to irreversible nerve conduction changes, whereas lesser pressures for shorter periods of time are less significant. There is more rapid resolution of electrophysiologic changes in the sensory nerves than in the motor nerves, which is consistent with resolution of pain more often than motor deficits following surgical decompression in patients being treated for symptomatic spinal stenosis. These studies also suggest there is more occurring than just mechanical compression. Ischemia also is created with arterial occlusion, compounded by venous pooling and stasis, further compromising nerve root function.[38-41]

Compression, besides the mechanical effect on the neural tissue and compression of the vasculature, also leads to nutritional alterations.[42-48] Cerebrospinal fluid (CSF) normally is a conduit of nutritional components to, and metabolic breakdown products from, the cauda equina. However, the percolation of the CSF around the neural elements is compromised by stenosis. The compression and lack of CSF alters the diffusion capabilities from the cells and axons. This alteration, coupled with the ischemia and lack of normal nutritional support and toxin removal, affects cell membrane permeability. The greater the level of compression, the longer the duration of compression, and the more levels involved (multisegmental), the greater the negative effect on the nerve roots of the cauda equina.

In the clinical setting Takahashi and associates[49] have introduced epidural catheters to measure pressure in asymptomatic and symptomatic individuals. Alterations in posture have a significant affect on cauda equina pressure. These pressures tend to increase when people stand or extend their spine, as well as with walking. These maneuvers also tend to increase leg symptoms in patients with spinal stenosis.

Anatomic and biomechanical effects can also jeopardize the nerve root. As the stenosis increases, particularly laterally, there can be tethering of the nerve roots as normal fluid nerve root motion is restrained.[50-52] Internal nerve root disruption can occur, altering the electrophysiologic function. A spinal nerve root normally moves 2 to 5 mm within a foramen. If the root is tethered or compromised, internal disruption can occur before failure is noted externally.

Perhaps the most important component leading to pain relates to inflammation.[53-55] A number of authors have shown that compression alone does not lead to pain unless it also is associated with an inflammatory reaction. Biochemical pain enhancers are produced with compression.[28,34,44] In animals, pain response such as increased foot (paw) hypersensitivity in the distribution of sensory nerves has been demonstrated when the neural elements are irritated. With compression across the DRG there is an associated increase in vasoactive proteins and an alteration in microvasculature with increased permeability, all leading to a further release of chemicals that can enhance the inflammatory reactions and, therefore, pain.[56-58]

The anatomy itself can help explain some of the variability of symptoms and signs noted in patients with spinal stenosis. Cadaveric and imaging studies have demonstrated the organized alignment of nerve fibers within the thecal sac.[59-61] In the cauda equina, the proximally numbered segments are layered more ventrally with the sacral roots the most dorsally situated as they course through the cauda equina. In addition, the motor components of the roots are anteromedial, and the larger sensory components more posterolateral at each segmental level within the thecal sac, as well as within the neuroforamen. Asymmetric compression may, therefore, lead to an irregularity in symptoms, depending on which neural components are affected.

The primary treatment of spinal stenosis, once symptoms start, is directed at attempting to decrease inflammation. In many cases the symptoms do improve, even though the compression itself is not altered. Surgery addresses the compression, reducing the pressure on the nerves and improving vascular flow. This indirectly decreases the progressive inflammatory effects. The latter are related to and/or compounded by mechanical compression, altered vascularity, decreased permeability with loss of localized nutritional support, release of local chemical constituents that further irritate the nerve root, increased edema and swelling, and, therefore, further compromise of the space available for the nerve roots and cauda equina.

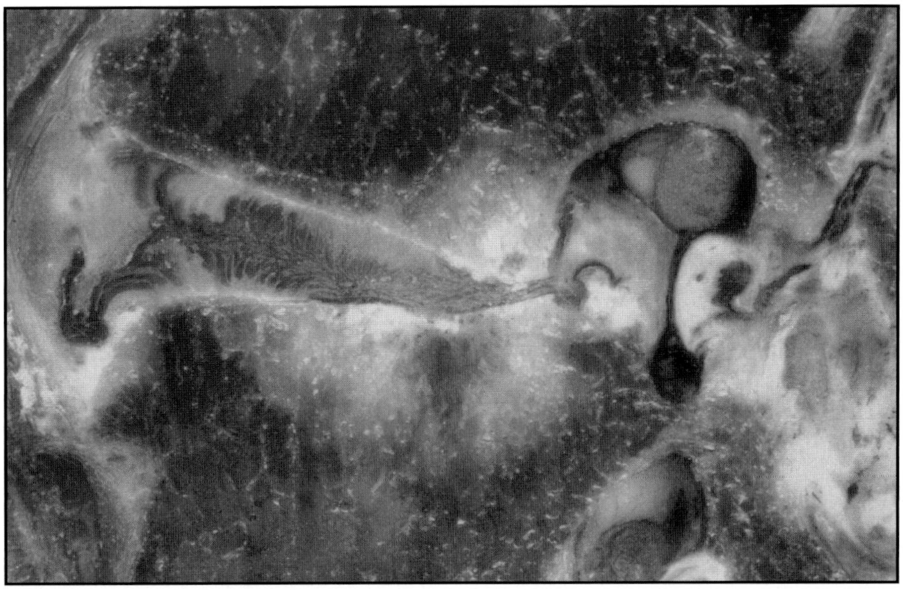

Fig. 7 Isthmic spondylolisthesis at L4-5 in a 44-year-old man. No clinical data were available in this case. This sagittal section runs through the medial border of the pedicle. At this level the beak of the pars interarticularis is displayed as it plunges into the interlaminar ligamentum flavum, causing it to mushroom anteriorly and into the lateral recess. The body of L4 is markedly rotated posteriorly, which appears to be facilitated by the severe internal disruption of the L4 disk. Its posterior anulus is partially detached superiorly from the apophyseal rim and allows the posterior anulus fibrosus to project posteriorly, virtually closing the lateral recess inferiorly. The extension-rotation of L4 causes the sharp lower rim of the pedicle to compress the ganglion.

Clinical Presentation

The important part of treatment, particularly surgical treatment, is patient selection. Because most humans eventually will have imaging studies consistent with spinal stenosis, the correct treatment (particularly if surgery is chosen) depends on identifying patients whose symptoms are consistent with their lumbar spine pathoanatomy.[62-70]

In spinal stenosis, women develop symptoms more often than do men.

This tends to occur in the age range of 65 to 70 years. A combination of congenital with degenerative changes occurs in a younger age group and is more difficult to treat (surgically, as well as nonsurgically).

Back pain tends to occur insidiously. Initially, it is often described as an ache or stiffness, and tends not to be disabling.

The leg pain is inconsistent and may be asymmetric. The symptoms may change in any one individual, depending on the activity, duration of symptoms, and so forth. The leg complaints may be described as numbness, tingling, cramping, weakness, or severe pain. The pain may be in the buttock and/or down the leg. It may involve any of a number of lumbar roots and vary from time to time. This inconsistency in symptoms may have led in previous eras to a diagnosis of a psychologic disorder or depression. In fact, it is consistent with the multilevel, often slightly asymmetric involvement from stenosis. The leg pains (occasionally back symptoms can be similar) tend to increase with walking and spine extension. They decrease somewhat with flexion. These individuals tend to do well using a shopping cart or squatting, as necessary, to relieve symptoms. They tend to do worse standing erect, and climbing stairs or inclines.

The neurologic symptoms may be sparse. There may be an alteration in deep tendon reflexes. Symmetric loss of ankle reflexes is common in older individuals. Asymmetric loss of either the ankle, knee, or posterior tibial tendon reflexes may suggest a spinal origin for patients' complaints. Frequently the only motor deficit is in the extensor hallicus longus or hip abductors (positive Trendelenburg test). This may only be noted with a stress-induced neurologic examination, which is performed by having patients walk repetitively in the hall until their symptoms occur, and then reexamining them. Marked weaknesses are rarely noted. Bowel and bladder loss is relatively rare. Because this is a gradual, symmetric narrowing, straight leg raising tests and tension signs usually are negative. Gait, at least in the initial phase, is usually normal. However, with walking and the beginning of pain and perhaps weakness, there may be an antalgic, or shuffling component to the gait pattern.

The differential diagnoses from spinal stenosis include vascular claudication and peripheral neuropathy. For leg pain related to vascular claudication, there tend to be symmetric reflexes (often bilaterally absent). The leg pain usually is described more as cramping with ambulation. Atrophic signs of the skin, including lower extremity hair loss, and most significantly, pulse asymmetry or loss of peripheral pulses can be noted. With neurogenic claudication (spinal stenosis) on the other hand, the pain tends to be related to back position. Pulses are symmetric and there usually is normal hair distribution on the lower extremities.

Individuals with peripheral neuropathy tend to have a stocking type of sensory deficit. They also may have other signs of systemic neurologic disorders. They may have a slap foot or steppage gait. A diagnosis frequently is made clinically and on electromyography and nerve conduction velocity studies. Occasionally, nerve (neural) or muscle biopsies are necessary.

The back pain complaints must be differentiated from pain caused by a tumor or infection. These pain complaints tend to increase over time, and are not relieved with rest. In addition, systemic signs may be noted. Patients with osteoporotic compression fractures may have back pain and some leg pain, consistent with stenosis. Radiographs, however, will help separate that diagnosis.

References

1. Arnoldi CC, Brodsky AE, Cauchoix J, et al: Lumbar spinal stenosis and nerve root entrapment syndromes: Definitions and classification. *Clin Orthop* 1976;115:4-5.
2. Kirkaldy-Willis WH, Paine KW, Cauchoix J, McIvor G: Lumbar spinal stenosis. *Clin Orthop* 1974;99:30-50.
3. Kirkaldy-Willis WH, Wedge JH, Yong-Hing K, et al: Pathology and pathogenesis of lumbar spondylosis and stenosis. *Spine* 1978;3:319-328.
4. Kirkaldy-Willis WH: The relationship of structural pathology to the nerve root. *Spine* 1984;9:49-52.
5. Verbiest H: A radicular syndrome from developmental narrowing of the lumbar vertebral canal. *J Bone Joint Surg Br* 1954;36:230-237.
6. Lindblom K, Rexed B: Spinal nerve injury in dorso-lateral protrusions of the lumbar disks. *J Neurosurg* 1948;5:413-432.
7. Coventry MB, Ghormley RK, Kernohan JW: The intervertebral disc: Its microscopic anatomy and pathology. Part III: Pathological changes in the intervertebral disc. *J Bone Joint Surg Am* 1945;27:460-474.
8. Naylor A: The biophysical and biochemical aspects of intervertebral disc herniation and degeneration. *Ann R Coll Surg Engl* 1962;31: 91-114.
9. Pearce RH, Grimmer BJ, Adams ME: Degeneration and the chemical composition of the human lumbar intervetebral disc. *J Orthop Res* 1987;5:198-205.
10. Coventry MB, Ghormley RK, Kernohan JW: The intervertebral disc: Its mircroscopic anatomy and pathology. Part II: Changes in the intervertebral disc concomitant with age. *J Bone Joint Surg Br* 1945;27:233-247.
11. Miller JA, Schmatz C, Schultz AB: Lumbar disc degeneration: Correlation with age, sex, and spine level in 600 autopsy specimens. *Spine* 1988;13:173-178.
12. Videman T, Malmivaara A, Mooney V: The value of the axial view in assessing discograms: An experimental study with cadavers. *Spine* 1987;12:299-304.
13. Eyre DR: Biochemistry of the intervertebral disc. *Int Rev Connect Tissue Res* 1979;8:227-291.
14. Eyring EJ: The biochemistry and physiology of the intervertebral disk. *Clin Orthop* 1969;67: 16-28.
15. Eyre DR, Muir H: Types I and II collagens in intervertebral disc: Interchanging radial distributions in annulus fibrosis. *Biochem J* 1976;157: 267-270.
16. Buckwalter JA, Pedrini-Mille A, Pedrini V, Tudisco C: Proteoglycans of human infant intervertebral disc: Electron microscopic and biochemical studies. *J Bone Joint Surg Am* 1985;67:284-294.
17. Gower WE, Pedrini V: Age-related variarion in protein-polysaccharides from human nucleus pulposus, annulus fibrosus, and costal cartilage. *J Bone Joint Surg Am* 1969;51:1154-1162.
18. Lipson SJ, Muir H: Experimental intervertebral disc degeneration: Morphologic and proteoglycan changes over time. *Arthritis Rheum* 1981;24:12-21.

19. Naylor A, Horton WG: The hydrophilic properties of the nucleus pulposus of the intervertebral disc. *Rheumatism* 1955;11:32-35.

20. Urban JP, McMullin JF: Swelling pressure of the lumbar intervetebral discs: Influence of age, spinal level, composition, and degeneration. *Spine* 1988;13:179-187.

21. Groebler LJ, Anderson PA, Novotny JE, et al: Etiology of spondylolisthesis: Assessment of the role played by lumbar facet joint morphology. *Spine* 1993;18:80-91.

22. Newman PH: Stenosis of the lumbar spine in spondylolisthesis. *Clin Orthop* 1976;115: 116-121.

23. Rosenberg NJ: Degenerative spondylolisthesis: Predisposing factors. *J Bone Joint Surg Am* 1975;57:467-474.

24. Garfin SR, Rydevik BL, Brown RA: Compressive neuropathy of spinal nerve roots: A mechanical or biological problem? *Spine* 1991;16:162-166.

25. Rydevik B, Brown MD, Lundborg G: Pathoanatomy and pathophysiology of nerve root compression. *Spine* 1984;9:7-15.

26. Pedowitz RA, Garfin SR, Massie JB, et al: Effects of magnitude and duration of compression on spinal nerve root conduction. *Spine* 1992;17:194-199.

27. Schonstrom N, Hansson T: Pressure changes following constriction of the cauda equina: An experimental study in situ. *Spine* 1988;13: 385-388.

28. Olmarker K: Spinal nerve root compression: Nutrition and function of the porcine cauda equina compressed in vivo. *Acta Orthop Scand* 1991;242(suppl):1-27.

29. Olmarker K, Rydevik B, Holm S, Bagge U: Effects of experimental graded compression on blood flow in spinal nerve roots: A vital microscopic study on the porcine cauda equina. *J Orthop Res* 1989;7:817-823.

30. Rydevik B, Lundborg G: Permeability of intraneural microvessels and perineurium following acute, graded experimental nerve compression. *Scan J Plast Reconstr Surg* 1977;11:179-187.

31. Rydevik B, Lundborg G, Bagge U: Effects of graded compression on intraneural blood flow: An in vivo study on rabbit tibial nerve. *J Hand Surg Am* 1981;6:3-12.

32. Rydevik B, Nordborg G: Changes in nerve function and nerve fibre structure induced by acute, graded compression. *J Neurol Neurosurg Psychiatry* 1980;43:1070-1082.

33. Rydevik BL, Pedowitz RA, Hargens AR, Swenson MR, Myers RR, Garfin SR: Effects of acute, graded compression on spinal nerve root function and structure: An experimental study of the pig cauda equina. *Spine* 1991;16:487-493.

34. Delamarter RB, Bohlman HH, Dodge LD, Biro C: Experimental lumbar spinal stenosis: Analysis of the cortical evoked potentials, microvasculature, and histopathology. *J Bone Joint Surg Am* 1990;72:110-120.

35. Olmarker K, Holm S, Rydevik B: Importance of compression onset rate for the degree of impairment of impulse propagation in experimental compression injury of the porcine cauda equina. *Spine* 1990;15:416-419.

36. Olmarker K, Rydevik B, Holms S: Edema formation in spinal nerve roots induced by experimental, graded compression: An experimental study on the pig cauda equina with special reference to differences in effects between rapid and slow onset of compression. *Spine* 1989;14: 579-563.

37. Olmarker K, Lind B, Holm S, Rydevik B: Continued compression increases impairment of impulse porpagation in experimental compression of the porcine cauda equina. *Neuro Orthop* 1991;11:75-81.

38. Parke WW, Gammell K, Rothman RH: Arterial vascularization of the cauda equina. *J Bone Joint Surg Am* 1981;63:53-62.

39. Parke WW, Watanabe R: The intrinsic vasculature of the lumbosacral spinal nerve roots. *Spine* 1985;10:508-515.

40. Watanabe R, Parke WW: Vascular and neural pathology of lumbosacral spinal stenosis. *J Neurosurg* 1986;64:64-70.

41. Yoshizawa H, Kobayashi S, Hachiya Y: Blood supply of nerve roots and dorsal root ganglia. *Orthop Clin North Am* 1991;22:195-211.

42. Olmarker K, Rydevik B: Single- versus double-level nerve root compression: An experimental study on the porcine cauda equina with analyses of nerve impulse conduction properties. *Clin Orthop* 1992;279:35-39.

43. Cornefjord M, Takahashi K, Matsui H, Olmarker K, Holms S, Rydevik B: Impairment of nutritional transport at double level cauda equina compression: An experimental study. *Neuro Orthop* 1992;13:107-112.

44. Olmarker K, Rydevik B, Hansson T, Holm S: Compression-induced changes of the nutritional supply to the porcine cauda equina. *J Spinal Disord* 1990;3:25-29.

45. Rydevik B, Holm S, Brown MD, Lundborg G: Diffusion from the cerebrospinal fluid as a nutritional pathway for spinal nerve roots. *Acta Physiol Scand* 1990;138:247-248.

46. Garfin SR, Cohen MS, Massie JB, et al: Nerve-roots of the cauda equina: The effects of hypotension and acute graded compression on function. *J Bone Joint Surg Am* 1990;72: 1185-1192.

47. Lind B, Massie JB, Lincoln T, Myers RR, Swenson MR, Garfin SR: The effects of induced hypertension and acute graded compression on impulse progagation in the spinal nerve roots of the pig. *Spine* 1993;18: 1550-1555.

48. Takahashi K, Olmarker K, Holm S, Porter RW, Rydevik B: Double-level cauda equina compression: An experimental study with continuous monitoring of intraneural blood flow in the porcine cauda equina. *J Orthop Res* 1993;11:104-109.

49. Takahashi K, Miyazaki T, Takino T, Matsui T, Tomita K: Epidural pressure measurements: Relationship between epidural pressure and posture in patients with lumbar spinal stenosis. *Spine* 1995;20:650-653.

50. Kwan MK, Rydevik B, Myers RR, Triggs K, Woo LY-Y, Garfin S: Biomechanical and histological assessment of human lumbosacral spinal nerve roots. *Trans Orthop Res Soc* 1989;14:348.

51. Smith SA, Massie JB, Chestnut R, Garfin SR: Straight leg raising: Anatomical effects on the spinal nerve root without and with fusion. *Spine* 1993;18:992-999.

52. Spencer DL, Irwin GS, Miller JA: Anatomy and significance of fixation of the lumbosacral nerve roots in sciatica. *Spine* 1983;8:672-679.

53. Cornefjord M, Olmarker K, Farley DB, Weinstein JN, Rydevik B: Neuropeptide changes in compressed spinal nerve roots. *Spine* 1995;20:670-673.

54. Olmarker K, Blomquist J, Stromberg J, Nannmark U, Thomsen P, Rydevik B: Inflammatogenic properties of nucleus pulosus. *Spine* 1995;20:665-669.

55. Olmarker K, Rydevik B, Nordborg C: Autologous nucleus pulposus induces neurophysiologic and histologic changes in porcine cauda equina nerve roots. *Spine* 1993;18: 1425-1432.

56. McLain RF, Weinstein JN: Ultrastructural changes in the dorsal root ganglion associated with whole body vibration. *J Spinal Disord* 1991;4:142-148.

57. Wall PD, Devor M: Sensory afferent impulses originate from dorsal root ganglia as well as from the periphery in normal and nerve injured rats. *Pain* 1983;17:321-339.

58. Weinstein J, Pope M, Schmidt R, Seroussi R: Neuropharmacologic effects of vibration on the dorsal root ganglion: An animal model. *Spine* 1988;13:521-525.

59. Cohen MS, Wall EJ, Brown RA, Rydevik B, Garfin SR: Cauda equina anatomy: II. Extrathecal nerve roots and dorsal root ganglia. Spine 1990;15:1248-1251.

60. Cohen MS, Wall EJ, Kerber CW, Abitbol JJ, Garfin SR: The anatomy of the cauda equina on CT scans and MRI. *J Bone Joint Surg Br* 1991;73:381-384.

61. Wall EJ, Cohen MS, Massie JB, Rydevik B, Garfin SR: Cauda equina anatomy: I. Intrathecal nerve root organization. *Spine* 1990;15:1244-1247.

62. Boden SD, Davis DO, Dina TS, Patronas NJ, Wiesel SW: Abnormal magnetic-resonance imaging scans of the lumbar spine in asymptomatic subjects: A prospective investigation. *J Bone Joint Surg Am* 1990;72:403-408.

63. Jensen MC, Brant-Zawadzki MN, Obuchowski N, Modic MT, Malkasian D, Ross JS: Magnetic resonance imaging of the lumbar spine in people without back pain. *N Engl J Med* 1994;331:69-73.

64. Modic MT, Masaryk T, Boumphrey F, Goormastic M, Bell G: Lumbar herniated disk disease and canal stenosis: Prospective evaluation by surface coil MR, CT, and myelography. *Am J Neuroradial* 1986;7:709-717.

65. Jonsson B, Stromqvist B: Symptoms and signs in degeneration of the lumbar spine: A prospective, consecutive study of 300 operated patients. *J Bone Joint Surg Br* 1993;75:381-385.

66. Johnsson K-E, Rosen I, Uden A: The natural course of lumbar spinal stenosis. *Clin Orthop* 1992;279:82-86.

67. Jonsson B, Stromqvist B: Symptoms and signs in degeneration of the lumbar spine: A prospective, consecutive study of 300 operated patients. *J Bone Joint Surg Br* 1993;75:381-385.

68. Katz JN, Dalgas M, Stucki G, et al: Degenerative lumbar spinal stenosis: Diagnostic value of the history and physical examination. *Arthritis Rheum* 1995;38:1236-1241.

69. Kirkaldy-Willis WH, Farfan HF: Instability of the lumbar spine. *Clin Orthop* 1982;165: 110-123.

70. Lipson S: Clinical diagnosis of spinal stenosis. *Semin Spine Surg* 1989;1:143-144.

16

Lumbar Spinal Stenosis: Treatment Options

Eeric Truumees, MD
Harry N. Herkowitz, MD

Nonsurgical Treatment Options

Because rapid symptomatic or functional decline is rare in patients with lumbar spinal stenosis, a course of nonsurgical management is recommended. Various nonsurgical modalities are often sufficient to control symptoms, and surgery may be deferred.[1,2] Regardless of the modalities ultimately selected, the patient should be actively involved in decision making and symptom management. Reassurance and education by way of books and videotapes are recommended.

Activity modification, including decreased lifting, twisting, and forward bending, is a mainstay in nonsurgical management. A period of relative rest may be advised for symptom flare-ups.[2] Although rest may temporarily control symptoms, exercise is another crucial element of management.[3] Exercise offers many benefits, including weight reduction, cardiopulmonary fitness, and release of endorphins. Stationary bicycle riding (while partially forward flexed), aquatic exercises, and partially unloaded treadmill exercises are well tolerated.[4]

A formal physical therapy program may pave the way for earlier recovery, decreased recurrence, and decreased disability and pain.[2,5] Hyperextension regimens should be avoided;[2,4,6,7] flexion exercises are preferred.[8,9] These exercises increase flexibility of lumbar soft tissues and hamstrings, provide for truncal stabilization, and help strengthen abdominal muscles, thereby helping to maintain a position of slight flexion.

A lumbar corset may decrease motion and at the same time reduce pain. Bracing may lead to weakness and is therefore controversial.[10,11] Muscle deconditioning must be carefully avoided with a concomitant exercise program.

Various medications such as acetaminophen and nonsteroidal anti-inflammatory drugs (NSAIDs) are frequently recommended in the treatment of lumbar spinal stenosis. However, in the elderly population, particular care must be taken relative to potential systemic complications such as gastrointestinal ulceration or impaired renal function. The newer class of COX-2 specific NSAIDs are not free of complications. Narcotics are occasionally prescribed for flare-ups; however, long-term narcotic use is to be avoided because it can lead to constipation, dependence, and impaired mental function.[10] Antidepressants used in low doses are occasionally helpful in promoting sleep and decreasing neurogenic and back pain.[12] Nasal calcitonin has been found to be helpful in mild cases.[13] Muscle relaxants and oral steroids are not recommended.[10,14]

Injection therapies are variably recommended in the sacroiliac joints, trigger points, and nerve root sleeves.[15] Epidural steroid injections are more common, yet also remain controversial.[16,17] Such injections may be helpful in the face of acute flare-ups, with significant radicular complaints, to allow institution of a nonsurgical treatment regimen including physical therapy, or in those for whom surgery is not an option.[18] Typically, three weekly injections of 80 mg Depo-Medrol and 0.5% xylocaine are given through the sacral hiatus. This approach avoids the technical difficulty of inserting a needle through the arthritic posterior elements of the spine, but may then miss symptoms from levels about the level of tightest stenosis. In two retrospective evaluations of the effectiveness of epidural steroid injections for lumbar spinal stenosis, 50% of patients experienced short-term pain relief.[19,20] Two reviews used meta-analysis, with differing conclusions. In one, a 14% improvement over the natural history of degenerative spinal disease was noted.[21] Another review of the use of epidural steroid injections in multiple trials found little support for the practice.[22] Epidural steroid injections may predict results of decompressive surgery.[23]

Other modalities of nonsurgical treatment of spinal stenosis include manipulation, acupuncture, stress reduction, ultrasound, transcutaneous electrical nerve stimulation units, thermal modalities, and traction. These modalities cannot be recommended based on available data.[24-28] In 1987, the Quebec Task Force on Spinal Disorders found no evidence for any nonsurgical approach in the treatment of lumbar spinal stenosis.[26] They did recommend orthoses, activity modification, traction, and exercise based on practice patterns and empirical evidence.

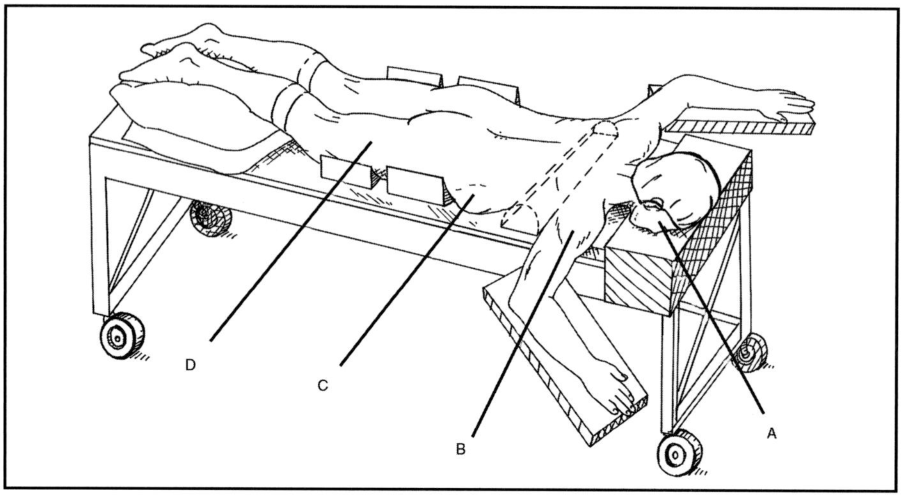

Fig. 1 Patient positioning is critical. Because these procedures are often lengthy, all bony prominences must be well padded. The eyes must be carefully padded (**A**). Careful attention to arm position will decrease the likelihood of postoperative brachial plexus palsy (**B**). Abdominal contents are allowed to hang free to decrease back pressure on the epidural venous plexus (**C**). The legs may be extended for a more normal lumbar lordosis (**D**). Here the final decompression will more closely mimic the standing position. (© William Beaumont Hospital, Royal Oak, MI)

Results of Nonsurgical Treatment

Very little objective evaluation of the various nonsurgical modalities has been done. In one series of 145 patients treated nonsurgically, 70% had significant symptomatic improvement, whereas 23% had mild improvement.[29] Johnsson and associates[30] followed 32 patients with lumbar spinal stenosis treated nonsurgically for a mean of 49 months. The pain was unchanged in 70%, improved in 15%, and worse in 15%. Atlas and associates[31] reported better results with surgery at 1 year in a prospective cohort study of surgically and nonsurgically treated patients with lumbar spinal stenosis. At 1 year, 15% of the nonsurgical group reported worse leg pain, while 20% had worse back pain.

Indications for Surgical Treatment

Except in the rare case of rapidly progressive neurologic deficits, surgery in patients with lumbar spinal stenosis is elective.[32,33] Indications include progressive neurologic deficit, intractable pain, and persistent impairment/functional limitations.[34-36] Because low back pain alone is not reliably alleviated, it alone is not an indication for surgery.[37-39] There is significant geographic variation in how these indications are applied.[40-43] Larequi-Lauber and associates[44] evaluated the appropriateness of surgical indications in 328 consecutive patients undergoing laminectomy for lumbar spinal stenosis. They found that in 38% of patients, surgical indications were inappropriate, particularly because of an inadequate trial of nonsurgical treatment.

There are no absolute contraindications to surgery. Although medical comorbidities significantly influence outcomes, age alone is not a contraindication.[36,45-47] However, patients without concordance of history, physical examination, and imaging data should be managed nonsurgically.

Principles of Surgical Management

The goals of surgery are increased function, decreased pain, and prevention of neurologic deficit progression. Central to achieving these goals is complete decompression of the neural elements. The extent of the decompression required is determined by the patient's pathoanatomy. Even with unilaterally symptomatic patients, unilateral surgery should be avoided in patients with radiographic evidence of bilateral stenosis. These patients will soon present with contralateral symptoms. Further, the number of levels involved should not be underestimated. Physical examination will often not allow localization to singular levels.[48]

Within the larger goal of obtaining a complete decompression, preservation of spinal stability is critical to the prevention of late failure. First, facet integrity may be maintained by undercutting with angled instruments. Second, protection of the pars will obviate postoperative fractures and incipient back pain and instability.[49] Third, unforeseen difficulties in decompression may require fusion in any patient undergoing a decompression. Therefore, all patients should be prepared for this possibility.

Before surgery, a complete medical and nutritional evaluation is recommended. For more extensive procedures, it remains our practice to encourage autologous blood donation. There are several other issues outside of the transmission of infectious viral diseases that make autologous blood transfusion preferable. These include the risk of unsuspected antibodies. In the operating room, a headlight and loupes or an operating microscope are valuable. Some authors use intraoperative monitoring to determine adequacy of decompression.[50] Others find that return of cerebrospinal fluid pulsation signals adequacy of decompression.[51] The patient is positioned prone or kneeling with the abdomen hanging free to decrease central venous pressure[52] (Fig. 1). Some authors recommend maintaining lumbar

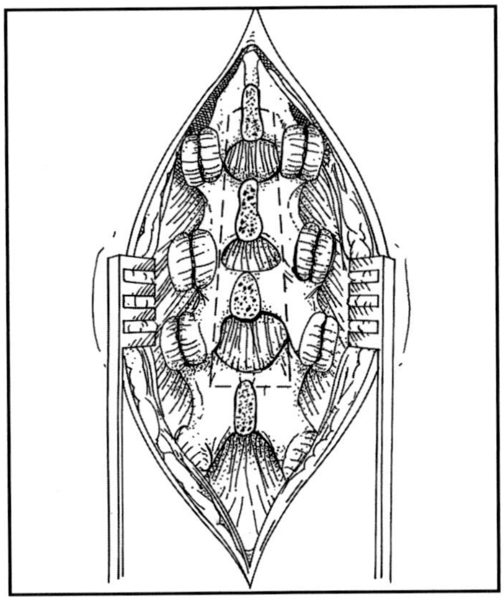

Fig. 2 Once the exposure has been completed, a radiograph is obtained to confirm spinal level. Then, the spinous processes from the inferior half of the superiormost and the superior half of the inferiormost levels to be decompressed are removed with double-action rongeurs. The entire spinous process of each intermediate level is removed. (© William Beaumont Hospital, Royal Oak, MI)

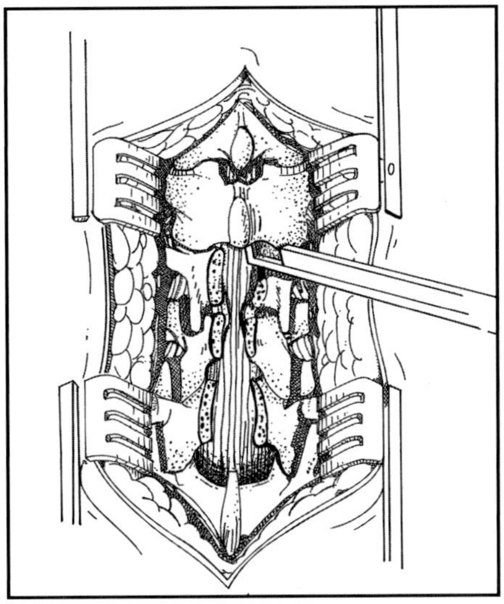

Fig. 3 Posteroanterior view demonstrating completed central decompression. The hypertrophic ligamentum flavum laterally causing continued compression is noted. (© William Beaumont Hospital, Royal Oak, MI)

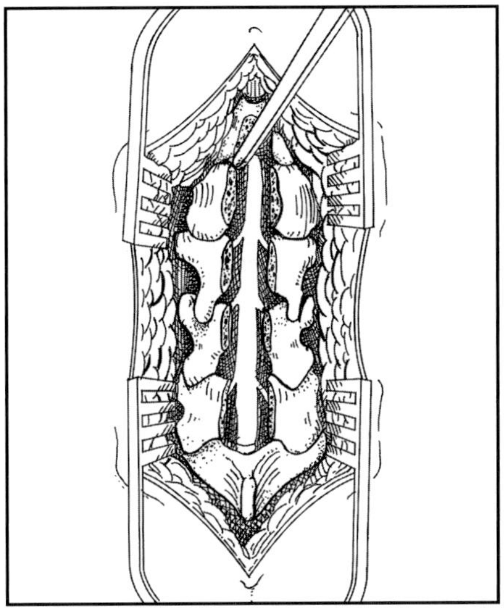

Fig 4 Posteroanterior view demonstrating lateral recess decompression. (© William Beaumont Hospital, Royal Oak, MI)

lordosis in that this positioning more closely emulates the symptomatic, standing position. Moreover, a fusion may then be undertaken in a more physiologically appropriate position. The disadvantage of this position is laminar shingling, which increases the difficulty of entering the canal.

Techniques of Surgical Decompression

Laminectomy remains the standard procedure for surgical decompression in lumbar spinal stenosis. Laminectomy begins with a central decompression. Herein, the inferior half of the superior spinous process and the superior half of the inferior spinous process are removed (along with all intermediate spinous processes) with a double-action rongeur (Fig. 2). A Leksell rongeur is then used to remove additional bone and soft tissue and to thin the laminae. A Kerrison rongeur is used to remove the remainder of the central laminae and flavum in a caudad to cephalad direction (Fig. 3).

Next, a decompression of the lateral recesses is undertaken by partial medial facetectomy (Fig. 4). To prevent destabilization, an undercutting technique with a 45° upbiting Kerrison rongeur is used. The decompression is taken out laterally to the pedicles (Fig. 5). Finally, the foramina are decompressed after the nerve roots are identified. The Kerrison rongeur is inserted dorsal to the roots and overlying spurs are removed. An angled dural separator or a ball-tip probe may be used to assess the adequacy of decompression. A 4-mm probe should pass without difficulty (Fig. 6). Finally, the root, when retracted with a Penfield dissector, should demonstrate 1 cm of medial displacement. Disk herniation is occasionally seen in conjunction with lumbar spinal stenosis. These herniations, if lateral or foraminal, may require removal. Central bulges alone are adequately decompressed with a laminectomy.[53]

Another common method of decompression is the laminotomy. Unilateral laminotomy has been advocated in certain patients with localized lateral recess stenosis and monoradicular complaints.[54] More often, however, a bilateral laminotomy is recommended as a spinous process- and ligament-sparing alternative to a complete laminectomy. This procedure is indicated if stenosis is limited to disk/facet joint level. It is contraindicated in patients with congenital stenosis and global narrowing. The role of laminotomy in patients with scoliosis and spondylolisthesis remains to be defined; however, posterior element preservation may minimize the risk of progression.[51] Disadvantages include increased technical difficulty, duration of surgery, and neurologic risk.

A patient undergoing laminotomy is positioned in the same manner as a laminectomy patient.[55] During the surgical approach to the spine, the supraspinous ligaments and spinous processes should be preserved. The inferior laminotomy is extended laterally to the base of the inferior facet. Then, a medial facetectomy of the inferior facet, including

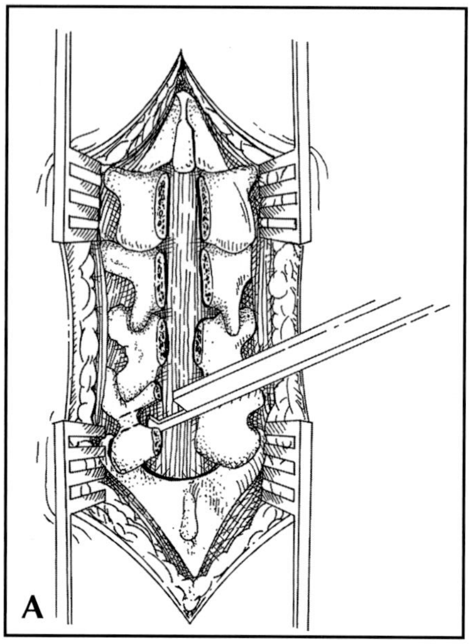

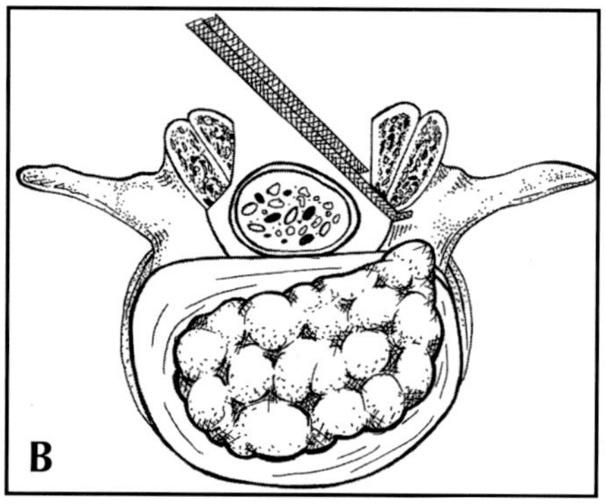

Fig. 5 A, Posteroanterior view demonstrating technique for foraminotomy. The Kerrison rongeur is passed over the nerve root into the foramen to allow decompression. Caution should be taken to prevent excessive pressure over the root. **B,** The axial view demonstrates a Kerrison rongeur used to perform an undercutting maneuver from the opposite side. (© William Beaumont Hospital, Royal Oak, MI)

undercutting of the laminae, is performed with a sharp osteotome. This maneuver exposes the underlying superior facet so that its medial portion can be removed using Kerrison rongeurs (Fig. 7). Others have described a similar procedure using high-speed burrs for facetectomies and undercutting of facet joints.[56]

Other, less commonly applied methods of decompression include the Ipsi-Contra procedure and lumbar canal expansive laminoplasty.[57,58]

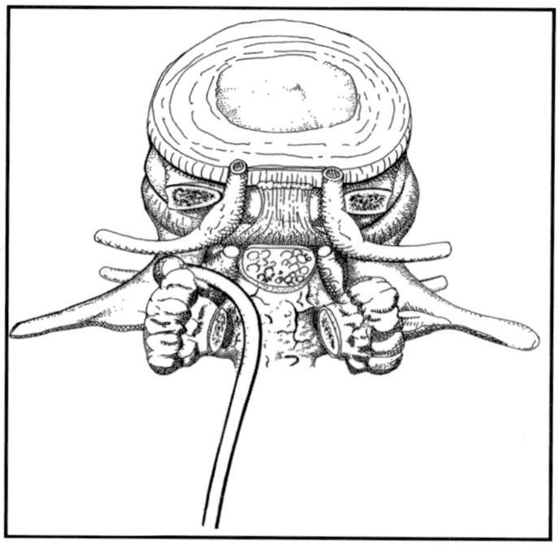

Fig. 6 Axial view of the completed decompression. Note that the probe passes easily out into the foramen. The undersurfaces of the facets and their associated osteophytes have been removed with an undercutting technique, thereby preserving the bulk of the facet itself. (© William Beaumont Hospital, Royal Oak, MI)

Results of Lumbar Canal Decompression

Most case series report greater than 85% good-to-excellent results after lumbar decompression for stenosis.[53,59-64] Verbiest[65] reviewed 91 of his patients with up to 20 years follow-up and noted complete relief of preoperative symptoms in 62 (68%); 29 had residual symptoms of which lumbago was the most frequent (47%). Herron and Mangelsdorf[66] reported on 140 patients of whom 80% had major improvement in leg pain. Another 11% had some improvement and 67% had major improvement in back pain. Female sex, compensation or litigation factors, no relief of symptoms from prior surgical procedures, or an objective postoperative sensory deficit predicted a poor outcome. Outcomes in patients with coexisting illnesses (osteoarthritis, cardiac disease, rheumatoid arthritis, chronic obstructive pulmonary disease) are less favorable.[39,40,67-69] Katz and associates[67] and later Jonsson and associates[70] have noted some deterioration of the early results of decompressive surgery over time. In Katz and associates' series, 17% of patients ultimately underwent a second procedure for instability or recurrent stenosis.

There are fewer series reporting outcomes of laminotomy procedures. However, most have reported 82% to 91% good-to-excellent results.[56,64,71] Postacchini and associates[72] assigned 67 patients with central lumbar stenosis to either multiple laminotomy or total laminectomy groups. In this series, some patients with severe stenosis were converted from laminotomy to laminectomy if inadequate decompression was performed, risk of neural injury was high, or too much bone was taken. After a 3.7-year follow-up, there were 78% good-to-excellent results reported in the laminectomy group and 81% in the multiple laminotomy group. The authors noted that the amount of blood loss was the same; however, duration of surgery and neurologic complications were increased with laminotomy. On the other hand, laminotomy patients had increased relief of back pain and no postoperative instability.

Fusion in the Treatment of Lumbar Spinal Stenosis

Although there appears to be a consensus that patients with lumbar spinal stenosis benefit from decompression if nonsurgical treatment fails, recommendations for fusion are less clearly established. The goals of fusion in these patients are elimination of motion at a painful degenerated segment, elimination of instability, prevention of progression of olisthesis, kyphosis, or scoliosis, or prevention of recurrent stenosis.

Ultimately, the decision to fuse is based on two factors: the preoperative condition of the spine and changes in the stability of the spine stemming from the decompression. Fusion has occcasionally been suggested for all patients undergoing decompression because of the difficulties in identifying unstable spines.[73,74]

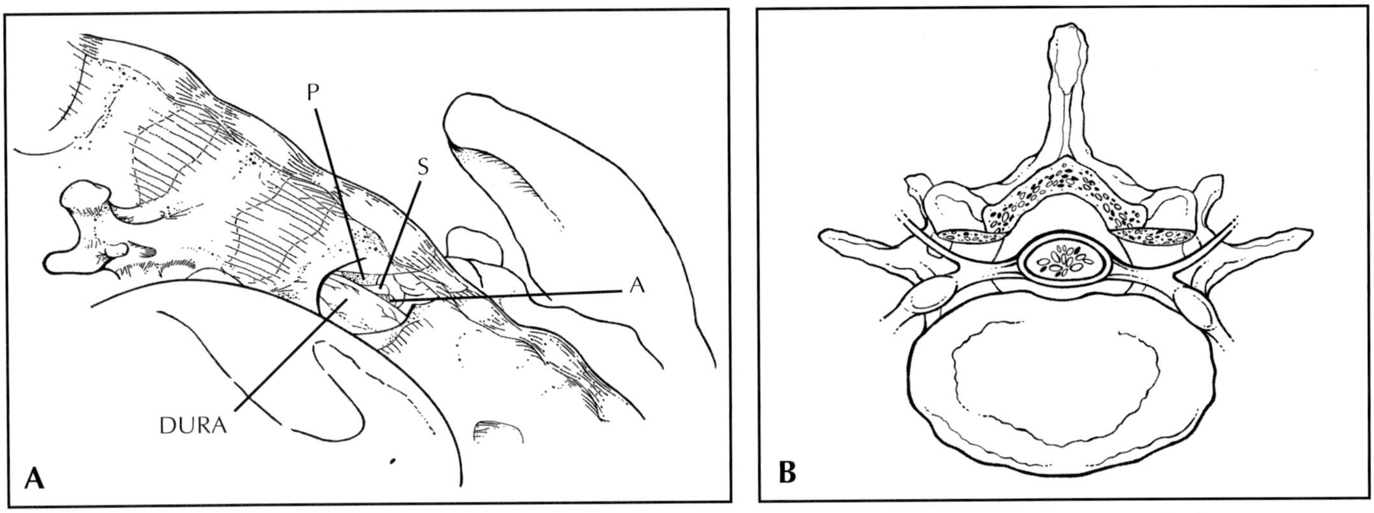

Fig. 7 A, An oblique view of a standard hemilaminotomy for decompression of central and lateral recess stenosis. Here, the ligamentum flavum and leading and trailing edges of the laminae have been removed. A dural retractor is used to protect the dura while a Kerrison rongeur is used to remove facet spurs. P = pedicle (nerve root may be compressed in this area); S = end plate spur; A = disk anulus (bulge may contribute to stenosis). **B,** The axial view demonstrates a sublaminar decompression performed from a laminotomy approach. Note that the medial aspects of the inferior facet of the superior level and the superior facet of the inferior level are removed. (© William Beaumont Hospital, Royal Oak, MI)

On the other hand, in one large series of patients undergoing wide decompression for stenosis, only 2% developed enough instability to require late fusion.[51]

Others argue that fusion increases morbidity with little added benefit and should rarely be required. Deyo and associates[75] reviewed 13,622 Medicare patients treated for lumbar spinal stenosis. Six percent of these patients underwent fusion after wide laminectomy. In fusion patients, complication rates were 1.9 times higher, transfusion rates were 5.8 times higher, nursing home placement was required 2.2 times more often, and the 6-week postoperative mortality was two times higher than in those undergoing decompression alone. Grob and associates[60] performed a randomized study of 45 patients with lumbar spinal stenosis without obvious signs of instability. They found no statistically significant difference in pain relief an average of 28 months of follow-up.

There is more support for routine fusion in patients with preoperative evidence of instability such as a degenerative spondylolisthesis or scoliosis. Here, decompression may accelerate deformity progression.[76] Yet, Herron and Trippi[77] argued that, with careful decompression, slips did not progress in their series of 24 patients. Even if the slip progresses, its effect on ultimate outcome was occasionally disputed.[66,77,78]

The emerging consensus, however, is to fuse spondylolisthetic segments in patients undergoing decompression for lumbar spinal stenosis.[79-85] Katz and associates[68] studied 105 patients with at least a 5 mm slip or 15° of scoliosis and found superior back pain relief at both 6 and 24 months in patients undergoing uninstrumented fusions versus patients undergoing either no fusion or instrumented fusions. Johnsson and associates[86] found that postoperative increases in listhesis were twice as common in patients with poor results. Herkowitz and Kurz[87] published a prospective study comparing decompressive laminectomy alone with decompressive laminectomy and intertransverse arthrodesis in 50 patients with single level spinal stenosis associated with degenerative spondylolisthesis. In their series the 90% good-to-excellent results in the fused group was a statistically significant improvement compared with the 44% good-to-excellent results in the nonfusion group.

When performing fusion on a patient who has degenerative spondylolisthesis, attempts to reduce the slip have been advocated. Such reduction is appealing in that restoration of the normal alignment may relieve anterior compression of the nerve roots, shorten the course of the nerve roots, and decrease the tension under which the fusion mass is placed. On the other hand, active, forceful reduction may increase the possibility of an intraoperative neurologic injury. Various techniques to achieve reduction have been described, including use of a sacral bar and Harrington distraction instrumentation[88] or a transpedicle screw and plate method.[89] Often, a two-level extension of the instrumentation to increase biomechanical stability of the construct is required.[90] Montgomery and Fischgrund[90] prospectively evaluated passive reduction in a series of patients undergoing decompressive laminectomy and fusion for degenerative spondylolisthesis. They found an average decrease in slip of 24% from the preoperative flexion view to the intraoperative prone lateral view. In many cases this passive reduction obviates the need for multilevel reconstructions of single-level slips and the danger of intraoperative reduction maneuvers in many cases.

Indications for fusion are even less clearly defined in patients with lumbar spinal stenosis and degenerative scoliosis.[91] Moreover, the additional surgery required to stabilize these multilevel deformities adds significant potential morbidity to the procedure. Most reports have focused on retrospective analysis of surgical technique without comparative reviews of the various options.[65]

It appears that not all degenerative scoliosis patients require fusion for stenosis symptoms. Decompression alone may suffice in patients with single root involvement when the facets can be preserved.[92] Indications for fusion include a large or progressive curve (> 35°), pain in the curve, loss of lumbar lordosis to the extent that it causes sagittal imbalance, and cardiopulmonary complications related to the curve (rare). In patients with radicular symptoms within the concavity of a curve, partial correction of the deformity with an instrumented fusion may be needed to reduce pedicular kinking.[93] Moreover, a curve demonstrating correctability on side bending will likely progress with laminectomy alone.[93] Careful consideration to fusion should be given in the presence of asymmetric tilt of single interspace (especially L4-5), lateral spondylolisthesis, or multiplanar instability.

Fusion may be required as a function of the decompression. The exact degree of instability engendered by a given decompression is difficult to predict. However, the prevailing wisdom has held that removal of one third to one half of both or all of one facet at a given level is tolerated.[71,94,95] Hazlett and Kinnard[96] reported on 33 patients undergoing unilateral or bilateral complete facet joint excision, many with concomitant disk excision. Only four showed signs of late instability and only two of these four had poor results. Grobler and associates[97] reported that progression of spondylolisthesis was more likely caused by facet joint orientation and dimensions than absolute amount of bone removed.

Recurrent stenosis at the same level or stenosis adjacent to a previously decompressed and fused segment also warrants fusion in that further compromise of the facet joints is usually needed for adequate decompression of restenotic patients.

Posterolateral fusion is sufficient in most patients with lumbar spinal stenosis. In addition, 360° fusions, via anteroposterior surgery or posterior lumbar interbody fusion, may be useful to increase correction and fusion rates in certain complex reconstruction situations. Whether instrumentation is required also remains controversial. The goals of instrumentation include deformity correction, spinal stabilization, improved rates of fusion, and reduced rehabilitation time. In patients with hyperlordosis or hyperkyphosis, improvement in the sagittal alignment through instrumented reduction and stabilization may improve outcome. On the other hand, instrumentation confers increased potential for complications, surgery time, and expense.

A pseudarthrosis may not represent a clinical failure.[98,99] Fischgrund and associates[100] reported the results of 68 patients with spinal stenosis and degenerative spondylolisthesis in a prospective study. The authors noted a significantly higher fusion rate (83%) in the instrumented group versus the noninstrumented group (45%). However, the clinical outcome was similar whether instrumentation was used or not. Bridwell and associates[101] found that uninstrumented fusion patients had significantly increased progression of their slips compared with instrumented patients.

The present indications for instrumented fusion include correction of a supple progressive scoliosis or kyphosis; or arthrodesis of two or more motion segments with a decompressive laminectomy; recurrent spinal stenosis with iatrogenic spondylolisthesis; transitional motion greater than 4 mm in flexion and extension and angular motion > 10° compared with adjacent levels; and revision for symptomatic pseudarthrosis.

Postoperative Care

The postoperative regimen is similar for all of the various surgical interventions described. The patient is mobilized to a chair the evening of surgery. Then, ambulation begins the next morning. Braces are typically not used. The patient should refrain from bending, lifting, or twisting for 6 to 12 weeks. Drains are removed on the first or second postoperative day. Most patients go home in 2 to 4 days as a function of extent of their procedure and medical comorbidities. Some elderly patients require inpatient rehabilitation. An office visit is undertaken at 2 weeks for wound check and staple removal. The occasional patient returns to physical therapy at 4 to 6 weeks for a two- to three-visit course to reinforce stretching and strengthening principles. NSAIDs are restricted in all fusion patients.

Complications

Ciol and associates[61] analyzed the data on 30,000 patients undergoing surgical treatment for lumbar spinal stenosis. Complications were divided into four groups: infectious, vascular, cardiopulmonary, and death. Mortality rates were related to age and the presence of comorbidities. In patients younger than age 75 years, the mortality rate was < 1%. In patients older than age 80 years, mortality rose to 2.3%. Complications were twice as frequent as well.

Another potential source of clinical failure is recurrent stenosis by way of laminar regrowth. Postachinni and Cinotti[102] reported on laminar regrowth after decompressive laminectomy for spinal stenosis. They reviewed 40 patients with average 8.6-year follow-up. A preoperative spondylolisthesis was present preoperatively in 16. Of these 16, 6 underwent laminectomy alone; 10 had an added arthrodesis. The authors found that those without arthrodesis had significantly poorer clinical outcome.

There are many potential causes for late-term failure of surgical decompression in lumbar spinal stenosis patients. Among these are recurrent stenosis at the decompressed level and degeneration with stenosis at segments adjacent to that previously treated.[103] In patients undergoing spinal fusion, changes in segmental stiffness may increase forces applied to adjacent segments, thereby accelerating degeneration. Alternatively, proprioceptive changes and postoperative weakness in the lumbar extensors may adversely influence the natural history of spinal stenosis. Both recurrent and adjacent segment stenosis may lead to recurrence of leg pain and pseudoclaudicatory symptoms.

References

1. Johnsson KE, Uden A, Rosen I: The effect of decompression on the natural course of spinal stenosis: A comparison of surgically treated and untreated patients. *Spine* 1991;16:615-619.
2. LaBan MM, Taylor RS: Conservative management of lumbar spinal stenosis, in Herkowitz HN, Garfin SR, Balderston RA, Eismont FJ, Bell GR, Wiesel SW (eds): *Rothman-Simeone: The Spine,* ed 4. Philadelphia, PA, WB Saunders, 1999, pp 806A-806F.
3. Davies JE, Gibson T, Tester L: The value of exercises in the treatment of low back pain. *Rheumatol Rehabil* 1979;18:243-247.
4. Fritz JM, Erhard RE, Vignovic M: A nonsurgical treatment approach for patients with lumbar spinal stenosis. *Phys Ther* 1997;77:962-973.
5. Mayer GT: Spine functional restoration, in Rothman RH, Simeone FA (eds): *The Spine,* ed 3. Philadelphia, PA, WB Saunders, 1992, vol 2, pp 1929-1944.
6. Cailliet R (ed): *Low Back Pain Syndrome,* ed 5. Philadelphia, PA, FA Davis, 1995.
7. Sikorski JM: A rationalized approach to physiotherapy for low-back pain. *Spine* 1985; 10:571-579.
8. Williams PC: Lesions of the lumbosacral spine: Acute traumatic destruction of the lumbosacral intervertebral disc. *J Bone Joint Surg Am* 1937;19:343-363.
9. Paine KW: Clinical features of lumbar spinal stenosis. *Clin Orthop* 1976;115:77-82.
10. Zdeblick TA: The treatment of degenerative lumbar disorders: A critical review of the literature. *Spine* 1995;20(suppl 24):126S-137S.
11. Frymoyer JW: Back pain and sciatica. *N Engl J Med* 1988;318:291-300.
12. Ward NG: Tricyclic antidepressants for chronic low-back pain: Mechanisms of action and predictors of response. *Spine* 1986;11:661-665.
13. Eskola A, Pohjolainen T, Alaranta H, Soini J, Tallroth K, Slatis P: Calcitonin treatment in lumbar spinal stenosis: A randomized, placebo-controlled, double-blind, cross-over study with one-year follow-up. *Calcif Tissue Int* 1992;50:400-403.
14. Basmajian JV: Acute back pain and spasm: A controlled multicenter trial of combined analgesic and antispasm agents. *Spine* 1989; 14:438-439.
15. Schwarzer AC, Aprill CN, Bogduk N: The sacroiliac joint in chronic low back pain. *Spine* 1995;20:31-37.
16. Cuckler JM, Bernini PA, Wiesel SW, Booth RE Jr, Rothman RH, Pickens GT: The use of epidural steroids in the treatment of lumbar radicular pain: A prospective, randomized, double-blind study. *J Bone Joint Surg Am* 1985;67:63-66.
17. Ferrante FM: Epidural steroids in the management of spinal stenosis. *Semin Spine Surg* 1989;1:177.
18. Benzon HT: Epidural steroid injections for low back pain and lumbosacral radiculopathy. *Pain* 1986;24:277-295.
19. Hoogmartens M, Morelle P: Epidural injection in the treatment of spinal stenosis. *Acta Orthop Belg* 1987;53:409-411.
20. Rosen CD, Kahanovitz N, Bernstein R, Viola K: A retrospective analysis of the efficacy of epidural steroid injections. *Clin Orthop* 1988;228:270-272.
21. Rapp SE, Haselkorn JK, Elam K, Deyo RA, Ciol MA: Abstract: Epidural injection in the treatment of low back pain: A meta-analysis. *Anesthesiology* 1994;(suppl A923):81.
22. Bigos SJ, Bower O, Braen G, Brown KC, Deyo RA, Haldeman S, et al: Acute low back problems in adults, in *Clinical Practice Guideline No 14: AHCPR Publication No: 95-0642.* Rockville, MD, Department of Health and Human Services, 1995.
23. Derby R, Kine G, Saal JA, et al: Response to steroid and duration of radicular pain as predictors of surgical outcome. *Spine* 1992;17(suppl 6):S176-S183.
24. Curtis P: Spinal manipulation: Does it work? *Occup Med* 1988;3:31-44.
25. Grieve GP (ed): *Mobilisation of the Spine: Notes on Examination, Assessment, and Clinical Method,* ed 4. Edinburgh, Scotland, Churchill Livingstone, 1984.
26. Scientific approach to the assessment and management of activity-related spinal disorders: A monograph for clinicians: Report of the Quebec Task Force on Spinal Disorders. *Spine* 1987;12(suppl 7):S1-S59.
27. Dimaggio A, Mooney V: Conservative care for LBP, What works? *J Musculoskeletal Med* 1987;4:27.
28. Pal B, Mangion P, Hossain MA, Diffey BL: A controlled trial of continuous lumbar traction in the treatment of back pain and sciatica. *Br J Rheumatol* 1986;25:181-183.
29. Onel D, Sari H, Donmez C: Lumbar spinal stenosis: Clinical/radiologic therapeutic evaluation in 145 patients: Conservative treatment or surgical intervention? *Spine* 1993;18:291-298.
30. Johnsson KE, Rosen I, Uden A: The natural course of lumbar spinal stenosis. *Clin Orthop* 1992;279:82-86.
31. Atlas SJ, Deyo RA, Keller RB, et al: The Maine Lumbar Spine Study: 1-year outcomes of surgical and nonsurgical management of lumbar spinal stenosis. *Spine* 1996;21:1787-1795.
32. Kirkaldy-Willis WH (ed): *Managing Low Back Pain.* New York, NY, Churchill Livingstone, 1983.
33. Van Akkerveeken P: Classification and treatment of spinal stenosis: History and classification on spinal stenosis, in Wiesel SW, Weinstein JN, Herkowitz HN, Dvorak J, Bell GR (eds): *The Lumbar Spine,* ed 2. Philadelphia, PA, WB Saunders, 1996, vol 2, pp 724-731.
34. Hanley EN Jr, Eskay ML: Degenerative lumbar spinal stenosis. *Adv Orthop Surg* 1985;8: 396-403.
35. Selby DK: When to operate and what to operate upon. *Orthop Clin North Am* 1983;14: 577-588.
36. Wiltse LL, Kirkaldy-Willis WH, Mclvor GW: The treatment of spinal stenosis. *Clin Orthop* 1976;115:83-91.
37. Grabias S: The treatment of spinal stenosis. *J Bone Joint Surg Am* 1980;62:308-313.
38. Hall S, Bartleson JD, Onofrio BM, Baker HL Jr, Okazaki H, O'Duffy JD: Lumbar spinal stenosis: Clinical features, diagnostic procedures, and results of surgical treatment in 68 patients. *Ann Intern Med* 1985;103:271-275.
39. Katz JN, Lipson SJ, Brick GW, et al: Clinical correlates of patient satisfaction after laminectomy for degenerative lumbar spinal stenosis. *Spine* 1995;20:1155-1160.
40. Ciol MA, Deyo RA, Howell E, Kreif S: An assessment of surgery for spinal stenosis: Time trends, geographic variations, complications and reoperations. *J Am Geriatr Soc* 1996;44: 285-290.

41. Katz JN: Lumbar spinal fusion: Surgical rates, costs, and complications. *Spine* 1995;20(suppl 24):78S-83S.

42. Taylor VM, Deyo RA, Cherkin DC, Kreuter W: Low back pain hospitalization: Recent United States trends and regional variations. *Spine* 1994;19:1207-1213.

43. Volinn E, Mayer J, Diehr P, Van Koevering D, Connell FA, Loeser JD: Small area analysis of surgery for low-back pain. *Spine* 1992;17: 575-581.

44. Larequi-Lauber T, Vader JP, Burnand B, et al: Appropriateness of indications for surgery of lumbar disc hernia and spinal stenosis. *Spine* 1997;22:203-209.

45. Fellrath RF Jr, Hanley EN Jr: The causes and management of pseudarthrosis following anterior cervical arthrodesis. *Semin Spine Surg* 1995;7:43-51.

46. Sanderson PL, Wood PL: Surgery for lumbar spinal stenosis in old people. *J Bone Joint Surg Br* 1993;75:393-397.

47. Spengler DM: Lumbar decompression for spinal stenosis: Surgical indications and technique, in Frymoyer JW, Ducker TB, Hadler NM, Kostuik JP, Weinstein JN, Whitecloud TS III (eds): *The Adult Spine: Principles and Practice.* New York, NY, Raven Press, 1991, vol 2, pp 1811-1819.

48. Katz JN, Dalgas M, Stucki G, Lipson SG: Degenerative lumbar spinal stenosis: Diagnostic value of the history and physical examination. *Arthritis Rheum* 1995;38: 1236-1241.

49. Rosen C, Rothman S, Zigler J, Capen D: Lumbar facet fracture as a possible source of pain after lumbar laminectomy. *Spine* 1991;16(suppl 6):S234-S238.

50. Herron LD, Trippi AC, Gonyeau M: Intraoperative use of dermatomal somatosensory-evoked potentials in lumbar stenosis surgery. *Spine* 1987;12:379-383.

51. Whiffen JR, Neuwirth MG: Spinal stenosis, in Bridwell KH, DeWald RL, Hammerberg KW, et al (eds): *The Textbook of Spinal Surgery,* ed 2. Philadelphia, PA, Lippincott-Raven, 1997, vol 2, pp 1561-1580.

52. DiStefano VJ, Klein KS, Nixon JE, Andrews ET: Intra-operative analysis of the effects of position and body habitus on surgery of the low back: A preliminary report. *Clin Orthop* 1974;99:51-56.

53. Garfin SR, Glover M, Booth RE, Simeone FA, Rothman RH: Laminectomy: A review of the Pennsylvania hospital experience. *J Spinal Disord* 1988;1:116-133.

54. Lee CK, Rauschning W, Glenn W: Lateral lumbar spinal canal stenosis: Classification, pathologic anatomy and surgical decompression. *Spine* 1988;13:313-320.

55. Lin PM: Internal decompression for multiple levels of lumbar spinal stenosis: A technical note. *Neurosurgery* 1982;11:546-549.

56. Young S, Veerapen R, O'Laoire SA: Relief of lumbar canal stenosis using multilevel subarticular fenestrations as an alternative to wide laminectomy: Preliminary report. *Neurosurgery* 1988;23:628-633.

57. diPierro CG, Helm GA, Shaffrey CI, et al: Treatment of lumbar spinal stenosis by extensive unilateral decompression and contralateral autologous bone fusion: Operative technique and results. *J Neurosurg* 1996;84:166-173.

58. Matsui H, Tsuji H, Sekido H, Hirano N, Katoh Y, Makiyama N: Results of expansive laminoplasty for lumbar spinal stenosis in active manual workers. *Spine* 1992;17 (suppl 3):S37-S40.

59. Getty CJ: Lumbar spinal stenosis: The clinical spectrum and the results of operation. *J Bone Joint Surg Br* 1980;62:481-485.

60. Grob D, Hunke T, Dvorak J: Degenerative lumbar spinal stenosis: Decompression with and without arthrodesis. *J Bone Joint Surg Am* 1995;77:1036-1041.

61. Ciol MA, Deyo RA, Howell E, Kreif S: An assessment of surgery for spinal stenosis: Time, trends, geographic variation, complications, and reoperations. *J Am Geriatr Soc* 1996;44:285-290.

62. Herkowitz HN, Garfin SR, Bell GR, Bumphrey F, Rothman RH: The use of computerized tomography in evaluating non-visualized vertebral levels caudad to a complete block on a lumbar myelogram: A review of thirty-two cases. *J Bone Joint Surg Am* 1987;69:218-224.

63. McNulty SE, Weiss J, Azad SS, Schaefer DM, Osterholm JL, Seltzer JL: The effect of the prone position on venous pressure and blood loss during lumbar laminectomy. *J Clin Anesth* 1992;4:220-225.

64. Nakai O, Ookawa A, Yamaura I: Long-term roentgenographic and functional changes in patients who were treated with wide fenestration for central lumbar stenosis. *J Bone Joint Surg Am* 1991;73:1184-1191.

65. Verbiest H: Results of surgical treatment of idiopathic developmental stenosis of the lumbar vertebral canal: A review of twenty-seven years' experience. *J Bone Joint Surg Br* 1977;59:181-188.

66. Herron LD, Mangelsdorf C: Lumbar spinal stenosis: Results of surgical treatment. *J Spinal Disord* 1991;4:26-33.

67. Katz JN, Lipson SJ, Larson MG, McInnes JM, Fossel AH, Liang MH: The outcome of decompressive laminectomy for degenerative lumbar stenosis. *J Bone Joint Surg Am* 1991;73:809-816.

68. Katz JN, Lipson SJ, Lew RA, et al: Lumbar laminectomy alone or with instrumented or noninstrumented arthrodesis in degenerative lumbar spinal stenosis: Patient selection, costs, and surgical outcomes. *Spine* 1997;22: 1123-1131.

69. Thalgott JS, Cotler HB, Sasso RC, LaRocca H, Gardner V: Postoperative infections in spinal implants: Classification and analysis. A multicenter study. *Spine* 1991;16:981-984.

70. Jonsson B, Annertz M, Sjoberg C, Stromqvist B: A prospective and consecutive study of surgically treated lumbar spinal stenosis: Part I. Clinical features related to radiographic findings. *Spine* 1997;22:2932-2937.

71. Aryanpur J, Ducker T: Multilevel lumbar laminotomies: An alternative to laminectomy in the treatment of lumbar stenosis. *Neurosurgery* 1990;26:429-433.

72. Postacchini F, Cinotti G, Perugia D, Gumina S: The surgical treatment of central lumbar stenosis: Multiple laminotomy compared with total laminectomy. *J Bone Joint Surg Br* 1993;75: 386-392.

73. Chen Q, Baba H, Kamitani K, Furusawa N, Imura S: Postoperative bone re-growth in lumbar spinal stenosis: A multivariate analysis of 48 patients. *Spine* 1994;19:2144-2149.

74. Hopp E, Tsou PM: Postdecompression lumbar instability. *Clin Orthop* 1988;227:143-151.

75. Deyo RA, Ciol MA, Cherkin DC, Loeser JD, Bigos SJ: Lumbar spinal fusion: A cohort study of complications, reoperations, and resource use in the Medicare population. *Spine* 1993;18:1463-1470.

76. Lombardi JS, Wiltse LL, Reynolds J, Widell EH, Spencer C III: Treatment of degenerative spondylolisthesis. *Spine* 1985;10:821-827.

77. Herron LD, Trippi AC: L4-5 degenerative spondylolisthesis: The results of treatment by decompressive laminectomy without fusion. *Spine* 1989;14:534-538.

78. Fitzgerald JA, Newman PH: Degenerative spondylolisthesis. *J Bone Joint Surg Br* 1976;58:184-192.

79. Caputy AJ, Luessenhop AJ: Long-term evaluation of decompressive surgery for degenerative lumbar stenosis. *J Neurosurg* 1992;77:669-676.

80. Dall BE, Rowe DE: Degenerative spondylolisthesis: Its surgical management. *Spine* 1985;10:668-672.

81. Feffer HL, Wiesel SW, Cuckler JM, Rothman RH: Degenerative spondylolisthesis: To fuse or not to fuse. *Spine* 1985;10:287-289.

82. Katz JN, Lipson SJ, Chang LC, Levine SA, Fossel AH, Liang MH: Seven- to 10-year outcome of decompressive surgery for degenerative lumbar spinal stenosis. *Spine* 1996;21:92-98.

83. Lehmann TR, Spratt KF, Tozzi JE, et al: Long-term follow-up of lower lumbar fusion patients. *Spine* 1987;12:97-104.

84. Smith DW, Lawrence BD: Vascular complications of lumbar decompression laminectomy and foraminotomy: A unique case and review of the literature. *Spine* 1991;16:387-390.

85. Farfan HF, Kirkaldy-Willis WH: The present status of spinal fusion in the treatment of lumbar intervertebral joint disorders. *Clin Orthop* 1981;158:198-214.

86. Johnsson KE, Redlund-Johnell I, Uden A, Willner S: Preoperative and postoperative instability in lumbar spinal stenosis. *Spine* 1989;14:591-593.

87. Herkowitz HN, Kurz LT: Degenerative lumbar spondylolisthesis with spinal stenosis: A prospective study comparing decompression with decompression and intertransverse process arthrodesis. *J Bone Joint Surg Am* 1991;73:802-808.

88. Zielke K, Strempel AV: Posterior lateral distraction spondylodesis using the two-fold sacral bar. *Clin Orthop* 1986;203:151-158.

89. Roy-Camille R, Saillant G, Mazel C: Internal fixation of the lumbar spine with pedicle screw plating. *Clin Orthop* 1986;203:7-17.

90. Montgomery DM, Fischgrund JS: Passive reduction of spondylolisthesis on the operating room table: A prospective study. *J Spinal Disord* 1994;7:167-172.

91. Nash CL Jr, Moe JH: A study of vertebral rotation. *J Bone Joint Surg Am* 1969;51:223-229.

92. Abitbol JJ, Dowling TJ, Benz RJ, Kostuik JP: Adult scoliosis, in Herkowitz HN, Garfin SR, Balderston RA, Eismont FJ, Bell GR, Wiesel SW (eds): *Rothman-Simeone: The Spine,* ed 4. Philadelphia, PA, WB Saunders, 1999, pp 809-834.

93. Garfin SR, Rydevik BL, Lipson SJ, et al: Spinal stenosis, in Rothman RH, Simeone FA (eds): *The Spine,* ed 3. Philadelphia, PA, WB Saunders, 1992, pp 791-857.

94. White AH, Wiltse LL: Postoperative spondylolisthesis, in Weinstein PR, Ehni G, Wilson CB (eds): *Lumbar Spondylolysis: Diagnosis, Management, and Surgical Treatment.* Chicago, IL, Year Book Medical Publishers, 1977, pp 184-194.

95. Boden SD, Martin C, Rudolph R, Kirkpatrick JS, Moeini SM, Hutton WC: Increase of motion between lumbar vertebrae after excision of the capsule and cartilage of the facets: A cadaver study. *J Bone Joint Surg Am* 1994;76:1847-1853.

96. Hazlett JW, Kinnard P: Lumbar apophyseal process excision and spinal instability. *Spine* 1982;7:171-176.

97. Grobler LJ, Robertson PA, Novotny JE, Ahern JW: Decompression for degenerative spondylolisthesis and spinal stenosis at L4-5: The effects on facet joint morphology. *Spine* 1993;18:1475-1482.

98. DePalma AF, Rothman RH: The nature of pseudarthrosis. *Clin Orthop* 1968;59:113-118.

99. Garfin SR, Herkowitz HN: Surgical management of spinal stenosis: Part II. Indications and surgical results of arthrodesis following spinal stenosis decompression, in Herkowitz HN, Garfin SR, Balderston RA, Eismont FJ, Bell GR, Wiesel SW (eds): *Rothman-Simeone: The Spine,* ed 4. Philadelphia, PA, WB Saunders, 1999, p 806M.

100. Fischgrund JS, Mackay M, Herkowitz HN, Brower R, Montgomery DM, Kurz LT: Degenerative lumbar spondylolisthesis with spinal stenosis: A prospective, randomized study comparing decompressive laminectomy and arthrodesis with and without spinal instrumentation. *Spine* 1997;22:2807-2812.

101. Bridwell KH, Sedgewick TA, O'Brien MF, Lenke LG, Baldus C: The role of fusion and instrumentation in the treatment of degenerative spondylolisthesis with spinal stenosis. *J Spinal Disord* 1993;6:461-472.

102. Postacchini F, Cinotti G: Bone regrowth after surgical decompression for lumbar spinal stenosis. *J Bone Joint Surg Br* 1992;74:862-869.

103. Truumees E, Fischgrund J, Herkowitz HN: Management of spinal stenosis adjacent to a previously treated segment. *Semin Spine Surg* 1999;11:282-291.

SECTION

4

Hip: Adult Reconstruction—Osteolysis and Osteotomy

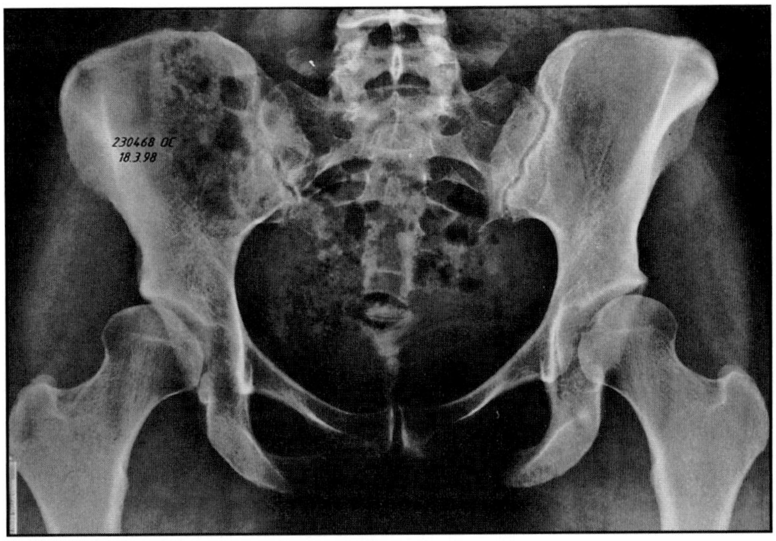

17 Bearing Surfaces in Total Hip Replacements: State of the Art and Future Developments

18 Cross-Linked Polyethylene: Why the Enthusiasm?

19 The Basic Science of Periprosthetic Osteolysis

20 Osteolysis of the Femur: Principles of Management

21 ***Symposium***
Basic Science of Bone Impaction Grafting

22 ***Symposium***
Acetabular Reconstruction With Bone Impaction Grafting: 20 Years of Experience ***(with video clip on enclosed CD)***

23 Rationale of Periacetabular Osteotomy and Background Work

24 Periacetabular Osteotomy: The Bernese Experience

25 Trochanteric Slide Osteotomy: Biomechanical Considerations

26 Osteotomies Around the Hip: Radiographic Planning and Postoperative Evaluation

17

Bearing Surfaces in Total Hip Replacements: State of the Art and Future Developments

Harry A. McKellop, PhD

Mechanisms, Damage, and Modes of Wear

To understand and compare the wear performance of bearing materials, it is convenient to define some key terms relating to the tribology of artificial joints. For joint replacements, it is most meaningful to define wear as the removal of material from the bearing surfaces in the form of wear particles, because the intensity of the biologic reaction is a function of the rate of release of this debris. This definition distinguishes wear from damage, which, as it is used in the orthopaedic literature, typically refers to visible changes in the surface of the bearings (polishing, scratching, etc)[1,2] that may or may not be accompanied by actual wear (Fig. 1).

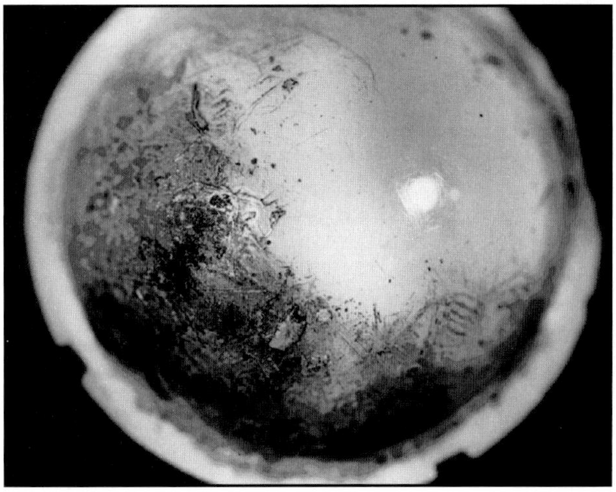

Fig. 1 Polyethylene acetabular cup worn in vivo (stained with ink to emphasize the morphology), showing highly polished area corresponding to high wear but low visible damage and damaged area (scratches, pits, and so forth) corresponding to low wear.

Wear is caused by fundamental mechanisms that include adhesion, abrasion, and fatigue.[3] Adhesive wear occurs if the bond strength of micro contacts, for example, between the polyethylene of the cup and the metal of the ball, exceeds the inherent strength of either material. Typically, polyethylene is pulled from the surface, forming fibrils and/or small pits. When adhesive wear occurs on a micron or submicron scale, the bearing surface still can appear highly polished to the eye.[4-7] Nevertheless, the billions of wear particles that are released into the tissues annually[6,8] are the driving force behind progressive osteolysis.[9-13]

Abrasive wear occurs when a hard projection on one surface cuts a scratch on the opposing surface during sliding. These projections can include the edge of an existing scratch, protruding carbides, embedded third-body particles, or even original contaminants that were exposed by the wear process itself. As with adhesive wear, abrasive scratching may be visible to the eye or, if it occurs on a microscopic scale, the surfaces may appear very smooth (undamaged), even though substantial wear has occurred. This wear is analogous to sanding a piece of wood with very fine sandpaper. The wood appears progressively smoother precisely because of the substantial amount of abrasive wear occurring. Fatigue wear is cracking, pitting, and/or delamination that is caused by cyclic stresses applied to the bearing surface. Again, this wear can occur on a micron scale, being nearly invisible to the eye, or on a millimeter scale, resulting in visible damage to the implant. Corrosion of a metal component and oxidation of a polyethylene component are not wear mechanisms per se, but they can substantially lower the wear resistance of the material.

Any number of these wear mechanisms may operate while the prosthesis is functioning in one of the following four distinct wear modes.[3,6] Mode 1 corresponds to articulation between two bearing surfaces only, which is necessary

The author or the departments with which he is affiliated have received something of value from a commercial or other party related directly or indirectly to the subject of this chapter.

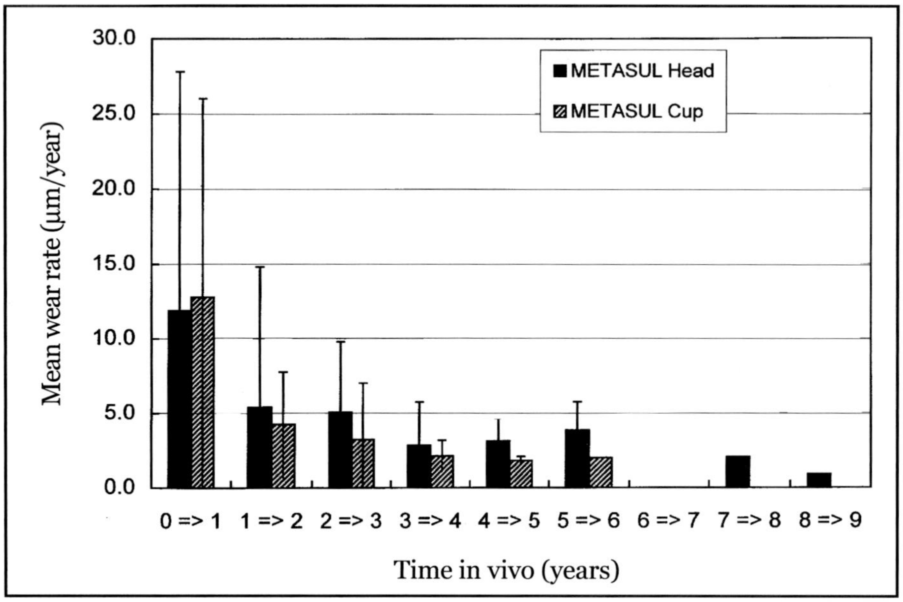

Fig. 2 Wear rate for retrieved, second-generation metal-metal hip prostheses. The decrease in wear rate after the initial wear-in phase has also been observed in hip simulator studies of metal-metal bearings. (Reproduced with permission from Rieker C, Kottig P, Schon R, Windler M, Wyss U: Clinical tribological performance of 144 metal-on-metal hip articulations, in Rieker C, Windler M, Wyss U (eds): *METASUL: A Metal-On-Metal Bearing.* Bern, Switzerland, Hans Huber, 1999, pp 83-91.)

for the prosthesis to function. Mode 2 corresponds to articulation between a bearing surface and a nonbearing surface; for example, if the femoral ball penetrates the polyethylene liner (after excessive mode 1 wear) and contacts the metal backing. Mode 3 wear corresponds to motion between two bearing surfaces, but with third-body abrasive contaminants present. Mode 4 wear corresponds to motion between two nonbearing surfaces, such as backside wear between the inside of a metal acetabular shell and the outside of the polyethylene liner or fretting of the Morse taper junction between the ball and the stem. Porous-coated prostheses that tend to shed particles are particularly susceptible to mode 3 wear, and the loaded interfaces between the components of a modular prosthesis provide additional opportunities for mode 4 wear. Furthermore, the debris produced in mode 4 may induce local osteolysis or it can migrate to the bearing surfaces, initiating mode 3 wear. Bearing surfaces for prosthetic joints should have high wear resistance under ideal conditions (mode 1) and adverse conditions (modes 2, 3, and 4).

Metal-on-Metal Bearings

The first widely used total hip replacements featured cobalt-chromium alloy bearing against itself, primarily the McKee-Farrar (Howmedica, Limerick, Ireland) design,[14] along with the Mueller (Sulzer AG, Winterthur, Switzerland), Ring (Downs, Ltd, Mitchham, England) and others.[15-18] Because of a relatively high rate of early failure, the first-generation metal-on-metal hips were largely supplanted by the Charnley prosthesis, which featured a stainless steel ball and a polyethylene socket.[19] However, in hindsight, it has become apparent that a large percentage of the early failures of the McKee-Farrar hips comprised implants from a single supplier and involved relatively thin acetabular shells and a small ball-cup clearance, possibly leading to distortion of the cups under physiologic loading, jamming, excessively high frictional torque, and rapid wear. Disregarding the early failures, the long-term survivorship of the early metal-on-metal designs has been comparable to that of the metal-on-polyethylene Charnley.[15,16,23,24] In particular, the steady-state wear rates have been on the order of a few micrometers per year[17,25,26] compared with the average of 100 to 200 µm of polyethylene wear per year typically reported for metal-on-polyethylene hips.[27-32]

In view of the growing awareness of the problem of extensive osteolysis caused by polyethylene wear debris, a number of second-generation metal-on-metal implants have been developed, including conventional total hips and surface replacements.[33-35] The first to be widely used clinically was the Metasul (Sulzer AG, Winterthur, Switzerland) hip,[16,36-38] which recently received United States Food and Drug Administration (FDA) approval for use in the United States. Hip simulator studies[39-42] and clinical retrievals[37,43,44] of modern metal-on-metal bearings also typically have shown steady-state wear rates on the order of a few micrometers per million cycles (with one million cycles being the equivalent of about 1 year's use in a patient of average activity[45]). It is also apparent that metal-on-metal implants have the ability to self-heal, that is, to polish-out isolated surface scratches caused by third-body particles or subluxation damage.[26,46] The overall clinical performance of second-generation metal-on-metal hips to date has been comparable to that of conventional metal-on-polyethylene hips and somewhat better than that of first-generation metal-on-metal hips.[37,47]

Clinical and laboratory wear studies have indicated that metal-on-metal implants often exhibit 10 to 20 times greater wear-in during the initial 1 to 2 years of clinical use (Fig. 2), or one to two million cycles in a hip simulator[37,39-41,43] In addition, some first-generation and second-generation metal-on-metal hips have exhibited extensive surface micropitting, possibly due to a fatigue-corrosion mechanism associated with the smaller carbides.[43,46,48] Although the high wear-in rate is a transitory phenomenon, and the presence of the micropits does not appear to be associated with a high wear rate,[43] they represent areas for potential improvement of metal-on-metal implants.

Table 1
Physical properties of alumina and zirconia[85]

Property	Alumina Sintered in air	Alumina Hipped	Zirconia (Y-TZP)
Grain size (μm)	3	1.8	< 0.5
Density (g/cm³)	≥ 3.96	≥ 3.98	> 6.00
Modulus (GPa)	380	380	210
Bending strength (Mpa)	> 500	> 500	> 950
Fracture toughness (MPa m$^{1/2}$)	4	4	8

Ceramic-on-Ceramic Implants

Alumina-on-Alumina Bearings

As with metal-on-metal bearings, the earliest designs of alumina-on-alumina hip bearings often experienced unacceptably high wear rates.[49-55] The United States' experience with ceramic-on-ceramic primarily involved the Autophor/Xenophor prostheses (Osteo, Selzach, Switzerland), which were first developed and used in Europe by Mittelmeier and Heisel.[50] The clinical results with the Autophor were subject to greater problems of pain, neck-socket impingement, ceramic fracture, and component loosening than for contemporary metal-on-polyethylene designs, and ceramic-on-ceramic implants were never widely used in the United States.[52,56] The causes of high wear included poor quality ceramic (by today's standards), edge contact of the cup on the ball due to inadequate range of motion and/or vertical cup placement, and other design shortcomings. For example, hips with a lateral opening smaller than 30° or larger than 55° and/or a high neck shaft angle (larger than about 140°) were at greater risk for neck socket impingement and/or high wear as a result of increased contact stress.[57]

Fortunately, the past two decades have seen substantial improvement in prosthesis design, implantation technique, and, most importantly, the quality of the alumina.[53,57-59] Changes in the latter have included higher purity, finer grain structure, and improved sintering techniques. Hip simulator studies and clinical retrievals have indicated that the steady-state wear rate of alumina-on-alumina bearings can be as low as 1 to 2 μm/yr.[60-64]

Modern alumina-on-alumina bearings are not, however, immune to high wear.[65-67] For example, in one study severe wear and osteolysis were reported in 22% of the patients after an average of only 7.7 years follow-up.[68] Although the causes of such unusually rapid wear in alumina-on-alumina bearings are a subject of continuing study,[57,69] these results emphasize the importance of observing proper surgical technique with ceramic-on-ceramic bearings.[53,58] For example, edge-chipping of ceramic balls or cups during insertion can be avoided by careful alignment of the components prior to assembly.[67,70]

Gross fracture of a ceramic bearing component in the patient is a catastrophic failure, and the surgeon performing the revision procedure can be faced with a difficult decision. If a new ceramic ball is placed on a damaged Morse taper, there is a much greater chance of fracture of the new ball.[71,72] On the other hand, if a metal ball is used in the revision, fragments of ceramic that are left in the tissues may subsequently become trapped between the ball and cup and initiate extremely rapid wear of the metal ball and massive metallosis. From the perspective of preventing wear, the safest option is to replace the femoral stem and use a new ceramic ball on a new taper; however, this can also be problematic if the stem is well fixed in the femur.

Fortunately, improvements in the quality of the alumina ceramic, particularly through hot isostatic pressing (Table 1), have led to a reduction in the rate of fracture to as low as one or two in 10,000 patients,[53,75,76] a risk that must be weighed against the potential benefits of very low wear and high biocompatibility of alumina-on-alumina bearings.

Ceramic-on-Ceramic Bearings Involving Zirconia

As the outside diameter of a femoral ball is reduced, for example, from 32 mm to 28 mm to 22 mm, the ball becomes progressively thinner adjacent to the Morse taper, and many surgeons are reluctant to use 22-mm diameter alumina balls. Due to its finer grain structure, yttria-stabilized zirconia ceramic (Y-TZP, where TZP refers to tetragonal zirconia polycrystals) is about 73% stronger than alumina (Table 1) and, therefore, provides a greater margin of safety, particularly with the smaller diameter balls.[77-79] For example, one survey reported only two fractures of zirconia balls out of 300,000 implanted.[80] However, at high temperatures in a wet environment, Y-TZP zirconia can undergo a phase transformation that substantially weakens the material and roughens the surface, degrading its wear properties.[81-83] Although zirconia is highly stable at physiologic temperature,[80,84] Y-TZP zirconia components should not be steam autoclaved.

To date, zirconia has been used primarily as a femoral ball articulating against an acetabular cup of polyethylene. The advisability of using Y-TZP zirconia balls against cups of alumina or zirconia is a subject of controversy. Laboratory studies using a washer-on-flat test configuration have reported severe wear of zirconia-on-zirconia and zirconia-on-alumina pairs,[85,86] possibly due to a temperature-induced degradation of the zirconia. In contrast, other investigators using a pin-on-disk machine[87] have observed very low wear of zirconia-on-alumina and zirconia-on-zirconia combinations. It seems likely that the differences in outcome of these studies were related to differences in the specimen configuration, the access of the lubricant to the bearing surfaces, and the type of lubricant used, resulting in substantial differences in the maximum temperatures generated. In particular, tests run in water gave severe wear of the zirconia, whereas tests run in serum did not. Thus, the clinical use of Y-TZP zirconia bearing against alumina or itself remains controversial, as do the optimal conditions for laboratory wear testing of ceramic-on-ceramic bearings.

Most recently, ceramics have been fabricated using a mixture of zirconia and alumina in various ratios. The resultant mixed-oxides materials appear to combine the high strength of zirconia with the thermal stability of alumina, and preliminary wear tests on a pin-on-disk machine and a hip joint simulator have indicated excellent wear resistance.[88-90] Although clinical trials have been underway in the United States for several years for alumina-on-alumina bearings, as yet, none of the ceramic-on-ceramic bearing combinations have received FDA approval.

Materials Bearing Against Polyethylene

Metal-on-Polyethylene Bearings

The metals used in conjunction with polyethylene principally have included stainless steel, cobalt-chromium alloy (in the vast majority), and titanium alloy. In some cases, the metal components have been surface hardened; for example, by nitriding or ion-implanting. In general, the wear rate of polyethylene against stainless steel has been comparable to that against cobalt-chrome alloy in laboratory tests[91,92] and in clinical use.[93-96] In contrast, although the wear rate of polyethylene against titanium alloy under clean conditions appears to be comparable to that with the other metals, the greater vulnerability of titanium alloy to abrasion by entrapped third-body particles can cause severe, runaway wear.[99-101] Hardening of the surface of the titanium alloy by techniques such as gas nitriding, solution nitriding, or ion implanting can markedly improve its resistance to abrasion by third-body particles, and good 10-year results have been reported for titanium nitride-hardened TiAlNb alloy balls used with polyethylene cups.[102] Nevertheless, if a hardened surface eventually is penetrated, severe wear of the underlying alloy still can be triggered.[101,103-105] Consequently, even hardened titanium alloys have seen limited clinical use as bearing surfaces.

The vast majority of metal-on-polyethylene bearings used in hip prostheses have involved cobalt-chrome alloy femoral balls, including cast or forged alloys, and the wear rate of this combination now forms the clinical baseline against which potentially improved bearing combinations are evaluated. As noted above, the *average* wear rate of the polyethylene against cobalt-chrome alloy is typically reported to be in the range of 0.1 to 0.2 mm/yr. However, it should be noted that this average includes those implants that have accelerated wear rates due to excessive third-body damage to the bearing surfaces, radiation-induced oxidative degradation of the polyethylene, or other causes.[30,105] Thus, the inherent wear rate of a polyethylene cup with a cobalt-chrome alloy ball under clean conditions (as are usually modeled in a hip simulator) is probably somewhat below the clinical average wear rate, possibly as low as 0.05 mm/yr.

Ion implanting and other surface hardening techniques also have been applied to cobalt-chromium alloy. Laboratory tests of hardened cobalt-chromium alloy have been reported to both markedly reduce wear and to increase wear of the opposing polyethylene,[105] and clinical results are not yet sufficient to resolve this contradiction. Whereas it seems likely that surface hardening of cobalt-chrome may improve its resistance to moderate amounts of third-body abrasion, the uncertainty of the advantage in general has limited its clinical application.

Ceramic-on-Polyethylene Bearings

Alumina and zirconia femoral balls have been used widely as bearing surfaces against polyethylene cups, and most clinical studies have shown substantially lower polyethylene wear rates than with metal balls, with the wear ratios ranging from 0.75 to as low as 0.25 with alumina balls.[53,105] A comparable advantage has been reported with zirconia against polyethylene.[106] However, in one recent radiographic study little difference was reported in the wear of polyethylene with alumina or metal balls,[96] as it was in one study of four retrieved alumina implants.[107] Unacceptably high rates of polyethylene wear, lysis, and loosening with an early type of zirconia ball were reported in another study.[82] Similarly, although the majority of the laboratory tests have indicated lower wear of polyethylene with alumina or zirconia than with metal,[105] in one hip simulator study slightly greater polyethylene wear was reported with alumina balls, but less with zirconia balls.[108]

Although the reasons for this disagreement among both clinical and laboratory studies are not clear, it may be due in part to the influence of third-body particles. That is, the greater hardness of ceramic balls renders them more resistant than metal balls to scratching by entrapped abrasive contaminants that can, in turn, accelerate the wear of the opposing polyethylene cup (wear mode 3). The differences in the relative wear rates in the various clinical studies might, therefore, reflect differences in the amount of third-body contamination, with those studies having relatively little such contamination showing comparable polyethylene wear rates for ceramic or metal balls (as in the laboratory tests run under clean conditions). Nevertheless, contamination by metal particles may be detrimental even with a ceramic ball, because the particles can adhere to the surface of the ceramic, effectively roughening it and, thereby, increasing abrasion of the polyethylene. Metal also can be transferred to the ceramic by contact against metallic components or instruments during surgery.[61] Regardless of the bearing material used, care must be taken to minimize the formation of abrasive contaminants in vivo, for example, by avoiding those porous coatings that are prone to shed particles.

Table 2
UHMWPE resins presently available[111]

Type	Supplier	Average Molecular Weight(10^6 g/mol)	Contains calcium stearate?
GUR 1150	Ticona*	5.5 to 6	Yes
GUR 1050	(Germany)	5.5 to 6	No
GUR 1120		3.5	Yes
GUR 1020		3.5	No
1900	Montell	4.4 to 4.9	No
1900 H	(USA)	> 4.9	No

*Ticona was formerly knows as Hoechst, and the Hoechst UHMWPEs produced in the USA prior to 1998 were GUR 4150/4050/4120/4020, with properties corresponding to the first four entries in the table, respectively

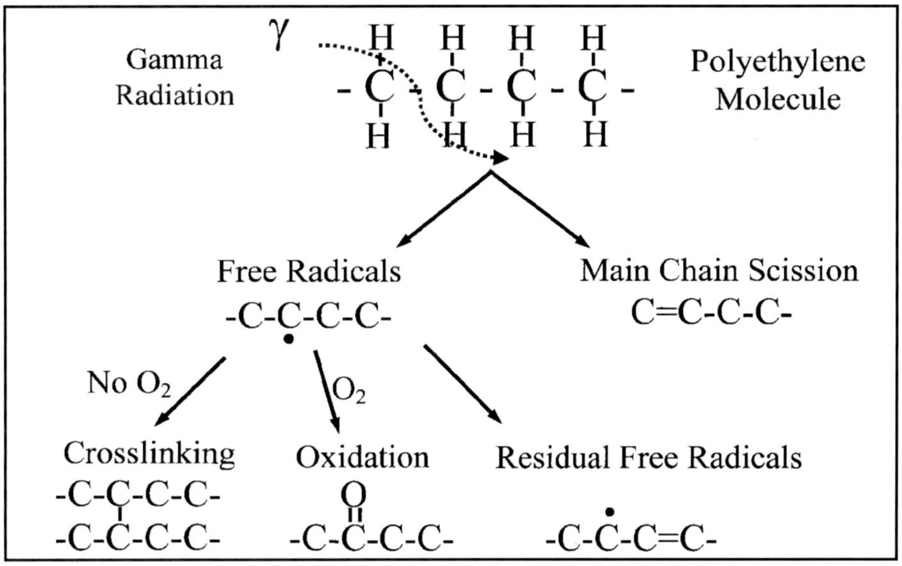

Fig. 3 Effect of radiation on the UHMWPE molecule. The radiation (gamma or electron-beam) causes chain scission and creates free radicals. In the absence of oxygen, the free radicals tend to form cross-links between adjacent molecules in the amorphous regions, improving wear resistance. Oxygen molecules present in the polyethylene, particularly near the surface, can combine with free radicals to cause chain scission, decreasing the strength, toughness, and wear resistance. Free radicals can remain trapped in the crystalline regions of the polyethylene for many years, eventually migrating to the amorphous regions and contributing to oxidative degradation. Free radicals can be neutralized very rapidly by heating above the "melt" temperature (crystalline-to-amorphous transition), or much more slowly by annealing below the melt temperature.

Improved Polyethylenes

Historic Polyethylenes and the Effects of Gamma-Air Sterilization

The ultra-high molecular weight polyethylenes (UHMWPEs) that were used for acetabular cups implanted during the past 30 years were fabricated from raw powder (also called resin) from a variety of manufacturers. Presently, there are just two suppliers[109-111] (Table 2). The powder is converted to solid form using one of three distinct methods. In the extrusion process, the polyethylene powder is driven by a ram through a heated nozzle, fusing the flakes into a continuous bar, typically several inches in diameter. The components are machined from the bar stock. In bulk compression molding, the powder is placed in a large mold and heated under pressure to fuse it into a block or sheet from which the final components are machined. In net-shape molding, the powder is placed in a metal mold having the desired shape of the implant and then fused under heat and pressure, such that little or no final machining is required.

The final step in any fabrication process was sterilization. Although ethylene oxide sterilization was used initially and gas plasma more recently,[112-114] the great majority of polyethylene components implanted during the past 25 years or more were sterilized by exposure to gamma radiation, with the dose

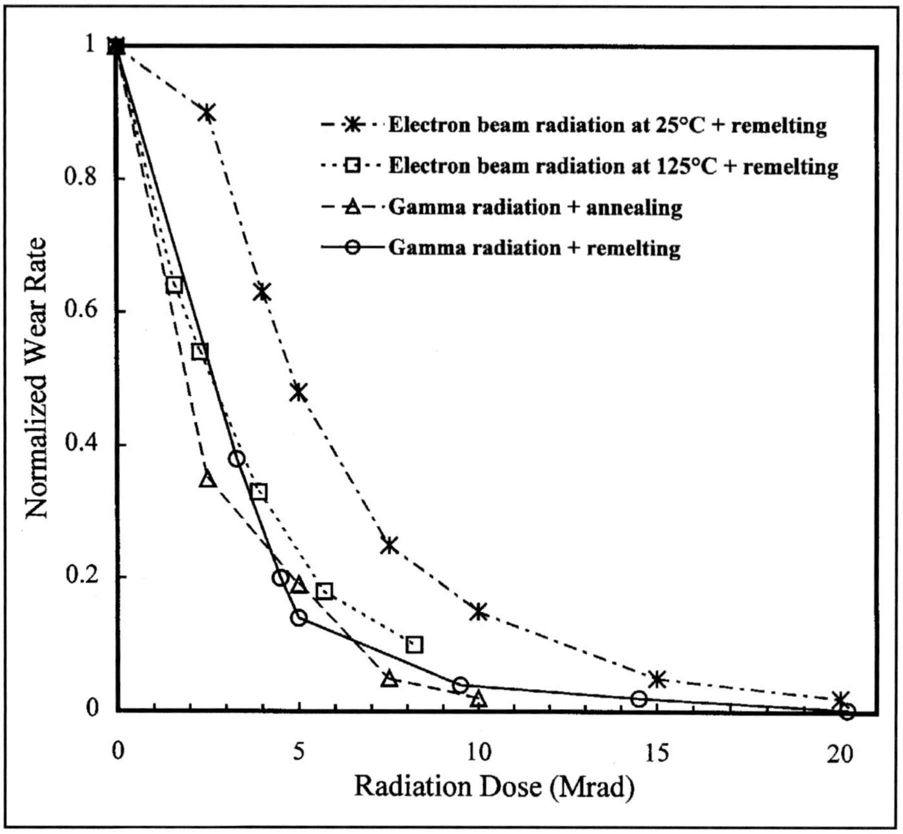

Fig. 4 Reduction in wear with increased level of cross-linking. The curves for the two gamma-radiation cross-linked polyethylenes were produced on hip joint simulators in two different laboratories.[118,119] The curves for the two electron-beam cross-linked polyethylenes were produced on a bidirectional pin-on-disk machine in a third laboratory.[120] Because two wear machines may produce different wear magnitudes for the same material due to differences in the applied load and/or the sliding distance per cycle, the original data were normalized by dividing by the wear rate for zero Mrad (no cross-linking) obtained in each test.

somewhere between 2.5 to 4 Mrads, and with the components sealed in air during irradiation and subsequent storage. Ethylene oxide and gas plasma sterilization have relatively little effect on the physical properties of polyethylene. In contrast, an extensive amount of research, particularly during the past 5 years, has shown that gamma sterilization in air, as well as extended storage in air, markedly affects the physical properties of UHMWPE components (Fig. 3). Near the surface of the component, free radicals generated by the radiation combine with oxygen that has diffused into the polymer during the period between fabrication and irradiation. Depending on how much oxygen is present, there could be immediate oxidative degradation and very little cross-linking of the surface layer. Beneath the level of diffused oxygen, free radicals generated by the radiation in the amorphous regions of the polyethylene rapidly combine to form cross-links. In contrast, free radicals generated in the crystalline regions are far less mobile but could eventually migrate to the amorphous regions and combine with any oxygen that had diffused to that level. This oxidative degradation of the polyethylene could continue for years during shelf-storage and, to a lesser extent,[115,116] during use in vivo. Oxidation leads to extensive chain-scission, weakening and embrittling the polyethylene, directly reducing its resistance to wear, delamination, and fracture. In addition, oxidation can indirectly reduce wear resistance by reducing the level of cross-linking.[117]

While, as discussed below, gamma-induced cross-linking can markedly improve the wear resistance of UHMWPE (Fig. 4), excessive cross-linking can adversely affect other physical properties such as ultimate strength, elongation, and fracture toughness.[118-121] However, studies of retrieved implants have demonstrated that weakening of the polyethylene due to immediate and long-term oxidation could be substantially greater than that due to the moderate level of cross-linking induced by the 2.5 to 4 Mrads used for routine sterilization.[115,122-127] Consequently, the alterations in the methods for fabricating and sterilizing UHMWPE components in the past few years have been directed at minimizing oxidative degradation while simultaneously optimizing the level of cross-linking to improve wear resistance.

Alternative Sterilization Techniques

In one approach to minimizing oxidative degradation, some manufacturers now sterilize the polyethylene components without irradiation, using either ethylene oxide or gas plasma.[111] Because these methods do not generate free radicals in the polyethylene, they completely avoid the potential for immediate and long-term oxidative degradation of the mechanical properties and wear resistance. However, because ethylene oxide or gas plasma do not induce cross-linking, they do not take advantage of its potential for improving the wear resistance of the polyethylene.

Other manufacturers continue to sterilize their implants with gamma radiation, but do so with the polyethylene components sealed in some type of low-oxygen atmosphere, including vacuum,[128] inert gas,[129] or with an oxygen scavenger.[130] In addition, one manufacturer anneals the polyethylene acetabular cups after sterilization by heating them in the nitrogen packaging at 37° to 50°C (well below the melt temperature of 135°C to avoid distorting the components) for about 6 days to reduce the level of residual free radicals that were induced by the gamma radiation.[131] These approaches can markedly reduce but not necessarily eliminate the oxidation that would otherwise occur during gamma sterilization and subsequent shelf-storage,[127,132] and the remaining free radicals may induce some oxidation during long-term use in vivo. Furthermore, because the level of cross-linking is determined by the 2.5- to 4-Mrad gamma radiation dose used to sterilize the components, the improvement in wear resistance (as exhibited in laboratory wear tests) relative to non-cross-linked polyethylene ranges from about 30% to 50%, compared to the 85% or more reduction achieved with elevated cross-linking doses.

In retrospective studies of shelf-stored and/or retrieved implants, some sets of components that were fabricated from block molded or net-shape molded polyethylene, gamma-sterilized, and stored in air have undergone substantially lower levels of oxidation than similarly treated extruded-machined components. It has been suggested that the molded polyethylene was more completely fused than typical extruded material, rendering it more resistant to diffusion of oxygen and, therefore, more resistant to immediate and long-term oxidative degradation, despite the presence of free radicals.[125,133] Consequently, several suppliers have reintroduced net-shape molding of components. Specialized molding techniques include hot-isostatic pressing of the polyethylene powder in an argon atmosphere[134] and special molding protocols that can provide polyethylene with a specified crystallinity and stiffness.[111,135] However, manufacturers no longer irradiate and store the polyethylene in air; therefore the marked differences in oxidation levels that occurred between molded and extruded-machined components in the past may not occur under current techniques of manufacturing and use. Furthermore, while molded polyethylene may have superior resistance to oxidation, this fabrication technique alone does not address cross-linking of the polyethylene to improve its wear resistance.

Clinical Studies of Polyethylenes With Elevated Levels of Cross-Linking

As noted above, the moderate level of cross-linking that was present in the vast majority of UHMWPE components implanted over the past three decades was an unintentional byproduct of the 2.5 to 4 Mrads of gamma radiation used to sterilize the components. Nevertheless, intentional cross-linking has long been used to improve the wear resistance of polyethylene in industrial applications; for example, as a lining for coal chutes. In addition, polyethylene acetabular cups that were intentionally cross-linked at levels much higher than occurs with routine sterilization were used in three clinical studies over the past 25 years. Grobbelaar and associates[136,137] cross-linked finished polyethylene acetabular cups by exposing them to 10 Mrads of gamma radiation. By irradiating the cups while immersed in acetylene gas, cross-linking in the outermost 300 μm was increased substantially above what would normally occur at 10 Mrads. No postirradiation thermal processing was done to reduce the residual free radicals. In anticipation of a lower wear rate, the cross-linked polyethylene was used with 30 mm diameter femoral balls to reduce the incidence of dislocation the investigators had experienced with 22-mm diameter heads. In a 14- to 21-year follow-up based on radiographs, Grobbelaar and associates[137]reported a "lack of measurable wear" in 56 of 64 cases, and only two revisions due to osteolysis.

Oonishi and associates[138] induced very high levels of cross-linking by exposing finished cups to 100 Mrads of gamma radiation, with the cups in air. As with Grobbelaar's method, there was no thermal treatment to extinguish free radicals. In a clinical follow-up from 6 to 8 years, Oonishi and associates[139]reported steady-state wear rates of 247 and 98 μm/yr for noncross-linked polyethylene cups bearing against cobalt-chrome and alumina heads, respectively, and 76 and 72 μm/yr for 100-Mrad cross-linked polyethylene cups bearing against stainless steel and alumina heads, respectively. Subsequently, Oonishi and associates[140] reported that against cobaltchrome heads, the long-term wear rates averaged 290 and 60 μm/yr for the noncross-linked cups and cross-linked cups, respectively. While this represented about a 79% reduction with cross-linking, the average wear rate for the noncross-linked cups in the study by Oonishi and associates[140] was substantially above the range of 100 to 200 μm/yr that typically has been reported for gamma-air sterilized polyethylene cups in clinical studies.[105]

More recently, Wroblewski and associates[141] chemically cross-linked polyethylene cups using a silane process. After an initial higher rate of penetration (possibly due to greater creep), the average steady-state wear rate in 19 patients with up to 8.3 years of follow-up was only 22 μm/yr for cross-linked cups bearing against alumina ceramic heads. While this rate was well below the clinical range for gamma-air cups, as with Oonishi's study, it was not clear how much of the advantage was due to head material rather than cross-linking. Nevertheless, the results of the three clinical studies were encouraging in that, despite any reduction in strength caused by the high levels of cross-linking, and despite the lack of thermal treatment to extinguish free radicals from the gamma-cross-linked materials,[137,138] none

Table 3
Comparison among new cross-linked thermally-stabilized polyethylenes

Name and Manufacturer	FDA Approved ? (June 2000)	Radiation Type and Dose	Thermal Stabilization	Final Sterilization	Manufacturer's Rationale
Marathon™ DePuy, Inc	Yes	Gamma radiation to 5 Mrads at room temperature	Remelted at 155°C for 24 hours	Gas plasma	5 Mrads gamma cross-linking provides about 85% wear reduction (well below the threshold for lysis) while preserving other mechanical properties. Remelting eliminates free radicals and prevents oxidative degradation.
XLPE™ Smith & Nephew-Richards, Inc	Yes	Gamma radiation to 5 Mrads at room temperature	Remelted at 150°C for two hours	Ethylene oxide	5 Mrads gamma to provide wear reduction (wear data not yet available), while preserving other mechanical properties. Remelting eliminates free radicals and prevents oxidation.
Longevity™ Zimmer, Inc	Yes	Electron beam radiation to 10 Mrads at room temperature	Remelted at 150°C for about two hours	Gas plasma	10 Mrads provides about 89% wear reduction. Remelting eliminates free radicals and prevents oxidation.
Durasul™ Sulzer, Inc	Yes	Electron beam radiation to 9.5 Mrads at 125°C	Remelted at 150°C for about two hours	Ethylene oxide	9.5 Mrads provides > 95% wear reduction. E-beam cross-linking at elevated temperature provides more wear reduction than E-beam at room temperature. Remelting eliminates free radicals and prevents oxidation.
Crossfire™ Stryker-Osteonics-Howmedica, Inc	Yes	Gamma radiation to 7.5 Mrads at room temperature	Annealed at about 120°C for a proprietary duration	Gamma at 2.5 to 3.5 Mrads while packaged in nitrogen	Depending on actual sterilization dose, total gamma cross-linking dose may vary from 10 to 11 Mrads, providing about 90% wear reduction. Annealing provides a different balance of material properties than remelting. Resultant material has substantial free radicals, but oxidation is limited by sterilization and storage in nitrogen.
Aeonian™ Kyocera, Inc	Approved in Japan; not yet in US	Gamma to 3.5 Mrads at room temperature	Annealed at 110°C for 10 hours	Gamma at 2.5 to 4 Mrads while packaged in nitrogen	Depending on actual sterilization dose, total gamma cross-linking dose may vary from 6 to 7.5 Mrads. Wear data not yet available. Annealing provides a different balance of material properties than remelting. Resultant material has substantial free radicals, but oxidation is limited by sterilization and storage in nitrogen.

(The processing parameters shown in this table were compiled from various publications and information provided by the manufacturers and are subject to modification.)

of the investigators reported fractures or other mechanical failures of their cross-linked cups.

Intentionally Cross-Linked, Thermally Stabilized Polyethylenes

Over the past few years, a number of laboratory wear simulations have demonstrated that the wear rate of UHMWPE cups decreases markedly with an increasing level of radiation-induced cross-linking.[118-120] Although the baseline wear rate differed among various wear machines due to systematic differences in the load, sliding distance per cycle, and other factors, the dose-wear curve was remarkably consistent among different laboratories and with different cross-linking techniques. The greatest reduction per Mrad occurred as the dose increased from zero to about 5 Mrads, with progres-sively less improvement at higher doses and no additional benefit after 15 to 20 Mrads (Fig. 4). While this dose-wear relationship was the basis for the recent development of a variety of intentionally-cross-linked polyethylenes, the developers have arrived at very different opinions regarding the appropriate dose and other processing parameters for optimizing the clinical performance of a polyethylene implant. The fabrication and characteristics of the new, intentionally-cross-linked polyethylenes are described in the following sections, and are summarized in Table 3.

Marathon Gamma Radiation-Cross-Linked and Remelted Polyethylene

In the Marathon (DePuy, Warsaw, IN) process,[119,142-144] extruded bars of UHMWPE are cross-linked by exposing them to 5 Mrads of gamma radiation. The bars are then heated to 155°C for 24 hours, followed by slow cooling to room temperature. When polyethylene is heated above the melt temperature, it is transformed from a partially crystalline solid to a totally amorphous solid. Because the uncombined free radicals that were generated during the gamma irradiation are trapped primarily in the crystalline regions,[145] heating above the melt temperature frees them to combine with each other, forming additional cross-links and, more importantly, minimizing the potential for long-term oxidative degradation.[119] The acetabular cup is then machined from the central portion of the cross-linked-remelted bar, thereby removing any surface-oxidized material, and is sterilized using gas plasma rather than gamma radiation to avoid increasing the level of cross-linking or reintroducing residual free radicals. In addition to reducing the wear under ideal, clean test conditions by about 85% (Fig. 4), Marathon has shown substantially less wear than noncross-linked polyethylene bearing against severely roughened femoral balls (that is, modeling third-body abrasive wear).[142] Comparable improved resistance to third-body abrasion has been demonstrated for two other cross-linked polyethylenes tested in hip simulators,[146,147] although greater wear of a cross-linked polyethylene was observed in one pin-on-plate test configuration.[148]

XLPE Gamma Radiation-Cross-Linked and Remelted Polyethylene

XLPE (Smith and Nephew Richards, Memphis, TN) is fabricated in much the same manner as Marathon, except that the final sterilization is done with ethylene oxide.[149]

Longevity Electron Beam-Cross-Linked and Remelted Polyethylene

In the Longevity (Zimmer, Warsaw, IN) process, compression molded sheets of UHMWPE are cross-linked by exposure to a 10-MeV electron beam.[150] After cross-linking, the polyethylene is heated above the melt temperature for about 2 hours to extinguish the free radicals and then machined into cups and sterilized with gas plasma.

Durasul Electron Beam-Cross-Linked and Remelted Polyethylene

The Durasul (Sulzer, Winterthur, Switzerland) process is similar to the Longevity process, with two exceptions. The polyethylene is machined into short segments or pucks that are cross-linked from both sides with a 10-MeV electron beam to a total of 9.5 Mrads, to increase the uniformity of the cross-linking. In addition, the pucks are preheated to about 125°C while being electron-beam cross-linked because comparative tests have indicated that this procedure provides greater wear resistance (Fig. 4) and less reduction in elongation to break and toughness than electron-beam cross-linking at room temperature.[151] For either process, because the electron beam drives the cross-linking energy into the polyethylene about 2,500 times faster than with gamma radiation (that is, in seconds rather than hours), which generates substantial heating of the polyethylene. After cross-linking, the Durasul cups are remelted to remove free radicals and sterilized with ethylene oxide.[152]

Crossfire Gamma-Cross-Linked and Annealed Polyethylene

In the Crossfire (Stryker-Howmedica Osteonics, Rutherford, NJ) process,[153] extruded bars of UHMWPE are cross-linked by exposure to 7.5 Mrads of gamma radiation. The bars are then annealed (rather than melted) by heating them to just below the melt temperature for a duration that is proprietary. Cups are then machined from the bars, sealed in nitrogen, and sterilized by exposure to an additional 2.5 to 3.5 Mrads of gamma radiation (that is, to a total gamma dose of 10 to 11 Mrads). No thermal treatment to extinguish free radicals is applied after the final gamma sterilization.

The developers of the Crossfire process prefer annealing to remelting of the polyethylene on the grounds that it induces less change in material morphology and material properties than does remelting.[153] However, as noted above, melting is used in the molding or extruding processes to fuse the UHMWPE powder into a solid form. Thus, it is not clear that remelting has a deleterious effect on the properties of the polymer. In addition, because crystalline regions remain in the polyethylene unless it is heated above the melt temperature, annealing is not as effective as remelting in extinguishing the residual free radicals. Consequently, Crossfire polyethylene that was artificially aged by being heated to 80°C in air for 3 weeks underwent substantial oxidative degradation of its strength and wear resistance.[154] In contrast, artificial aging has negligible effect on radiation-cross-linked polyethylenes that have been remelted to extinguish the residual free radicals[154,155] As with other current gamma-sterilized polyethylenes, however, the manufacturer of Crossfire implants recommends that they be shelf-stored in the nitrogen-filled package, and for only a limited duration prior to implantation. In view of this, the developers argue that any oxidative degradation of Crossfire implants will be far less than historically occurred with polyethylene components that were irradiated and stored in air, or for artificially aged implants, such that the residual free radicals will have negligible effect on the clinical performance of the implants.[153] Careful clinical follow-up will be required to resolve these issues.

Aeonian Gamma-Cross-Linked and Annealed Polyethyene

Except for the use of a lower range of cross-linking dose (Table 3), the rationale and processing of Aenoian (Kyocera, San Diego, CA) parallels that for Crossfire.

Optimum Method for Cross-Linking

The optimum amount of cross-linking to use is also a subject of current debate. Because increasing the level of cross-linking causes a progressively greater reduction in some mechanical properties, such as ultimate strength, ductility, fracture toughness, and fatigue strength,[119,121,144] one extreme is to avoid cross-linking altogether (for example, by simply sterilizing with ethylene oxide or gas plasma). This avoidance is to retain the maximum values of strength, elongation, and fracture toughness, despite the fact that it results in substantially higher wear of the polyethylene.

Among those who advocate cross-linking, the particular dose used represents that manufacturer's approach to balancing reduced wear against the need to maintain other mechanical properties well above that needed for acceptable clinical performance. Those using the high levels of cross-linking (9.5 to 11 Mrads, Table 3), about 3 to 4 times the typical dose used historically to sterilize polyethylene components, maintain that these high levels are justified to obtain the additional 5% to 10% improvement in wear over that provided by a moderate dose (Fig. 4), despite the corresponding reduction in other physical properties. In contrast, advocates of a moderate cross-linking dose, such as 5 Mrads (Table 3), maintain that the corresponding reduction in wear to 85% below that of a noncross-linked polyethylene, if realized clinically, will be sufficient to avoid an osteolytic reaction in even the most active patients, without unnecessarily reducing other physical properties.

Clearly, it is not desirable to use a dose that will result in mechanical failure of the polyethylene components. However, it is important to recall several facts when considering the likelihood of failure of a cross-linked cup in vivo: (1) the vast majority of polyethylene cups implanted in the past were moderately cross-linked at gamma doses ranging from 2.5 to 4 Mrads; (2) irradiation was done in air and without the benefit of postirradiation thermal treatment, such that many of these cups were subject to immediate and long-term oxidative degradation; and (3) this poststerilization oxidative degradation caused a much greater loss in strength than the moderate level of cross-linking that was induced by the gamma sterilization.[126,133] Despite their being moderately cross-linked, very few cups used in the past 20 to 30 years fractured in vivo and, when fracture did occur, it was strongly associated with oxidative degradation of the polymer.[156] It is reasonable, therefore, to predict that an acetabular cup that is moderately cross-linked and adequately stabilized against oxidative degradation will be less likely to fracture than the gamma-air sterilized and oxidized cups that have been the clinical standard for the past three decades.

On the other hand, there is questionable justification for increasing the level of cross-linking substantially above that which is necessary to reduce the wear below the threshold for clinically significant lysis.[157] For example, in a 7-year minimum follow-up, Xenos and associates[158] and others[159] reported that, after 4 to 7.2 years, those patients without lysis averaged a total radiographic wear depth of only 0.8 mm, while patients with lysis averaged 1.2 mm. Consistent with this, Nashed and associates[160] reported no lysis in a group of patients with a hip prosthesis that averaged 0.1 mm/yr or less, 31% in a group averaging 0.13 mm/yr, 24% in a group averaging 0.17 mm/yr, and 87% in a group averaging 0.25 mm/yr. Wan and Dorr[161] found that osteolysis was more

Table 4
Overall advantages and disadvantages of current bearing choices

Bearing Combination	Potential Advantages	Potential Disadvantages
Alumina on alumina	Usually very low wear High biocompatability	Sometimes high wear Component fracture Higher cost Technique sensitive surgery
Cobalt-chrome on cobalt-chrome	Usually very low wear Can self-polish moderate surface scratches	Question of long-term local and systemic reactions to metal debris and/or ions
Hardened cobalt chrome on polyethylene	Some additional protection against third-body abrasion	Hardened layer can wear off Higher cost
Ceramic on polyethylene	Lower wear of polyethylene than with conventional metal-polyethylene Some additional protection against third-body abrasion	Component fracture Difficulty of revision (that is, if Morse taper is damaged) Higher cost
Polyethylene sterilized with ethylene oxide or gas plasma	No short- or long-term oxidation	No cross-linking so doesn't minimize polyethylene wear
Polyethylene sterilized with gamma in low-oxygen	Some cross-linking, some wear reduction	Polyethylene wear not minimized Residual free radicals (long-term oxidation?)
Cross-linked, thermally-stabilized polyethylene	Minimal polyethylene wear rate No short- or long-term oxidative degradation	Newest of low-wear bearing combinations, only early clinical results available Questions remain regarding optimum cross-linking level and optimum method for thermal stabilization (Table 3)

likely to be present in hips with polyethylene wear depths exceeding 0.2 mm/yr.

Together, these studies show that clinically significant osteolysis is very rare in patients with polyethylene acetabular cups wearing less than about 0.1 mm (100 μm) per year. As noted above, while the inherent wear rate of UHMWPE (absent substantial oxidative degradation) may fall in the range of 0.05 to 0.1 mm/yr in a patient with average activity, the most active patients walk three to four times the average,[45] which would be sufficient to increase the wear rate of conventional polyethylene to as much as 0.4 mm/yr, well into the range for clinical osteolysis. In contrast, the 85% reduction provided by 5 Mrads of cross-linking (Fig. 4) would reduce the wear rate in such active patients to 0.06 mm/yr or less, well below the threshold for lysis. Although increasing the dose as high as 10 Mrads provides some additional reduction in wear (Fig. 4), this also increases the risk of introducing new problems that were not encountered with the historic maximum of 4 Mrads used for routine sterilization of polyethylene components. Again, resolving these controversies will require close monitoring of the clinical performance of the new polyethylenes over the coming years.

Summary

Because the UHMWPE components fabricated by the historic process of gamma-sterilization in air are no longer marketed, a surgeon who wishes to continue performing joint replacement surgery must choose among the new polyethylenes, or he or she may choose a modern metal-metal or ceramic-ceramic bearing, each of which has its potential advantages and disadvantages (Table 4). Ultimately, it is the responsibility of the surgeon to assess the risk-benefit ratios of each of the new bearing combinations and make an informed and wise choice among them.

References

1. Rostoker W: The appearacnces of wear on poyethylene: A comparison of in vivo an in vitro wear surfaces. *J Biomed Mater Res* 1978;12:317-335.
2. Hood RW, Wright TM, Burstein AH: Retrieval analysis of total knee prostheses: A method and its application to 48 total condylar prostheses. *J Biomed Mater Res* 1983;17:829-842.
3. McKellop HA: Wear modes, mechanisms, damage, and debris: Separating cause from effect in the wear of total hip replacements, in Galante JO, Rosenberg AG, Callaghan JJ (eds): *Total Hip Revision Surgery.* New York, NY, Raven Press, 1995, pp 21-39.
4. Cooper JR, Dowson D, Fisher J: Macroscopic and microscopic wear mechanisms in ultra-high molecular weight polyethylene. *Wear* 1993;162:378-384.
5. Jasty M, Bragdon C, Jiranek W, Chandler H, Maloney W, Harris WH: Etiology of osteolysis around porous-coated cementless total hip arthroplasties. *Clin Orthop* 1994;308:111-126.
6. McKellop HA, Campbell P, Park SH, et al: The origin of submicron polyethylene wear debris in total hip arthroplasty. *Clin Orthop* 1995;311:3-20.
7. Wang A, Stark C, Dumbleton JH: Mechanistic and morphological origins of ultra-high molecular weight polyethylene wear debris in total joint replacement prostheses. *Proc Inst Mech Eng [H]* 1996;210:141-155.
8. Clarke IC, Kabo JM: Wear in total hip replacement, in Amstutz HC (ed): *Hip Arthroplasty.* New York, NY, Churchill Livingstone, 1991, pp 535-553.
9. Willert HG, Semlitsch M: Reactions of the articular capsule to wear products of artificial joint protheses. *J Biomed Mater Res* 1977;11:157-164.
10. Goldring SR, Jasty M, Roelke MS, Rourke CM, Bringhurst FR, Harris WH: Formation of a synovial-like membrane at the bone-cement interface: Its role in bone resorption and implant loosening after total hip replacement. *Arthritis Rheum* 1986;29:836-842.
11. Howie DW, Vernon-Roberts B, Oakeshott R, Manthey B: A rat model of resorption of bone at the cement-bone interface in the presence of polyethylene wear particles. *J Bone Joint Surg Am* 1988;70:257-263.
12. Schmalzried TP, Jasty M, Harris WH: Periprosthetic bone loss in total hip arthroplasty: Polyethylene wear debris and the concept of the effective joint space. *J Bone Joint Surg Am* 1992;74:849-863.
13. Amstutz HC, Campbell P, Kossovsky N, Clarke IC: Mechanism and clinical significance of wear-debris induced osteolysis. *Clin Orthop* 1992;276:7-18.
14. McKee GK, Watson-Farrar J: Replacement of arthritic hips by the McKee-Farrar prosthesis. *J Bone Joint Surg Br* 1966;48:245-259.
15. Amstutz HC, Grigoris P: Metal on metal bearings in hip arthroplasty. *Clin Orthop* 1996;329(suppl):11-34.
16. Schmidt M, Weber H, Schon R: Cobalt chromium molybdenum metal combination for modular hip prostheses. *Clin Orthop* 1996;329(suppl):35-47.
17. Willert HG, Buchhorn GH, Gobel D, et al: Wear behavior and histopathology of classic cemented metal on metal hip endoprostheses. *Clin Orthop* 1996;329(suppl):160-186.
18. Scott ML, Lemons JE: The wear characteristics of Sivash/SRN Co-Cr-Mo THA articulating surfaces, in Jacobs JJ, Craig TL (eds): *Alternative Bearing Surfaces in Total Joint Replacement.* West Conshohocken, PA, ASTM, 1998, pp 159-172.
19. Charnley J, Cupic Z: The nine and ten year results of the low-friction arthroplasty of the hip. *Clin Orthop* 1973;95:9-25.
20. Walker PS, Salvati E, Hotzler RK: The wear on removed McKee-Farrar total hip prostheses. *J Bone Joint Surg Am* 1974;56:92-100.
21. Semlitsch M, Streicher RM, Weber H: Long-term results with meta/metal pairings in artificial hip joints, in Buchhorn G, Willert HG (eds): *Technical Principles, Design, and Safety of Joint Implants.* Seattle, WA, Hogrefe & Huber, 1994, pp 62-67.
22. Poggie RA: A review of the effects of design, contact stress, and materials on the wear of metal-on-metal hip prostheses, in Jacobs JJ, Craig TL (eds): *Alternative Bearing Surfaces in Total Joint Replacement.* West Conshohocken, PA, ASTM, 1998, pp 47-54.
23. Jacobsson S-A, Djerf K, Wahlstrom O: A comparative study between McKee-Farrar and Charnley arthroplasty with long-term follow-up periods. *J Arthroplasty* 1990;5:9-14.
24. Schmalzried TP, Szuszczewicz ES, Akizuki KH, Petersen TD, Amstutz HC: Factors correlating with long term survival of McKee-Farrar total hip prostheses. *Clin Orthop* 1996;329(suppl)48-59.
25. Kothari M, Bartel DL, Booker JF: Surface geometry of retrieved McKee-Farrar total hip replacements. *Clin Orthop* 1996;329(suppl):141-147.
26. McKellop H Park, S-H, Chiesa R, et al: In vivo wear of three types of metal on metal hip prostheses during two decades of use. *Clin Orthop* 1996;329(suppl):128-140.
27. Griffith MJ, Seidenstein MK, Williams D, Charnley J: Socket wear in Charnley low friction arthroplasty of the hip. *Clin Orthop* 1978; 137:37-47.
28. Rimnac CM, Wilson PD Jr, Fuchs MD, Wright TM: Acetabular cup wear in total hip arthroplasty. *Orthop Clin North Am* 1988;19:631-636.
29. Shih CH, Lee PC, Chen JH, et al: Measurement of polyethylene wear in cementless total hip arthroplasty. *J Bone Joint Surg Br* 1997;79:361-365.
30. Schmalzried TP, Dorey FJ, McKellop H: The multifactorial nature of polyethylene wear in vivo. *J Bone Joint Surg Am* 1998;80:1234-1243.
31. Sochart DH: Relationship of acetabular wear to osteolysis and loosening in total hip arthroplasty. *Clin Orthop* 1999;363:135-150.

32. Yamaguchi M, Hashimoto Y, Akisue T, Bauer TW: Polyethylene wear vector in vivo: A three-dimensional analysis using retrieved acetabular components and radiographs. *J Orthop Res* 1999;17:695-702.

33. Wagner M, Wagner H: Preliminary results of uncemented metal on metal stemmed and resurfacing hip replacement arthroplasty. *Clin Orthop* 1996;329(suppl):78-88.

34. Schmalzried TP, Fowble VA, Ure KJ, Amstutz HC: Metal on metal surface replacement of the hip: Technique, fixation, and early results. *Clin Orthop* 1996;329(suppl):106-114.

35. McMinn D, Treacy R, Lin K, Pynsent P: Metal on metal surface replacement of the hip: Experience of the McMinn prosthesis. *Clin Orthop* 1996;329(suppl):89-98.

36. Rieker C, Windler M, Wyss U (eds): *METASUL: A Metal-On-Metal Bearing.* Bern, Switzerland, Hans Huber, 1999.

37. Weber BG: Experience with the Metasul total hip bearing system. *Clin Orthop* 1996;329(suppl):69-77.

38. Dorr LD, Hilton KR, Wan Z, Markovich GD, Bloebaum R: Modern metal on metal articulation for total hip replacements. *Clin Orthop* 1996;333:108-117.

39. Streicher RM, Semlitsch M, Schon R, Weber H, Rieker C: Metal-on-metal articulation for artificial hip joints: Laboratory study and clinical results. *Proc Inst Mech Eng [H]* 1996;210:223-232.

40. Medley JB, Chan FW, Krygier JJ, Bobyn JD: Comparison of alloys and designs in a hip simulator study of metal on metal implants. *Clin Orthop* 1996;329(suppl):148-159.

41. Chan FW, Bobyn JD, Medley JB, Krygier JJ, Tanzer M: Wear and lubrication of metal-on-metal hip implants. *Clin Orthop* 1999;369:10-24.

42. Rieker C, Weber H, Schon R, Windler M, Wyss U: Development of the METASUL articulations, in Rieker C, Windler M, Wyss U (eds): *METASUL: A Metal-On-Metal Bearing.* Bern, Switzerland, Hans Huber, 1999, pp 15-21.

43. Rieker C, Kottig P, Schon R, Windler M, Wyss U: Clinical tribological performance of 144 metal-on-metal hip articulations, in Rieker C, Windler M, Wyss U (eds): *METASUL: A Metal-On-Metal Bearing.* Bern, Switzerland, Hans Huber, 1999, pp 83-91.

44. Campbell P, McKellop H, Alim R, et al: Metal-on-metal hip replacements: Wear performance and cellular response to wear particles, in Disegi JA, Kennedy RL, Pilliar R (eds): *Cobalt-base Alloys for Biomedical Applications.* West Conshohocken, PA, ASTM, 1999, pp 193-209.

45. Schmalzried TP, Szuszczewicz ES, Northfield MR, et al: Quantitative assessment of walking activity after total hip or knee replacement. *J Bone Joint Surg Am* 1998;80:54-59.

46. Park S-H, McKellop H, Lu B, Chan F, Chiesa R: Wear morphology of metal-metal implants: Hip simulator tests compared with clinical retrievals, in Jacobs JJ, Craig TL (eds): *Alternative Bearing Surfaces in Total Joint Replacement.* West Conshohocken, PA, ASTM, 1998, pp 129-143.

47. Dorr LD, Wan Z, Longjohn DB, Dubois B, Murken R: Total hip arthroplasty with use of the Metasul metal-on-metal articulation: Four to seven-year results. *J Bone Joint Surg Am* 2000;82:789-798.

48. Walker PS (ed): Friction and wear of artificial joints, in *Human Joints and Their Artificial Replacements.* Springfield, IL, Charles C Thomas, 1977, pp 368-442.

49. Boutin P, Christel P, Dorlot JM, et al: The use of dense alumina-alumina ceramic combination in total hip replacement. *J Biomed Mater Res* 1988;22:1203-1232.

50. Mittelmeier H, Heisel J: Sixteen-years' experience with ceramic hip prostheses. *Clin Orthop* 1992;282:64-72.

51. Nizard RS, Sedel L, Christel P, Meunier A, Soudry M, Witvoet J: Ten-year survivorship of cemented ceramic-ceramic total hip prosthesis. *Clin Orthop* 1992;282:53-63.

52. Clarke IC: Role of ceramic implants: Design and clinical success with total hip prosthetic ceramic-to-ceramic bearings. *Clin Orthop* 1992;282:19-30.

53. Clarke IC, Willmann G: Structural ceramics in orthopedics, in Cameron HU (ed): *Bone Implant Interface.* St. Louis, MO, Mosby Year Book, 1994, pp 203-252.

54. Garcia-Cimbrelo E, Martinez-Sayanes JM, Minuesa A, Munuera L: Mittelmeier ceramic-ceramic prosthesis after 10 years. *J Arthroplasty* 1996;11:773-781.

55. Meunier A, Nizard R, Bizot P, Sedel L: Clinical results of alumina-on-alumina couple in total hip replacement, in Jacobs JJ, Craig TL (eds): *Alternative Bearing Surfaces in Total Joint Replacement.* West Conshohocken, PA, ASTM, 1998, pp 213-234.

56. Mahoney OM, Dimon JH III: Unsatisfactory results with a ceramic total hip prosthesis. *J Bone Joint Surg Am* 1990;72:663-671.

57. Walter A: On the material and the tribology of alumina-alumina couplings for hip joint prostheses. *Clin Orthop* 1992;282:31-46.

58. Richter HG, Willmann G, Weick K: Improving the reliability of the ceramic-on-ceramic wear couple in THR, in Jacobs JJ, Craig TL (eds): *Alternative Bearing Surfaces in Total Joint Replacement.* West Conshohocken, PA, ASTM, 1998, pp 173-185.

59. Ueno M, Amino H, Okimatu H, Oonishi H: Wear, friction, and mechanical investigation and development of alumina-to-alumina combination total hip joint in Imura S, Wada M, Omori H (eds): *Joint Arthroplasty.* Tokyo, Japan, Springer, 1999, pp 119-131.

60. Willmann G: Ceramics for total hip replacement: What a surgeon should know. *Orthopedics* 1998;21:173-177.

61. Willmann G, Brodbeck A, Effenberger H, et al: Investigation of 87 retrieved ceramic femoral heads, in Puhl W (ed): *Bioceramics in Orthopaedics: New Applications.* Stuttgart, Germany, Ferdinand Enke Verlag, 1998, pp 13-18.

62. Taylor SK: In-vitro wear performance of a contemporary alumina:alumina bearing couple under anatomically-relevant hip joint simulation, in Sedel S, Willmann G (eds): *Reliability and Long-term Results of Ceramics in Orthopaedics.* Stuttgart, Germany, Georg Thieme Verlag, 1999, pp 85-90.

63. Fisher J, Ingham E, Stone MH, et al: Wear and debris generation in artificial hip joints, in Sedel L, Willmann G (eds): *Reliability and Long-term Results of Ceramics in Orthopaedics.* Stuttgart, Germany, Georg Thieme Verlag, 1999, pp 78-81.

64. Oonishi H, Nishida M, Kawanabe K, et al: In-vitro wear of Al2O3/Al2O3 implant combination with over 10 million cycles duration. *Trans Orthop Res Soc* 1999;24:50.

65. Winter M, Griss P, Scheller G, Moser T: Ten- to 14-year results of a ceramic hip prosthesis. *Clin Orthop* 1992;282:73-80.

66. Nevelos JE, Fisher J, Ingham E, Doyle C, Nevelos AB: Examination of alumina ceramic components from Mittelmeier total hip arthroplasties. *Trans Orthop Res Soc* 1998;23:219.

67. Bergman NR, Young DA: The rationale, short-term outcome and early complications of a ceramic couple in total hip arthroplasty, in Sedel L, Willmann G (eds): *Reliability and Long-term Results of Ceramics in Orthopaedics.* Stuttgart, Germany, Georg Thieme Verlag, 1999, pp 52-56.

68. Yoon TR, Rowe SM, Jung ST, Seon KJ, Maloney WJ: Osteolysis in association with a total hip arthroplasty with ceramic bearing surfaces. *J Bone Joint Surg Am* 1998;80:1459-1468.

69. Boehler M, Knahr K, Plenk H Jr, Walter A, Salzer M, Schreiber V: Long-term results of uncemented alumina acetabular implants. *J Bone Joint Surg Br* 1994;76:53-59.

70. Fuchs GA: 2-4 year clinical results with a ceramic-on-ceramic articulation in a new modular THR-system, in Willmann G, Zweymuller K (eds): *Bioceramics in Hip Joint Replacement: Proceedings 5th International CeramTec Symposium,* Stuttgart. Germany, Georg Thieme, 2000, pp 39-46.

71. Allain J, Goutallier D, Voisin MC, Lemouel S: Failure of a stainless-steel femoral head of a revision total hip arthroplasty performed after a fracture of a ceramic femoral head: A case report. *J Bone Joint Surg Am* 1998;80:1355-1360.

72. Sedel L: Revision strategy for ceramic implant failures, in Sedel L, Willmann G (eds): *Reliability and Long-Term Results of Ceramics in Orthopaedics.* Stuttgart, Germany, Georg Thieme Verlag, 1999, pp 75-76.

73. Kempf I, Semlitsch M: Massive wear of a steel ball head by ceramic fragments in the polyethylene acetabular cup after revision of a total hip prosthesis with fractured ceramic ball. *Arch Orthop Trauma Surg* 1990;109:284-287.

74. Frohling M, Zichner L, Koch R: Revisionsstrategie bei der verwendung von keramikköpfen, in Sedel L, Willmann G (eds): *Reliability and Long-term Results of Ceramics in Orthopaedics.* Stuttgart, Germany, Georg Thieme Verlag, 1999, pp 72-74.

75. Fritsch EW, Gleitz M: Ceramic femoral head fractures in total hip arthroplasty. *Clin Orthop* 1996;328:129-136.

76. Piconi C, Labanti M, Magnani G, Caporale M, Maccauro G, Magliocchetti G: Analysis of a failed alumina THR ball head. *Biomaterials* 1999;20:1637-1646.

77. Christel P, Meunier A, Heller M, Torre JP, Peille CN: Mechanical properties and short-term in-vivo evaluation of yttrium-oxide-partially-stabilized zirconia. *J Biomed Mater Res* 1989;23:45-61.

78. Drouin JM, Cales B, Chevalier J, Fantozzi G: Fatigue behavior of zirconia hip joint heads: Experimental results and finite element analysis. *J Biomed Mater Res* 1997;34:149-155.

79. Cales B, Stefani Y: Yttria-stabilized zirconia for improved orthopaedic prostheses, in Wise DL, Trantolo DJ, Yaszemski MJ, Gresser JD, Schwartz ER (eds): *Encyclopedic Handbook of Biomaterials and Bioengineering Part B: Applications.* New York, NY, Marcel Dekker, 1995, pp 415-452.

80. Piconi C, Maccauro G: Zirconia as a ceramic biomaterial. *Biomaterials* 1999;20:1-25.

81. Birkby I, Harrison P, Stevens R: The effect of surface transformation on the wear behavior of zirconia TZP ceramics. *J European Ceramics Soc* 1989;5:37-45.

82. Piconi C, Burger W, Richter HG, et al: Y-TZP ceramics for artificial joint replacements. *Biomaterials* 1998;19:1489-1494.

83. Allain J, Le Mouel S, Goutallier D, Voison MC: Poor eight-year survival of cemented zirconia-polyethylene total hip replacements. *J Bone Joint Surg Br* 1999;81:835-842.

84. Cales B, Stefani Y, Lilley E: Long-term in vivo and in vitro aging of a zirconia ceramic used in orthopaedy. *J Biomed Mater Res* 1994;28:619-624.

85. Fruh HJ, Willmann G, Pfaff HG: Wear characteristics of ceramic-on-ceramic for hip endoprostheses. *Biomaterials* 1997;18:873-876.

86. Willmann G, Fruh HJ, Pfaff HG: Wear characteristics of sliding pairs of zirconia (Y-TZP) for hip endoprostheses. *Biomaterials* 1996;17:2157-2162.

87. Cales B, Chevalier J: Wear behavior of ceramic pairs compared on different testing configurations. in Jacobs JJ, Craig TL (eds): *Alternative Bearing Surfaces in Total Joint Replacement.* West Conshohocken, PA, ASTM, 1998, pp 186-196.

88. Affatato S, Testoni M, Cacciari GL, Toni A: Mixed-oxides prosthetic ceramic ball heads: Part 2. Effect of the ZrO2 fraction on the wear of ceramic on ceramic joints. *Biomaterials* 1999;20:1925-1929.

89. Affatato S, Testoni M, Cacciari GL, Toni A: Mixed oxides prosthetic ceramic ball heads: Part 1. Effect of the ZrO2 fraction on the wear of ceramic on polyethylene joints. *Biomaterials* 1999;20:971-975.

90. Kaddick C, Pfaff HG: Wear study in the alumina-zirconia system, in Sedel L, Willmann G (eds): *Reliability and Long-Term Results of Ceramics in Orthopaedics.* Stuttgart, Germany, Georg Thieme Verlag, 1999, pp 96-101.

91. McKellop H, Clarke I, Markolf K, Amstutz H: Friction and wear properties of polymer, metal, and ceramic prosthetic joint materials evaluated on a multichannel screening device. *J Biomed Mater Res* 1981;15:619-653.

92. Lancaster JG, Dowson D, Isaac GH, Fisher J: The wear of ultra-high molecular weight polyethylene sliding on metallic and ceramic counterfaces representative of current femoral surfaces in joint replacement. *Proc Inst Mech Eng [H]* 1997;211:17-24.

93. Bankston AB, Faris PM, Keating EM, Ritter MA: Polyethylene wear in total hip arthroplasty in patient-matched groups: A comparison of stainless steel, cobalt chrome, and titanium-bearing surfaces. *Arthroplasty* 1993;8:315-322.

94. Wroblewski BM: Wear of the high-density polyethylene socket in total hip arthroplasty and its role in endosteal cavitation. *Proc Inst Mech Eng [H]* 1997;211:109-118.

95. Furman BD, Lee CL, Block A, Lefebvre FK, Li S: A comparison of directly molded and machined retrieved acetabular cups of a single design. *Trans Orthop Res Soc* 1998;23:50.

96. Devane PA, Horne JG: Assessment of polyethylene wear in total hip replacement. *Clin Orthop* 1999;369:59-72.

97. McKellop HA, Sarmiento A, Schwinn CP, Ebramzadeh E: In vivo wear of titanium-alloy hip prostheses. *J Bone Joint Surg Am* 1990;72:512-517.

98. McKellop H, Rostlund T, Ebramzadeh E, Sarmiento A: Wear of titanium alloy in laboratory tests and in retrieved human joint replacements, in Brown SA, Lemons JE (eds): *Medical Applications of Titanium and Its Alloys: The Material and Biological Issues.* West Conshohocken, PA, ASTM, 1996, pp 266-293.

99. Agins HJ, Alcock NW, Bansal M, et al: Metallic wear in failed titanium-alloy total hip replacements: A histological and quantitative analysis. *J Bone Joint Surg Am* 1988;70:347-356.

100. Lombardi AV Jr, Mallory TH, Vaughn BK, Drouillard P: Aseptic loosening in total hip arthroplasty secondary to osteolysis induced by wear debris from titanium-alloy modular femoral heads. *J Bone Joint Surg Am* 1989;71:1337-1342.

101. McKellop HA, Rostlund TV: The wear behavior of ion-implanted Ti-6A1-4V against UHMW polyethylene. *J Biomed Mater Res* 1990;24:1413-1425.

102. Semlitsch M, Willert HG: Clinical wear behaviour of ultra-high molecular weight polyethylene cups paired with metal and ceramic ball heads in comparison to metal-on-metal pairings of hip joint replacements. *Proc Inst Mech Eng [H]* 1997;211:73-88.

103. Davidson JA, Poggie RA, Mishra AK: Abrasive wear of ceramic, metal, and UHMWPE bearing surfaces from third-body bone, PMMA bone cement, and titanium debris. *Biomed Mater Eng* 1994;4:213-229.

104. Mishra AK, Davidson JA, Poggie RA, Kovacs P, FitzGerald TJ: Mechanical and tribological properties and biocompatibility of diffusion hardened T-13Nb-13Zr: A new titanium alloy for surgical implants, in Brown SA, Lemons JE (eds): *Medical Applications of Titanium and Its Alloys: The Material and Biological Issue.* West Conshohocken, PA, ASTM, 1996, pp 96-112.

105. Sauer WL, Anthony ME: Predicting the clinical wear performance of orthopaedic bearing surfaces, in Jacobs JJ, Craig TL (eds): *Alternative Bearing Surfaces in Total Joint Replacement.* West Conshohocken, PA, ASTM, 1998, pp 1-29.

106. Willmann G: New generation ceramics, in Willmann G, Zweymüller K (eds): *Bioceramics in Hip Joint Replacement: Proceedings of the 5th International CeramTec Symposium.* Stuttgart, Germany, Georg Thieme, 2000, pp 127-135.

107. Bragdon CR, O'Connor DO, Lowenstein JD, et al: Comparison of volumetric wear using 22mm, 26mm and 32mm femoral heads using a new hip simulator. *Trans Orthop Res Soc* 1998;23:53.

108. McKellop H, Lu B, Benya P:Friction, lubrication and wear of cobalt-chromium, alumina and zirconia hip prostheses compared on a joint simulator. *Trans Orthop Res Soc* 1992;17:402.

109. Li S, Burstein AH: Ultra-high molecular weight polyethylene: The material and its use in total joint implants. *J Bone Joint Surg Am* 1994;76:1080-1090.

110. Lewis G: Polyethylene wear in total hip and knee arthroplasties. *J Biomed Mater Res* 1997;38:55-75.

111. Kurtz SM, Muratoglu OK, Evans M, Edidin AA: Advances in the processing, sterilization, and cross-linking of ultra-high molecular weight polyethylene for total joint arthroplasty. *Biomaterials* 1999;20:1659-1688.

112. Fisher J, Reeves EA, Isaac GH, Saumm KA, Sanford WM: Comparison of the wear of aged and non-aged ultrahigh molecular weight polyethylene sterilized by gamma irradiation and by gas plasma, in *Fifth World Biomaterials Congress: Programme and Transactions.* Toronto, Canada, University of Toronto Press, 1996, p 971.

113. Goldman M, Pruitt L: Comparison of the effects of gamma radiation and low temperature hydrogen peroxide gas plasma sterilization on the molecular structure, fatigue resistance, and wear behavior of UHMWPE. *J Biomed Mater Res* 1998;40:378-384.

114. McNulty DE, Hastings RS, Swope SW, Huston DE:Sterilization methods and artificial aging of UHMWPE resins: The relation between resilience and oxidation. *Trans Orthop Res Soc* 1999;24:821.

115. Sutula LC, Collier JP, Saum KA, et al: Impact of gamma sterilization on clinical performance of polyethylene in the hip. *Clin Orthop* 1995;319:28-40.

116. Furman BD, Reish T, Li S: The effect of implantation on the oxidation of ultra high molecular weight polyethylene, in Merchant RE (ed): *Transactions: Twenty-Third Annual Meeting of the Society for Biomaterials.* Minneapolis, MN, Society for Biomaterials, 1997, p 427.

117. Pienkowski D, Patel A, Lee KY, et al: Solubility changes in shelf-aged ultra-high molecular weight polyethylene acetabular liners. *J Long Term Eff Med Implants* 1999;9:273-288.

118. Wang A, Essner A, Polineni VK, Stark C, Dumbleton JH: Lubrication and wear of ultra-high molecular weight polyethylene in total joint replacements. *Tribology* 1998;31:17-33.

119. McKellop H, Shen FW, Lu B, Campbell P, Salovey R: Development of an extremely wear-resistant ultra high molecular weight polyethylene for total hip replacements. *J Orthop Res* 1999;17:157-167.

120. Muratoglu OK, Bragdon CR, O'Connor DO, et al: Unified wear model for highly cross-linked ultra-high molecular weight polyethylenes (UHMWPE). *Biomaterials* 1999;20:1463-1470.

121. Gillis AM, Schmieg JJ, Bhattacharyya S, Li S:An independent evaluation of the mechanical, chemical and fracture properties of UHMWPE cross-linked by 34 different conditions, in LaBerge M, Agrawal C, Mauli CM (eds): *Transactions: Twenty-Fifth Annual Meeting of the Society for Biomaterials.* Minneapolis, MN, Society of Biomaterial, 1999, p 216.

122. Roe RJ, Grood ES, Shastri R, Gosselin CA, Noyes FR: Effect of radiation sterilization and aging on ultrahigh molecular weight polyethylene. *J Biomed Mater Res* 1981;15:209-230.

123. Eyerer P, Ke YC: Property changes of UHMW polyethylene hip cup endoprostheses during implantation. *J Biomed Mater Res* 1984;18: 1137-1151.

124. Premnath V, Harris WH, Jasty M, Merrill EW: Gamma sterilization of UHMWPE articular implants: An analysis of the oxidation problem. Ultra high molecular weight poly ethylene. *Biomaterials* 1996;17:1741-1753.

125. Gillis AM, Furman BD, Li S: Influence of ultra high molecular weight polyethylene resin type and manufacturing method on real time oxidation. *Trans Orthop Res Soc* 1998;23:360.

126. Collier JP, Bargmann LS, Currier BH, Mayor MB, Currier JH, Bargmann BC: An analysis of Hylamer and polyethylene bearings from retrieved acetabular components. *Orthopedics* 1998;21:865-871.

127. Edidin A, Muth J, Spiegelberg S, Schaffner S: Sterilization of UHMWPE in nitrogen prevents oxidative degradation for more than ten years. *Trans Orthop Res Soc* 2000;25:1.

128. Greer KW, Schmidt MB, Hamilton JV: The hip simulator wear of gamma-vacuum, gamma-air, and ethylene oxide sterilized UHMWPE following a severe oxidative challenge. *Trans Orthop Res Soc* 1998;23:52.

129. Streicher RM: Influence of ionizing irradiation in air and nitrogen for sterilization of surgical grade polyethylene for implants. *Radiat Phys Chem* 1988;31:693-698.

130. Bapst JM, Valentine RH, Vasquez R: Wear simulation testing of direct compression molded UHMWPE irradiated in oxygenless packaging, in Merchant RE (ed): *Transactions: Twenty-Third Annual Meeting of the Society for Biomaterials.* Minneapolis, MN, Society for Biomaterials, 1997, p 72.

131. Sun DC, Wang A, Stark C, Dumbleton JH: The concept of stabilization in UHMWPE, in *Fifth World Biomaterials Congress: Programme and Transactions.* Toronto, Canada, University of Toronto Press, 1996, p 195.

132. McKellop H, Shen FW, Lu B, Campbell P, Salovey R: The effect of sterilization method and other modifications on the wear resistance of acetabular cups of ultra-high molecular weight polyethylene: A hip simulator study. *J Bone Joint Surg Am,* in press.

133. Currier BH, Currier JH, Collier JP, Mayor MB: Effect of fabrication method and resin type on performance of tibial bearings. *J Biomed Mater Res* 2000;53:143-51.

134. *"Arcom® Processed Polyethylene. A Technical Report."* Warsaw, IN, Biomet, 1996.

135. Walsh H, Gillis A, Furman B, Li S: Factors that determine the oxidation resistance of molded 1900: Is it the resin or the molding? *Trans Orthop Res Soc* 2000;25:543.

136. Grobbelaar CJ, du Plessis TA, Marais F: The radiation improvement of polyethylene prostheses: A preliminary study. *J Bone Joint Surg Br* 1978;60:370-374.

137. Grobbelaar CJ, Weber FA, Spirakis A, et al: Clinical experience with gamma irradiation-cross-linked polyethylene: A 14 to 20 year follow-up report. *SA Bone Joint & Joint Surg* 1999;9:140-147.

138. Oonishi H, Takayama Y, Tsuji E: Improvement of polyethylene by irradiation in artificial joints. *Radiat Phys Chem* 1992;39:495-504.

139. Oonishi H, Takayama Y, Tsuji E: The low wear of cross-linked polyethylene socket in total hip prostheses, in Wise DL, Trantolo DJ, Altobelli DE, Yaszemski MJ, Gresser JD, Schwartz ER (eds): *Encyclopedic Handbook of Biomaterials and Bioengineering: Part A. Materials.* New York, NY, Marcel Dekker, 1995, pp 1853-1868.

140. Oonishi H, Saito M, Kadoya Y: Wear of high-dose gamma irradiated polyethylene in total joint replacement: Long term radiological evaluation. *Trans Orthop Res Soc* 1998;23:97.

141. Wroblewski BM, Siney PD, Fleming PA: Low-friction arthroplasty of the hip using alumina ceramic and cross-linked polyethylene: A ten-year follow-up report. *J Bone Joint Surg Br* 1999;81:54-55.

142. McKellop H, Shen F-W, DiMaio W, Lancaster JG: Wear of gamma-cross-linked polyethylene acetabular cups against roughened femoral balls. *Clin Orthop* 1999;369:73-82.

143. DiMaio WG, Lilly WB, Moore WC, Saum KA: Low wear, low oxidation radiation cross-linked UHMWPE. *Trans Orthop Res Soc* 1998;23:363.

144. Hastings RS, Huston DE, Reber EW, DiMaio WG: Knee wear testing of a radiation cross-linked and remelted UHMWPE, in LaBerge M, Agrawal C, Mauli CM (eds): *Transactions: Twenty-Fifth Annual Meeting of the Society for Biomaterials.* Minneapolis, MN, Society for Biomaterials, 1999, p 328.

145. Bhateja SK, Duerst RW, Martens JA, Andrews EH: Radiation-induced enhancement of crystallinity in polymers. *J Macromol Sci-Revs Chem Phys* 1995;C35:581-659.

146. Essner A, Polineni VK, Wang A, Stark C, Dumbleton JH: Effect of femoral head surface roughness and cross-linking on the wear of UHMWPE acetabular cups, in Goodman SB (ed): *Transactions: Twenty-Fourth Annual Meeting of the Society for Biomaterials.* Minneapolis, MN, Society of Biomaterials, 1998, p 4.

147. Laurent MP, Yao JQ, Gilbertson LN, Swarts DF, Crowninshield RD: Wear of highly cross-linked UHMWPE acetabular liners under adverse conditions, in *Trans Sixth World Biomaterials Congress.* 2000, p 874.

148. Endo MM, Barbour PSM, Barton DC, et al: Comparative wear and debris generation of cross-linked and non-cross-linked ultrahigh molecular weight polyethylene under three different femoral counterface conditions, in *Trans Sixth World Biomaterials Congress.* 2000, p 836.

149. Greenwald AS, Ries MD, DuncanCP, Jacobs JJ, Stulberg BN: Abstract: New polys for old: Contribution or caveat? *67th Annual Meeting Proceedings.* Rosemont, IL, American Academy of Orthopaedic Surgeons, 2000, p 278.

150. Laurent MP, Yao JQ, Bhambri SK, et al: High cycle wear of highly cross-linked UHMWPE acetabular liners evaluated in a hip simulator. *Trans Orthop Res Soc* 2000;25:567.

151. Muratoglu OK, Bragdon CR, O'Connor DO, et al: The effect of temperature on radiation cross-linking of UHMWPE for use in total hip arthroplasty. *Trans Orthop Res Soc* 2000;25:547.

152. Muratoglu OK, Harris WH, Delaney J, et al: The development of an in vitro hip simulator model for fatigue failure: Application to conventional and highly cross-linked UHMWPE. *Trans Orthop Res Soc* 2000;25:548.

153. Manley MT, Capello WN, D'Antonio JA, Taylor SK, Wang A: Abstract: Reduction in wear in total hip replacement: Highly crosslinked polyethylene acetabular liners versus ceramic/ceramic bearings. *67th Annual Meeting Proceedings.* Rosemont, IL, American Academy of Orthopaedic Surgeons. 2000, p 275.

154. Muratoglu OK, Bragdon CR, O'Connor DO, et al: The comparison of the wear behavior of four different types of cross-linked acetabular components. *Trans Orthop Res Soc* 2000;25:566.

155. Streicher RM: Ionizing irradiation for sterilization and modification of high molecular weight polyethylenes. *Plastics and Rubber Processing and Applications* 1988;10:221-229.

156. Walsh HA, Furman BD, Naab S, Li S: Role of oxidation in the clinical fracture of acetabular cups. *Trans Orthop Res Soc* 1999;24:845.

157. McKellop HA: Wear assessment, in Callaghan JJ, Rosenberg AG, Rubash HE (eds): *The Adult Hip.* Philadelphia, PA, Lippincott-Raven, 1998, pp 231-246.

158. Xenos JS, Hopkinson WJ, Callaghan JJ, Heekin RD, Savory CG: Osteolysis around an uncemented cobalt chrome total hip arthroplasty. *Clin Orthop* 1995;317:29-36.

159. Devane PA, Bourne RB, Rorabeck CH, MacDonald S, Robinson EJ: Measurement of polyethylene wear in metal-backed acetabular cups II: Clinical application. *Clin Orthop* 1995;319:317-326.

160. Nashed RS, Becker DA, Gustilo RB: Are cementless acetabular components the cause of excess wear and osteolysis in total hip arthroplasty? *Clin Orthop* 1995;317:19-28.

161. Wan Z, Dorr LD: Natural history of femoral focal osteolysis with proximal ingrowth smooth stem implant. *J Arthroplasty* 1996;11:718-725.

18

Cross-Linked Polyethylene: Why the Enthusiasm?

William H. Harris, MD

Introduction

The remarkable interest in highly cross-linked polyethylene for use in total hip replacement (THR) surgery is driven by two compelling features of the current THR scene: (1) the pervasive, deleterious, adverse role of periprosthetic osteolysis on the intermediate and long-term results of THR surgery and (2) the dramatic improvement in wear resistance and oxidation resistance that selected new highly cross-linked polyethylenes display in hip simulator testing. In this chapter, each of these two driving forces will be examined.

Periprosthetic Osteolysis

Attention clearly has been focused on the scope of the osteolysis problem, not only in THR surgery, but also in other total joint surgery such as total knee, total elbow, and total shoulder replacement. Archibeck and associates (chapter 19) have described the molecular biology underlying the macrophage reaction to submicrometer particulate debris (primarily submicrometer polyethylene) and the resulting activation of osteoclasts, which leads to periprosthetic osteolysis.

That the impact of periprosthetic osteolysis is the leading motivation supporting the use of a highly cross-linked polyethylene for THR surgery is shown in two recent publications concerning widely used total hip implants. These articles describe the incidence of periprosthetic osteolysis at 10 years follow-up after their implantation. Because this type of lysis is uncommon before 5 years after surgery, and the lytic lesions progressively increase in both size and prevalence with increasing time, 10-year results are far more valuable than results of shorter-term studies.

Clohisy and Harris[1] reported that the incidence of femoral periprosthetic osteolysis was 60% at an average of 10 years after use of the Harris-Galante femoral component (Zimmer, Warsaw, IN). Hellman and associates[2] found there was a 61% overall incidence of periprosthetic osteolysis 10 to 12 years after insertion of the Omnifit cementless femoral component (Osteonics, Allendale, NJ) when used with the dual geometry acetabular component (Osteonics, Allendale, NJ). Moreover, by 10 to 12 years, 17% of hips had had revision surgery for periprosthetic osteolysis.

In addition, there has been a high incidence of osteolysis at the follow-up of the APR I implant[3] (Sulzer Medica, Austin, TX) and with use of the AML implant (DePuy, Warsaw, IN) combined with the trispike AML cementless acetabular component[4] (DePuy, Warsaw, IN). But these reports do not stand alone.

All of these concerns about osteolysis become magnified when the data on late loosening of cemented acetabular components are added. Schmalzried and associates[5] showed that the mechanism of loosening of cemented acetabular components in most cases also is periprosthetic osteolysis—the slower, linear form that leads to the radiolucent zone between the cement and the bone and eventually to component loosening. Thus, in most cases, the high incidence of acetabular component loosening and of revision for aseptic loosening must be added to the list of THR failures that are directly attributable to periprosthetic osteolysis. For example, Schulte and associates[6] found a 48% prevalence of loose or loose and revised acetabular components in the 18-year study of Johnston's cases; Barrack and associates[7] found 50% loose or revised cemented sockets at 12 years in patients younger than 51 years of age, and Raut and associates[8] reported a high incidence of failure of fixation among 386 cemented acetabular components at 5.5 years inserted at revision surgery.

These data clearly show that the dominant, single most important, long-term issue in THR surgery is periprosthetic osteolysis.[9-12] To these reports must be added the cases of periprosthetic femoral fracture, which almost always are a result, in part at least, of periprosthetic osteolysis. Moreover, the marked complexity of the revision surgery on both the femur and acetabulum that results from severe lysis is another manifestation of the price paid for this complication.

The author or the departments with which he is affiliated have received something of value from a commercial or other party related directly or indirectly to the subject of this chapter.

These extensive problems are caused mainly by wear of the polyethylene. However, the mechanical complication from wear must be added to the periprosthetic osteolytic processes caused by the wear. Wroblewski[13] has emphasized these issues as a result of his long-term experience with THR surgery, noting the decreased range of motion as the head penetrates into the polyethylene, the increasing late dislocation rate attributable to extensive wear, the increased torsional forces applied to the cement-bone interface because of the penetration of the femoral head, and such issues as polyethylene fracture and socket disruption.

If the failures of THRs as a result of femoral lysis, pelvic lysis, acetabular component loosening caused by lysis, femoral component loosening caused or abetted by lysis, spontaneous fractures secondary to lysis, and the mechanical problems that follow marked penetration of the femoral head into the polyethylenes are added together, the toll on THR surgery caused by polyethylene wear clearly is seen to be overwhelming. In addition, the cost, complications, and surgical complexities that loss of bone stock from lysis add to the difficulties in revision surgery must be considered.

Polyethylene wear and the resulting periprosthetic osteolysis constitute the number one problem in THR surgery; therefore, they constitute the number one motivation supporting the need for a highly cross-linked wear-resistant polyethylene.

Highly Cross-Linked Polyethylenes

What are the features of the new highly cross-linked polyethylenes that address the wear issue? To understand the special features of the new highly cross-linked polyethylenes, it is necessary to be aware of the striking advances in basic science that lie behind this development. Over the past 20 years and especially the past decade, marked progress has been made in understanding (1) the mechanism of wear of polyethylene in the hip, (2) how to reduce wear, (3) what causes oxidation,[14] (4) how to reduce oxidation, and (5) the duration over which testing should be completed. This progress has led to improved testing methods.

Wang and associates[15] and Bragdon and associates[16] reported that the molecular structure of portions of the surface of the worn areas of retrieved acetabular components was oriented in the direction of principal motion, namely flexion and extension. Others[14,17-19] have reported similar findings. This large scale molecular reorientation makes the polyethylene more resistant to wear in that direction (unidirectional wear) but vulnerable to wear in crossing directions.[16] This finding is important because the development of a bidirectional pin-on-disk wear tester, most pin-on-disk wear testing was done using unidirectional wear machines. These tests did not produce a wear mechanism or wear rates equivalent to those occurring in the hip in vivo. Poly II and Hylamer were tested on such machines. They were introduced based on tests that were less sophisticated than current tests and without published hip simulator data. Neither of these materials proved to be advantageous in patient use.

Not only was this observation of the surface reorientation of the polyethylene important in leading to improvements in proper testing of candidate materials, it also suggested a way to reduce wear. If the polyethylene could be heavily cross-linked, perhaps it would not reorient and, thus, would be less vulnerable to wear. Heavily cross-linked polyethylene has been shown by many contemporary tests to have improved wear resistance. This finding confirms the indication that for reduced wear, the material must be more heavily cross-linked.

Major advances also have occurred in the understanding of polyethylene oxidation. It is caused by the radiation that, in addition to creating cross-links, breaks some chains (chain scission) and leaves behind free radicals that can oxidize later. The residual free radicals cause the slow, progressive, delayed oxidation of the polyethylene. It is now known that the free radicals can be reduced by heating the material at temperatures below its melt temperature and can be eliminated (reduced below detection levels) by heating the material above its melt temperature. It is upon these scientific advances that the new highly cross-linked polyethylenes are based.

The cross-linking that dramatically reduces the wear of ultra-high molecular weight polyethylene (UHMWPE) can be achieved by exposure to either gamma irradiation or electron-beam irradiation or gamma radiation. The reduction in wear is related directly to the extent of radiation up to about 10 Mrad. Beyond that level, the increase in wear reduction becomes much less while the compromise in the mechanical properties of the polyethylene becomes greater. Thus, it is necessary to ensure that all processing of the UHMWPE (radiation and heat treatment) is done in a way that maintains its mechanical properties within the standards of the American Society for Testing of Materials (ASTM), the United States Food and Drug Administration (FDA), and the International Organization for Standardization (ISO).

The new, more heavily cross-linked UHMWPE with FDA approval can be considered under two headings: (1) partial versus fuller cross-linking and (2) with versus without residual free radicals.

A cross-linked material that has been irradiated to slightly above conventional sterilization levels (2.5 to 4.5 Mrad) is Marathon (DePuy, Warsaw, IN), which is gamma irradiated to 5 Mrad and contains no detectable free radicals. In hip simulator tests, this material has reduced wear compared with nonirradiated UHMWPE but, in hip simulator tests, it has measurable wear. More extensively cross-linked materials are listed in Table 1.

Durasul (Sulzer Medica, Austin, TX) and Longevity (Zimmer, Warsaw, IN) are irradiated with electron beams and then melted. They are nearly fully cross-linked and contain no detectable free radicals. Crossfire (Stryker-Howmedica Osteonics, Rutherford, NJ) is gamma irradiated at 7.5 Mrad, heated below its melting point, and then gamma irradiated further with a sterilizing dose of 2.5 Mrad. It contains free radicals.

Hip simulator testing often is done using different simulators, different rates of testing, and different lubricants. Therefore, direct comparison of actual numbers reported for the wear rates may not be fully representative. In hip simulator testing, Marathon and Crossfire wear at discernible levels, reported at about 6 mg per million cycles, which is less than conventional polyethylene. Durasul and Longevity have been tested in hip simulators to 27 and 30 million cycles each, and after these extensive tests the machining marks are still visible on the contact area. Machining marks are about 10-µm high, and their visibility after 20 million cycles or more suggests that the total cumulative wear is under 10 µm, which virtually is no detectable wear. Gravimetric testing and coordinate measuring machine analysis have indicated that wear of these two materials has been below the detectable level or nearly so.[20]

Crossfire oxidizes because it contains free radicals, but Marathon, Longevity, and Durasul do not oxidize. All of these materials have properties that are somewhat reduced compared with conventional UHMWPE, but all property values of these materials are within the ASTM, FDA, and ISO standards and superior to the material properties of Himont 1900, a successful UHMWPE used for over 20 years.[21] All of these materials are FDA approved, and all have successfully passed FDA inspection evaluation in terms of creep, locking mechanisms, and backside wear. An important caveat is that most of these materials have minimal in vivo data. It remains to be seen if the in vivo behavior will mimic the bench testing.

There is one additional feature of Durasul and Longevity. In all the testing for these two electron beam irradiated, melted, and highly cross-linked materials, increasing the head diameter does not increase wear. Therefore, with these materials, many surgeons have gone back to using only the largest head size possible. For most cases, it is the 32-mm head diameter. The return to the 32-mm head has contributed to the enthusiasm for the use of these materials.

In addition, extensive hip simulator tests of Durasul have shown that there is little or no detectable wear with a 38-mm head or with a 46-mm head. This material now has FDA approval for use with these larger heads. The larger heads have substantially improved range of motion and stability and have reduced tendency for dislocation. Some surgeons now use only 32-mm or 38-mm heads. It is satisfying to do a THR and have the range of motion and stability of a small bipolar reconstruction.

Summary

If these materials behave in vivo as they do in vitro and if no unexpected complications occur, periprosthetic osteolysis should be reduced, the duration of THR success should be greater, and the percentage of complications should be lower. Femoral loosening, socket loosening, and pelvic and femoral lysis should be reduced. There should be fewer revisions and dislocations and a greater range of motion.

Table 1
Extensively cross-linked UHMWPEs

Material	Radiation Dose (Mrad)	Free Radical
Durasul	9.5	no
Longevity	10	no
Crossfire	10	yes

If these improvements come to pass, use of the new materials may be an important advance in THR surgery.

References

1. Clohisy JC, Harris WH: The Harris-Galante uncemented femoral component in primary total hip replacement at 10 years. *J Arthroplasty* 1999;14:915-917.
2. Hellman EJ, Capello WN, Feinberg JR: Omnifit cementless total hip arthroplasty: A 10-year average followup. *Clin Orthop* 1999;364:164-174.
3. Dorr LD, Lewonowski K, Lucero M, Harris M, Wan Z: Failure mechanisms of anatomic porous replacement I cementless total hip replacement. *Clin Orthop* 1997;334:157-167.
4. Beauchesne R, Engh CA, Knezevich S, Suthers K, Kukita Y: Roentgenographic evaluation of the AML porous coated acetabular component: A six year minimum follow-up study. *Orthop Transact* 1993;16:834.
5. Schmalzried TP, Kwong LM, Jasty MJ, et al: The mechanism of loosening of cemented acetabular components in total hip arthroplasty: Analysis of specimens retrieved at autopsy. *Clin Orthop* 1992;274:60-78.
6. Schulte KR, Callaghan JJ, Kelley SS, Johnston RC: The outcome of Charnley total hip arthroplasty with cement after a minimum twenty-year follow-up: The results of one surgeon. *J Bone Joint Surg Am* 1993;75:961-975.
7. Barrack RL, Mulroy RD Jr, Harris WH: Improved cementing techniques and femoral component loosening in young patients with hip arthroplasty: A 12-year radiographic review. *J Bone Joint Surg Br* 1992;74:385-389.
8. Raut VV, Siney PD, Wroblewski BM: Cemented revision for aseptic acetabular loosening: A review of 387 hips. *J Bone Joint Surg Br* 1995;77:357-361.
9. Harris WH: The problem is osteolysis. *Clin Orthop* 1995;311:46-53.
10. Harris WH: Osteolysis and particle disease in hip replacement: A review. *Acta Orthop Scand* 1994;65:113-123.
11. Willert H: Tissue reactions to plastic and metallic wear products of joint endoprostheses, in Gschwend N, Debrunner HU (eds): *Total Hip Prosthesis*. Bern, Switzerland, Hans Huber Press, 1976.
12. Mirra JM, Amstutz HC, Matos M, Gold R: The pathology of the joint tissues and its clinical relevance in prosthesis failure. *Clin Orthop* 1976;117:221-240.

13. Wroblewski BM: Wear and loosening of the socket in the Charnley low-friction arthroplasty. *Orthop Clin North Am* 1988;19:627-630.

14. Sutula LC, Collier JP, Saum KA, et al: Impact of gamma sterilization on clinical performance of polyethylene in the hip. *Clin Orthop* 1995;319:28-40.

15. Wang A, Sun DC, Stark C, Dumbleton JH: Wear mechanism of ultra high molecular weight polyethylene knee and total joint replacements. *Wear* 1995;181:241-249.

16. Bragdon CR, O'Connor DO, Lowenstein JD, Syniuta WD: The importance of multidirectional motion for the wear of polyethylene in the hip, in *Fifth World Biomaterials Congress: Programme and Transactions*. Toronto, Canada, University of Toronto Press, 1996.

17. Blunn GW, Joshi AB, Lilley PA, et al: Polyethylene wear in unicondylar knee prostheses: 106 retrieved Marmor, PCA, and St Georg tibial components compared. *Acta Orthop Scand* 1992;63:247-255.

18. Cooper JR, Dowson D, Fisher J: Macroscopic and microscopic wear mechanisms in ultra high molecular weight polyethylene. *Wear* 1993;162:378-384.

19. Cooper JR, Dowson D, Fisher J: Birefringent wear of polyethylene specimens in acetabular cups. *Wear* 1991;151:391-402.

20. Muratoglu OK, Bragdon CR, O'Connor DO, Delaney J, Jasty M Harris WH: Comparison of the wear behavior and oxidation resistance of four different types of crosslinked acetabular components. *J Arthroplasty*, in press.

21. Currier BH, Currier JH, Collier JP, Mayor MB: Effect of fabrication method and resin type on performance of tibial bearings. *J Biomed Mater Res* 2000;53:143-151.

19

The Basic Science of Periprosthetic Osteolysis

Michael J. Archibeck, MD
Joshua J. Jacobs, MD
Kenneth A. Roebuck, PhD
Tibor T. Glant, MD, PhD

Total joint replacement has been very successful and cost-effective in restoring function and mobility to millions of patients worldwide since its advent more than 30 years ago. With improvements in prophylaxis against infection, the fatigue strength of the components, and skeletal fixation, wear and its sequelae have become the primary limitation to joint replacement longevity.[1] Initially termed "cement disease,"[2] osteolysis is believed to be a biologic response not only to polymethylmethacrylate but also to a variety of particles that may originate at several locations around a joint replacement. These include the articulating surfaces, modular component interfaces, fixation surfaces, and devices used for adjuvant fixation.[3]

Recent research has been directed at understanding the biologic cascade of events that is initiated by particulate debris and results in periprosthetic bone loss. Clinically, periprosthetic osteolysis can lead to aseptic loosening of components, massive bone loss that renders revision surgery substantially more complex, and periprosthetic pathologic fracture (Fig. 1). The current understanding of osteolysis with regard to the sources of wear, the morphology of wear particles, and the biologic response to wear particles according to findings reported in cell culture, tissue explant, and animal studies is presented here.

One or more of the authors or the departments with which they are affiliated have received something of value from a commercial or other party related directly or indirectly to the subject of this chapter.

Sources of Periprosthetic Wear Debris

The generation of particulate debris after total joint arthroplasty can occur as a result of two processes: wear and corrosion. Wear has been defined as the removal of material from the prosthesis in the form of debris.[4] The fundamental mechanisms of wear include adhesion, abrasion, and fatigue.[5] The mechanical conditions under which the prosthesis is functioning when wear occurs have been classified as modes of wear.[4] Mode 1 refers to the generation of wear debris that occurs with motion between the two bearing surfaces as intended by the designers. Mode 2 refers to a primary bearing surface rubbing against a secondary surface in a manner not intended by the designers (for example, a femoral head articulating with an acetabular shell following wear-through of the polyethylene). Mode 3 refers to two primary bearing surfaces with interposed third-body particles (such as bone, cement, metal, and so on). Mode 4 refers to two nonbearing surfaces rubbing together (such as back-sided wear of an acetabular liner, fretting of the Morse taper, stem-cement fretting, and so on).[3] While several modes of wear often occur simultaneously, mode 1 accounts for the

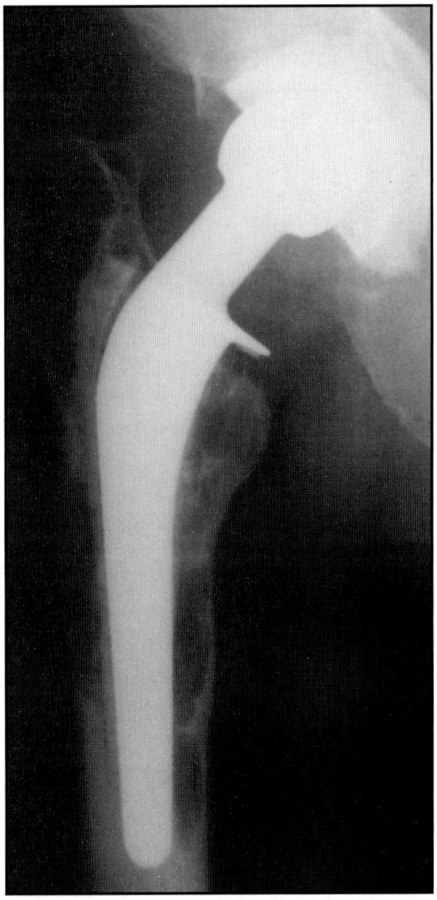

Fig. 1 Radiograph demonstrating extensive osteolysis in the proximal part of the femur in a patient with a cemented total hip replacement.

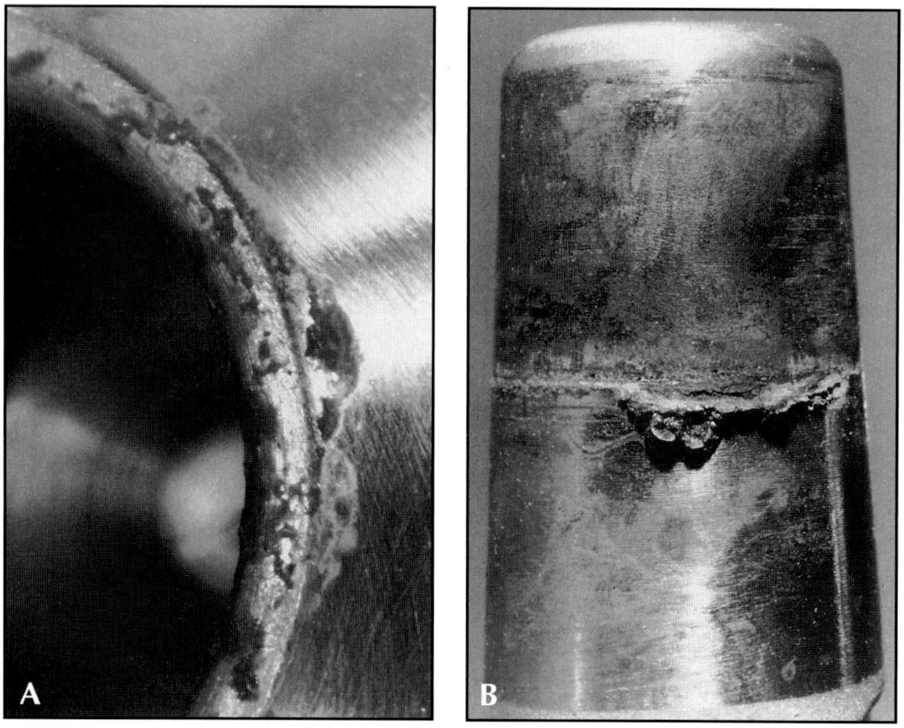

Fig. 2 A, Photograph of chromium orthophosphate hydrate-rich corrosion products around the rim of the bore of a cobalt-chromium-alloy femoral head that was coupled with a titanium-alloy stem (magnification ×7). **B**, Photograph of chromium orthophosphate hydrate-rich corrosion products circumscribing the neck of a cobalt-chromium-alloy femoral component, just distal to the head-neck junction (magnification ×5). (Reproduced with permission from Urban RM, Jacobs JJ, Gilbert JL, Galante JO: Migration of corrosion products from modular hip prostheses: Particle microanalysis and histopathological findings. *J Bone Joint Surg Am* 1994;76:1345-1359.)

majority of wear in well-functioning hip or knee replacements.[5]

Corrosion is an electrochemical process in which metal ions are released from an implant surface. Corrosion products can be generated from any metal surface, but they most commonly originate from metal-on-metal modular interfaces, such as the head-neck junction in both mixed-metal or similar-metal femoral stems in total hip replacements[6] (Fig. 2). The particles are metal-salt precipitates of these ions that form in the surrounding aqueous environment. Fine particulate debris of chromium phosphate corrosion products is often observed in the periprosthetic tissues of specimens retrieved at revision.[6] Chromium phosphate corrosion products from the modular junction have been found in sites remote from the hip joint as well.[6]

The most common particle in the periprosthetic tissues is polyethylene, which is predominantly generated by means of mode 1 wear. The remaining particles in the periprosthetic tissues include polymethylmethacrylate, cobalt alloy, and titanium alloy particles. In much smaller volumes, silicates and stainless steel particles are also seen; these most likely represent contaminants from surgical tools, supplemental fixation wires, or remnants from surface processing. Wear debris can gain access to all periprosthetic regions that are accessible to joint fluid.[7,8] This so-called effective joint space[8] is dependent on many variables, including component design and implantation techniques. The concentration of wear particles within periprosthetic tissues can extend into billions per gram of tissue.[8-13]

Morphology of Wear Particles

It has recently been recognized that most wear particles are less than 1 μm in size. As light microscopy resolution is limited by the wavelength of visible light (0.4 to 0.7 μm), submicrometer particles cannot be well visualized with these techniques. As such, the volume of particulate polyethylene debris was greatly underestimated in many of the early studies of periprosthetic tissues. Numerous research groups recently established techniques for the isolation, separation, and characterization of particles within periprosthetic tissues.[11-14] These techniques typically involve digestion of periprosthetic tissue with proteolytic enzymes and a strong acid or alkali. Particles can be separated with use of density-gradient centrifugation and characterized with an automated particle analyzer. With these techniques, the mean size of polyethylene particles has been found to be approximately 0.5 μm, with more than 90% of the particles less than 1 μm in size.[11,12]

Studies of wear debris from periprosthetic tissues characterized by scanning electron microscopy have demonstrated that 70% to 90% of the recovered particles are submicrometer polyethylene particles, with a mean size of about 0.5 μm.[10,11,13,14] These particles vary in shape, with spheroid forms being the most common, but fibrillar and globular shapes are also present (Fig. 3). The morphologic characteristics of polyethylene particles after total hip arthroplasty are different from those after total knee arthroplasty. Submicrometer particles are more prevalent in tissues around total hip replacements than in those around total knee replacements.[10,15,16] In hip replacements, microabrasion and microadhesion produce polyethylene particles that are primarily less than 1 μm in lerlgth.[4] In total knee replacements, decreased conformity and differing motion patterns result in higher contact stresses and more prevalent fatigue-type wear, leading to much larger polyethylene wear particles.[17,18]

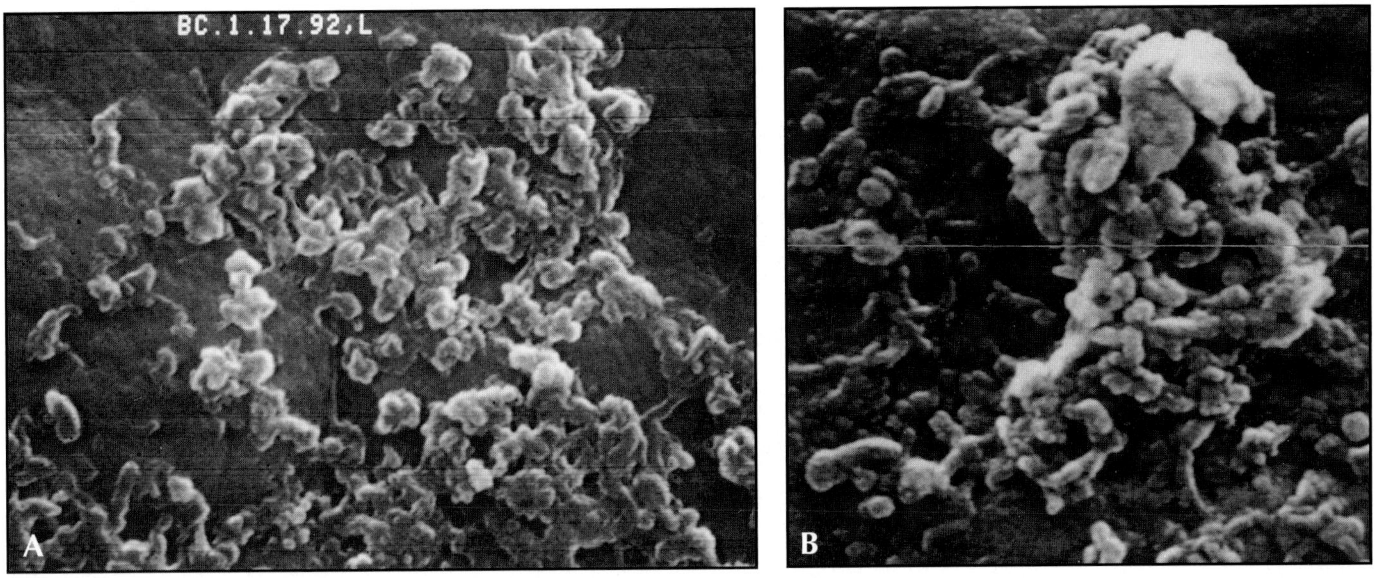

Fig. 3 Photomicrographs of polyethylene particles isolated from tissues, showing spheroids (**A**) and clusters of finer particles with bridging fibrils (**B**). (Reproduced with permission from Shanbhag AS, Jacobs JJ, Glant TT, Gilbert JL, Black J, Galante JO: Composition and morphology of wear debris in failed uncemented total hip replacement. *J Bone Joint Surg Br* 1994;76:60-67.)

Biologic Response to Particulate Debris

Background

In 1977, Willert and Semlitsch[19] were among the first to hypothesize that aseptic loosening of joint replacements was caused by the local macrophage response to wear debris. Goldring and associates[20] subsequently described the synovial-like character of the bone-implant interface in patients with a loose total hip replacement and demonstrated that the cells within the membrane had the capacity to produce large amounts of the so-called bone-resorbing factors PGE_2 (prostaglandin E_2) and collagenase. While these initial reports concerned cemented implants, similar processes have been identified in association with cementless implants.[8,21,22] Since then, a plethora of studies have documented the release of a variety of mediators of bone resorption from periprosthetic tissues in tissue culture. More recently, molecular biologic tools have been used to study tissue samples retrieved from patients with osteolysis. Techniques including immunohistochemistry, in situ hybridization, and quantitative polymerase chain reaction have provided powerful tools to elucidate the basic biology of loosening.[23]

Size, Composition, and Concentration of Particles

A number of investigators have examined the effects of particle size, composition, and dose on cell response. With regard to size, Horowitz and associates[21] demonstrated that polymethylmethacrylate particles that are phagocytosable (less than approximately 7μm in size) stimulate macrophage activation and release of tumor necrosis factor-α (TNF-α), while larger particles do not.[21] Gelb and associates,[24] using an air pouch model in rats, found that small (less than 20 μm), irregularly shaped polymethylmethacrylate particles produced a greater inflammatory reaction than did larger (50 to 350 μm) particles as expressed by the release of TNF-α, neutral metalloprotease, and PGE_2. Catelas and associates,[25] using a macrophage cell-culture line and particles of ceramic and polyethylene, found that cytotoxicity increased with the size and concentration of particles of greater than 2 μm.[25] Smaller particles (0.6 μm) caused limited cell mortality only at higher concentrations. Goodman and associates[26] examined the histologic effects of different sizes of polyethylene particles implanted into rabbit tibiae and found that the larger particles (mean, 67 μm) produced more fibrous encapsulation than did smaller particles.

The composition of the particles also has been shown to affect cellular responses. Haynes and associates[27] studied the in vitro response of human monocytes to particles of cobalt-chromium-molybdenum, stainless steel, and titanium-aluminum-vanadium of a similar size. Stainless-steel and cobalt-chromium-molybdenum particles were toxic, while titanium-aluminum-vanadium particles did not affect cell viability. With regard to the release of proinflammatory cytokines, titanium-aluminum-vanadium particles were the strongest stimulators of interleukin-6 (IL-6) and PGE_2 release, while all particles induced the release of TNF-α and IL-1β.[27] Catelas and associates[25] found no difference in cell mortality and release of TNF-α when Al_2O_3 and ZrO_2 particles were compared. They found release of TNF-α in response to polyethylene to be greater than that in response to ceramics. Shanbhag and associates[28] found that polyethylene particles were less toxic to cells than were polymethylmethacrylate particles. Glant and associates[29] studied the effect of titanium and polymethylmethacrylate particles on macrophage IL-1 and PGE_2 secretion and bone-resorbing activity. In the initial study, titanium particles were found to be the most stimulatory. This effect was most marked when there were about 10 to 15 particles per cell and only when the particles were of phagocytosable size (1 to 3 μm). In a subsequent study, different macrophage populations (peritoneal macrophages and the transformed macrophage cell-lines P388D and IC-21) were found to respond differently to these particles.[30] The peritoneal macrophages responded to titanium particles with significantly enhanced bone-resorbing activity ($P < 0.01$), while polymethylmethacrylate elicited this effect to a greater extent in the P388D and IC-21 cell lines.[30] In a rabbit model, Kubo and associates[31] found that the material composition was more strongly correlated (regression analysis, $P < 0.09$) with histiocyte reaction than were particle size and total surface area. They found the reaction to be greatest around particles of polyethylene (11 μm), cobalt-chromium (0.03 and 3.9 μm), stainless steel (3.9 μm), and titanium alloy (0.03 μm). Less response was identified around larger polyethylene particles (99 μm), larger titanium-alloy particles (3.9 μm), and alumina ceramics (3.9 μm).[31] Cobalt-chromium, titanium, and polyethylene particles have been used to challenge peripheral blood monocytes as well.[28,32] Metallic particles were more stimulatory for PGE_2, IL-1α, IL-1β, TNF-α, and IL-6α than were polyethylene particles.

The concentration of particulate debris to which a macrophage is exposed has been shown to alter its response as well. Catelas and associates[25] demonstrated increasing phagocytosis with increasing concentrations of particles of up to 2 μm in size. Phagocytosis of larger particles (up to 4.5 μm) reached a plateau independent of size and concentration that suggested a saturation of phagocytosis possibly dependent on the volume of particles ingested.[25] In a more recent study, Catelas and associates[33] found macrophage apoptotic cell death to be both size- and concentration-dependent, reaching a plateau at a concentration of more than 150 particles per macrophage for both ceramic and polyethylene particles. Shanbhag and associates[34] used the concept of surface-area ratio to standardize the particle challenge in a study of macrophage response to titanium and polystyrene particles. With use of weight percent, volume percent, or number of particles, a nonuniform challenge may result if particles of varying densities and sizes are compared. They found that the macrophage response to particulate debris was dependent on particle size, composition, and dose as given by surface-area ratio.[34]

Thus, the bioreactivity of particles has been shown to depend on their size, composition, and concentration. Most studies have suggested that particles of phagocytosable sizes are the most stimulatory and that higher doses elicit more response (often up to a saturation level). At this time, it is not possible to generalize about the role of composition, as all particle types (metal, polymer, and ceramic) can elicit a cell response, which varies with the cell type and the specific response measured (such as cell toxicity, proinflammatory cytokine release, and so on). It is clear that particle production can lead to bone resorption, but currently it is not possible to determine which particle types will have the least clinical effect.

Cell and Organ-Culture Studies

Macrophages and/or other cell lines cultured with particles in vitro have added to our understanding of the events that lead to bone resorption in response to particulate debris. Cell-culture studies have demonstrated that particulate wear debris from prosthetic materials or bone cement (less than 12 to 15 μm in size) are phagocytosed by macrophages and these activated cells release various mediators. Of the numerous cellular mediators released, IL-1, IL-6, TNF-α, and PGE_2 are believed to be among the most important components capable of inducing cell proliferation, promoting osteoclast formation, and stimulating osteoclasts in order to resorb the adjacent bone.[2,29,35-37] Other factors involved in bone resorption include the enzymes responsible for the catabolism of the organic component of bone. These include the matrix metalloproteinases collagenase and stromelysin.[38] Although cytokines secreted by the macrophage may directly lead to the stimulation of osteoclastic bone resorption, the intermediary role of other cells, such as osteoblasts and fibroblasts, has recently been identified.[21,23]

An earlier study identified the toxic effects of many of these particles on cultured macrophages.[39] Cobalt-chromium alloy particles were found to lead to altered phagocytic activity and cell death.[39] Shanbhag and associates[28,34] demonstrated that cell death increased with increasing dosages of particles.

Although toxic to macrophages, these same particles have the ability to activate macrophage production of proinflammatory cytokines at lower doses. In their studies, Glant and associates[29,30] demonstrated the release of PGE_2 and IL-1 from cultured macrophages in response to polymethylmethacrylate and titanium particles. Horowitz[40] identified TNF-α as a primary mediator released by particle-activated macrophages. TNF-α stimulates osteoblasts to produce granulocyte-macrophage colony-stimulating factor and IL-6, both of which stimulate recruitment of additional macrophages, osteoclasts, and other inflammatory cells into the area. TNF-α was also found to stimulate the release of PGE_2 by osteoblasts, which, in turn, activates osteoclastic bone resorption. Nakashima and associates[41] found increased monocyte/macrophage expression of C-C chemokines, which primarily function as chemoattractants, in response to polymethylmethacrylate and titanium alloy particles. Pollice and associates[42] used an in vitro rat osteoclast precursor model to investigate the role of activated macrophages in bone resorption. They found that bone resorption was mediated, in part, by factors secreted by osteoblasts responding to activated macrophages.

Fibroblasts have been studied in cell culture as well. Maloney and associates[43] exposed cultured bovine synovial fibroblasts to particulate metallic debris. The effects of the metallic particles on the synthesis and secretion of proteolytic enzymes and on cell proliferation and viability were examined. At high concentrations of particles, all particles were toxic and caused a decrease in proteolytic and collagenolytic activity. Titanium elevated the level of lysosomal enzyme hexosaminidase except at high concentrations. Scanning electron microscopy demonstrated that the morphologic response was typical of active fibroblasts.[43] In a study by Yao and associates,[38] synovial fibroblasts and fibroblasts that had been isolated from interfacial membranes of patients with a failed total hip replacement were challenged with titanium particles. Both types of fibroblasts responded with elevated expressions of collagenase, stromelysin, and, to a much lesser extent, the tissue inhibitor of metalloproteinase (TIMP). Manlapaz and associates[44] demonstrated that introduction of titanium-alloy particles resulted in direct activation of fibroblasts and release of proinflammatory mediators (IL-6 and PGE_2) and fibroblast growth factor. In addition, collagenase activity increased.

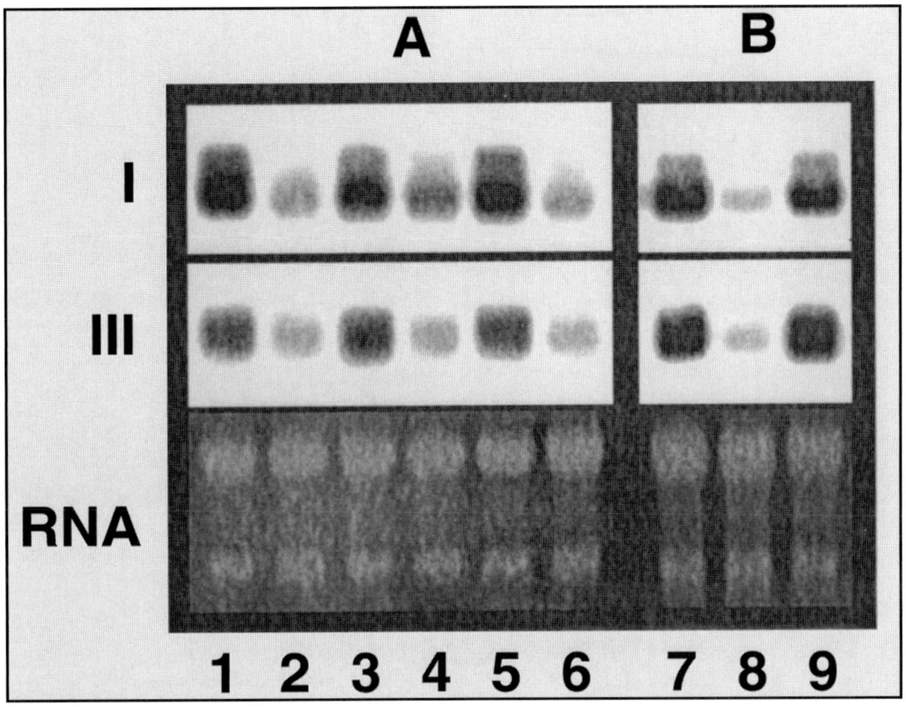

Fig. 4 Autoradiograph of Northern blot analysis, showing the expression of mRNAs for procollagen α_1(I) and α_2(III) in human MG-63 osteoblast-like cells incubated for 48 hours with various particles at a concentration of 0.05%. The lowest panel shows the responses of corresponding RNAs. **A**, The cells were untreated (lane 1) or treated with small (1- to 3-μm) titanium particles (lane 2), large (21- to 85-μm) titanium particles (lane 3), small (1.14 ± 0.007-μm) polystyrene particles (lane 4), large (21.1 ± 4.09-μm) polystyrene particles (lane 5), or small (0.7- to 1.3-μm) silver particles (lane 6). **B**, The cells were incubated for 48 hours without titanium particles (lane 7), with small (1- to 3-μm) titanium particles (lane 8), or with particle-free medium in which small titanium particles had been preincubated alone without cells (lane 9). (Reproduced with permission from Yao J, Szabo G; Jacobs JJ, Kuettner KE, Glant TT: Suppression of osteoblast function by titanium particles. *J Bone Joint Surg Am* 1997;79:107-112.)

Ongoing work in the area of cellular signal transduction pathways has begun to elucidate the basic molecular mechanisms by which particles induce cellular (osteoblast, osteoclast, macrophage, and fibroblast) response. A recent study showed upregulation of TNF-α and IL–6 expression in macrophages in the absence of phagocytosis, suggesting that cell membrane-particle interactions are sufficient to initiate macrophage activation.[45,46] The nuclear transcription factors nuclear factor-kappa B (NF-κB) and nuclear factor-interleukin-6 (NF-IL-6) are key upstream intermediaries in this process.[45] Other work has shown that the initial response of osteoblasts to particulate metallic debris includes phosphorylation of protein tyrosine kinase pathways and activation of NF-κB.[46]

Normal bone maintenance relies on the balance of bone formation and bone resorption. While the abovementioned investigations have, for the most part, focused on the bone resorption limb of this cascade, more recent studies have examined the effect of particles on bone formation. Yao and associates found that both titanium and polystyrene particles smaller than 3 μm suppressed the

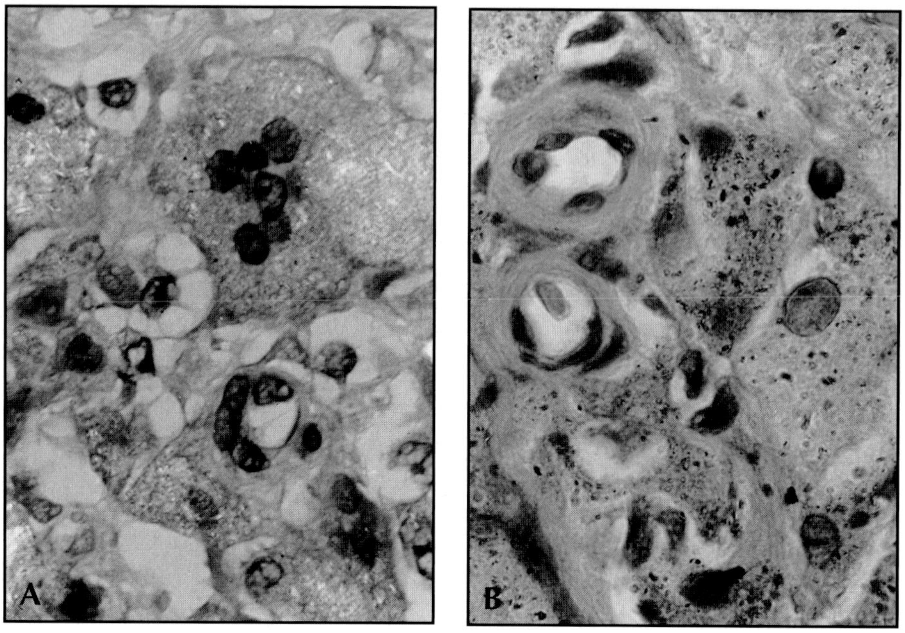

Fig. 5 Photomicrographs of periprosthetic interfacial tissue removed from patients with failed cementless (**A**) and cemented (**B**) total hip replacements. Numerous submicrometer birefringent particles that are most likely polyethylene (**A**) and dark metal particles (**B**) are seen within the cells (original magnification, ×50). (Reproduced with permission from Glant TT, Jacobs JJ, Mikecz K, et al: Particulate-induced prostaglandin- and cytokine-mediated bone resorption in an experimental system and in failed joint replacements. *Am J Ther* 1996;3:27-41.)

expression of the genes that code for collagen type I and type III precursor molecules. The suppression of these genes was related to the size but not to the composition of the particles. The biosynthesis of both type I and type III collagen also was decreased in an osteoblastic cell line that had been treated with titanium particles[47] (Fig. 4). Studies, from other laboratories, performed with use of a bone-chamber model have shown diminished bone ingrowth in the presence of particulate degradation products.[48] The amount of bone ingrowth was greatest in the control specimens, moderately decreased in the presence of high-density-polyethylene particles, and greatly decreased in the presence of cobalt-chromium particles.[48]

Tissue Explant Studies

The histopathologic features of the periprosthetic membrane have been studied extensively. Common findings in cases of aseptic loosening or osteolysis include a fibrous stroma, abundant macrophages, foreign-body giant cells, and wear debris[20,36] (Fig. 5). As mentioned previously, the majority of particles are submicrometer in size and require electron microscopy for visualization and quantitation. Larger nonphagocytosable particles (more than 30 μm) generate a foreign-body reaction with surrounding giant cells. The quantity of macrophages and the presence of radiographic osteolysis have been associated with the amount of particulate debris.[8] Analysis of these membranes has demonstrated the presence of many biochemical mediators of inflammation, cellular recruitment, and bone resorption.

PGE_2 was one of the first mediators to be identified in tissues surrounding loose implants. Many studies of this membrane have identified high levels of PGE_2 capable of causing bone resorption.[20] Goodman and associates[36] demonstrated that the levels of PGE_2 in the membranes of loose implants were significantly elevated compared with the levels in the membranes of implants that were not loose ($P < 0.05$). Cila and associates[49] found that the degree of prosthetic loosening was associated with significantly higher levels of periprosthetic PGE_2 activity ($P < 0.01$). Dorr and associates[35] found no difference in the levels of IL-1, PGE_2, and collagenase when periprosthetic membranes from failed titanium-alloy and cobalt-chromium-alloy components were compared. Kim and associates[22] analyzed membranes from failed hip prostheses inserted without cement and found a histologic appearance similar to that described for membranes from failed cemented implants. They found some biochemical mediators, including collagenase, IL-1, and PGE_2, in these membranes as well. Chiba and associates[50] studied interfacial tissues from failed cementless total hip replacements with and without femoral osteolysis and found a greater activity of IL-1, TNF-α, and IL-6 in hips with osteolysis than in those without osteolysis. Goodman and associates,[51] using immunohistochemistry and in situ hybridization techniques on periprosthetic membranes, demonstrated the presence of increased quantities of macrophages, T-lymphocyte subgroups, and IL-1 and IL-6 expression in osteolytic lesions around cemented implants. In the vicinity of cementless implants, osteolysis was associated with elevated levels of T-lymphocyte subgroups and TNF-α, suggesting different biologic mechanisms of loosening for cemented and cementless implants. Jiranek and associates[23] used in situ hybridization techniques to identify the cellular components of the periprosthetic membrane. Those authors demonstrated that the membrane consists predominantly of macrophages, fibroblasts, and, less commonly, T-lymphocytes (less than 10%). Nucleic acid probes used in that same study demonstrated IL-1β mRNA to be expressed primarily in macrophages. IL-1β protein was identified on both macrophages and fibroblasts, suggesting that the protein was bound by both cell types but was secreted predominantly by macrophages. Platelet-derived growth-factor transcripts were found in both macrophages and fibroblasts.[23]

Other species identified in periprosthetic tissues from loose implants include matrix metalloproteinases (MMPs) that act to degrade the extracellular matrix. In a recent study of the membranes from failed cementless total hip replacements, Vidovszky and associates[52] compared tissue from osteolytic regions with that from nonosteolytic regions and found that the expression of collagenase, gelatinase, and stromelysin (MMP-1, MMP-2, and MMP-11) was elevated in the membranes from the osteolytic regions. Takagi and associates[53] demonstrated elevated production of MMP-2 and induction of MMP-9 in tissue extracts from both the interface tissues between bone and implants and the pseudocapsular tissues around loose implants. Ishiguro and associates[54] found elevated expression of MMPs and tissue inhibitors of metalloproteinase from tissues around loose cemented total hip replacements. Other substances recently identified in tissue-explant studies include mesenchymal collagenase,[55] elastase,[56] cathepsin G,[57] nitrous oxide synthase mRNA,[58] and C-C chemokines (chemoattractants).[41]

Analysis of synovial fluid from patients with a loose hip prosthesis has demonstrated the presence of similar chemical mediators. Sabokbar and Rushton[59] found elevation in the levels of PGE_2, IL-6, IL-8, and multiple adhesion molecules in the synovial fluid around loose implants compared with the levels in the synovial fluid around controls. Kim and associates[60] found elevation in the levels of IL-6, soluble IL-6 receptor (sIL-6R), and tartrate-resistant acid phosphatase (TRAP) in joint fluid from failed total hip replacements. They also demonstrated that, compared with controls, this joint fluid was able to significantly stimulate osteoclastic bone resorption on dentin slices ($P < 0.05$).

Bone-resorbing cytokines and other factors have also been studied in the serum of patients with aseptic loosening of a total hip replacement. Granchi and associates[61] found an elevation in the level of serum granulocyte-macrophage colony-stimulating factor, while the levels of IL-6 and TNF-α were not significantly elevated. Serum IL-1β levels were found to be higher in patients who had a titanium-aluminum-vanadium cemented prosthesis.

Animal Studies

The use of animal models has allowed researchers to perform well-controlled studies, with standardized models, to elucidate the complex biologic response of both bone and soft tissues to particles. When implanted in bulk form, medical polymers and metals are surrounded by an incomplete fibrous-tissue layer.[62] When implanted in particle form, these same materials induce an inflammatory reaction, including the infiltration of macrophages, foreign body giant cells, and fibrous tissue similar to that seen around loose implants.[26,62]

Animal models of osteolysis have been developed as well. Howie and associates[63] demonstrated osteolysis after injection of polyethylene particles around an acrylic plug placed in the femora of rats. Spector and associates[64] developed a canine model of aseptic loosening by loosely implanting a femoral component into a bed of preinserted cement particles. They isolated and cultured periprosthetic cells from these animals and found an elevated secretion of IL-1 and PGE_2. The secretion of these mediators paralleled the radiographic appearance of loosening. The PGE_2 response was partially suppressed by in vitro administration of naproxen. Goodman and associates[65] used New Zealand rabbits to demonstrate the process of aseptic loosening of a poorly cemented tibial hemiprosthesis. Subsequent tissue-culture supernatants from this model demonstrated elevated PGE_2 levels in association with loose implants. Gelb and associates[24] used a subcutaneous air-pouch rat model to quantitatively demonstrate the in vivo effects of the size, morphology, and surface area of polymethylmethacrylate particles on the acute inflammatory response. Kubo and associates[31] evaluated the response to a variety of particles (namely ultra-high molecular weight polyethylene, cobalt-chromium, alumina ceramics, stainless steel, and titanium-aluminum-vanadium) of differing sizes by inserting a polymethylmethacrylate plug with a groove for particle placement into rabbit femora. They found a marked histiocytic response around particles of ultra-high molecular weight polyethylene (11 μm), stainless steel (3.9 μm), and cobalt-chromium (3.9 μm). A less intense histiocytic response was found surrounding particles of alumina ceramics and titanium (3.9 μm for each).[31]

Turner and associates[66] reported on aseptic loosening of cemented total hip prostheses in a canine model. They found thick fibrous and granulomatous membranes at the failed cement-bone interface with sheets of histiocytes and occasional foreign-body giant cells. They identified granulomatous cortical erosions with evidence of particulate debris. Dowd and associates[67] also used an in vivo canine hip arthroplasty model to study the effects of motion and particles. The prosthesis was designed with a reservoir for particles. In addition, a midshaft ball joint allowed motion between the proximal and distal portions of the prosthesis. The histologic and biochemical characteristics of the experimentally induced membranes were similar to those of tissues retrieved at revision surgery. This model has been implemented in other investigations.[68] Merkel and associates[69] recently used a murine model to investigate the in vivo response to particles. The model involved subperiosteal exposure of the cranium with placement of particles directly on the surface of the bone. With use of this model, they investigated genetically engineered mice that were deficient in TNF-α receptors and found that these mice were protected from the particle-induced bone resorption seen in wild mice.

Pharmacologic Intervention in Particulate-Induced Bone Resorption

The goal in gaining a better understanding of the mechanism of osteolysis is to reduce wear-related complications after joint arthroplasty. Investigators are approaching this goal with efforts both to reduce particle generation and to inhibit the biologic response to particulate debris. Currently, intensive research and development activities are directed toward reducing the production of particulate debris by polyethylene bearing materials and so-called hard-on-hard bearings. As these activities are beyond the scope of this review, we present a summary of the preliminary in vitro and animal studies directed at the pharmacologic modification of the adverse host response to particulate debris.

Horowitz and associates,[70] in a rat calvaria/macrophage co-culture model, studied the effects of indomethacin, anti-TNF-α antibody, and disodium pamidronate on bone resorption that is induced by macrophages exposed to bone-cement particles. They found that indomethacin inhibited the production of PGE_2 but not the release of TNF-α or calcium. Anti-TNF antibodies neutralized the presence of TNF to undetectable levels but did not affect release of PGE_2 or calcium. In contrast, the addition of disodium pamidronate was effective in inhibiting the release of calcium, indicating decreased bone resorption. Haynes and associates[71] treated macrophages with drugs that prevent a decrease in pH within phagosomes. This treatment significantly reduced the toxicity of cobalt-chromium particles ($P < 0.05$) and reduced the levels of PGE_2 and IL-6 release induced by titanium particles ($P < 0.005$). Glant and associates[72] demonstrated a partial inhibitory effect of indomethacin and misoprostol on the bone resorption activity of cultured cells from the interfacial membranes of failed total hip replacements. Shanbhag and associates[68] used a canine total hip replacement model to study the efficacy of an oral bisphosphonate for inhibition of wear-debris-mediated bone resorption. They demonstrated a reduction in the frequency of radiographic periprosthetic radiolucencies, while the levels of PGE_2 and IL-1 remained elevated in cultures of tissue from the sites of these implants. Blaine and associates[32] found that cyclic adenosine monophosphate (cAMP) agonists inhibited the release of TNF-α by titanium-stimulated peripheral monocytes, while cAMP antagonists enhanced the production of TNF-α. Dobai and associates[73] demonstrated suppressed collagen gene expression and diminished collagen synthesis induced by particulate debris in bone marrow-derived osteoblasts. It was found that these effects were reversed by pretreatment of the osteoblasts with 1,25-dihydroxyvitamin D_3 ($1,25(OH)_2D_3$). Clearly, human trials are needed before any of these potential pharmacological treatments are recommended for clinical use.

Other Possible Factors in the Etiology of Osteolysis

Recently, the role of elevated intra-articular pressure in the development of osteolysis has been studied.[74] Computer simulations and direct measurements have demonstrated fluid pressures in the hip or knee to be elevated to as high as 700 mm Hg with activity. Van der Vis and associates[75] found that a pressure of 200 mm Hg applied for 2 weeks in a rabbit bone-chamber model caused massive bone resorption under the pressurized area. The histologic findings were similar to those in areas of periprosthetic osteolysis, with large quantities of macrophages. With fluctuating pressures (between 50 and 150 mm Hg), bone resorption was also present but to a lesser degree.[76] Histologically, bone resorption was preceded by osteocyte death. Van der Vis and associates,[77] using a similar rabbit model, found that compression of a fibrous membrane interposed between bone and a prosthesis can lead to resorption of the underlying bone primarily because of osteocyte death and subsequent resorption of dead bone tissue. They thought that this finding might explain the observation that early migration of a hip or knee prosthesis is predictive of clinical loosening of the prosthesis.

Aspenberg and Herbertsson[78] used a rat model to determine the role of motion in periprosthetic bone resorption. A titanium plug was inserted through a plate into a milled depression in the cortex. After use of motion of the flat titanium surface and/or application of particles to the milled depression, they concluded that mechanical stimuli were of primary importance in prosthetic loosening and that particles may modulate the later stages of the process.

The role of hypersensitivity in periprosthetic osteolysis has yet to be established. Evans[79] was one of the first to suggest that metal sensitivity may contribute to aseptic loosening. He found that 9 of 14 patients who had loose metal-on-metal implants demonstrated cutaneous sensitivity to one or more of the components of the alloys. In subsequent studies, however, metal hypersensitivity was not found to be associated with loosening.[80,81]

Gil-Albarova and associates[82] investigated lymphocyte-mediated immune response to polymethylmethacrylate in patients with a failed cemented total hip replacement. Patch tests of reactivity to polymethylmethacrylate were positive in 50% (13) of 26 patients. However, they found no difference in patch-test reactivity between patients who had a granulomatous loosening pattern and those who had a nongranulomatous loosening pattern. Wooley and associates[83] studied in vitro cellular immune responses to particulate cobalt-chromium alloy and polymethylmethacrylate in patients before and after total joint replacement. They found an elevated proliferative cellular response to polymethylmethacrylate and metallic particles in patients examined before revision surgery and in those evaluated after a primary joint replacement. These immune responses were more marked in patients with aseptic loosening and were diminished following revision for loosening. They concluded that specific cellular responses to polymethylmethacrylate and/or cobalt-chromium-alloy particles may be associated with loose or painful prostheses.

Santavirta and associates[84] cultured peripheral blood mononuclear cells with polymethylmethacrylate particles and found induction of inflammatory mononuclear cell migration and adhesion leading to a nonspecific lymphocyte reaction. They concluded that polymethylmethacrylate is essentially immunologically inert. In a subsequent study, they used a human lymphocyte culture protocol to identify the biocompatibility of ultra-high molecular weight polyethylene particles.[85] Polyethylene did not cause an increase in lymphocyte DNA synthesis and did not stimulate the expression of major histocompatibility complex class II antigen or IL-2 receptor CD25. Santavirta and associates concluded that ultra-high molecular weight polyethylene, while inducing a foreign-body reaction, was relatively immunologically inert. Jiranek and associates[86] examined the response induced by injections of particulate polymethylmethacrylate into four strains of mice, one of which was immunocompetent and three of which had different levels of lymphocyte dysfunction. The granulomas were similar among the strains, with a paucity or absence of lymphoid cells. They concluded that, in mice, there is a lymphocyte-independent pathway of macrophage activation in response to particles. Overall, findings reported in the literature conflict with regard to the role of specific immune responses in association with aseptic loosening and osteolysis. Clearly, additional work in this area is needed.

Summary

Despite improvements in the techniques, materials, and fixation of total joint replacements, wear and its sequelae continue to be the main factors limiting the longevity and clinical success of arthroplasty. Since Charnley[87] first recognized aseptic loosening in the early 1960s, a tremendous amount of information has been gained on the basic science of osteolysis. Tissue explant, animal, and cell culture studies have allowed development of an appreciation of the complexity of cellular interactions and chemical mediators involved in these processes. Cellular participants have been shown to include the macrophage, osteoblast, fibroblast, and osteoclast. The plethora of chemical mediators that are responsible for the cellular interactions and effects on bone primarily include PGE_2, TNF-α, IL-1, and IL-6. Recent and ongoing work in the field of signaling pathways will continue to advance our understanding of the mechanisms of periprosthetic bone loss. Although initial animal studies are promising for the development of possible pharmacologic agents for the treatment and prevention of osteolysis, well controlled human trials are required.

References

1. Harris WH: The problem is osteolysis. *Clin Orthop* 1995;311:46-53.
2. Jones LC, Hungerford DS: Cement disease. *Clin Orthop* 1987;225:192-206.
3. McKellop H, Park SH, Chiesa R, et al: In vivo wear of 3 types of metal on metal hip prostheses during 2 decades of use. *Clin Orthop* 1996;329(suppl):S128-S140.
4. McKellop HA, Campbell P, Park SH, et al: The origin of submicron polyethylene wear debris in total hip arthroplasty. *Clin Orthop* 1995;311:3-20.
5. Schmalzried TP, Callaghan JJ: Current concepts review: Wear in total hip and knee replacements. *J Bone Joint Surg Am* 1999;81:15-136.
6. Urban RM, Jacobs JJ, Gilbert JL, Galante JO: Migration of corrosion products from modular hip prostheses: Particle microanalysis and histopathological findings. *J Bone Joint Surg Am* 1994;76:1345-1359.
7. Schmalzried TP, Akizuki KH, Fedenko AN, Mirra J: The role of access of joint fluid to bone in periarticular osteolysis: A report of four cases. *J Bone Joint Surg Am* 1997;79:447-452.
8. Schmalzried TP, Jasty M, Harris WH: Periprosthetic bone loss in total hip arthroplasty: Polyethylene wear debris and the concept of the effective joint space. *J Bone Joint Surg Am* 1992;74:849-863.
9. Hicks DG, Judkins AR, Sickel JZ, Rosier RN, Puzas JE, O'Keefe RJ: Granular histiocytosis of pelvic lymph nodes following total hip arthroplasty: The presence of wear debris, cytokine production, and immunologically activated macrophages. *J Bone Joint Surg Am* 1996;78:482-496.
10. Hirakawa K, Bauer TW, Stulberg BN, Wilde AH: Comparison and quantitation of wear debris of failed total hip and total knee arthroplasty. *J Biomed Mater Res* 1996;31:257-263.
11. Maloney WJ, Smith RL, Schmalzried TP, Chiba J, Huene D, Rubash H: Isolation and characterization of wear particles generated in patients who have had failure of a hip arthroplasty without cement. *J Bone Joint Surg Am* 1995;77:1301-1310.
12. Margevicius KJ, Bauer TW, McMahon JT, Brown SA, Merritt K: Isolation and characterization of debris in membranes around total joint prostheses. *J Bone Joint Surg Am* 1994;76:1664-1675.
13. Shanbhag AS, Jacobs JJ, Glant TT, Gilbert JL, Black J, Galante JO: Composition and morphology of wear debris in failed uncemented total hip replacement. *J Bone Joint Surg Br* 1994;76:60-67.
14. Campbell P, Ma S, Yeom B, McKellop H, Schmalzried TP, Amstutz HC: Isolation of predominantly submicron-sized UHMWPE wear particles from periprosthetic tissues. *J Biomed Mater Res* 1995;29:127-131.
15. Horikoshi M, Macaulay W, Booth RE, Crossett LS, Rubash HE: Comparison of interface membranes obtained from failed cemented and cementless hip and knee prostheses. *Clin Orthop* 1994;309:69-87.

16. Schmalzried TP, Jasty M, Rosenberg A, Harris WH: Polyethylene wear debris and tissue reactions in knee as compared to hip replacement prostheses. *J Biomater Appl* 1994;5:185-190.

17. Wright TM, Rimnac CM, Stulberg SD, Mintz L, Tsao AK, Klein RW, McCrae C: Wear of polyethylene in total joint replacements: Observations from retrieved PCA knee implants. *Clin Orthop* 1992;276:126-134.

18. Collier JP, Mayor MB, McNamara JL, Surprenant VA, Jensen RE: Analysis of the failure of 122 polyethylene inserts from uncemented tibial knee components. *Clin Orthop* 1991;273:232-242.

19. Willert H G, Semlitsch M: Reactions of the articular capsule to wear products of artificial joint prostheses. *J Biomed Mater Res* 1977;11:157-164.

20. Goldring SR, Schiller AL, Roelke M, Rourke CM, O'Neil DA, Harris WH: The synovial-like membrane at the bone-cement interface in loose total hip replacements and its proposed role in bone lysis. *J Bone Joint Surg Am* 1983;65:575-584.

21. Horowitz SM, Doty SB, Lane JM, Burstein AH: Studies of the mechanism by which the mechanical failure of polymethylmethacrylate leads to bone resorption. *J Bone Joint Surg Am* 1993;75:802-813.

22. Kim KJ, Chiba J, Rubash HE: In vivo and in vitro analysis of membranes from hip prostheses inserted without cement. *J Bone Joint Surg Am* 1994;76:172-180.

23. Jiranek WA, Machado M, Jasty M, et al: Production of cytokines around loosened cemented acetabular components: Analysis with immunohistochemical techniques and in situ hybridization. *J Bone Joint Surg Am* 1993;75:863-879.

24. Gelb H, Schumacher HR, Cuckler J, Ducheyne P, Baker DG: In vivo inflammatory response to polymethylmethacrylate particulate debris: Effect of size, morphology, and surface area. *J Orthop Res* 1994;12:83-92.

25. Catelas I, Huk OL, Petit A, Zukor DJ, Marchand R, Yahia L: Flow cytometric analysis of macrophage response to ceramic and polyethylene particles: Effects of size, concentration, and composition. *J Biomed Mater Res* 1998;41:600-607.

26. Goodman SB, Fornasier VL, Lee J, Kei J: The histological effects of the implantation of different sizes of polyethylene particles in the rabbit tibia. *J Biomed Mater Res* 1990;24:517-524.

27. Haynes DR, Boyle SJ, Rogers SD, Howie DW, Vernon-Roberts B: Variation in cytokines induced by particles from different prosthetic materials. *Clin Orthop* 1998;352:223-230.

28. Shanbhag AS, Jacobs JJ, Black J, Galante JO, Glant TT: Human monocyte response to particulate biomaterials generated in vivo and in vitro. *J Orthop Res* 1995;13:792-801.

29. Glant TT, Jacobs JJ, Molnar G, Shanbhag AS, Valyon M, Galante JO: Bone resorption activity of particulate-stimulated macrophages. *J Bone Min Res* 1993;1071-1079.

30. Glant TT, Jacobs JJ: Response of three murine macrophage populations to particulate debris: Bone resorption in organ cultures. *J Orthop Res* 1994;12:720-731.

31. Kubo T, Sawada K, Hirakawa K, Shimizu C, Takamatsu T, Hirasawa Y: Histiocyte reaction in rabbit femurs to UHMWPE, metal, and ceramic particles in different sizes. *J Biomed Mater Res* 1999;45:363-369.

32. Blaine TA, Pollice PF, Rosier RN, Reynolds PR, Puzas JE, O'Keefe RJ: Modulation of the production of cytokines in titanium-stimulated human peripheral blood monocytes by pharmacological agents: The role of cAMP-mediated signaling mechanisms. *J Bone Joint Surg Am* 1997;79:1519-1528.

33. Catelas I, Petit A, Zukor DJ, Marchand R, Yahia L, Huk OL: Induction of macrophage apoptosis by ceramic and polyethylene particles in vitro. *Biomaterials* 1999;20:625-630.

34. Shanbhag AS, Jacobs JJ, Black J, Galante JO, Glant TT: Macrophage/particle interactions: Effect of size, composition and surface area. *J Biomed Mater Res* 1994;28:81-90.

35. Dorr LD, Bloebaum R, Emmanual J, Meldrum R: Histologic, biochemical, and ion analysis of tissue and fluids retrieved during total hip arthroplasty. *Clin Orthop* 1990;261:82-95.

36. Goodman SB, Chin RC, Chiou SS, Schurman DJ, Woolson ST, Masada MP: A clinical-pathologic-biochemical study of the membrane surrounding loosened and nonloosened total hip arthroplasties. *Clin Orthop* 1989;244:182-187.

37. Shanbhag AS, Jacobs JJ, Black J, Galante JO, Glant TT: Cellular mediators secreted by interfacial membranes obtained at revision total hip arthroplasty. *J Arthroplasty* 1995;10:498-506.

38. Yao J, Glant TT, Lark MW, et al: The potential role of fibroblasts in periprosthetic osteolysis: Fibroblast response to titanium particles. *J Bone Min Res* 1995;10:1417-1427.

39. Rae T: A study on the effects of particulate metals of orthopaedic interest on murine macrophages in vitro. *J Bone Joint Surg Br* 1975;57:444-450.

40. Horowitz S: Particulate debris and osteolysis, in Lotke P, Garino J (eds): *Revision Total Knee Arthroplasty*. Philadelphia, PA, Lippincott-Raven, 1999, pp 31-41.

41. Nakashima Y, Sun D-H, Trindade MCD, et al: Induction of macrophage C-C chemokine expression by titanium alloy and bone cement particles. *J Bone Joint Surg Br* 1999;81:155-162.

42. Pollice PF, Silverton SF, Horowitz SM: Polymethylmethacrylate-stimulated macrophages increase rat osteoclast precursor recruitment through their effect on osteoblasts in vitro. *J Orthop Res* 1995;13:325-334.

43. Maloney WJ, Smith RL, Castro F, Schurman DJ: Fibroblast response to metallic debris in vitro: Enzyme induction, cell proliferation, and toxicity. *J Bone Joint Surg Am* 1993;75:835-844.

44. Manlapaz M, Maloney WJ, Smith RL: In vitro activation of human fibroblasts by retrieved titanium alloy wear debris. *J Orthop Res* 1996;14:465-472.

45. Nakashima Y, Sun D-H, Trindade MC, et al: Signaling pathways for tumor necrosis factor-a and interleukin-6 expression in human macrophages exposed to titanium-alloy particulate debris in vitro. *J Bone Joint Surg Am* 1999;81:603-615.

46. Roebuck KA, Jacobs JJ, Glant TT: New horizons in orthopaedic research: Elucidation of cellular signal transduction pathways. *J Bone Joint Surg Am* 1999;81:599-602.

47. Yao J, Szabo G, Jacobs JJ, Kuettner KE, Glant TT: Suppression of osteoblast function by titanium particles. *J Bone Joint Surg Am* 1997;79:107-112.

48. Goodman S, Aspenberg P, Song Y, et al: Tissue ingrowth and differentiation in the bone-harvest chamber in the presence of cobalt-chromium-alloy and high-density-polyethylene particles. *J Bone Joint Surg Am* 1995;77:1025-1035.

49. Cila E, Alpaslan AM, Melli M, Tokgozoglu AM: Prostaglandin E2 activity in the synovial-like membrane. *J Arthroplasty* 1994;9:67-71.

50. Chiba J, Rubash HE, Kim KJ, Iwaki Y: The characterization of cytokines in the interface tissue obtained from failed cementless total hip arthroplasty with and without femoral osteolysis. *Clin Orthop* 1994;300:304-312.

51. Goodman SB, Huie P, Song Y, et al: Cellular profile and cytokine production at prosthetic interfaces. Study of tissues retrieved from revised hip and knee replacements. *J Bone Joint Surg Br* 1998;803:531-539.

52. Vidovszky TJ, Cabanela ME, Rock MG, Berry DJ, Morrey BF, Bolander ME: Histologic and biochemical differences between osteolytic and nonosteolytic membranes around femoral components of an uncemented total hip arthroplasty. *J Arthroplasty* 1998;13:320-330.

53. Takagi M, Konttinen YT, Lindy O, et al: Gelatinase/type IV collagenases in the loosening of total hip replacement endoprostheses. *Clin Orthop* 1994;306:136-144.

54. Ishiguro N, Ito T, Kurokouchi K, et al: mRNA expression of matrix metalloproteinases and tissue inhibitors of metalloproteinase in interface tissue around implants in loosening total hip arthroplasty. *J Biomed Mater Res* 1996;32: 611-617.

55. Santavirta S, Sorsa T, Konttinen YT, Saari H, Eskola A, Eisen AZ: Role of mesenchymal collagenase in the loosening of total hip prosthesis. *Clin Orthop* 1993;290:206-215.

56. Takagi M, Konttinen, YT, Santavirta S, et al: Elastase activity, uninhibited by alpha 1-antitrypsin, in the periprosthetic connective matrix around loose total hip prostheses. *J Orthop Res* 1995;13:296-304.

57. Takagi M, Konttinen YT, Santavirta S, Kangaspunta P, Suda A, Rokkanen P: Cathepsin G and alpha 1-antichymotrypsin in the local host reaction to loosening of total hip prostheses. *J Bone Joint Surg Am* 1995;77:16-25.

58. Pearson ML, Goodman SB, Huie P, Sibley RK: Inducible nitric oxide synthase messenger RNA levels in hip periprosthetic tissue: A preliminary study. *J Biomed Mater Res* 1998;40:419-424.

59. Sabokbar A, Rushton N: Role of inflammatory mediators and adhesion molecules in the

pathogenesis of aseptic loosening in total hip arthroplasties. *J Arthroplasty* 1995;10:810-816.

60. Kim KJ, Hijikata H, Itoh T, Kumegawa M: Joint fluid from patients with failed total hip arthroplasty stimulates pit formation by mouse osteoclasts on dentin slices. *J Biomed Mater Res* 1998;43:234-240.

61. Granchi D, Verri E, Ciapetti G, et al: Bone-resorbing cytokines in serum of patients with aseptic loosening of hip prostheses. *J Bone Joint Surg Br* 1998;80(suppl 5):912-917.

62. Goodman SB, Fornasier VL, Kei J: The effects of bulk versus particulate polymethylmethacrylate on bone. *Clin Orthop* 1988;232:255-262.

63. Howie DW, Vernon-Roberts B, Oakeshott R, Manthey B: A rat model of resorption of bone at the cement-bone interface in the presence of polyethylene wear particles. *J Bone Joint Surg Am* 1988;70:57-263.

64. Spector M, Shortkroff S, Hsu H-P, Lane N, Sledge CB, Thornhill TS: Tissue changes around loose prostheses. A canine model to investigate the effects of an antiinflammatory agent. *Clin Orthop* 1990;261:140-152.

65. Goodman SB, Chin RC, Magee FP: Prostaglandin E2 production by the membrane surrounding loose and fixated cemented tibial hemiarthroplasties in the rabbit knee. *Clin Orthop* 1992;284:283-287.

66. Turner TM, Urban RM, Sumner DR, Galante JO: Revision, without cement, of aseptically loose, cemented total hip prostheses: Quantitative comparison of the effects of four types of medullary treatment on bone ingrowth in a canine model. *J Bone Joint Surg Am* 1993;75:845-862.

67. Dowd JE, Schwendeman LT, et al: Aseptic loosening in uncemented total hip arthroplasty in a canine model. *Clin Orthop* 1995;319:106-121.

68. Shanbhag AS, Hasselman CT, Rubash HE: Inhibition of wear debris mediated osteolysis in a canine total hip arthroplasty model. *Clin Orthop* 1997;344:33-43.

69. Merkel KD, Erdmann JM, McHugh KP, Abu-Amer Y, Ross FP, Teitelbaum SL: Tumor necrosis factor-alpha mediates orthopedic implant osteolysis. *Am J Pathol* 1999;154:203-210.

70. Horowitz SM, Algan SA, Purdon MA: Pharmacologic inhibition of particulate-induced bone resorption. *J Biomed Mater Res* 1996; 31:91-96.

71. Haynes DR, Rogers SD, Howie DW, Pearcy MJ, Vernon-Roberts B: Drug inhibition of the macrophage response to metal wear particles in vitro. *Clin Orthop* 1996;323:316-326.

72. Glant TT, Jacobs JJ, Mikecz K, et al: Particulate-induced prostaglandin- and cytokine-mediated bone resorption in an experimental system and in failed joint replacements. *Am J Ther* 1996;3:27-41.

73. Dobai JG, Chandrasekaran R, Yao J, et al: Suppressed collagen gene expression and diminished collagen synthesis induced by particulate wear debris in bone marrow-derived osteoblasts are reversed by 1,25(OH)2D3. *Trans Orthop Res Soc* 1999;24:898.

74. Aspenberg P, Van der Vis H: Migration, particles, and fluid pressure: A discussion of causes of prosthetic loosening. *Clin Orthop* 1998;352:75-80.

75. Van der Vis HM, Aspenberg P, Marti RK, Tigchelaar W, Van Noorden CJ: Fluid pressure causes bone resorption in a rabbit model of prosthetic loosening. *Clin Orthop* 1998;350:201-208.

76. Van der Vis H, Aspenberg P, de Kleine R, Tigchelaar W, van Noorden CJ: Short periods of oscillating fluid pressure directed at a titanium-bone interface in rabbits lead to bone lysis. *Acta Orthop Scandinavica* 1998;69:5-10.

77. Van der Vis HM, Aspenberg P, Tigchelaar W, Van Noorden CJ: Mechanical compression of a fibrous membrane surrounding bone causes bone resorption. *Acta Histochem* 1999;101:203-212.

78. Aspenberg P, Herbertsson P: Periprosthetic bone resorption: Particles versus movement. *J Bone Joint Surg Br* 1996;78(suppl 4):641-646.

79. Evans EM: Metal sensitivity as a cause of bone necrosis and loosening of the prosthesis in total joint replacement. *J Bone Joint Surg Br* 1974;56(suppl 4):626-642.

80. Rooker GD, Wilkinson JD: Metal sensitivity in patients undergoing hip replacement: A prospective study. *J Bone Joint Surg Br* 1980;62(suppl 4):502-505.

81. Brown GC, Lockshin MD, Salvati EA, Bullough PG: Sensitivity to metal as a possible cause of sterile loosening after cobalt-chromium total hip-replacement arthroplasty. *J Bone Joint Surg Am* 1977;59:164-168.

82. Gil-Albarova J, Lacleriga A, Barrios C, Canadell J: Lymphocyte response to polymethylmethacrylate in loose total hip prostheses. *J Bone Joint Surg Br* 1992;74(suppl 6):825-830.

83. Wooley P, Petersen S, Song Z, Nasser S: Cellular immune responses to orthopaedic implant materials following cemented total joint replacement. *J Orthop Res* 1997;15:874-880.

84. Santavirta S, Konttinen Y, Bergroth V, Gronblad M: Lack of immune response to methyl methacrylate in lymphocyte cultures. *Acta Orthop Scand* 1991;62:29-32.

85. Santavirta S, Nordström D, Metsärinne K, Konttinen YT: Biocompatibility of polyethylene and host response to loosening of cementless total hip replacement. *Clin Orthop* 1993;297:100-110.

86. Jiranek W, Jasty M, Wang JT, et al: Tissue response to particulate polymethylmethacrylate in mice with various immune deficiencies. *J Bone Joint Surg Am* 1995;77:1650-1661.

87. Charnley J: *Low Friction Arthroplasty of the Hip: Theory and Practice*. New York, NY, Springer, 1979, pp 41-65.

20

Osteolysis of the Femur: Principles of Management

Michael J. Dunbar, MD, FRCSC
Hugh R.L. Blackley, MB, ChB, FRACS
Robert B. Bourne MD, FRCSC

Introduction

Osteolysis, or aseptic loosening, remains the primary reason for long-term failure of total hip arthroplasty (THA).[1,2] Because the number of THAs performed annually is projected to increase by at least 40% in the next three decades,[3] a concomitant increase in the number of hip arthroplasty patients presenting with periprosthetic osteolysis can be anticipated. Therefore, it is important for orthopaedic surgeons to be familiar with this topic.

However, confusion persists regarding fundamental concepts such as nomenclature, and debate continues over pathophysiology and issues of patient management. This chapter will focus primarily on management issues, with the aim of providing a balanced overview.

Nomenclature

The terms "osteolysis" and "aseptic loosening" are often used interchangeably when describing bone loss in association with THA. Sinha and associates[4] point out that the distinction between terms is partly historical and more associated with the different patterns of bone loss seen with cemented and noncemented femoral components. More specifically, aseptic loosening initially referred to the progressive natural history of linear radiolucency associated with previously well-fixed cemented femoral components that led to impending or frank loosening of the prosthesis.[5,6] The term's current connotation is that interfacial bone loss has resulted in a loose implant. This bone loss may be either linear or scalloped. Osteolysis was initially defined as an area of focal radiolucency at the implant-bone or cement-bone interface.[7] This term implies that despite the bone loss, the implant is stable. Linear radiolucencies may progress into focal areas of osteolysis, and focal osteolytic areas may progress until the fixation of either cemented or noncemented components fails. Clearly, there is considerable overlap in the terminology, indicating that both terms represent a spectrum of the same pathologic process.[8,9] Therefore, this chapter will adopt the more precise terminology used by Sinha and associates.[4] Linear osteolysis will refer to what was previously termed aseptic loosening, and focal osteolysis will refer to large scalloped or expansile lesions. The term osteolysis used in isolation can refer to either linear or focal osteolysis.

One or more of the authors or the departments with which they are affiliated have received something of value from a commercial or other party related directly or indirectly to the subject of this chapter.

Pathophysiology

A detailed discussion of the pathophysiology of femoral osteolysis is beyond the scope of this chapter. The reader is instead referred to previous review chapters on this subject.[4,10] Nevertheless, because some aspects of the pathophysiology are important in the management of osteolysis, they warrant discussion.

Particles have been widely attributed as the cause of osteolysis associated with THA.[11-15] Sources of particles include suboptimal polyethylene,[16] modular acetabular components with suboptimal locking mechanisms and/or incomplete backside contact,[17,18] titanium femoral heads,[19,20] 32-mm diameter femoral heads,[21,22] corrosion products and fretting from modular head-neck designs,[17,23] femoral prosthesis burnishing,[24] braided cables,[25] and cement[11,26] (Fig. 1) (Table 1). Particles can interfere with the bearing surfaces and exacerbate wear of the low-friction tribologic coupling, a process that is referred to as third-body wear. Periprosthetic regions that are accessible to joint fluid, and subsequently particles, constitute the effective joint space.[13] Well-fixed noncemented femoral prostheses that have a circumferential porous coat effectively limit the effective joint space.[27] The same is true for intact cement mantles with the appropriate prosthesis.[28,29]

The clinical significance of particles, third-body wear, and effective joint space in the management of femoral osteolysis relates to treatment issues. The effective revision should address these issues directly by eliminating particle generators and reducing the effective joint space.

Although the hypothesis that particles cause osteolysis is essentially an orthopaedic paradigm in North America,

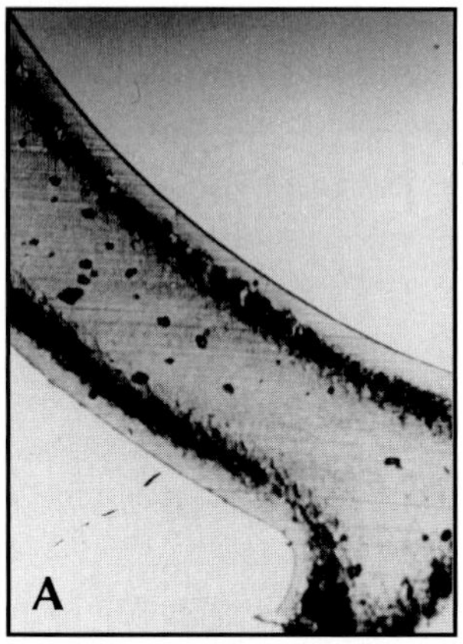

Fig. 1 Sources of particle debris in THA. **A**, Cross-section of polyethylene from an acetabular component demonstrating subsurface laminar oxidation. **B**, Metal acetabular shell with polyethylene liner. Note the considerable polyethylene wear and the fretting at the locking interface (*arrows*). **C**, Cross-section of a metal-backed acetabular component demonstrating poor contact with the polyethylene liner (*arrows*). **D**, Titanium femoral head with advanced asymmetrical wear. **E**, Significant abrasion of a femoral component (*arrows*).

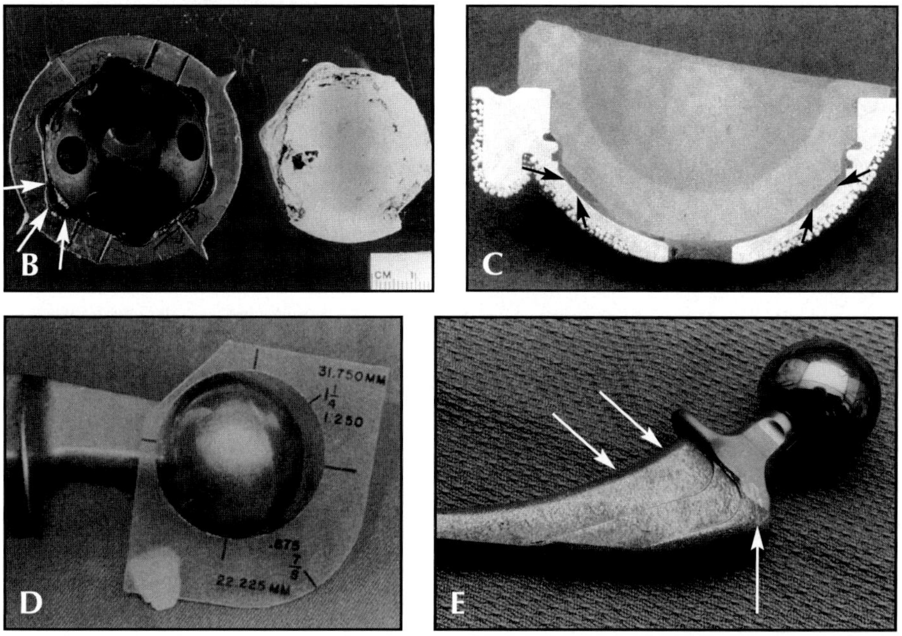

Table 1
Particle generators in THA

Polyethylene
Oxidized secondary to sterilization technique
Poor locking mechanisms in modular cups
Poor contact with counterface wear in modular cups
Titanium femoral heads
32-mm femoral heads
Corrosion or fretting at the head-neck taper
Burnishing of the femoral component
Bone cement
Braided cables

this view is not universal. Some authors believe that the effect of fluid pressure transmitted through the effective joint space is the primary cause for osteolysis and that particles play a secondary role, if any.[29-36]

Clinical Presentation

Osteolysis is the silent disease of orthopaedics and its presentation can be variable.[37] Initially, patients have no clinical symptoms despite radiographic evidence of osteolysis and can remain completely asymptomatic, even in the presence of substantial bone loss.[26,38] Symptoms usually do not occur until the bone loss has reached the point of causing implant loosening, implant failure (fracture), or periprosthetic fracture. However, before any of these events have occurred, patients may present with pain secondary to synovitis induced by wear debris.

When implant loosening, implant failure, or periprosthetic fracture has occurred, the chief presenting symptom is typically pain. In the case of femoral osteolysis, the pain is usually localized to the thigh; pain in the groin or buttocks is more often associated with acetabular pathology. Pain caused by femoral component loosening is typically associated with activity, especially ambulation, and abates with rest. Night pain is uncommon, but it can occur. A periprosthetic fracture typically has a sudden onset of pain brought about with activity. The patient cannot bear weight on the extremity and continues to have pain with rest. The presentation of pain associated with fracture of the prosthesis may vary between sudden onset of continuous pain with inability to bear weight and more gradual onset of activity-related pain that is relieved with rest. The variation in presentation depends on the location of the fracture and the degree to which the resulting mechanically functional aspect of the prosthesis is supported by host bone and/or cement.

Signs associated with implant loosening and implant fracture may include shortening of the extremity and external rotation. During the physical examination, it may be possible to piston the implant within the femoral canal. This test must be performed carefully, especially in the presence of substantial bone loss. The proximal extremity remains aligned without swelling and the incision remains dry and nonerythematous. Periprosthetic fractures may also be associated with external rotation and shortening, but there is usually deformity in the proximal extremity with swelling and pain to direct palpation. An algorithm for the clinical presentation of femoral osteolysis is presented in Figure 2.

Radiographic Presentation

The radiographic presentation of femoral osteolysis is also variable and depends on the access of wear debris to the periprosthetic interface,[13] which in turn depends on the design of the implant and mode of fixation. The pattern is slightly different for both cemented and noncemented implants.

In cemented femoral implants, the development of either focal or linear osteolysis depends primarily on the access of particulate debris and fluid to the periprosthetic environment. Early cementing techniques (first generation) were associated with circumferential osteolysis.[5,11] More modern and improved cementing techniques (second and third generations) have resulted in a substantial reduction in this finding.[39,40] The improved cement mantle is believed to form an effective seal around the implant, restricting the access of fluid and particulate debris generated in the joint.[29] Stem micromotion and cement fractures are also reduced with an improved cementing technique, resulting in a reduction in particle generation. This mechanism can explain the occurrence of proximal focal osteolysis; however, the stem tip osteolysis commonly seen in cemented stems is more difficult to explain.

Anthony and associates[41] have proposed that the high intra-articular pressures generated during the gait cycle force particles and fluid along the cement-implant interface into the distal region where focal osteolysis occurs. Recently, Crawford and associates[28,29] substantiated this theory. An alternative hypothesis by Maloney and Woolson[42] states that local cement debris causes these regions of distal focal osteolysis. They observed that 60% of these distal lesions were associated with a defect in the cement or a thin cement mantle. Histologic examination of tissue retrieved from these regions showed particulate polymethylmethacrylate, supporting the theory that the poorly constructed cement mantle fractured, leading to the production of local cement debris and subsequent focal osteolysis.

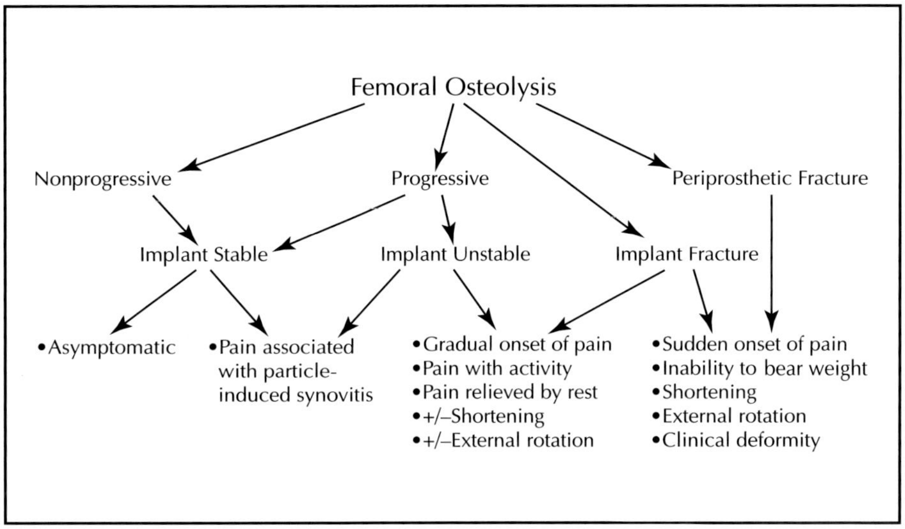

Fig. 2 Algorithm for the clinical presentation of femoral osteolysis.

In noncemented stems, the design features of the implant appear to play a significant role in the radiologic appearance of osteolysis.[27] Implants with patch porous coating or incomplete titanium mesh designs have smooth channels that provide low-resistance pathways for debris and fluid to travel, resulting in mid- to distal focal osteolysis in up to 50% of these stems.[43,44] Designs with circumferential porous coating provide an effective seal against distal migration of debris and fluid, provided that ingrowth occurs.[27] In these designs, the radiographic appearance is of focal osteolysis localized to the greater and lesser trochanter, because this is the area the debris can access.[45,46] However, if ingrowth fails to occur, debris and fluid can gain access to the diaphysis through the noningrowth regions, which has been demonstrated in certain proximally porous-coated stems that did not achieve bone ingrowth where mid and distal osteolysis has occurred.[47] When circumferential bone ingrowth does not occur, so-called fibrous tissue ingrowth stabilization may result, with reactive lines adjacent to the implant. This fibrous tissue may provide a partial barrier to fluid and debris from the joint space. If osteolysis does occur, it tends to be of the linear type, producing an expanding linear line around the component with progressive loss of diaphyseal bone.[6,48]

Differential Diagnosis

Osteolysis is rare within the first 2 years after surgery.[49] Examples in the literature are generally associated with poor components or techniques.[50-54] Infection should be considered in patients presenting with linear or focal osteolysis within this time period. After this early period, infection persists as an important differential diagnosis in the face of radiologic osteolysis. Unfortunately, infection can mimic aseptic osteolysis both radiographically and clinically. Even after a thorough diagnostic evaluation, the distinction between aseptic and septic osteolysis is sometimes difficult to make. Therefore, infection should always be included in the differential diagnosis for periprosthetic femoral osteolysis.

Periprosthetic femoral osteolysis resulting from other causes occurs less often (Table 2). Periprosthetic metastatic carcinoma is a well-described clinical

Table 2
Differential diagnosis for periprosthetic femoral osteolysis

Infection
Metastatic carcinoma
Multiple myeloma
Paget's disease
Lymphoma
Age-related osteoporosis
Stress shielding
Fracture
Idiopathic bone loss
Premature cement mantle failure

entity that can easily be confused with focal osteolysis, often resulting in delays of appropriate oncologic treatment.[55] Multiple myeloma has also been reported to appear as multiple focal osteolytic lesions around a noncemented femoral component.[56] In addition, lymphoma and Paget's disease should be considered in the differential diagnosis, especially given the typical age of hip arthroplasty patients. Stress shielding, age-related bone loss, premature cement mantle failure, and cortical stress fracture should also be considered. Idiopathic bone loss is a very rare cause of osteolysis, particularly in the elderly patient.

Clinical Investigations

History

The work-up for periprosthetic femoral osteolysis begins, as always, with a thorough history. The history of present illness should first be directed at the suspected hip. Symptoms in or around the hip should be elicited. If pain is a component of the presentation, then the onset, location, intensity, and temporal pattern should be determined, especially the presence of nighttime thigh pain. Provoking events, such as weight bearing or activity, as well as palliating events, such as rest and analgesic use, should also be investigated. To objectively quantify patient pain, the type, dose, and frequency of analgesic use should be quantified. The physician must exclude referred sources of pain when obtaining radiographs to investigate hip pain and periprosthetic osteolysis in a patient. Possible sources of referred pain include intra-abdominal, intrapelvic, retroperitoneal, spinal, and inguinal pathology. The physician should ask specific questions pertaining to infection, such as the presence of fevers or chills, wound erythema or drainage, or recent remote foci of infection such as urinary tract infection or major dental manipulation. Questions regarding recent trauma should also be asked. The history of the prosthesis, including time implanted and preoperative diagnosis, should be established, along with a history of complications, including wound problems and revisions. A chart review helps establish the surgical environment in which the prosthesis was implanted (for example, laminar flow and body exhaust suits), antibiotic prophylactic regimen, the implanting surgeon's level of experience, and the type of materials and components used, such as titanium or 32-mm heads and precoated femoral stems. A careful review of body systems is warranted to rule out referred pain, primary or metastatic cancers, or metabolic bone disease.

Physical Examination

The physical examination should begin with an observation of the gait pattern. Hip abductor strength (Trendelenburg sign) should next be tested with the patient in the standing position. Next, with the patient lying comfortably, the general attitude of the extremity should be inspected and leg lengths should be measured. The incision should be examined carefully for signs of infection, including erythema, induration, and breakdown. The joint should be put through a passive and active range of motion so that provocation of pain or signs of instability can be observed. Muscle strength should be assessed. The neurovascular status of the extremity should be determined and an examination of remote joints and the spine should be performed. A general abdominal examination should be performed on patients who have pain.

Additional Investigations

Aseptic linear or focal periprosthetic osteolysis is a diagnosis of exclusion. As mentioned earlier, sepsis is the major differential to aseptic osteolysis. Therefore, this section shall concentrate on investigations that primarily distinguish aseptic osteolysis from septic osteolysis. Special investigations required in the diagnosis of other conditions will not be covered here. The physician must have a high index of suspicion for the more rare disease processes that may mimic periprosthetic osteolysis. Any findings in the history or physical examination that raise the possibility of one of these diagnoses warrants further investigation.

Plain Radiographs The first tests usually available to the orthopaedic surgeon are the anteroposterior and lateral radiographs of the hip. However, the specificity of plain radiographic examination in distinguishing aseptic and septic causes of osteolysis is low. Serial radiographs obtained over a period of time assist in this capacity. Gradual progression of periprosthetic osteolysis with an obvious source of particle generation and increased effective joint space are more likely to represent aseptic osteolysis. In contrast, a previously well-fixed component with no obvious source of particle generation and a rapid onset of osteolysis is more likely to represent infection.

Blood Work A white blood cell (WBC) count, erythrocyte sedimentation rate (ESR), and C-reactive protein (CRP) analysis should be done on all patients in whom the suspicion of infection is raised. Results of these tests should be carefully assessed in patients with inflammatory disorders, collagen vascular disease, malignancies, recent trauma or surgery, remote infections, or an immunocompromised status. An increase in the

WBC count suggests infection; however, patients with a chronic infection may have a normal WBC count. The sensitivity of the test has been reported to be 20%, the specificity 96%, the positive predictive value (ppv) 50%, and the negative predictive value (npv) 85%.[57] An ESR greater than 30 mm/h can be considered elevated.[57,58] The sensitivity of the test has been reported to be 82%, the specificity 85%, the ppv 58%, and the npv 95%.[57] The CRP analysis is perhaps a more sensitive test for infection than the ESR. The CRP levels return to baseline levels within 3 weeks of the index operation, as opposed to more than 40 weeks for the ESR.[59] The sensitivity has been reported as 96%, the specificity 92%, the ppv 74%, and the npv 99%.[57] None of these tests in isolation will yield pathognomonic results for infection. Instead, the results are more useful in ruling out infection, as indicated by the high npv in each. The results of all tests must be considered together and combined with the history and physical examination.

Other Imaging Modalities At this stage, if the diagnosis of infection cannot be excluded, we believe that the most appropriate next step is to perform a hip aspiration. Other investigations have been recommended, including MRI, technetium Tc 99m, Indium-111, gallium-67, and immunoglobulin G bone scans. These tests are expensive, sometimes difficult to obtain, difficult to interpret with hip arthroplasty, and add little to the diagnostic algorithm.[60-62] A more detailed discussion of these issues can be found in a previous review by Spangehl and associates.[57]

Hip Aspiration Hip aspirations are performed under fluoroscopic guidance with sterile technique. Administration of antibiotics should cease 3 weeks prior to aspiration. An arthrogram is performed to ensure that the needle is in the joint. A localized pooling of contrast material may suggest an abscess. A local anesthetic with antibiotic preservatives should not be used. Ideally, three samples are drawn and sent for immediate culture. If results of all three samples are positive for the same organism, then a diagnosis of infection is made. If only two cultures are positive for the same organism, the results are assessed with respect to the history, physical examination, and the previous investigations. If the index of suspicion for infection before the aspiration is high, the aspiration results are considered positive. If not, the aspiration is repeated. If only one culture is positive, the aspiration is repeated. Spangehl and associates[57] provide a more detailed description of the hip aspiration technique. A sensitivity of 86%, specificity of 94%, ppv of 67%, and an npv of 98% have been reported using this technique.[57]

Intraoperative Investigations

Even if all of the above mentioned investigations fail to exclude the diagnosis of infection, tissue should be obtained for frozen section at the time of revision surgery. Ideally, tissue should be acquired from the pseudocapsule, retroacetabular space, and the femoral canal. We prefer to collect at least five soft-tissue specimens. All samples should be labeled and sent for immediate assessment to an experienced pathologist. Five polymorphonuclear leukocytes (PMNL) per high-powered field has been advocated as suggestive of infection.[63] In an effort to improve the specificity of this test, some authors have recommended that 10 PMNLs per high-powered field should indicate infection.[64] We instead rely on the pathologist's assessment as to whether acute or chronic inflammation is present. This assessment is more precise than relying on the number of PMNLs and has worked well over the years. The surgeon must establish a good working relationship with the pathology group that will be interpreting the results.

Tissue and swabs should be collected from the surgical site and sent for culture and sensitivity; however, the results of these tests will not be available to guide the intraoperative management of the patient.

Principles of Clinical Management

Several considerations must be taken into account when managing the patient with osteolysis. The first practical consideration is whether the patient is symptomatic or asymptomatic. The decision to operate is easier, for both surgeon and patient, if the patient is symptomatic. This decision is related in part to the degree of pain as well as other factors. Generally, after other causes of pain have been excluded, a symptomatic patient will have a loose component. The next issue is determining which component(s) is loose. Sometimes this is obvious; however, more often it is difficult to determine whether at least one of the components is loose.

Harris and associates[7] have assigned three categories of radiologic criteria of cemented stem stability. If there is evidence of subsidence or radiolucency at the stem-cement interface, cement mantle fracture, or a stem fracture, the stem is considered definitely loose. A complete cement-bone radiolucent line indicates that the stem is probably loose. If there is a cement-bone radiolucent line greater than 50% but less than 100%, the stem is possibly loose. These definitions must be carefully applied to prostheses that are designed to subside.[65] Because of a greater variety of designs and modes of loosening in noncemented stems, categories of looseness are not as well defined. In porous-coated components, successful bone ingrowth signs include endosteal spot welds, an absence of reactive lines, proximal stress shielding, and an increase in cortical density at the stem tip.[66] Definite loosening is demonstrated by progressive implant migration greater than 2 mm, especially if it occurs more than 6 months postoperatively.[67] A potentially unstable implant is demonstrated by widening circumferential radiolucencies, divergent reactive lines, the absence of proximal stress shielding, shedding of the porous beads, calcar hypertrophy, and pedestal formation. Similar criteria apply for cemented and noncemented acetabular cups,[6,68] but these criteria may be even less reliable than on the femoral side.[68] A good general rule for surgery is to plan to revise the loose component, but have all the equipment available to revise the other component if it also is found to be loose intraoperatively.

In the asymptomatic patient, the decision to operate is more difficult, and many factors need to be considered. These factors include the patient's age, activity level and medical status, the location of the lesion, its size, and the likelihood that it will progress to the extent of causing significant complications. Most osteolysis is progressive,[69] although the rate of progression is variable, and some lesions remain static for years.[70] These lesions rarely have been reported to regress.[71] It is prudent to consider all lesions as progressive until proven otherwise. Serial radiographic examinations every 3 to 6 months help document progression. Surgery is usually indicated if the lesion is large and progressive, particularly if it is eroding the cortex adjacent to the distal aspect of the stem. However, patient factors, especially medical risk, play an important role in the analysis of benefit versus risk. Knowledge of the implant's predilection to osteolysis and the location of osteolysis can be useful, particularly in the noncemented implant. For example, in extensively porous-coated ingrown stems, the osteolytic lesions occur primarily in Gruen zones 1 and 7 (the greater and lesser trochanter) and do not result in loosening.[45,46] Occasionally, these lesions have resulted in fractures of the greater trochanter.[72] A well-fixed stem is difficult to remove and often causes further bone loss. In this scenario, curettage and grafting of the lesions, retention of the stem, and exchange of the femoral head and acetabular liner may be appropriate, although there are no long-term data on this technique. In the asymptomatic elderly, the sedentary, or the medically unfit patient, simple observation of these lesions is a reasonable approach.

Patch-coated components that allow the joint fluid to reach the diaphysis present with more distal osteolysis, which tends to be progressive, causing diaphyseal bone loss and eventual loosening.[71,73,74] These stems should be revised, preferably before structural defects become so advanced that large allografts are needed or periprosthetic fracture occurs. Cavitary lesions at and distal to the stem should be revised early because of the increased risk of periprosthetic fracture in this location. The pattern of osteolysis is also important. Linear osteolysis tends to lead to earlier symptomatic loosening. Local expansile osteolysis extending away from the implant into the corticocancellous bone tends to result in greater bone loss before loosening and symptoms occur. Linear and local expansile osteolyses are usually more difficult to revise and have the greater potential for fracture. The physician must be aware that assessment with plain radiographs often underestimates the amount of bone loss.

In addition to curettage and grafting the lesion and/or revising the stem, the source of the debris, the so-called particle generators, should be removed or at least modified. Modification includes acetabular revision or minimally changing the polyethylene in well-fixed cups. Those cups with a history of a poor locking mechanism causing wear debris should probably be revised even if they are well ingrown. Titanium heads should be replaced with cobalt-chromium-molybdenum (Co-Cr-Mo) heads and downsized to 28- or 26-mm diameters. Damaged modular heads should be exchanged. Revision of monoblock titanium stems and stems with a damaged Morse taper should be considered.

Classification of Femoral Osteolysis

There are numerous revision classifications, most of which are based on the femoral bone deficiency. The American Academy of Orthopaedic Surgeons classification is one of the more popular and comprehensive.[75] According to this system, type I includes segmental defects, type II includes cavitary defects, and type III includes combined segmental and cavitary defects. Malalignment, stenosis, and discontinuity characterize types IV, V, and VI, respectively. Each category is also assigned a level and a grade. Level I lesions are proximal to the inferior aspect of the lesser trochanter, level II lesions extend up to 10 cm distal to the lesser trochanter, and level III lesions are distal to this. Grade I indicates minimum bone loss, grade II indicates moderate bone loss, and grade III indicates the need for structural bone grafting in order for the revision to be successful. Although useful, we find this classification rather complex for everyday surgical planning in revision surgery. We tend to revert to a simple but practical classification based on the cancellous bone quality and the intactness of the cortical tube (Table 3). Our classification is useful because it relates to the type of revision implant that can be used. Generally, the amount of bone loss and the location dictates the type of revision component used and the surgical technique. However, this decision is also influenced by patient factors, such as age and activity level, and whether the implant is well-fixed. Removal of well-ingrown noncemented implants can cause substantial bone loss.

Preoperative Planning

Preoperative planning is a critical determinant for a successful postoperative outcome and its importance cannot be overemphasized. Ideally, this planning should take place the week before the surgery with the key members of the surgical team present. The first principle in planning is to establish the mode of failure, including a final review of the relevant history, physical examination, and laboratory tests to ensure that

Table 3
Bourne-Rorabeck classification of femoral bone deficiency

Defect Type	Bone Description Cancellous	Cortical
1	Intact	Intact
2	Deficient	Intact
3	Deficient	Deficient
4	Absent	Absent

infection has been ruled out. Only by identifying the mechanism of failure can deliberate steps be taken to ensure that the same situation is not recreated postoperatively. Next, the assessment of the bony defects is made to assist in the selection of implants and the method of fixation. Again, we find the simple classification proposed here useful in this capacity. Surgical exposure options are discussed, and special emphasis is placed on whether extended surgical exposures will be required in order to achieve the preoperative goals. Resources are also assessed at this time to determine if special equipment or prosthetic components will be required. We recommend developing a primary plan, and two contingency plans at this time for both anticipated and unanticipated complications, especially if the removal of the prosthesis results in a higher class of defect. We refer to these as plans A, B, and C. A treatment algorithm is outlined in Figure 3.

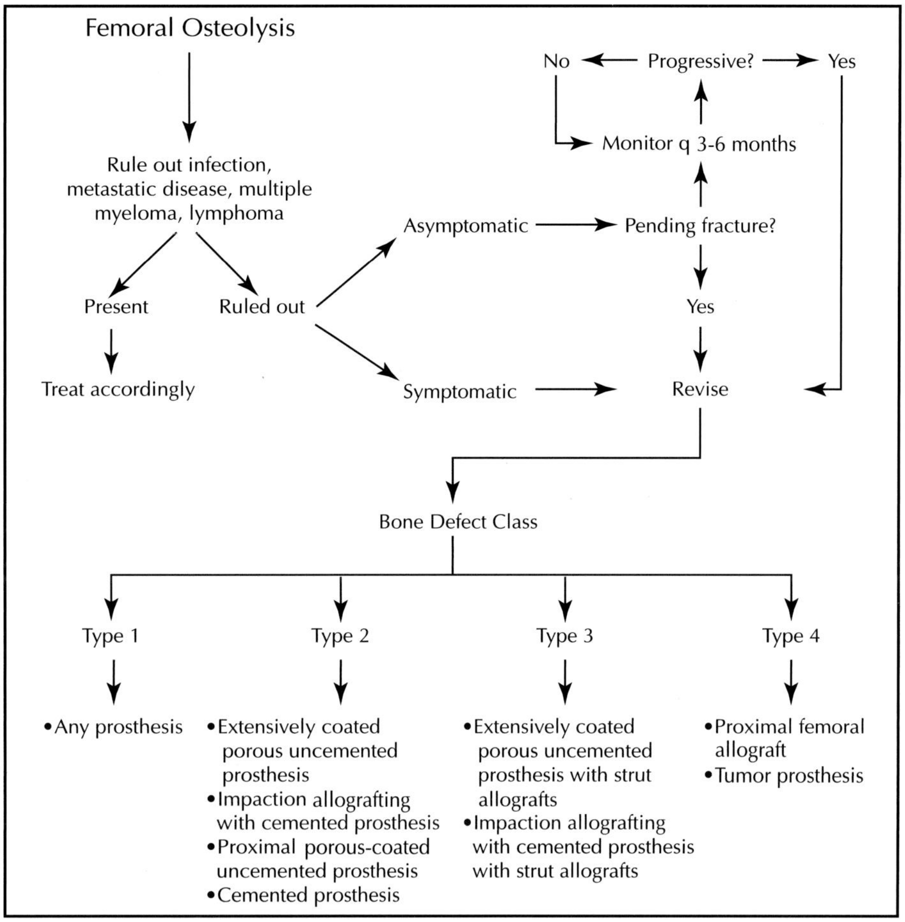

Fig. 3 Algorithm for the management of femoral osteolysis.

Surgical Treatment and Results

Type 1: Intact Cancellous Bone and Cortical Tube

In patients with an undamaged femoral cortical tube and well-preserved cancellous bone, virtually any primary stem, cemented or noncemented, can be used. Typically, this type of defect is seen after a failed surface replacement arthroplasty of a press-fit endoprosthesis. The surgeon can approach this case like any other primary femoral arthroplasty. Generally, the results are similar to a primary arthroplasty (Fig. 4).

Type 2: Deficient Cancellous Bone and an Intact Cortical Tube

This type of femoral revision is more common. The femoral tube is intact but the cancellous bone is deficient so that it will not adequately support a primary femoral component (Fig. 5). Typically, this pattern is seen with linear osteolysis around a cemented stem, resulting in loss of cancellous bone and subsequent implant loosening. Occasionally, the pattern may be seen in a noncemented implant that has failed to obtain bony ingrowth. The cortical tube remains intact with removal of the implant. However, the proximal cancellous bone is inadequate to allow successful interdigitation of cement or bone ingrowth using primary femoral implants. Treatment options include a cemented prosthesis, a proximally porous-coated noncemented prosthesis, an extensively coated porous prosthesis, and impaction allografting with a cemented prosthesis.

The results of recementing into the cancellous bone with early cementing techniques have been disappointing; re-revision or impending failure rates of nearly 40% occurred at a mean of less than 5 years.[67,76] Results were even worse if patients had undergone a previous revision. Kavanagh and Fitzgerald[77] reported a 50% clinical or radiographic failure at an average 3-year follow-up. These poor results are believed to be related to the poor bone cement interface secondary to the smooth endosteal femoral surface. The Swedish Hip Registry reported a re-revision or radiographically loose implant in 38% of 202 patients at 7 years follow-up using early cementing techniques.[78] With better

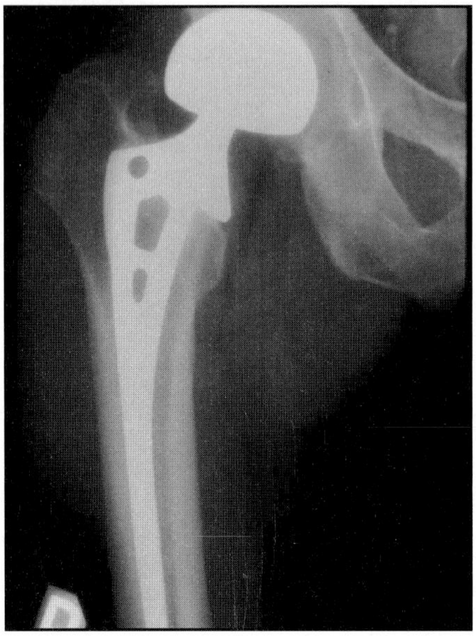

Fig. 4 Type 1 femoral defect with cancellous and cortical bone mostly intact.

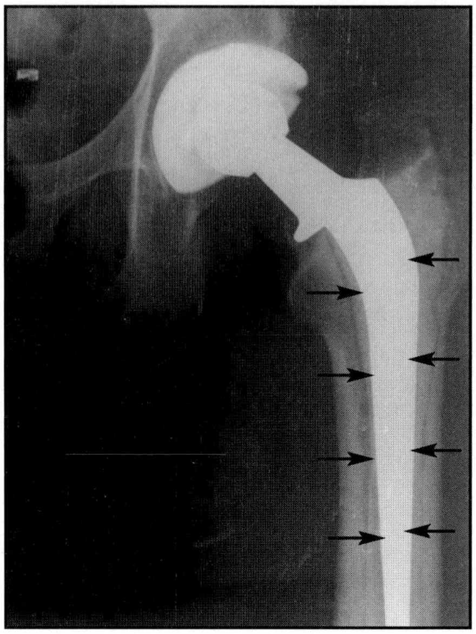

Fig. 5 Type 2 femoral defect. Circumferential osteolysis around the cement mantle is noted (*arrows*).

cementing techniques and the use of longer stems to obtain cement fixation in the distal undamaged cancellous bone, the results have improved. Mulroy and Harris[39] reported a combined loosening and femoral revision rate of 26% in 43 consecutive patients at an average 15 years follow-up. The best results are in patients older than 60 years.[39]

The results of proximal porous-coated stems in this type of deficiency are variable and depend first on the ability to obtain an initial stable fit and then bone ingrowth. Good results are often difficult if there is significant loss of cancellous bone and distortion of the proximal anatomy. Hedley and associates[79] reported a 9.5% loosening rate with the porous coated anatomic stem after 1 year, while Harris and associates[80] reported a 4% rate after a minimum 2-year period with the Harris-Galante component. If the metaphyseal damage extends to the diaphysis, distal rotational stability added to a proximally fixed component or a distally fixed component is required. Results using these components have been superior and are discussed in the next section.

An alternative method of revision is to reconstitute the cancellous bone with impaction grafting. Gie and associates[81] reported good early results with this technique in 56 hips at 18 to 49 months, while Elting and associates[82] reported similar results in an additional 56 hips between 2 and 5 years. Although this technique shows promise, and retrieval and histologic data confirm bone reconstruction, there are some concerns. These concerns include the lack of long-term studies, the high complication rate (such as femoral fracture), a steep learning curve, and the incidence of severe subsidence and its significance.[83-85] However, the technique is a very useful addition to the list of surgical options. The major indication of its use for many surgeons is the patient who needs bone stock restoration and in whom distal fixation is difficult to achieve. This patient is typically younger than age 65 with a large (greater than 20 mm diameter) patulous diaphysis and in whom less than 4 cm of diaphyseal fit can be obtained or in whom proximal stress shielding or thigh pain from modulus mismatch are major concerns.

Type 3: Deficient Cancellous Bone and Cortical Tube

Type 3 defects typically are seen with expansile osteolysis where cortical erosion has occurred (Fig. 6, *A*) or where the osteolysis has become so advanced that a periprosthetic fracture has occurred (Fig. 7). Removal of a well-fixed noncemented component can result in accidental or intentional cortical tube defect, transforming a type 2 defect into a type 3 defect. Treatment options for type 3 defects include an extensively coated porous prosthesis, calcar replacing prosthesis, impaction allografting with cemented prosthesis (Fig. 6, *B* and *C*), and long-stem cemented revisions, all with or without cortical strut graft augmentation.

Because of the deficiencies in the proximal femur, distal stabilization of the implant is important. If a cemented component is used, it should pass the most distal cortical defect by at least two to three cortical diameters.[86] Defects in the cortex make obtaining adequate cement pressurization difficult, and cement can extrude into the soft tissues. Often, to gain adequate fixation, the long-stem femoral component must extend distal to the isthmus of the femur. In the region of the metaphyseal flare, the effectiveness of the cement restrictor is decreased; therefore, therefore, effective cement pressurization is reduced. In the presence of significant cortical bone loss, these cemented revisions can be very difficult to perform and even more difficult to revise. Even with modern cementing techniques, the incidence of revision or radiographic loosening is 15% at a mean of 9.4 years[87] and 22% at 11.9 years.[88] In patients with extensive osteolysis and in young or high-demand patients, other techniques should probably be considered.

Another option is the reconstruction of the cortical tube with wire mesh

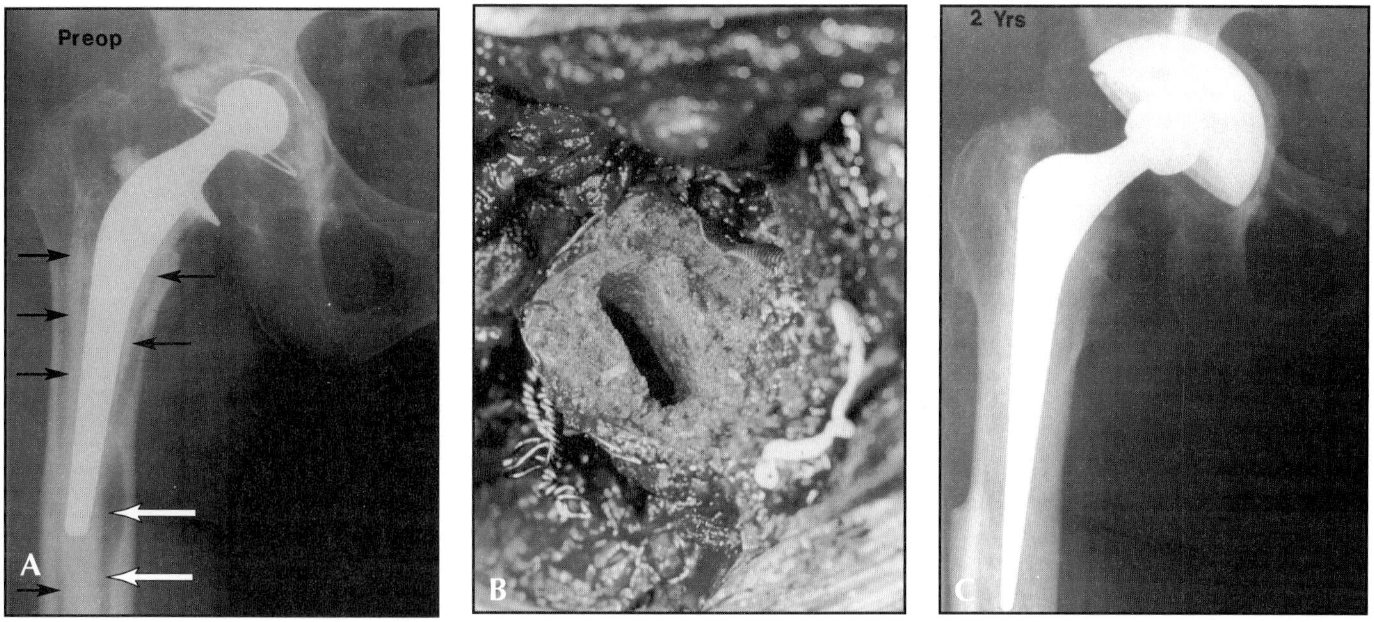

Fig. 6 Type 3 femoral defect. **A,** Cemented femoral component with circumferential osteolysis (*black arrows*) and a focal area of cortical deficiency (*white arrows*). **B,** Intraoperative photograph of the same femur after the impaction allografting. **C,** Radiograph obtained 2 years after surgery shows a successful impaction allograft revision with cemented stem and strut allograft.

or allograft struts followed by restoration of the cancellous bone with impaction grafting. This technique, as discussed above, has good early to intermediate results but there is a steep learning curve for the physician performing it. For this technique to be suitable, femoral defects include a proximal segmental defect that can be easily converted into a contained defect and a distal defect that can be bypassed by the stem. However, the indications for using this technique are being expanded to include larger and more diaphyseal defects.[83-85] Such distal defects, particularly at the stem tip, are associated with a higher risk of postoperative fracture[82] and subsidence.[83] The originators of the technique have expressed concern about the expanding indications and its use in advanced bone loss.[89]

The inability to obtain proximal fit and initial stability with proximally stabilized components has led to the concept of obtaining initial implant stability with diaphyseal fit. This fit can be obtained with a fully coated porous surface or distal fluting. The results of revision with a fully porous coated stem have been good for the intermediate term. Moreland and Bernstein[90] reported a femoral re-revision rate of 4% and a mechanical loosening rate of 4% in 175 patients with a mean follow-up of 5 years. Paprosky and Krishnamurthy[91] reported a re-revision rate of 6% at a mean follow-up of 5.8 years in a series of 311 patients with severe proximal bone loss. More recently, Engh and associates[92] reported on the revision of 21 symptomatically loose porous-coated femoral components replaced with Anatomic Medullary Locking Stems (DePuy, Warsaw, IN). At 6.3 years follow-up, the average preoperative Harris Hip Score had doubled, none of the femoral components had shown radiographic or clinical signs of repeat loosening, and none had been rerevised.

Bone deficiencies can be treated a number of ways. Significant calcar deficiencies are best restored with a calcar-replacing prosthesis, as opposed to calcar allografts. Allan and associates[93] noted that 50% of calcar allografts less than 3 cm long underwent significant radiographic resorption at an average of 36

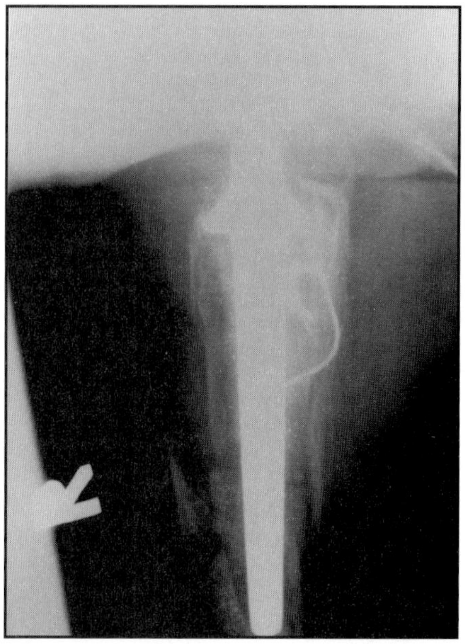

Fig 7 Lateral radiograph of a type 3 femur with extensive osteolysis and associated periprosthetic fracture.

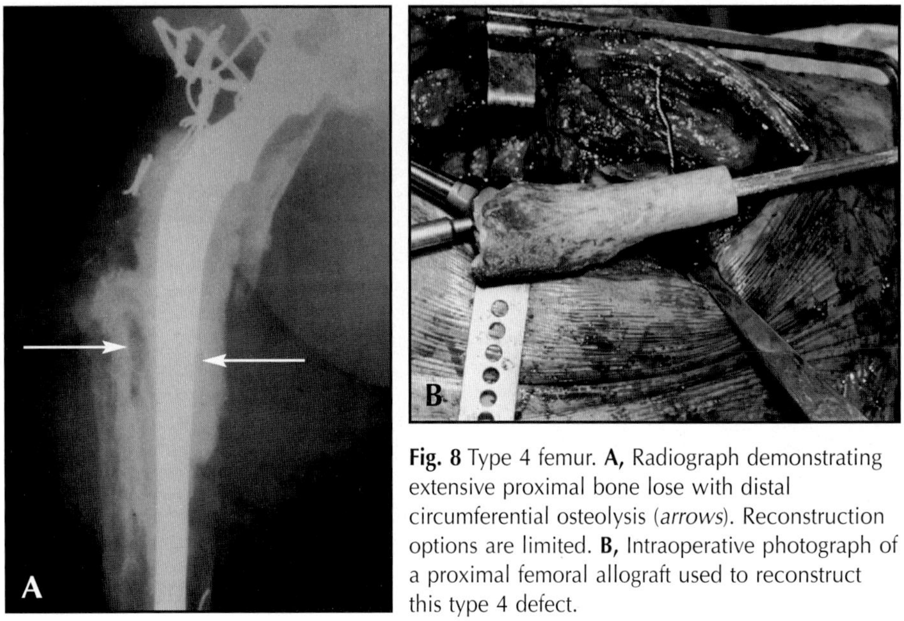

Fig. 8 Type 4 femur. **A,** Radiograph demonstrating extensive proximal bone lose with distal circumferential osteolysis (*arrows*). Reconstruction options are limited. **B,** Intraoperative photograph of a proximal femoral allograft used to reconstruct this type 4 defect.

months. Contained bone defects can be filled with morcellized allograft bone, and noncircumferential structural defects can be restored with strut allografts. Hozack and associates[94] monitored 154 femoral osteolytic defects radiographically in 59 total hip revision arthroplasties treated with fully porous coated revision stems. At 2 to 5 years follow-up, 27 defects had stabilized, 65 had regressed, and 62 healed. The response of the lesion did not appear to be related to the cancellous allografting. Slow remodeling around a well-fixed porous ingrowth stem was noted. A number of authors have reported on the success of cortical strut allografts.[27,95] Head and associates[95] reported 98% of onlay cortical struts united with radiologic evidence of revascularization in a series of 174 patients.

Type 4: Absent Cancellous Bone and Cortical Tube

This type of deficiency is the least common and is usually found in the patient who has undergone multiple revisions (Fig. 8, *A*). Fortunately, in most revisions there is enough diaphysis for 4 to 6 cm of diaphyseal "scratch" fit, and the proximal deficiency is such that it can be reconstructed, often with strut allografts. However, in patients with a type 4 deficiency, there is insufficient bone into which to secure an implant. One option in such a situation is to use a long-stem prosthesis cemented into a proximal or distal femoral allograft (Fig. 8, *B*). This implant/allograft construct is then prefit into the native distal femoral canal. The host-graft junction consists of a step cut stabilized by the stem and strut allografts held with cerclage wires and autologous bone grafting to encourage union. Another option in the deficient bone with a tumor is to replace it with a custom prosthesis. Both these options have high complication rates; however, in many patients they are the only solution to severe osteolytic bone loss.

The general indications for an allograft-implant composite are circumferential bone loss greater than 5 cm in a femur that will not support distal fixation. Clinically, this situation is most commonly seen with multiply revised femoral components, failed tumor prostheses, failed distal fixation of long-stemmed revision prostheses (cemented or noncemented), and femurs with insufficient diaphysis to allow 5 cm of ingrowth or femurs that are too deficient or patulous for impaction grafting.

Gross and associates[96] reported on 168 proximal femoral allografts with an average follow-up of 4.8 years and a re-revision rate of 10%, predominantly because of infection, graft nonunion, or dislocation. More recently, the same group reported on 63 revision hip arthroplasties with a proximal femoral allograft-prosthesis construct with an average follow-up of 11 years. The mean size of the allograft was 15 cm (range, 10 to 22 cm). The allograft-prosthesis composite survivorship was 87%. No failures occurred as a result of allograft resorption.[97]

The use of a metal component as a substitute for missing bone resulting from a tumor or custom prosthesis has some disadvantages. These disadvantages include instability because of poor soft-tissue attachment;[98,99] late fatigue fracture;[100] early loosening because of a stem that is only distally fixed;[101] severe stress shielding and difficulty with fixation especially in the large diameter or short diaphysis.[102,103] Finally, these "megaprostheses" are very difficult to revise, resulting in further destruction of the host bone stock and soft-tissue attachments.[104]

Malkani and associates[105] reported a survivorship of 73% at 11 years in 49 patients with a proximal femoral replacement prosthesis used for failed THAs with massive proximal bone loss. At 12 years, the survivorship with revision as the end point was 64%.[98] However, dislocation was a significant problem in 11 of the hips. The authors recommend limiting the use of a proximal femoral replacement prosthesis to the elderly and inactive patient.

Future Directions

Outcome studies associated with the Swedish Hip Arthroplasty Registry have effected a fourfold reduction in the revision rate over the last 15 years by identifying patient and prostheses risk factors and the efficacy of improved surgical techniques.[1] The establishment of other national arthroplasty registries has the potential to lower revision rates in the host countries as well as contributing to collective orthopaedic knowledge.

Pharmacotherapy with bisphosphonates has shown some promise in treating osteolysis. Alendronate has been shown to supress bone turnover and can be successful in the treatment of Paget's disease.[106] The application of alendronate in animal models of osteolysis has produced differing results. Wang and associates[107] demonstrated short-term inhibition of a particle-induced osteolytic canine model. Astrand and Aspenberg,[108] however, found no inhibition of bone resorption in an instability-induced osteolytic rat model. Bisphosphonates, including alendronate, will continue to be tested in this application and may ultimately play a role in the management of osteolysis.

The number of hip arthroplasties performed in the United Kingdom over the next 30 years is estimated to increase by 40%.[3] This estimation is attributed to demographic changes in the population and does not account for a continuous increase in the threshold for hip arthroplasty surgery, which is likely. Therefore, regardless of improvement in surgical technique or prosthesis design, the establishment of national arthroplasty registries, or advances in pharmacotherapy, the orthopaedic surgeon will continue to be confronted for the foreseeable future with difficult revision hip arthroplasties involving various degrees of periprosthetic osteolysis.

Summary

Femoral osteolysis is and will remain an important cause of THA failures. The presentation is initially radiographic and patients may or may not become symptomatic. If so, pain is the most common symptom. Infection is the most common differential diagnosis and must be excluded. Osteolysis is usually progressive and may eventually lead to loss of implant fixation, implant fracture, or periprosthetic fracture. Multiple factors influence the decision to revise a femoral component, including the degree and type of bone loss, the rate at which it is progressing, the potential for fracture, the degree of symptoms, especially pain, and the activity level and general health of the patient. There are many options for revising failed femoral stems, each with varying degrees of success. The choice of technique and prosthesis used in the revision can be guided by a simple bone defect classification presented in this chapter. Revision of femoral components in these patients can be fraught with complications and poor results; hence, the importance of preoperative planning cannot be overemphasized.

References

1. Herberts P, Malchau H: How outcome studies have changed total hip arthroplasty practices in Sweden. *Clin Orthop* 1997;344:44-60.
2. Malchau H, Herberts P, Ahnfelt L: Prognosis of total hip replacement in Sweden: Follow-up of 92,675 operations performed 1978-1990. *Acta Orthop Scand* 1993;64:497-506.
3. Birrell F, Johnell O, Silman A: Projecting the need for hip replacement over the next three decades: Influence of changing demography and threshold for surgery. *Ann Rheum Dis* 1999;58:569-572.
4. Sinha RK, Shanbhag AS, Maloney WJ, Hasselman CT, Rubash HE: Osteolysis: Cause and effect. *Instr Course Lect* 1998;47:307-320.
5. Gruen TA, McNeice GM, Amstutz HC: "Modes of failure" of cemented stem-type femoral components: A radiographic analysis of loosening. *Clin Orthop* 1979;141:17-27.
6. Hodgkinson JP, Shelley P, Wroblewski BM: The correlation between the roentgenographic appearance and operative findings at the bone-cement junction of the socket in Charnley low friction arthroplasties. *Clin Orthop* 1988;228:105-109.
7. Harris WH, Schiller AL, Scholler JM, Freiberg RA, Scott R: Extensive localized bone resorption in the femur following total hip replacement. *J Bone Joint Surg Am* 1976;58:612-618.
8. Kim KJ, Rubash HE, Wilson SC, D'Antonio JA, McClain EJ: A histologic and biochemical comparison of the interface tissues in cementless and cemented hip prostheses. *Clin Orthop* 1993;287:142-152.
9. Shanbhag AS, Jacobs JJ, Black J, Galante JO, Glant TT: Cellular mediators secreted by interfacial membranes obtained at revision total hip arthroplasty. *J Arthroplasty* 1995;10:498-506.
10. Rubash HE, Sinha RK, Maloney WJ, Paprosky WG: Osteolysis: Surgical treatment. *Instr Course Lect* 1998;47:321-329.
11. Willert HG, Bertram H, Buchhorn GH: Osteolysis in alloarthroplasty of the hip: The role of bone cement fragmentation. *Clin Orthop* 1990;258:108-121.
12. Amstutz HC, Campbell P, Kossovsky N, Clarke IC: Mechanism and clinical significance of wear debris-induced osteolysis. *Clin Orthop* 1992;276:7-18.
13. Schmalzried TP, Jasty M, Harris WH: Periprosthetic bone loss in total hip arthroplasty: Polyethylene wear debris and the concept of the effective joint space. *J Bone Joint Surg Am* 1992;74:849-863.
14. Rubash HE, Sinha RK, Shanbhag AS, Kim SY: Pathogenesis of bone loss after total hip arthroplasty. *Orthop Clin North Am* 1998;29:173-186.
15. Maloney WJ, Smith RL, Castro F, Schurman DJ: Fibroblast response to metallic debris in vitro: Enzyme induction cell proliferation, and toxicity. *J Bone Joint Surg Am* 1993;75:835-844.
16. Sutula LC, Collier JP, Saum KA, et al: Impact of gamma sterilization on clinical performance of polyethylene in the hip. *Clin Orthop* 1995;319:28-40.
17. Bobyn JD, Tanzer M, Krygier JJ, Dujovne AR, Brooks CE: Concerns with modularity in total hip arthroplasty. *Clin Orthop* 1994;298:27-36.
18. Mulliken BD, Bourne RB, Rorabeck CH, Nayak N: Results of the cementless Mallory-Head primary total hip arthroplasty: A 5 to 7 year review. *Iowa Orthop J* 1996;16:20-34.
19. Lombardi AV Jr, Mallory TH, Vaughn BK, Drouillard P: Aseptic loosening in total hip arthroplasty secondary to osteolysis induced by wear debris from titanium-alloy modular femoral heads. *J Bone Joint Surg Am* 1989;71:1337-1342.
20. Buly RL, Huo MH, Salvati E, Brien W, Bansal M: Titanium wear debris in failed cemented total hip arthroplasty: An analysis of 71 cases. *J Arthroplasty* 1992;7:315-323.
21. Hirakawa K, Bauer TW, Stulberg BN, Wilde AH, Secic M: Characterization and comparison of wear debris from failed total hip implants of different types. *J Bone Joint Surg Am* 1996;78:1235-1243.
22. Devane PA, Horne JG, Martin K, Coldham G, Krause B: Three-dimensional polyethylene wear of a press-fit titanium prosthesis: Factors influencing generation of polyethylene debris. *J Arthroplasty* 1997;12:256-266.
23. Urban RM, Jacobs JJ, Gilbert JL, Galante JO: Migration of corrosion products from modular hip prostheses: Particle microanalysis and histopathological findings. *J Bone Joint Surg Am* 1994;76:1345-1359.
24. Jasty M, Bragdon C, Jiranek W, Chandler H, Maloney W, Harris WH: Etiology of osteolysis around porous-coated cementless total hip arthroplasties. *Clin Orthop* 1994;308:111-126.
25. Hop JD, Callaghan JJ, Olejniczak JP, Pedersen DR, Brown TD, Johnston RC: Contribution of cable debris generation to accelerated polyethylene wear. *Clin Orthop* 1997;344:20-32.

26. Maloney WJ, Jasty M, Rosenberg A, Harris WH: Bone lysis in well-fixed cemented femoral components. *J Bone Joint Surg Br* 1990;72:966-970.

27. Emerson RH Jr, Sanders SB, Head WC, Higgins L: Effect of circumferential plasma-spray porous coating on the rate of femoral osteolysis after total hip arthroplasty. *J Bone Joint Surg Am* 1999;81: 1291-1298.

28. Crawford RW, Psychoyios V, Gie G, Ling R, Murray D: Incomplete cement mantles in the sagittal femoral plane: An anatomical explanation. *Acta Orthop Scand* 1999;70:596-598.

29. Crawford RW, Evans M, Ling RS, Murray DW: Fluid flow around model femoral components of differing surface finishes: In vitro investigations. *Acta Orthop Scand* 1999;70:589-595.

30. Aspenberg P, van der Vis H: Fluid pressure may cause periprosthetic osteolysis: Particles are not the only thing. *Acta Orthop Scand* 1998;69:1-4.

31. Aspenberg P, Van der Vis H: Migration, particles, and fluid pressure: A discussion of causes of prosthetic loosening. *Clin Orthop* 1998;352: 75-80.

32. Aspenberg P: Letter: Wear and osteolysis in total joint replacements. *Acta Orthop Scand* 1998;69:435-436.

33. Mjöberg B: Theories of wear and loosening in hip prostheses: Wear-induced loosening vs loosening-induced wear. A review. *Acta Orthop Scand* 1994;65:361-371.

34. Robertsson O, Wingstrand H, Kesteris U, Jonsson K, Onnerfalt R: Intracapsular pressure and loosening of hip prostheses: Preoperative measurements in 18 hips. *Acta Orthop Scand* 1997;68:231-234.

35. van der Vis H, Aspenberg P, de Kleine R, Tigchelaar W, van Noorden CJ: Short periods of oscillating fluid pressure directed at a titanium-bone interface in rabbits lead to bone lysis. *Acta Orthop Scand* 1998;69:5-10.

36. Van der Vis HM, Aspenberg P, Marti RK, Tigchelaar W, Van Noorden CJ: Fluid pressure causes bone resorption in a rabbit model of prosthetic loosening. *Clin Orthop* 1998;350:201-208.

37. Engh GA, Ammeen DJ: Clinical manifestations of a sometimes silent disease. *Orthopedics* 1999;22:799-801.

38. Maloney WJ, Jasty M, Harris WH, Galante JO, Callaghan JJ: Endosteal erosion in association with stable uncemented femoral components. *J Bone Joint Surg Am* 1990;72:1025-1034.

39. Mulroy WF, Harris WH: Revision total hip arthroplasty with use of so-called second-generation cementing techniques for aseptic loosening of the femoral component: A fifteen-year-average follow-up study. *J Bone Joint Surg Am* 1996;78:325-330.

40. Mulroy RD Jr, Harris WH: The effect of improved cementing techniques on component loosening in total hip replacement: An 11-year radiographic review. *J Bone Joint Surg Br* 1990;72:757-760.

41. Anthony PP, Gie GA, Howie CR, Ling RS: Localised endosteal bone lysis in relation to the femoral components of cemented total hip arthroplasties. *J Bone Joint Surg Br* 1990;72:971-979.

42. Maloney WJ, Woolson ST: Increasing incidence of femoral osteolysis in association with uncemented Harris-Galante total hip arthroplasty: A follow-up report. *J Arthroplasty* 1996;11:130-134.

43. Bobyn JD, Jacobs JJ, Tanzer M, et al: The susceptibility of smooth implant surfaces to periimplant fibrosis and migration of polyethylene wear debris. *Clin Orthop* 1995;311:21-39.

44. Wan Z, Dorr LD: Natural history of femoral focal osteolysis with proximal ingrowth smooth stem implant. *J Arthroplasty* 1996;11:718-725.

45. Engh CA, Hooten JP Jr, Zettl-Schaffer KF, et al: Porous-coated total hip replacement. *Clin Orthop* 1994;298:89-96.

46. Zicat B, Engh CA, Gokcen E: Patterns of osteolysis around total hip components inserted with and without cement. *J Bone Joint Surg Am* 1995;77:432-439.

47. Heekin RD, Callaghan JJ, Hopkinson WJ, Savory CG, Xenos JS: The porous-coated anatomic total hip prosthesis, inserted without cement: Results after five to seven years in a prospective study. *J Bone Joint Surg Am* 1993;75:77-91.

48. Stauffer RN: Ten-year follow-up study of total hip replacement. *J Bone Joint Surg Am* 1982;64: 983-990.

49. Buechel FF, Drucker D, Jasty M, Jiranek W, Harris WH: Osteolysis around uncemented acetabular components of cobalt-chrome surface replacement hip arthroplasty. *Clin Orthop* 1994;298:202-211.

50. Dowd JE, Cha CW, Trakru S, Kim SY, Yang IH, Rubash HE: Failure of total hip arthroplasty with a precoated prosthesis: 4- to 11-year results. *Clin Orthop* 1998;355:123-136.

51. Unwin AJ, Stiles PJ: Early failure of titanium alloy femoral components: A quantitative radiological analysis of osteolytic and granulomatous change. *J R Soc Med* 1993;86:460-463.

52. Morscher EW, Hefti A, Aebi U: Severe osteolysis after third-body wear due to hydroxyapatite particles from acetabular cup coating. *J Bone Joint Surg Br* 1998;80:267-272.

53. Marr DS, Rosenthal DI, Cohen GL, Tomford WW: Rapid postoperative osteolysis in Paget disease: A case report. *J Bone Joint Surg Am* 1994;76:274-277.

54. Vaughn BK, Dameron TB Jr, Bauer TW, Mochida Y, Akisue T, Eberle RW: Early osteolysis following total hip arthroplasty with use of a Hylamer liner in combination with a modular ceramic femoral head: A case report. *J Bone Joint Surg Am* 1999;81:1446-1449.

55. Schmidt AH, Walker G, Kyle RF, Thompson RC Jr: Periprosthetic metastatic carcinoma: Pitfalls in the management of two cases initially diagnosed as osteolysis. *J Arthroplasty* 1996;11:613-619.

56. Shaw JA: Multiple myeloma: A differential consideration for osteolysis surrounding total hip arthroplasties. *J Arthroplasty* 1995;10: 397-400.

57. Spangehl MJ, Masri BA, O'Connell JX, Duncan CP: Prospective analysis of preoperative and intraoperative investigations for the diagnosis of infection at the sites of two hundred and two revision total hip arthroplasties. *J Bone Joint Surg Am* 1999;81:672-683.

58. Thoren B, Wigren A: Erythrocyte sedimentation rate in infection of total hip replacements. *Orthopedics* 1991;14:495-497.

59. Shih LY, Wu JJ, Yang DJ: Erythrocyte sedimentation rate and C-reactive protein values in patients with total hip arthroplasty. *Clin Orthop* 1987;225:238-246.

60. Brause BD: Infections associated with prosthetic joints. *Clin Rheum Dis* 1986;12:523-536.

61. Fehrman DA, McBeath AA, DeSmet AA, Tuite MJ: Imaging barium-free bone cement. *Am J Orthop* 1996;25:172-174.

62. Reing CM, Richin PF, Kenmore PI: Differential bone-scanning in the evaluation of a painful total joint replacement. *J Bone Joint Surg Am* 1979;61:933-936.

63. Mirra JM, Amstutz HC, Matos M, Gold R: The pathology of the joint tissues and its clinical relevance in prosthesis failure. *Clin Orthop* 1976;117:221-240.

64. Lonner JH, Desai P, Dicesare PE, Steiner G, Zuckerman JD: The reliability of analysis of intraoperative frozen sections for identifying active infection during revision hip or knee arthroplasty. *J Bone Joint Surg Am* 1996;78: 1553-1558.

65. Huiskes R, Verdonschot N, Nivbrant B: Migration, stem shape, and surface finish in cemented total hip arthroplasty. *Clin Orthop* 1998;355:103-112.

66. Engh CA, Glassman AH, Griffin WL, Mayer JG: Results of cementless revision for failed cemented total hip arthroplasty. *Clin Orthop* 1988;235: 91-110.

67. Callaghan JJ, Salvati EA, Pellicci PM, Wilson PD Jr, Ranawat CS: Results of revision for mechanical failure after cemented total hip replacement, 1979 to 1982: A two to five-year follow-up. *J Bone Joint Surg Am* 1985;67: 1074-1085.

68. O'Neill DA, Harris WH: Failed total hip replacement: Assessment by plain radiographs, arthrograms, and aspiration of the hip joint. *J Bone Joint Surg Am* 1984;66:540-546.

69. Smith E, Harris WH: Increasing prevalence of femoral lysis in cementless total hip arthroplasty. *J Arthroplasty* 1995;10:407-412.

70. Learmonth ID, Hussell JG, Grobler GP: Unpredictable progression of osteolysis following cementless hip arthroplasty: 24 femoral components followed for 6-10 years. *Acta Orthop Scand* 1996;67:245-248.

71. Tanzer M, Maloney WJ, Jasty M, Harris WH: The progression of femoral cortical osteolysis in association with total hip arthroplasty without cement. *J Bone Joint Surg Am* 1992;74: 404-410.

72. Heekin RD, Engh CA, Herzwurm PJ: Fractures through cystic lesions of the greater trochanter: A cause of late pain after cementless total hip arthroplasty. *J Arthroplasty* 1996;11: 757-760.

73. Goetz DD, Smith EJ, Harris WH: The prevalence of femoral osteolysis associated with components inserted with or without cement in total hip replacements: A retrospective matched-pair series. *J Bone Joint Surg Am* 1994;76:1121-1129.

74. Martell JM, Pierson RH III, Jacobs JJ, Rosenberg AG, Maley M, Galante JO: Primary total hip reconstruction with a titanium fiber-coated prosthesis inserted without cement. *J Bone Joint Surg Am* 1993;75:554-571.

75. D'Antonio J, McCarthy JC, Bargar WL, et al: Classification of femoral abnormalities in total hip arthroplasty. *Clin Orthop* 1993;296:133-139.

76. Kavanagh BF, Ilstrup DM, Fitzgerald RH Jr: Revision total hip arthroplasty. *J Bone Joint Surg Am* 1985;67:517-526.

77. Kavanagh BF, Fitzgerald RH Jr: Multiple revisions for failed total hip arthroplasty not associated with infection. *J Bone Joint Surg Am* 1987;69:1144-1149.

78. Stromberg CN, Herberts P, Palmertz B: Cemented revision hip arthroplasty: A multicenter 5-9-year study of 204 first revisions for loosening. *Acta Orthop Scand* 1992;63:111-119.

79. Hedley AK, Gruen TA, Ruoff DP: Revision of failed total hip arthroplasties with uncemented porous-coated anatomic components. *Clin Orthop* 1988;235:75-90.

80. Harris WH, Krushell RJ, Galante JO: Results of cementless revisions of total hip arthroplasties using the Harris-Galante prosthesis. *Clin Orthop* 1988;235:120-126.

81. Gie GA, Linder L, Ling RS, Simon JP, Slooff TJ, Timperley AJ: Contained morselized allograft in revision total hip arthroplasty: Surgical technique. *Orthop Clin North Am* 1993;24: 717-725.

82. Elting JJ, Mikhail WE, Zicat BA, Hubbell JC, Lane LE, House B: Preliminary report of impaction grafting for exchange femoral arthroplasty. *Clin Orthop* 1995;319:159-167.

83. Leopold SS, Berger RA, Rosenberg AG, Jacobs JJ, Quigley LR, Galante JO: Impaction allografting with cement for revision of the femoral component: A minimum four-year follow-up study with use of a precoated femoral stem. *J Bone Joint Surg Am* 1999;81:1080-1092.

84. Masterson EL, Masri BA, Duncan CP: The cement mantle in the Exeter impaction allografting technique: A cause for concern. *J Arthroplasty* 1997;12:759-764.

85. Meding JB, Ritter MA, Keating EM, Faris PM: Impaction bone-grafting before insertion of a femoral stem with cement in revision total hip arthroplasty: A minimum two-year follow-up study. *J Bone Joint Surg Am* 1997;79:1834-1841.

86. Panjabi MM, Trumble T, Hult JE, Southwick WO: Effect of femoral stem length on stress raisers associated with revision hip arthroplasty. *J Orthop Res* 1985;3:447-455.

87. Raut VV, Siney PD, Wroblewski BM: Revision for aseptic stem loosening using the cemented Charnley prosthesis: A review of 351 hips. *J Bone Joint Surg Br* 1995;77:23-27.

88. Katz RP, Callaghan JJ, Sullivan PM, Johnston RC: Results of cemented femoral revision total hip arthroplasty using improved cementing techniques. *Clin Orthop* 1995;319:178-183.

89. Ling RS: Letter: Femoral component revision using impacted morsellised cancellous graft. *J Bone Joint Surg Br* 1997;79:874-875.

90. Moreland JR, Bernstein ML: Femoral revision hip arthroplasty with uncemented, porous-coated stems. *Clin Orthop* 1995;319:141-150.

91. Paprosky WG, Krishnamurthy A: Five to 14-year follow up on cementless femoral revisions. *Orthopedics* 1996;19:765-768.

92. Engh CA, Culpepper WJ II, Kassapidis E: Revision of loose cementless femoral prostheses to larger porous coated components. *Clin Orthop* 1998;347:168-178.

93. Allan DG, Lavoie GJ, McDonald S, Oakeshott R, Gross AE: Proximal femoral allografts in revision hip arthroplasty. *J Bone Joint Surg Br* 1991;73:235-240.

94. Hozack WJ, Bicalho PS, Eng K: Treatment of femoral osteolysis with cementless total hip revision. *J Arthroplasty* 1996;11:668-672.

95. Head WC, Malinin TI, Mallory TH, Emerson RH Jr: Onlay cortical allografting for the femur. *Orthop Clin North Am* 1998;29:307-312.

96. Gross AE, Hutchison CR, Alexeeff M, Mahomed N, Leitch K, Morsi E: Proximal femoral allografts for reconstruction of bone stock in revision arthroplasty of the hip. *Clin Orthop* 1995;319:151-158.

97. Blackley HRL, Davis AM, Hutchinson CR, et al: Proximal femoral allografts for reconstruction of bone stock in revision arthroplasty of the hip: A nine to fifteen-year follow-up. *J Bone Joint Surg Am*, in press.

98. Malkani AL, Settecerri JJ, Sim FH, Chao EY, Wallrichs SL: Long-term results of proximal femoral replacement for non-neoplastic disorders. *J Bone Joint Surg Br* 1995;77:351-356.

99. Haentjens P, De Boeck H, Opdecam P: Proximal femoral replacement prosthesis for salvage of failed hip arthroplasty: Complications in a 2-11 year follow-up study in 19 elderly patients. *Acta Orthop Scand* 1996; 67:37-42.

100. Renard AJ, Veth RP, Schreuder HW, Schraffordt Koops H, van Horn J, Keller A: Revisions of endoprosthetic reconstructions after limb salvage in musculoskeletal oncology. *Arch Orthop Trauma Surg* 1998;117:125-131.

101. Shin DS, Weber KL, Chao EY, An KN, Sim FH: Reoperation for failed prosthetic replacement used for limb salvage. *Clin Orthop* 1999;358: 53-63.

102. Morris HG, Capanna R, Del Ben M, Campanacci D: Prosthetic reconstruction of the proximal femur after resection for bone tumors. *J Arthroplasty* 1995;10:293-299.

103. Aribindi R, Barba M, Solomon MI, Arp P, Paprosky W: Bypass fixation. *Orthop Clin North Am* 1998;29:319-329.

104. Clarke HD, Berry DJ, Sim FH: Salvage of failed femoral megaprostheses with allograft prosthesis composites. *Clin Orthop* 1998;356:222-229.

105. Malkani AL, Sim FH, Chao EY: Custom-made segmental femoral replacement prosthesis in revision total hip arthroplasty. *Orthop Clin North Am* 1993;24:727-733.

106. Lombardi A: Treatment of Paget's disease of bone with alendronate. *Bone* 1999;24(suppl 5):59S-61S.

107. Wang X, Shanbhag AS, Rubash HE, Agrawal CM: Short-term effects of bisphosphonates on the biomechanical properties of canine bone. *J Biomed Mater Res* 1999;44:456-460.

108. Astrand J, Aspenberg P: Alendronate did not inhibit instability-induced bone resorption: A study in rats. *Acta Orthop Scand* 1999;70:67-70.

21

SYMPOSIUM

Basic Science of Bone Impaction Grafting

B. Willem Schreurs, MD, PhD
Thomas J.J.H. Slooff, MD, PhD
Pieter Buma, PhD
Nico Verdonschot, PhD

Introduction

This chapter will discuss the scientific basis of bone impaction grafting and will describe the background of the technique, in vitro and in vivo experimental data, and animal and human histology of bone impaction grafting. Clinical application to acetabular and femoral reconstruction and the clinical results with impacted bone grafts are presented in chapter 22.

Background

Large bone defects in patients with a failed total hip prosthesis present a new clinical challenge to the orthopaedic surgeon; since the 1970s, the number of patients has gradually increased. Although initially these defects were filled with bone cement, it soon became clear that the failure rate of this technique was unacceptably high, especially in those patients with poor bone quality.[1-3] In 1979, we started to apply bone impaction grafting to the acetabular side in patients with failed acetabular cups. Our technique was based on studies by Hastings and Parker[4] and McCollum and Nunley.[5] Hastings and Parker[4] used autogenous morcellized cancellous bone grafts to fill the defect in protrusion caused by rheumatoid arthritis. Next, they applied a metal mesh on top of the bone grafts, which were regularly placed and inserted, then a cemented cup. McCollum and Nunley[5] used autogenous corticocancellous bone wafers to fill acetabular defects in patients with primary protrusio acetabuli and to reconstruct failed cup arthroplasty. To prevent penetration of bone cement into the bone grafts, an absorable gelatin sponge was used as a barrier between the bone graft and cement. In patients with medial wall defects, a metal reinforcement ring was used.

One or more of the authors or the departments with which they are affiliated have received something of value from a commercial or other party related directly or indirectly to the subject of this chapter.

We believe that the technique of using bone grafts to fill defects is very attractive because lost bone stock is reconstructed in a physiological way. We made modifications to the technique by using firm impaction of substantial cancellous autografts and allografts in combination with a cemented revision total hip replacement. The goals of the technique are to restore bone stock loss; reconstruct the acetabulum at the original center of rotation; transform a segmental defect into a cavitary defect using metal meshes; stabilize the bone graft using impactors and a vigorous impaction technique; use standard prosthetic components with bone cement; and use a standardized, uniform surgical technique.

Slooff and associates[6] reported the preliminary clinical results of bone impaction grafting and cement on the acetabular side, and all the acetabular reconstructions in revision cases were recently reviewed.[7] Long-term results were good with a survival rate of 94% for aseptic loosening after an average follow-up of 11.8 years.

Based on clinical experience on the acetabular side, some crude femoral reconstructions were performed in the 1980s. Intramedullary bone grafting was applied independently at the orthopaedic centers in Exeter and Nijmegen. In early 1987, the Exeter group began to use the technique on the femoral side on a regular basis, with the femoral stem as an impactor.[8] The Nijmegen group was the first to perform basic research into this subject.[9-11] A special set of instruments was developed in 1988 to facilitate reproducible reconstruction with this grafting technique. In a goat model the use of this technique in combination with a cemented and a noncemented stem was studied. The X-Change Femoral Revision System was developed in 1990 based on experiences in both Exeter and Nijmegen.

Basic Mechanical Data on Morcellized Bone Grafts

The mechanical behavior of impacted morcellized bone chips was characterized in a confined compression test.[12] It was hypothesized that the initial stability of the reconstruction and the effectiveness of

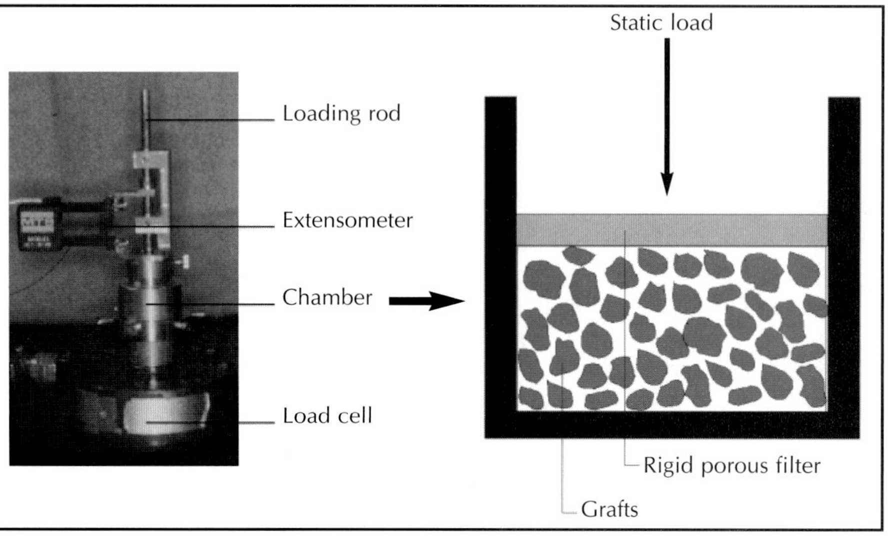

Fig. 1 Overview of the creep-test loading apparatus (*left*) and in detail a schematic of the container with a porous filter on top of the grafts (*right*).

later revitalization and incorporation would depend on the mechanical integrity of the graft. The objective of this study was to document the time-dependent properties of the morcellized graft material. This information was expected to be useful to clinical application of the material and to studies on implant migration or joint design optimization. The graft was considered to be a porous, permeable solid structure filled with fluid. This enabled determination of the compressive modulus of the matrix and its permeability to fluid flow. Testing was performed using a special container, while load was applied dynamically with the maximal treadmill stress (MTS) loading machine using a dynamic load (Fig. 1). During testing, large irreversible deformations were caused by flow-independent creeping behavior due to rolling and sliding of the bone chips. Mean permeability was 8.82×10^{-12} m^4/Ns (SD, 43%) and the compressive mode was 38.7 MPa (SD, 34%). A creeping law could capture the irreversible deformations. We concluded that clinical application of morcellized bone grafts would be subject to permanent postoperative deformation. The permeability of the graft material was relatively high compared with, for example, human cartilage. The confined compression modulus was relatively low compared to cancellous bone of the same apparent density. It was hypothesized that prostheses used in revision surgery must be designed to accommodate both viscoelastic and permanent deformations in the graft without causing interface loosening. The type of stem is of special interest; for example, a double-tapered smooth stem can easily gain secondary stability after some subsidence.

Brewster and associates[13] considered compacted bone to be a friable particulate aggregate and used an established engineering theory to predict the outcome of their experiments, assuming that more irregular particle size would be beneficial. They investigated four different bone mills, which produced particles of 2 to 4 mm. It was concluded that the bone mills produced particles that were too uniform. The research group also determined the effect of impaction on the size of the bone graft particles by using them for femoral reconstruction with the standard impaction technique. The average size of these relatively small particles remained unchanged relative to nonimpacted chips. However, it was unclear whether this would also be the case for the larger bone chips that are often used in the acetabulum. The authors concluded that the size of the chips from these four mills was not affected when the donor femoral heads were still frozen. Osteoporotic femoral heads produced similar chip sizes, but fewer particles were obtained from each specimen.

In Vitro Testing of Cup Stability After Impaction Grafting

One of the most important parameters that can influence prosthetic stability after impaction bone grafting is bone chip size. The stability of acetabular cups in fresh frozen human pelvic bones was studied after acetabular reconstruction with bone impaction grafting.[14] Bone chips were prepared from fresh frozen femoral heads in two different ways: a rongeur nibbled relatively large bone chips (average chip diameter 9.2 mm; SD = 0.8 mm), and a bone mill produced smaller chips (average chip diameter 2.0 mm; SD = 0.5 mm). The acetabula of the human pelvic bones were overreamed and bilateral symmetrical cavitary superomedial defects were made. On one pelvic bone, paired tests were done with large and small chips. Impaction was performed with metal impactors of different sizes. After reconstruction, cups were implanted with bone cement under cement pressurization. Two surgeons experienced with the technique performed the implantations. Next the bones were tested with an MTS machine using a dynamic load with maximum 1,500 N directed in the superomedial direction. Roentgen stereophotogrammetric analysis (RSA) was used to calculate the migration of the cups. The size of the bone chips had a significant effect on migration; smaller chips led to greater migration, which was significant at the end of the loading phase. Closer analysis of the results revealed that only one of the surgeons had induced the effects of graft size on migration. With the larger chip size, the amount of stability achieved by the two surgeons was similar. This surgeon-dependent effect may be explained by the degree of impaction. The surgeon who achieved greater stability with the smaller chips used significantly more graft material than the other surgeon to fill a defect of the same size; this applied to both the larger and smaller chips. Apparently, the amount of graft material had a significant effect when the smaller chips were used, and no effect when the larger chips were used. This indicates that the surgical technique may be of greater importance when small-size bone chips are used. Initially, the Exeter group used smaller chips for acetabular reconstruction, which proved to be associated with less successful clinical results (R. Ling, MD, Exeter, WI, 1998, personal communication). Therefore, the use of bone chips between 0.7 and 1.0 cm for acetabular reconstruction is strongly recommended in order to reproduce the results.

In Vitro Testing of Femoral Stability After Impaction Grafting

An in vitro goat model was used to investigate the stability of cemented femoral stems versus noncemented hydroxyapatite (HA) coated femoral stems that were immediately inserted in combination with an intramedullary femoral impaction reconstruction technique.[9-11] In a loading experiment, displacement of the stems relative to the bone was determined with RSA. The most striking movements were axial rotations (cemented stems, up to 2.1°; noncemented stems, up to 6.8°) and subsidence (cemented stems, up to 0.5 mm; noncemented stems, up to 2.9 mm). Slipping and compaction of the grafts were the predominant causes of these motions. It was concluded that better stability was achieved with the cemented stems, probably because of cement penetration into the graft layer. The graft reconstruction definitely could not provide enough stability for noncemented stems; this might be because the used noncemented stems are designed with rounded, not sharp, edges. Sharp edges might generate a better initial stability.

Eldridge and associates[15] studied the effect of bone chip size on the stability of the stem using three different sizes of bone chips. Large chips (5 mm) prepared by hand with an osteotome produced better stability than chips prepared by conventional bone mills. Wallace and associates[16] analyzed the effects of chip size after several preparation techniques: manual nibbling, manual milling, and power milling with five different machines. The majority of particles had a diameter of 3.5 mm or smaller. In another study by Wallace and associates,[17] it was concluded that maximum femoral stability could be obtained by using particles larger than 4.5 mm. It was also suggested that larger bone particles would lead to enhanced stem stability.[18] However, on the femoral side, the dimensions of the intramedullary canal limit the size of the chips. Larger chips can only be applied in the more proximal part of the femur.

Malkani and associates[19] studied the stability of collarless cemented stems in paired human femora. Primary cementing of the stem was studied as well as a revision situation in which all the trabecular bone was removed first and the femur was overreamed. Bone impaction grafting was performed next. Both situations were tested in a loading device and showed less than 1 mm subsidence (primary, average 0.27 mm; revision, average 0.52 mm). It was concluded that revision of the femoral component with morcellized cancellous graft restored the integrity of the femur and provided immediate stability of the implant.

Berzins and associates[20] compared the stability of primary cemented stems, primary noncemented stems, and stems cemented within an impacted particulate allograft. The stability of the stems with impaction grafting was no more or no less than that of the primary cemented and the primary noncemented stems. In addition, they showed that noncemented stems exhibited the largest micromotions. They also studied the effect of increased cement pressure on the stability of the stems within the allografts. Although pressurization of the cement led to greater cement penetration into the graft bed, this did not at all influence the fixation strength of the cement-allograft reconstruction.

Chassin and associates[21] studied the feasibility of performing bone impaction grafting after extended trochanteric osteotomy, a technique that facilitates component removal on the femoral side. They reconstructed a femur cadaver model after osteotomy by applying cables and wires. It was concluded that the stability of the cemented allograft impaction construction was comparable to that in a control construction, which consisted of similar impacted cadaveric reconstruction without osteotomy. In 1998, Hellman and associates[22] reported two cases with nonunion of the osteotomy after impaction grafting. One reason might be that extensively porous-coated stems were used in contrast with the cemented stems in the previous study.

Extensive cortical defects are major problems in revision surgery. The femoral impaction technique in combination with metal meshes fixed with cerclage wires can be used to close these segmental defects. Strut grafting, such as onlay grafts, can also be used. It is suggested that these strut grafts provide better initial stability after closure of the defect: however, we could find no data on this subject. Therefore, using a goat model, the initial stability of the Exeter sheep prosthesis was studied after bridging a medial femoral defect with either a strut graft or mesh in the femur (Fig. 2). Four groups of five femurs were tested. In group 1, the prosthesis was placed in femurs with an intact cortical wall in combination with bone impaction grafting. In the other three groups, a reproducible medial segmental defect was made. In group 2, the defect was not supported; in group 3, the defect was reconstructed with a metal mesh, and in group 4, the defect was reconstructed with a cortical

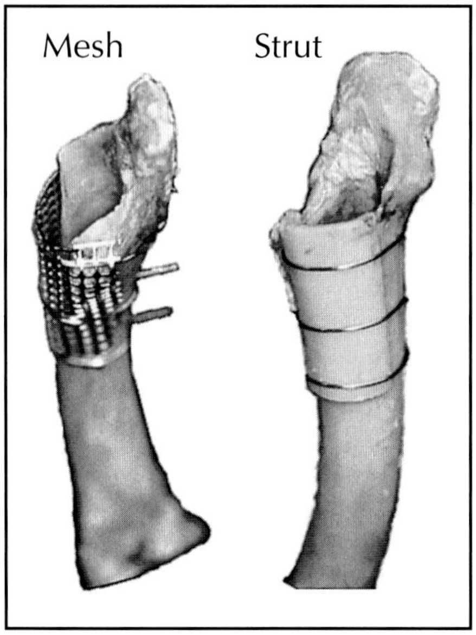

Fig. 2 Femur with medial cortical defect bridged by a mesh or a strut graft.

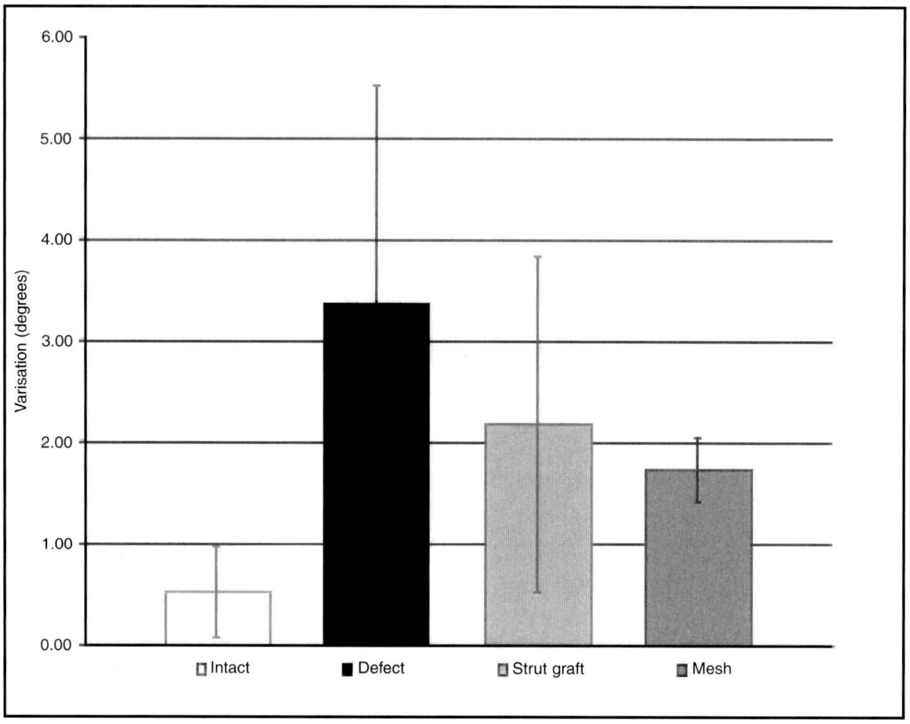

Fig. 3 Movement of the stem in medial direction (varisation) in degrees for an intact femur, a defect femur, and after reconstruction with a strut graft and a metal mesh.

onlay graft. The cerclage wires in groups 3 and 4 were positioned at similar locations. In a dynamic loading experiment, the micromotions of the stem were calculated with RSA. During the experiment, all group 2 femurs failed, with a very reproducible failure mechanism, so the size of the defect was critical for stem stability. There were no failures in group 3 or in the strut graft group 4. It was concluded that bridging a medial defect in the femur was beneficial to the stability of the implanted stem (Fig. 3). There were no significant differences between the results of the strut grafts and those of mesh reconstruction. However, the standard deviation was larger in the strut group, which indicates that stability was more reproducible when meshes were used.

The Application of Alternative Biomaterials With Impaction Grafting

All of our clinical experience is based on the application of fresh frozen femoral head bone grafts. However, there are other processed bone or even biomaterials that have been used to bone reconstruct defects. Data on the influence of these materials when used for bone impaction grafting are lacking. Therefore, we adapted the model of Giesen and associates[12] to compare the mechanical behavior of impacted bone grafts with that of biomaterials, bovine xenografts, and human freeze-dried bone available on the market. In this study, the hypothesis was formulated that the (bio)materials should approach the mechanical behavior of human bone grafts in order to produce clinical success. Time-dependent deformational behavior, stiffness and viscoelasticity were studied, and HA/tricalcium phosphate particles were tested. Different sized particles with different porosities and HA:tricalcium phosphate ratios were used. It was concluded that although it is possible to manufacture all kinds of biomaterials, it may be very difficult to mimic the mechanical behavior of morcellized bone grafts. The most important difference seemed to be that human bone grafts exhibit viscoelastic behavior. The xenografts and freeze-dried bone grafts showed some elastic recovery, whereas their mechanical data were fairly comparable with fresh frozen bone. Although the application of biomaterials seems to be very attractive if bone grafts are unavailable, the surgeon should exercise great caution. It may be worthwhile to consider using a mixture of bone grafts and biomaterials if a compromise has to be made because too little bone graft material is available. However, extensive data (research is currently in progress) are required before biomaterials can be applied clinically.

Animal Experiments and Histologic Data

Although it was suggested at the end of the 1980s that direct contact between bone graft and cement would interfere with graft incorporation,[23,24] Roffman and associates[25,26] already reported on this subject in 1982 and 1983. In a dog model, they studied the viability and osteogenity of bone coated with bone cement.[25] They used corticocancellous strips of autogenous bone placed around osteotomies in the canine femur. Next, the grafts were covered with polymethylmethacrylate (PMMA) bone cement. The authors concluded that despite the contact between the graft and PMMA, the grafts retained their viability and healing was observed. In another dog model, protrusio acetabuli was created with a segmental medial wall defect.[26] This defect was filled with autogenous bone chips and covered with bone cement. Histologic evaluation at 6 months showed a viable graft with bone remodeling up to the bone cement.

Schimmel and associates[27] used a goat model to establish the mechanical stability and the incorporation capacity of acetabular grafts. A defect in the acetabulum was created and it was reconstructed with morcellized grafts and a cemented cup. Postoperative performance of the reconstruction was followed both histologically and biomechanically. Histology showed consolidation of the graft with the host bone bed within 3 weeks. In the subsequent period, a front of vascular sprouts had infiltrated the graft. Graft resorption, woven bone deposition, and subsequent remodeling resulted in a new trabecular structure. This structure contained only scarce remnants of the original dead graft material after 24 weeks. At the graft-cement interface, graft resorption and new bone formation had resulted in areas of direct vital bone-cement contact. Locally, a soft-tissue interface was present. After longer follow-up periods, progressive interface formation and loosening of the cups were found in most animals. Mechanical testing showed that the stability of the reconstruction increased during the first 12 postoperative weeks. Thereafter, the stability decreased, probably because of soft-tissue formation at the graft-cement interface. It was concluded that cemented morcellized allografts have a high capacity to incorporate. Initial cup stability was adequate to provoke graft incorporation. To apply this grafting technique to the femoral side, a special set of instruments were developed to facilitate reconstruction in a reproducible way in 1988. In an in vitro study on goat femurs, cemented and noncemented femoral HA-coated stems in combination with impaction grafting were compared. Initial stability was determined in a loading experiment with RSA.[9,28] The initial stability of the cemented stems was better than that of the noncemented stems, probably because of cement penetration. However, the design of the noncemented stems probably was not optimal for this application. Displacement of the two stems was predominantly nonelastic, but after unloading, some elastic recovery was seen. Next, both stem designs were implanted in goats and both mechanical and histologic studies were done 6 and 12 weeks after implantation.[10] Mechanical testing of the cemented stem showed increased stability relative to the initial stability immediately after implantation; there was no difference in stability between the 6 and 12 weeks group. Histologically, revascularization and resorption of the graft were evident, but not yet complete. Bone apposition and bone resorption resulted in a mixture of graft and new bone formation. Failure rates in the noncemented stems were higher, but the stems that were successful were very stable. Histologically, revascularization and remodeling were seen in all animals in the form of a mixture of remnants of grafts and new bone.

To study the influence of loading on morcellized bone graft incorporation, we developed a new goat model in which a subcutaneous pressure implant was used.[29] This device can generate controlled loading conditions onto a fixed amount of bone graft in the distal femur. The goal was to assess the in vivo effects of mechanical stimuli on the incorporation process of impacted morcellized bone grafts and to assess what happens to the incorporated graft during the longer term. In a pilot study, 20 goats were divided into three groups: nonloaded, 2 MPa loading, and 4 MPa loading (1 Hz, 1 h/day). Investigations were performed after 3, 6, and 12 weeks. Specimens were studied for quantitative bone density using quantitative computed tomography (QCT) and histomorphometry. Three goats were lost to follow-up due to complications. At 12 weeks, after complete incorporation of the bone graft, QCT bone density measurements and histomorphometric analysis of the histology have revealed a difference between the three groups. There was a high density of incorporated bone in the 4 MPa specimens, but reduced density in the nonloaded specimens.

In a separate experiment, we studied the effect of loading on the speed of graft incorporation. Grafts were nonloaded or loaded with 3 MPa. Specimens were examined after 5 weeks. Irrespective of loading or nonloading, a front of vascular fibrous tissue with macrophages and osteoclasts had invaded and resorbed the dead bone graft. Osteoblasts had deposited new woven bone on the graft remnants and in the interstitial tissues. Surprisingly, no statistical differences were found in the areas of incorporated bone between the situations with and without loading. This means that load plays a minor role during the initial phase of bone graft incorporation. Other factors related to the trauma induced by the surgery or immunologic conditions are much more important.

In a nonloaded bone chamber experiment in a rat model, Tagil and Aspenberg[30] recently compared the ingrowth of impacted cancellous bone grafts to that of unimpacted allografts. Impaction of the grafts was done with 25 or 2,500 MPa. In the unimpacted controls, bone ingrowth was 30% higher than that in the 25 MPa and the 2,500 MPa impaction groups. They concluded that impaction seemed to inhibit osteoconduction, although this might be not a disadvantage in the clinical situation.

Human Mechanical Data

Clinical Experience With Migration of the Cup After Revision of the Acetabulum With Impacted Morcellized Bone Grafts

Although we have studied the long-term outcome of acetabular reconstruction with impaction bone grafts in primary total hip arthroplasty (THA) and revision THA in long-term follow-up has been studied,[7,31,32] it was not possible to interpret migration of the cup on our radiographs. Acetabular migration of less than 4 to 6 mm cannot be detected on conventional radiographs.[33] In an RSA study on cemented versus noncemented acetabular cup revision with impacted bone allografts, Herberts and associates[34] concluded that impacted allografts did not significantly compromise the early stability of the acetabular revisions, even when the cup was resting on 50% or more allograft bone. The medioproximal migration of noncemented cups was between 0.2 and 6.5 mm; in cemented cups, migration was between 0.2 and 2.2 mm. Patients with rheumatoid arthritis were at risk for increased migration. No information was reported about the type and size of the bone chips.

Ornstein and associates[35] presented RSA data on 21 hip revisions with impacted bone chips and a cemented cup. The patients were followed up for 2 years. The chips had an average diameter of 3 mm and had been produced by a bone mill from fresh frozen femoral heads. All but one component migrated a distance of between 0.5 and 6.4 mm in the proximal direction during follow-up. This migration exceeded that observed after cemented acetabular revision. Seven of the 21 components were still migrating at 1.5 to 2 years follow-up. Additional RSA data are needed to clarify when these components will stop their migration. Some of the patients in our long-term study showed migrations of up to 13 mm in the immediate postoperative period, but this migration stabilized shortly afterward and did not influence the long-term outcome.

Clinical Experience With Migration of the Stem After Revision With Impacted Morcellized Bone Grafts

An obvious problem with the bone impaction bone grafting technique is instability of the stem within a reconstructed bone. Although there have been several reports, it is difficult to interpret the results, because of the different types of prosthesis used and the lack of information about the type of bone grafts used (for example, fresh frozen, irradiated, freeze-dried). So far, it is unknown whether alternative stems will produce results comparable with those from polished, tapered, collarless stems. Given the basic mechanical data on impacted bone grafts,[12] problems can be expected when using different stem designs.

Excessive subsidence was observed in two out of five studies in which this technique was used with a polished, tapered, colorless stem. Meding and associates[36] observed subsidence in 38% of the cases, with an average subsidence of 10.1 mm (4 to 31 mm). Eldridge and associates[37] studied subsidence in 79 patients; 9 (11%) showed massive subsidence. In contrast, Gie and associates[8] reported subsidence of less than 4 mm in 45 out of the 56 revisions in his original study. Mikkelsen and Horlyck[38] observed an average subsidence of less than 1 mm in a series of 22 patients with impacted bone grafts. Ornstein and associates[39] reported on the results of an RSA study on 16 consecutive femoral revisions. Although there was initial subsidence in most cases, it was stabilized within 2 years. At our own clinic, we studied subsidence in 33 revision cases with an average follow-up of 5.2 years (3 to 8 years). Excluding one patient with a nonrecognized intraoperative fracture, which subsided by 15 mm, the average subsidence in the entire group was 2.6 mm.

Karrholm and associates[40] performed RSA on 24 consecutive nonpolished cemented stems. The average subsidence was 0.32 mm after 2 years. At 3 years follow-up, no further subsidence was observed, indicating stabilization.

Human Histology

Heekin and associates[41] studied the outcome of morcellized allografts on the acetabular side in three retrieval cases at 18 months, 53 months, and 83 months after surgery. At 18 months, remodeling was incomplete, with revascularization of only 4 mm; however, more incorporation was seen over time. At 83 months, the graft was almost completely incorporated. This observation contrasted sharply with a report by Hooten and associates[42] on two graft retrievals in which structural bulk allografts had been used for acetabular reconstruction. Although the patients had good clinical results and the radiographs showed healing of graft to host bone, microscopically there was only a limited degree of bony union. Revascularization extended for no more than 2 mm into the structural graft. Even after 48 months, allograft revascularization and remodeling were minimal.

In 1996, the histology of acetabular reconstructions with bone impaction grafting following revision THA was studied in 8 patients.[43] Most of the reconstructed defects were cavitary, and two had combined cavitary-segmental defects. The number of femoral heads used for reconstruction varied from one to three. Reoperation after revision of the acetabulum was necessary for deep infection in three patients, recurrent subluxation in one, and excision of ectopic bone in one. The biopsies during these procedures were obtained using a Yanshini needle. The process of bone graft incorporation was found to be similar to that observed in various animal studies:

a front of fibrovascular tissue had invaded the graft.[10,11,27,29] More recently we re-reviewed all the available biopsy samples prepared for histologic investigation from acetabular reconstructions. Now, histologic specimens were available from 24 biopsies on 20 patients. Only biopsies from acetabular reconstructions with bone impaction grafting according to our technique were included. The follow-up period was between 3 and 170 months. Most revisions had been performed with fresh frozen allograft bone from the local bone bank. Histology was performed on undecalcified bone specimens. The biopsy sections were scored semiquantitatively according to the following three phase definitions: (1) nonvascularized graft remnants, surrounded/not surrounded with fibrous tissue; (2) actively incorporating graft bone with revascularization; and (3) newly formed trabecular bone, surrounded by normal, fibrotic, or necrotic marrow. In addition, special findings such as cartilage remnants and newly formed fibrocartilage were scored. Although the degree of incorporation varied among the specimens, a clear trend could be recognized. Remnants of graft material could be distinguished clearly on the basis empty osteocyte lacunae (Fig. 4, *D*). At 3 months, there was already some graft incorporation. In the biopsy specimens taken at 4 and 5 months, a front of revascularization was visible (Fig. 4, *A*). This revascularization front could be recognized on the basis of vital soft tissue. During the passage of this front, osteoclasts were removing bone graft (Fig. 4, *B*), while osteoblasts were producing osteoid and woven bone on the remnants of the graft, in the interstitial space and on fibrin cloths (Fig. 4, *C*). The specimens obtained 8 to 30 months after revision showed different stages of graft incorporation. At 8 and 9 months, various amounts of graft were embedded in a new trabecular structure. Initially, the newly formed bone was of the woven bone type (Fig. 4, *D*). The bone close to the graft-cement interface contained mostly woven bone, indicating that the revascularization and remodeling front arrived later at this location. In the biopsies obtained at 15, 22, and 28 months, graft remnants were extremely scarce in the newly formed bone. In the specimens obtained after a longer follow-up, no woven bone was found and the bone had been completely remodeled into normal vital lamellar trabecular bone, which did not contain any graft remnants (Fig. 4, *E* and *F*). In one patient with secondary osteoarthritis caused by congenital hip dysplasia, the cup had been implanted at the original center of rotation, bringing the cup about 5 cm distally. This patient subsequently developed sciatic problems; 15 months after reconstruction, the sciatic nerve was explored and a needle biopsy from the acetabulum was taken. Because of persistent complaints, the hip was reoperated 28 months after reconstruction and a higher hip center was created while removing a large part of the original reconstruction. All the bone specimens from this patient showed a normal lamellar structure with little or no graft remnants. Graft and woven bone remnants were only present at locations where very dense trabecular or cortical bone had formed, for instance at the margins of the new acetabular wall.

Some specimens obtained between 59 and 79 months showed areas of nonincorporated graft remnants, in most cases surrounded by vital fibrotic tissue and very often coated with a dark material of unknown nature (Fig. 4, *H*). However, four out of the five patients underwent revision because of aseptic loosening of the cup. All of the grafts with a follow-up of 10 years or longer had become completely incorporated. Only the tissue surrounding the new bone differed in these cases; some showed necrotic or fibrotic marrow. Interface fibrosis and normal fibrotic tissue with or without macrophages containing wear particles of various origin were found at the graft-cement interface in these cases (Fig. 4, *G*). In a number of biopsies, particularly those prepared with a bone mill, large nonincorporated cartilage fragments were found (Fig. 4, *I*).

Ling and associates[44] performed the first histologic study on impacted bone grafts in femoral reconstruction. A retrieval case was studied 3.5 years after reconstruction. Although morcellized bone graft had only been used to fill two large cortical defects, the basic technique was considered to be the same. The allograft chips impacted in the cortical defects had largely been replaced by viable cortical bone, whereas the interface between the cement and bone tissue resembled that seen after primary cemented arthroplasty.

Nelissen and associates[45] obtained biopsy specimens from the proximal femur of four patients with a follow-up of 11 to 27 months after femoral impaction grafting. They observed three relatively ill-defined zones: an inner zone consisting of bone cement, fibrous tissue, and partially necrotic trabeculae; a middle zone with viable trabecular bone; and an outer zone with a viable cortex. Their results demonstrated bone remodeling and at least partial restoration of bone stock in the proximal part of the femur.

Ullmark and Linder[46] reported on a retrieval case 6 months after femoral reconstruction. Most of the transplanted areas were revascularized. Proximally, a large proportion of the new bone had formed peripherally, but a substantial amount of fibrous tissue had embedded graft pieces closer to the cement.

In contrast with the acetabular side, the fate of impacted bone grafts on the femoral side is not yet clear. More human data are needed. Also, the potential for revascularization is more limited than on the acetabular side, because of the cortical bone surrounding the

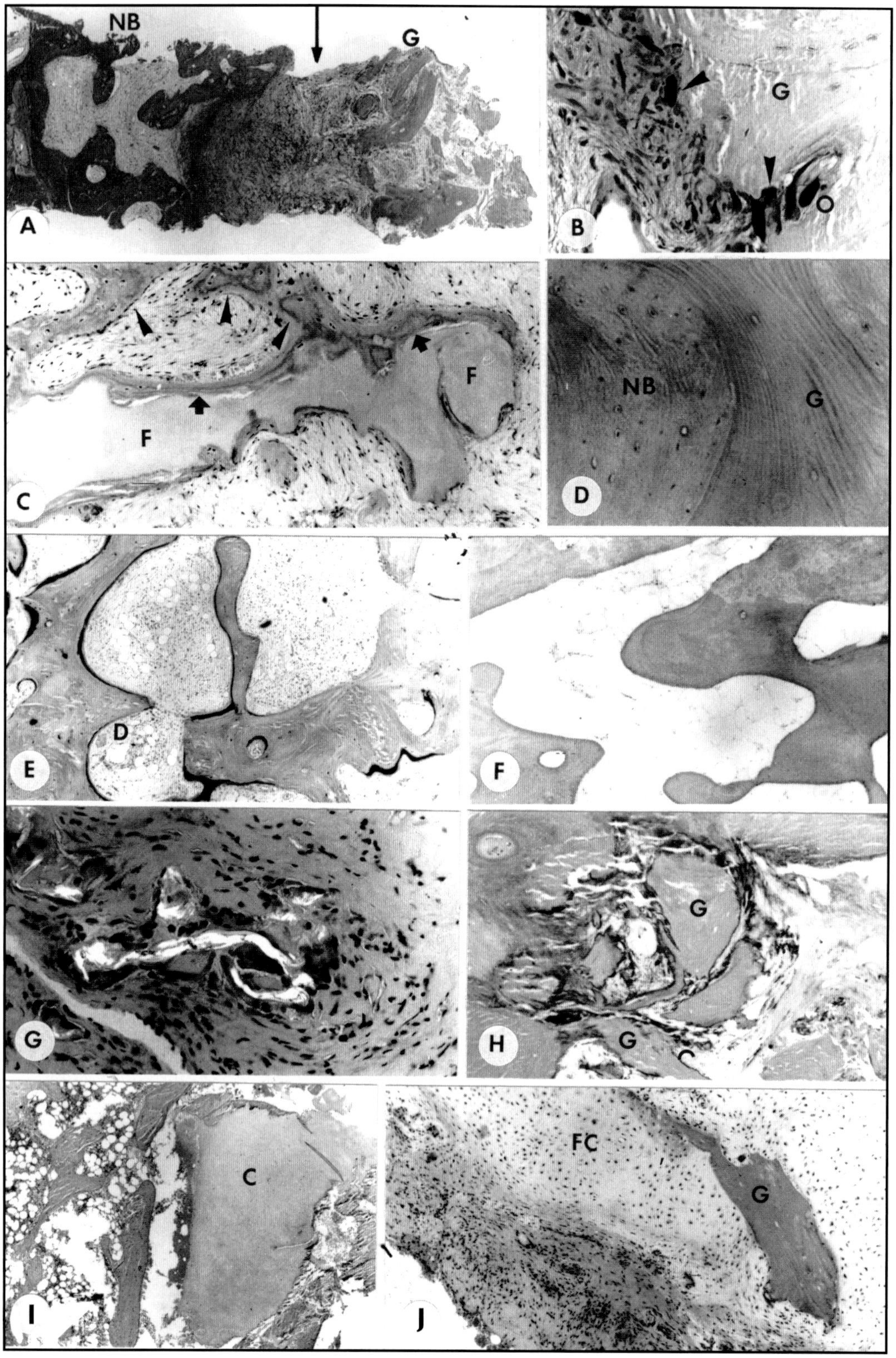

Fig. 4 Histology of human acetabular impaction grafting. **A**, Biopsy with revascularization front. Graft (G) is nonvascularized impacted bone graft, arrow indicates location of revascularization, NB indicates location with new bone formation. Hematoxylin and eosin, ×15. **B**, Osteoclastic *(arrows)* resorption of graft bone (G). O indicates osteoclasts. Acid phosphatase, ×100 **C**, New bone formation *(arrows)* on fibrin cloths (F) and free in stroma tissue *(arrowheads)*. Hematoxylin and eosin, ×50. **D**, Mixture of woven bone (NB) and graft remnants (G). Hematoxylin and eosin, ×100. **E** and **F**, Newly formed trabecular structure after completion of the incorporation process. **E**, Goldner-Masson and trichrome. **F**, Hematoxylin and eosin, ×50. **G**, Giant cells loaded with polyethylene particles in the interface of aseptically loosened acetabular reconstruction. Hematoxylin and eosin, ×120. **H**, Nonincorporated graft remnants in biopsy with long-term follow-up. Hematoxylin and eosin, ×30. **I**, Cartilage remnant (C) in partially incorporated graft. Hematoxylin and eosin, ×25. **J**, Fibrocartilage (FC) in interface between cement layer and incorporate graft. Hematoxylin and eosin, ×80.

impacted bone. The often-used releases of the femur will further hamper revascularization.

Summary and Recommendations

More is known about the clinical application of bone impaction grafting than the graft's basic behavior. Based on the good long-term clinical results of impaction bone grafting on the acetabular side and the promising midterm data on the femoral side, this technique is becoming more popular. An additional advantage of this technique is that it is possible to reconstruct bone stock loss in a physiological way. However, more basic knowledge about this technique is needed.

Surgeons performing bone impaction grafting should be highly trained. The technique is not easy and it is imperative that the grafts be impacted very vigorously, on both the acetabular and femoral sides.

It is essential that load from the cup is directly transmitted to the grafted area. Thus, in our view, the use of morcellized bone grafts in combination with a reconstruction ring is different from the original technique of bone impaction grafting. Although good long-term results have been reported with this technique[47] it is considered to be a different reconstruction method on the acetabular side. Another potential problem is that some surgeons use acetabular reamers in reverse to impact the morcellized bone grafts. Mechanical tests suggest that the mechanical stability is inferior to that after impaction bone grafting with vigorous impaction.

Until more data become available, we recommend following the original technique of bone impaction grafting on the acetabular and femoral sides as closely as possible. On the acetabular side, this means the application of large trabecular fresh frozen bone chips with a diameter of 7 to 10 mm in combination with a cemented cup. On the femoral side, the use of a bone mill is mandatory. Chip size should be 2 to 4 mm. We only have experience with a smooth, double-tapered cemented stem.

References

1. Amstutz HC, Ma SM, Jinnah RH, Mai L: Revision of aseptic loose total hip arthroplasties. *Clin Orthop* 1982;170:21-33.
2. Kavanagh BF, Ilstrup DM, Fitzgerald RH Jr: Revision total hip arthroplasty. *J Bone Joint Surg Am* 1985;67:517-526.
3. Retpen JB, Varmarken JE, Rock ND, Jensen JS: Unsatisfactory results after repeated revision of hip arthroplasty: 61 cases followed for 5 (1-10) years. *Acta Orthop Scand* 1992;63:120-127.
4. Hastings DE, Parker SM: Protrusio acetabuli in rheumatoid arthritis. *Clin Orthop* 1975;108:76-83.
5. McCollum DE, Nunley JA: Bone grafting in acetabular protrusio: A biologic buttress, in Nelson CL (ed): *The Hip: Proceedings of the Sixth Open Scientific Meeting of the Hip Society, 1978*. St. Louis, MO, CV Mosby, 1978, pp124-146.
6. Slooff TJ, Huiskes R, van Horn J, Lemmens AJ: Bone grafting in total hip replacement for acetabular protrusion. *Acta Orthop Scand* 1984;55:593-596.
7. Schreurs BW, Slooff TJ, Buma P, Gardeniers JW, Huiskes R: Acetabular reconstruction with impacted morsellised cancellous bone graft and cement: A 10- to 15-year follow-up of 60 revision arthroplasties. *J Bone Joint Surg Br* 1998;80:391-395.
8. Gie GA, Linder L, Ling RS, Simon JP, Slooff TJ, Timperley AJ: Impacted cancellous allografts and cement for revision total hip arthroplasty. *J Bone Joint Surg Br* 1993;75:14-21.
9. Schreurs BW, Huiskes R, Slooff TJJH: The initial stability of hip prosthesis in combination with femoral intramedullary bonegraft, in Odgaard A, Kjaersgaard-Andersen P, Sojbjerg JO (eds): *European Biomechanics: Proceedings of the 7th Meeting of the European Society of Biomechanics.* Aarhus, Denmark, European Society of Biomechanics, 1990, p A14.
10. Schreurs BW, Buma P, Huiskes R, Slagter JL, Slooff TJ: Morsellized allografts for fixation of the hip prosthesis femoral component: A mechanical and histological study in the goat. *Acta Orthop Scand* 1994;65:267-275.
11. Schreurs BW, Huiskes R, Buma P, Slooff TJ: Biomechanical and histological evaluation of a hydroxyapatite-coated titanium femoral stem fixed with an intramedullary morsellized bone grafting technique: An animal experiment on goats. *Biomaterials* 1996;17:1177-1186.
12. Giesen EB, Lamerigts NM, Verdonschot N, Buma P, Schreurs BW, Huiskes R: Mechanical characteristics of impacted morsellised bone grafts used in revision of total hip arthroplasty. *J Bone Joint Surg Br* 1999;81:1052-1057.
13. Brewster NT, Gillespie WJ, Howie CR, Madabhushi SP, Usmani AS, Fairbairn DR: Mechanical considerations in impaction bone grafting. *J Bone Joint Surg Br* 1999;81:118-124.
14. Verdonschot N, Schreurs BW, Van Unen JMJ, Slooff TJJH, Huiskes R: Cup stability after acetabulum reconstruction with morsellized grafts is less surgical dependent when larger grafts are used. *Trans Orthop Res Soc* 1999;24:867.
15. Eldridge JDJ, Hubble MJW, Nelson K, Smith EJ, Learmonth ID: Abstract: The effect of bone chip size on initial stability following femoral impaction grafting. *J Bone Joint Surg Br* 1997;79(suppl 3):364.
16. Wallace IW, Ammon PR, Beave RJ: Abstract: How should bone be milled? *J Bone Joint Surg Br* 1997;79(suppl 3):365-366.
17. Wallace IW, Ammon PR, Day R, Lee DA, Beaver RJ: Abstract: Does size matter? An investigation into the effects of particle size on impaction grafting in vitro. *J Bone Joint Surg Br* 1997:79(suppl 3):366.
18. Kuiper JH, Merry JC, Cheah K, Richardson JB: Graft composition influences early mechanical stability in impaction grafting. *Transactions of the 6th Congress of the European Orthopaedic Research Society 1996, Bergen, Norway*. Marburg, Germany, European Orthopaedic Research Society, 1996, p 45.
19. Malkani AL, Voor MJ, Fee KA, Bates CS: Femoral component revision using impacted morsellised cancellous graft: A biomechanical study of implant stability. *J Bone Joint Surg Br* 1996;78:973-978.
20. Berzins A, Sumner DR, Wasielewski RC, Galante JO: Impacted particulate allograft for femoral revision total hip arthroplasty: In vitro mechanical stability and effects of cement pressurization. *J Arthroplasty* 1996;11:500-506.
21. Chassin EP, Silverton CD, Berzins A, Rosenberg AG: Implant stability in revision total hip arthroplasty: Allograft bone packing following extended proximal femoral osteotomy. *J Arthroplasty* 1997;12:863-868.
22. Hellman EJ, Capello WN, Feinberg JR: Nonunion of extended trochanteric osteotomies in impaction grafting femoral revisions. *J Arthroplasty* 1998;13:945-949.
23. Hungerford DS, Jones LC: The rationale of cementless revision of cemented arthroplasty failures. *Clin Orthop* 1988;235:12-24.
24. Samuelson KM, Freeman MA, Levack B, Rassmussen GL, Revell PA: Homograft bone in revision acetabular arthroplasty: A clinical and radiographic study. *J Bone Joint Surg Br* 1988;70:367-372.
25. Roffman M, Silbermann M, Mendes DG: Viability and osteogenicity of bone graft coated with methylmethacrylate cement. *Acta Orthop Scand* 1982;53:513-519.

26. Roffman M, Silbermann M, Mendes DG: Incorporation of bone graft covered with methylmethacrylate onto the acetabular wall. *Acta Orthop Scand* 1983;54:580-583.

27. Schimmel JW, Buma P, Versleyen D, Huiskes R, Slooff TJ: Acetabular reconstruction with impacted morselized cancellous allografts in cemented hip arthroplasty: A histological and biomechanical study on the goat. *J Arthroplasty* 1998;13:438-448.

28. Schreurs BW, Huiskes R, Slooff TJJH: The initial stability of cemented and non-cemented femoral stems fixated with a bone grafting technique. *Clin Mater* 1994;16:105-110.

29. Lamerigts NM, Buma P, Huiskes R, Schreurs W, Gardeniers J, Slooff TJ: Incorporation of morsellized bone graft under controlled loading conditions: A new animal model in the goat. *Biomaterials* 2000;21:741-747.

30. Tagil M, Aspenberg P: Impaction of cancellous bone grafts impairs osteoconduction in titanium chambers. *Clin Orthop* 1998;352:231-238.

31. Rosenberg WJ, Schreurs BW, Waal Malefijt MC de, Veth RPH, Slooff TJJH: Impacted morsellized bone grafting and cemented primary total hip arthroplasty for acetabular protrusion in patients with rheumatoid arthritis. *Acta Orthop Scand* 2000;71:143-146.

32. Welten MLM, Schreurs BW, Buma P, Verdonschot N, Slooff TJJH: Acetabular reconstruction with impacted morsellized cancellous autograft and cemented total hip arthroplasty. *J Arthroplasty,* in press.

33. Karrholm J, Herberts P, Hultmark P, Malchau H, Nivbrant B, Thanner J: Radiostereometry of hip prostheses: Review of methodology and clinical results. *Clin Orthop* 1997;344:94-110.

34. Herberts P, Hultmark P, Karrholm J, Malchau H: Fixation of cemented and cementless acetabular revisions treated with impacted cancellous allograft, in Bach CS (ed): *6th Instructional Course EFORT,* Copenhagen, Denmark, EFORT, 1998, p 18.

35. Ornstein E, Franzen H, Johnsson R, Sandquist P, Stefansdottir A, Sundberg M: Migration of the acetabular component after revision with impacted morselized allografts: A radiostereometric 2-year follow-up analysis of 21 cases. *Acta Orthop Scand* 1999;70:338-342.

36. Meding JB, Ritter MA, Keating EM, Faris PM: Impaction bone-grafting before insertion of a femoral stem with cement in revision total hip arthroplasty: A minimum two-year follow-up study. *J Bone Joint Surg Am* 1997;79:1834-1841.

37. Eldridge JD, Smith EJ, Hubble MJ, Whitehouse SL, Learmonth ID: Massive early subsidence following femoral impaction grafting. *J Arthroplasty* 1997;12:535-540.

38. Mikkelsen SS, Horlyck E: Abstract: Evaluation of femoral hip arthroplasty revisions using impacted cancellous bone grafting. *Acta Orthop Scand* 1997;68(suppl 274):39.

39. Ornstein E, Sandqvist P, Sundberg M, Franzen H, Johnsson R: Abstract: 1.5-year prosthetic migration after hip revision with impacted morselized allograft: A RSA study. *Acta Orthop Scand* 1997;68(suppl 274):9.

40. Karrholm J, Hultmark P, Carlsson L, Malchau H: Subsidence of a non-polished stem in revisions of the hip using impaction allograft: Evaluation with radiostereometry and dual-energy x-ray absorptiometry. *J Bone Joint Surg Br* 1999;81:135-142.

41. Heekin RD, Engh CA, Vinh T: Morselized allograft in acetabular reconstruction: A postmortem retrieval analysis. *Clin Orthop* 1995;319:184-190.

42. Hooten JP Jr, Engh CA, Heekin RD, Vinh TN: Structural bulk allografts in acetabular reconstruction: Analysis of two grafts retrieved at post-mortem. *J Bone Joint Surg Br* 1996;78:270-275.

43. Buma P, Lamerigts N, Schreurs BW, Gardeniers J, Versleyen D, Slooff TJ: Impacted graft incorporation after cemented acetabular revision: Histological evaluation in 8 patients. *Acta Orthop Scand* 1996;67:536-540.

44. Ling RS, Timperley AJ, Linder L: Histology of cancellous impaction grafting in the femur: A case report. *J Bone Joint Surg Br* 1993;75:693-696.

45. Nelissen RG, Bauer TW, Weidenhielm LR, LeGolvan DP, Mikhail WE: Revision hip arthroplasty with the use of cement and impaction grafting: Histological analysis of four cases. *J Bone Joint Surg Am* 1995;77:412-422.

46. Ullmark G, Linder L: Histology of the femur after cancellous impaction grafting using a Charnley prosthesis. *Arch Orthop Trauma Surg* 1998;117:170-172.

47. Schatzker J, Wong MK: Acetabular revision: The role of rings and cages. *Clin Orthop* 1999;369:187-197.

22

SYMPOSIUM

Acetabular Reconstruction With Bone Impaction Grafting: 20 Years of Experience

B. Willem Schreurs, MD, PhD
Jean W.M. Gardeniers, MD, PhD
Thomas J.J.H. Slooff, MD, PhD

Introduction

Total hip arthroplasty (THA) is one of the most innovative and successful procedures in modern medicine. As a result, millions of people have been able to resume normal activities after the procedure. However, failure can be expected over the long term. The main complication of a failed THA is the osteolysis induced by aseptic loosening. Additional loss of bone stock is unavoidable during revision surgery because of the procedures necessary to remove the prosthesis. The loss of periprosthetic bone stock, therefore, is a key problem to be addressed during revision surgery.

With acetabular reconstruction, the loosening process often results in a cavitary defect, but in the more serious cases, segmental wall defects will also develop. Many acetabular reconstruction techniques have been described with cemented and noncemented cups. Controversy still exists about the best approach to these bone stock deficiencies. We use tightly impacted morcellized cancellous allografts in combination with a cemented cup in all patients with acetabular bone stock loss, both in primary and revision THA.

In 1979 at our institution, the University Medical Center Nijmegen, bone impaction grafting was started on the acetabular side in patients with bone stock loss. This technique is based on studies presented by Hastings and Parker[1] and McCollum and Nunley,[2] with modifications.

The main modifications we have made to their techniques are the use of larger fragments of trabecular bone and very vigorous impaction of the graft fragments. Rings are not used, relying instead on the stability of the cement-graft reconstruction. It is believed that bone cement does not harm incorporation of the bone graft.

This chapter will focus on the indications, preoperative planning, surgical technique, and long-term results of the method. The scientific background of this reconstruction technique is discussed in chapter 21, Basic Science of Bone Impaction Grafting.

One or more of the authors or the departments with which they are affiliated have received something of value from a commercial or other party related directly or indirectly to the subject of this chapter.

Indications

This technique is used in patients with acetabular bone stock loss who are scheduled for total hip reconstruction (primary and revision). In primary total hip reconstruction with simple protrusio, the autogenous femoral head is used as the source of bone chips, sometimes in combination with trabecular bone from the proximal femur. However, in patients with severe bone stock deficiencies (for example, congenital hip dysplasia) femoral head allografts are used in combination with meshes in primary THA to reconstruct the defects and restore the original center of rotation.

The main indication for revision arthroplasty is progressive loss of periprosthetic bone stock due to osteolysis. In most patients, this is accompanied by return of the pain and increasing physical disability. In our opinion, regular follow-up of patients with hip implants is mandatory to prevent disastrous situations, although this can sometimes be difficult. Since the 1970s, we have been following a standard protocol after primary THA at our institution to prevent excessive loss of bone stock. Radiographic signs of loosening often precede complaints from the patient. Serial radiographs are obtained to monitor changes in the position of the hip components and the cement, and bone stock loss. Sometimes surgery has to be considered even before clinical symptoms appear.

In patients with bone stock loss, it is essential to detect the reason for failure. A history of wound healing problems after implantation is an important factor.

A thorough physical examination should include laboratory blood tests. Good quality plain radiographs should be obtained in three views (anteroposterior, axial, and abduction-external). These radiographs can be used to evaluate the severity of the anatomic distortion, the location and extent of bone lysis and, if appropriate, the bone cement distribution.

It should be realized that the bone stock defects and acetabular distortions observed during surgery are often much more severe than the preoperative radiographs suggest. If septic loosening is suspected on plain radiographs, technetium scanning and gamma-immunoglobulin scintigraphy, if appropriate, can be used to exclude infection as the cause of loosening. To obtain bacterial cultures in suspect cases, needle biopsy is performed on the hip joint. Sometimes nuclear arthrography or administration of bupivacaine to the hip can help to confirm loosening of an implant.

Surgical Technique

We routinely use the posterolateral approach with the patient in the lateral decubitus position. Correct preoperative positioning of the patient is essential and is the sole responsibility of the surgeon. The patient is stabilized on the operating table with pubic and lumbar pads. In time-consuming operations, these pads are used in combination with a vacuum mattress.

This approach enables extensive exposure of the acetabulum and proximal femur, so that trochanteric osteotomy is seldom necessary. Draping should facilitate an incision that can be extended to the region of the anterior-superior iliac spine, and care should be taken to ensure free movement of the extremity and provide a clear view of the posterior, lateral, and anterior aspects of the hip joint.

In revision surgery, the major landmarks and the sciatic nerve must be identified to understand the local anatomy, because it may have been disturbed during previous surgery and by scarring. Suitable landmarks are the tip of the greater trochanter, the lesser trochanter, the tendinous part of the gluteus maximus muscle, and the borders of the medius and minimus gluteal muscles; extensive exposure is essential. Aspiration of the hip joint can be performed to obtain joint fluid for Gram staining and culture. We attempt to open the hip joint while conserving the posterior part of the hip capsule. By using stay sutures in this tissue, the sciatic nerve can be protected from direct trauma. Before dislocating the hip joint, the proximal part of the femur is extensively exposed and carefully mobilized to prevent fracturing the femur, which is often very weak. Sometimes it may be necessary to apply preventive cerclage wires around the femur to prevent accidental fracture. After dislocation, the femoral component is removed. Very wide exposure of the entire socket is achieved and all scar tissue is removed. Next, the cup is removed, taking care to avoid any additional bone damage. Biopsy specimens from the acetabular and femoral interface tissues are obtained and sent for frozen sectioning and bacterial culture. At this stage systemic perioperative antibiotics are administered. **(CD-22.1)**

The medial wall of the acetabulum is meticulously examined for segmental defects (Fig. 1, *A*). It is also imperative to determine the strength of the medial wall. If weakness is suspected, a medial wall mesh might be considered to prevent fracture during the vigorous impaction (Fig. 1, *B*). The complete rim is exposed so that the peripheral wall may be examined for segmental defects.

To restore normal hip biomechanics, we always attempt to reconstruct the cup at the original center of rotation. In most instances, the transverse ligament can be located at the caudal part of the acetabulum; it is used as a reference point for positioning the cup. A trial cup is inserted using the ligament as a reference, and the extent of the peripheral wall defect is established. Damage to the superior gluteal muscles and the nerve can be prevented by subperiosteal dissection. Next, the muscles are elevated from the bone to facilitate positioning of the meshes. These meshes should preferably be placed on the outer side of the acetabular rim (Fig. 1, *B*). Using special scissors and clamps, the flexible metal meshes are trimmed and adapted to conform with the peripheral wall defects. They can be fixed with screws or, at locations with very thin cortical bone, cerclage wires. In patients with extensive peripheral wall defects, it is sometimes impossible to achieve stability with the mesh on the outer side of the acetabulum. In these special circumstances, the mesh can be applied to the inner side and fixed with more central screws.

After all the soft tissue interface remnants have been removed, a small acetabular reamer is used to remove the sclerotic cortical bone. This action produces a freshly bleeding trabecular bone bed, which is essential for incorporation of the impacted bone graft. In patients with extreme sclerotic areas, multiple drill holes should be made to create a bleeding host bone bed and promote vascular invasion into the graft.

Medial wall defects can also be covered by a metal mesh. In most instances, adequate stability of the mesh can be achieved without screw fixation. However, the use of one or two very short screws can prevent problems. After closing the segmental wall defects in this manner, the acetabulum is contained and the situation has been converted into a cavitary defect. The foundations have been laid for bone impaction grafting.

Preparation of the Bone Graft

All of our long-term data are based on the use of fresh-frozen femoral heads that were obtained from our local bone

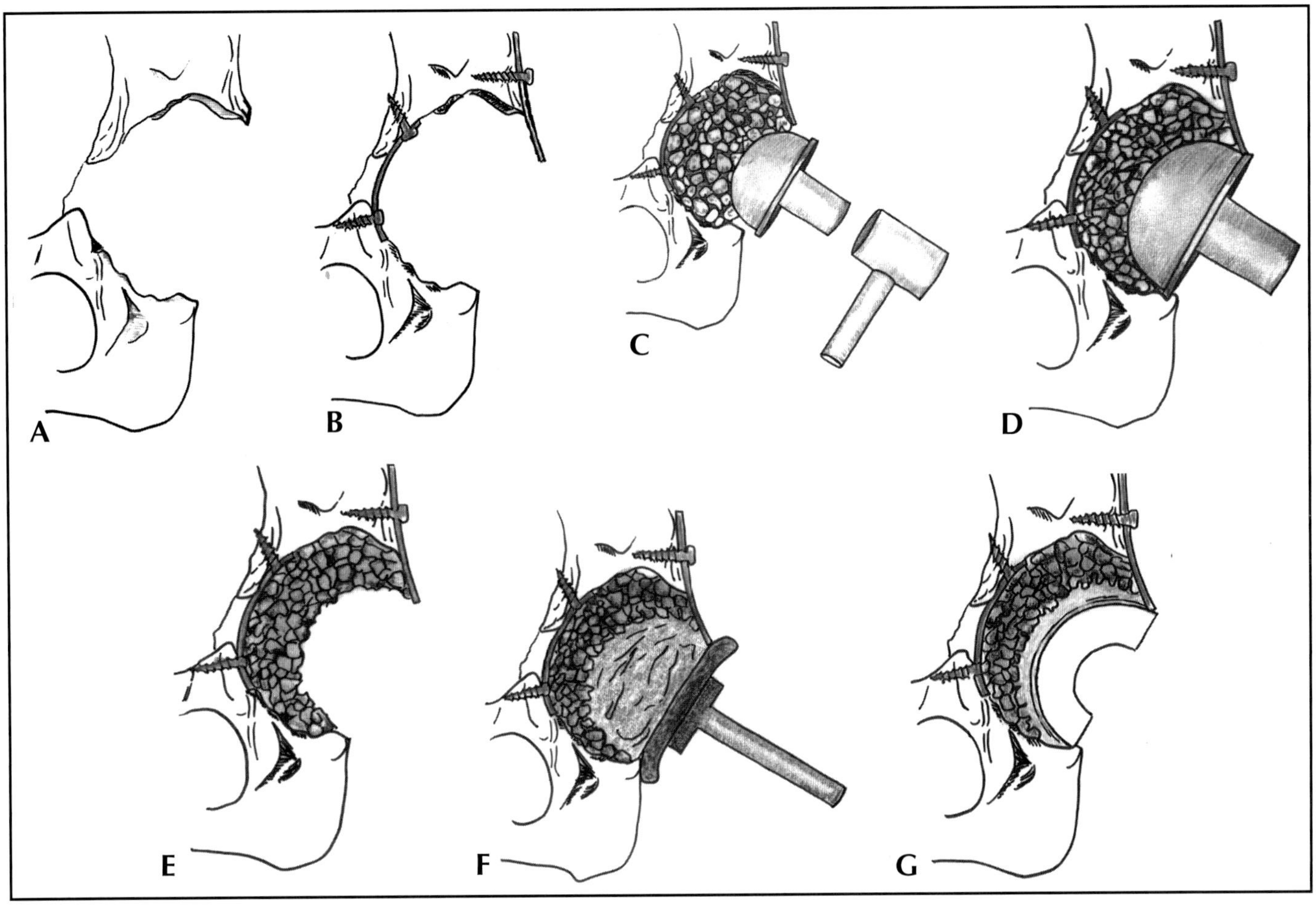

Fig. 1 A, Schematic of a hip with both a medial segmental defect and a peripheral superolateral rim defect after removal of the failed cup. **B**, The medial wall defect is closed by a metal mesh that can be fixed with screws, although this is not always necessary. The superolateral rim defect is closed by a metal mesh on the outer side of the acetabulum. This mesh must always be fixed with at least three screws. Next, a cavitary defect is created. A trial cup prosthesis inside the acetabulum is very helpful for positioning the lateral mesh at the right position. **C**, The cavitary defect is filled layer by layer with bone chips. **D**, It is essential that these bone grafts be impacted using a hammer and several diameters of impactors. **E**, After optimal impaction the impactors can be removed without collapse of the construction. A trial prostheses can be inserted to check the position. It is advised that a graft thickness of at least 5 mm be created. **F**, Cement is injected and pressurized to facilitate cement penetration into the graft. **G**, Final situation after inserting the cup.

bank. We have no experience with processed or irradiated bone. The femoral head is stored at -80°C and is only used after testing the donor at donation and at 6 months after donation. The femoral head is thawed, cleaned of all soft tissues, and divided into four parts. Morcellized grafts are produced by hand, using a bone nibbler. The inclusion of cartilage remnants from the femoral head cartilage is avoided, if possible.

Alternatively, a specially designed bone mill can be used, which produces fairly large bone chips. We recommend a chip size of 7 to 10 mm; most commercially available bone mills produce substantially smaller bone chips (2 to 4 mm), which are not recommended for impaction acetabular reconstruction.[3,4]

Acetabular Reconstruction Technique

The acetabular bone bed is cleaned using pressure lavage and the acetabulum is packed with bone chips. First, the small cavities are filled, then the entire socket, layer by layer. The bone chips are vigorously impacted using special instruments and a hammer (Fig. 1, *C* and *D*). If there is any danger of fracturing the weak medial wall, a metal mesh should be used to support this structure, but the force of impaction should not be reduced. A small impactor should be used initially, progressing to larger ones. When the impaction technique has been performed correctly, the graft layer will be stable in the acetabulum after removal of the impactor (Fig. 1, *E*). The defect is filled layer by layer, until the planned cup position has been achieved. A substantial layer of bone material at least 5 mm thick must be accumulated; otherwise, the graft may become saturated with bone cement during the process. The last impactor should be 4 mm larger than the proposed cup size to create a sufficiently large mantle of cement. The position of the socket should be brought down to the level of the transverse ligament. After impaction, the preexisting enlarged acetabular diameter will have been reduced to standard size. Pressure lavage is never used on the bone graft before cementation. During preparation of the antibiotic-loaded bone cement, pressure is maintained on the graft with the impactor last used. After insertion, the bone cement is pressurized to obtain good interdigitation with the graft (Fig. 1, *F*). Next, the cup is guided into position and held in place with a pusher until the cement has polymerized (Fig. 1, *G*).

Postoperative Care

Postoperative treatment includes anticoagulation therapy and systemic antibiotics for 24 hours. Immediately after the operation, indomethacin is administered for 7 days to prevent heterotopic ossification. Mobilization of the patient is individualized according to the extent of the original defects. In the presence of simple cavitary defects, the patient is mobilized within 2 days with partial weight bearing on crutches. Patients with more extensive original defects are mobilized after 2 weeks with partial weight bearing. In contrast with our earlier reports, only patients with a complete defect in the superolateral wall are allowed 6 weeks of bed rest. All of the patients are kept on crutches for 3 months.

Clinical Results

Acetabular Reconstruction in Primary THA

In 1984, we reported our short-term results on bone impaction grafting in 40 patients with 43 acetabular reconstructions; 21 were performed in primary cases, and 22 were revision cases after failed THA.[5] After a 2-year follow-up there had been no revisions, but radiolucent lines were visible in five instances. However, to evaluate the validity of this technique, we analyzed several groups of patients over the long term.

The outcome of the application of impacted morcellized bone grafts in primary THA was recently studied.[6] Between 1979 and 1986, 72 acetabular reconstructions were performed in 66 patients. At review, 10 patients have been lost to follow up, leaving 61 hips in 56 patients. The indication for THA was primary osteoarthritis (n = 25 hips), secondary osteoarthritis (n = 18), or rheumatoid arthritis (n = 18). Eleven patients (12 hips) had died within 10 years after the operation; none of them had undergone revision surgery. Follow-up was 10 years or longer (10 to 17 years, average 12 years) in 49 hips (45 patients). Defects were classified according to D'Antonio and associates[7] as cavitary in 81% and combined in 19% of the cases. Femoral head autografts had been used in all but three patients. At an average of 12 years' follow-up, four revisions had been performed: one for septic loosening (1.5 years after primary surgery) and three for aseptic loosening (after 7, 12, and 17 years). There were three radiographic failures, but these patients had only mild complaints at review. It was concluded that the survival rate for aseptic loosening of primary THA was 94% at 10 to 17 years' follow-up after bone impaction grafting.

The results with this technique were reviewed in patients with rheumatoid arthritis, because the outcome of total hip replacement patients with rheumatoid arthritis was worse than that in patients with osteoarthritis.[8] In patients with rheumatoid arthritis and preexisting acetabular bone stock deficiency, the results are expected to be even worse. Rosenberg and associates[9] studied the outcome of 36 primary THAs performed in 31 patients with rheumatoid arthritis and protrusio acetabuli. At review, 3 had been lost to follow-up and 12 had died within 8 years after the operation. None of the deceased patients had undergone revision. Data on 16 patients (20 hips) that had been gathered over an average follow-up of 12 years were reviewed. Revision had been performed for aseptic loosening of the acetabular component in two hips at 6.5 and 8 years after primary surgery, respectively. The survival rate of THA in this group of patients was 90%, according to the Kaplan-Meier analysis. The bone impaction technique can be considered of great value in patients with protrusio acetabuli caused by rheumatoid arthritis.

As a result of increasing experience, we decided to use this method for all acetabular reconstructions in patients with congenital hip dysplasia. In comparison with the previous study, the extent of the acetabular bone stock defects was far greater. Data were available on a group of 25 patients who had undergone acetabular reconstruction, with an average follow-up of 5 years. One patient had undergone revision of the acetabular reconstruction at 2 years after the operation because of severe pain caused by stretching of the sciatic nerve. We reconstructed the acetabulum and applied a higher center of rotation. In three patients, a radiolucent line was visible immediately after the operation, in zone 1 according to DeLee and Charnley's classifications,[10] but none was progressive.

Acetabular Reconstruction in Revision THA

The impaction method in acetabular revision surgery was reviewed.[11] Between 1979 and 1986, 62 acetabular reconstructions had been performed at

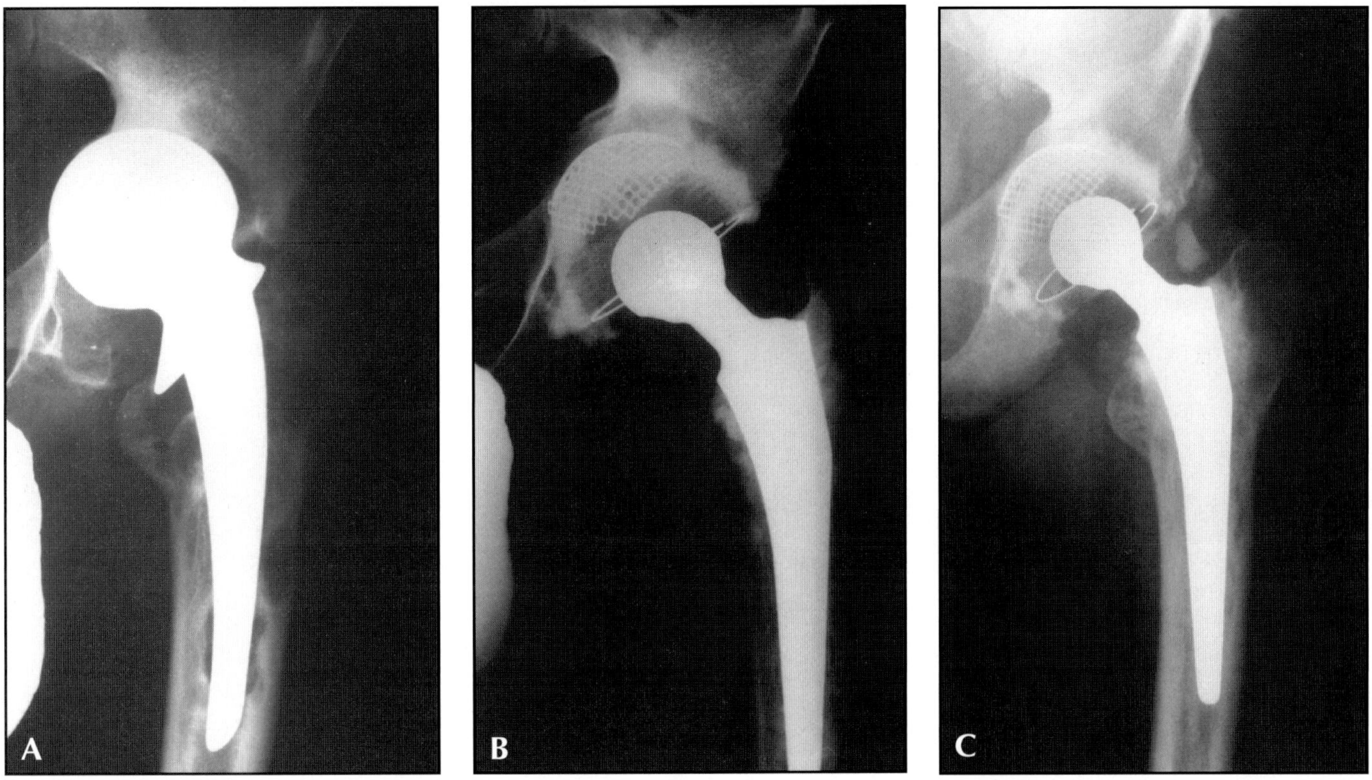

Fig. 2 A, Radiograph of a 36-year-old patient with a protrusion of a femoral head prosthesis that was inserted 6 years after femoral head necrosis. **B**, Radiograph obtained after reconstruction with bone impaction grafting in which a metal mesh was used to close the medial wall defect. **C**, Last available follow-up 19 years after the reconstruction. There is no migration and no sign of loosening. Note the homogeneous structure of the bone graft.

our institute in 58 patients with failed hip prostheses. Two hips were lost to follow-up, leaving data on 56 patients (60 hips). Fifteen patients had died, but none had undergone a re-revision. The indication for revision was aseptic loosening in 56 hips and septic loosening in 4 hips; 2 hips had previous revisions, once and twice, respectively. There were 13 men and 43 women with a mean age at operation of 59.1 years (range, 23 to 82). Defects were classified as cavitary in 37 hips and combined cavitary/segmental defects in 23 hips (10 central segmental and 13 peripheral wall defects). At review after an average of 11.8 years (10 to 15 years), the mean Harris hip score was 85 (range, 53 to 100). Re-revisions had been done in 5 hips: 2 for culture-proven septic loosening after 3 and 6 years and 3 for aseptic loosenings after 6, 9, and 12 years. Radiologic loosening was observed in four hips with progressive radiolucent lines in three zones according to the DeLee and Charnley classification. However, most hips were radiologically very stable, even in young patients with a long follow-up (Figs. 2 and 3). The survival rate for aseptic loosening of revision THA surgery was 94% at a mean follow-up of nearly 12 years.

The outcome of primary and revision THA in young patients with bone stock loss is unfavorable. We studied 42 acetabular reconstructions over the long term; impacted morcellized bone grafts and a cemented THA had been performed in patients younger than age 50 years at surgery (21 to 49 years; average, 37.9 years).[12] Reconstruction was performed in 23 primary THAs (19 patients) and 19 revision THAs (18 patients). Three patients (4 hips) had died within 10 years after the operation without revision and 3 patients were untraceable. Data were available on 35 hips (31 patients), with a mean follow-up of 12.7 years (range, 10 to 17 years). At review, revision of the acetabular reconstruction had been performed in 4 hips: 1 for septic loosening after 2 years and 3 for aseptic loosening after 7, 11, and 12 years, respectively. The overall THA survival rate after 12.7 years was 89%; excluding the hip with septic loosening, the THA survival rate for hips with aseptic loosening was 91%. It can therefore be concluded that acetabular reconstruction with impacted morcellized bone grafts and cement gives satisfactory long-term results, even in patients younger than age 50 years.

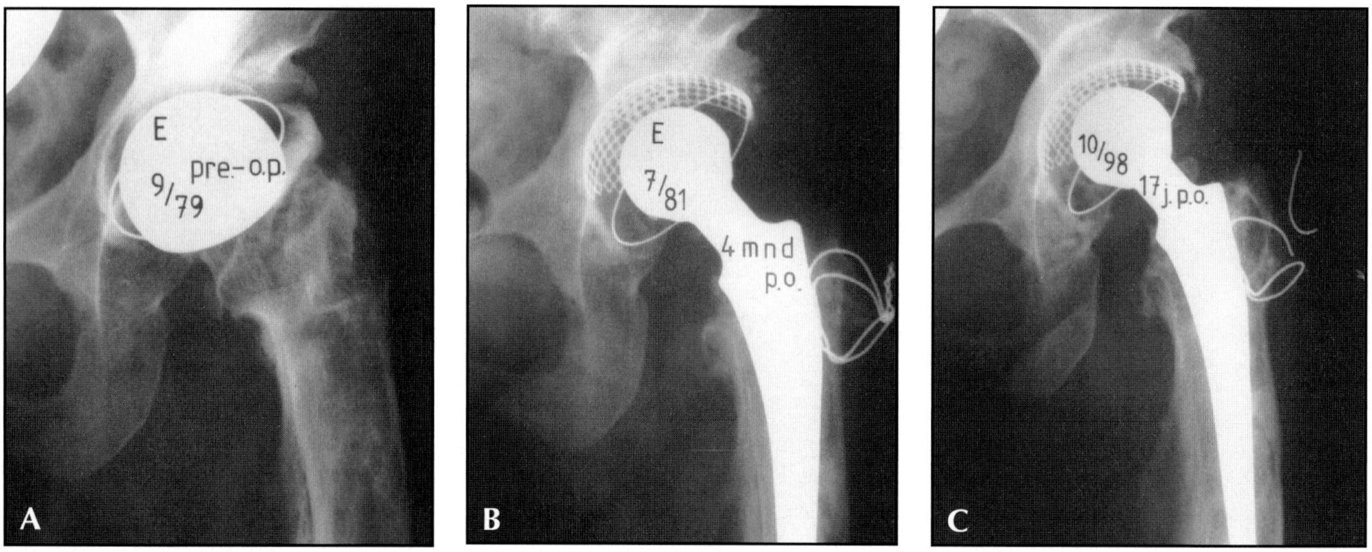

Fig. 3 A, Radiograph of a 23-year-old woman with a failed resurfacing prosthesis that was inserted for severe secondary osteoarthritis after neonatal septic arthritis. **B**, Radiograph obtained 4 months after reconstruction of the cavitary defect with impacted bone grafts. A metal mesh is positioned on top of the graft as a kind of metal backing. (The metal mesh on top of the graft is currently not recommended.) **C**, After 17 years of follow-up, there is no sign of impending failure. There is some wear but no radiolucent lines in a clinically well-performing hip.

Discussion and Recommendations

The process of aseptic loosening results in bone stock loss caused by osteolysis, both with cemented and noncemented cups. This leads to widening of the acetabulum and weakening of the pelvic bone bed. The implant becomes progressively more unstable and the patient often complains of pain and impaired function.

Revision arthroplasty on the acetabular side is still a controversial issue among orthopaedic surgeons. A variety of reconstructive techniques have been proposed. In revision surgery, it must be decided how to cope with the bone stock loss, how to restore the original center of rotation, and how to achieve stability of the new implant. In addition, it is difficult to compare the outcome of the different techniques because several methods have been used to classify the preexisting bone stock defect.[13] Therefore, more uniformity in classification is required.

Cemented fixation in revisions is less effective in the presence of bone stock loss and it is impossible to achieve adequate cement interdigitation under these conditions in the remaining sclerotic host bone, especially when the bone stock loss is extensive.[14-18] However, this method can be considered in elderly patients with limited life expectancy. In the presence of large rim defects, several types of reinforcement rings have been used in combination with bone grafting and cement. Although reports at midterm follow-up are acceptable,[19-21] there are some concerns. This rigid metal reinforcement is prone to fail over time because of the mismatch between the more elastic pelvic bone and the rigid metal shell. Besides, it should be stressed that the use of morcellized bone grafts in combination with metal reinforcement rings is a totally different method from that of acetabular reconstruction with impacted morcellized bone grafts. We believe that it is essential that these impacted bone grafts are loaded, because load protection by a metal shell hampers the process of graft incorporation. After failure of a metal ring, the defect can be expected to be larger than the original one, therefore, the surgical problems at that reconstruction will be even more challenging.

Structural femoral head autografts and allografts have been used to reconstruct large acetabular rim defects. However, long-term results showed a failure rate of 29% after a mean follow-up of 16.5 years.[22] It was concluded that the clinical outcome was not predictable and that graft resorption occurred. The explanation is probably incomplete incorporation of these structural grafts. Hooten and associates[23] reported the results of two graft retrievals after structural bulk allografts had been used for acetabular reconstruction. Although the patients had good clinical results and the radiographs showed incorporation between the graft and the host bone, microscopically there was only limited bony union. Revascularization extended for no more than 2 mm into the structural graft. Even after 48 months, allograft revascularization and remodeling were minimal.

Some reports on cementless acetabular components showed promising short-term and intermediate results.[24,25] These cementless components were very often supplemented by bone grafts: particulate bone grafting successfully restored the bone stock loss in cavitary and noncontained medial wall defects. In cavitary defects and in defects with more than 80% of the acetabular rim intact, the results were excellent at midterm follow-up. The results of the use of noncemented cups in combination with more severe rim defects were unclear. Morsi and associates[26] showed a success rate of 86% after an average of 7.1 years in patients with type 2A defects in which the involvement is less than 50% of the acetabulum. This gives rise to serious concern regarding the long-term results of noncemented acetabular revision in more extensive defects. Another cause of concern is the severe osteolysis over the longer term (> 10 years) seen after the use of some noncemented cups for primary reconstruction. If osteolysis also occurs in revision cases, the outcome will probably be unfavorable. Very large noncemented implants have been used in the presence of extensive bone stock loss. Although a large jumbo cup or a double bubble cup can be used to reconstruct the original center of rotation, long-term success rates of these procedures have not been reported.

We believe that a biologic technique should be used to reconstruct skeletal defects, and we now have more than 20 years of experience with bone impaction grafting in combination with cement. Long-term data are available on primary THA with preexisting bone stock loss and acetabular revisions.[6,9,11] Although the cup survival rate declines in time at 10 to 15 years' follow-up, the results are favorable. The application of this technique to larger segmental defects is technically far more demanding. In general, certain surgically-related factors play the greatest role in the success or failure of a revision procedure. Therefore, before acetabular reconstruction with impaction grafting and cement is begun, the surgeon should become as familiar as possible with the clinical, technical, and scientific details of this reconstruction method. It is important to be aware that a wide exposure is essential to facilitate the application of the meshes to contain peripheral segmental defects. Preparation of the bone graft material is also important. The bone graft was never washed after impaction. Although washing may be possible using a sieve to protect the bone graft and this procedure may facilitate cement intrusion into the graft, a potential drawback is that a lot of potentially important biologic factors (for example, bone morphogenetic protein, growth factors, etc) may be diluted or washed out.

The stability of acetabular cups after reconstruction with impaction bone grafting in fresh-frozen human pelvises was studied.[27] Bone chips were prepared from fresh-frozen femoral heads in two different ways: one part was nibbled by a rongeur (average chip size 9.2 mm, SD = 0.8 mm), while the other part was produced by a bone mill (average chip size 2.0 mm, SD = 0.5 mm). The acetabulae of the fresh-frozen human pelvic bones were overreamed and symmetrical bilateral cavitary superomedial defects type 2 (American Academy of Orthopaedic Surgeons classification) were made. In one pelvic bone, paired tests were done with large and small chips. Two surgeons experienced with the technique performed the implantations. The size of the bone chips had a significant effect on stability. When large bone chips were used, the outcome was more predictable, consistent and less surgeon-dependent. Therefore, the use of bone chips between 0.7 and 1.0 cm for acetabular reconstruction is strongly recommended because the outcome is more reproducible.

Concern has been expressed about cement coming into contact with impacted morcellized bone graft material. However, Roffman and associates[28,29] already showed that contact with bone cement did not impair incorporation of the bone graft. This was confirmed in two goat models in which the outcome of bone impaction grafting on the acetabular and femoral sides was studied.[30,31] Heekin and associates[32] reported incorporation in retrievals after morcellized bone grafting. In 1996, the histology of acetabular reconstruction with bone impaction grafting in 8 instances of THA cases was reported.[33] More recently, we have re-reviewed all the biopsy specimens obtained for histologic investigation of acetabular reconstructions. (unpublished data, 2000). This new series contains a number of larger biopsies. Histology specimens were available on 25 biopsies from 20 patients. The follow-up period was between 3 and 170 months. Most revisions were performed with fresh-frozen allograft bone from the local bone bank. Although the degree of incorporation between the specimens differed widely, a clear trend was visible. Remnants of graft material could be easily recognized on the basis of empty osteocyte lacunae. At 3 months, large amounts of the graft had already become incorporated and occasionally some enchondral ossification was seen. In the biopsy specimens obtained at 4 and 5 months, a front of revascularization had penetrated through the graft and could be recognized on the basis of vital soft tissue. During the passage of this front, osteoclasts removed bone graft and osteoblasts produced osteoid and woven bone on the remnants of the graft and in the interstitial space. The biopsy specimens obtained at 8 to 30 months showed various stages of graft incorporation. At 8 and 9 months, varying amounts of graft had become embedded in a new trabecular structure. Initially, the newly formed bone was of the woven type. The most woven bone was present at the graft-cement interface. In the specimens obtained after longer follow-up, relatively less woven bone was seen and large areas had become remodeled into normal vital lamellar trabecular bone. In the specimens obtained at 15, 22, and 28 months, graft remnants in the newly formed bone were extremely scarce. Surprisingly, the specimens that were obtained between 59 and 79 months' follow-up showed larger areas of graft remnants, with or without fibrotic tissue. However, four out of five specimens had been revised because of aseptic loosening of the cup. At follow-up of 10 years or longer, the grafts had become completely incorporated.

Bone impaction grafting is very suitable for acetabular reconstruction in primary and revision surgery. It provides a biologic solution for acetabular bone stock loss. However, the method is technically highly demanding and great care must be taken to fully understand the principles of the technique.

References

1. Hastings DE, Parker SM: Protrusio acetabuli in rheumatoid arthritis. *Clin Orthop* 1975;108:76-83.
2. McCollum DE, Nunley JA: Bone grafting in acetabular protrusio: A biologic buttress, in Nelson CL (ed): *The Hip: Proceedings of the Sixth Open Scientific Meeting of the Hip Society*. St Louis, MO, CV Mosby, 1978, pp 124-146.
3. Brewster NT, Gillespie WJ, Howie CR, Madabhushi SP, Usmani AS, Fairbairn DR: Mechanical considerations in impaction bone grafting. *J Bone Joint Surg Br* 1999;81:118-124.
4. Wallace IW, Ammon PR, Beave RJ: Abstract: How should bone be milled? *J Bone Joint Surg Br* 1997;79(suppl III):S365-366.
5. Slooff TJ, Huiskes R, van Horn J, Lemmens AJ: Bone grafting in total hip replacement for acetabular protrusion. *Acta Orthop Scand* 1984;55:593-596.
6. Welten MLM, Schreurs BW, Buma P, Verdonschot N, Slooff TJJH: Acetabular reconstruction with impacted morsellized cancellous auto graft and cemented total hip arthroplasty. *J Arthroplasty*, in press.
7. D'Antonio JA, Capello WN, Borden LS, et al: Classification and management of acetabular abnormalities in total hip arthroplasty. *Clin Orthop* 1989;243:126-137.
8. Malchau H, Herberts P: Abstract: Re-revision after total hip replacement: A re-revision-risk study of 160,000 primary and 11,500 revision total hip replacements (THR). *65th Annual Meeting Proceedings.* Rosemont, IL, American Academy of Orthopaedic Surgeons, 1998, p 323.
9. Rosenberg WW, Schreurs BW, de Waal Malefijt MC, Veth RP, Slooff TJ: Impacted morsellized bone grafting and cemented primary total hip arthroplasty for acetabular protrusion in patients with rheumatoid arthritis: An 8- to 18-year follow-up study of 36 hips. *Acta Orthop Scand* 2000;71:143-146.
10. DeLee JG, Charnley J: Radiological demarcation of cemented sockets in total hip replacement. *Clin Orthop* 1976;121:20-32.
11. Schreurs BW, Slooff TJ, Buma P, Gardeniers JW, Huiskes R: Acetabular reconstruction with impacted morsellised cancellous bone graft and cement: A 10- to 15- year follow-up of 60 revision arthroplasties. *J Bone Joint Surg Br* 1998;80:391-395.
12. Schreurs BW, van Tienen TG, Buma P, Verdonschot N, Gardeniers JWM, Slooff TJJH: Favorable results of acetabular reconstruction with impacted morsellized bone grafts in patients younger than 50 years: A 10 to 18 year follow up study. *Acta Orthop Scand*, in press.
13. Campbell DG, Masri BA, Garbuz DS, Duncan CP: Acetabular bone loss during revision total hip replacement: Preoperative investigation and planning. *Instr Course Lect* 1999;48:43-56.
14. Kavanagh BF, Ilstrup DM, Fitzgerald RH Jr: Revision total hip arthroplasty. *J Bone Joint Surg Am* 1985;67:517-526.
15. Retpen JB, Varmarken JE, Rock ND, Jensen JS: Unsatisfactory results after repeated revision of hip arthroplasty: 61 cases followed for 5 (1-10) years. *Acta Orthop Scand* 1992;63:120-127.
16. Stromberg CN, Herberts P, Ahnfelt L: Revision total hip arthroplasty in patients younger than 55 years old: Clinical and radiologic results after 4 years. *J Arthroplasty* 1988;3:47-59.
17. Kershaw CJ, Atkins RM, Dodd CA, Bulstrode CJ: Revision total hip arthroplasty for aseptic failure: A review of 276 cases. *J Bone Joint Surg Br* 1991;73:564-568.
18. Raut VV, Siney PD, Wroblewski BM: Cemented revision for aseptic acetabular loosening: A review of 387 hips. *J Bone Joint Surg Br* 1995;77:357-361.
19. Berry DJ, Muller ME: Revision arthroplasty using an anti-protrusio cage for massive acetabular bone deficiency. *J Bone Joint Surg Br* 1992;74:711-715.
20. Schatzker J, Wong MK: Acetabular revision: The role of rings and cages. *Clin Orthop* 1999;369:187-197.
21. Gill TJ, Sledge JB, Muller ME: The Burch-Schneider anti-protrusio cage in revision total hip arthroplasty: Indications, principles and long-term results. *J Bone Joint Surg Br* 1998;80:946-953.
22. Shinar AA, Harris WH: Bulk structural autogenous grafts and allografts for reconstruction of the acetabulum in total hip arthroplasty: Sixteen-year-average follow-up. *J Bone Joint Surg Am* 1997;79:159-168.
23. Hooten JP Jr, Engh CA, Heekin RD, Vinh TN: Structural bulk allografts in acetabular reconstruction: Analysis of two grafts retrieved at post-mortem. *J Bone Joint Surg Br* 1996;78:270-275.
24. Padgett DE, Kull L, Rosenberg A, Sumner DR, Galante JO: Revision of the acetabular component without cement after total hip arthroplasty: Three to six-year follow-up. *J Bone Joint Surg Am* 1993;75:663-673.
25. Silverton CD, Rosenberg AG, Sheinkop MB, Kull LR, Galante JO: Revision of the acetabular component without cement after total hip arthroplasty: A follow-up note regarding results at seven to eleven years. *J Bone Joint Surg Am* 1996;78:1366-1370.
26. Morsi E, Garbuz D, Gross AE: Revision total hip arthroplasty with shelf bulk allografts: A long-term follow-up study. *J Arthroplasty* 1996;11:86-90.
27. Verdonschot N, Schreurs BW, Van Unen JMJ, Slooff TJJH, Huiskes R: Cup stability after acetabulum reconstruction with morsellized grafts is less surgical dependent when larger grafts are used. *Trans Orthop Res Soc* 1999;24:867.
28. Roffman M, Silbermann M, Mendes DG: Viability and osteogenicity of bone graft coated with methylmethacrylate cement. *Acta Orthop Scand* 1982;53:513-519.
29. Roffman M, Silbermann M, Mendes DG: Incorporation of bone graft covered with methylmethacrylate onto acetabular wall: An experimental study. *Acta Orthop Scand* 1983;54:580-583.
30. Schreurs BW, Buma P, Huiskes R, Slagter JL, Slooff TJ: Morsellized allografts for fixation of the hip prosthesis femoral component: A mechanical and histological study in the goat. *Acta Orthop Scand* 1994;65:267-275.
31. Schimmel JW, Buma P, Versleyen D, Huiskes R, Slooff TJ: Acetabular reconstruction with impacted morselized cancellous allografts in cemented hip arthroplasty: A histological and biomechanical study on the goat. *J Arthroplasty* 1998;13:438-448.
32. Heekin RD, Engh CA, Vinh T: Morselized allograft in acetabular reconstruction: A post-mortem retrieval analysis. *Clin Orthop* 1995;319:184-190.
33. Buma P, Lamerigts N, Schreurs BW, Gardeniers J, Versleyen D, Slooff TJ: Impacted graft incorporation after cemented acetabular revision: Histological evaluation in 8 patients. *Acta Orthop Scand* 1996;67:536-540.

Reference to Video

Sloof T, Gardeniers JWM: Acetabular reconstruction with impacted grafting and cement. *Total Hip Arthroplasty, Management of Acetabular Bone Loss.* Nijmegen, The Netherlands, 1995.

23

Rationale of Periacetabular Osteotomy and Background Work

Michael Leunig, MD
Klaus A. Siebenrock, MD
Reinhold Ganz, MD

Osteoarthrosis of the hip is frequently caused by mechanical abnormalities, for example, residual deformity from developmental hip disease such as acetabular dysplasia.[1] Untreated acetabular dysplasia is the most common cause of secondary osteoarthrosis[2,3] arising from pathological joint-loading forces.[4] It has been reported to cause secondary osteoarthrosis by the age of 50 years in 25% to 50% of patients.[5,6] In order to improve the prognosis for the hip in this relatively young cohort of patients, pelvic osteotomies have recently been introduced to improve the abnormal anatomic conditions and reduce the load across the hip joint.[7]

Pathomechanisms

In acetabular dysplasia, intrinsically normal intra-articular soft-tissue structures are exposed to loading forces that physically exceed their tolerance level, resulting in anatomic deformities and damage to the hip joint. For example, deficient acetabular coverage of the femoral head has been related to osteoarthrosis,[8,9] whereas the orientation of the femoral head plays a less important role.[10] The resulting instability and anterolateral migration of the femoral head leads to chronic shear stresses at the acetabular margin. The acetabular labrum initially hypertrophies in order to maintain the femoral head within the joint. If the chronic shear stresses persist, the labral "soft-tissue compensation" fails, and the labrum is torn off the acetabular rim, sometimes with an osseous fragment.[11] Histomorphologically, the labrum shows myxoid degeneration of its fibrocartilage structure and adjacent ganglion formation within the bone or soft tissues.[11] In addition to increased femoral head instability resulting from secondary labral lesions, the joint-sealing function, which is required for sufficient cartilage lubrication and distribution of joint pressures,[12,13] is lost.[14] Labral alterations are known to represent an early precursor of osteoarthrosis of the hip.[8,11,15] In this mechanically compromised situation, elevation of joint contact pressures at the acetabular rim is directly related to the onset of cartilage degeneration.[4] As a consequence, an adaptive increase in the anterolateral subchondral bone density occurs in these insufficiently contained hips.[9]

Therapeutic Options

Although prosthetic replacement of the hip has a predictably good functional outcome in the elderly, the longevity of prosthetic replacement in young patients has been notably inconsistent.[16,17] Artificial prosthetic surfaces with the mechanical properties and durability of articular cartilage have yet to be found.[7] Prosthetic replacement therefore remains the treatment of choice for most patients with inflammatory disease and for patients who are not expected to outlive their implant. However, its use in the younger, more physically active patient remains controversial, especially if the cause of the osteoarthrosis is mechanically correctable.[18,19] Since arthrodesis is not indicated for bilateral hip disease and this procedure is frequently unacceptable to the patient, alternative methods with which to prevent the hip from failing have been pursued.[20] There is an increasing body of evidence that the prognosis for the hip can be substantially improved by joint-preserving osteotomies in which the emphasis has shifted from the proximal part of the femur to the pelvis.[21-23]

Principles of Pelvic Osteotomy

The goal of pelvic osteotomy is to change the pathologic mechanical environment that leads to secondary osteoarthrosis. In patients with acetabular dysplasia, this might be achieved by improving coverage or congruity, or both, through either of two basic mechanisms. Either the pelvic osteotomy increases femoral head coverage by augmentation of the acetabular

Table 1
Characteristics of pelvic reorientation osteotomies

Study	Closeness of Osteotomy to Acetabulum	Types of Osteotomy	Physis Crossed
Salter[30]	Distant	Single	No
Sutherland and Greenfield[33]	Distant	Double	No
Hopf[34]	Distant	Double	No
LeCoeur[31]	Distant	Triple	No
Steel[32]	Distant	Triple	No
Tonnis and associates[35,36]	Close	Triple	No
Carlioz and associates[37]	Close	Triple	No
Nishio[38]	Close	Spherical	Yes
Eppright[39]	Close	Spherical	Yes
Wagner[40]	Close	Spherical	Yes
Ninomiya and Tagawa[41]	Close	Spherical	Yes
Kuznenko and Adiev[42]	Close	Translocation	Yes
Ganz and associates[43]	Close	Periacetabular	Yes

roof or it changes the spatial orientation of the acetabulum (Table 1).

Augmentation Procedures

Procedures such as the Chiari osteotomy[24] and the shelf procedure[25,26] reduce joint-loading forces by augmenting the main weight-bearing area of the joint. With both methods, osseous coverage can be reproducibly improved, and the superior aspect of the capsule undergoes metaplastic transformation to fibrocartilage. However, the labrum remains within the main weight-bearing area and is subjected to chronic shear stresses. Nishina and associates[27] reported a 50% rate of failure of the Chiari osteotomy in patients with acetabular dysplasia when the preoperative arthrogram showed evidence of a labral lesion. Moreover, compared with hyaline cartilage, fibrocartilage has inferior mechanical characteristics for withstanding axial loading. Also, optimal coverage, particularly in the posterolateral quadrant of the acetabulum, is not achieved.[28] While augmentation procedures can provide reliable pain relief for some years, they should be regarded as salvage procedures.[29]

Reorientation Procedures

These procedures change the orientation of the acetabular articular surface, thereby correcting the anterolateral deficiency. In the vast majority of hips with acetabular dysplasia, there is sufficient articular surface in the posteroinferior quadrant to allow reorientation procedures. These provide greater surface area for load-bearing while maintaining stability of the joint. In reorientation procedures, coverage is achieved with hyaline cartilage supported by subchondral bone, which has optimal mechanical qualities for weight bearing. Reorientation procedures include single, double, and triple osteotomies as well as spherical and periacetabular osteotomies. The Bernese periacetabular osteotomy redirects the acetabulum into a mechanically more appropriate position, thereby decreasing shear forces and load at the acetabular rim. This chapter focuses on the Bernese periacetabular osteotomy for reorientation of the acetabulum with an emphasis on the rationale for its development.

Rationale for the Bernese Periacetabular Osteotomy

Mechanics

The dysplastic acetabulum can be reoriented by a single innominate osteotomy such as that described by Salter.[30] While this may be beneficial in children, the degree of correction that is possible in adolescents and adults is limited by the age-related increase in the stiffness of the symphysis pubis. Moreover, this osteotomy retroverts and lateralizes the joint because of a hinged angulation of the acetabulum around a fixed axis. The dysplastic hip joint is usually relatively lateralized. Additional lateralization and distalization is undesirable, as it further increases adverse joint reactive forces. As a result, a variety of double and triple osteotomies and periacetabular osteotomies have been developed in an attempt to improve the degree and accuracy of correction.

LeCoeur[31] was the first to perform a technique for triple osteotomy of the pelvis. His method, and the one described later by Steel,[32] divides the ilium, pubis, and ischium distant to the joint. Improvements in coverage with this osteotomy are limited by the size of the fragment and by the muscular and ligamentous attachments, especially the strong sacropelvic ligaments. The double osteotomy technique of Sutherland and Greenfield[33] consists of an anterior pelvic osteotomy in addition to an innominate osteotomy close to the symphysis pubis. Hopf[34] recommended a double osteotomy variant through the floor of the true acetabulum in hips with higher subluxation.

Acetabular reorientation has been substantially increased by the juxta-articular triple osteotomy of Tonnis and associates.[35,36] This technique avoids the sacropelvic ligaments, which usually limit the mobility of the osteotomized fragment. A similar technique was proposed by Carlioz and associates.[37] These osteotomies may result in a defect between the osteotomized fragment and the ischium if major corrections are performed. They may often require special efforts for stabilization, such as use of a spica cast. Nishio,[38] Eppright,[39] Wagner,[40] and Ninomiya and Tagawa[41] described the so-called dial, or spherical, osteotomy in the periacetabular region. The osteotomy described by Eppright is barrel-shaped along the anterior-posterior axis, allowing for excellent lateral coverage but only a limited amount of anterior coverage. Kuznenko and Adiev[42] described a translocation osteotomy in which the acetabulum is cut into the shape of a funnel, with the apex situated inside the pelvis. The more spherical osteotomies provide good lateral and anterior coverage but are limited with regard to the correction of version and mediolateral displacement.

On the basis of mechanical as well as biologic considerations, and in light of the limitations of previous techniques, a new pelvic osteotomy, the Bernese periacetabular osteotomy,[43] was developed in 1983. The polygonally-shaped juxta-articular osteotomy respects the vascular blood supply to the acetabular fragment. It facilitates extensive acetabular reorientation, including correction of version and mediolateral displacement, and it can be combined with a femoral osteotomy. The posterior column remains mechanically intact, which protects the sciatic nerve and enables minimal internal fixation as well as early mobilization. The dimensions of the true pelvis remain unchanged, permitting unimpaired vaginal delivery,[44] an important aspect that is less favorable with all other nonspherical osteotomies. All steps of the acetabular osteotomy are performed with use of the modified Smith-Petersen approach.[45] An anterior joint capsulotomy provides information about and treatment options for lesions of the acetabular rim and, more importantly, allows control of an impingement-free range of motion.

In contrast to distant pelvic osteotomies, the Bernese periacetabular osteotomy and the spherical osteotomies cross the posterior line of the triradiate cartilage. Therefore, these osteotomies are not indicated if growth potential remains within this physis, because growth abnormalities could result from its premature closure.[46]

Biological Characteristics

There are some concerns regarding the vascularity of the acetabular fragment with juxta-articular (spherical) osteotomies. Although vascular compromise has not been described, as it was after Hopf's double osteotomy,[34] there is the potential of separating the acetabular fragment from the acetabular artery. Since, after spherical osteotomies, the acetabular fragment relies on the blood supply provided through the acetabular artery and the capsule, a simultaneous capsulotomy should not be performed. The conception of the Bernese periacetabular osteotomy ensured the preservation of the blood supply to the acetabular fragment.[46,47]

Clinical and Radiographic Assessment

Establishing the diagnosis is straightforward in cases of clinical and radiographic end-stage disease, whereas it is much more difficult to assess incipient disease. However, patients with incipient disease are the ones who benefit the most from a joint-preserving procedure, especially when there are no radiographic signs of secondary osteoarthrosis.

History

The majority of patients presenting with symptoms related to an underlying lesion of the acetabular rim[11] are young adults in their second, third, or fourth decade of life. The primary symptom is a sharp, knife-like pain in the groin that subsides as acutely as it presents. Prolonged sitting or walking can exacerbate the pain. Symptoms of acetabular dysplasia range from early fatigue to clear weakness of the abductors, with irritation over the greater trochanter. The pain can be reproduced by activities that involve forced hip flexion, adduction, and internal rotation, including rapid descent of stairs (particularly on a circular staircase), breaststroke swimming, entering or exiting a motor vehicle, tennis, and soccer. The catching phenomenon appears to be similar to that caused by meniscal disease of the knee and occasionally requires manipulation of the lower limb, usually in the form of a "shaking-free" movement. As the symptoms increase in frequency, residual pain may result in a slight limp.

Physical Examination

A complete physical examination includes assessment of gait, limb length, muscle power, and range of motion as well as special tests. An antalgic gait will be evident immediately after an acute episode of locking. A positive Trendelenburg gait and sign indicate underlying abductor weakness. A full (or even increased) range of motion is normal in early hip dysplasia and will begin to decrease with the onset of secondary osteoarthrosis. There is a clunk in some dysplastic hips with deficient anterior coverage. As the extremity is externally rotated, the active iliopsoas tendon snaps over the prominent femoral head, producing a normally pain-free snapping or clunking sensation. This is eliminated by placing the limb in neutral or internal rotation.

There are specific clinical tests that are used to examine underlying hip disease and abnormalities of the surrounding osseous and soft-tissue structures. A suspicion of a lesion of the acetabular rim[11,48] is best confirmed by the impingement test (Fig.1, *A*). With the patient supine, the hip is internally rotated as it is passively flexed to about 90° and adducted. Flexion and adduction leads to the approximation of the femoral neck and the acetabular rim. Additional internal rotation ind-uces shearing forces at the labrum, which is similar to the knee meniscus, causing

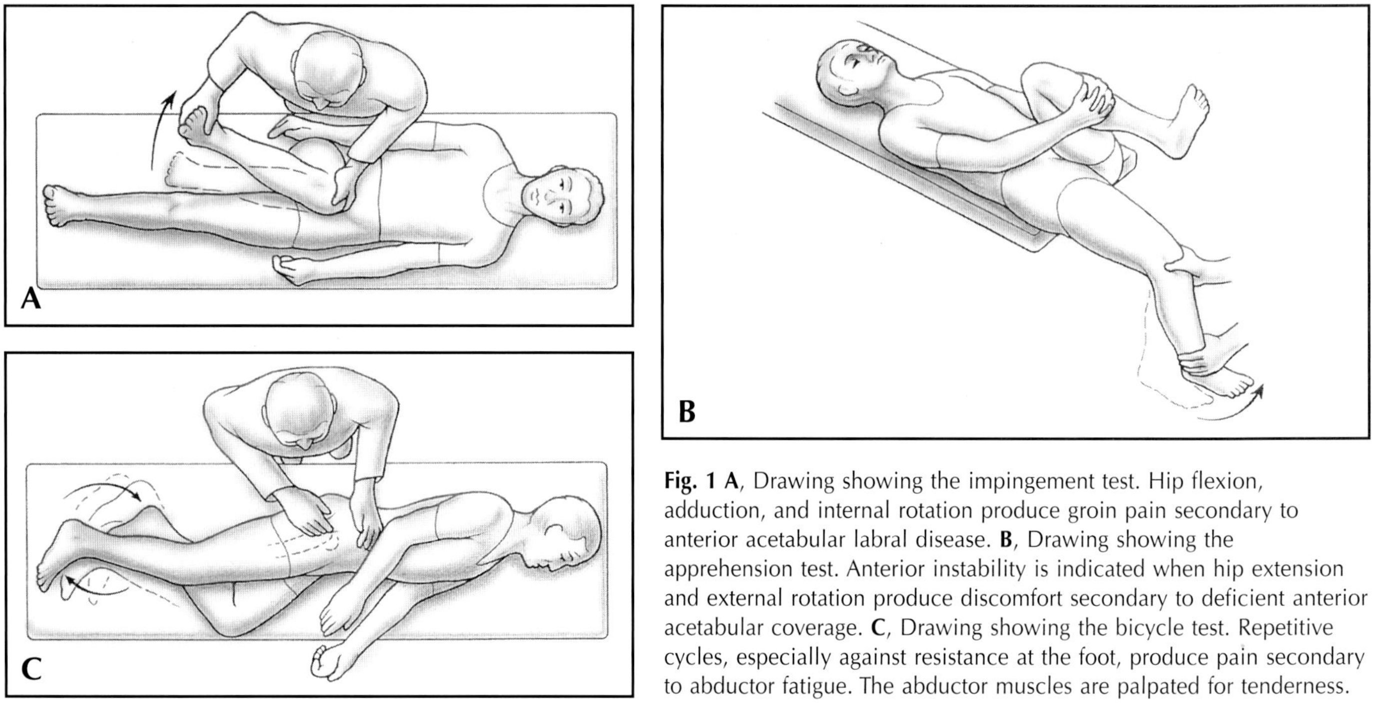

Fig. 1 A, Drawing showing the impingement test. Hip flexion, adduction, and internal rotation produce groin pain secondary to anterior acetabular labral disease. **B**, Drawing showing the apprehension test. Anterior instability is indicated when hip extension and external rotation produce discomfort secondary to deficient anterior acetabular coverage. **C**, Drawing showing the bicycle test. Repetitive cycles, especially against resistance at the foot, produce pain secondary to abductor fatigue. The abductor muscles are palpated for tenderness.

stimulation of the nerve endings. This will elicit sharp groin pain if the labrum is torn or degenerated. Less frequently, patients may have a positive apprehension test for symptomatic anterior instability (Fig. 1, *B*). With this test, the patient lies supine and the hip is extended, abducted, and externally rotated. Discomfort and a sense of instability are produced secondary to deficient anterior acetabular coverage of the femoral head. In a very thin patient, this external rotation in extension can produce a mass in the inguinal region, referred to as the lump sign,[15] which represents the femoral head pushing against the anterior aspect of the hip capsule. Patients may also reveal troch-anteric irritation on the bicycle test (in the lateral position), reflecting abductor muscle insufficiency (Fig. 1, *C*). This test is performed by placing the patient in the lateral position, with the affected hip up; a bicycle-pedaling maneuver is then performed as the lateral and posterior margins of the trochanter are palpated. Increasing the load on the pedaling foot may exacerbate the pain. Tenderness is most commonly palpated along the posterior border of the gluteus medius muscle. With direct palpation over the trochanteric bursa, the examiner may feel crepitus, which the patient may have previously des-cribed as a sensation of "sand in the joint."

Conventional Radiography

An orthograde standing anteroposterior radiograph and a false-profile radiograph of the pelvis are made for each patient, to assess hip joint biomechanics[49,50] and to check for the presence of osteoarthrosis.[51] The anteroposterior radiograph allows visualization of the three innominate bones, the caudad part of the lumbar spine, the sacrum, the coccyx, and the proximal fourth of both femora (Fig. 2, *A*). The false-profile radiograph permits evaluation of the anterior portion of the acetabular roof and the amount of anterior coverage of the femoral head (Fig. 2, *B*). For this projection, the patient stands with the affected hip against the radiographic cassette and the pelvis rotated 65° from the plane of the radiographic film, maintaining the ipsilateral foot parallel. The beam is then centered on the femoral head, perpendicular to the cassette. Finally, anteroposterior abduction radiographs are used to assess the joint congruency achievable with reorientation of the acetabulum and the potential need for a concomitant femoral intertrochanteric osteotomy (Fig. 2, *C*).

Magnetic Resonance Arthrography

Magnetic resonance arthrography is a widely accepted method for imaging of the hip joint. It has a high sensitivity and specificity for the detection of various processes such as avascular necrosis of the femoral head, transient bone marrow edema, occult trauma, neoplasm, and infection. Expanding applications and the development of new techniques have allowed improved visualization of intra-articular and periarticular joint structures, especially the acetabular labrum and the cartilage sur-

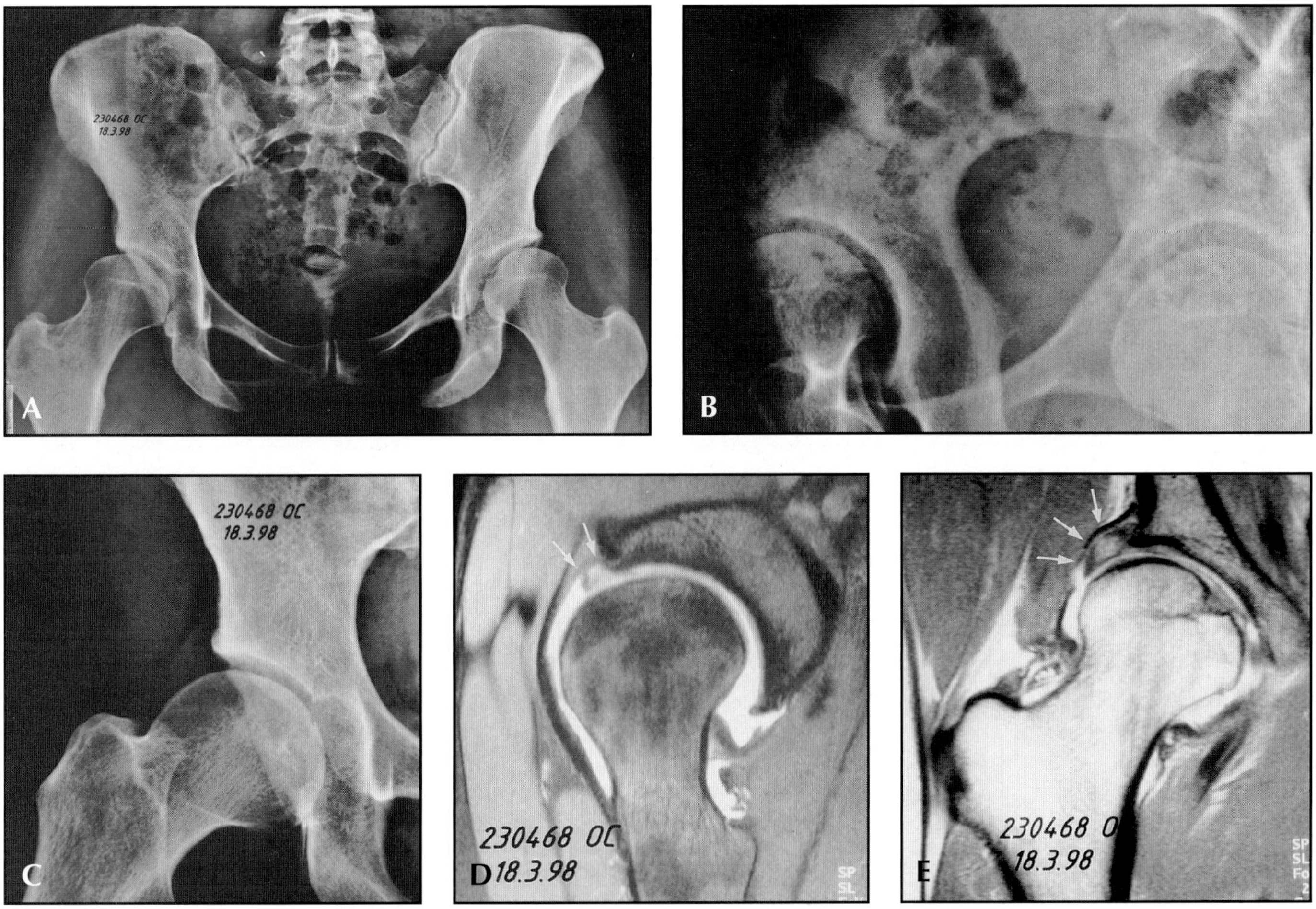

Fig. 2 A hip with insufficient acetabular coverage of the right femoral head. **A**, Anteroposterior radiograph showing osseous landmarks and soft-tissue planes. **B**, False-profile radiograph revealing decreased anterior coverage by the acetabulum. **C**, Anteroposterior abduction radiograph showing good joint congruency. **D** and **E**, Magnetic resonance arthrography depicting a hypertrophied labrum at the anteromedial and lateral parts of the acetabular rim *(arrows)*.

face of the hip. These techniques include high field-strength MRI and use of surface coils. The development of new imaging protocols and the use of intra-articular gadolinium-diethylenetriamine pentaacetic acid as a contrast agent have improved intra-articular soft-tissue contrast. In addition to standard T1- and T2-weighted sagittal oblique and coronal oblique images, magnetic resonance arthrography includes proton-weighted radial sequencing of the acetabulum,[52] which allows the imaging to be initiated at the center of the femoral head and to continue in a plane that proceeds radially. The acetabular and femoral articular cartilage, as well as the labrum, are visualized orthogonal to the radius of curvature.

With these modifications, magnetic resonance arthrography has been shown to be extremely helpful in detecting labral lesions (Fig. 2, *D* and *E*), including tears, degenerative changes, and cyst and ganglion formation,[53-57] with the latter frequently predating any degenerative changes.[11] Moreover, this technique enables a better assessment of the cartilage damage, which is always more extensive than it appears on conventional radiographs.[58]

Current Indications for the Bernese Periacetabular Osteotomy

The most frequent indication for the Bernese periacetabular osteotomy is symptomatic acetabular dysplasia in an adolescent or adult. The lower age limit is determined by whether the patient has open triradiate cartilage of the acetabulum. The upper age limit is determined by the degree of secondary osteoarthrosis and whether the morbidity, risk, and individual prognosis associated with the procedure are worse than those associated with a total hip arthroplasty. Contraindications include high subluxation

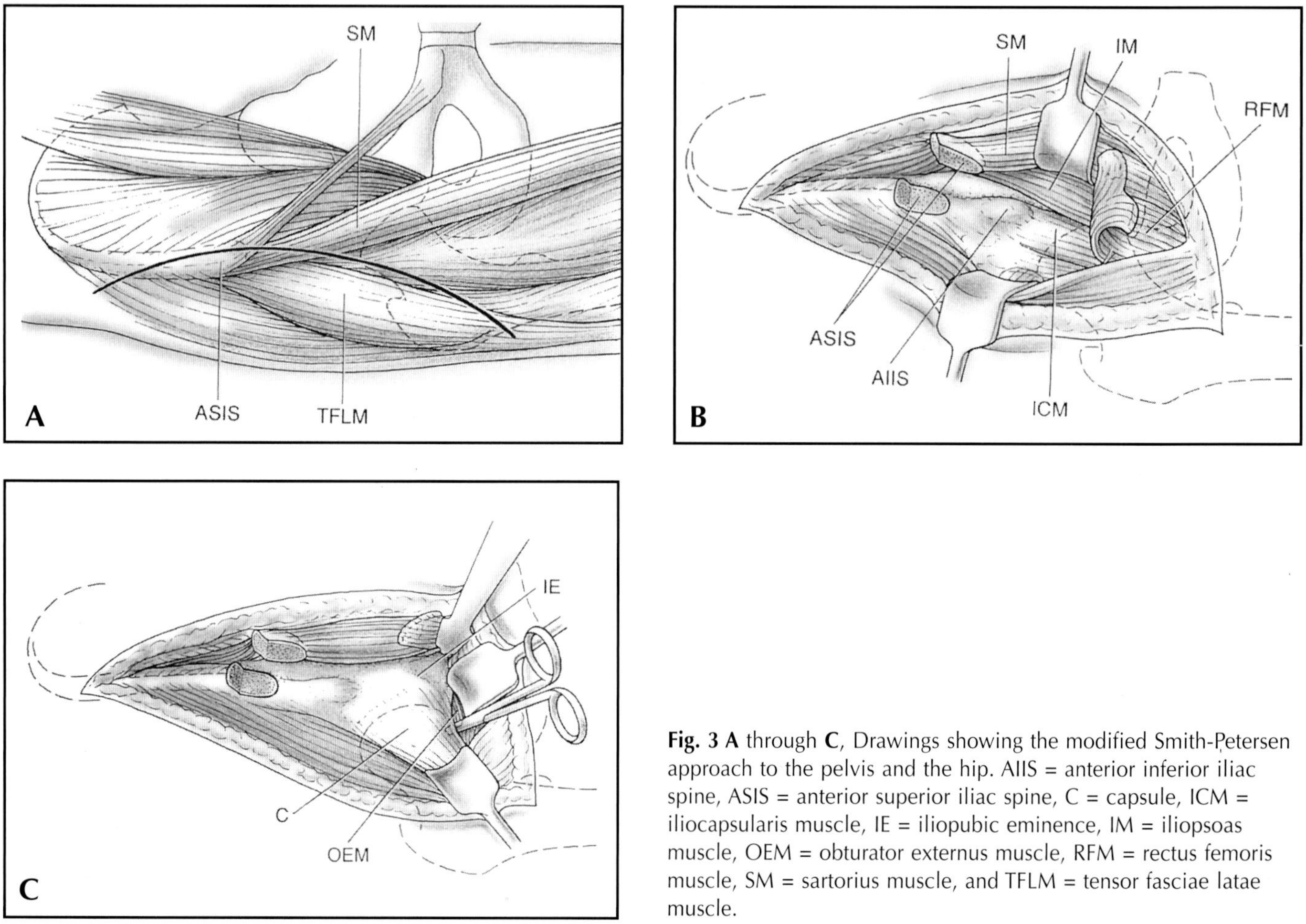

Fig. 3 A through **C**, Drawings showing the modified Smith-Petersen approach to the pelvis and the hip. AIIS = anterior inferior iliac spine, ASIS = anterior superior iliac spine, C = capsule, ICM = iliocapsularis muscle, IE = iliopubic eminence, IM = iliopsoas muscle, OEM = obturator externus muscle, RFM = rectus femoris muscle, SM = sartorius muscle, and TFLM = tensor fasciae latae muscle.

with the femoral head articulating with a secondary acetabulum, complete dislocation, end-stage (grade 3) osteoarthrosis,[50] and a radius of the acetabulum that is smaller than that of the femoral head with the possibility of worsening of the congruity after the reorientation. The latter can be assessed on a preoperative anteroposterior abduction radiograph. It is important also to be aware of functional incongruities such as impingement between the femoral head-neck junction and the acetabular rim, as is seen when the anterior head-neck offset is insufficient. These situations might be encountered in a Perthes-like hip with resulting secondary acetabular dysplasia. General aspects such as the patient's chronological and biological age, the status of adjacent joints (the knee and spine), the body habitus, the level of activity, and the functional goals also have to be considered in the decision regarding the performance of an osteotomy.

Approach for the Bernese Periacetabular Osteotomy

For the Bernese periacetabular osteotomy, the ilioinguinal, direct anterior, combined anterior-posterior, and modified Smith-Petersen approaches have been described.[43,59,60] Since 1993, we have used the modified Smith-Petersen approach, which does not necessitate stripping of the abductors.[45,60] The incision is curved, starting at the anterior third of the os ilium, crossing the anterior superior iliac spine, and running fifteen centimeters distally, crossing the tensor fasciae latae muscle (Fig. 3, *A*). The anterior superior iliac spine is osteotomized, with preservation of the attachment of the sartorius muscle and the inguinal ligament to protect the lateral cutaneous femoral nerve. The osteotomized fragment, including the iliacus muscle, is mobilized medially (Fig. 3, *B*). This is performed by placing the hip in 45° of flexion to release muscular tension. Between the tensor fasciae latae and the rectus femoris, both heads of the rectus femoris are identified. The indirect head is tenotomized, and the direct head is separated from the anterior inferior iliac spine. Together with the iliocapsularis muscle, this flap is mobilized medially.[61] Distally, the iliopectineal bursa is

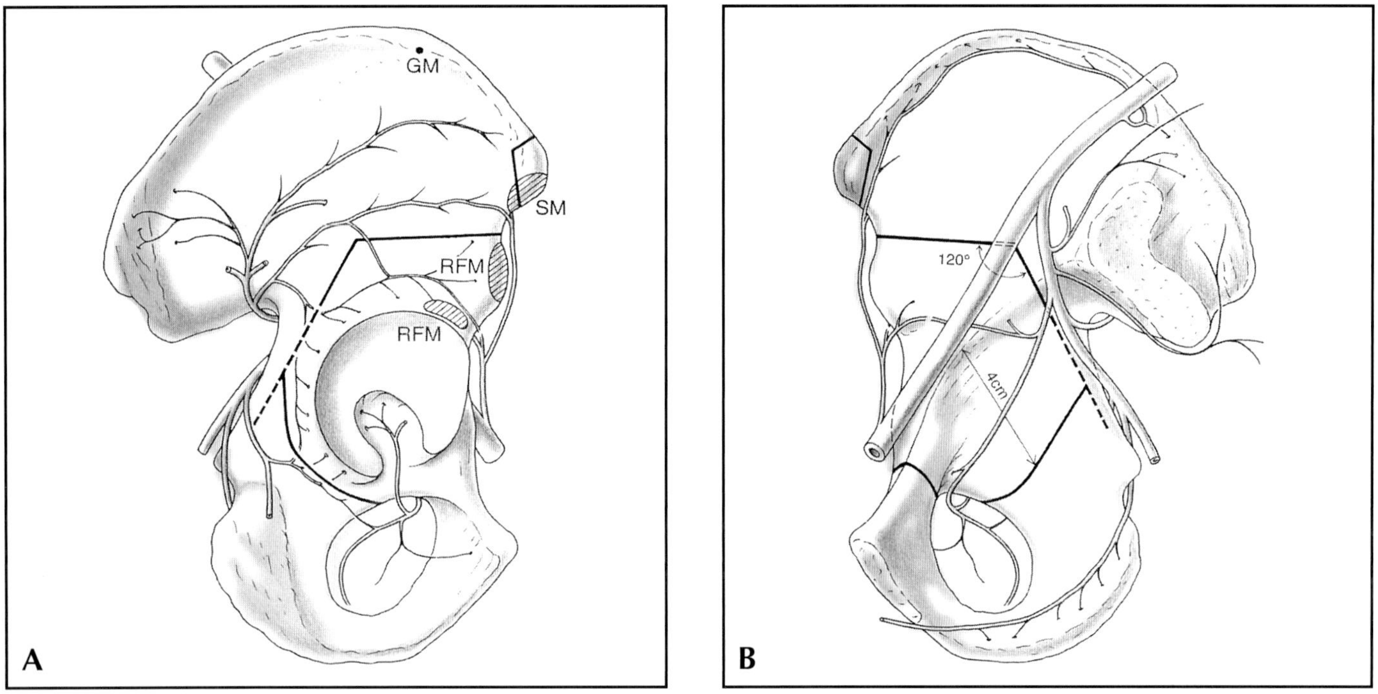

Fig. 4 Drawings showing the vascularity to the acetabulum and the sequence of osteotomies at the external (**A**) and internal (**B**) pelvic surface. The abductors are not detached from the external iliac wing. GM = gluteus medius tubercle, RFM = rectus femoris muscle (direct and indirect heads), and SM = sartorius muscle.

opened to identify the iliopectineal eminence (Fig. 3, *C*). Lateral to this, the gap between the capsule and the psoas tendon anteriorly, and that between the capsule and the obturator externus muscle more posteriorly, are identified. This allows access to the ischium. The abductor muscles are elevated from the iliac wing only at the level of the horizontal part of the superior acetabular osteotomy. A blunt retractor protecting the soft tissues is inserted through this tunnel, in a posterior direction, into the greater sciatic notch. Medially, the strong periosteum over the quadrilateral surface is elevated by a blunt retractor, which is placed on the base of the ischial spine, thus protecting the medially located obturator and external iliac neurovascular bundles.

Technique of the Bernese Periacetabular Osteotomy

The individual correction remains the most difficult part of this procedure.[45] Therefore, current attention is focused on the narrow range between undercorrection and overcorrection, with the latter possibly causing impingement between the femoral neck and the acetabular rim. When overcorrection is extensive, the acetabular notch becomes part of the loaded area. To prevent malcorrection, CT-based preoperative planning and computer-guided intraoperative navigation have been shown to be promising, with the latter still under clinical evaluation.[62,63]

After identification of the pubis, ischium, and ilium, the five steps of the Bernese periacetabular osteotomy can be performed (Fig. 4, *A* and *B*). The first step is the incomplete osteotomy of the ischium. With the hip in flexion and after palpation to determine the ischial location and size, a specially angled chisel is inserted distal to the acetabulum, between the capsule and the tendon of the psoas and the obturator externus muscle. The osteotomy starts at the infracotyloid groove with a depth of 15- to 25-mm, incompletely separating the ischial bone. Care must be taken not to injure the sciatic nerve, and fluoroscopy may be used to monitor this step.

The second step is the complete osteotomy of the pubic bone, with maintenance of slight flexion and adduction of the hip to prevent damage to the neurovascular structures of the thigh. After subperiosteal preparation of the pubic bone, two blunt retractors are placed around the anterior ramus to protect the obturator nerve and vessels. The centrally inclined oblique osteotomy is performed medial to the iliopectineal eminence.

The third step is the chevron-shaped supra-acetabular osteotomy, which is performed with the hip joint kept in slight flexion and adduction. At present, this osteotomy, consisting of two parts, is performed more proximally than it was in the first description of this procedure.[43] An oscillating saw is used to begin the cut at the inferior border of the osteotomized anterior superior iliac spine and directed transversely, ending approximately 1 cm proximal to the iliopectineal line. The second, posterior part is performed with a chisel and is directed inferiorly toward the ischial spine at an angle of 110° to 120° to the anterior osteotomy. A 1-cm bone bridge is kept between the inferior border and the greater sciatic notch. A 5-mm Schanz screw is inserted into the anterior inferior iliac spine parallel to the supra-acetabular osteotomy in the acetabular fragment; this provides a good lever for mobilization of the fragment. Care must be taken not to perforate the joint. With distal traction and tilt on the Schanz screw, the supra-acetabular osteotomy gap is opened and a lamina spreader is inserted into the posterior part of the gap. Opening the spreader leads to a fracture propagation of the posterior osteotomy toward the ischial spine. Sometimes, additional gentle blows on an osteotome directed toward the ischial spine are required to promote this propagation.

The fourth step is the retroacetabular osteotomy. This is performed after subperiosteal preparation of the quadrilateral surface 4 cm beneath the iliopectineal line, at an angle of approximately 30° toward the quadrilateral surface. For this cut, a special chisel is used while steady traction is applied with use of the Schanz screw and the lamina spreader within the supra-acetabular osteotomy site. By maintaining tension, this step produces the fifth step of the osteotomy, a controlled fracture of the incompletely osteotomized ischium (the first cut).

Performance of the osteotomies as described above avoids compromise of the vascularity to the periacetabular fragment. The blood flow to the periacetabular fragment is supplied by three main sources entering the bone on the external surface of the pelvis. The acetabular branch of the obturator artery supplies the acetabular notch, the entire subchondral bone, the anterior wall, and the labrum. The inferior branch of the superior gluteal artery penetrates the gluteus minimus, following the course of the piriformis muscle, and supplies the roof of the acetabulum and the posterior wall as well as parts of the capsule and the labrum. Terminal branches of the inferior gluteal artery and the internal pudendal artery supply the ischial bone and the posterior wall. In order not to endanger the branches of the superior gluteal artery running within the gluteus minimus, the surgeon dissects this muscle from the external iliac wing only in an area big enough to facilitate the supra-acetabular osteotomy. The osteotomy of the ischium may separate the fragment from the blood supply coming from the inferior gluteal artery and the internal pudendal artery; however, anastomoses with the obturator system and the medial femoral circumflex artery remain intact and usually provide adequate perfusion.[64]

The acetabular fragment is completely mobilized, and the necessary correction is performed. After provisional fixation of the fragment with Kirschner wires, an orthograde anteroposterior pelvic radiograph is made to evaluate the correction. Image-intensifier or radiographic assessment of the treated side alone is insufficient. For judgment of the correction, radiographic landmarks such as the orientation of the acetabular roof, the position of the head relative to the ilioischial line, the position of the radiographic teardrop, the anterior and posterior aspects of the acetabular rim, and Shenton's line are evaluated. While radiographs are made and processed, an anterior capsulotomy is performed. The joint is inspected for intra-articular lesions (labral, cartilaginous, and osseous) and, if necessary, these lesions are addressed.

Labral tears can range in size from a very small microdetachment to one involving 50% of the circumferential attachment.[55] The lesion is ususally located in the anterosuperior quadrant of the acetabular rim and can resemble a bucket-handle tear of a knee meniscus. The next most common lesion is an intrasubstance degeneration with an intact outer surface but an undersurface rupture into a degenerative focus. Less commonly, the labrum will be attached to a free osseous fragment from the acetabular rim. An unstable labrum (intrasubstance lesion) might be resected or, if an osseous fragment of sufficient size is attached to it, it can be refixed. Small and stable tears are left untreated. Cartilage damage observed in these hips ranges from superficial erosions through cartilage flakes to full-thickness defects, which are treated by resection and sometimes drilling of the subchondral bone. If current limitations are overcome, cartilage transplantation might be a promising future adjunctive approach in the reconstruction of these lesions.

Cyst or ganglion formation is frequently found in these hips. Soft-tissue ganglia are removed, and cysts within bone are curetted and filled with cancellous bone. Even more important is an assessment of the range of motion after correction, which has to be of sufficient amplitude for flexion and internal rotation to be free of impingement. Often, the anterior head-neck contour in dysplastic hips is flat and therefore may lead to impingement with the acetabular rim after correction. If necessary, the superomedial offset of the femoral neck should be optimized by the creation of a substantial step-off at the head-neck junction.

After the correct reorientation is seen on the intraoperative radiograph, definitive fixation of the fragment to the ilium is performed with three 3.5-mm screws placed in the supra-acetabular area in a triangular configuration. The polygonal shape of the osteotomy with the posterior column left intact and the avoidance of soft-tissue stripping of the abductors enhance stabilization of the reoriented fragment; thus, early mobilization and rehabilitation are facilitated.

Perioperative Care

Preoperatively, two to three units of autologous blood is obtained. Intraoperatively, a cell-saver system is used. The operation is performed under spinal, peridural, or general anesthesia, with the patient supine on a radiolucent table and the side of the operation draped free.

During the first 48 hours postoperatively, the patient remains in bed with the leg in a positioning device for pain relief. After the drains are removed, the patient is allowed to walk using crutches. For the first 8 weeks, the maximum allowed load on the hip joint is restricted to 5 to 10 kg. Active flexion of the hip joint is prohibited for 6 weeks to protect the reattached sartorius and rectus femoris muscles. Prophylaxis against deep vein thrombosis is achieved with use of low molecular weight heparin. Because of the careful dissection technique with use of a scalpel only, prophylaxis against heterotopic ossification is not necessary. Eight weeks postoperatively, the patient is assessed clinically and radiographically. By then, healing is usually sufficient for full weight bearing, and full muscular strengthening can be started.

Summary

The Bernese periacetabular osteotomy is a joint-preserving procedure used after growth plate closure to correct acetabular coverage and stabilize the femoral head. The polygonal, juxta-articular osteotomy respects the vascular blood supply to the acetabular fragment and facilitates an extensive acetabular reorientation. It achieves improvement of the insufficient coverage of the femoral head, reduction of mediolateral displacement, and correction of the version of the fragment. All osteotomies are performed through the modified Smith-Petersen approach, which also allows for an anterior capsulotomy. Joint inspection not only provides information on lesions of the rim but also facilitates the control of an impingement-free range of motion after the correction. The posterior column remains partially intact, allowing minimal internal fixation of the acetabular fragment and early mobilization similar to that after an intertrochanteric osteotomy. Because the majority of this patient population consists of young women, it is important to note that the dimensions of the true pelvis and thus the potential for future vaginal delivery are preserved.

References

1. Aronson J: Osteoarthritis of the young adult hip: Etiology and treatment. *Instr Course Lect* 1986;35:119-128.
2. Solomon L, Schnitzler CM: Pathogenetic types of coxarthrosis and implications for treatment. *Arch Orthop Trauma Surg* 1983;101:259-261.
3. Stulberg SD, Cordell LD, Harris WH, Ramsey PL, MacEwen GD: Unrecognized childhood hip disease: A major cause of idiopathic osteoarthritis of the hip, in *The Hip: Proceedings of the Third Open Scientific Meeting of the Hip Society*. St. Louis, MO, CV Mosby, 1975, pp 212-228.
4. Hadley NA, Brown TD, Weinstein SL: The effects of contact pressure elevations and aseptic necrosis on the long-term outcome of congenital hip dislocation. *J Orthop Res* 1990;8:504-513.
5. Cooperman DR, Wallensten R, Stulberg SD: Post-reduction avascular necrosis in congenital dislocation of the hip: Long-term follow-up study of 25 patients. *J Bone Joint Surg Am* 1980;62:247-258.
6. Cooperman DR, Wallensten R, Stulberg SD: Acetabular dysplasia in the adult. *Clin Orthop* 1983;175:79-85.
7. Millis MB, Murphy SB, Poss R: Osteotomies about the hip for the prevention and treatment of osteoarthrosis. *J Bone Joint Surg Am* 1995;77:626-647.
8. Harris WH: Etiology of osteoarthritis of the hip. *Clin Orthop* 1986;213:20-33.
9. Pauwels F (ed): *Biomechanics of the Normal and Diseased Hip: Theoretical Foundation, Technique, and Results of Treatment: An Atlas*. Berlin, Germany, Springer-Verlag, 1976.
10. Kitaoka HB, Weiner DS, Cook AJ, Hoyt WA Jr, Askew MJ: Relationship between femoral anteversion and osteoarthritis of the hip. *J Pediatr Orthop* 1989;9:396-404.
11. Klaue K, Durnin CW, Ganz R: The acetabular rim syndrome: A clinical presentation of dysplasia of the hip. *J Bone Joint Surg Br* 1991;73:423-429.
12. Takechi H, Nagashima H, Ito S: Intra-articular pressure of the hip joint outside and inside the limbus. *Nippon Seikeigeka Gakkai Zasshi* 1982;56:529-536.
13. Weber W, Weber E: Ueber die Mechanik der menschlichen Gehwerkzeuge nebst Beschreibung eines Versuches über das Herausfallen des Schenkelkopfes aus der Pfanne im luftverdünnten Raum. *Ann Phys Chem* 1837;40:1-13.
14. Ferguson SJ, Bryant JT, Ganz R, Ito K: The acetabular labrum seal: A poroelastic finite element model. *Clin Biomech* 2000;15:463-468.
15. Dorrell JH, Catterall A: The torn acetabular labrum. *J Bone Joint Surg Br* 1986;68:400-403.
16. Sedel L: Long-term results of cemented total hip arthroplasty in patients 45 years old or younger: A 16-year follow-up study. *J Arthroplasty* 1995;9:453-456.
17. Woolson ST, Murphy MG: Wear of the polyethylene of Harris-Galante acetabular components inserted without cement. *J Bone Joint Surg Am* 1995;77:1311-1314.
18. Buckwalter JA, Lohmander S: Operative treatment of osteoarthrosis: Current practice and future development. *J Bone Joint Surg Am* 1994;76:1405-1418.
19. Chandler HP, Reineck FT, Wixson RL, McCarthy JC: Total hip replacement in patients younger than thirty years old: A five-year follow-up study. *J Bone Joint Surg Am* 1981;63:1426-1434.
20. Radin EL: Osteoarthrosis: What is known about prevention. *Clin Orthop* 1987;222:60-65.
21. Millis MB, Kaelin AJ, Schluntz K, Curtis B, Hey L, Hall JE: Spherical acetabular osteotomy for treatment of acetabular dysplasia in adolescents and young adults. *J Pediatr Orthop B* 1994;3:47-53.
22. Siebenrock KA, Schöll E, Lottenbach M, Ganz R: Bernese periacetabular osteotomy. *Clin Orthop* 1999;363:9-20.
23. Trousdale RT, Ekkernkamp A, Ganz R, Wallrichs SL: Periacetabular and intertrochanteric osteotomy for the treatment of osteoarthrosis in dysplastic hips. *J Bone Joint Surg Am* 1995;77:73-85.
24. Chiari K: Beckenosteotomie zur Pfannendachplastik. *Wien Med Wochenschr* 1953;103:707-709.
25. König F: Üeber die Berechtigung fruhzeitiger blutiger Eingriffe bei subcutanen Knochenbruchen. *Archf Klin Chir Berl* 1905;76:725-777.
26. Lance M: Constitution d'une butee osteoplastique dans les luxations et subluxations congenitales de la hanche. *Presse Med* 1925;33: 945-948.

27. Nishina T, Saito S, Ohzono K, Shimizu N, Hosoya T, Ono K: Chiari pelvic osteotomy for osteoarthritis: The influence of the torn and detached acetabular labrum. *J Bone Joint Surg Br* 1990;72:765-769.

28. Klaue K, Sherman M, Perren SM, Wallin A, Looser C, Ganz R: Extra-articular augmentation for residual hip dysplasia: Radiological assessment after Chiari osteotomies and shelf procedures. *J Bone Joint Surg Br* 1993;75: 750-754.

29. White RE Jr, Sherman FC: The hip-shelf procedure: A long-term evaluation. *J Bone Joint Surg Am* 1980;62:928-932.

30. Salter RB: Innominate osteotomy in the treatment of congenital dislocation and subluxation of the hip. *J Bone Joint Surg Br* 1961;43: 518-539.

31. LeCoeur P: Corrections des défaults d'orientation de l'articulation coxo-femorale par ostéotomie de l'isthme iliaque. *Rev Chir Orthop Reparatrice Appar Mot* 1965;51:211-212.

32. Steel HH: Triple osteotomy of the innominate bone. *J Bone Joint Surg Am* 1973;55:343-350.

33. Sutherland DH, Greenfield R: Double innominate osteotomy. *J Bone Joint Surg Am* 1977;59:1082-1091.

34. Hopf A: Hip acetabular displacement by double pelvic osteotomy in the treatment of hip joint dysplasia and subluxation in young people and adults. *Z Orthop Ihre Grenzgeb* 1966;101:559-586.

35. Tonnis D, Behrens K, Tscharani F: A modified technique of the triple pelvic osteotomy: Early results. *J Pediatr Orthop* 1981;1:241-249.

36. Tonnis D, Behrens K, Tscharani F: A new technique of triple osteotomy for turning dysplastic acetabula in adolescents and adults. *Z Orthop Ihre Grenzgeb* 1981;119:253-265.

37. Carlioz H, Khouri N, Hulin P: Triple juxtacotyloid osteotomy. *Rev Chir Orthop Reparatrice Appar Mot* 1982;68:497-501.

38. Nishio A: Transposition osteotomy of the acetabulum in the treatment of congenital dislocation of the hip. *J Jpn Orthop Assoc* 1956;30:483.

39. Eppright RH: Abstract: Dial osteotomy of the acetabulum in the treatment of dysplasia of the hip. *J Bone Joint Surg Am* 1975;57:1172.

40. Wagner H: Osteotomies for congenital hip dislocation, in *The Hip: Proceedings of the Fourth Open Scientific Meeting of the Hip Society*. St. Louis, MO, CV Mosby, 1976, pp 45-66.

41. Ninomiya S, Tagawa H: Rotational acetabular osteotomy for the dysplastic hip. *J Bone Joint Surg Am* 1984;66:430-436.

42. Kuznenko WW, Adiev TM: The translocation of the hip joint in the treatment of secondary arthritis in hip dysplasia in the adult. *Orthop Travmatol* 1977;6:70.

43. Ganz R, Klaue K, Vinh TS, Mast JW: A new periacetabular osteotomy for the treatment of hip dysplasias: Technique and preliminary results. *Clin Orthop* 1988;232:26-36.

44. Flückiger G, Eggli S, Kosina J, Ganz R: Birth after peri-acetabular osteotomy. *Orthopäde* 2000;29:63-67.

45. Hussell JG, Mast JW, Mayo KA, Howie DW, Ganz R: A comparison of different surgical approaches for the periacetabular osteotomy. *Clin Orthop* 1999;363:64-72.

46. Damsin JP, Lazennec JY, Gonzales M, Guerin-Surville H, Hannoun L: Arterial supply of the acetabulum in the fetus: Application to periacetabular surgery in childhood. *Surg Radiol Anat* 1992;14:215-221.

47. Howe WW Jr, Lacey T II, Schwartz RP: A study of the gross anatomy of the arteries supplying the proximal portion of the femur and the acetabulum. *J Bone Joint Surg Am* 1950;32:856-866.

48. MacDonald SJ, Garbuz D, Ganz R: Clinical evaluation of the symptomatic young adult hip. *Semin Arthroplasty* 1997;8:3-9.

49. Lequesne M, deSeze S: Le faux profil du bassin: Nouvelle incidence radiographique pour l'étude de la hanche: Son utilité dans les dysplasies et les differentes cexopathies. *Rev Rhum* 1961;28:643-652.

50. Tonnis D: The prearthrotic deformity as origin of coxarthrosis: Radiographic measurements and their value in the prognosis. *Z Orthop Ihre Grenzgeb* 1978;116:444-446.

51. Trousdale R, Ekkernkamp A, Ganz R: Plain radiographs of the adult hip. *Semin Arthroplasty* 1997;8:10-19.

52. Horii M, Kubo T, Hirasawa Y: Radial MRI of the hip with moderate osteoarthritis. *J Bone Joint Surg Br* 2000;82:364-368.

53. Cotten A, Boutry N, Demondion X, et al: Acetabular labrum: MRI in asymptomatic volunteers. *J Comput Assist Tomogr* 1998;22:1-7.

54. Lecouvet FE, Vande Berg BC, Malghem J, et al: MR imaging of the acetabular labrum: Variations in 200 asymptomatic hips. *AJR Am J Roentgenol* 1996;167:1025-1028.

55. Leunig M, Werlen S, Ungersböck A, Ito K, Ganz R: Evaluation of the acetabular labrum by MR arthrography. *J Bone Joint Surg Br* 1997;79:230-234.

56. Petersilge CA: Current concepts of MR arthrography of the hip. *Semin Ultrasound CT MR* 1997;18:291-301.

57. Petersilge CA, Haque MA, Petersilge WJ, Lewin JS, Lieberman JM, Buly R: Acetabular labral tears: Evaluation with MR arthrography. *Radiology* 1996;200:231-235.

58. Werlen S, Porcellini B, Ungerböck A: Magnetic resonance imaging of the hip joint. *Semin Arthroplasty* 1997;8:20-26.

59. Letournel E: The treatment of acetabular fractures through the ilioinguinal approach. *Clin Orthop* 1993;292:62-76.

60. Millis MB, Murphy SB: The Boston concept: Peri-acetabular osteotomy with simultaneous arthrotomy via direct anterior approach. *Orthopäde* 1998;27:751-758.

61. Ward WT, Fleisch ID, Ganz R: Anatomy of the iliocapsularis muscle: Relevance to surgery of the hip. *Clin Orthop* 2000;374:278-285.

62. Klaue K, Wallin A, Ganz R: CT evaluation of coverage and congruency of the hip prior to osteotomy. *Clin Orthop* 1988;232:15-25.

63. Nolte LP, Langlotz F, Klaue K, Stucki M, Ganz R: Advancement in pelvic osteotomies by means of computer assistance. *Semin Arthroplasty* 1997;8:108-113.

64. Gautier E, Ganz K, Krügel N, Gill T, Ganz R: Anatomy of the medial femoral circumflex artery and its surgical implications. *J Bone Joint Surg Br* 2000;82:679-683.

24

Periacetabular Osteotomy: The Bernese Experience

Klaus A. Siebenrock, MD
Michael Leunig, MD
Reinhold Ganz, MD

Introduction

The periacetabular osteotomy (PAO) developed in 1983 provides the ability to reorient severe dysplastic acetabula in adults and adolescents with closed physes. Advantages of this technique are: the fragment has great mobility as a result of cuts close to the acetabulum; pelvic stability is maintained because the posterior column is preserved, requiring less fixation of the acetabular fragment; and the shape of the true pelvis essentially is preserved. The first PAO was performed in April 1984. Since then more than 700 PAOs have been performed at our institution. Increasing experience over time has led to some changes in assessment and surgical technique. Surgical exposure of the outer iliac wing has been limited. More emphasis is placed on balancing the anterior and posterior coverage of the femoral head at reorientation of the acetabulum. Intraoperative joint revision is done routinely with specific attention to potential impingement of the anterosuperior femoral head-neck junction against the acetabular rim. This area now is trimmed, usually after acetabular reorientation.

Improved understanding of this rather complex pathology will increase patients' benefit from a joint-preserving procedure that can be judged only after many years and even decades. For that reason, the results of the first 75 PAOs, reported in the original description of this technique[1] in 1988, have been analyzed 10 years or more after initial surgery.

Table 1
Previous surgeries on 23 affected hip joints

Previous Surgery	Number of Hip Joints
Intertrochanteric osteotomies (IO)	9
Combined pelvic osteotomy and IO	8
Pelvic osteotomies	4
Shelfplasty and IO	2

(Reproduced with permission from Siebenrock KA, Schöll E, Lottenbach M, Ganz R: Bernese periacetabular osteotomy. *Clin Orthop* 1999;363:9-20.)

Patients and Methods

Seventy-five PAOs were performed in 63 patients between April 1984 and December 1987. The male to female ratio was 1:3.4, and the average age of the patients was 29.3 years (13 to 56 years). An underlying neurologic disease was found in six hip joints, a posttraumatic acetabular deficiency was found in two, and a proximal femoral focal dysplasia was seen in another two. Twenty-three hips (31%) had undergone previous surgery for dysplasia (Table 1). Thirty-seven hips (50%) were classified as group III dysplasia according to Severin,[2] representing dysplastic hips without subluxation of the femoral head. Thirty-three hips (44%) were classified as group IV with femoral head subluxation, four hips (5%) represented group V with a secondary acetabululm, and one hip (1%) was classified as group II dysplasia. All patients had pain at time of surgery, and in 55 patients (73%) ambulation was restricted.

Radiographic evaluations were performed on a standard anteroposterior (AP) pelvis view and a false profile view according to Lequesne and de Sèze.[3] Dysplasia was measured using the lateral center edge (LCE) angle according to Wiberg,[4] the anterior center edge (ACE) angle according to Lequesne and de Sèze,[3] and the acetabular index described by Tönnis[5] for the obliquity of the acetabular roof. Lateralization of the femoral head was measured by the distance between the medial edge of the femoral head and the ilioischial line. The distance was measured before and after surgery and compared with normal contralateral hips. Instances of Shenton's line were recorded pre- and postoperatively. At the time of surgery radiographs were graded for osteoarthritis according to the criteria of Tönnis.[5] Grade 1 is represented by a widened sclerosis zone and minimal osteophytes, grade 2 by a moderate loss of joint width and cysts, and grade 3 by

Table 2
Preoperative and postoperative radiographic variables

Variable	Preoperative	Postoperative
Mean LCE angle	6° (–24° to 25°)	34° (10° to 55°)
Mean ACE angle	4° (–20° to 24°)	26° (12° to 50°)
Acetabular index	26° (12° to 50°)	6° (–15° to 18°)
Lateralization	16 mm (6 to 30 mm)	10 mm (–9 to 24 mm)
Shenton's line intact	39%	62%

(Reproduced with permission from Siebenrock KA, Schöll E, Lottenbach M, Ganz R: Bernese periacetabular osteotomy. *Clin Orthop* 1999;363:9-20.)

Table 3
D'Aubigne score[6] before and after surgery

Points	Preoperative (n = 58)	Postoperative (n = 58)
Total*	14.6 (7 to 17)	16.3 (12 to 18)
Pain*	3.9 (2 to 5)	5.3 (3 to 6)
Ambulation*	4.9 (1 to 6)	5.6 (4 to 6)
Motion	5.8 (4 to 6)	5.4 (3 to 6)

* Differences statistically significant ($P < 0.0001$)

(Reproduced with permission from Siebenrock KA, Schöll E, Lottenbach M, Ganz R: Bernese periacetabular osteotomy. *Clin Orthop* 1999;363:9-20.)

degenerative findings with a joint space less than 1 mm.

The clinical evaluation included recording of pain level, ambulatory status, and range of motion. The results for the three subgroups scored according to the system of D'Aubigné and Postel[6] and the overall evaluation were recorded. The impingement test, which is performed in forced flexion, internal rotation, and adduction,[7] was used to test for an acetabular rim lesion, usually represented by an anterosuperior labral and adjacent cartilage lesion. Surgery was performed using the technique described earlier by the senior author.[1] After reorientation of the acetabulum, an intraoperative radiograph was taken routinely. Thereby, an additional intertrochanteric osteotomy was judged to be necessary to improve joint congruency in 16 hips. An abduction osteotomy was performed in 13 hips, an adduction osteotomy in 2, and an extension osteotomy in 1. In 7 of the 13 abduction osteotomies, this was done to reverse the effect of a previous adduction osteootomy. Surgery time averaged 3.5 hours (range 2 to 5 hours), blood loss averaged 2,000 cc (range 750 to 4,500 cc), and a mean of four red blood cell units were required (range 1 to 11 units).

Minimum follow-up (10 years) could be obtained in 71 cases (95%) at an average of 11.3 years (range 10 to 13.8 years). One patient with bilateral osteotomy (2.5%) died during the observation period 6 years after the PAO. Two patients (2.5%) were lost to follow-up early after the osteotomy.

Radiographic Results

The LCE and ACE angles and the acetabular index improved significantly after surgery. Shenton's line was interrupted preoperatively in 40 of 66 available radiographs (61%) and postoperatively in 25 cases (38%). Preoperative lateralization of the femoral head averaged 16 mm on the affected side (range 6 to 30 mm) compared to 11 mm on the unaffected hips (range –3 to +18 mm) and to 10 mm (range –9 to +24 mm) postoperatively. All these differences were statistically significant with a P value between 0.001 and 0.0001. The results are summarized in Table 2.

Fifty-eight (82%) of the 71 hips that underwent surgery had a preserved hip joint at an average follow-up of 11.3 years. Thirteen hips were revised subsequently to either a total hip arthroplasty (12 hips) or a hip fusion. These procedures were performed at an average of 6.1 years (range 1 to 13.2 years) after the PAO. In 4 of these hips, total hip replacement was done after an interval of 10 years or more.

Clinical Results

The average D'Aubigné score increased from 14.6 points (range 7 to 17) preoperatively to 16.3 points (range 12 to 18 points) at last follow-up in the 58 preserved hip joints ($P < 0.0001$). There was a significant improvement in pain and ambulation. The range of motion decreased in most hips, especially for flexion and internal rotation (Table 3). In 6 of the 58 hips, the D'Aubigné score was less than 15 points, ranging from 12 to 14 points. Thus, a total of 52 (73%) of the 71 surgically corrected hip joints were preserved and rated clinically as good or excellent (Fig. 1).

Osteoarthritis

The immediately preoperative radiographs from 55 patients with a preserved hip joint were available and could be graded for osteoarthritis (OA). In 27 hips (49%), there were no signs of OA and 46 (84%) had no or grade 1 OA. At last follow-up, 44 hips (80%) had no or grade 1 OA (Table 4). In 14 hips (25%), there was progression of degenerative signs including 10 hips with progression from no to grade 1 OA. Each of four hips had a radio-

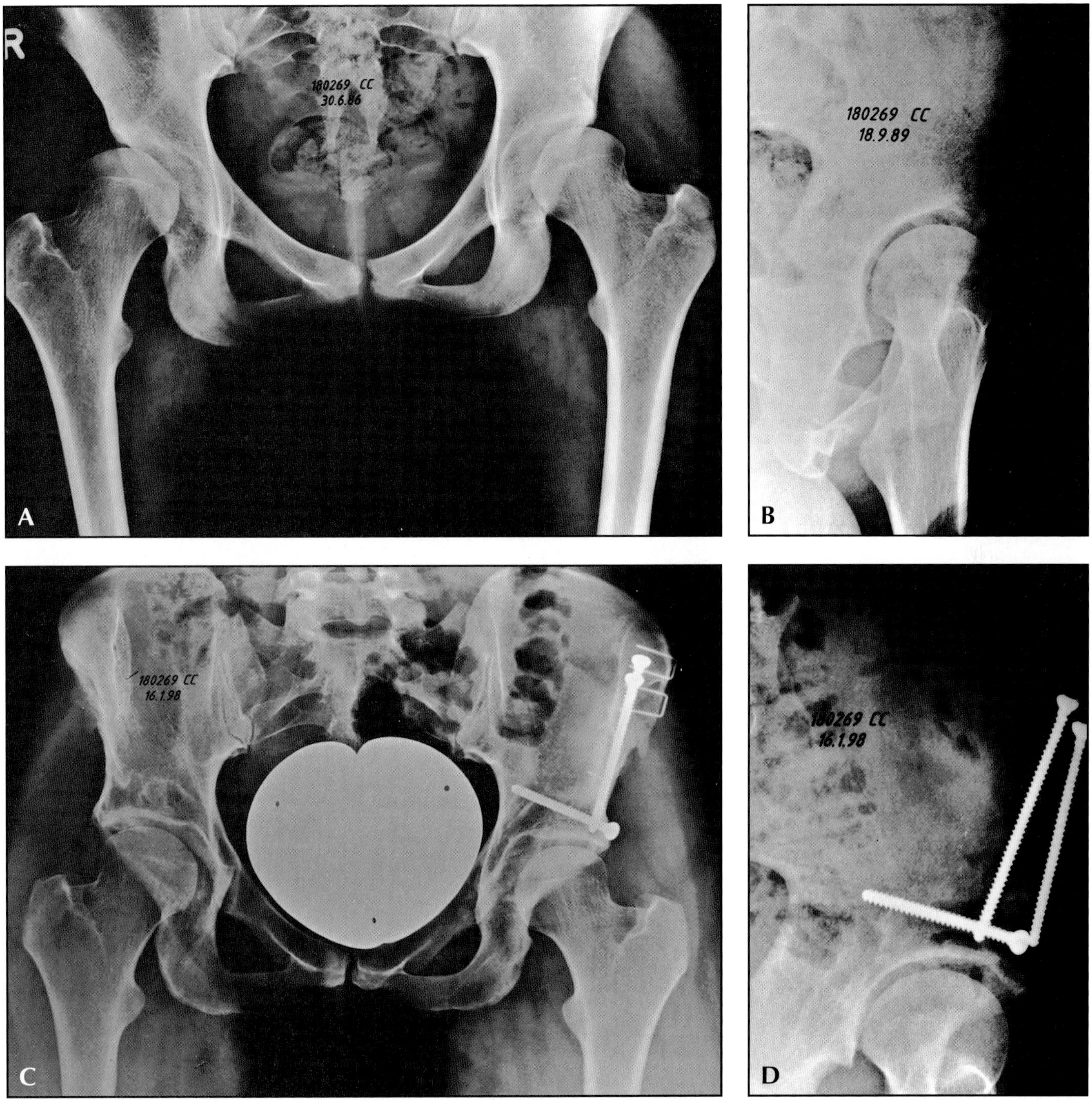

Fig. 1 A, AP radiograph obtained from a 17-year-old girl with symptomatic bilateral hip dysplasia with femoral head subluxation. **B,** The false-profile view of the left side, showing severely deficient anterior coverage. AP pelvic radiograph (**C**) and false-profile view (**D**) 9 and 12 years after surgery with an excellent clinical result on both sides.

graphic improvement of one grade. Complete preoperative radiographic documentation was available in 11 of 13 patients with nonpreserved hip joints. Six (55%) of these hip joints had grade 2 OA prior to surgery (Table 5). Five (10%) of a total of 51 hips with no or grade 1 OA were not preserved, whereas, six (46%) of a total of 13 hips joints with grade 2 OA were replaced at last follow-up. A statistically significant correlation with an unsatisfactory clinical outcome in patients with advanced OA after a PAO has been reported. At a mean follow-up of 4 years, eight of nine

Table 4
Tönnis[5] grading of OA before surgery and at last follow-up in 55 patients with preserved hip joints

OA	Grade 0	Grade 1	Grade 2	Grade 3
(n=55)*				
Preoperative	27 (49%)	19 (34%)	7 (13%)	2 (4%)
Last follow-up	18 (33%)	26 (47%)	8 (15%)	3 (5%)

*Three cases with incomplete radiographs are not included

(Reproduced with permission from Siebenrock KA, Schöll E, Lottenbach M, Ganz R: Bernese periacetabular osteotomy. *Clin Orthop* 1999;363:9-20.)

Table 5
Tönnis[5] grading of OA before surgery in 11 patients with replaced hip joints

OA	Grade 0	Grade 1	Grade 2	Grade 3
(n=11)*				
Preoperative	1 (9%)	4 (36%)	6 (55%)	—

*Two cases with incomplete radiographs are not included

(Reproduced with permission from Siebenrock KA, Schöll E, Lottenbach M, Ganz R: Bernese periacetabular osteotomy. *Clin Orthop* 1999;363:9-20.)

patients with grade 3 OA had a Harris hip score of less than 70 points.[8]

Labral Lesions

Labral lesions were detected in 15 hips (21%) during joint revision surgery, although arthrotomy was not done routinely in the early period. A positive impingement test on the initial physical examination, which was present in 27 (38%) of 71 hip joints, has been found over the years to be closely correlated with acetabular rim pathology[7] and detectable labral lesions on magnetic resonance arthrography.[9] The 15 hip joints with labral lesions detected by arthrotomy were correlated with a significantly worse outcome. The labral lesions were left untreated in 12 hips in the present series. Resuturing the torn labrum in 2 cases failed and led to joint revision with later resection of the labrum.

Additional Intertrochanteric Osteotomy

A simultaneous intertrochanteric osteotomy was performed in 16 hips (21%) as a second step after the PAO. The decision was predominantly based on the intraoperative radiographs after the acetabular correction was performed, although it was possible to suspect additional benefit from an intertrochanteric osteotomy on preoperative radiographs. Intraoperative imaging routinely included an AP pelvis view. An abduction or adduction view was taken to simulate the effects of an additional intertrochanteric osteotomy in hips with insufficient joint congruency, joint space width, or femoral head coverage, despite adequate acetabular correction. Thirteen of the 16 hips underwent an abduction osteotomy. An adduction osteotomy was performed in two hips and an extension osteotomy in one. Seven of the 13 abduction osteotomies, however, were performed to reverse the effects of former adduction osteotomies.

Prognostic Factors

The Wilcoxon signed rank sum test was used to evaluate the significance of differences between preoperative and postoperative clinical and radiographic variables. Patient groups with different variables (eg, preoperative OA, labral tear) were compared using the Mann-Whitney U-test. Logistic regression analysis of the different variables was used to detect independent factors that might indicate prognostic relevance. Significant variables predicting negative outcome were older age at surgery ($P > 0.0001$), presence and grade of OA ($P < 0.0001$), and presence of a labral lesion ($P < 0.001$). A low ACE angle after correction and an acetabular index after correction outside of the range of 0° to 10° were also correlated to less favorable outcome ($P < 0.0058$).

Complications

All major complications in these series occurred during the first 18 osteotomies. They included an intra-articular osteotomy in two hips. In one patient, the joint was replaced by a total hip arthroplasty 19 months later. A fair result was seen in the other patient who died in a traffic accident 6 years later. Three hips underwent a re-osteotomy. In two hips, this was due to loss of correction with too-early weight bearing, and in one it was due to too extensive lateralization of the fragment. Dorsal subluxation of the femoral head occurred in 3 hips, with lack of posterior coverage postoperatively. In two of these hips, a subsequent dorsal shelfplasty was performed. One transient femoral nerve palsy was observed in this series. There was no damage to major blood vessels. Significant heterotopic ossifications with restricted motion occurred in four patients (5.6%). Subsequent successful resection of ectopic bone was performed in two of them. In one patient nonunion of an osteotomy site was seen at the pubis with a large gap after an extreme correction. Consolidation did not occur despite subsequent autogenous bone grafting. All subsequent surgeries are listed in Table 6. An extensive study about the complications in 508 PAOs was performed by Hussell and associates.[10]

Discussion

The study represents the results in a heterogenous, predominantly adult patient group with variable features and degrees of hip dysplasia, including patients with underlying neurologic pathology, a high number of previous surgeries (31%), advanced OA changes (23%), and four patients (5%) with a false acetabulum. It also represents the early learning curve with a new surgical technique, which is underlined by the fact that the major complications occurred in the first 18 osteotomies. Nevertheless, the results after a minimal follow-up of 10 years are encouraging, with 87% of hip joints lasting over a minimal period of ten years and 82% of the hip joints preserved at the last follow-up. A good to excellent clinical result was seen in 73% of the hips at that time.

Table 6
Subsequent surgeries after periacetabular osteotomy

Type	Description	Number of Hips
Major surgeries	Revision of hip joint	2
	Shelfplasty	2
	Reosteotomy	3
	Total hip arthroplasty (+1 hip fusion)	13
Minor surgeries	Screw removal from pelvis	14
	Additional removal of femoral plate	7
	Intertrochanteric osteotomy	5
	Resection of heterotopic ossification	2
	Bone grafting of pubis	1
Total	(38 patients)	49

(Reproduced with permission from Siebenrock KA, Schöll E, Lottenbach M, Ganz R: Bernese periacetabular osteotomy. *Clin Orthop* 1999;363:9-20.)

Comparison with the results of other reconstructive techniques for hip dysplasia in adults is difficult because there are only a few results with a 10-year or longer follow-up. The single osteotomy described by Salter[11] may be efficient for minor corrections in childhood, but does not have the potential for correct spatial reorientation in major deficiencies in adults.[12] This lack also exists for the osteotomies in which the pubic or ischial cuts are distant from the acetabululm.[13,14] After acetabular reorientation with the triple osteotomy, according to Tönnis and associates[5,15] the LCE angle still was less than 20° in up to 26%, and the ACE angle measured less than 20° in up to 39% of the hips with Severin grade 3 or 4 dyslpasia.[5,15] Good to excellent results were seen in 85% at an average follow-up of 7.7 years, rated by a different scoring system. Thirty-six percent of the patients were younger than 18 years old. Younger age is a significant prognostic factor for favorable outcome, as has been shown in the present study and by other authors.[15-19]

Spherical or dial osteotomies have been described by several authors.[18,20,21] Ninomiya[22] reported on 41 patients with a rotational acetabular osteotomy at a mean follow-up of 7.9 years. Corrected angles showed a large variation with a postoperative LCE angle ranging from −20° to 50° and an acetabular index ranging from −15° to 35°. Twenty-nine percent showed progression of OA, and good/excellent results were described in 76%. Recently published long-term results for 145 hips with an average follow-up of 13 years, showed good and excellent results in 68%.[23] Marked progression of OA was seen in 26.5% of 68 hip joints after spherical reorientation according to Schramm and associates[24] at a follow-up ranging from 2 to 25 years (mean 11.2 years). The Chiari technique and its modifications rely on the formation of secondary fibrocartilage in the weight-bearing zone.[25] The correction potential is limited in regard to balancing anterior and posterior coverage. Postoperative LCE and ACE angles vary considerable according to the applied techniques, with a correction of the LCE angle to an average of 25° to 41°.[16,26,27] After a minimal follow-up of 10 years, progression of OA was in the range of 20% to 79%, varying with different osteotomy angles and levels and age of the patients. Good to excellent results were reported in the range of 55% to 75%, defined by different criteria and also varying with the surgical technique; typically there were better results in very young patients.[16,19,26]

Compromised blood supply and osteonecrosis of the acetabular fragments after performing a PAO was a concern in the early period. However, anatomic studies have shown that this technique can be applied safely.[1,28] In the present series, persistent sclerotic density of the supra-acetabular region in a single case was interpretated as partial osteonecrosis of the acetabular fragment. This was seen in one of the two hip joints with an intra-articular osteotomy and occurred in the patient who died 6 years later. Modifications of the surgical exposure of the outer iliac wing, with less muscle stripping, further decreased the risk for compromised acetabular blood supply and the postoperative recovery time of this muscle group without ectopic ossifications. The abductor muscles are no longer detached from the outer iliac wing but are tunnelled at the level of the horizontal part of the iliac osteotomy. A blunt retractor protecting the soft tissues is inserted in a posterior direction through this tunnel into the greater sciatic notch. For many years, no routine prophylaxis against heterotopic ossifications has been given. In a series of more than 500 PAOs, revision for resection of heterotopic ossification was necessary in less than 1%.[10]

The need for an additional intertrochanteric osteotomy depends on several factors, including extrusion index of the femoral head, abnormal femoral anteversion angles, and a deformed femoral head and signs of OA.[7,29] The most significant predictive factor, however, was a previous adduction osteotomy.[29] Adduction osteotomies alone are insufficient for correction of hip dysplasia in most cases, because only the usually less-involved femoral side is addressed. Over the years there has been an essential decrease in the number of combined intertrochanteric osteotomies and PAOs. This decrease may partially be due to the decreased number of corrections attempted through an intertrochanteric osteotomy alone. In addition, our increased experience with acetabular corrections and the awareness of negative effects caused by overcorrection, especially by creating an overabundant anterosuperior coverage, have led to a more restrictive attitude toward additional intertrochanteric osteotomies.

Advanced OA changes are correlated with unfavorable clinical results for the PAO and other reconstructive procedures.[8,16-19] The decision for performing a joint-perserving procedure has to be based on the sum of all the patient's individual, clinical, and radiographic variables, taking into account, especially, the patient's age and treatment alternatives. The hips of the two patients with grade 3 OA in the current study were preserved at last follow-up. In adolescents and young adults, total hip arthroplasty does not represent a sound procedure for a painful hip, because it implies bony reconstruction of the socket, shorter prosthesis survival and subsequent increasingly complex surgeries in an active young population.[30-35]

Over the years it has become evident that labral lesions and acetabular rim fractures as consequences of an overload to the dysplastic rim[7] are more frequently encountered than had been expected. Clinical examination and more frequent indications for MR arthrography provide very sensitive tests for detection of acetabular rim lesions that could be verified by routine intraoperative capsulotomy.[9] A labral lesion in the dysplastic hip indicates the onset of an anterolateral migration of the femoral head, leading to pressure-point loading and more rapid degeneration of the acetabular cartilage.[7,36] Degeneration and thinning of adjacent cartilage next to a labral lesion in dysplastic hips also was demonstrated recently by an magnetic resonance arthrography study.[37]

In patients with long-standing symptoms, intra-articular degenerative changes are frequently far more advanced than had been believed. Conventional radiography is insufficient to demonstrate these changes and, to our minds, depicts only degenerative changes in a stage that probably should no longer be called early. Reorientation of the acetabular fragment reduces the load on the acetabular rim and torn labrum. Resection of the labrum initially may be necessary only in extended lesions, and refixation of an osseous acetabular rim lesion seems beneficial in large lesions.[38,39] The present study underlined the clinical importance of resection and refixation, revealing a significantly worse outcome in the presence of a labral lesion. Regarding only the 48 hip joints of the present study with no or grade 1 OA and without a known labral lesion, a good or excellent outcome was found in 42 hip joints (88%). Unfavorable prognosis due to rapid progression of OA in dysplastic hips with a labral tear has also been observed earlier.[36]

The study also revealed an unexpected finding that led to the awareness of the potential danger of a critically limited clearance after reorientation. This problem is caused by overcorrection or, more frequently, by the shape of the anterior head-neck junction with little or no offset in many dysplastic hips. At last follow-up, 17 (29%) of the 58 patients with a preserved hip joint had a positive impingement test, which was a new finding in 7 of them. Impingement of the femoral head and neck against the anterosuperior acetabular rim with new labral lesions after correction could be identified in 5 patients undergoing hip-joint revision for newly developed impingement signs.[40] As a consequence, routine arthrotomy during a PAO now includes visual control of hip joint motion and impingement. Impingement in flexion and internal rotation with adequate acetabular correction can be remedied by trimming the anterosuperior head and neck until a range of motion necessary for daily activities is obtained. Furthermore, a lateral approach to the hip joint for performing a simultaneous PAO and joint revision with femoral head subluxation has been developed. This procedure is reserved for hips with a pathologic morphology of the proximal femur such as a short neck and/or hips in which the head diameter does not essentially exceed the neck diameter. These hips are associated with increased risk for impingement during flexion and rotation.

The understanding of an optimal correction has considerably improved over time, especially with regard to evaluation of the anterior coverage from an AP pelvis view taken during surgery. Developmental hip dysplasia, however, does not represent a unique entity but, rather, a pathoanatomic situation with a wide variance in shape and orientation of the acetabulum including retroversion and potential abnormal morphologies of the proximal femur.[12,41] The range between insufficient, normal, and overcoverage is rather small and is influenced by a multitude of factors. Isolated, radiographically measured angles may be less helpful than the combined evaluation of all radiographic parameters together. It is a balancing of the maloriented horseshoe-shaped acetabular cartilage over the femoral head that leads to an optimal use of a limited area of hyaline cartilage for weight bearing. Improvements in surgical technique, introduction of magnetic resonance arthrography, routine joint inspection, and eventual trimming of the anterosuperior femoral head and neck, together with an improved understanding of what is believed to be an optimal correction should further decrease wrong indications, unfavorable outcome, and complications.

References

1. Ganz R, Klaue K, Vinh TS, Mast JW: A new periacetabular osteotomy for the treatment of hip dysplasias: Technique and preliminary results. *Clin Orthop* 1988;232:26-36.
2. Severin E: Contribution to the knowledge of congenital dislocation of the hip joint: Late results of closed reduction and arthrographic studies of recent cases. *Acta Chir Scand* 1941;63(suppl):7-142.
3. Lequesne M, de Sèze S: Le faux profil du bassin. Nouvelle incidence radiographique pour l'étude de la hanche: Son utilité dans les dysplasies et les differentes coxopathies. *Rev Rhum Mal Osteoartic* 1961;28:643-652.
4. Wiberg G: Studies on dysplastic acetabula and congenital subluxation of the hip joint: With special reference to the compliction of osteoarthritis. *Acta Chir Scand* 1939;58(suppl): 5-135.
5. Tönnis D (ed): *Congenital Dysplasia and Dislocation of the Hip in Children and Adults.* Berlin, Germany, Springer-Verlag, 1987.
6. D'Aubigné RM, Postel M: Functional results of hip arthroplasty with acrylic prosthesis. *J Bone Joint Surg Am* 1954;36:451-475.
7. Klaue K, Durnin CW, Ganz R: The acetabular rim syndrome: A clinical presentation of dysplasia of the hip. *J Bone Joint Surg Br* 1991;73:423-429.
8. Trousdale RT, Ekkernkamp A, Ganz R, Wallrichs SL: Periacetabular and intertrochanteric osteotomy for the treatment of osteoarthrosis in dysplastic hips. *J Bone Joint Surg Am* 1995;77:73-85.
9. Leunig M, Werlen S, Ungersböck A, Ito K, Ganz R: Evaluation of the acetabular labrum by MR arthrography. *J Bone Joint Surg Br* 1997;79:230-234.
10. Hussell JG, Rodriguez JA, Ganz R: Technical complications of the Bernese periacetabular osteotomy. *Clin Orthop* 1999;363:81-92.
11. Salter RB: Innominate osteotomy in the treatment of congential dislocation and subluxation of the hip. *J Bone Joint Surg Br* 1961;43:518-539.
12. Murphy SB, Kijewski PK, Millis MB, Harless A: Acetabular dysplasia in the adolescent and young adult. *Clin Orthop* 1990;261:214-223.
13. Steel HH: Triple osteotomy of the innominate bone. *J Bone Joint Surg Am* 1973;55:343-350.
14. Sutherland DH, Moore M: Clinical and radiographic outcome of patients treated with double innominate osteotomy for congenital hip dysplasia. *J Pediatr Orthop* 1991;11:142-148.
15. Tönnis D, Arning A, Bloch M, Heinecke A, Kalchschmidt K: Triple pelvic osteotomy: Part B. *J Pediatr Orthop* 1994;3:54-67.
16. Calvert PT, August AC, Albert JS, Kemp HB, Catterall A: The Chiari pelvic osteotomy: A review of the long-term results. *J Bone Joint Surg Br* 1987;69:551-555.
17. Millis MB, Murphy SB, Poss R: Osteotomies about the hip for the prevention and treatment of osteoarthritis. *J Bone Joint Surg Am* 1995;77:626-647.
18. Wagner H: Osteotomies for congenital hip dislocation, in *The Hip: Proceedings of the Fourth Open Scientific Meeting of the Hip Society.* St Louis, MO, CV Mosby, 1976, pp 45-66.
19. Windhager R, Pongracz N, Schönecker W, Kotz R: Chiari osteotomy for congenital dislocation and subluxation of the hip: Results after 20 to 34 years follow-ups. *J Bone Joint Surg Br* 1991;73:890-895.
20. Eppright RH: Abstract: Dial osteotomy of the acetabulum in the treatment of dysplasia of the hip. *J Bone Joint Surg Am* 1975;57:1172.
21. Ninomiya S, Tagawa H: Rotational acetabular osteotomy for the dysplastic hip. *J Bone Joint Surg Am* 1984;66:430-436.
22. Ninomiya S: Rotational acetabular osteotomy for the severly dysplastic hip in the adolescent and adult. *Clin Orthop* 1989;247:127-137.
23. Nakamura S, Ninomiya S, Takatori Y, Morimoto S, Umeyama T: Long-term outcome of rotational acetabular osteotomy: 145 hips followed for 10-23 years. *Acta Orthop Scand* 1998;69:259-265.
24. Schramm M, Pitto RP, Bär K, Meyer M, Rohn E, Hohmann D: Prophylaxis of secondary osteoarthrosis with spherical osteotomy in residual acetabular dysplasia: Analysis of predictive factors of success. *Arch Orthop Trauma Surg* 1999;119:418-422.
25. Chiari K: Beckenosteotomie zur Pfannendachplastik. *Wein Med Wochenschr.* 1953;103:707-709.
26. Lack W, Windhager R, Kutschera HP, Engel A: Chiari pelvic osteotomy for osteoarthritis secondary to hip dysplasia. *J Bone Joint Surg Br* 1991;73:229-234.
27. Matsuno T, Ichioka Y, Kaneda K: Modified Chiari pelvic osteotomy: A long-term follow-up study. *J Bone Joint Surg Am* 1992;74:470-478.
28. Damsin JP, Lazennec JY, Gonzales M, Guerin-Surville H, Hannoun L: Arterial supply of the acetabulum in the fetus: Application to periacetabular surgery in childhood. *Surg Radiol Anat* 1992;14:215-221.
29. Hersche O, Casillas M, Ganz R: Indications for intertrochanteric osteootomy after periacetabular osteotomy for adult hip dysplasia. *Clin Orthop* 1998;347:19-26.
30. Booth RE Jr: The closing circle: Limitations of total joint arthroplasty. *Orthopedics* 1994;17: 757-759.
31. Buckwalter JA, Lohmander S: Operative treatment of osteoarthrosis: Current practice and future development. *J Bone Joint Surg Am* 1994;76:1405-1418.
32. Chandler HP, Reineck FT, Wixson RL, McCarthy JC: Total hip replacement in patients younger than thirty years old: A five-year follow-up study. *J Bone Joint Surg Am* 1981;63: 1426-1434.
33. Dorr LD, Takei GK, Conaty JP: Total hip arthroplasties in patients less than forty-five years old. *J Bone Joint Surg Am* 1983;65: 474-479.
34. Istrup DM, Nolan DR, Beckenbaugh RD, Coventry MB: Factors influencing the results in 2012 total hip arthroplasties. *Clin Orthrop* 1973;95:250-262.
35. Kavanagh BF, Ilstrup DM, Fitzgerald RH Jr: Revision total hip arthroplasty. *J Bone Joint Surg Am* 1985;67:517-526.
36. Dorrell JH, Catterall A: The torn acetabular labrum. *J Bone Joint Surg Br* 1986;68:400-403.
37. Hasegawa Y, Fukatsu H, Matsuda T, Iwase T, Iwata H: Magnetic resonance imaging in osteoarthrosis of the dysplastic hip. *Arch Orthop Trauma Surg* 1996;115:243-248.
38. Mast JW, Mayo KA, Chosa E, Berlemann U, Ganz R: The acetabular rim fracture: A variant of the acetabular rim syndrome. *Semin Arthroplasty* 1997;8:97-101.
39. Pitto RP, Klaue K, Ganz R: Labrum lesions and acetabular dysplasia in adults. *Z Orthop Ihre Grenzgeb* 1996;134:452-456.
40. Myers SR, Eijer H, Ganz R: Anterior femoroacetabular impingement after periacetabular osteotomy. *Clin Orthop* 1999;363: 93-99.
41. Reynolds D, Lucas J, Klaue K: Retroversion of the acetabulum: A cause of hip pain. *J Bone Joint Surg Br* 1999;81:281-288.

25

Trochanteric Slide Osteotomy: Biomechanical Considerations

Derek Plausinis, MASc, MD
Fares S. Haddad, BSc, MCH (Orth), FRCS
Thomas R. Oxland, PhD
Clive P. Duncan, MD, FRCSC

Introduction

Revision total hip arthroplasty often requires wide exposure of the hip joint. Osteotomy of the greater trochanter has long been used as an effective technique for gaining surgical access. With the classic trochanteric osteotomy popularized by Charnley, significant shear loads are generated by the unopposed pull of the abductors on the osteotomized trochanter. The trochanteric slide osteotomy was developed as an alternative to the classic trochanteric osteotomy to facilitate stable trochanteric fixation and reduce the incidence of nonunion. The trochanteric slide osteotomy preserves the attachment of the vastus lateralis to the greater trochanter. In doing so, the insertion of the abductors remains in continuity with the origin of the vastus lateralis, and a compressive load is generated across the osteotomy. In addition to improved acetabular exposure, elevation of the vastus lateralis facilitates exposure of the upper femur. This allows for removal of previous fixation hardware or corrective osteotomies and, when needed, can permit exposure of the medullary canal through controlled perforations or fenestrae. The trochanteric slide was first devised by Mercati and associates[1] in 1972, and the details of the surgical technique have been described in the literature.[1-5]

Knowledge of the biomechanics of the osteotomized greater trochanter is limited to the study of the classic (Charnley) osteotomy. Moreover, the stability of fixation of the osteotomized trochanter has been studied only for uniaxial loading of the classic trochanteric osteotomy.[6-9] For trochanteric slide osteotomies, no theoretical or experimental studies have been reported that quantitatively model the pull of both the glutei and the vastus lateralis. Although we can apply the results of the experimental studies on classic trochanteric osteotomies to determine the most rigid construct for fixing the trochanteric fragment, these results are not applicable to selecting appropriate fixation for the trochanteric slide. Trochanteric slides have inherent stability because of the vastus pull on the trochanter, and the surgeon may be able to use alternative, less rigid fixation methods that offer lower complication rates. For instance, it has been established that the cable grip system provides more rigid fixation for classic trochanteric osteotomies than do various wiring techniques.[7-8] However, studies have demonstrated a significant rate of cable fraying and fragmentation[10] and an increased incidence of acetabular loosening secondary to cable debris.[11] Trochanteric wires and knots also have been implicated as a cause of trochanteric bursitis.[12] Because the trochanteric slide osteotomy is inherently more stable than the classic trochanteric osteotomy, it may be possible to decrease the fixation required and thus reduce complications of osteotomy fixation devices. However, the present knowledge on the exact loads acting at the interface of trochanteric slide osteotomies is limited.

This chapter aims to theoretically quantify the compressive and shear loads acting on the osteotomized trochanter for trochanteric slide osteotomies. The important variables contributing to the stability of the osteotomized greater trochanter will be delineated.

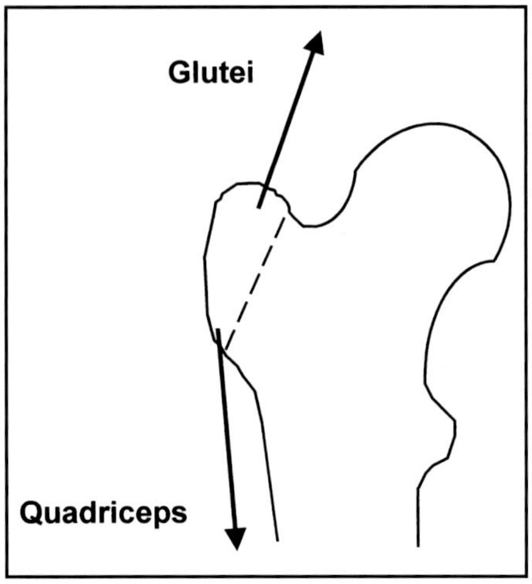

Fig. 1 Idealized abductor and quadriceps actions are shown on a trochanteric slide osteotomy. The glutei act at an angle of approximately 23° from the vertical,[14,20] and the vastus lateralis portion of the quadriceps acts at an angle of approximately 8° from the vertical, in line with the femur.[20]

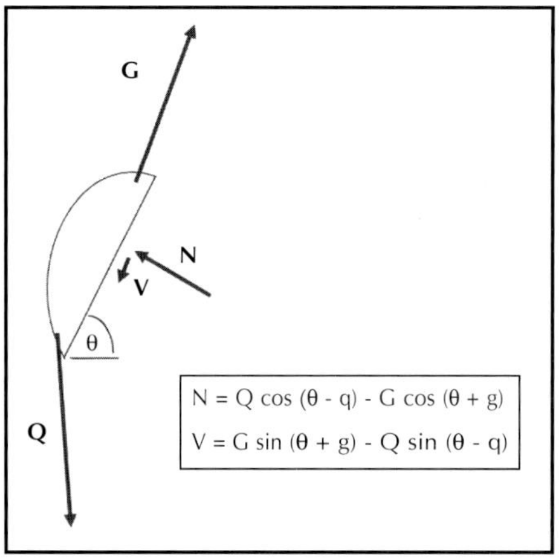

Fig. 2 Free-body diagram of the greater trochanter. The pull of the glutei, G, is at an angle *g* from the vertical and the pull of the vastus lateralis, *Q*, is at an angle *q* from the vertical. The corresponding reactions for equilibrium are the normal (compressive) force N and the shear force V acting on the plane of the osteotomy.

Biomechanical Model

Single Limb Support Period of Gait

The literature contains a large body of data on various aspects of hip biomechanics. Much of the recent literature is based on the extensive theoretical and experimental considerations reported by Pauwels.[13,14] Using theory[14-17] and experimental results of joint reaction forces,[18] it is possible to predict the magnitude and direction of the net abductor force pulling on the greater trochanter. In the case of a classic Charnley trochanteric osteotomy, the trochanteric fixation devices must withstand loads that are simply the result of the pull of the abductors.

Biomechanical analysis of loads acting just distal to the greater trochanter are less well understood. Pauwels[14] theorized that in stance, tensile and compressive stresses in the femur are significantly reduced by the tension-band effect of the vastus lateralis and the iliotibial tract. This theory was substantiated by anatomic considerations and photoelastic experiments. More recently, gait studies using electromyography have demonstrated that innervation of the hip abductors and knee extensors is nearly synchronous during walking, both qualitatively and quantitatively.[19]

In 1993, Heimkes and associates[20] used Pauwels' theory[14] to study the loads acting about the juvenile hip. Pauwels demonstrated that growth plates are oriented in a plane perpendicular to the net force, where shear forces are minimal. Heimkes and associates[20] used this principle to calculate the magnitude of the forces acting distally on the trochanteric apophysis by assuming that there were no shear forces acting along the physis. They further substantiate the model using the aforementioned gait studies as evidence[19] and citing the fact that in the pediatric population, any displaced fractures of the greater trochanter are amenable to conservative treatment and can be fully stressed soon after injury. In addition, the apophysis of the greater trochanter rarely avulses.[20]

It is interesting to note the similarities between the biomechanics of the trochanteric apophysis in the juvenile hip[20] and the biomechanics of the trochanteric slide osteotomy in the adult hip. To investigate this point, a two-dimensional model of the forces on the greater trochanter can be constructed (Fig. 1). The corresponding free-body diagram of the osteotomized greater trochanter is shown in Figure 2. In this model, G represents the tension of the glutei, and Q is the vastus lateralis component of the quadriceps. These muscle forces are balanced by reactions acting on the osteotomy interface. N is the normal (or compressive) force and V is the shear force acting on the plane of the osteotomy. Theta (θ) is the angle the osteotomy makes with the horizontal. In the case of the juvenile hip, θ indicates the inclination of the physis, which is approximately 52° from the horizontal and is age independent.[20] In the juvenile hip model described earlier, Heimkes and associates calculated that Q equals 3.23 times body weight and G equals 2.32 times body weight in one-legged stance. Recall that the juvenile hip model assumes that along the plane of the physis, the shear force (V) should be negligible and the net reaction force purely compressive (N). This is an assumption that implies that if a trochanteric slide osteotomy is made in the same plane as the fused physis, and if the abductors and the vastus lateralis act synchronously in the ratio Q/G of 1.39 (3.23/2.32), then there is no shear force acting along the plane of the osteotomy.

The trochanteric slide osteotomy, however, differs somewhat from the juvenile hip model. The angle of the osteotomy, θ, may not have the same orientation as the plane of the fused physis. In addition, the magnitude of pull of the quadriceps may be affected by inability to preserve the entire vastus attachment during a difficult revision procedure, or by postoperative muscle inhibition. To study the mechanics of the trochanteric slide, the model described previously for the osteotomized greater trochanter can be used (Fig. 2). The normal (N) and shear

(V) loads acting on the plane of the osteotomy may be calculated by noting that for equilibrium of the greater trochanter, the sum of all forces in any direction must be equal to zero. The equations for the reactions N and V are shown in Figure 2. The glutei act at an angle of approximately 23° from the vertical[14,20] and the vastus lateralis portion of the quadriceps acts at an angle of approximately 8° from the vertical, in line with the femur.[20]

The magnitude of the pull of the abductors, G, may be more substantial than 2.32 times body weight used in the juvenile hip model.[20] Several investigators have estimated the magnitude of the pull of the abductors using theoretical and experimental techniques, and these results have been summarized in the study by Bergmann and associates.[18] Based on measurements of in vivo instrumented hip prostheses, the peak reaction force at the hip joint would be approximately 3.5 times body weight for a walking speed of 4 km/h.[18] Using the anatomic data given in Pauwels' model of the hip,[14] the corresponding maximum pull of the glutei would be 2.73 times body weight. For the numerical analysis in our study, the anticipated maximum pull of the glutei was selected to be G_{max} = 3 times body weight. If G and Q act synchronously in the ratio Q/G = 1.39 as produced by Heimkes and associates[20] for the juvenile hip, then Q_{max} = 4.17 times body weight.

Effect of Osteotomy Angle

As described by the juvenile hip model, at an osteotomy angle of 52° the shear force is predicted to be zero. When the osteotomy angle differs from 52°, the compressive and shear force at the osteotomy interface will vary. This variation in forces at the osteotomy interface with different osteotomy angles can be predicted using the theoretical model (Fig. 2). Figure 3 illustrates this result over a practical range of osteotomy angles with G = 3 times

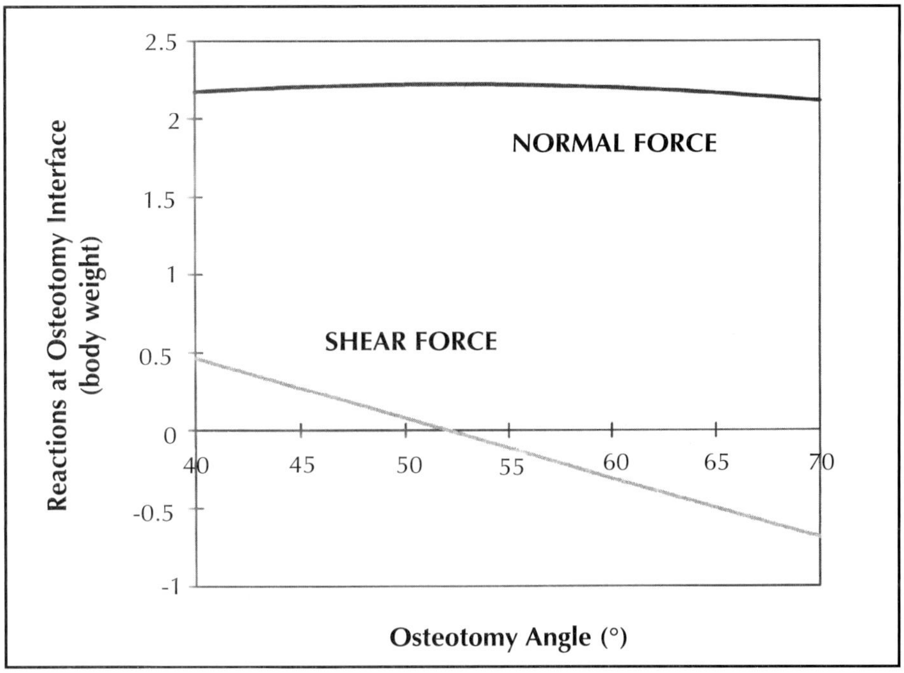

Fig. 3 Normal and shear forces as a function of the osteotomy angle with a constant gluteal force (G = 3 times body weight) and a constant quadriceps force (Q = 4.17 times body weight). The normal (compressive) force changes very little over a practical range of osteotomy angles, and the shear force remains relatively small.

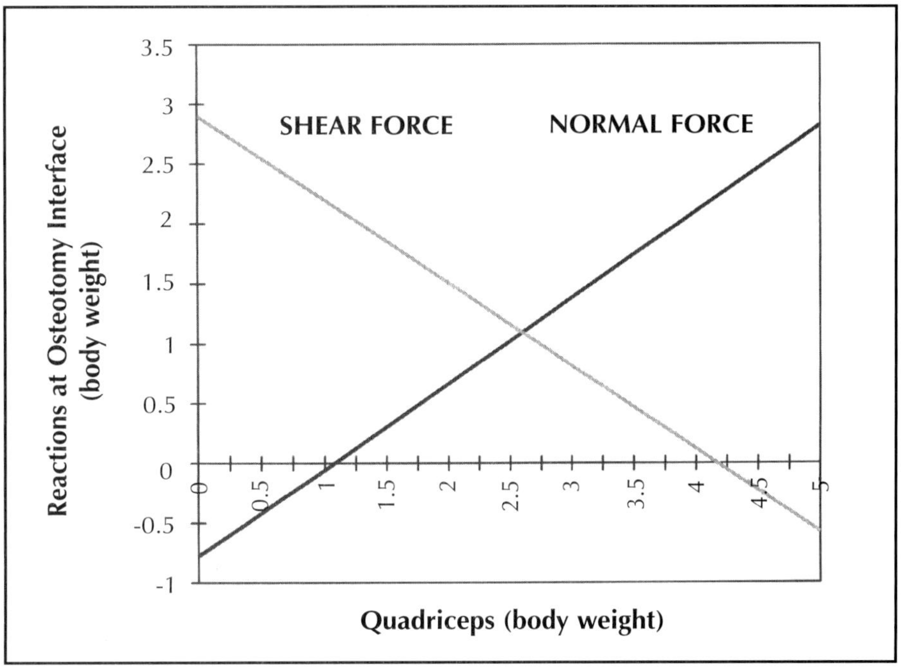

Fig. 4 Normal and shear forces as a function of the strength of the vastus lateralis for the case G = 3 times body weight and θ = 52°. As the quadriceps decreases in strength, compression across the osteotomy decreases and shear forces increase significantly.

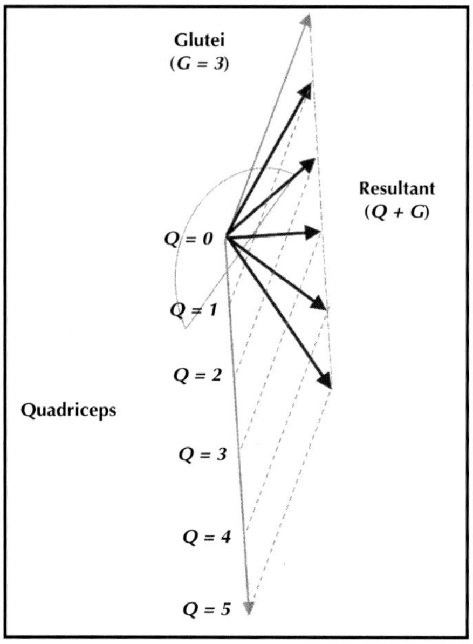

Fig. 5 Resultant force (Q + G) for variations in pull of the vastus lateralis (Q) with a constant gluteal force (G = 3 times body weight). Forces are in units of body weight. Note that Q = 0 is the same situation as the classic (Charnley) osteotomy, where the resultant force produces both shear and tensile forces at the osteotomy interface.

body weight and Q = 4.17 times body weight. Note that for an osteotomy angle measured from the horizontal in the range from 40° to 70°, the compressive load (N) practically remains constant, and the shear force (V) remains relatively small compared with the compressive load.

Effect of Variation in Magnitude of Vastus Pull

Consider the case where the quadriceps force on the greater trochanter is less than expected because of inability to preserve the entire vastus attachment during a difficult revision procedure or because of postoperative muscle inhibition. For a fixed osteotomy angle (θ = 52°) and a constant abductor force (G = three times body weight), the model predicts that the normal and shear forces vary in direct proportion to the quadriceps force (Q) as shown in Figure 4. These results demonstrate a substantial increase in shear force and a decrease in compressive force across the osteotomy as the pull of vastus is weakened. Figure 5 illustrates this effect in vector format using parallelograms to determine the resultant (net) force acting on the greater trochanter. Of particular note is that the normal force becomes tensile when the quadriceps force drops below approximately one time body weight. This is the situation for a classic (Charnley) osteotomy.

Effect of Friction

Given that there are compressive loads across the osteotomy in most cases, a frictional force will exist to counteract the shear forces. The magnitude of this friction force is the product (μN) of the coefficient of static friction, designated by μ, and the normal force (N) acting across the osteotomy. The shear load (V) at the point where the unrestrained osteotomy is about to slip may then may given by this frictional force (μN). Substituting the frictional force into the model (Fig. 2) allows for the estimation of the minimum quadriceps pull required to prevent slip of the osteotomized greater trochanter, $(Q/G)_{min} = [\sin(\theta + g) + \mu \cos(\theta + g)]/[\sin(\theta - q) + \mu \cos(\theta - q)]$.

For the frictionless case ($\mu = 0$), the quadriceps to glutei ratio 1.39 is calculated for the values of θ, *q*, and *g* used earlier. If we consider a very high coefficient of friction ($\mu = 0.5$), then the minimum quadriceps to glutei ratio to prevent shear slippage of the trochanter falls to 1.04, implying that only 75% (1.04/1.39) of the expected quadriceps pull is required to prevent relative motion of the greater trochanter.

An in vitro experimental study using osteotomized pig femora calculated a static coefficient of friction of 0.46[21] for diaphyseal bone. In reality, the coefficient of friction would be expected to be highly variable because the surface geometry of the osteotomized greater trochanter varies significantly among revision cases, and surface properties in vivo and in vitro may be quite different.

Effect of Active Abduction

Patient activity will have a significant effect on the loads across the osteotomy. It is the current practice at our institution to restrict patients from performing active abduction beyond neutral for 6 weeks. This practice can be justified using the theoretical model. Consider the case of a patient performing active hip abduction. As the hip is abducted, the angle between the vector pull of the glutei and the vastus increases, and consequently, the vector sum of these forces yields a smaller resultant force across the osteotomy. This concept is illustrated using vectors in Figure 6. Quantitatively, this can be modeled using the equations in Figure 2. Because the osteotomy angle (θ) is fixed with respect to the alignment of femur (angle *q*), active abduction may simply be modeled by decreasing the angle that the glutei make with the vertical (*g*). The net effect of abduction on shear and compressive loads across the osteotomy is shown in Figure 7. With active hip abduction, the compressive force across the osteotomy decreases and the shear force increases.

Loads Acting Outside the Coronal Plane

Comparatively less is known about loads on the greater trochanter acting out of the coronal plane. Pauwels[14] considered a biomechanical analysis of the hip in the transverse plane; however, this model included the activity of all the external rotators of the femur balanced with the dynamic loads generated during walking. No theoretical consideration was given to model the glutei or the vastus, and, therefore, the results cannot be extended to the trochanteric slide. In addition, there appears to be no literature documenting the combined activity of the quadriceps and the glutei during active internal rotation, flexion, or extension of the hip.

The only experimental results in the literature are for uniaxial loading of the classic osteotomy in the coronal plane, with anteroposterior motion of the trochanter recorded during hip flexion and extension cycles.[7,9] These experimental models were developed to test fixation devices for the classic trochanteric osteotomies and do not account for pull of the vastus as in the trochanteric slide.

The literature does provide us with good anatomic data on the muscles crossing the hip joint.[22] It is possible to develop a model of the anterior one third of the glutei and the vastus lateralis acting on the greater trochanter using the work of Dostal and associates.[15] However, no literature is available to indicate the relative pull of the glutei and the vastus lateralis during active internal rotation or flexion of the hip.

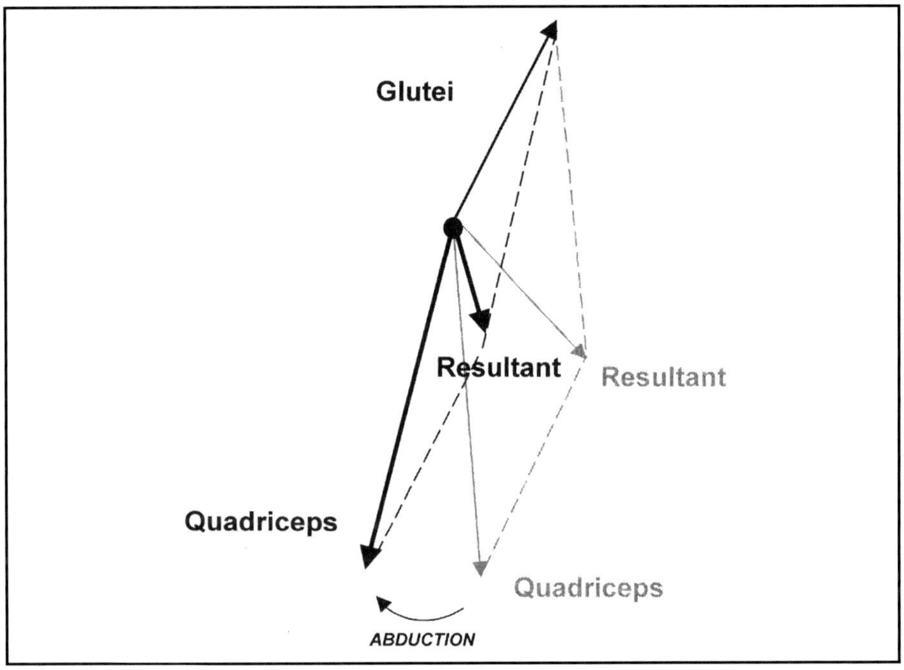

Fig. 6 Effect of active abduction. The vectors in thin lines represent the forces and the resultant force in one-legged stance. As the hip is abducted, the resultant force decreases in magnitude as shown by the vectors in thick lines.

Discussion

The theory presents the concept of inherent stability of the trochanteric slide osteotomy. For the single limb support period of gait, the theory suggests that when the glutei and the vastus lateralis act synchronously, the shear loads across the osteotomy are negligible. The magnitude of the stabilizing compressive loads changes very little over a practical range of osteotomy angles (40° to 70°), and the corresponding shear loads are small (Fig. 3). The theory would then predict that only minimal fixation is required for trochanteric slide osteotomies. However, if the quadriceps muscle is not fully functional, as would be the case for postoperative muscle inhibition or a difficult revision procedure requiring some soft-tissue stripping, then significant shear loads can be generated (Figs. 4 and 5). This may account for clinical observation that if the trochanter from a slide osteotomy displaces postoperatively, it tends to migrate proximally.[2,3,12,23-25]

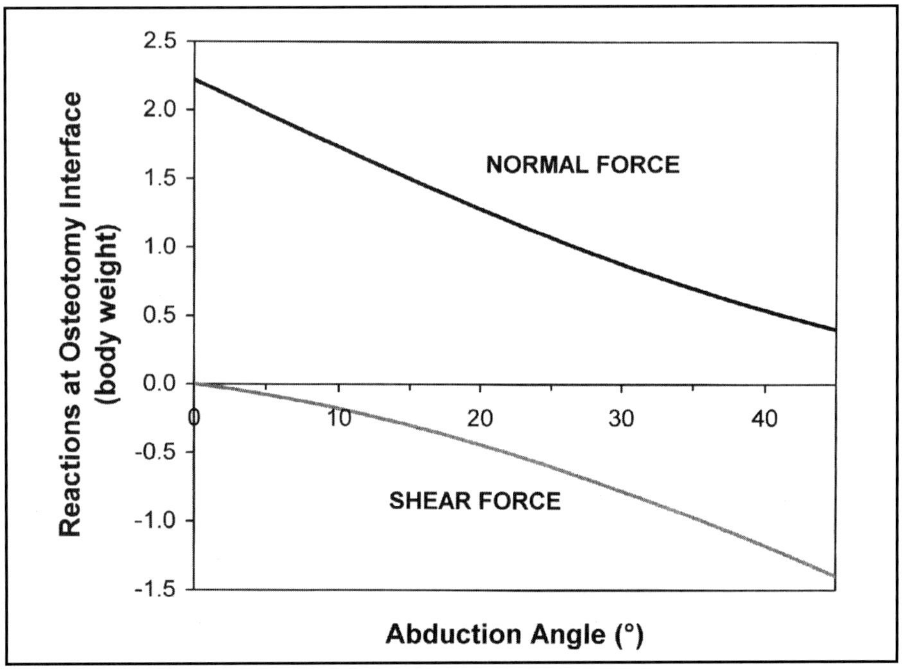

Fig. 7 Effect of abduction on normal and shear forces for G = 3 times body weight and Q = 4.17 times body weight. As the leg is abducted the normal (compressive) loads at the osteotomy interface decreases and shear forces increase.

In addition to the quadriceps reducing shear on the osteotomized trochanter, the presence of high compressive loads will produce a stabilizing frictional force at the interface. The in vivo coefficient of friction, however, remains unknown. With a very high coefficient of friction of 0.5, frictional forces alone can stabilize the trochanter if the quadriceps function does not fall below 75% of the predicted value.

The theory also supports the practice of restricting active abduction in the post-operative period. Active abduction alters the magnitude and direction of vastus and glutei pull (Fig. 6), with a corresponding decrease in the stabilizing compressive loads and an increase in the shear loads at the osteotomy interface (Fig. 7).

Although the results are encouraging in terms of illustrating the inherent stability of the trochanteric slide osteotomy with a fully intact vastus lateralis, the theory is limited to a two-dimensional analysis. Little is known from theory and experiments about the magnitude of shear loads in the anteroposterior direction; however, this does not appear to be a clinically significant mode of failure.[2,3,12,23-26] The compressive and shear loads for complex hip movement such as rising from a chair remain unknown, and the results are thus limited to normal gait.

As with many clinical results on the classic Charnley osteotomy of the greater trochanter,[5] the limited clinical outcomes reported with the trochanteric slide osteotomies have variable results.[2,3,12,23-26] Recent preliminary clinical reports of trochanteric slide osteotomies for revision procedures have been supportive of the theoretical concept of inherent stability.[25,26] A nonunion rate of 3% was reported in a series with the trochanter repaired using a wiring technique,[25] and a nonunion rate of 9% was reported for cable grip fixation in another series.[26] McCarthy and associates[26] comment that the rate of nonunion fell from 9% to 4% when bone to bone apposition was achieved at the time of surgery.

Union of the greater trochanter will be influenced by many factors. Based on our theoretical model, we hypothesize that the quality of the attachment of the vastus lateralis to the greater trochanter at the end of the surgical procedure is likely to be the most significant factor influencing the stability of the repaired trochanter. It may be possible to minimize the fixation required, and thus decrease the complications of trochanteric osteotomy, when the attachment of the vastus lateralis to the greater trochanter is maximally preserved.

References

1. Mercati E, Guary A, Myquel C, Bourgeon A: A postero-external approach to the hip joint: Value of the formation of a digastric muscle. *J Chir (Paris)* 1972;103:499-504.
2. English TA: The trochanteric approach to the hip for prosthetic replacement. *J Bone J Surg Am* 1975;57:1128-1133.
3. Glassman AH, Engh CA, Bobyn JD: A technique of extensile exposure for total hip arthroplasty. *J Arthroplasty* 1987;2:11-21.
4. Masri BA, Campbell DG, Garbuz DS, Duncan CP: Seven specialized exposures for revision hip and knee replacement. *Orthop Clin North Am* 1998;29:229-240.
5. Silverton CD, Rosenberg AG: Management of the trochanter, in Callaghan JJ, Rosenberg AG, Rubash HE (eds): *The Adult Hip*. Philadelphia, PA, Lippincott-Raven, 1998, pp 1269-1294.
6. Markolf KL, Hirschowitz DL, Amstutz HC: Mechanical stability of the greater trochanter following osteotomy and reattachment by wiring. *Clin Orthop* 1979;141:111-121.
7. Dall DM, Miles AW: Re-attachment of the greater trochanter: The use of the trochanter cable-grip system. *J Bone Joint Surg Br* 1983;65:55-59.
8. Hersh CK, Williams RP, Trick LW, Lanctot D, Athanasiou K: Comparison of the mechanical performance of trochanteric fixation devices. *Clin Orthop* 1996;329:317-325.
9. Charnley J (ed): *Low Friction Arthroplasty of the Hip: Theory and Practice*. Berlin, Germany, Springer-Verlag, 1979.
10. Silverton CD, Jacobs JJ, Rosenberg AG, Kull L, Conley A, Galante JO: Complications of a cable grip system. *J Arthroplasty* 1996;11: 400–404.
11. Kelley SS, Johnston RC: Debris from cobalt-chrome cable may cause acetabular loosening. *Clin Orthop* 1992;285:140-146.
12. Glassman AH: Complications of trochanteric osteotomy. *Orthop Clin North Am* 1992; 23:321-333.
13. Pauwels F (ed): *Biomechanics of the Normal and Diseased Hip: Theoretical Foundation, Technique, and Results of Treatment: An Atlas*. Berlin, Germany, Springer-Verlag, 1976.
14. Pauwels F (ed): *Biomechanics of the Locomotor Apparatus: Contributions on the Functional Anatomy of the Locomotor Apparatus*. Berlin, Germany, Springer-Verlag, 1980.
15. Dostal WF, Soderberg GL, Andrews JG: Actions of hip muscles. *Phys Ther* 1986;66:351-361.
16. Delp SL, Maloney W: Effects of hip center location on the moment-generating capacity of the muscles. *J Biomech* 1993;26:485-499.
17. Antolic V, Iglic A, Herman S, et al: The required resultant abductor force and the available resultant abductor force after operative changes in hip geometry. *Acta Orthop Belg* 1994;60:374-377.
18. Bergmann G, Graichen F, Rohlmann A: Hip joint loading during walking and running, measured in two patients. *J Biomech* 1993;26:969-990.
19. Rab GT: Muscle, in Rose J, Gamble JG (eds): *Human Walking*, ed 2. Baltimore, MD, Williams & Wilkins, 1994, pp 101-121.
20. Heimkes B, Posel P, Plitz W, Jansson V: Forces acting on the juvenile hip joint in the one-legged stance. *J Pediatr Orthop* 1993;13:431-436.
21. Tillett ED, von Fraunhofer JA, Seligson D: Coefficient of static friction at pig femoral osteotomies: The role of anatomic reduction and compression on the value of the coefficient. *J Biomed Eng* 1989;11:107-110.
22. Dostal WF, Andrews JG: A three-dimensional biomechanical model of hip musculature. *J Biomech* 1981;14:803-812.
23. Lindgren U, Svenson O: A new transtrochanteric approach to the hip. *Int Orthop* 1988;12:37-41.
24. Schneeberger AG, Murphy SB, Ganz R: The trochanteric flip osteotomy. Orthopaedics and Traumatology, Issue 1, 1997. Die digastrische trochanterosteotomie, Operative Orthopadie und Traumatologie, Vol 9, Issue 1, pp 1-15, 1997.
25. Langlais F, Lambotte JC, Thomazeau H, Dreano T, Sevestre FX: Digastric trochanter osteotomy for complex THR. *4th Congress of the European Federation of National Associations of Orthopaedics and Traumatology (EFORT)*. Brussels, 1999.
26. McCarthy JC, Bono JV, Turner RH, Kremchek TE, Lee J: Abstract: The outcome of trochanteric reattachment in revision THR with a cable grip system with mean 6-year follow-up. *66th Annual Meeting Proceedings*. Rosemont, IL, American Academy of Orthopaedic Surgeons, 1999, p 58.

26

Osteotomies Around the Hip: Radiographic Planning and Postoperative Evaluation

Fares S. Haddad, BSc, MCH (Orth), FRCS
Donald S. Garbuz, MD, MHSc, FRCSC
Clive P. Duncan, MD, FRCSC

Introduction

A wide range of treatments is available for the dysplastic adolescent and adult hip. These include arthroscopic procedures on the hip joint, a number of femoral and pelvic osteotomies, and total hip arthroplasty. Procedures that lead to anatomic correction of the dysplasia are very attractive because they potentially restore relatively normal biomechanics and may delay or avert later degenerative change. Foremost among these are reorientation periacetabular osteotomies and the Bernese periacetabular rotational osteotomy, in particular.[1-3]

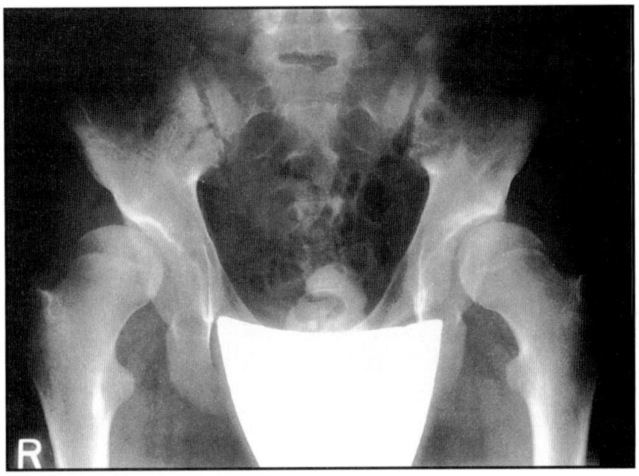

Fig. 1 Weight-bearing AP radiograph showing bilateral dysplastic hips. The erect posture accentuates the dysplasia and more clearly defines the surgical challenge.

The aims of imaging before any osteotomy around the hip must be to confirm the diagnosis; to assess any associated degenerative changes; to quantify the severity of the dysplasia and, hence, identify the appropriate management pathway; to facilitate surgical planning and procedures; and to evaluate the outcomes of treatment. The primary aim of the Bernese periacetabular osteotomy is to recreate relatively normal anatomy and biomechanics in an attempt to improve the long-term prognosis of the hip joint by achieving optimum coverage and containment of the femoral head. Such a multiplanar osteotomy requires careful planning[4,5] because the precise anatomic abnormality needs to be defined as clearly as possible, and there is a potential for overcorrection.[6] Moreover, methods to determine the degree of correction obtained are also necessary and will be important in the interpretation of long-term data on the efficacy of this intervention.

This chapter will summarize the methods available for the preoperative, surgical, and postoperative imaging of the adult dysplastic hip and will detail the authors' preferred protocol for the radiographic evaluation of periacetabular osteotomies.

Plain Radiographs

A number of methods have been devised for quantification of acetabular dysplasia in adults. Plain radiographs traditionally have been, and still remain, the primary imaging modality for both detection and quantification. At least two recent outcome studies after acetabular osteotomies[7,8] have relied solely on indices obtained from the anteroposterior (AP) pelvic radiograph to quantitatively evaluate preoperative dysplasia and postoperative results. Plain radiographs alone are often sufficient to allow diagnosis and guide management. A number of views may be required, however.

The AP view of the pelvis usually is obtained with the patient lying supine and the feet (hips) internally rotated 15°. Internal rotation makes up for some, if not all, of the anteversion of the femoral neck, and allows better observation of the femoral neck and greater trochanter. This view usually allows an assessment of the bony architecture of the pelvic

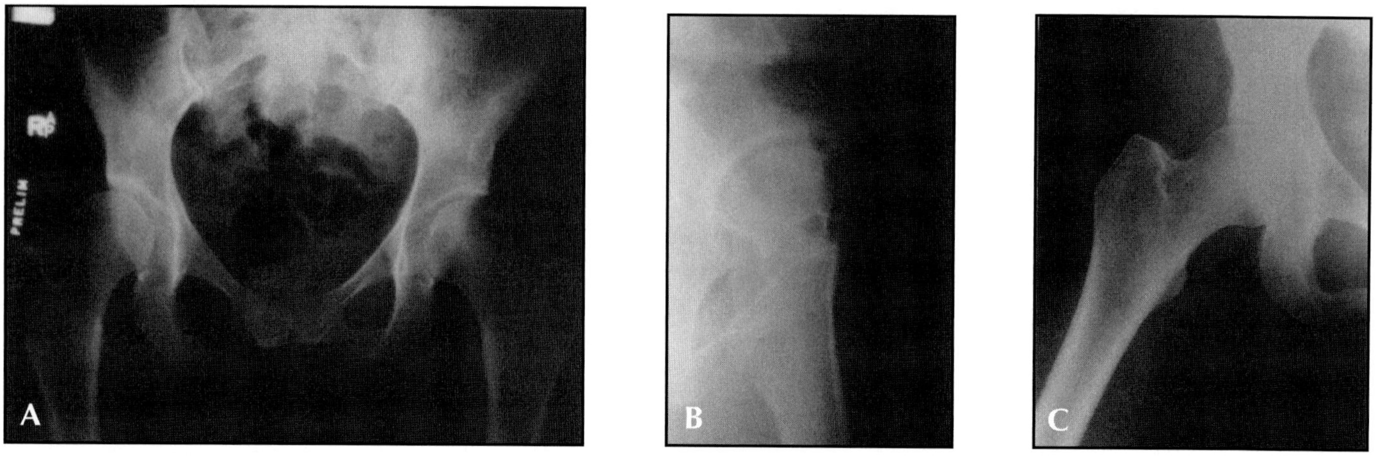

Fig. 2 A, AP radiograph of the pelvis showing a dysplastic right hip. **B**, A false-profile view showing anterior uncovering. **C**, Abduction view showing a satisfactory congruent reduction.

bones, the sacrum, the lower lumbar spine, and the proximal femora. The joint space can also be assessed, although more subtle abnormalities are better picked up by weight-bearing films. Weight-bearing films allow an assessment of the hip as it bears load and give a preliminary assessment of femoral head position, acetabular development, and any obvious subluxation or dislocation. Subtle proximal and lateral subluxation of the femoral head also are accentuated. The weight-bearing AP view of the pelvis also provides a very useful guide to any leg-length discrepancy and is less expensive than full-length scanograms (Fig. 1). An AP view centered on the hip in question, alone, may provide more detail but is not usually necessary.

Lateral radiographs of the pelvis are rarely useful in evaluating hip dysplasia. True lateral and oblique (frog-lateral) views of the hip joint are useful in confirming apparent acetabular anteversion or retroversion, but generally are used to assess proximal femoral deformity and to look for femoral neck lesions. Likewise, Judet views are not normally part of our assessment of the potentially dysplastic hip.

The false profile view described by Lequesne and de Seze[9] allows evaluation of the ventral portion of the acetabular roof and helps to determine the anterior coverage of the femoral head. This view is obtained with the patient standing with the affected hip on the cassette with the pelvis rotated 65° from the plane of the radiographic film and with the ipsilateral foot parallel to the film. The beam is centered on the femoral head perpendicular to the cassette.

Functional views are very useful for the assessment of the dysplastic hip. These give an impression of the reducibility of any subluxation or dislocation and a clearer idea of the congruency of the hip joint.[10,11] With the patient supine and the pelvis orthograde, radiographs are taken in maximal abduction and internal rotation and in maximal adduction and external rotation. These films allow an assessment of the joint space and of articular congruity at the extremes of motion and are particularly helpful in planning proximal femoral osteotomies. These data can also be obtained functionally through a full range of motion with the use of hip arthrography and real-time screening.

Dunn[12] has described a plain radiographic method of assessing femoral neck anteversion, but this method has been superseded by CT scans of the proximal femur and femoral condyles. Johnston and associates[13] used a modified pelvic inlet view to estimate femoral head coverage and concentricity without the need for more complex imaging modalities such as CT scans, but this view has not been widely adapted.

It is our practice to obtain a weight-bearing AP view of the pelvis, a false-profile view, and a functional view in abduction as our initial assessment of suspected hip dysplasia (Fig. 2). The center edge angle (CEA), ventral inclination angle (VCA), and Tönnis angle are also helpful. The abduction view confirms that the hip reduces, that it can be covered, and that the articulation becomes congruent. These views allow an estimate of the severity of hip dysplasia, of femoral head sphericity, and of the precence of any degenerative changes.

Many measurements are described on pelvic radiographs in an effort to quantify acetabular dysplasia. Only a small number of these are used in day-to-day practice. We try to get a general impression of the presence or absence of dysplasia and of degenerative changes, and we take measurements of lateral and anterior coverage, of acetabular opening, and of the extent of any dislocation or subluxation.[14,15]

General Review

The initial radiographic review includes an assessment of the pelvis as a whole and, in particular, an inspection of the size, rotation, and symmetry of the hemipelves and proximal femora. Shenton's line also is assessed, because discontinuity in the absence of trauma suggests hip dysplasia. The presence of an acetabular rim fracture may be suggestive of lateral overload.[16] The hip joint space and the presence of any degenerative changes also are assessed. These can be graded according to a number of scales. We use that of Tönnis[17] in which grade 0 shows no osteoarthritis, grade 1 sclerosis and minimal osteophytes, grade 2 moderate loss of joint space and cysts, and grade 3 degenerative changes with a joint space of less than 1 mm. Long-term review suggests that rotational acetabular osteotomy gives favorable results only if there is little or no osteoarthritis. This suggestion is supported by medium-term,[18] and long-term[19] follow-up data.

Lateral Cover

The CEA of Wiberg is measured on the AP radiograph of the pelvis. This is the angle subtended by a line from the center of the femoral head to the lateral acetabular margin, and a vertical line from the center of the femoral head.[14,20-22] It is otherwise known as the lateral CEA, and is greater than 25° in nondysplastic hips.

Anterior Cover

The corresponding angle on the false profile views of Lequesne and de Seze,[9] the anterior CEA, is measured by drawing a vertical line from the center of the femoral head and a second line from the center of the femoral head to the anterior acetabular margin. The angle between these lines is known as the VCA and is greater than 20° in normal hips.

Acetabular Dysplasia

There are a number of indices of acetabular dysplasia or obliquity. The Tönnis angle or the acetabular index of the weight-bearing zone is obtained by drawing a horizontal line at the level of the sourcil and a second line from this point to the lateral acetabular margin.[17] This is very similar to the acetabular roof obliquity described by Massie and Howorth.[23] The normal range in nondysplastic hips is 10° ± 2°. Likewise, the acetabular angle of Sharp[24] is the angle between a horizontal line joining the teardrops and and a line drawn from the ipsilateral teardrop to the outer edge of the acetabular roof.

The anterior and posterior rims of the mouth of the acetabulum can be followed on an AP radiograph of the pelvis. These give an indication of acetabular version that can also be confirmed by CT scans. If the anterior line crosses the posterior line (the crossover sign) or if the posterior line is medial to the center of the femoral head (the posterior wall sign) the acetabulum is retroverted. In some cases, these may be the only abnormal plain radiographic indices.[25,26]

Femoral Head Displacement

The acetabular head index or the acetabular index of depth to width described by Heyman and Herndon[27] is calculated on the AP radiograph of the pelvis. This index is the ratio of the horizontal distance of the femoral head with satisfactory cover to the total width of the femoral head. It also is known as the percentage femoral head coverage.[7]

The femoral head extrusion index is the ratio of of the horizontal extent of that part of the femoral head that lies lateral to the edge of the acetabulum to the total horizontal width of the femoral head. The head lateralization index is the ratio of the distance from the center of the teardrop to the medial border of the femoral head relative to that from the center of the teardrop to the middle of the symphysis pubis.[8,28]

Lateralization of the femoral head can be measured as the distance between the medial edge of the femoral head and the ilioischial line. In a similar manner, cranialization can be measured as the distance from the inferior edge of the femoral head to the posteroinferior edge of the acetabulum.[1,15] Other indices include the distance of the femoral head from the midline.[29] The peak to edge distance is the distance from the apex of the acetabular weight-bearing dome to the lateral edge of the acetabulum.[4]

Klaue and associates[16] also assessed the ratio of the radius of the femoral head and that of the acetabulum and the distance between the center of the femoral head and the center of the acetabulum. They also measured "e lat," the distance from the tear drop to the medial edge of the femoral head, as an index of lateral subluxation.

Femoral Anatomy

An assessment of the neck shaft angle is a useful indicator of the need for adjunctive femoral osteotomy as well as periacetabular reorientation.[2] Reliance on any of these indices should be tempered by the understanding that there may be considerable interobserver and intraobserver measurement variation as recently has been illustrated by Portinaro and associates[30] for the acetabular index in children and by Werier and associates[31] for the CEA and VCA. Moreover, de Kleuver and associates[32] undertook radiostereometric analysis of the acetabular reorentiation achieved by triple pelvic osteotomy in six cadavers. Their data correlated very poorly with the interpretation of plain radiographs. On the other hand, Nelitz and associates[33] recently investigated the reliability of most of these parameters, and found a high intraobserver and interobserver reliability for the CEA, the acetabular angle of Sharp, the Tönnis angle, the acetabular head index, the neck shaft angle, and lateral subluxation.

Although plain radiographs remain the primary means by which we diagnose acetabular dysplasia, they are of limited benefit in quantifying the

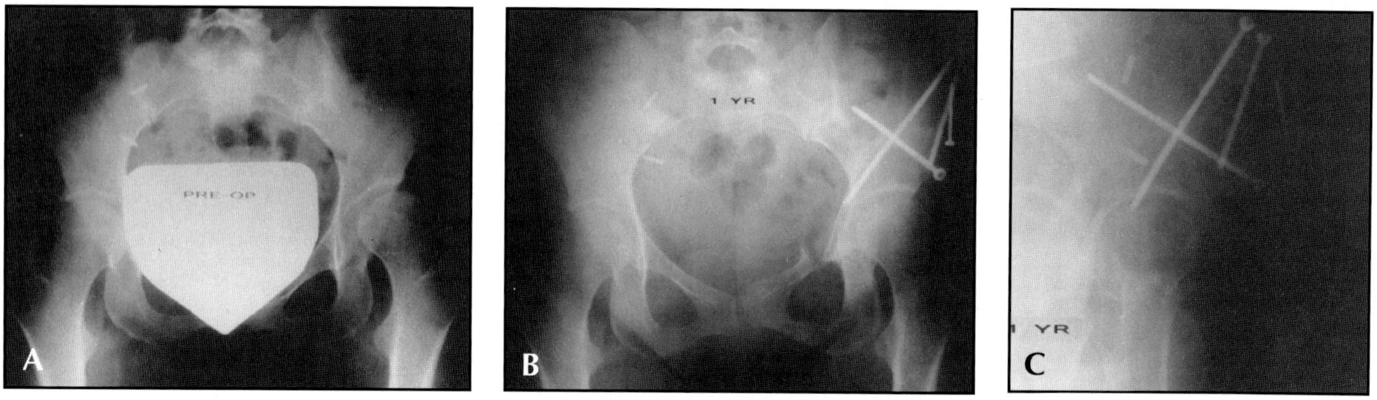

Fig. 3 A, AP radiograph of the pelvis before periacetabular osteotomy. **B**, AP and **C**, false-profile radiographs of the pelvis and left hip 1 year after periacetabular osteotomy showing bone union with improved coverage.

exact degree and precise location of the acetabular deficiency. Complicated mathematical estimations of acetabular coverage have been derived from plain radiographs, but these methods are complex and make a number of assumptions regarding the geometry of the hip joint.[14,34] Konishi and associates described the estimation of three-dimensional (3-D) acetabular coverage using only an AP radiograph of the hip.[6,34] This technique assumes that the acetabulum and femoral head are spherical and congruent, and it is very susceptible to errors produced by alterations in positioning and X-ray beam divergence. It is also very complex and time consuming and requires computer equipment and digitizers not commonly available in hospital departments. Chosa and associates[14] have used the CEA on the AP and false profile views to define a mathematical formula for acetabular coverage. This formula is based on the same assumptions as Konishi's technique and has similar drawbacks, although it has good potential for large screening studies and for obtaining an estimation of coverage with relatively low radiation exposures.

Plain radiographs or fluoroscopy are also used for the intraoperative assessment of periacetabular osteotomies. Plain radiographs are much more useful because they allow the whole pelvis to be seen in direct contrast to the limited local view afforded by fluoroscopy. The acetabular roof should be horizontal, the femoral head should be congruous and centered beneath the acetabular roof, the version must not be overcorrected because overcorrection can lead to excessive posterior uncovering (in neutral version, the two limbs of the anterior and posterior walls meet at the superolateral corner of the acetabulum), the femoral head should be medialized to between 5 and 15 mm of the ilioischial line, and Shenton's line should normalize (Fig. 3). Intraoperative radiographs allow a very good assessment of lateral coverage but not of anterior and posterior coverage. Crockarell and associates[35] recommend covering one third of the radiographic surface area of the femoral head on the intraoperative AP radiograph to obtain a satisfactory anterior correction.

Computed Tomography Scans

Plain radiographs allow a reasonable qualitative assessment of acetabular coverage, but are severely limited by the lack of 3-D information, by the overlap of bony structures,[13] and by potential errors.[13,17,30] Interest has recently centered on the use of CT.[4,5,36-41] Techniques for 3-D CT (3DCT) allow accurate visualization of the bony anatomy and permit accurate angular and linear measurements in an infinite number of planes.[42,43] The use of CT scans allows the measurement of a number of variables, such as femoral neck-shaft angle, femoral anteversion, and acetabular anteversion, that are more difficult to interpret accurately from plain radiographs alone.[36,37]

CT is an ideal modality for assessment of acetabular coverage, because it provides 3-D information with high-spatial resolution.[41,42,44,45] Klaue and associates[4] performed CT scans with the patients supine, with the iliac crests level in the transverse plane, the knees extended, and the legs and feet parallel and together. Four millimeter slices were taken through the acetabular roof and joint. Using these films, the contours of the acetabular roof, of the surrounding part of the pelvis, and of the femoral head were digitized. The center of the femoral head was used to divide it into four quadrants. The contours could then be superimposed on a computer and an intersection diagram created to estimate femoral head coverage. The method of Murphy and associates[46,47] involves construction of surface contour maps of the acetabular surface and femoral head (derived from axial images) from which the acetabular orientation can be determined and manipulated. Femoral head containment is defined in terms of anterior, lateral, and posterior (center edge) angles. The anterior and posterior angles are measured in a transverse plane and are not analagous to the CEA of Wiberg, which is measured in a vertical plane. Anda[48] suggested that the terms anterior and posterior acetabular sector angles should be used rather than anterior and posterior CEAs. These pioneering techniques have proved very useful but the analyses are time consuming, and specialized computer and graphics equipment are required.

We have devised a simple and reproducible 3DCT technique for the measurement of acetabular coverage in adults.[49,50] This technique is simple to learn (learning time approximately 30 minutes) and relatively rapid to perform (approximately 20 minutes per hip). The CT scanning is performed using a GE HiLight Scanner (GE Medical Systems, Milwaukee, WI). The subjects are positioned supine on the scanning table with the midline of the body aligned with the central axis of the scanning table. The hips are fully extended and the feet stabilized with the hips in 15° of external rotation. Care is taken to avoid pelvic tilt and hip or knee flexion. Helical 3-mm CT sections are performed at a pitch of 1:1 (kV 120, mA 300, field-of-view 38 to 42 cm, standard algorithm) through both acetabula and femoral heads. The helical CT data are reconstructed at 1-mm intervals. The scan data are transferred to a 3-D workstation (Advantage Windows Workstation, GE Medical Systems). Using the automated 3-D bone reconstruction program, a surface-shaded 3-D model of the pelvis is obtained (Fig. 4).

This 3-D program automatically discards all soft-tissue signals and produces a surface-shaded image of the bony structures. Like most similar techniques, this method assumes femoral head sphericity. This precondition usually is satisfied by patients undergoing periacetabular osteotomies because their femoral heads are either spherical or near spherical. It is therefore possible to simultaneously view the axial, coronal, and sagittal images, and to manually place a cursor at the center of the femoral head. Vertical planar images are then obtained through the center of the femoral head at various rotations from 0° (anterior acetabular margin) through 90° (lateral acetabular margin) to 180° (posterior acetabular margin). The acetabular margin is defined as the edge of the smooth subchondral bone surface. The CEA is measured at 10° rotational increments around the acetabular rim. For example, the CEA angle at 90° corresponds to the classic CEA of Wiberg on an AP radiograph of the pelvis. The data are then presented graphically, with the CEA on the y-axis and the rotational position on the x-axis.

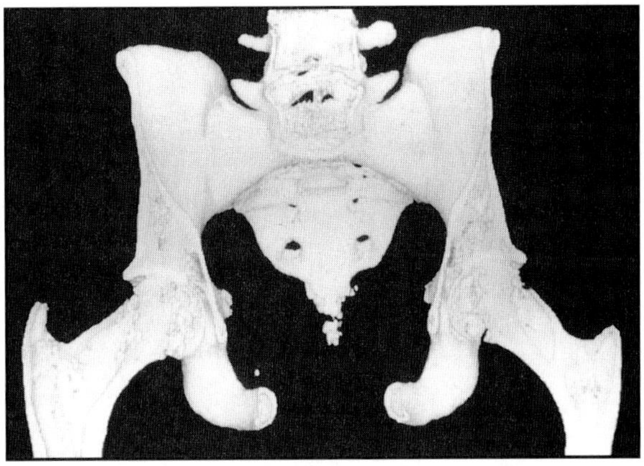

Fig. 4 Cross-sectional view of a 3DCT surface shaded model of a human pelvic phantom.

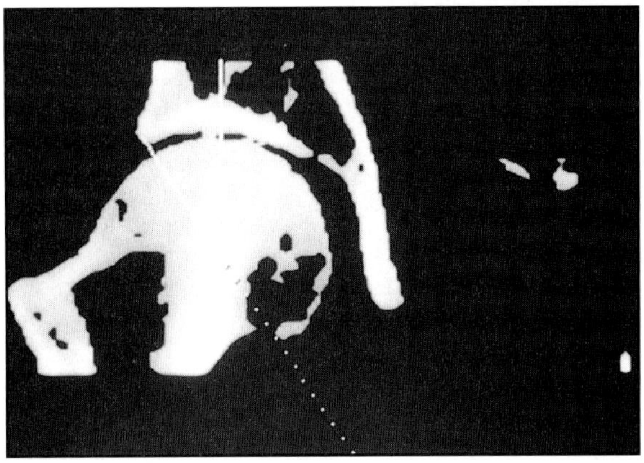

Fig. 5 Coronal planar image through the center of the femoral head. The CEA is measured as the angle between the vertical axis and the line connecting the femoral head center to the lateral acetabular margin. The 90° position corresponds to the classic CEA of Wiberg on the AP pelvis radiograph.

Normative data were derived from 15 normal hips in 12 subjects (aged 19 to 49 years, mean 34.2 years) who underwent thin section CT scans for the evaluation of contraletral acetabular fractures (9 patients) or for the assessment of soft-tissue abnormalities (3 patients, 6 hips). These data, and their reliability, validity, and reproducibilty have been published.[50] The intraobserver variability of using this technique for hip dysplasia has also been assessed using six randomly selected patients with dysplastic hips. The average measurement error was 2.4° (range 0° to 4.3°). This measurement error was greatest in the posterior portion of the acetabulum.

To allow the assessment of global and regional dysplasia severity, dysplasia indices are quantified. The dysplasia

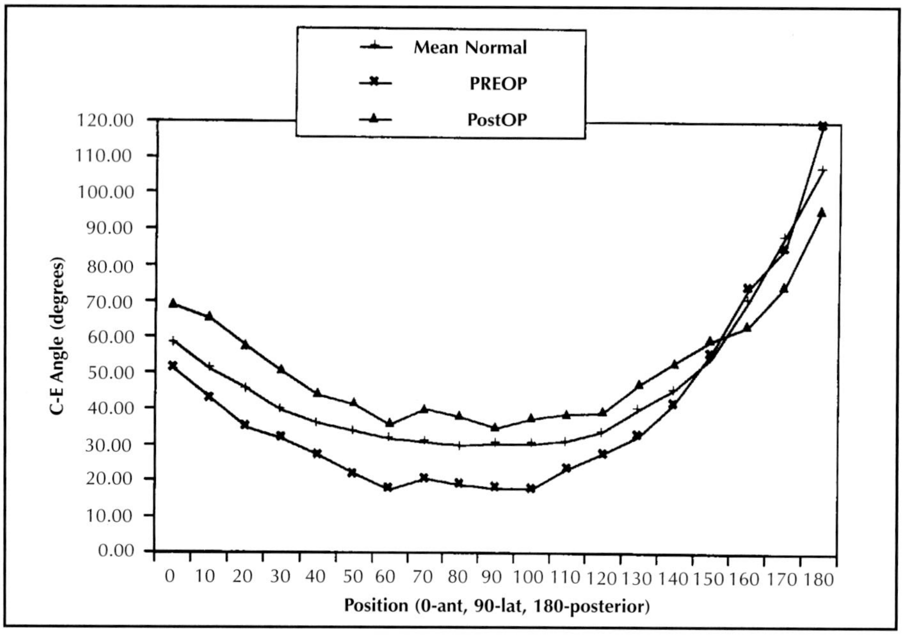

Fig. 6 Graph of preoperative and postoperative coverage compared with normal controls. This curve is used to determine the degree of correction required and to assess whether the correction had been achieved postoperatively. (Reproduced with permission from Haddad FS, Garbuz DS, Duncan CP, Janzen DL, Munk PL: CT evaluation of periacetabular osteotomies. *J Bone Joint Surg Br* 2000;82:526-531.)

indices are based on the area under the curve on a graph of CEA versus position along the acetabular rim. The indices are calculated as a ratio (dyplastic hip/normal mean data). Global coverage is defined as the area under the curve from 0° to 180° positions, anterolateral coverage from the 0° to 40° rotational positions, lateral coverage from the 50° to 120° positions, and posterolateral coverage from the 130° to 180° positions. The dysplasia indices are most useful in allowing easy comparison between patients and between preoperative and postoperative acetabular coverage. We ultimately may be able to categorize groups of acetabular dysplasia patients on the basis of these indices.

The data obtained are easily presented both as images (Fig. 5) and in graphic form (Fig. 6) and give a clearer indication of the coverage obtained than plain radiographic indices. For each patient, the preoperative graphic recording is compared with that of the control group and used to plan the correction performed at the time of surgery. The correction is defined in terms of angular coverage of the femoral head required in any single plane at the time of surgery. This is far easier to reproduce and measure at the time of surgery than other parameters such as surface area coverage because the femoral head is not routinely exposed. The use of angular coverage measurements also corrects for variations in patient size; normal surface area coverage measurements are difficult to obtain because of the variable size of the articular surface of the femoral head.

All the described CT techniques have limitations. They are not ideally suited to patients with nonspherical femoral heads, because the center of the femoral head cannot be defined precisely, and this lack of precision leads to increased measurement variability. Malalignment of the pelvis on the CT scanner gantry also creates measurment errors. Although lateral pelvic tilt can easily be controlled by assessing the AP scout image, the vertical tilt (that is, lumbosacral lordosis or kyphosis) is difficult to control or measure and may introduce error into our measurements. Abel and associates[36] have shown however that 3-D reformatting overcomes some of these errors.

CT techniques are evolving constantly. They are increasingly used for surgical modeling and simulation,[51,52] are essential prerequisites to computer-guided surgical navigation,[53-55] and have the potential for examining cartilage thickness and determining its impact on preoperative planning and postoperative outcomes.[56] Hipp and associates[57] used 3DCT scan data to calculate joint contact pressures and advocate their technique for the planning of acetabular reorientation surgery with a view to obtaining the best possible joint pressure distribution after surgery.

Magnetic Resonance Imaging

There is concern about the gonadal radiation dose inherent in thin-section CT of the acetabulum, especially because most of adult acetabular dysplasia patients are women of child-bearing age. At this time, however, no alternative, radiation-free imaging methods have been developed to quantify acetabular dysplasia. MRI has some potential advantages for the measurement and assessment of acetabular dysplasia, including its multiplanar imaging capability and the absence of ionizing radiation. MRI cuts can be digitized in the same way as CT scan slices to produce 3-D surface reconstructions. MRI may ultimately be used in a similar way and would have the potential for dynamic weight-bearing studies; however, it remains expensive and is not readily available in our center.

At present MRI is useful for detecting labral tears and ganglia and for the assessment of articular cartilage. The management of intra-articular ganglia and labral lesions in the presence of acetabular dysplasia is controversial because reorientation of the acetabulum with the resulting improved biomechanics may resolve the problem without the need for arthrotomy.

Computer-Assisted Surgery

Although very clear information can be obtained from plain radiographs and CT scans, it is difficult to link the surgical plan directly to intraoperative findings and procedures. Computer assistance has helped to bridge this gap both through the use of 3-D imaging techniques and through the introduction of image interactive free-hand navigation of surgical instruments.

Nolte and associates[55] use a 3-D differentiated reconstructive imaging technique whereby selected points of interest are marked on slices of CT hardcopies. These points are then digitized and a triangular or quadrangular algorithm applied to obtain a wire-frame reconstruction that can be tiled and smoothed. The resulting reconstruction can be manipulated to allow preoperative simulation and assessment of the effects of different surgical procedures on femoral head coverage and congruency. The 3-D reconstructions also can be used to create image-based templates that can be used as guides at the time of surgery.[58]

The most exciting advance has been the introduction of computer assistance at the time of surgery. Preinserted percutaneously placed cortical screws and easily defined anatomic landmarks are identified on preoperative CT scans and are incorporated into a 3-D reconstruction. These points are then identified at the time of surgery and digitized using an optoelectronic camera system. This step allows matching between the surgical object (the pelvis) and the virtual image (on screen) and allows the surgical navigation of specially designed tools with markers that allow quasi real-time identification of their positions. This system gives exact and easily understandable feedback of the location and orientation of the osteotomes.

Langlotz and associates[54] reported the use of computer assistance for 12 periacetabular osteotomies. There were slight increases in surgery time and blood loss compared to standard cases but the use of this system changed the direction of the pubic osteotomy, which previously had risked joint penetration more. The authors believe that computer assistance increased the accuracy and safety of periacetabular osteotomy, and that it had potential to decrease the use of intraoperative radiographs in such procedures. The future potential of image guidance includes less invasive approaches to such interventions, fewer technical complications, and a facilitation of the surgical learning curve. We are not aware of any data on whether computer-assisted surgery has any effect on clinical outcome.

Summary

The management of the dysplastic hip represents a clinical and a technical challenge. There is a great deal of variation in the degree and direction of acetabular dysplasia, and the accurate determination of femoral head coverage is difficult. It is, therefore, important to measure and plan any osteotomy based on each patient's unique acetabular anatomy. A clear understanding of the underlying anatomic abnormalities is vital so that reconstruction can be appropriately planned. This understanding is facilitated by an appreciation of the imaging techniques available and their correct application.

The initial imaging of the dysplastic hip is based on plain radiographs. These determine the diagnosis of dysplasia and give a good indication of its severity and of the degree of congruency, instability, and degenerative change. A number of indices have been defined on these radiographs to facilitate surgical planning and to evaluate surgical outcomes. Moreover, plain radiographs or fluoroscopy are usually the only modalities accessible during surgery.

More complex imaging is necessary to define any associated lesions and to quantify the acetabular deficiency more accurately. Multiplanar imaging using CT scans and computer reconstructions reduces the need for complex spatial interpretation, facilitates preoperative planning, and allows preoperative simulation. The availability of more powerful computers has extended the use of these techniques to intraoperative surgical navigation.

Continued progress and development of imaging techniques will further determine the type and degree of correction required for each hip and will help to stratify dysplastic hips for outcomes assessment. Ultimately, it will help orthopaedic surgeons to evaluate whether the success or failure of osteotomies around the hip are intrinsic to the techniques used or to the primary disease process or are related to the surgeon's failure to create a more normal biomechanical environment for the hip.

Acknowledgments

One of the authors (FSH) was supported by the John Charnley and BOA/Wishbone trusts and by the Norman Capener Traveling Fellowship.

References

1. Ganz R, Klaue K, Vinh TS, Mast JW: A new periacetabular osteotomy for the treatment of hip dysplasias: Technique and preliminary results. *Clin Orthop* 1988;232:26-36.
2. Hersche O, Casillas M, Ganz R: Indications for intertrochanteric osteotomy after periacetabular osteotomy for adult hip dysplasia. *Clin Orthop* 1998;347:19-26.

3. Wedge JH: Osteotomy of the pelvis for the management of hip disease in young adults. *Can J Surg* 1998;38(suppl 1):S25-32.

4. Klaue K, Wallin A, Ganz R: CT evaluation of coverage and congruency of the hip prior to osteotomy. *Clin Orthop* 1988;232:15-25.

5. Millis MB, Murphy SB: Use of computed tomographic reconstruction in planning osteotomies of the hip. *Clin Orthop* 1992;274:154-159.

6. Mieno T, Konishi N, Hasegawa Y, Genda E: Three-dimensional evaluation of acetabular coverage of the femoral head in normal hip joints and hip joints with acetabular dysplasia. *Nippon Seikeigeka Gakkai Zasshi* 1992;66:11-22.

7. McCarthy JJ, Fox JS, Gurd AR: Innominate osteotomy in adolescents and adults who have acetabular dysplasia. *J Bone Joint Surg Am* 1996;78:1455-1461.

8. Shindo H, Igarashi H, Taneda H, Azuma H: Rotational acetabular osteotomy for severe dysplasia of the hip with a false acetabulum. *J Bone Joint Surg Br* 1996;78:871-877.

9. Lequesne M, de Seze S: False profile of the pelvis: A new radiographic incidence for the study of the hip: Its use dysplasias and different coxopathies. *Rev Rhum Mal Osteoartic* 1961;28:643-652.

10. Matta JM, Stover MD, Siebenrock K: Periacetabular osteotomy through the Smith-Petersen approach. *Clin Orthop* 1999;363:21-32.

11. Nakamura S, Ninomiya S, Takatori Y, Morimoto S, Umeyama T: Long-term outcome of rotational acetabular osteotomy: 145 hips followed for 10-23 years. *Acta Orthop Scand* 1998;69:259-265.

12. Dunn DM: Anteversion of the neck of the femur: A method of measurement. *J Bone Joint Surg Br* 1952;34:181-186.

13. Johnston CE II, Wenger DR, Roberts JM, Burke SW, Roach JW: Acetabular coverage: Three-dimensional anatomy and radiographic evaluation. *J Pediatr Orthop* 1986;6:548-558.

14. Chosa E, Tajima N, Nagatsuru Y: Evaluation of acetabular coverage of the femoral head with anteroposterior and false profile radiographs of the hip joint. *J Orthop Sci* 1997;2:378-290.

15. Murphy SB, Ganz R, Muller ME: The prognosis in untreated dysplasia of the hip: A study of radiographic factors that predict the outcome. *J Bone Joint Surg Am* 1995;77:985-989.

16. Klaue K, Durnin CW, Ganz R: The acetabular rim syndrome: A clinical presentation of dysplasia of the hip. *J Bone Joint Surg Br* 1991;73:423-429.

17. Tönnis D: Normal values of the hip joint for the evaluation of X-rays in children and adults. *Clin Orthop* 1976;119:39-47.

18. Trousdale RT, Ganz R: Periacetabular and intertrochanteric osteotomy for the treatment of osteoarthrosis in dysplastic hips. *J Bone Surg Am* 1995;77:73-85.

19. Siebenrock KA, Scholl E, Lottenbach M, Ganz R: Bernese periacetabular osteotomy. *Clin Orthop* 1999;363:9-20.

20. Fredensborg N: The CE angle of normal hips. *Acta Orthop Scand* 1976;47:403-405.

21. Mandal S, Bhan S: The centre-edge angle of Wiberg in the adult Indian population. *J Bone Joint Surg Br* 1996;78:320-321.

22. Wiberg G: Shelf operation in congenital dysplasia of the acetabulum and in subluxation and dislocation of the hip. *J Bone Joint Surg Am* 1953;35:65-80.

23. Massie WK, Howorth MB: Congenital dislocation of the hip: Part 1. Method of grading results. *J Bone Joint Surg Am* 1950;32:519-531.

24. Sharp IK: Acetabular dysplasia: The acetabular angle. *J Bone Joint Surg Br* 1961;43:268-272.

25. Reynolds D, Lucas J, Klaue K: Retroversion of the acetabulum: A cause of hip pain. *J Bone Joint Surg Br* 1999;81:281-288.

26. Tonnis D, Heinecke A: Acetabular and femoral anteversion: Relationship with osteoarthritis of the hip. *J Bone Joint Surg Am* 1999;81:1747-1770.

27. Heyman CH, Herndon CH: Legg-Perthes Disease: A method for the measurement of the roentgenographic result. *J Bone Joint Surg Am* 1950;32:767-778.

28. Ninomiya S, Tagawa H: Rotational acetabular osteotomy for the dysplastic hip. *J Bone Joint Surg Am* 1984;66:430-436.

29. Trumble SJ, Mayo KA, Mast JW: The periacetabular osteotomy: Minimum 2-year follow-up in more than 100 hips. *Clin Orthop* 1999;363:54-63.

30. Portinaro NM, Murray DW, Bhullar TP, Benson MK: Errors in measurement of acetabular index. *J Pediatr Orthop* 1995;15:780-784.

31. Werier JM, Garbuz D, Younger ASE, Masri BA, Janzen DL, Duncan CP: Abstract: The reliability of the centre edge angle and false profile view in assessing hip dysplasia. *J Bone Joint Surg Br* 1998;80(suppl 1):9.

32. de Kleuver M, Huiskes R, Kauer JM, Veth RP: Three-dimensional displacement of the hip joint after triple pelvic osteotomy: A post-mortem radiostereometric study. *Acta Orthop Scand* 1998;69:585-589.

33. Nelitz M, Guenther KP, Gunkel S, Puhl W: Reliability of radiological measurements in the assessment of hip dysplasia in adults. *Br J Radiol* 1999;72:331-334.

34. Konishi N, Mieno T: Determination of acetabular coverage of the femoral head with use of a single anteroposterior radiograph: A new computerized technique. *J Bone Joint Surg Am* 1993;75:1318-1333.

35. Crockarell J Jr, Trousdale RT, Cabanela ME, Berry DJ: Early experience and results with the periacetabular osteotomy: The Mayo Clinic experience. *Clin Orthop* 1999;363:45-53.

36. Abel MF, Sutherland DH, Wenger DR, Mubarak SJ: Evaluation of CT scans and 3-D reformatted images for quantitative assessment of the hip. *J Pediatr Orthop* 1994;14:48-53.

37. Abel MF, Wenger DR, Mubarak SJ, Sutherland DH: Quantitative analysis of hip dysplasia in cerebral palsy: A study of radiographs and 3-D reformatted images. *J Pediatr Orthop* 1994;14:283-289.

38. Azuma H, Taneda H, Igarashi H, Fujioka M: Preoperative and postoperative assessment of rotational acetabular osteotomy for dysplastic hips in children by three-dimensional surface reconstruction computed tomography imaging. *J Pediatr Orthop* 1990;10:33-38.

39. Kim HT, Wenger DR: Location of acetabular deficiency and associated hip dislocation in neuromuscular hip dysplasia: Three-dimensional computed tomographic analysis. *J Pediatr Orthop* 1997;17:143-151.

40. Roach JW, Hobatho MC, Baker KJ, Ashman RB: Three-dimensional computer analysis of complex acetabular insufficiency. *J Pediatr Orthop* 1997;17:158-164.

41. Sutherland CJ, Bresina SJ, Gayou DE: Use of general purpose mechanical computer assisted engineering software in orthopaedic surgical planning: Advantages and limitations. *Comput Med Imaging Graph* 1994;18:435-442.

42. Kuszyk BS, Heath DG, Bliss DF, Fishman EK: Skeletal 3-D CT: Advantages of volume rendering over surface rendering. *Skeletal Radiol* 1996;25:207-214.

43. Martinez CR, Di Pasquale TG, Helfet DL, Graham AW, Sanders RW, Ray LD: Evaluation of acetabular fractures with two- and three-dimensional CT. *Radiographics* 1992;12:227-242.

44. Conway WF, Totty WG, McEnery KW: CT and MR imaging of the hip. *Radiology* 1996;198:297-307.

45. Delaunay S, Dussault RG, Kaplan PA, Alford BA: Radiographic measurements of dysplastic adult hips. *Skeletal Radiol* 1997;26:75-81.

46. Murphy SB, Kijewski PK, Millis MB, Harless A: Acetabular dysplasia in the adolescent and young adult. *Clin Orthop* 1990;261:214-223.

47. Murphy SB, Millis MB, Hall JE: Surgical correction of acetabular dysplasia in the adult: A Boston experience. *Clin Orthop* 1999;363:38-44.

48. Anda S: Letter: Acetabular dysplasia in the adolescent and young adult. *Clin Orthop* 1993;286:308-310.

49. Haddad FS, Garbuz DS, Duncan CP, Janzen DL, Munk PL: The CT evaluation of periacetabular osteotomies. *J Bone Joint Surg Br* 2000;82:526-531.

50. Janzen DL, Aippersbach SE, Munk PL, et al: Three-dimensional CT measurement of adult acetabular dysplasia: Technique, preliminary results in normal subjects, and potential applications. *Skeletal Radiol* 1998;27:352-358.

51. Gerber JD, Ney DR, Magid D, Fishman EK: Simulated femoral repositioning with three-dimensional CT. *J Comput Assist Tomogr* 1991;15:121-125.

52. Radermacher K, Portheine F, Anton M, et al: Computer assisted orthopaedic surgery with image based individual templates. *Clin Orthop* 1998;354:28-38.

53. Langlotz F, Bachler R, Berlemann U, Nolte LP, Ganz R: Computer assistance for pelvic osteotomies. *Clin Orthop* 1998;354:92-102.

54. Langlotz F, Stucki M, Bachler R, et al: The first twelve cases of computer assisted periacetabular osteotomy. *Comput Aided Surg* 1997;2:317-326.

55. Nolte LP, Langlotz F, Klaue K, Stucki M, Ganz R: Advancements in pelvic osteotomies by means of computer assistance. *Semin Arthroplasty* 1997;8:108-113.

56. Kawabe K, Konishi N: Three-dimensional modeling of cartilage thickness in hip dysplasia. *Clin Orthop* 1993;289:180-185.

57. Hipp JA, Sugano N, Millis MB, Murphy SB: Planning acetabular redirection osteotomies based on joint contact pressures. *Clin Orthop* 1999;364:134-143.

SECTION

5

Hip: Adult Reconstruction—Unstable Total Hip Arthroplasty

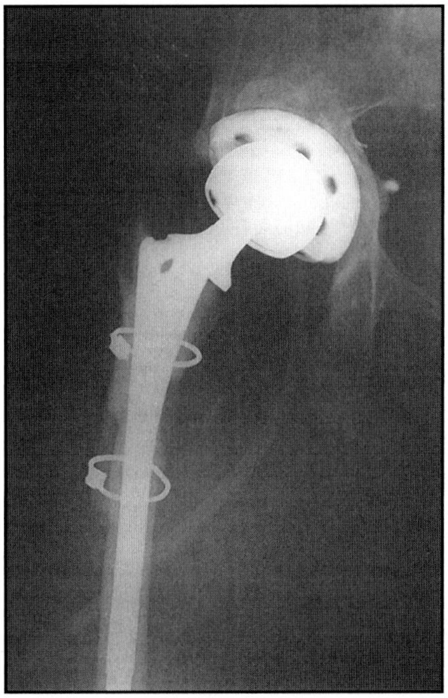

27 Unstable Total Hip Arthroplasty: Detailed Overview

28 The Effect of Component Design on Range of Motion to Impingement in Total Hip Arthroplasty ***(with video clip on enclosed CD)***

29 The Use of a Constrained Acetabular Component for Recurrent Dislocation

30 The Unstable Total Hip Arthroplasty: The Role of Postoperative Bracing

27

Unstable Total Hip Arthroplasty: Detailed Overview

Daniel J. Berry, MD

Introduction

Dislocation is one of the most common complications of total hip arthroplasty (THA). Hip dislocation is a disturbing event for the patient and a frustrating problem for the surgeon and is associated with pain, morbidity,[1] and expense. Despite the increasing sophistication of THA implants and techniques, the problem of dislocation remains common, and although specific techniques may reduce the rate of dislocation, there is as yet no evidence that the overall prevalence has declined. Dislocation usually is treated nonsurgically initially, but recurrent dislocation usually requires surgical treatment. To date, most reports indicate that reoperation for recurrent instability carries with it a disconcertingly high chance of failure but, with better understanding of dislocation and improved technologies to treat dislocation, the success rate of surgical treatment probably can be improved. This chapter reviews the epidemiology of hip dislocation, measures that may be taken to avoid dislocation, and methods available to treat the dislocation.

Epidemiology

The prevalence of dislocation after THA varies widely, from 0.3% to 10% or more in different series.[2-6] In several large series the rate is 2% to 3%.[7-10] The rate in any specific series depends on many factors, including patient mix, the surgeon's experience,[11] and the surgical approach. It is clear that the reported prevalence of hip dislocation is higher if a specific program is in place at an institution to identify all patients who dislocate because many dislocations are not treated at the institution where the THA surgery was performed. Furthermore, the reported prevalence of dislocation is higher if patients are followed for longer periods of time, because first-time dislocations continue to occur for the life of the arthroplasty.

Risk Factors for Dislocation

Hip dislocation is well documented to be more common in specific demographic groups and is suspected to be more common in several others. Patient gender has an effect on the rate of dislocation: several series have shown women have a higher rate of dislocation than men.[9,10,12-15] Age at surgery appears to affect the risk of dislocation, with older patients at higher risk than younger patients, although the correlation between age and dislocation is not yet proven.[16-18] The reasons for a higher rate of dislocation in older patients may include a greater risk of falls, poorer soft tissues, and, perhaps, a greater incidence of confusion and noncompliance with dislocation precautions.

The underlying diagnosis leading to THA has an effect on dislocation risk. Patients treated with THA for a diagnosis of hip fracture are at high risk.[19-21] Advanced age, poorer or damaged muscles, greater propensity for falls, and altered proximal femoral anatomy probably all play a role in the increased risk of dislocation in these patients. The rate of dislocation in patients treated with THA for developmental dysplasia of the hip is elevated in some series.[21] In these patients, poorer muscle strength, bone deformity, and alterations from normal implant position may increase the risk.

Associated medical conditions and comorbidities also affect the risk of dislocation. Dislocation is more common in patients with neuromuscular conditions that lead to weakness in muscles around the hip or contractures around the hip.[4,22-25] Cognitive dysfunction increases the rate of hip dislocation, probably because impaired cognition leads to less compliance with hip dislocation precautions.[18,24]

Revision hip arthroplasty is associated with a considerably higher risk of dislocation than primary THA.[26] The main reasons for higher risk of dislocation after revision THA are compromised abductor muscles and bone loss that leads to compromises in implant location and orientation.

Chronology of Dislocation

Many authors[8,9,27,28] have reported that the majority of dislocations, on the order of 50% to 75%, occur in the first few months after THA. However, two studies[15,29] found that over 60% of dislocations occurred more than 4 to 5 weeks after surgery. Clearly, first-time dislocations continue indefinitely after a THA, and the longer patients are followed, the greater number that are identified late. Dislocations that occur in the first few months after THA, before the soft tissues have healed, are less likely to be recurrent than those that occur later according to most,[9,27] but not all,[29] authors. Late dislocation of a previously stable THA may be related to trauma or chronic changes around the hip (such as increased laxity of the pseudocapsule with time),[12] deteriorating muscle strength, or wear or deformation of the acetabular polyethylene.

Prevention of Dislocation

Measures to prevent dislocation can be divided into three main categories: preoperative measures, intraoperative measures, and postoperative measures.

Preoperative Measures

Some dislocation problems can be avoided by preoperatively identifying patients at high risk for dislocation and applying appropriate preventive measures. Knowledge of the epidemiologic factors discussed in the previous section helps the surgeon identify demographic groups at high risk for dislocation. Occasional patients may be at such high risk for dislocation that THA is considered contraindicated. Some patients with no preoperative abductor function, severe neuromuscular problems, or severe substance abuse or cognitive problems fall into this category. More commonly, patients will be recognized to be at increased risk for dislocation but nevertheless will be considered candidates for THA. Under these circumstances the surgeon may use a surgical exposure or implants that provide some protection against dislocation. For example, an elderly patient with Parkinson's disease, marked flexion contracture of the hip, and a diagnosis of subcapital hip fracture and little hip arthritis might be treated with an anterolateral approach rather than a posterolateral approach and a hemiarthroplasty rather than a THA.

Careful preoperative planning with implant templates helps prevent instability problems. Templating allows the surgeon to predict the optimal location and orientation of implants relative to bony landmarks of the pelvis and femur and predicts the proper level of femoral neck osteotomy. Importantly, preoperative templating allows the surgeon to choose implants that will restore leg length, femoral offset, and soft-tissue tension.

Intraoperative Measures

Approach Surgical approach affects the risk of dislocation. Multiple series have shown a higher risk of dislocation is associated with a posterior approach compared to an anterolateral approach.[2,14,15,30-35] The main reason for the difference is that in the posterior approach, the capsule and short external rotators that otherwise would provide posterior hip stability and act as a check rein to excessive hip internal rotation are taken down. There are also other reasons; inadequate acetabular component anteversion is more common with the posterior approach because the femur can interfere with socket insertion, leading to insufficient anteversion, and because when the patient is in the lateral position the pelvis tends to roll forward, creating the illusion of increased acetabular anteversion. Enhanced repair of the posterior soft tissues may reduce the risk associated with the posterior approach; recently a series in which preservation and meticulous repair of the posterior capsule and short external rotators was used demonstrated a low incidence of early postoperative dislocation.[36] Although the posterior approach has been associated with a higher dislocation rate, it also has advantages; the most important is that the abductor mechanism is not violated. The choice of exposure should be left to the surgeon's preference based on familiarity with each approach and the specifics of a given patient's situation. For patients at high risk for posterior dislocation, an anterolateral approach may reduce the risk.

Implant Orientation Implant orientation is one of the most important factors under the surgeon's control that strongly influences dislocation risk.[2-4,6,8,10,12,31,37-39] Many series have demonstrated the importance of implant orientation for hip stability, and the orientation of both the acetabular component and femoral component are important. The classic article by Lewinnek and associates[39] showed that excess cup abduction or too little or too much cup forward flexion (hereafter called anteversion) increased the risk of hip instability. Barrack and associates (chapter 28) further refined the optimal cup position using a virtual reality computer model. They found the optimal cup position was approximately 45° of abduction and 20° of anteversion. Excessively abducted cups, that is, cups too vertical in orientation, lead to an increased risk of lateral hip dislocation with hip abduction. Insufficient abduction (that is, cups too horizontal in orientation) leads to less hip range of motion free of impingement in extension-external rotation and flexion-internal rotation. Insufficient anteversion increases the risk of posterior dislocation, whereas excessive anteversion increases the risk of anterior dislocation.

Femoral component orientation also plays a role in hip dislocation risk, but fewer studies have examined this factor because true femoral component version is difficult to measure radiographically without CT. One study showed femoral malposition to be a common source of hip instability.[7] The optimal femoral implant position appears to be about 15° of anteversion in most cases.

Acetabular and femoral component position have an additive influence on hip stability. Thus, modest additive malposition of both components may produce instability while modest malposition of one component may be partially compensated by the other.

Implant Location The location (as opposed to orientation) of the acetabular and femoral components affect hip stability. The location influences stability because it determines the likelihood of bony and soft tissue impingement, the efficiency of the abductor muscles, and the tension of the soft tissues. Marked socket medialization increases the likelihood of impingement of the femur against the pelvis, particularly in hip flexion and internal rotation, and can reduce the soft tissue tension in the hip unless a femoral stem with extra femoral offset is used. Markedly superior socket positioning increases the risk of impingement of the femur against the ischium in hip adduction, extension, and external rotation, and superior socket position also reduces the hip abductor tension if the leg is shortened. Thus, for primary hip replacements in the absence of bony deformity, hip stability can be optimized by avoiding excessively medial or superior placement of the socket.

Implant Choice Bipolar hemiarthroplasties appear to have a lower rate of dislocation than THA, probably because of the large outside diameter of the bipolar implant and the biarticular nature of the implant. These characteristics probably are the reason for a much lower reported hip instability risk for patients with femoral neck fractures treated with a bipolar arthroplasty when compared with THA.[40] For most patients with arthritic hips, however, resurfacing of the acetabulum with a fixed socket is preferred to optimize clinical results and pain relief.

A number of implant-related factors affect hip stability; these include femoral component offset, femoral component head-to-neck diameter ratio, femoral component neck geometry, and acetabular component design.[41,42] Although theoretically all these factors should affect hip stability, to date, proof in clinical series is lacking, probably because dislocation is a multifactorial problem and multiple confounding factors make it difficult to prove that a specific design factor affects hip stability. Nevertheless, if specific design features may improve hip stability, it is reasonable for the surgeon to consider using them, provided they have no major drawbacks.

Femoral offset is the horizontal distance from the center of the femoral canal to the center of the femoral head. The reproduction of femoral offset helps restore soft-tissue tension and reduces the hip-joint reactive force. Implants with increased femoral offset are an important recent design advance that for many patients better restore hip mechanics and, hopefully, will improve hip stability without excessive leg lengthening. The main drawback of higher offset femoral implants is increased torsional and bending stress on the femoral implant.

Increasing femoral component head diameter theoretically increases hip stability[41,43] by increasing the femoral head displacement necessary to cause dislocation. Increasing the femoral head-to-neck diameter ratio also should increase hip stability by increasing the arc of hip motion that can occur free of prosthetic impingement. Despite these theoretical advantages, clinical series have not shown a strong correlation between femoral head size and hip stability.[6,7,9,15,32,38,44] Large femoral head sizes do have a major disadvantage: increased volumetric polyethylene wear that can lead to increased periprosthetic osteolysis. Balancing the risks of instability and volumetric polyethylene wear, most surgeons prefer 28-, 26-, or 22-mm head sizes in most situations. However, the advantages of larger femoral head sizes may outweigh their disadvantages in specific patients at high risk for dislocation.

For a given femoral head size, the head-to-neck diameter ratio can be improved by reducing (within the constraints of material strength) the prosthetic femoral neck diameter. Neck geometries with a narrow anterior-posterior profile also help maintain implant strength while optimizing range of motion free of implant impingement. A better head-to-neck ratio is maintained by avoiding extra-long modular femoral heads that have reinforcing skirts on the neck. Good preoperative planning will allow the surgeon to choose a sufficiently high femoral neck osteotomy level and an implant with sufficient neck length and offset to minimize the need for skirted modular femoral heads.

Elevated acetabular rim liners also affect hip stability, and different types of elevated rims are made by different manufacturers.[13] Some change the orientation of the face of the socket, while others provide an extended wall on one side of the socket. The two types of rim elevation are not identical; however, they both reorient the arc of hip stability but usually do not increase its magnitude.[45] Placement of an elevation posteriorly increases posterior stability at the expense of anterior stability, and placement of an elevation anteriorly increases anterior stability at the expense of posterior stability. Elevated rims can at times create prosthetic impingement and actually cause dislocation.[46] In one of the few clinical studies on the subject, Cobb and associates[47] found elevated liners provided a statistically significantly decreased likelihood of dislocation in patients treated with a primary THA using a posterior approach (but not an anterior approach) and in patients treated with revision THA.

Postoperative Measures

Postoperative patient education can help prevent dislocation. It is helpful for both the surgeon and physical therapists to emphasize the importance of hip dislocation precautions before the patient is discharged from the hospital after THA. Patients benefit from instruction on how to get in and out of chairs, bed, and automobiles, and how to put on shoes and socks safely. Prophylactic postoperative hip guide braces also can reduce the risk of dislocation in high-risk patients.

Treatment of Dislocation

The choice of surgical or nonsurgical treatment of hip dislocation depends on whether the dislocation is recurrent, the chronology of the dislocation relative to the hip arthroplasty, and patient-specific factors.

Closed Reduction

Most dislocations that occur early after THA and most first or second dislocations are managed nonsurgically with closed reduction. Exceptions to this include dislocations associated with failed implants, dislocations associated with marked component malposition, and dislocations that cannot be reduced by closed means. During closed reduction, care needs to be taken to avoid implant dislodgment or modular implant disassembly.[48] Usually, some form of immobilization is used to reduce the risk of early redislocation; this immobilization can take the form of either a cast or a brace. Hip braces can minimize hip adduction and limit hip flexion. A hip spica cast provides even more constraint to motion, but, because it hinders ambulation and sitting, this treatment is reserved for very unstable hips.

The results of closed reduction followed by bracing or casting are available in a limited number of patients. Dorr and Wan[49] found 10 of 12 hips treated with a hip guide brace for 4 to 6 weeks became stable, and Clayton and Thirupathi[50] reported success in seven of nine patients treated with longer term bracing. Ritter[6] reported success in three of five hips treated with a hip spica cast. Bracing or casting are likely to be successful in treating first dislocations not associated with a clear-cut mechanical problem with the arthroplasty, but are less successful when the dislocation is recurrent. Stewart[51] found five of five first time dislocations were treated successfully with a brace, but only three of eight recurrent dislocations were treated successfully.

The optimal duration of bracing or cast immobilization following dislocation is not known. For most patients 6 to 12 weeks after dislocation is a reasonable length of time that allows soft tissues disrupted by the dislocation to heal. Recurrent episodes of dislocation will usually require surgical treatment, although when strong medical or orthopaedic contraindications to surgery exist, prolonged nonsurgical treatment with bracing is an option.

Surgical Treatment

Surgical treatment of hip instability is estimated to be required after about 1% of THAs. This means that recurrent dislocation is probably the most frequent reason for early reoperation after THA. Although surgical treatment usually can solve a dislocation problem, the surgeon should not be complacent about this operation; in several of the largest series the redislocation rate after reoperation for hip instability was 20% to 40%.[52,53] These sobering statistics mean that historically, reoperation for instability has carried with it the highest likelihood of failure of any commonly performed reoperation after THA, including reoperation for infection. With improved understanding of hip dislocation, surgeons have become better at identifying the problems that lead to dislocation and solving them. Furthermore, powerful new technologies have become available to treat dislocation problems that once would not have been solvable. It is hoped that the rate of success now can be improved markedly.

When surgical management of dislocation is contemplated, an organized approach to analyzing the problem aids treatment. The surgeon first must understand the direction of dislocation: anterior, posterior, or directly lateral. When possible, this direction should be determined by a true lateral radiograph taken when the hip is dislocated. A detailed discussion about the hip position that led to dislocation also helps identify the direction of dislocation.

The surgeon should make every effort to understand the etiology of dislocation by considering the differential diagnosis of problems that lead to hip instability (Table 1). A discussion with the patient to determine cognitive or behavioral problems that contributed to dislocation, a careful physical examination aimed at determining leg length and abductor strength, and good-quality radiographs of the hip arthroplasty to determine implant stability and orientation[54,55] are all important parts of this evaluation. The etiology of a hip dislocation cannot always be identified, but, whenever possible, it is important, because understanding the cause leads to more directed and successful treatment.[11,52]

Component Malposition

When the main problem leading to hip instability is component malposition, the treatment is usually component reorientation (Fig. 1). Acetabular malposition is treated by reorienting the socket. Excess cup abduction, excess cup anteversion, or insufficient cup anteversion all can be treated by socket repositioning. Daly and Morrey[52] reported an 81% success rate (22 of 28 hips) when an unstable hip with insufficient acetabular component anteversion was revised by socket repositioning.

Elevated rim liners for modular sockets, or socket wall additions that are attached to nonmodular sockets with screws,[32,56-59] produce small adjustments in relative cup position. Placement of an elevated liner with the elevated hood laterally reduces the relative cup abduction; placement of an elevated rim posteriorly produces more cup anteversion; and placement anteriorly, less relative cup anteversion. The amount of reorientation of the safe zone of hip motion provided by elevated rim liners is modest, and they do not correct major abnormalities in acetabular component position. Fehring and associates[60] reported a high rate of failure when the only measure applied to treat recurrent instability was modular liner and modular head exchange. In a selected group of 29 patients treated in this manner, 16 (55%) had at least one redislocation in the study period.

Table 1
Differential diagnosis of hip dislocation after THA

Component malposition
Socket
Stem
Both socket and stem
Inadequate soft-tissue tension
Unrestored leg length/femoral offset
Excessively lax soft tissues
Impingement
Bone of femur against pelvis
Soft tissue or heterotopic bone interposed between femur and pelvis
Prosthetic femoral neck on acetabular component
Abductor mechanism deficiency
Abductor muscle deficiency due to poor healing, loss of substance, or superior gluteal nerve damage
Trochanteric osteotomy or fracture with proximal migration
Patient compliance problems
Cognitive
Behavioral
Substance abuse
Neuromuscular deficiency

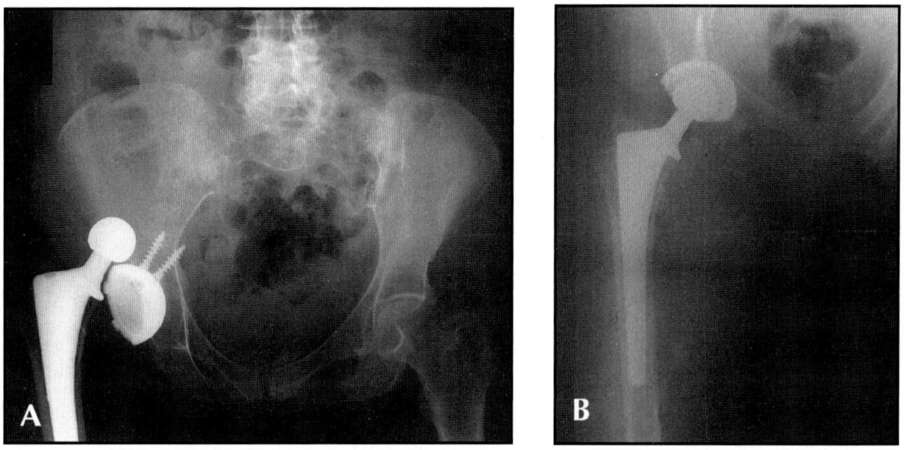

Fig. 1 A, AP pelvis radiograph of a patient with acetabular component malposition causing recurrent dislocation. **B,** AP hip radiograph after the acetabular component was revised to a less abducted position, thereby restoring hip stability.

Marked abnormalities in stem version can be treated with femoral component revision. However, revision of a well-fixed femoral component can be a major undertaking and can lead to substantial bone loss; thus, the surgeon must determine whether directed treatment of the problem (femoral component revision) is the best choice or whether the problem can be solved by compensating for the suboptimal femoral position in other ways.

Soft-Tissue Tension Insufficiency

The treatment of insufficient soft-tissue tension caused by lax but present soft tissues depends on its etiology and the implants in place. If the etiology is inadequate restoration of femoral offset or leg length, the soft tissues may be retensioned by increasing the femoral length or offset (by exchanging components). If modular implants are in place, then a modular femoral head can be exchanged to a longer size. Modular "offset" or "lateralized" acetabular liners move the hip center of rotation laterally and inferiorly and increase the tension of the soft-tissue sleeve. If implants are not modular or if modular implants cannot provide a sufficient increase in soft-tissue tension, then the femoral component can be revised. Alternatively, trochanteric advancement can tension the abductor sleeve and thus improve hip stability. Ekelund[61] reported success with this technique in 19 of 21 patients, and Kaplan and associates[62] reported success with this technique in 17 of 21 patients. In both reports, a prerequisite for this form of treatment was satisfactory implant position. A disadvantage of trochanteric osteotomy is the risk that trochanteric nonunion, if it should occur, can cause an instability problem to worsen. Several factors determine the best method of restoring soft-tissue tension, including the desired leg length, whether the implants are modular, consideration of the pros and cons of long modular femoral heads with reinforcing skirts, and the suitability for advancement of the patient's trochanteric bone quality and abductors.

Impingement

Impingement can cause dislocation because the impingement source acts as a fulcrum levering the femoral head out of the socket. The impingement source can be the femur against the pelvis, interposed soft tissue, heterotopic bone, a migrated greater trochanter fragment, or the prosthetic neck against the prosthetic acetabulum. Impingement between the greater trochanter and pelvis with hip flexion and internal rotation may be treated either by excising some of the anterior greater trochanter or by removing hypertrophic soft tissues between the femur and pelvis in the region of the anterior capsule and the reflected head of the rectus femoris. Impingement between the femur and the ischium with the leg in extension, adduction, and external rotation can be treated by removing a small amount of prominent ischium or removing hypertrophic posterior inferior capsule or scar. Prosthetic impingement of the femoral neck against the acetabular component occurs with implant malposition, with a poor head-to-neck-diameter ratio, or when an acetabular component design has a very elevated rim. Prosthetic impingement is treated

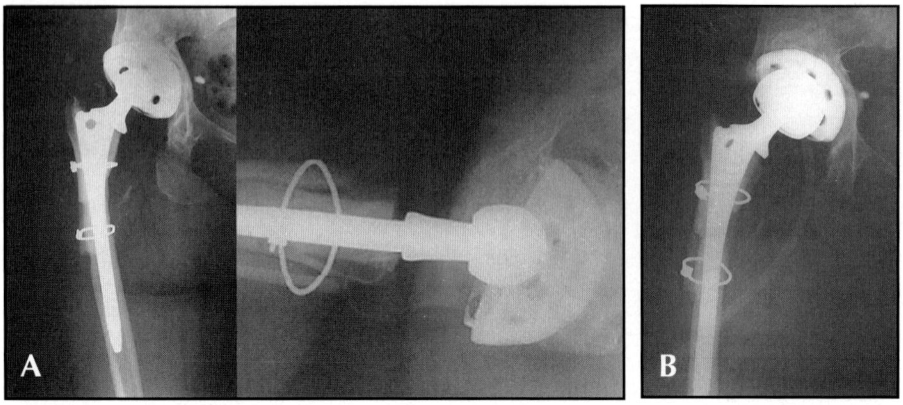

Fig. 2 A, AP and lateral hip radiographs of a patient with proximal femoral allograft, deficient abductors, and recurrent hip instability despite good implant position. **B,** AP hip radiograph after revision to a nonconstrained tripolar device using a custom, large-inside-diameter polyethylene liner.

by improving the implant position, optimizing the head-to-neck ratio, or removing an elevated acetabular rim liner.

Abductor Muscle Deficiency

The abductors normally contribute to hip stability by forming a dynamic sleeve around the hip. When the abductors are deficient or dysfunctional, the risk of hip instability is increased markedly. Abductor deficiency can be caused by trauma, failure of abductor or greater trochanteric healing after previous operations, or superior gluteal nerve dysfunction. Regardless of the etiology, abductor muscle insufficiency is one of the most difficult-to-solve causes of hip instability.

Fracture or nonunion of the greater trochanter with proximal migration leads to insufficiency of the abductor mechanism. Woo and Morrey[15] demonstrated that the dislocation rate increased from 2.8% to 17.6% when the trochanter failed to unite and migrated proximally. Reattachment of the greater trochanter can successfully restore continuity of the abductor mechanism and hip stability; however, trochanteric reattachment may not be possible when the trochanteric fragment is dysvascular or small, or the trochanteric bed (the proximal lateral femur) is markedly deficient. Sometimes the greater trochanter can be advanced to healthy host bone by "pie crusting" tight scar and tendons of the abductor mechanism or by detaching the abductor mechanism from the proximal lateral ileum and advancing it distally on the superior gluteal neurovascular pedicle.

Abductor insufficiency also can result from the abductors failing to heal to the trochanter after an anterolateral approach to the hip. When the remaining abductors are of sufficient quality to allow reattachment, abductor repair sometimes can restore hip stability.[63] When the abductors cannot be repaired because of marked loss of abductor substance, severe scarring, or gluteal nerve damage, other measures to restore hip stability, such as constrained implants, must be considered.

Multifactorial Instability Problems

Many patients have some combination of implant malposition, impingement, or soft-tissue tension problems that together lead to instability. In these circumstances, combined measures aimed at solving in turn each of the contributing problems may be successful.

Conversion of THA to a Bipolar Femoral Head or Constrained Acetabular Component

The directed treatment methods discussed above are most effective when a specific problem leading to instability can be identified and solved. Unfortunately, the etiology of an instability problem cannot always be diagnosed, and, furthermore, some problems cannot be treated successfully by standard means. For such instability problems conversion to a bipolar femoral head or to a constrained acetabular component may be considered.

Conversion to Bipolar Femoral Head

Conversion of a conventional THA to a bipolar arthroplasty can restore hip stability.[64] Limited results of the technique have been reported. Zelicof and Scott[65] reported that all of 11 hips revised for instability were stabilized by conversion to a bipolar arrangement, and an 81% success rate (22 of 27 hips) in restoring hip stability was reported by Parvizi and Morrey.[66] The main disadvantage of conversion to a bipolar femoral head is that the mobile head articulates directly with acetabular bone and can cause pain and bone erosion; these problems are more likely when there is marked preexisting acetabular bone loss.

A bipolar or large-diameter monopolar head also can be articulated with a large inside diameter custom-made polyethylene liner of an acetabular component (Fig. 2). This approach gains the stability advantages of a bipolar head or very large head size while avoiding its main drawback—direct articulation of a mobile femoral head surface with bone. The technique requires a sufficiently large socket diameter to allow a custom-made large-inside-diameter polyethylene bearing surface to be inserted. Limited results of conversion to a tripolar arrangement (bipolar against a large-inside-diameter socket) have been reported. Grigoris and associates[67] reported that all of eight hips treated for instability with this method became stable.

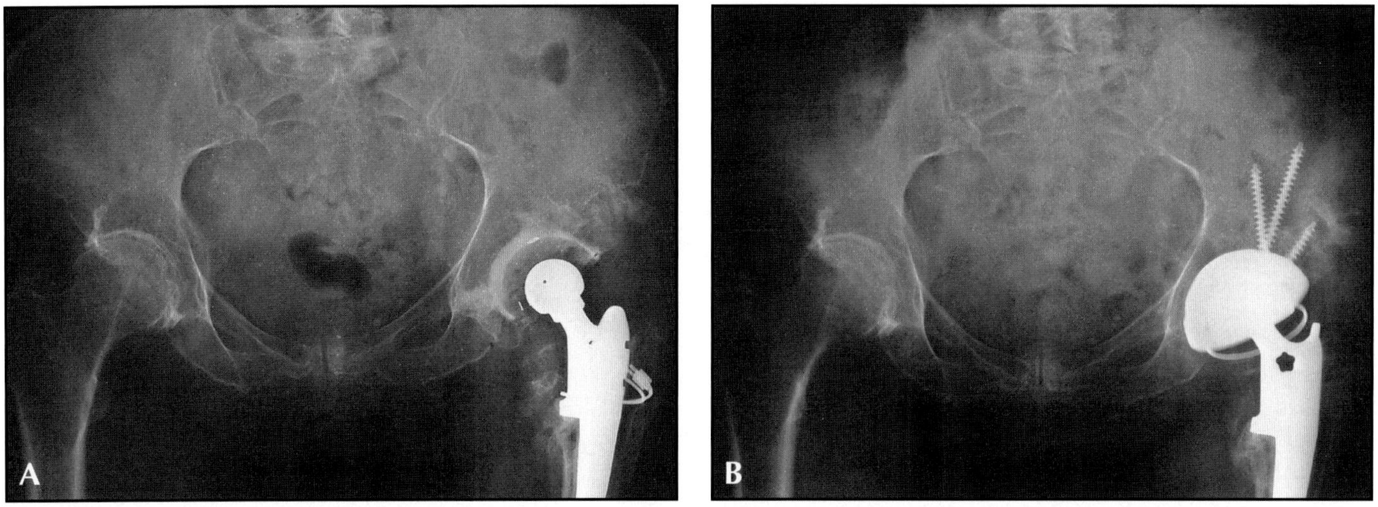

Fig. 3 A, AP pelvis radiograph of an elderly patient with recurrent hip instability after THA for an intertrochanteric hip fracture. The abductors were deficient. **B,** AP pelvis radiograph after the acetabular component was revised to a constrained tripolar component.

Constrained Implants These implants, which capture the femoral head, provide a powerful solution to manage many previously untreatable hip problems[30] (Figs. 3 and 4). These devices mostly have supplanted bipolar implants as a means of treating difficult instability problems. The advantages of these devices, however, come at a cost. Constrained implants have the potential to transmit high loads, which would otherwise lead to hip dislocation, to implant interfaces; these loads can lead to implant loosening (Fig. 5, *A*) or implant disassembly (Fig. 5, *B*). Most constrained liners provide less hip range of motion free of prosthetic impingement; repetitive impingement can lead to fatigue failure of the locking mechanism (Fig. 5, *C*). Constrained implants also have a risk of increased polyethylene wear and, potentially, osteolysis because of component impingement or multiple large-diameter metal-on-polyethylene articulating surfaces. Finally, if dislocation occurs when a constrained socket is in place, open reduction usually is required.

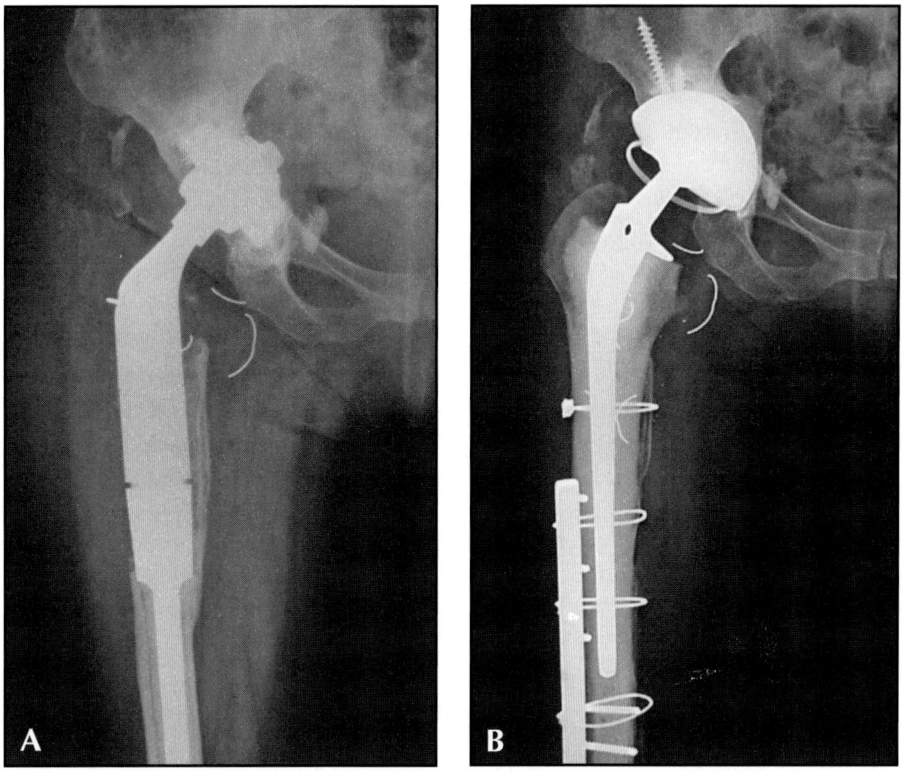

Fig. 4 A, AP hip radiograph of a patient with recurrent hip instability and failed tumor prosthesis. **B,** AP hip radiograph after revision to a constrained tripolar socket. The femur was revised to an allograft prosthetic composite.

There is considerable variability in constrained implant designs. Different designs provide different levels of constraint and are subject to different modes of failure. The three main types of constrained implants are snap-fit sockets, sockets with constraint provided by a metal locking ring around the periphery of a polyethylene insert, and constrained tripolar devices. Snap-fit designs provide

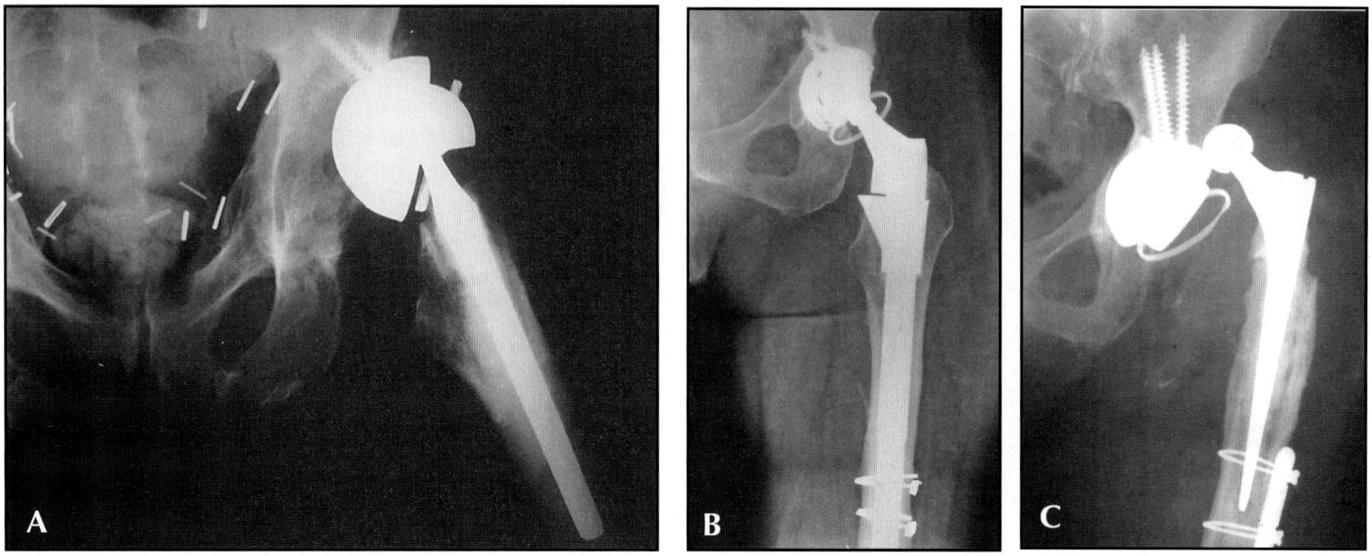

Fig. 5 A, AP hip radiograph demonstrating failure of a constrained uncemented socket at the implant-bone interface. **B**, AP hip radiograph demonstrating disassembly of the locking ring of a constrained socket. **C**, AP hip radiograph of a constrained socket that failed due to prosthetic impingement. The prosthetic femoral neck impinged on the locking ring (note deformation of the ring), leading to locking ring failure and dislocation.

less constraint than the other two design types. Constrained modular designs with locking rings can fail by disassembly of the locking ring,[68] dislocation of the head from the liner, or failure at the socket-bone, bone-cement, implant-cement, or polyethylene liner-shell interfaces. Failures can occur by acute overload or fatigue failure of the captured head locking mechanism. Anderson and associates[69] reported the results of 21 constrained S-ROM sockets (DePuy, Johnson & Johnson, Warsaw, IN); 18 of these were placed for recurrent instability. At a minimum of 2 years after surgery six had redislocated, and failures occurred at both the liner-shell interface and the head-liner interface. Lombardi and associates[70] reported 28 of 31 hips with previous instability treated with the same constrained socket were stable at a minimum of 2 years. Using a constrained tripolar device (Howmedica Osteonics, East Rutherford, NJ), Goetz and associates[71] reported a 96% (54 of 56 hips) success rate in 56 hips revised specifically for hip instability. In that series, the constrained tripolar was used selectively for difficult instability problems in patients with a history of an average of six dislocations each. In 46 hips the tripolar component was placed without cement, and in 10 it was placed with cement (in four of which it was cemented into a well-fixed, porous-coated shell). One of the two failures occurred at the cement-metal interface of a constrained liner cemented into the metal-backed shell of another manufacturer, and the other failure occurred at the implant-bone interface of an uncemented socket.

The indications for use of constrained acetabular implants continue to evolve, and there are differing opinions about the indications for use of these devices. As a general rule, the threshold for using constrained implants is higher in younger than older patients because of the worrisome consequences of polyethylene wear and implant impingement in younger patients. Constrained implants are most helpful in the following situations: (1) patients who have failed well-done attempts to solve an instability problem without constrained implants; (2) patients in whom the etiology of instability cannot be delineated, a situation in which the failure rate of other treatment methods is high; (3) patients with cognitive problems who cannot comply with reasonable dislocation precautions; (4) patients with deficient abductors (Figs. 4 and 5); (5) patients in whom the application of any other technique to gain stability carries a greater potential for problems or complications than would a constrained implant; and (6) some patients, particularly elderly or low-activity individuals, with reasonably well-positioned implants and a well-ingrown porous uncemented modular socket that is compatible with a constrained off-the-shelf or custom-made implant. (In this situation, constraint represents an expeditious, low-risk solution to a difficult problem. In the same patients, cementing a constrained liner into the well-fixed shell could be considered if a constrained liner were not available.)

Constrained implants should not be used when the bone quality is too poor for solid fixation of the implant to bone because constrained implants produce higher interface stresses. Constrained implants also should not be used to compensate for hopelessly malpositioned implants.

Summary

Hip dislocation is one of the most common complications of THA. Good preoperative planning, good postoperative patient education, accurate intraoperative component positioning, rigorous intraoperative testing of hip stability, and good repair of soft tissues during closure all help prevent dislocation. Early postoperative dislocations and first or second dislocations usually are treated with closed reduction and a hip guide brace or hip spica cast, but when dislocation becomes recurrent, surgical treatment usually is needed. When possible, surgical treatment is based on identifying and treating a specific problem leading to the dislocation, such as implant malposition, inadequate soft-tissue tension, or impingement. In selected circumstances, constrained implants or bipolar or tripolar implants provide powerful tools to restore hip stability.

References

1. Chandler RW, Dorr LD, Perry J: The functional cost of dislocation following total hip arthroplasty. *Clin Orthop* 1982;168:168-172.
2. Eftekhar NS: Dislocation and instability complicating low friction arthroplasty of the hip joint. *Clin Orthop* 1976;121:120-125.
3. Etienne A, Cupic Z, Charnley J: Postoperative dislocation after Charnley low-friction arthroplasty. *Clin Orthop* 1978;132:19-23.
4. Morrey BF: Instability after total hip arthroplasty. *Orthop Clin North Am* 1992;23:237-248.
5. Rao JP, Bronstein R: Dislocations following arthroplasties of the hip: Incidence, prevention, and treatment. *Orthop Rev* 1991;20:261-264.
6. Ritter MA: Dislocation and subluxation of the total hip replacement. *Clin Orthop* 1976; 121:92-94.
7. Fackler CD, Poss R: Dislocation in total hip arthroplasties. *Clin Orthop* 1980;151:169-178.
8. Garcia-Cimbrelo E, Munuera L: Dislocation in low-friction arthroplasty. *J Arthroplasty* 1992; 7:149-155.
9. Ali Khan MA, Brakenbury PH, Reynolds IS: Dislocation following total hip replacement. *J Bone Joint Surg Br* 1981;63:214-218.
10. Kristiansen B, Jorgensen L, Holmich P: Dislocation following total hip arthroplasty. *Arch Orthop Trauma Surg* 1985;103:375-377.
11. Hedlundh U, Ahnfelt L, Hybbinette CH, Weckstrom J, Fredin H: Surgical experience related to dislocations after total hip arthroplasty. *J Bone Joint Surg Br* 1996;78:206-209.
12. Coventry MB: Late dislocations in patients with Charnley total hip arthroplasty. *J Bone Joint Surg Am* 1985;67:832-841.
13. Nicholas RM, Orr JF, Mollan RA, Calderwood JW, Nixon JR, Watson P: Dislocation of total hip replacements: A comparative study of standard, long posterior wall and augmented acetabular components. *J Bone Joint Surg Br* 1990;72:418-422.
14. Turner RS: Postoperative total hip prosthetic femoral head dislocations: Incidence, etiologic factors, and management. *Clin Orthop* 1994;301:196-204.
15. Woo RY, Morrey BF: Dislocations after total hip arthroplasty. *J Bone Joint Surg Am* 1982;64:1295-1306.
16. Ekelund A, Rydell N, Nilsson OS: Total hip arthroplasty in patients 80 years of age and older. *Clin Orthop* 1992;281:101-106.
17. Newington DP, Bannister GC, Fordyce M: Primary total hip replacement in patients over 80 years of age. *J Bone Joint Surg Br* 1990;72: 450-452.
18. Woolson ST, Rahimtoola ZO: Risk factors for dislocation during the first 3 months after primary total hip replacement. *J Arthroplasty* 1999; 14:662-668.
19. Gregory RJ, Gibson MJ, Moran CG: Dislocation after primary arthroplasty for subcapital fracture of the hip: Wide range of movement is a risk factor. *J Bone Joint Surg Br* 1991;73:11-12.
20. Lee BP, Berry DJ, Harmsen WS, Sim FH: Total hip arthroplasty for the treatment of an acute fracture of the femoral neck: Long-term results. *J Bone Joint Surg Am* 1998;80:70-75.
21. Mallory TH, Lombardi AV Jr, Fada RA, Herrington SM, Eberle RW: Dislocation after total hip arthroplasty using the anterolateral abductor split approach. *Clin Orthop* 1999;358:166-172.
22. Hedlundh U, Fredin H: Patient characteristics in dislocations after primary total hip arthroplasty: 60 patients compared with a control group. *Acta Orthop Scand* 1995;66:225-228.
23. Hedlundh U, Karlsson M, Ringsberg K, Besjakov J, Fredin H: Muscular and neurologic function in patients with recurrent dislocation after total hip arthroplasty: A matched controlled study of 65 patients using dual-energy x-ray absorptiometry and postural stability tests. *J Arthroplasty* 1999;14:319-325.
24. Paterno SA, Lachiewicz PF, Kelley SS: The influence of patient-related factors and the position of the acetabular component on the rate of dislocation after total hip replacement. *J Bone Joint Surg Am* 1997;79:1202-1210.
25. Pierchon F, Pasquier G, Cotten A, Fontaine C, Clarisse J, Duquennoy A: Causes of dislocation of total hip arthroplasty: CT study of component alignment. *J Bone Joint Surg Br* 1994;76:45-48.
26. Berry, DJ: Dislocation, in Steinberg ME, Garino JP (eds): *Revision Total Hip Arthroplasty*. Philadelphia, PA, Lippincott-Williams & Wilkins, 1999, pp 463-481.
27. Lindberg HO, Carlsson AS, Gentz C-F, Pettersson H: Recurrent and non-recurrent dislocation following total hip arthroplasty. *Acta Orthop Scand* 1982;53:947-952.
28. Williams JF, Gottesman MJ, Mallory TH: Dislocation after total hip arthroplasty: Treatment with an above-knee hip spica cast. *Clin Orthop* 1982;171:53-58.
29. Joshi A, Lee CM, Markovic L, Vlatis G, Murphy JC: Prognosis of dislocation after total hip arthroplasty. *J Arthroplasty* 1998;13:17-21.
30. Browne AO, Sheehan JM: Trochanteric osteotomy in Charnley low-friction arthroplasty of the hip. *Clin Orthop* 1986;211:128-133.
31. Horwitz BR, Rockowitz NL, Goll SR, et al: A prospective randomized comparison of two surgical approaches to total hip arthroplasty. *Clin Orthop* 1993;291:154-163.
32. McCollum DE, Gray WJ: Dislocation after total hip arthroplasty: Causes and prevention. *Clin Orthop* 1990;261:159-170.
33. Roberts JM, Fu FH, McClain EJ, Ferguson AB Jr: A comparison of the posterolateral and anterolateral approaches to total hip arthroplasty. *Clin Orthop* 1984;187:205-210.
34. Unwin AJ, Thomas M: Dislocation after hemiarthroplasty of the hip: A comparison of the dislocation rate after posterior and lateral approaches to the hip. *Ann R Coll Surg Engl* 1994;76:327-329.
35. Vicar AJ, Coleman CR: A comparison of the anterolateral, transtrochanteric, and posterior surgical approaches in primary total hip arthroplasty. *Clin Orthop* 1984;188:152-159.
36. Pellicci PM, Bostrom M, Poss R: Posterior approach to total hip replacement using enhanced posterior soft tissue repair. *Clin Orthop* 1998;355:224-228.
37. Carlsson AS, Gentz CF: Postoperative dislocation in the Charnley and Brunswik total hip arthroplasty. *Clin Orthop* 1977;125:177-182.
38. Dorr LD, Wolf AW, Chandler R, Conaty JP: Classification and treatment of dislocations of total hip arthroplasty. *Clin Orthop* 1983; 173:151-158.
39. Lewinnek GE, Lewis JL, Tarr R, Compere CL, Zimmerman JR: Dislocations after total hip-replacement arthroplasties. *J Bone Joint Surg Am* 1978;60:217-220.
40. Barnes CL, Berry DJ, Sledge CB: Dislocation after bipolar hemiarthroplasty of the hip. *J Arthroplasty* 1995;10:667-669.

41. Brien WW, Salvati EA, Wright TM, Burstein AH: Dislocation following THA: Comparison of two acetabular component designs. *Orthopedics* 1993;16:869-872.

42. Scifert CF, Brown TD, Pedersen DR, Callaghan JJ: A finite element analysis of factors influencing total hip dislocation. *Clin Orthop* 1998;355:152-162.

43. Kelley SS, Lachiewicz PF, Hickman JM, Paterno SM: Relationship of femoral head and acetabular size to the prevalence of dislocation. *Clin Orthop* 1998;355:163-170.

44. Hedlundh U, Ahnfelt L, Hybbinette CH, Wallinder L, Weckstrom J, Fredin H: Dislocations and the femoral head size in primary total hip arthroplasty. *Clin Orthop* 1996;333:226-233.

45. Krushell RJ, Burke DW, Harris WH: Elevated-rim acetabular components: Effect on range of motion and stability in total hip arthroplasty. *J Arthroplasty* 1991;6:S53-S58.

46. Graham GP, Jenkins AI, Mintowt-Czyz W: Recurrent dislocation following hip replacement: Brief report. *J Bone Joint Surg Br* 1988;70:675.

47. Cobb TK, Morrey BF, Ilstrup DM: The elevated-rim acetabular liner in total hip arthroplasty: Relationship to postoperative dislocation. *J Bone Joint Surg Am* 1996;78:80-86.

48. Star MJ, Colwell CW Jr, Donaldson WF III, Walker RH: Dissociation of modular hip arthroplasty components after dislocation: A report of three cases at differing dissociation levels. *Clin Orthop* 1992;278:111-115.

49. Dorr LD, Wan Z: Causes of and treatment protocol for instability of total hip replacement. *Clin Orthop* 1998;355:144-151.

50. Clayton ML, Thirupathi RG: Dislocation following total hip arthroplasty: Management by special brace in selected patients. *Clin Orthop* 1983;177:154-159.

51. Stewart HD: The hip cast-brace for hip prosthesis instability. *Ann R Coll Surg Engl* 1983;65:404-406.

52. Daly PJ, Morrey BF: Operative correction of an unstable total hip arthroplasty. *J Bone Joint Surg Am* 1992;74:1334-1343.

53. Fraser GA, Wroblewski BM: Revision of the Charnley low-friction arthroplasty for recurrent or irreducible dislocation. *J Bone Joint Surg Br* 1981;63:552-555.

54. Ackland MK, Bourne WB, Uhthoff HK: Anteversion of the acetabular cup: Measurement of angle after total hip replacement. *J Bone Joint Surg Br* 1986;68:409-413.

55. Magilligan DJ: Calculation of the angle of anteversion by means of horizontal lateral roentgenography. *J Bone Joint Surg Am* 1956;38:1231-1246.

56. Bradbury N, Milligan GF: Acetabular augmentation for dislocation of the prosthetic hip: A 3 (1-6)-year follow-up of 16 patients. *Acta Orthop Scand* 1994;65:424-426.

57. Mogensen B, Árnason H, Jónsson GT: Socket wall addition for dislocating total hip: Report of two cases. *Acta Orthop Scand* 1986;57:373-374.

58. Olerud S, Karlström G: Recurrent dislocation after total hip replacement: Treatment by fixing an additional sector to the acetabular component. *J Bone Joint Surg Br* 1985;67:402-405.

59. Watson P, Nixon JR, Mollan RA: A prosthesis augmentation device for the prevention of recurrent hip dislocation: A preliminary report. *Clin Orthop* 1991;267:79-84.

60. Fehring TK, Griffin WL, Mason JB, McCoy TH, Earll MD: Abstract: Failure of bloodless revision of the unstable total hip. *67th Annual Meeting Proceedings.* Rosemont, IL, American Academy of Orthopaedic Surgeons, 2000, p 151.

61. Ekelund A: Trochanteric osteotomy for recurrent dislocation of total hip arthroplasty. *J Arthroplasty* 1993;8:629-632.

62. Kaplan SJ, Thomas WH, Poss R: Trochanteric advancement for recurrent dislocation after total hip arthroplasty. *J Arthroplasty* 1987; 2:119-124.

63. Weber M, Berry DJ: Abductor avulsion after primary total hip arthroplasty: Results of repair. *J Arthroplasty* 1997;12:202-206.

64. Ries MD, Wiedel JD: Bipolar hip arthroplasty for recurrent dislocation after total hip arthroplasty: A report of three cases. *Clin Orthop* 1992;278:121-127.

65. Zelicof SB, Scott RD: Abstract: Conversion to bipolar arthroplasty for the treatment of recurrent total hip dislocations: A two- to- seven-year follow-up study. *59th Annual Meeting Proceedings*. Rosemont, IL, American Academy of Orthopaedic Surgeons, 1992, p 69.

66. Parvizi J, Morrey BF: Abstract: Bipolar hip arthroplasty as a salvage for intractable recurrent instability of the hip. *67th Annual Meeting Proceedings*. Rosemont, IL, American Academy of Orthopaedic Surgeons, 2000, p 315.

67. Grigoris P, Grecula MJ, Amstutz HC: Tripolar hip replacement for recurrent prosthetic dislocation. *Clin Orthop* 1994;304:148-155.

68. Fisher DA, Kiley K: Constrained acetabular cup disassembly. *J Arthroplasty* 1994;9:325-329.

69. Anderson MJ, Murray WR, Skinner HB: Constrained acetabular components. *J Arthroplasty* 1994;9:17-23.

70. Lombardi AV Jr, Mallory TH, Kraus TJ, Vaughn BK: Preliminary report on the S-ROM™ constraining acetabular insert: A retrospective clinical experience. *Orthopedics* 1991;14:297-303.

71. Goetz DD, Capello WN, Callaghan JJ, Brown TD, Johnston RC: Salvage of total hip instability with a constrained acetabular component. *Clin Orthop* 1998;355:171-181.

28

The Effect of Component Design on Range of Motion to Impingement in Total Hip Arthroplasty

Robert L. Barrack, MD
Robert L. Thornberry, MD
Michael D. Ries, MD
Carlos Lavernia, MD
Evangelos Tozakoglou, PhD

Introduction

Measurement of range of motion (ROM) is a part of the standard evaluation of the results of hip replacement.[1] Patients' responses to questions regarding function have been found to correlate closely with measured ROM of the hip.[2] A number of factors determine the ROM that is achieved following hip replacement. The interaction of component position and component geometry are two factors under the surgeon's control that determine the arc of motion that occurs prior to impingement.[3]

In the 1980s, with the widespread use of cementless components, the modular design was used for most femoral and acetabular components. This led to a proliferation of femoral head and acetabular liner designs. The effect of these various design features on the arc of motion to impingement has not been carefully examined. At extremes of motion the prosthetic femoral neck can impinge on the polyethylene liner. If the prosthetic femoral neck impinges on the liner within the physiologic arc of motion, a number of deleterious effects can occur. Motion and therefore function may be limited.

One or more of the authors or the departments with which they are affiliated have received something of value from a commercial or other party related directly or indirectly to the subject of this chapter.

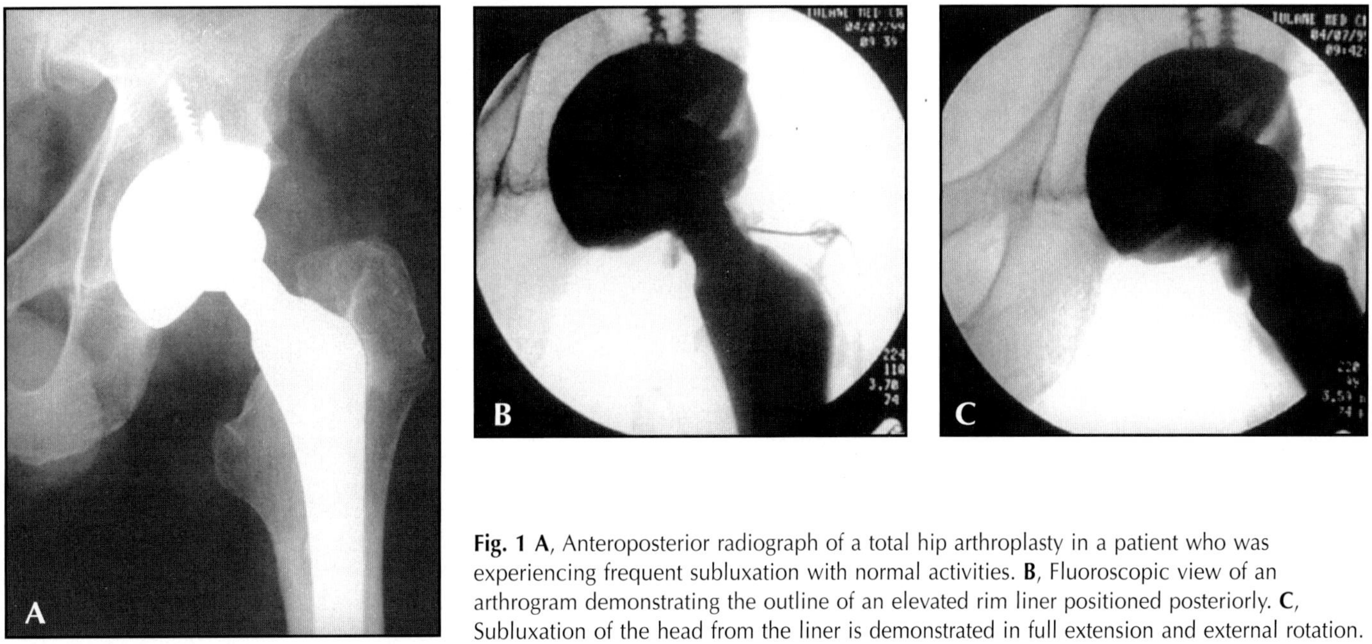

Fig. 1 A, Anteroposterior radiograph of a total hip arthroplasty in a patient who was experiencing frequent subluxation with normal activities. **B**, Fluoroscopic view of an arthrogram demonstrating the outline of an elevated rim liner positioned posteriorly. **C**, Subluxation of the head from the liner is demonstrated in full extension and external rotation.

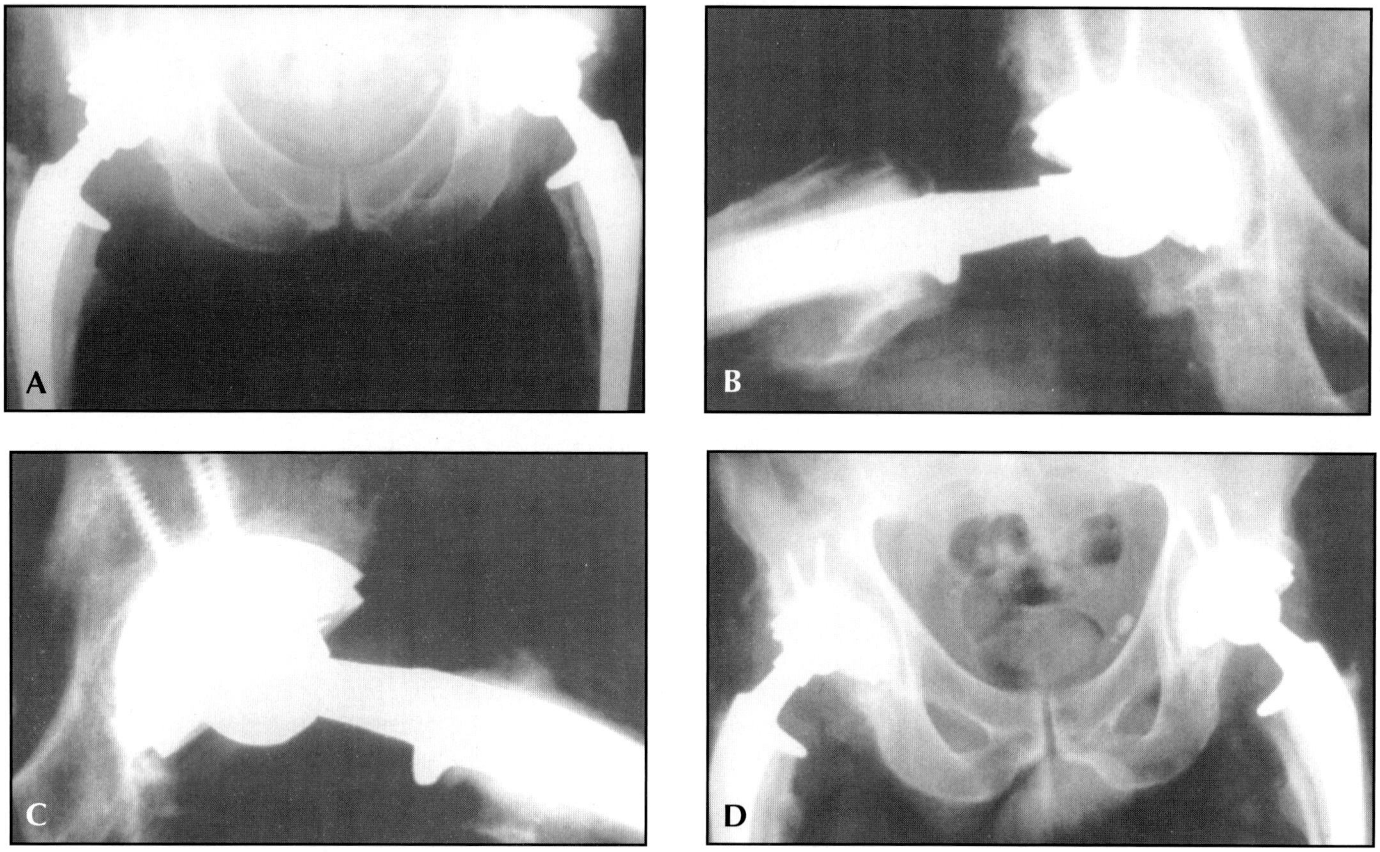

Fig. 2 A, Anteroposterior radiograph of a patient who has had bilateral total hip replacements with a skirted modular head on the right and a nonskirted head on the left. **B**, Frog lateral view of the right hip demonstrating close proximity and possible contact of the skirt with the polyethylene liner. **C**, The same view of the nonskirted head shows clearance between the neck and the liner. **D**, The side with the skirted head subsequently had dislodgement of the liner from the shell, requiring a revision procedure.

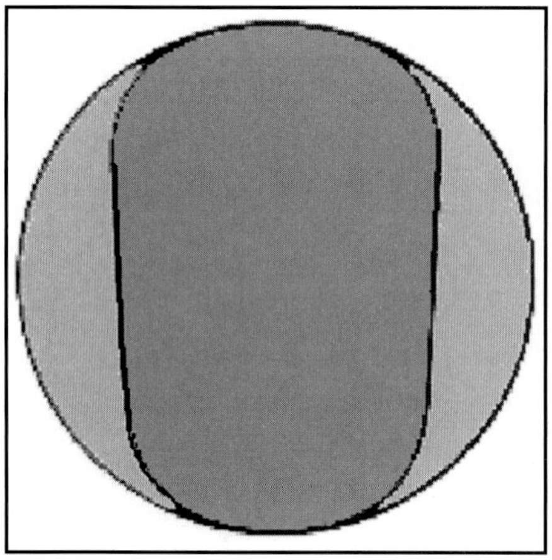

Fig. 3 Cross-section schematic comparing a trapezoidal neck cross section with a circular neck cross section.

Excessive polyethylene wear might result from repeated impingement of the neck on the liner. The increased wear could lead to osteolysis. Metal debris could be abraded from the femoral neck from the repeated impact, which could also accelerate polyethylene wear by a third body mechanism. The femoral neck could lever on the liner, leading to subluxation or dislocation (Fig. 1). The eccentric load on the rim of the liner could contribute to acetabular loosening or alternatively to dislodgement of the modular liner (Fig. 2). Given the numerous potential negative effects of component impingement, a study was undertaken to quantify the arc of motion to impingement obtained with various designs of modular femoral head and acetabular liners.

Materials and Methods

ROM to impingement was studied with a virtual reality hip simulator, which records the maximum motion of the hip joint in any direction until impingement occurs between the femoral and acetabular components. Different femoral neck geometries and acetabular component liner types were studied to determine the effect of variations in implant geometry and design on ROM to impingement in total hip arthroplasty. The femoral components tested included a circular and noncircular neck geometry (Fig. 3). The acetabular components tested included two different elevated lip liner geometries (Fig. 4). The implant geometries tested were chosen to represent features of currently used total hip components. Each femoral and acetabular component was digitized using a Microscribe 3DX digitizer (Comsoft, Inc, San Jose, CA) and Verisketch for Lightwave 3D software (Newtek Inc, San

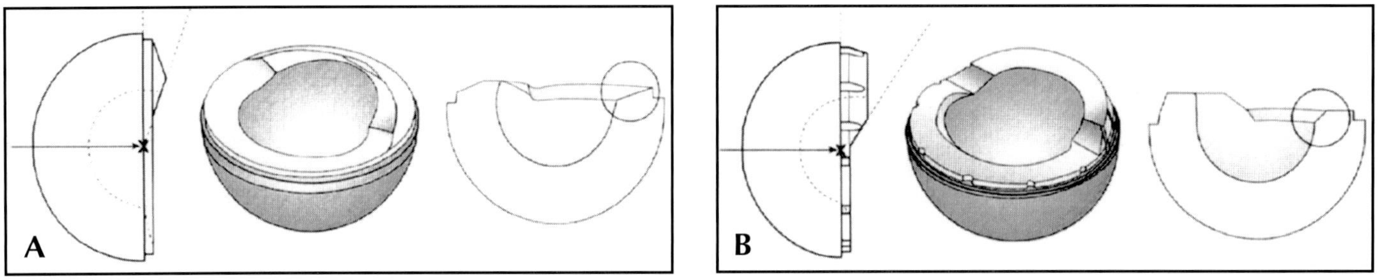

Fig. 4 Schematic of liner types. **A,** Liner type with a relatively low angle, wide chamfer zone. **B,** Liner type with a higher angle, more narrow chamfer zone.

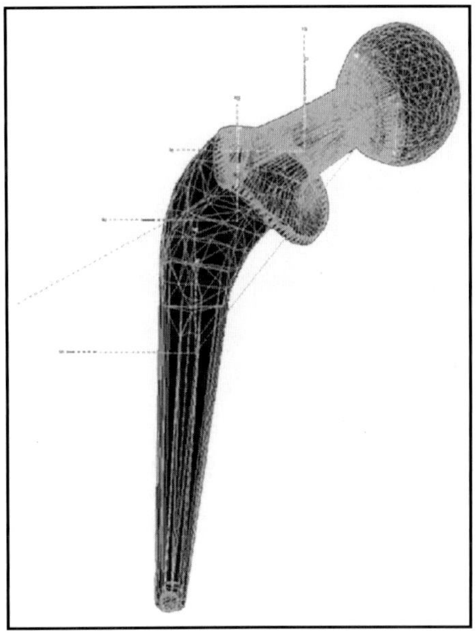

Fig. 5 Computer-generated model that resulted from digitizing one of the components tested.

Antonio, TX) to a stated accuracy of 0.23 mm.[4] During the digitization process, each component was held in a vice while the tip of the digitizer traced its geometry. When a point on the surface of the component was digitized, its coordinate was entered into the program's database. The software was used to create surfaces from the digitized points. The accuracy of replication of the three-dimensional implant shape depended on the number of points selected on the surface of the implant. In our model, the average number of selected points per component was 750. From these points an average of 1,200 triangles were generated to represent the surface of the component (Fig. 5).

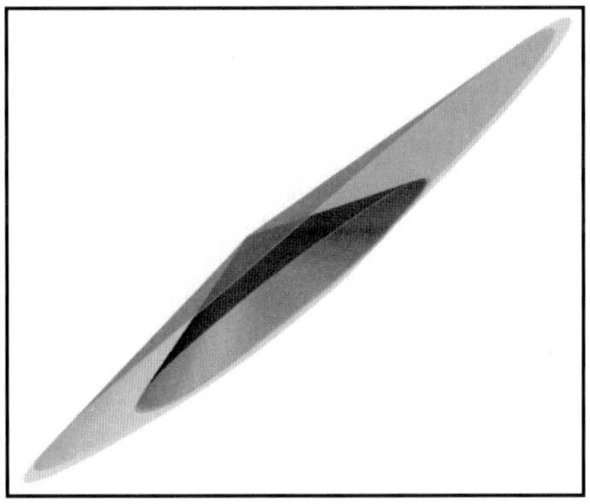

Fig. 6 Cone of motion obtained from the computer animation of two different component combinations.

The digitized components were then entered in Lightwave 3D virtual reality software. Using the software, the components could be placed within a digitized skeleton at any orientation. The femoral component was then animated while the acetabular component remained fixed to simulate motion of the hip until impingement occurred between the neck of the component and the liner. The animation software was used to simulate ROM in six directions (flexion, extension, abduction, adduction, internal rotation, and external rotation) representing motion in the sagittal (flexion-extension), coronal (abduction-adduction), and transverse (internal-external rotation) planes. Selected measurements were compared with a benchtop model and they were found to be accurate within 5°.[5] The maximum motion to impingement in each direction was combined with the maximum motion to impingement in the other two planes to create an overall arc of motion. The arc of motion, represented by a cone, illustrates the maximum ROM to impingement for the combined directions of motion (Fig. 6). An example of an animation comparing two component types is demonstrated. **(CD-28.1)**

The acetabular components were positioned at 45° of abduction and 20° of anteversion. The stems were positioned at 15° of anteversion and neutral varus-valgus alignment. The center of elevation for the elevated hip liners was midway between the posterior and superior quadrants.

Testing was then repeated by mixing the different neck and acetabular geometries to determine the relative influence of implant design features on ROM to impingement. The effect of femoral head size on ROM to impingement was also assessed by comparing 28- and 32-mm diameter femoral heads.

Two types of acetabular liners were modeled and tested. Both were elevated rim liners. In one there was a low angle and relatively high distance between the inner and outer edge of the liner (a so-called wide chamfer), while in the other there was a steeper angle and shorter distance (a narrow chamfer) (Fig. 4). Femoral neck designs included both a circular and a trapezoidal neck. Modular heads with and without skirts were compared. Finally, the effect of changing from

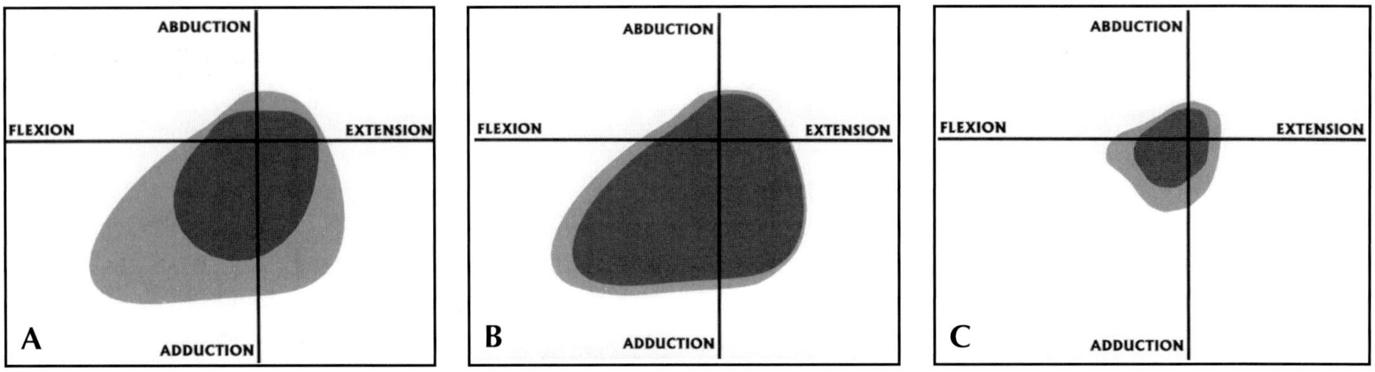

Fig. 7 The cone of motion is demonstrated graphically for two different component combinations. **A,** The combination of a circular neck with a narrow angle chamfer zone liner results in markedly less motion to impingement (dark shading) compared to a trapezoidal neck with a wide chamfer zone liner (lighter shading). **B,** Changing from a 28-mm head (dark shading) to a 32-mm head (lighter shading) resulted in a 7° increase in flexion prior to impingement. **C,** A large circular taper had a dramatically decreased ROM to impingement (lighter shading) that was even further diminished by having a skirted modular head (darker shading)

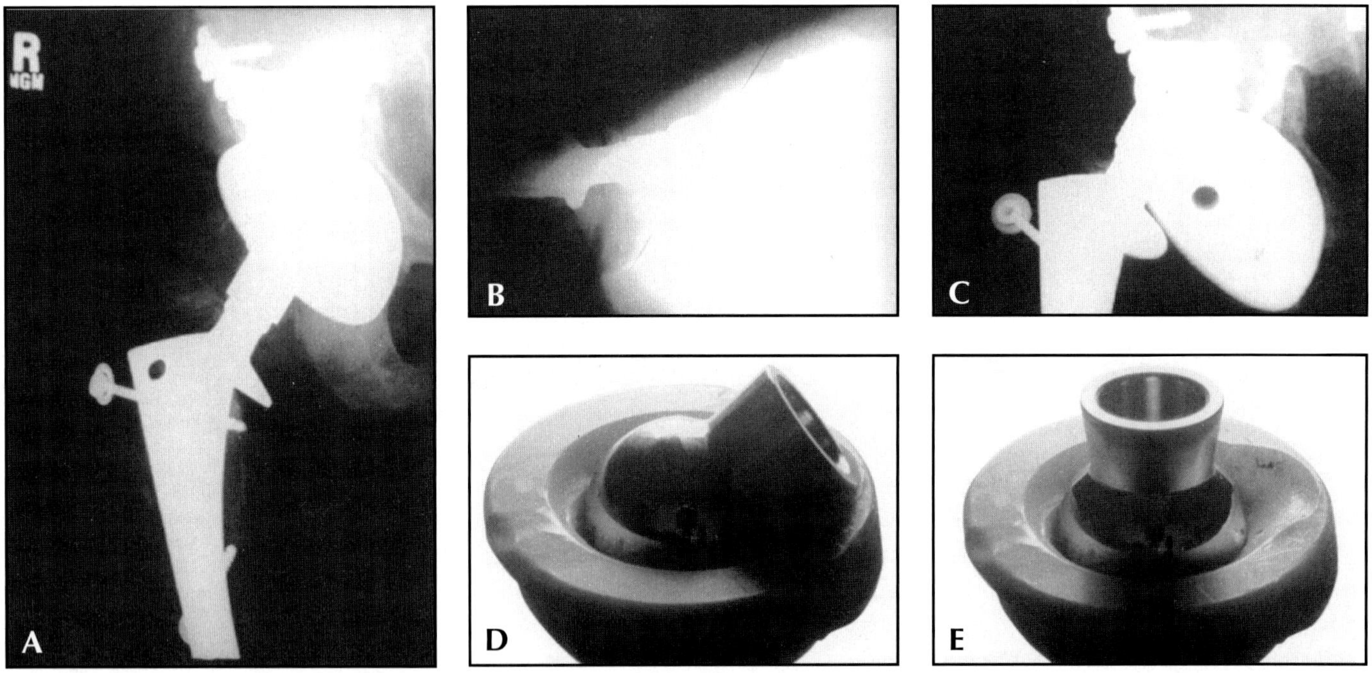

Fig. 8 Postoperative radiographs of a patient who underwent a THA following traumatic arthritis. Anteroposterior (**A**) and lateral (**B**) views show components in acceptable position. However, the patient was experiencing recurrent anterior dislocations (**C**). The components retrieved at surgery indicated that the skirted head was impinging on the elevated rim liner posteriorly (**D**), leading to dislocation as well as excessive polyethylene wear (**E**).

a 28- to a 32-mm head was quantified with all other parameters held constant.

Results

The maximal arc of motion was achieved with the combination of a trapezoidal neck with a wide chamfer elevated rim liner. Combining a circular neck with a narrow chamfer liner results in a markedly reduced arc of motion. The difference between the combination of a trapezoidal neck cross section and a wide chamfer angle liner to the combination of a circular neck and a narrow chamfer angle is dramatic (Fig. 7, *A*). When the area of the cone of motion was quantified, the difference was more than twofold. Changing from a 28- to a 32-mm head increased flexion to impingement by 7° (Fig. 7, *B*). The least motion to impingement was observed with a large (14/16) circular neck. This was further diminished with the addition of a skirted head (Fig. 7, *C*).

Discussion

The results of the present study indicate that design details have a dramatic effect on the ROM that can be achieved before the femoral head component and acetabular liner make contact and impede further motion. The effects are additive and if a number of suboptimal features are combined, component impingement within the normal physiologic range for daily activities can be anticipated.[6] There are a number of options available for design features of modular femoral heads and acetabular liners and certain choices are clearly preferable to others in terms of maximizing motion. On the acetabular side, an elevated rim liner with a low angle and wide chamfer zone outperformed the high angle, narrow chamfer zone option. The latter design could possibly have some advantage when a metal shell is placed in a suboptimal position. In the position modeled in this study, however, this design did not do well. On the femoral side, the optimal combination was a trapezoidal cross-sectional geometry without a skirt and a 32-mm head. The advantage of such a large head, however, must be balanced against the thinner polyethylene and increased volumetric wear that accompanies its use. In the revision situation, however, large shell sizes are often used and polyethylene thickness is therefore not an issue. A lower activity level is also probable and stability is often a concern. In such a scenario, increasing head size to 32 mm can be expected to give between 6° of additional flexion before component impingement occurs.

The effect of component design has previously been evaluated with cadaver models and protractors or goniometers.[7,8] Skirted heads and elevated rim liners were predicted to restrict motion.[7,8] Cobb and associates,[9] however, showed a lower incidence of dislocation with an elevated rim liner. That was one specific design, however; the present study shows that there are substantial differences between designs, and conclusions from results from one liner type therefore should not be generalized to all elevated rim liner designs. In addition, dislocation is only one of several potential consequences of component impingement. There is at least one study that indicates that increased polyethylene wear and osteolysis is a more common result. Urquhart and associates[10] reported the presence of a skirted femoral head was the single factor that had the greatest correlation with a higher polyethylene wear rate. Skirts were also associated with a higher incidence of osteolysis. Dislocation was not mentioned as being associated with the presence of a skirt, although skirted necks can clearly contribute to both increased wear as well as instability (Fig. 8).

Another retrieval study pointed to the potential importance of component impingement following total hip arthroplasty. Yamaguchi and associates[11] examined 104 retrieved acetabular components and found peripheral indentations in 41 (39%) consistent with the occurrence of chronic impingement. Those components that displayed evidence of impingement were more likely to have a higher degree of wear as well as an abnormal pattern of wear defined by multiple wear vectors, implying that the impingement was altering the normal wear path of the femoral head against the liner. These liners were of the high angle, narrow chamfer zone variety that demonstrated less arc of motion to impingement in the present study. The abnormal wear pattern was more common with smaller heads (26 mm), emphasizing the additive nature of femoral and acetabular design features.

The current study does have some notable limitations. There are numerous causes of instability, such as soft-tissue laxity and muscle weakness, that are not considered in this model. There are also other types of impingement that are not accounted for such as impingement of the trochanter on the pelvis or impingement of the femoral neck on peripheral osteophytes or soft tissue. In addition, the components were ideally positioned in these computer animations and the findings are therefore specific for components that are in the orientation described in this study.

It seems clear, however, that the details of component design can have a profound potential effect on the arc of motion prior to impingement. Component impingement within the expected arc of motion of normal activities clearly can lead to a number of complications and should be avoided if possible. Many of these designs emerged when there was a rapid transition to modular components and the potential negative effects were probably not appreciated or anticipated. Currently, there is more widespread understanding of the importance of these design details. Many orthopaedic manufacturers have recently changed the designs of their femoral necks, modular heads, and modular liners. Surgeons should be aware of these design issues because many new modular heads will not be compatible with previous femoral stem trunions. A similar situation will exist with modular acetabular liners. Awareness of these design details allows for careful intraoperative attention to the interaction of these design parameters as well as the assessment of this aspect of components that are being considered for clinical use.

References

1. Harris WH: Traumatic arthritis of the hip after dislocation and acetabular fractures: Treatment by mold arthroplasty. An end-result study using a new method of result evaluation. *J Bone Joint Surg Am* 1969;51:737-755.
2. McGrory BJ, Freiberg AA, Shinar AA, Harris WH: Correlation of measured range of hip motion following total hip arthroplasty and responses to a questionnaire. *J Arthroplasty* 1996;11:565-571.
3. Chandler DR, Glousman R, Hull D, et al: Prosthetic hip range of motion and impingement: The effects of head and neck geometry. *Clin Orthop* 1982;166:284-291.

4. *Microscribe 3DX User Manual.* San Jose, California, Immersion Corporation.

5. Kummer FJ, Shah S, Iyer, S, DiCesare PE: The effect of acetabular cup orientations on limiting hip rotation. *J Arthroplasty* 1999;14:509-513.

6. Johnston RC, Smidt GL: Hip motion measurements for selected activities of daily living. *Clin Orthop* 1970;72:205-215.

7. Gondi G, Roberson JR, Ganey TM, Shahriari A, Hutton WC: Impingement after total hip arthroplasty related to prosthetic component selection and range of motion. *J South Orthop Assoc* 1997;6:266-272.

8. Krushell RJ, Burke DW, Harris WH: Range of motion in contemporary total hip arthroplasty: The impact of modular head-neck components. *J Arthroplasty* 1991;6:97-101.

9. Cobb TK, Morrey BF, Ilstrup DM: The elevated-rim acetabular liner in total hip arthroplasty: Relationship to postoperative dislocation. *J Bone Joint Surg Am* 1996;78:80-86.

10. Urquhart AG, D'Lima DD, Venn-Watson E, Colwell CW Jr, Walker RH: Polyethylene wear after total hip arthroplasty: The effect of a modular femoral head with an extended flange-reinforced neck. *J Bone Joint Surg Am* 1998;80:1641-1647.

11. Yamaguchi M, Bauer TW, Hashimoto Y: Three-dimensional analysis of multiple wear vectors in retrieved acetabular cups. *J Bone Joint Surg Am* 1997;79:1539-1544.

Reference to Video

Barrack R: *Range of Motion (Hip).* New Orleans, LA, 2000.

29

The Use of a Constrained Acetabular Component for Recurrent Dislocation

Gary S. Shapiro, MD
Daniel Weiland, MD
Thomas P. Sculco, MD
Douglas E. Padgett, MD
Paul M. Pellicci, MD

Introduction

Dislocation is a recognized complication following total hip arthroplasty (THA). Conservative management of a first-time dislocation is usually successful with an orthosis or cast, in conjunction with patient education.[1] If an etiology is identified and dislocation does not become chronic, surgical correction is frequently successful. Recurrent dislocations, which are frustrating to both the patient and the surgeon, may occur despite diligent conservative and surgical effort. Repeat dislocation occurs in as many as 33% of patients[2] (Fig. 1).

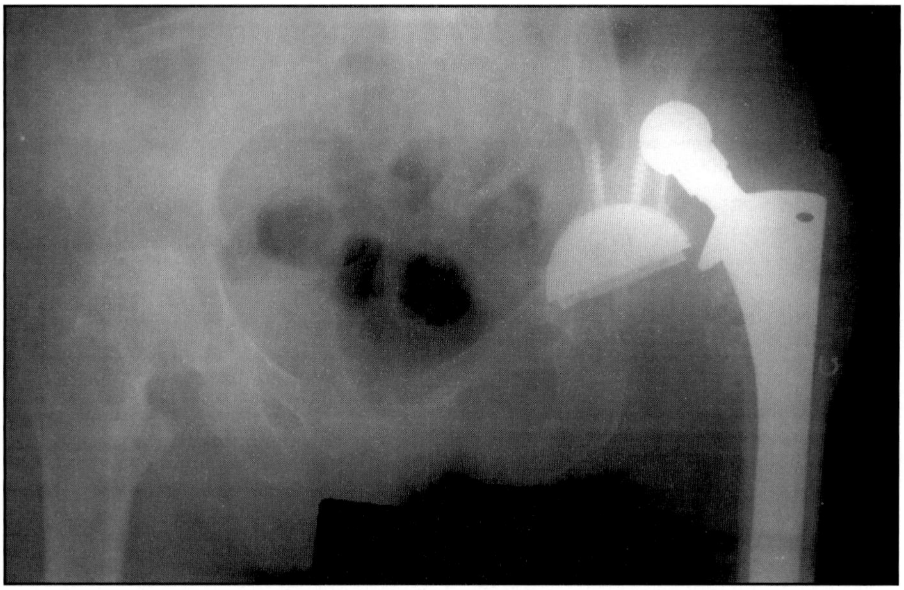

Fig. 1 Anteroposterior radiograph showing a dislocated left THA.

Surgical Options

Procedures described to treat instability include reorientation of the femoral or acetabular position, trochanteric reattachment or advancement, capsulorrhaphy, use of an elevated acetabular liner, conversion to a bipolar prosthesis, lengthening of the femoral neck, and resection arthroplasty. The use of a constrained acetabular cup system has been reported in the literature with favorable results.[3-5]

Preoperative Workup

Patients should be evaluated for potential causes of instability, which include excessive tissue laxity, component malposition, poor motor control, dementia, and muscle deficiency. If a cause can be identified, it should be corrected without the use of constraints. Once the decision to proceed is made, several preoperative measures must be checked.

True anteroposterior pelvis and lateral radiographic views of the affected hip should be obtained, as well as the operative report from any previous surgery to help the surgeon plan the surgery. The surgeon must know the size, model, and manufacturer of the existing shell. Additionally, the femoral component should be checked for compatibility of head size and taper of the neck. Both the femoral and acetabular components should be assessed for stability, and the surgeon must be prepared to exchange loose components at the time of surgery. The Omnifit constrained liner (Osteonics, Allendale, NJ) is not compatible with other acetabular components; therefore, the issue of how to proceed with well-fixed acetabular shells from other

Table 1
Breakdown of noncemented and cemented components in 85 hips

Noncemented (53)	
New Osteonics press-fit cup with new liner (group 1)	49
Exchange to constrained liner with previous Osteonics shell (group 2)	4
Cemented (32)	
Constrained liner cemented into a well-fixed press-fit cup from a different manufacturer (group 3)	16
Constrained liner cemented directly into the acetabulum (group 4)	8
Osteonics cup cemented into the acetabulum with a constrained liner snapped into place (group 5)	8

manufacturers will arise. The surgeon must be prepared to remove components while using bone conservation techniques. In the presence of poor bone stock, the surgeon may have to cement the liner into an existing shell.

Authors' Experience

We reviewed 87 constrained total hip replacements for treatment of recurrent dislocation in 84 patients (GS Shapiro MD, et al, New York, NY, unpublished data, 2000). Of these, 85 hips had adequate follow-up. The patients' average age was 75 years, and the average follow-up period was 58 months. Most patients had undergone at least one revision. The indication for constraint was instability without an identifiable etiology, with or without gross abductor insufficiency. All patients had been managed previously with an abduction brace. Despite conservative treatment, patients had an average of four dislocations. Table 1 shows the breakdown of noncemented and cemented components in these patients.

The primary goal of treatment was to place the cup without cement, unless there was significant bone loss or a poor biologic environment. All patients with noncemented fixation in this series received supplemental fixation with two 6.5-mm cancellous screws. The liners cemented into existing shells were scored with a high-speed burr to roughen the surface for cement fixation. All femoral components were cemented.

The posterolateral approach was used with all patients under hypotensive epidural anesthesia. The capsule and short external rotators were reapproximated to their anatomic positions. The patients were divided into the following five groups for analysis (Fig. 2): (1) new (Osteonics) press-fit cup with a new liner; (2) exchange to constrained liner with previous Osteonics shell; (3) constrained liner cemented into a well-fixed press-fit cup from a different manufacturer; (4) constrained liner cemented directly into the acetabulum; and (5) Osteonics cup cemented into the acetabulum with a constrained liner snapped into place.

Noncemented acetabular components were evaluated for loosening. Fixation by bone ingrowth was defined as no migration and no formation of a circumferential radiolucent line; stable fibrous ingrowth as formation of a circumferential radiolucent line; and unstable fibrous ingrowth as definite migration or progression in the width of a previously noted circumferential radiolucent line.

Cemented acetabular components were assessed by observing the quality of the cement-bone interface in each of the three zones defined by DeLee and Charnley.[6] Definite loosening was defined as migration of the component or the presence of any new fracture in the cement mantle; probable loosening as the presence of a circumferential radiolucent line around the entire component at the bone-cement interface; and possible loosening as the presence of a radiolucent line around 50% to 99% of the component at the bone-cement interface.

Zones described by Gruen and associates[7] were evaluated for osteolysis. Subsidence was measured using the method of Loudon and Charnley.[8] Loosening of cemented femoral components was classified according to criteria set by Harris and associates.[9] Definite loosening was defined as subsidence of the femoral component, fracture of the cement or stem, or the presence of a radiolucent line not seen on early postoperative radiographs at the interface between the stem of the prosthesis and the cement. Probable loosening was defined as the presence of a continuous radiolucent line along the entire bone-cement interface. Possible loosening was defined as the presence of a radiolucent line that encompassed more than 50% but less than 100% the circumference of the stem at the bone-cement interface on at least one radiograph.

Clinical Results

Clinical and radiologic evaluation was performed on 82 patients (85 hips) at a minimum of 3 years' follow-up. Two patients who were lost to follow-up had died; however, no instability had been noted prior to death. The charts of 12 patients who had died after being followed for a minimum of 3 years (range, 3 to 8 years) were reviewed for the most recent examination, and family members were contacted to determine the function of the hip immediately before death. Of the 82 patients, 51 used no assistive device, 10 used a walker, and 21 used a cane for ambulation. At the time of the latest follow-up, there was no pain in 52 hips, mild pain in 22, moderate pain in 8, and severe pain in 3. A trochanteric nonunion from previous operations caused discomfort in 10 patients.

Femoral Components All 36 femoral components inserted at the time of conversion to a constrained system were stable at the time of the latest radiographic follow-up, with no significant osteolysis

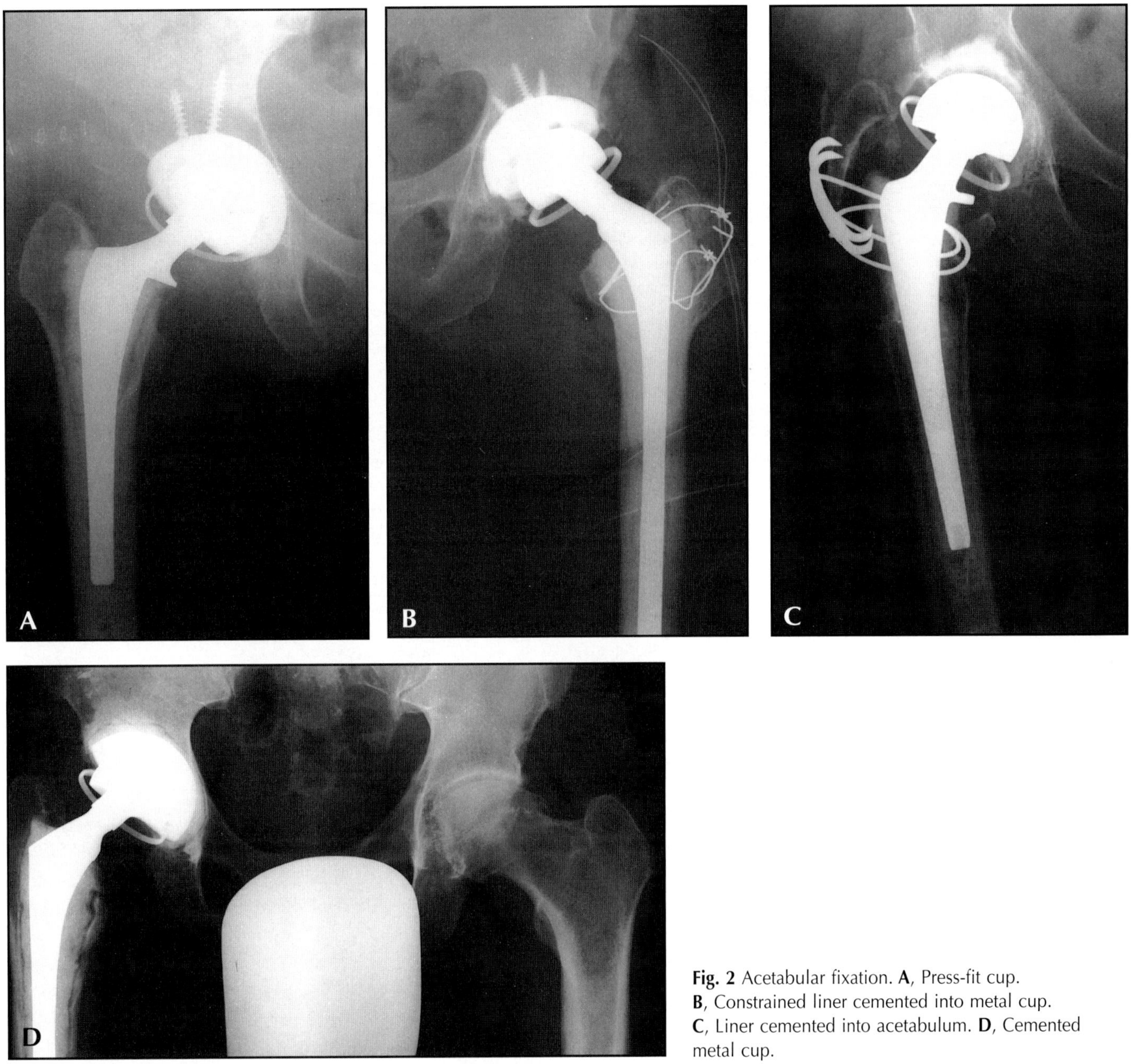

Fig. 2 Acetabular fixation. **A**, Press-fit cup. **B**, Constrained liner cemented into metal cup. **C**, Liner cemented into acetabulum. **D**, Cemented metal cup.

or progression of radiolucent lines around the femoral components. The type of fixation of the acetabular component made no difference in femoral component wear.

One of the 49 existing cemented femoral components required revision concomitantly with an acetabular shell after 19 months. The patient had massive bone loss surrounding both components at the time of the index procedure, and, although the femoral component was not grossly loose, fixation was suspect. Of the remaining 48 femoral components, 45 were stable, 2 were possibly loose, and 1 was definitely loose at the time of the latest follow-up. There was no significant osteolysis or progression of radiolucent lines around the femoral components.

Acetabular Components No acetabular osteolysis was noted regardless of the implant technique. The progression of radiolucent lines was less than 1 mm, with the exception of cemented metal cups. Progression of radiolucent lines with cemented cups was 1.5 mm at an average of 53 months.

Of the 49 hips in group 1 (Table 1), two acetabular components were revised. One had aseptic loosening of the shell (at 41 months), which was revised with a

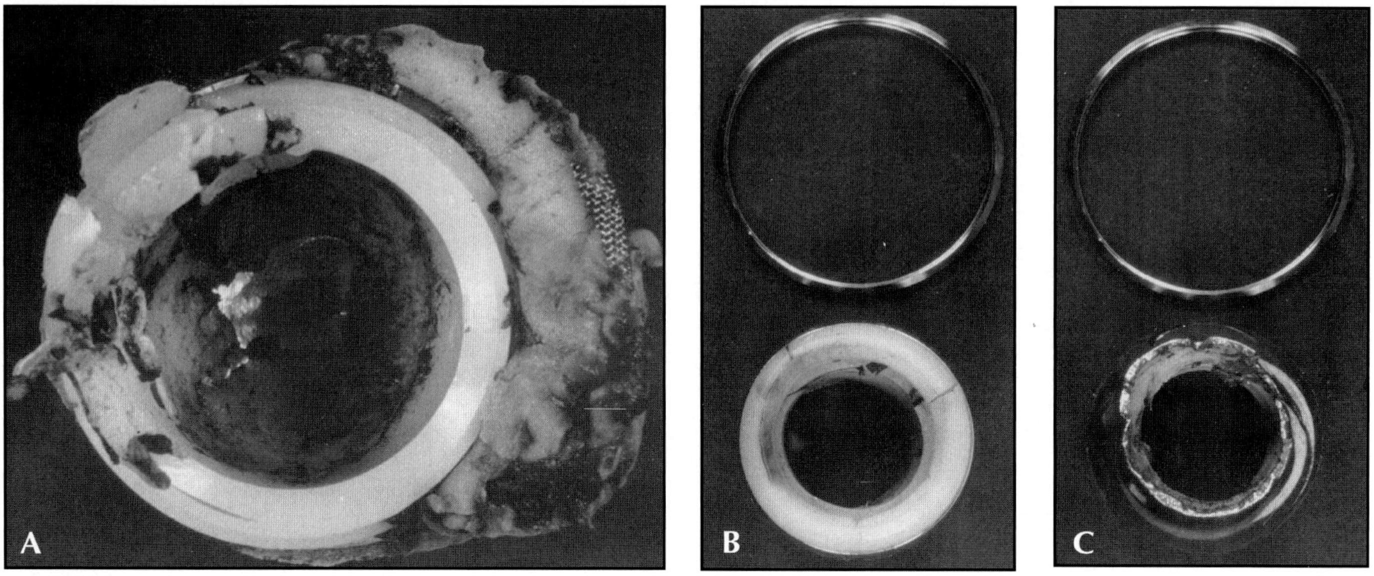

Fig. 3 A through **C**, Clinical photographs showing a failed implant.

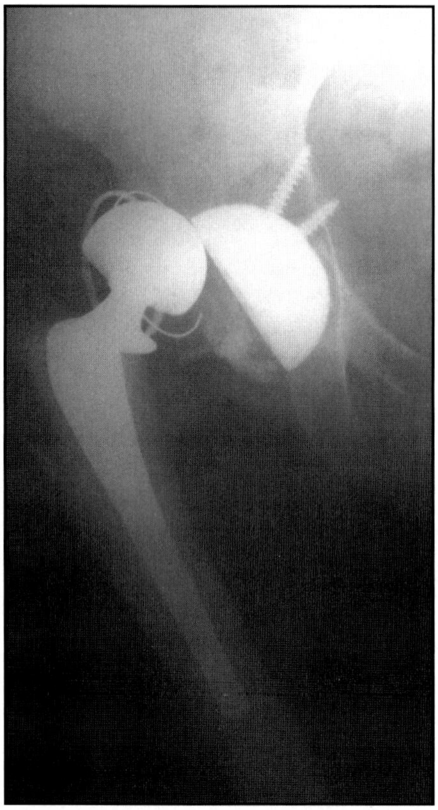

Fig. 4 Dissociation of liner that had been cemented into cup.

press-fit shell. Excessive wear of the polyethylene was seen in one liner at 50 months and was revised on an elective basis (Fig. 3). The 4 hips in group 2 were fixed by bone ingrowth at the latest follow-up. In group 3, two of 16 hips failed (at 20 and 29 months) by dissociation of the liner (Fig. 4). Both hips were revised to a press-fit shell with a constrained liner snapped in place. All components were fixed by bone ingrowth at the latest follow-up. All eight hips in group 4 were stable at the time of the latest follow-up. In group 5, two of the eight metal-backed cups cemented into the acetabulum had to be revised as a result of aseptic loosening (at 19 and 39 months). At the time of the latest follow-up, 11 components had no evidence of loosening, 3 had possible loosening, and 2 had probable loosening.

Complications

A dislocation secondary to dissociation of the liner from the shell occurred in two hips. Revision of three acetabular components and one femoral component was necessary because of aseptic loosening. Revision because of excessive wear of the constrained liner was necessary in one acetabular component. Overall, two dislocations occurred in 85 hips (2.4%), seven components were revised (8.2%), and one deep infection was treated with suppression (1.1%).

Discussion

The incidence of hip dislocation following THA ranges from 0.5% to 10% in primary THA and up to 28% in revision THA.[3,10-15] Most hip dislocations occur less than 3 months after surgery. Early dislocations are commonly a result of soft-tissue laxity prior to healing of the pseudocapsule of the hip.[12] Williams and associates[14] reported 70% of dislocations occurred within the first month after surgery.

Previous surgery, particularly revision surgery, is a predisposing factor and places the hip at significant risk for dislocation. Williams and associates[14] demonstrated an increase in the dislocation rate from 0.6% in primary procedures to 20% in revision surgery. Morrey[1] found a threefold increase in the dislocation rate from 2% to 6.3%. Evidence suggests that prevention of hip dislocation begins with the surgical approach. The posterior approach appears to place the hip at greater risk when compared with the anterolateral approach.[3,16] Loss of posterior capsular restraints and injury to the abductor mechanism are the most likely causes of this finding. The surgeon must weigh the risks and benefits of the excellent exposure afforded by the posterior approach against an increased rate of postoperative dislocation. Trochanteric osteotomy (although frequently implicated as a cause of instability) has not been conclusively shown to cause problems unless a nonunion results in abductor insufficiency. Injury to the abductors can have a significant impact on stability of the hip.

Component positioning is the most significant factor in surgical technique impacting on the dislocation rate. Malposition of components is the most frequent etiology of hip instability and accounts for at least 40% of hip instability cases.[12,14] Fackler and Poss[11] noted that 44% of patients with hip instability had component malposition compared to 6% of controls.

Patient compliance is of great importance during the postoperative period. Noncompliant patients and those with poor muscle control are at a higher risk of dislocation. Patient education is helpful in emphasizing positional restrictions and most patients will abide by long-term restrictions to prevent dislocation. Despite good intentions, a small percentage of patients continue to sustain recurrent dislocations. Revision because of instability was necessary in 1% of patients at the Mayo Clinic.[15]

Initial management typically includes relocation of the hip and use of a motion-limiting hip abduction orthosis or cast. Success rates ranging from 63% to 83% have been reported after cast or brace immobilization for dislocated THA.[1,10] Chronic instability occurs in up to 33% of dislocations.[1,2] In some situations, an etiology for the dislocation can be identified. Assessment of component orientation, myofascial tension, abductor function, range of motion, bony or soft-tissue impingement, patient noncompliance, and direction of dislocation are crucial.

Daly and Morrey[17] outlined the surgical success rates for instability at the Mayo Clinic. A 70% success rate was noted when the etiology of the instability could be clearly identified. When the etiology was unclear, the success rate dropped to 33% to 50%. Many procedures to correct chronic dislocation have been described in the literature. Improved hip stability may be accomplished by trochanteric advancement procedures, or by overcorrecting the femoral/acetabular component position, through a mechanical block, or by creating a bony or synthetic shelf.

Constrained acetabular components can predictably control the stability of the hip in cases of chronic instability in failed cases of bracing or other procedures. These components do not limit the use of secondary procedures such as trochanteric advancement. The secondary procedures might further protect the hip and help to avoid extreme situations in which the cup is actually restraining the hip.

Constraint is very attractive in patients with chronic instability. The control and limitation of excessive motion provide security to the patient and surgeon. The concern lies with increasing stresses imparted to the bone-cement or component-cement interface in cemented components and the bone-prosthesis interface in noncemented components, in addition to stresses imparted to the component itself. Problems related to failure have occurred in constrained and semiconstrained systems for the shoulder, elbow, knee, and ankle.

The acetabular component holds the head within the socket using polyethylene constraints and might be described as tripolar in its design (Fig. 5). The constraint system in the Osteonics acetabular system is similar to a bipolar femoral head. The femoral head snaps into a polyethylene shell with an inner diameter of 22, 28, or 32 mm and is free to rotate.

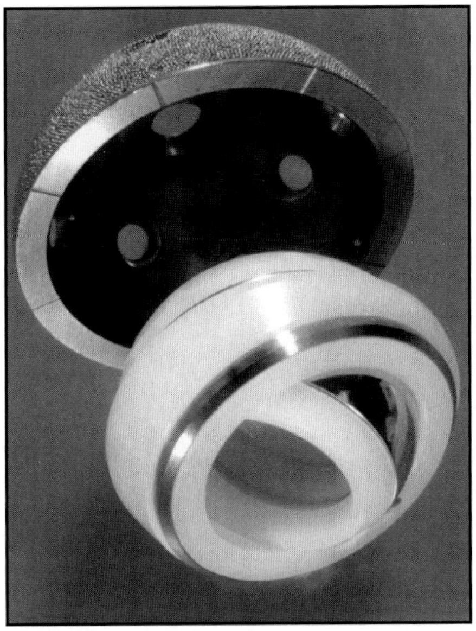

Fig. 5 The Osteonics (Allendale, New Jersey) constrained system.

This shell in turn can rotate within the true polyethylene liner of the acetabulum. The shell is available in sizes ranging from 50 to 70 mm. The inner polyethylene shell is restricted from dislocating from the acetabulum because the size of its circumferential arc is larger than the introitus of the extended walls of the true polyethylene liner.

A systematic preoperative approach to revision acetabular surgery is essential to predictably produce successful results. In situations with advanced degrees of bone loss, large segment allograft or ring devices may need to be used. In situations where extensive allograft bone is used to reconstruct major defects, noncemented acetabular reconstruction may be inappropriate because of the poor biologic environment for fixation to cadaveric bone, and fixation with cement is recommended.[12,18]

Migration of porous press-fit cups is less than with cemented metal cups.[19,20] Increased rates of complete radiolucency, migration, and revision of cemented metal-backed cups have been shown.[21-27] Our series showed significant increases in wear rates with cemented metal-backed cups.

The ability to remove the previously placed implant depends on the method of fixation, integrity of fixation, and association with periprosthetic bone loss. The key is to minimize bone loss and avoid iatrogenic bone destruction by using proper instruments for removal and demonstrating patience. The hips in which the constrained liner was roughened and cemented into a metal-backed cup did poorly; two of 16 hips dissociated at an average of 20 months. The tensile load on the cement might cause additional failures as time increases.

Goetz and associates[4] reported on 56 constrained acetabular components (Osteonics) in patients with recurrent dislocation followed on an average of 52 months. Of these patients, 36% had severe mental impairment, and 4% had a subsequent dislocation necessitating a revision. Revision because of aseptic loosening was needed in one acetabular and one femoral component. Overall, 16% of patients required repeat surgery, and one of two cemented liners failed in the series.

In 1991, Lombardi and associates[5] reported on 55 patients with the S-ROM (DePuy/Johnson & Johnson, Warsaw, IN) acetabular insert with a subsequent dislocation rate of 9%. The mechanism of failure of the device is unclear.[5] Kaper and Bernini[28] observed failure of 4 of 12 S-ROM constrained systems. Failure in two systems occurred by a lever-out mechanism in which the femoral head became disengaged from the polyethylene. Fracture of the constraining ring caused dislocation in two others. Fisher and Kiley[29] reported two failures with the S-ROM. The S-ROM device has less pull-out force and torque than the Osteonics constrained system. Pull-out and lever-out strength for the S-ROM device are 300 lb and 150 in/lb, respectively. Pull-out and lever-out strength for the Osteonics system are 514 lb and 450 in/lb, respectively. (GS Shapiro, MD, et al, New York, NY, unpublished data, 2000).

Anderson and associates[3] reported a 71% success rate in preventing dislocation with the S-ROM constrained system in 21 patients. The six dislocations that occurred were at an average of 10 months. Modes of failure included dissociation of the liner and disengagement of the femoral head from the liner.[3]

A constrained acetabular component is a useful surgical option in patients in whom other treatable causes of dislocation are excluded and control cannot be obtained conservatively. The component is also a reasonable option in primary settings in which dislocation is likely due to patient dementia, deficient musculature, and poor muscle control. The constrained system does not limit the use of secondary procedures that might further protect the hip. The system may be used in massive revision cases, in which the components will be predictably unstable.

Accelerated loosening of the bone-cement and cement-metal interfaces and catastrophic component failure are all potential problems with the constrained system. Additionally, dislocation requires an open reduction. In our series, we have not seen excessive wear rates leading to failure in most patients. Although the long-term results of progressive loosening are not known, the short-term results are encouraging based on the literature and our own results. The revision rate of 8.2% far exceeds other options in this group of patients.

References

1. Morrey BF: Instability after total hip arthroplasty. *Orthop Clin North Am* 1992;23:237-248.
2. Ali Khan MA, Brakenbury PH, Reynolds ISR: Dislocation following total hip replacement. *J Bone Joint Surg Br* 1981;63:214-218.
3. Anderson MJ, Murray WR, Skinner HB: Constrained acetabular components. *J Arthroplasty* 1994;9:17-23.
4. Goetz DD, Capello WN, Callaghan JJ, Brown TD, Johnston RC: Salvage of a recurrently dislocating total hip prosthesis with use of a constrained acetabular component: A retrospective analysis of fifty-six cases. *J Bone Joint Surg Am* 1998;80:502-509.
5. Lombardi AV Jr, Mallory TH, Kraus TJ, Vaughn BK: Preliminary report on the S-ROM constraining acetabular insert: A retrospective clinical experience. *Orthopedics* 1991;14: 297-303.
6. DeLee JG, Charnley J: Radiological demarcation of cemented sockets in total hip replacement. *Clin Orthop* 1976;121:20-32.
7. Gruen TA, McNeice GM, Amstutz HC: "Modes of failure" of cemented stem-type femoral components: A radiographic analysis of loosening. *Clin Orthop* 1979;141:17-27.
8. Loudon JR, Charnley J: Subsidence of the femoral prosthesis in total hip replacement in relation to the design of the stem. *J Bone Joint Surg Br* 1980;62:450-453.
9. Harris WH, McCarthy JC Jr, O'Neill DA: Femoral component loosening using contemporary techniques of femoral cement fixation. *J Bone Joint Surg Am* 1982;64:1063-1067.
10. Eftekhar NS: Dislocation and instability complicating low friction arthroplasty of the hip joint. *Clin Orthop* 1976;121:120-125.
11. Fackler CD, Poss R: Dislocation in total hip arthroplasties. *Clin Orthop* 1980;151:169-178.
12. Berry DJ, Muller ME: Revision arthroplasty using an anti-protrusio cage for massive acetabular bone deficiency. *J Bone Joint Surg Br* 1992;74:711-715.
13. Kristiansen B, Jorgensen L, Holmich P: Dislocation following total hip arthroplasty. *Arch Orthop Trauma Surg* 1985;103:375-377.
14. Williams JF, Gottesman MJ, Mallory TH: Dislocation after total hip arthroplasty: Treatment with an above-knee hip spica cast. *Clin Orthop* 1982;171:53-58.
15. Hedlundh U, Ahnfelt L, Hybbinette CH, Wallinder L, Weckstrom J, Fredin H: Dislocations and the femoral head size in primary total hip arthroplasty. *Clin Orthop* 1996;333:226-233.
16. Woo RY, Morrey BF: Dislocations after total hip arthroplasty. *J Bone Joint Surg Am* 1982;64:1295-1306.
17. Daly PJ, Morrey BF: Operative correction of an unstable total hip arthroplasty. *J Bone Joint Surg Am* 1992;74:1334-1343.
18. Hooten JP Jr, Engh CA Jr, Engh CA: Failure of structural acetabular allografts in cementless revision hip arthroplasty. *J Bone Joint Surg Br* 1994;76:419-422.
19. Nivbrant B, Karrholm J, Onsten I, Carlsson A, Snorrason F: Migration of porous press-fit cups in hip revision arthroplasty: A radiostereometric 2-year follow-up study of 60 hips. *J Arthroplasty* 1996;11:390-396.

20. Ritter MA, Keating EM, Faris PM, Brugo G: Metal-backed acetabular cups in total hip arthroplasty. *J Bone Joint Surg Am* 1990; 72: 672-677.

21. Cates HE, Faris PM, Keating EM, Ritter MA: Polyethylene wear in cemented metal-backed acetabular cups. *J Bone Joint Surg Br* 1993;75:249-253.

22. Ritter MA: Dislocation and subluxation of the total hip replacement. *Clin Orthop* 1976; 121:92-94.

23. Harris WH, Penenberg BL: Further follow-up on socket fixation using a metal-backed acetabular component for total hip replacement: A minimum ten-year follow-up study. *J Bone Joint Surg Am* 1987;69:1140-1143.

24. Zicat B, Engh CA, Gokcen E: Patterns of osteolysis around total hip components inserted with and without cement. *J Bone Joint Surg Am* 1995;77:432–439.

25. Weber KL, Callaghan JJ, Goetz DD, Johnston RC: Revision of a failed cemented total hip prosthesis with insertion of an acetabular component without cement and a femoral component with cement: A five- to eight-year follow-up study. *J Bone Joint Surg Am* 1996;78:982-994.

26. Wixson RL, Stulberg SD, Mehlhoff M: Total hip replacement with cemented, uncemented, and hybrid prostheses: A comparison of clinical and radiographic results at two to four years. *J Bone Joint Surg Am* 1991;73:257-270.

27. Hernandez JR, Keating EM, Faris PM, Meding JB, Ritter MA: Polyethylene wear in uncemented acetabular components. *J Bone Joint Surg Br* 1994;76:263-266.

28. Kaper BP, Bernini PM: Failure of a constrained acetabular prosthesis of a total hip arthroplasty: A report of four cases. *J Bone Joint Surg Am* 1998;80:561-565.

29. Fisher DA, Kiley K: Constrained acetabular cup disassembly. *J Arthroplasty* 1994;9:325-329.

30

The Unstable Total Hip Arthroplasty: The Role of Postoperative Bracing

Kyle F. Baldwin, DPT
Lawrence D. Dorr, MD

Introduction

The unstable total hip arthroplasty (THA) is problematic for both the patient and the surgeon. An unstable THA can be a painful condition that can lead to a patient's mental and functional decline. In addition, the surgeon and the rehabilitation team are presented with the challenge of appropriately managing the hip instability, preventing further hip dislocation, and ensuring hip joint function.

The posterior surgical approach for performing a THA means that the patient must comply with the established hip precautions during the 6 to 8 weeks after surgery. These precautions are: no hip adduction past the midline of the body, no hip internal rotation, and no hip flexion greater than 90°. It is important to caution patients both before and after surgery about moving the operated hip into one or a combination of these positions in order to decrease the risk of hip dislocation after THA.[1] It is particularly important to point out the dangers of arising from a low chair. In doing so, patients attempt to move their center of gravity anterior over their base of support, which subsequently places the operated hip into too much flexion (Fig. 1). The patient also tends to internally rotate the hip during this task. This position of increased flexion and internal rotation puts the patient at greatest risk for a posterior hip dislocation.[2-4] Additionally, the influence of the muscular contractions of the hip during such an activity should not be ignored. As the position of the hip approaches more flexion, the force vector of the gluteus maximus encourages a more direct posterior translation of the femoral head.[2] This increases the stress to the posterior capsule and is likely to be a contributing factor to dislocation of the femoral head. Dislocation always causes a capsular defect (Fig. 1).

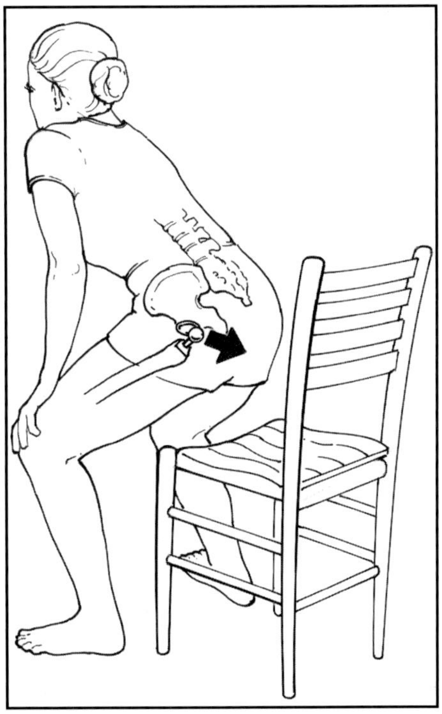

Fig. 1 The patient positions self in too much hip flexion when rising from the chair. The arrow indicates the direction of the femoral head dislocation from the cup.

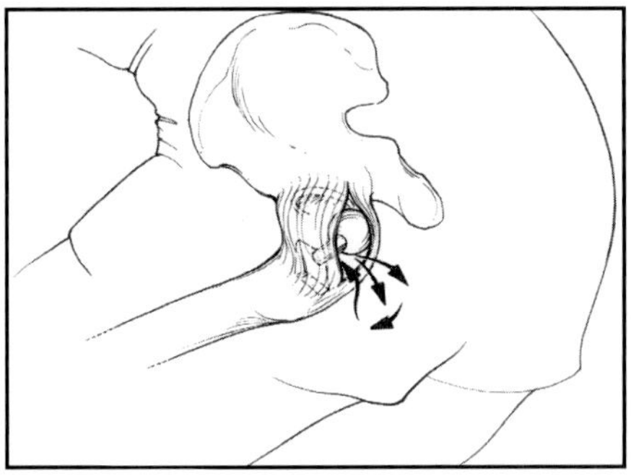

Fig. 2 Posterolateral view of the left hip demonstrating the fluid movement in and out of the capsular defect with motion of the joint.

Causes of Instability

Dorr and associates[5] established a classification system of dislocations of THA. This classification consists of three categories: instability caused by incorrect patient position (with impingement as a probable contributor to this cause), soft-tissue imbalance, and component malposition. In some patients a fourth category, a combination of soft-tissue imbalance and component malposition, occurs.[6] Postoperative bracing/casting (including that after closed reduction) is used most successfully when hip instability is caused by soft-tissue imbalance or dislocation resulting from incorrect

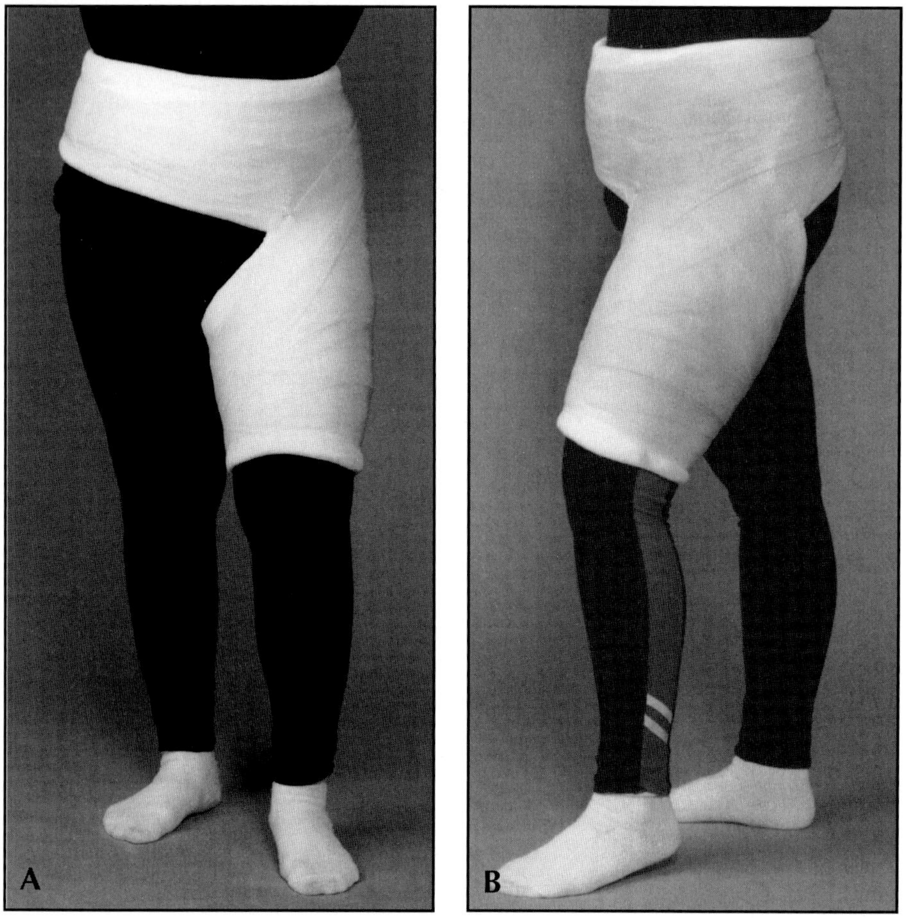

Fig. 3 The hip spica cast. **A**, Anterior view. **B**, Lateral view.

patient positioning. The patient with a severely unstable hip from soft-tissue imbalance or component malposition in whom dislocation occurs should undergo revision immediately. The diagnosis of excessive instability is easily made by performing a closed reduction of the dislocation under anesthesia and then moving the hip through the entire range of motion (ROM). If dislocation occurs within 10° of internal rotation when hip flexion is at 90°, or within 20° of external rotation with the leg in full extension, then the hip has such excessive instability that the patient should undergo revision. In our experience, if the patient does not have an easily dislocated THA, then a cast or brace should be applied because all causes of dislocation have some success with this treatment. The expected success of closed reduction without the need for reoperation in hips with positional instability was 45%; in those with component malposition, 35%. In hips with soft-tissue imbalance, closed reduction was successful in 17%, and in those hips with component malposition and soft-issue imbalance there was a 17% success rate.[6]

Certainly, the best treatment for the unstable THA is prevention. The components must be appropriately sized and positioned, and must have the appropriate balance of the surrounding soft tissues. The creation of the correct hip length and offset, and balance of the contracted tissues[7] provides the best chance for the patient to recover the ROM needed for function and activities of daily living (ADL) without instability of the hip. In order to heal, an intact capsular scar requires stability of the hip, including the muscle balance, or else excessive fluid in the hip can prevent a capsular scar. The combination of increased fluid, capsular defect, and hip motion makes healing of the surgery site difficult.[8] Motion of the hip acts as a pump to move fluid in and around the joint. This pumping motion can prevent the capsular defect from healing (Fig. 2). If a THA has too much slack in the surrounding musculature, the muscular sling that helps stabilize the joint against instability may be inadequate.

Soft-tissue imbalance of the hip can be confirmed with radiographs and the physical examination of the patient. Muscle weakness can be demonstrated on physical examination with a weak sidelying abduction test[6] or by observation of the gait pattern. If the length-tension relationship of the hip abductors is inadequate, the patient is likely to have a Trendelenburg gait pattern. This type of gait pattern is uncomfortable for the patient and increases energy consumed during gait.[9] It also leads to further disuse of the hip abductors and decreased protection of hip stability. It has been demonstrated that the correct function of the hip abductors is the key to successful functional mobility following THA.[9]

Failure of the capsular scar to form after THA, or failure of a capsular defect to heal after a dislocation, will increase the prevalence of dislocation even with correct component position. The normal hip joint contains approximately 2.7 mL of fluid.[10] The unstable THA has excessive chronic joint fluid that can perpetuate capsular defects, particularly if in conjuction with excessive joint movements. This capsular insufficiency is a type of soft-tissue imbalance that cannot be identified without an arthrogram. This capsular insufficiency is usually identified at reoperation for dislocation and is characterized by the presence of a smooth cystic lining surrounding the extent of the capsular defect, and fluid collection.

Capsular insufficiency allows fluid to continue to move in and out of the defect, keeping the defect patent (Fig. 2). A hip abduction brace or pantaloon cast may be used as external support for capsular healing. Application of a locked brace or a pantaloon cast restricts ROM of the joint, prevents the fluid from pumping, and provides an environment for capsular healing. Healing of the capsule promotes internal stability for the joint.

Capsular Healing

The hip joint capsule is primarily composed of collagen types I, III, and V.[8] Type I collagen is the most prevalent form and accounts for 90% of the collagen in the body.[8] Type III collagen is found mostly in embryonic connective tissue and in adults in the deep dermis, blood vessels, and wounds.[11] The healing of collagen is of immediate clinical relevance because it will be a major contributor to the stability of the hip joint.[12] Tissue creep and resilience are needed to withstand load over time and to return the tissue to its original shape after injury. Both tissue creep and resilience depend on the number and distribution of the collagen fibers.[11] Postoperatively (or postdislocation), the capsular repair process proceeds based on available blood supply, enzymes, hormones, and mechanical stress.[13] The first collagen to be produced in the reparative phase is highly disorganized and has poor wound strength.[8,9] It is for this reason that patients must comply with the precautions indicated for THA. Collagen in this stage of repair is mainly type III; conversion to type I occurs when stress and strain are placed across the healing tissue of the capsule.[8,13] This stress and strain is known to assist in alignment of connective tissue during the repair phase.[13]

Total hip replacements that are unstable have a capsular defect and may have soft-tissue imbalance. Positive mechanical stress to collagen is a variable that can be altered to assist healing.[8,13] The collagen fibers align themselves in a direction that can best accommodate stress. Additionally, the response to stress causes the wound to produce more collagen tissue. In contrast, random collagen fibers not under stress/strain may not be signaled to form as dense a network of collagen as that of a controlled movement environment.[8,13] If the hip is placed in a hip abduction brace that allows up to 45° of motion, then this controlled movement will provide a significant stimulus for collagen synthesis and repair, as well as protect against end range of movements that could sabotage the integrity of the healing wound site.[13] Additionally, having a stop on the abduction brace at 45° provides protection against excessively high intracapsular pressure, which can help promote fluid resorption that must occur for collagen fibers to become dense and heal in the line of stress.[14-16] Fluid absorption and early maturation of tissue healing should occur within 6 weeks. However, if concomitant muscle weakness is present, the brace should remain until the sidelying abduction test shows strong abduction, which may require 3 months of physical therapy and exercise.

Postoperative Bracing

The Hip Pantaloon Cast

The pantaloon cast is certainly the most cumbersome method of immobilization for the patient, but it provides the highest degree of external stability. This cast should be used with patients who are not entirely compliant with hip precautions or who have weight-bearing restrictions such as excessive alcohol intake, advanced age, and physical or mental disability. This cast should also be used for the patient who has a known serious soft-tissue imbalance, such as shortening of the hip as observed on radiographs, or nonunion of the greater trochanter.[6] Additionally, the cast is used after a trochanteric osteotomy has been performed for surgical exposure or to help reestablish the correct length/tension relationship of the hip abductors, because failure of the trochanter to heal after it is transferred for treatment of dislocation usually signals failure of the treatment. The pantaloon cast is applied so that the patient's hip is fixed at 30° to 35° of hip flexion, 10° of hip abduction, and neutral rotation (Fig. 3).

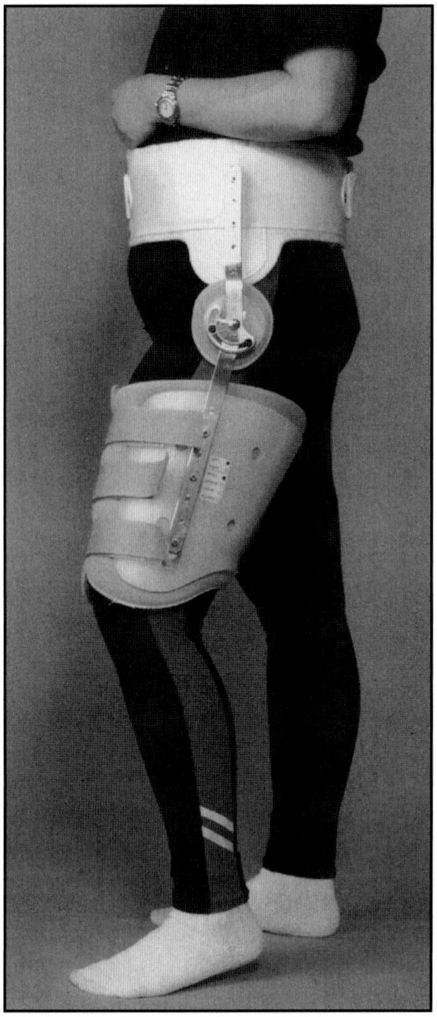

Fig. 4 Static hip abduction brace (lateral view). Note the position of the hip hinge, locked at 30° to 35° of flexion.

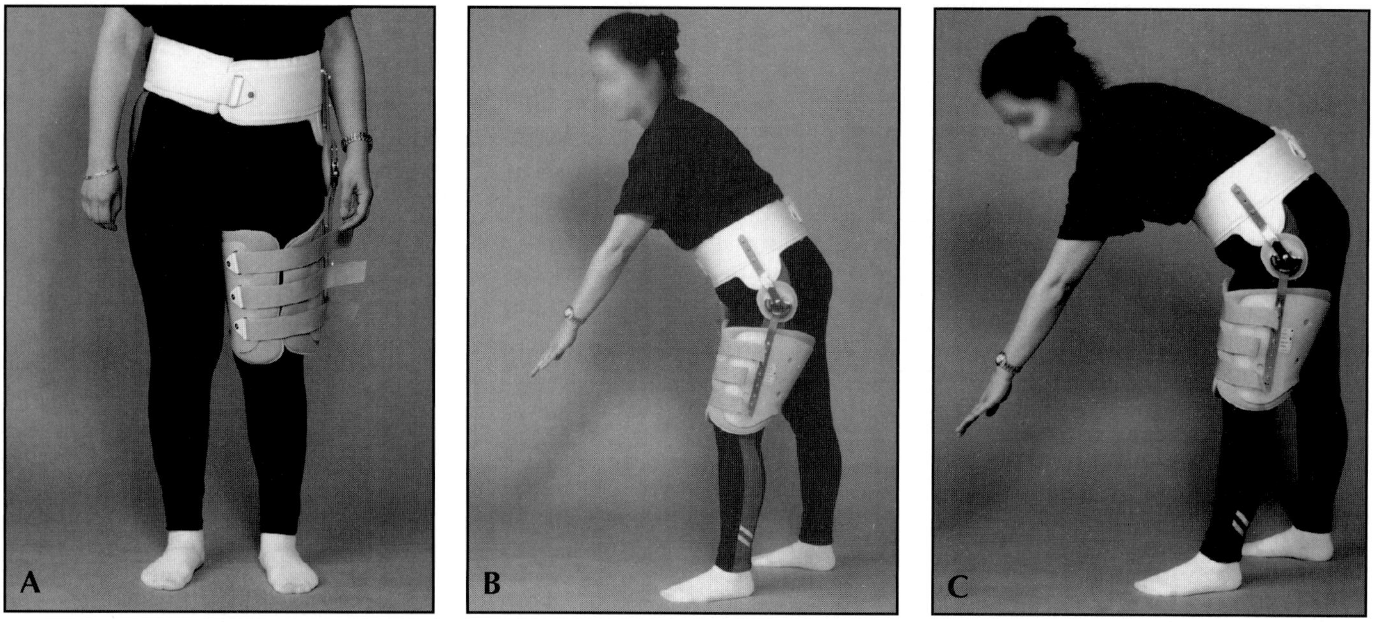

Fig. 5 Dynamic hip abduction brace. **A**, Anterior view, zero degrees of flexion. **B**, Lateral view, with hinge blocked at 45° of flexion. **C**, Lateral view demonstrating that the brace will allow approximately 10° to 15° more flexion when stressed during functional activities.

There should be adequate clearance with the cast for personal hygiene and toileting. The cast is usually necessary for 6 weeks. The patient is trained by the physical therapy staff to move into and out of bed, ambulate, and perform ADL within the constraints of the cast. The patient may be allowed full weight bearing on the involved lower extremity if no specific contraindication (such as trochanteric osteotomy) is involved. Full weight bearing with the cast is helpful in ensuring muscle use and thereby helping to promote muscle strength.[17]

The Hip Abduction Brace

The stabilizing forces of a THA have been described as component position, muscular co-contractions, soft-tissue balance, and the joint capsule.[6,7,14] Following THA or any hip joint trauma, it has been demonstrated that intracapsular pressures are significantly increased secondary to increased amounts of fluid.[10,14-16,18] Additionally, these pressures are also influenced by joint position.[14,19] Schwarz and associates[15] reported that the highest intracapsular pressures were achieved at internal and external rotation of the hip. This is important when considering the tissue mechanics of the healing joint. Therefore, application of the hip abduction brace helps control the mechanics of the joint to assist in healing by minimizing internal and external rotation.

The hip abduction brace can be used to control motion either statically or dynamically. The static hip abduction brace has the hinge locked to effectively allow no motion (although there always is some motion that occurs). The static brace is used for the compliant patient who has muscle weakness, component malposition, or positional instabilities. The advantage of the fixed brace versus the cast is that the patient may remove the brace to shower and after 3 weeks of use, remove it at night and use only a pillow between the legs. The hinge of the brace is locked at 30° to 35° of flexion with 10° of abduction and neutral rotation (Fig. 4). The dynamic hip abduction brace allows motion and can be used more successfully for the patient who has only a positional instability.[6] This brace should only allow zero to 45° of hip flexion ROM and should be positioned at 10° of hip abduction and neutral rotation (Fig. 5, *A*). Even though the hinge is blocked at 45° of flexion (Fig. 5, *B*) it is expected that the patient can actually achieve 10° to 15° more hip flexion in the brace (Fig. 5, *C*), thereby with the brace having an end range of approximately 60° of flexion. This arc of motion provides a good margin of safety for the patient with positional instability, allows controlled movement to promote collagen alignment, and protects the patient who may forget the established hip precautions. Therefore, the patient should wear the brace whenever out of bed. The noncompliant patient with THA instability should be instructed to wear the brace at all times, except when showering. Finally, the patient should be instructed that the brace is used to promote healing and provide physical and mental constraints, but does not guarantee prevention of dislocation.

The patient should be cautioned against overexertion during ADL so as to avoid muscle fatigue. They may resume their daily routine around the house, but should avoid any activity or movements that will stress their already unstable joint or perpetuate joint inflammation.[18]

Consequences of Immobilization

Immobilization can be used successfully to control ROM around the joint and protect the soft tissues, but there are concerns with the application of these devices. Restricted motion of the joint results in disuse of the muscles, leading to muscular atrophy.[17] The gluteal muscles are affected specifically and it is these muscles that provide the most important stability of the joint. The casted patient is less mobile than other patients who have had THA, and for this reason they are more likely to develop disuse weakness. Disuse weakness is contrary to one of the principles of providing stability for the joint, which is muscle strength. Therefore, it is necessary to instruct the casted patient to perform isometric exercises for the hip. For example, patients should perform three sets of 10 repetitions, twice daily, for each of the following exercises: isometric gluteal sets, quadriceps sets, and hamstring sets. Each repetition/contraction should be 3 to 5 seconds in duration.[17] Additionally, ankle pumping 10 times per hour while awake will guard against deep vein thrombosis. With these exercises, the patient can hope to maintain some degree of muscle tone and feel more comfortable. The advantage of these isometric exercises is that the patient will have a greater degree of control of the hip once the cast is removed. This will make the hip more stable for walking and other functional mobility. Patients with a brace can participate in supervised physical therapy that is focused on increasing muscle strength and control of the joint.

Summary

Control of the unstable THA can be problematic, but conservative management with casting and bracing can assist the patient in gaining stability, both externally and internally. The application of such appliances does not negatively affect the ultimate function of the hip and can prevent further surgical intervention.

References

1. Anderson R: Closed reduction of posterior hip dislocation. *Am J Orthop* 1999;28:401.
2. Hodge WA, Fijan RS, Carlson KL, Burgess RG, Harris WH, Mann RW: Contact pressures in the human hip joint measured in vivo. *Proc Natl Acad Sci USA* 1986;83:2879-2883.
3. Lewin R: Pressures measured in live hip joint. *Science* 1986;232:1192-1193.
4. Scifert CF, Brown TD, Pedersen DR, Callaghan JJ: A finite element analysis of factors influencing total hip dislocation. *Clin Orthop* 1998;355: 152-162.
5. Dorr LD, Wolf AW, Chandler R, Conaty JP: Classification and treatment of dislocations of total hip arthroplasty. *Clin Orthop* 1983;173: 151-158.
6. Dorr LD, Wan Z: Causes of and treatment protocol for instability of total hip replacement. *Clin Orthop* 1998;355:144-151.
7. Longjohn D, Dorr LD: Soft tissue balance of the hip. *J Arthroplasty* 1998;13:97-100.
8. Weiss EL: Connective tissue in wound healing, in McCulloch JM, Kloth LC, Feedar JA (eds): *Wound Healing: Alternatives in Management*, ed 2. Philadelphia, PA, FA Davis, 1995, pp 17-31.
9. Chandler RW, Dorr LD, Perry J: The functional cost of dislocation following total hip arthroplasty. *Clin Orthop* 1982;168:168-172.
10. Moss SG, Schweitzer ME, Jacobson JA, et al: Hip joint fluid: Detection and distribution at MR imaging and US with cadaveric correlation. *Radiology* 1998;208:43-48.
11. Burgeson RE: The collagens of skin. *Curr Probl Dermatol* 1987;17:61-65.
12. Wright V, Johns RJ: Physical factors concerned with the stiffness of normal and diseased joints. *Bull Johns Hopkins Hosp* 1960;106:215-231.
13. Haukipuro K, Melkko J, Risteli L, Kairaluoma MI, Risteli J: Connective tissue response to major surgery and postoperative infection. *Eur J Clin Invest* 1992;22:333-340.
14. Wingstrand H, Wingstrand A, Krantz P: Intracapsular and atmospheric pressure in the dynamics and stability of the hip. *Acta Orthop Scand* 1990;61:231-235.
15. Schwarz N, Leixnering M, Hopf R, Jantsch S: Pressure-volume ratio in human cadaver hip joints. *Arch Orthop Trauma Surg* 1988;107: 322-325.
16. Wingstrand H, Egund N, Forsberg L: Sonography and joint pressure in synovitis of the adult hip. *J Bone Joint Surg Br* 1987;69:2 54-256.
17. Scully RM, Barnes MR, Canfield JS, Moffat M, Shepard KF (eds): *Physical Therapy*. Philadelphia, PA, JB Lippincott, 1989, pp 224-225.
18. Koski JM, Anttila P, Hamalainen M, Isomaki H: Hip joint ultrasonography: Correlation with intra-articular effusion and synovitis. *Br J Rheumatol* 1990;29:189-192.
19. Wingstrand H, Egund N, Carlin NO, Forsberg L, Gustafson T, Sunden G: Intracapsular pressure in transient synovitis of the hip. *Acta Orthop Scand* 1985;56:204-210.

SECTION

6

Hip: Adult Reconstruction—Complex Primary Total Hip Arthroplasty

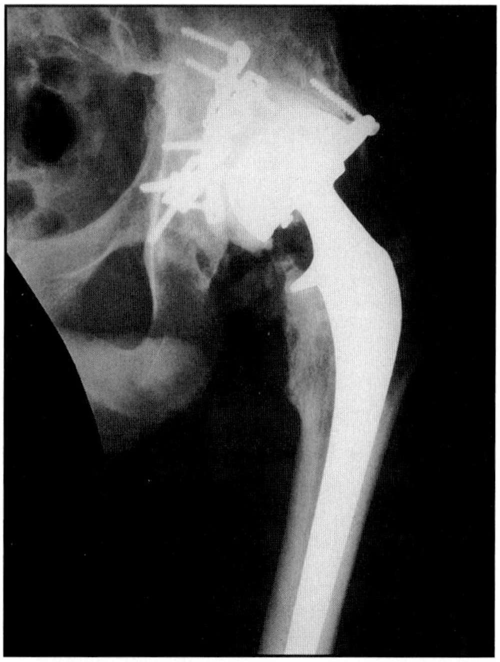

31 Conversion of Hip Arthrodesis to Total Hip Arthroplasty

32 Total Hip Replacement for the Dislocated Hip

33 Primary Total Hip Arthroplasty After Infection

34 Primary Total Hip Arthroplasty After Acetabular Fracture

31

Conversion of Hip Arthrodesis to Total Hip Arthroplasty

Kostas P. Panagiotopoulos, MD, BSc
Graham M. Robbins, MD
Bassam A. Masri, MD, FRCSC
Clive P. Duncan, MD, FRCSC

Introduction

Arthrodesis of the hip was first performed by Heusner in 1885 for congenital dislocation of the hip. Historically, this procedure has been carried out for tuberculosis, septic arthritis, developmental dysplasia, slipped capital femoral epiphysis, destructive osteoarthritis, and posttraumatic arthritis.[1,2]

A variety of techniques have been introduced, including intra-articular and extra-articular procedures with and without internal fixation. In addition, ankylosis of the hip may occur spontaneously as a result of infectious and noninfectious arthritic conditions.[1]

In the era of total hip arthroplasty (THA), hip arthrodesis has limited indications. Infection as a reason for arthrodesis is now less common, accounting for less than 20% in more recent reports.[3-8] Moreover, the success of THA, even in young patients, has led to an increasing reluctance by patients to accept hip arthrodesis. The ideal candidate for a hip arthrodesis today is a young, heavy male, working as a manual laborer, who has advanced degeneration of the hip.

One or more of the authors or the departments with which they are affiliated have received something of value from a commercial or other party related directly or indirectly to the subject of this chapter.

Table 1
Pain in other joints after hip arthrodesis

Study	Lower Back	Ipsilateral Knee	Contralateral Knee	Contralateral Hip
Sponseller et al[19]	57% (30 of 53)	45% (24 of 53)	26% (14 of 53)	17% (9 of 53)
Callaghan et al[17]	61% (17 of 28)	57% (16 of 28)		32% (9 of 28)
Sofue et al[18]	65% (26 of 40)	30% (12 of 40)	13% (5 of 40)	13% (5 of 40)
Perugia et al[20]	50%	76% (39 of 51)	33% (17 of 51)	25%

Outcomes of Arthrodesis

There have been several studies focused on the results of hip arthrodesis, both spontaneous and surgical. Failure to achieve bone union has been one of the most common complications of this procedure. Before the introduction of internal fixation, rates of pseudarthrosis were over 20%.[1,2,9-11] However, with the introduction of internal fixation and modification of techniques and fixation devices, nonunion rates have decreased substantially.[3,12-14]

In 1966, Schneider[8] introduced the cobra head plate as a means of achieving hip arthrodesis. The use of this plate with and without an innominate osteotomy has produced fusion rates as high as 100%.[3,4,7,15,16]

A number of studies have clearly documented the long-term effects of a hip arthrodesis.[17-19] It has been found that patients generally have suprisingly little limitation in their activities of daily living. Bending, prolonged sitting, and various sports were most affected.[8,28] Most patients were able to walk 1 mile and were able to continue with their occupation, including manual labor.[17,19] Hip arthrodesis also has been associated with some difficulty with sexual intercourse, the concern being more prevalent in females.[17-19]

The effect of a hip arthrodesis on other joints also has been documented. Back pain is the most prevalent, ranging from 50% to 65%.[17-20] The pain generally is exacerbated by activity or prolonged sitting or standing. Radicular symptoms are uncommon. Radiographic changes of the lumbar spine are highly prevalent in many patients several years (10 to 35 years) after hip arthrodesis (Table 1).

Knee pain frequently is found late after a hip arthrodesis. Discomfort in the ipsilateral knee is present in 30% to 76% of patients,[17-20] while only 13% to 33% experience pain in the contralateral knee[18-20] (Table 1). Most patients experienced the discomfort with prolonged sitting, standing, or stair climbing. Laxity of the ipsilateral knee in various planes has been documented after hip fusion,

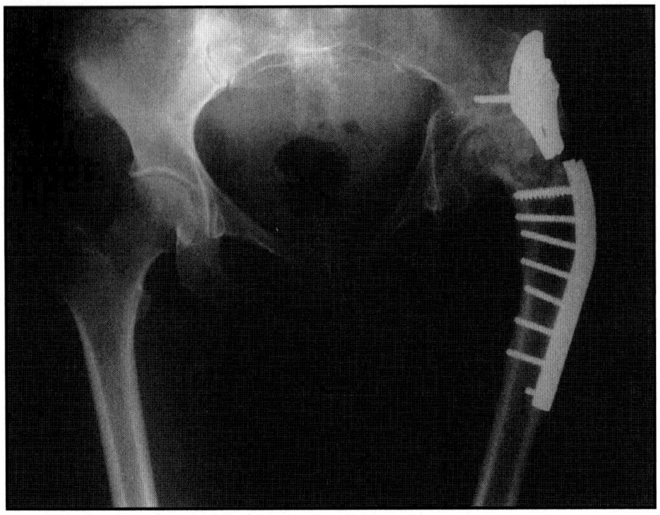

Fig. 1 Painful pseudarthrosis is one indication for conversion to a THA.

particularly when the arthrodesed hip is in abduction.[17,19]

Contralateral hip pain occurs in 13% to 32% of patients after at least 20 years with a hip arthrodesis,[17-20] with corresponding degenerative radiographic changes. This pain may be more progressive in patients with preexisting degenerative changes in the hip.[18]

After hip arthrodesis, patients have a limp when walking. In over half of the patients, the limp is moderate to severe.[17] In addition, a substantial limb-length inequality (ranging from 2.9 to 3.9 cm)[21,22] is frequently present after hip fusion. Gore and associates[23] have reviewed the gait patterns in patients who have a unilateral hip fusion. Their results have demonstrated a shorter step length with an overall wider-based gait and slower cadence. The lumbar spine; contralateral hip; and ipsilateral knee, foot, and ankle all compensate for the arthrodesed hip. Despite these adaptations of other joints, Waters and associates[24] found an overall decrease in walking speed, a reduction of gait efficiency to only 53%, and an increase in oxygen consumption.

Other complications after hip arthrodesis include infection (0 to 18%)[1,6,8-11] and fracture of the femur (4% to 19%).[3,6,10,11,16,19] With the introduction of internal fixation such as the cobra head plate, patients can be mobilized much earlier,[16] and hip spica immobilization is required much less frequently.

Indications for Conversion of Arthrodesis

Currently, the most common indications to convert an arthrodesed hip to a THA include disabling low back pain, ipsilateral knee pain, or contralateral hip pain; a painful pseudarthrosis; or a malpositioned hip with associated loss of function.[22,25,26] In addition, because of the widespread appreciation of the results of hip replacement and the feasibility of converting a hip fusion to a mobile arthroplasty, in the senior author's experience an increasing number of patients are less likely to accept arthrodesis as a treatment option, and more patients with an existing hip fusion are demanding conversion to a hip replacement because of lack of motion. Another indication for takedown of a hip fusion, particularly if it is in poor position, is to allow a knee replacement on the ipsilateral side. Fewer patients with a hip fusion are willing to accept its inconvenience and associated symptoms elsewhere. Consequently, it is unlikely that we will witness future studies with the long-term data that have been collected in the past.[17,19] Patients today are unwilling to accept the long-term functional effects of arthrodesis on their activities of daily living.

Preoperative Clinical Assessment

When assessing a patient before conversion of a hip arthrodesis, it is important to establish the symptoms and functional difficulties that are being attributed to the hip. A thorough history must be taken to document the patient's current and desired activity levels as well as any comorbid conditions. It is essential to determine the source of the patient's discomfort and decide whether this is amenable to improvement by conversion of the arthrodesis to a THA.

The physician must be aware of the original diagnosis leading to the hip arthrodesis. Specifically, any prior infection in the hip would alert the examiner to ensure that active infection is ruled out before embarking on a conversion procedure. The examiner should obtain a history of any prior wound infection or prolonged wound drainage. The wound should be carefully examined for any evidence of inflammation or drainage. Laboratory investigations should include a C-reactive protein and erythrocyte sedimentation rate. If there is any concern or history of wound infection, a bone scan may be considered. Intraoperatively, the surgeon may obtain tissue samples if there are concerns about wound inspection.[27] Hardinge and associates[21] did obtain intraoperative specimens during the conversion procedure; however, obtaining intraoperative cultures has not been a routine practice in the literature.

When examining the patient, the orthopaedist must determine whether a pseudarthrosis is present and whether this is the cause of the patient's symptoms (Fig. 1). The position of the hip arthrodesis should be determined as well as a clinical measure of leg-length

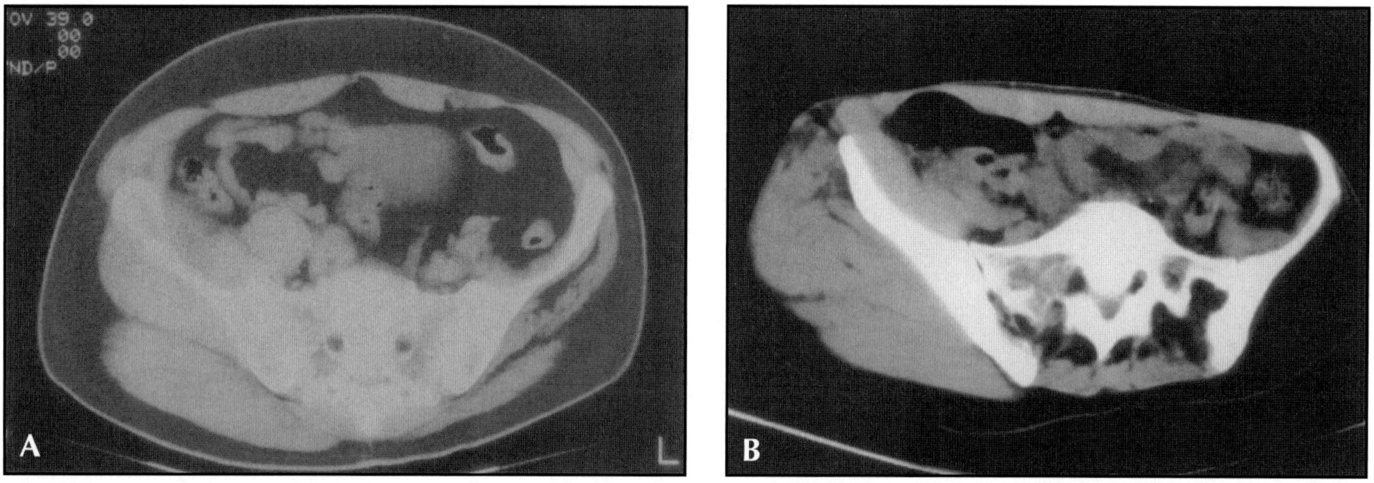

Fig. 2 Preoperative CT scan can be useful in the assessment of the abductor muscles, which are usually atrophied (**A**) but may be absent if the original procedure was due to poliomyelitis (**B**).

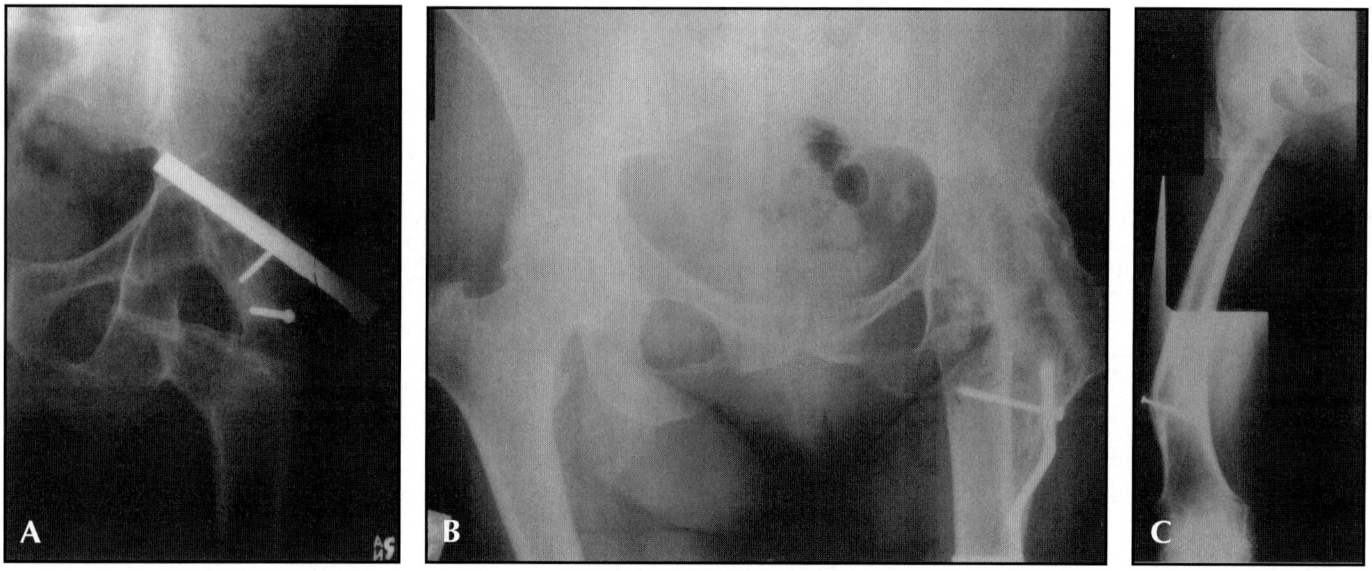

Fig. 3 A and **B,** Portions of a long leg film. It is important to consider the influence of preexisting deformity on the surgical technique. Radiographs of the entire femur (**C**) may be required.

discrepancy. It is essential to establish whether the patient has functioning abductors. The examiner should place a hand over the gluteus medius and ask the patient to actively abduct the leg. Electromyography has been used to evaluate the abductors but its usefulness has not been established.[20,28] Weak abductors may be associated with a poorer functional outcome postoperatively.[20] A preoperative CT scan can be used to assess the quality of the abductors as well as to determine the presence of a pseudoarthrosis (Fig. 2). Thorough examination of the lumbar spine, contralateral hip, and both knees should be carried out as well.

Preoperative Radiographic Evaluation

The preoperative radiographs should include an AP radiograph of the pelvis and true lateral radiograph of the affected hip and femur. Clinical measurement of the leg-length inequality may be difficult, especially if the arthrodesis is malpositioned, and a long leg film will allow more accurate assessment, demonstrate the overall limb alignment, and identify any other deformity present (Fig. 3). If there is concern regarding the acetabular bone stock, Judet views or CT scans should be considered. CT scans also can

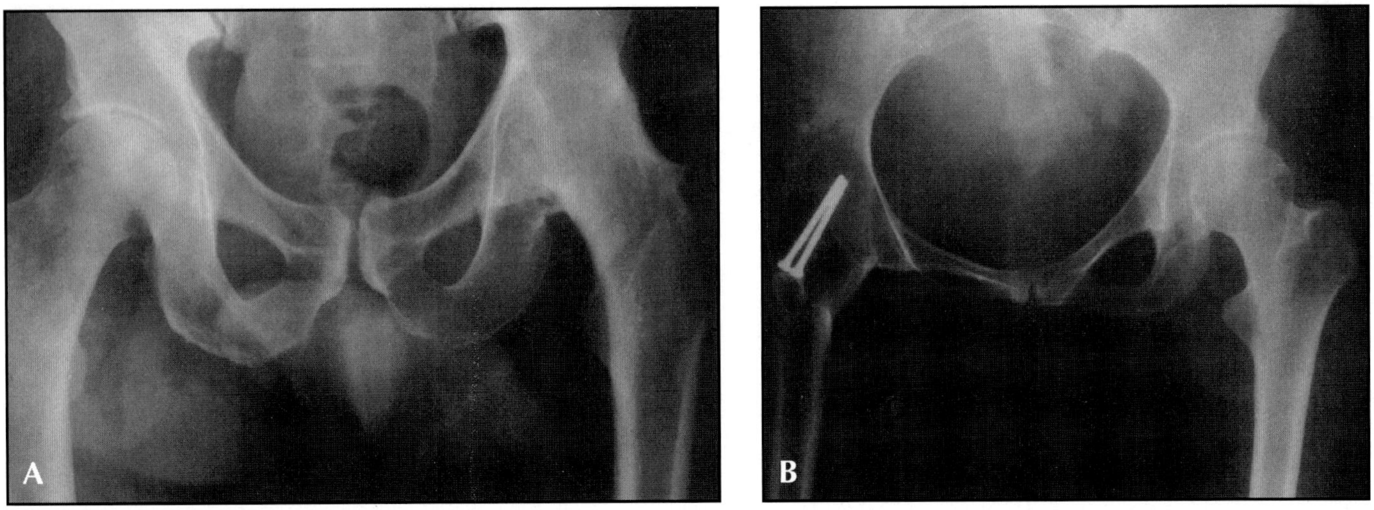

Fig. 4 The technical details of conversion are more straightforward following spontaneous fusion in adults (**A**) than after surgical fusion in children (**B**) because the anatomy is less distorted, the leg lengths are relatively equal, and the sciatic nerve is not shortened.

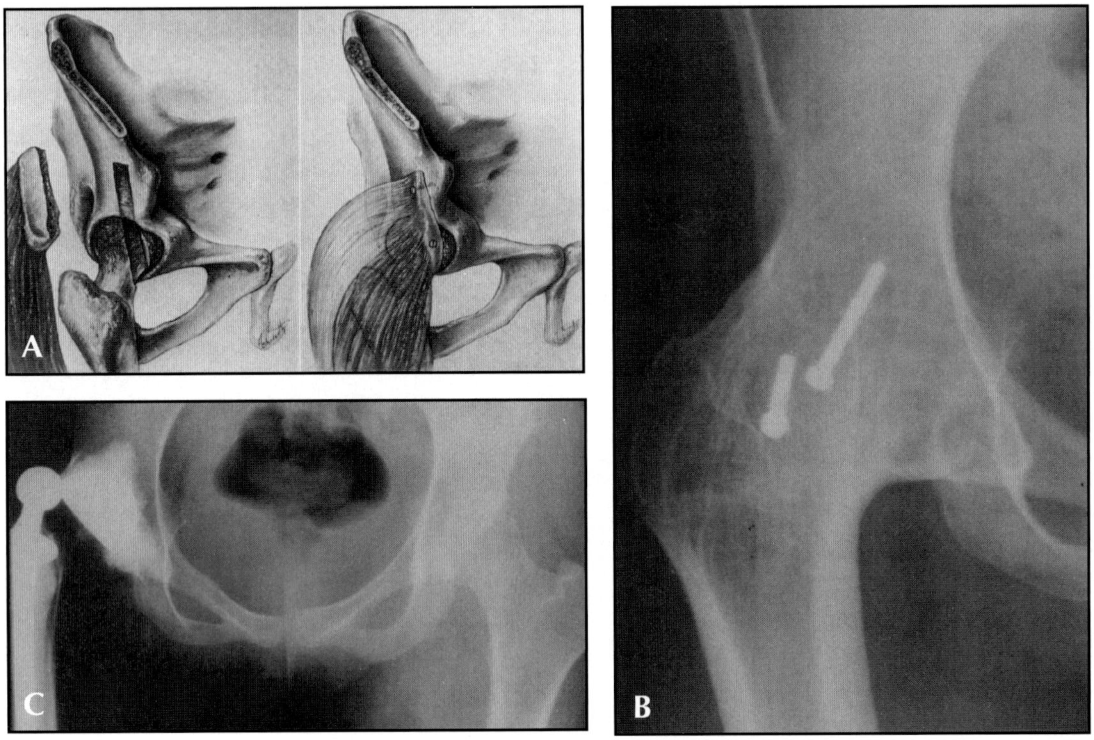

Fig. 5 A, Schematic representation of the Davis technique, which uses an iliac crest muscle pedicle graft to achieve an iliofemoral arthrodesis. The graft is secured with two screws. (Reproduced with permission from Davis JB: The muscle-pedicle bone graft in hip fusion. *J Bone Joint Surg Am* 1954;36:790-799.) **B,** Radiographic appearance of the "two-screw danger sign" suggesting anterior abductor mass deficiency. **C,** Subsequent postoperative anterior dislocation.

demonstrate the presence or absence of the abductors and the degree of atrophy (Fig. 2).

Many procedures have been used to perform hip arthrodesis, and the surgeon undertaking these conversions should have a sound understanding of the techniques that have been used, the different radiographic appearances, and the specialized equipment that may be needed to remove obsolete or unusual fixation hardware. Different techniques may substantially alter the anatomy of the hip, affecting the technical aspects of a THA. The position of any internal fixation implant should accurately be established to facilitate planning of the surgical approaches. The surgeon must understand the difference between a surgical ankylosis in childhood versus a spontaneous ankylosis in adulthood with reference to distortion of anatomy and leg-length discrepancy, as well as sciatic nerve length and mobility (Fig. 4).

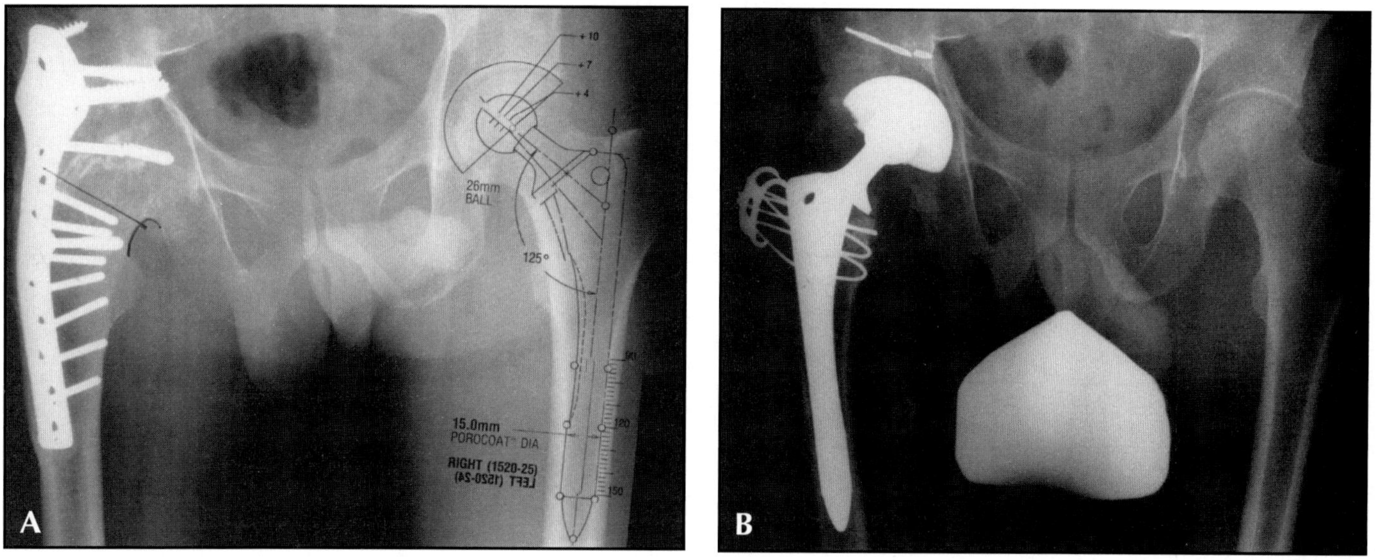

Fig. 6 A, A screw hole can be used to guide the location and line of the femoral neck osteotomy. The "pubofemoral arch" can also be used to guide the femoral cut. If the anatomy is not distorted, the opposite side may be used to template the size of the components. **B,** Postoperative radiograph.

The surgeon should specifically be alerted to the radiographic appearance of anterior extra-articular screw fixation, the "two-screw danger sign." This pattern of fixation was used in the Thompson[13] and Davis[29] techniques of hip arthrodesis as a means of securing a substantial anterior iliac crest bone graft, with the attached abductors, across the hip joint. This commonly led to substantial anterior abductor deficiency and to risk of postoperative instability (Fig. 5).

Several landmarks can be identified on the preoperative radiographs that will facilitate the conversion of the distorted anatomy of an arthrodesis to a correctly orientated hip arthroplasty. An assessment of the size and position of the greater trochanter if present may provide initial orientation. If an implant such as a cobra plate is present, the screw holes provide useful landmarks for the location of the osteotomy. The inferior arch of the neck or pubofemoral arch is also useful in guiding the femoral neck osteotomy (Fig. 6).

If the arthrodesis occurred in adult years, the opposite side usually is normal and may be templated to assess the optimum implant sizes. The templates should then be checked on the arthrodesed side to ensure that the distorted anatomy will accommodate them and that an offset sufficient to prevent impingement has been chosen (Fig. 6).

Surgical Technique

The authors operate with the patient in the lateral decubitus position. A lateral incision that curves posteriorly by 20° in its proximal half is preferred, but will be dictated by previous incisions, the surgical plan, and the location of internal fixation implants. Intraoperative fluoroscopy may be necessary to help locate the implants. In addition, the surgeon should have available a wide variety of screwdrivers and metal cutters to help remove various internal fixation devices. Separate attention needs to be given to extra-articular bridges of bone seen in various types of arthrodesis, such as the Brittain procedure (Fig. 7).

If the greater trochanter is present, a trochanteric osteotomy with gentle elevation and proximal retraction of the abductors provides optimal exposure and prevents further violation of the abductors. Care must be taken to preserve the superior gluteal bundle. After clearance of the soft tissue overlying the arthrodesis, an in situ osteotomy of the femoral neck is performed; its location is based on the preoperative plan (Figs. 6, *A* and 8). Further soft-tissue release of the proximal femur will improve exposure.

Acetabular preparation begins at the center of the cut surface of the femoral neck if this is in keeping with the preoperative plan. The teardrop is not easily located because it is buried beneath bone. However, its location can be estimated by locating the superior rim of the obturator foramen (Fig. 9). The acetabulum is carefully deepened medially and expanded with sequential reamers, paying close attention to the thickness of the anterior and posterior columns throughout. Even in cases with apparently normal anatomy, errors in cup placement are easily made. It is therefore recommended that an intraoperative AP radiograph be obtained

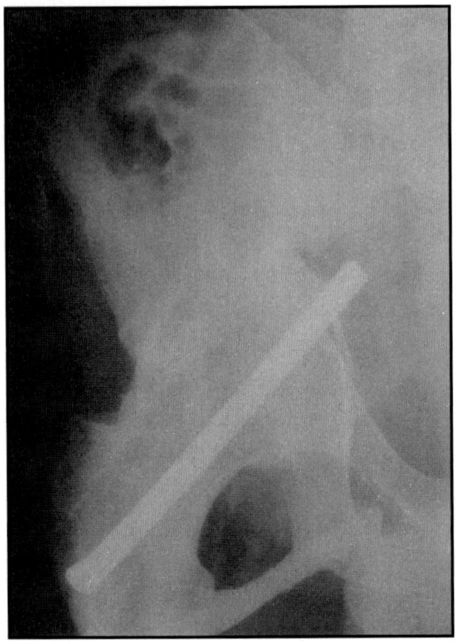

Fig. 7 In the Brittain procedure, the ischiofemoral bridge needs to be taken down as well.

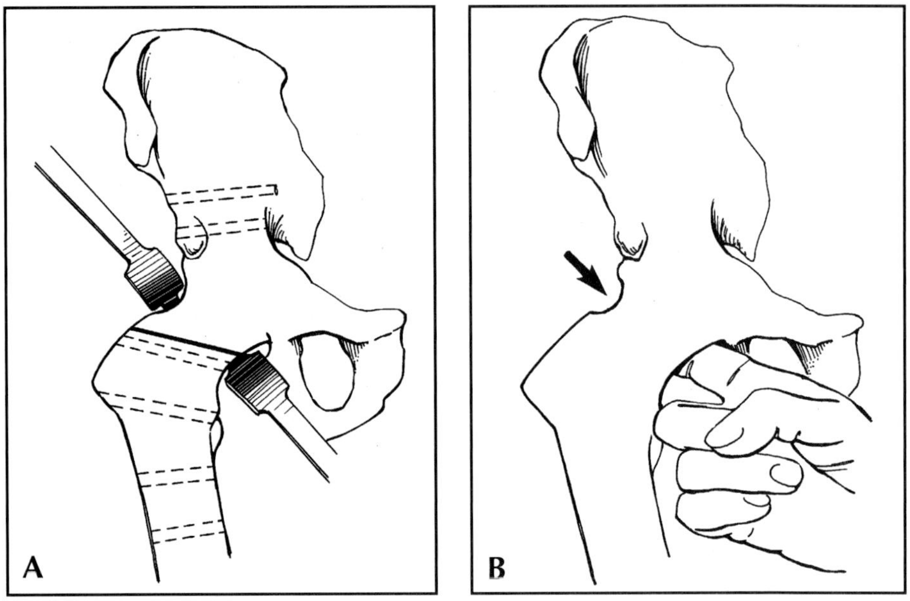

Fig. 8 Intraoperatively, the surgeon may use the screw holes of the implant to help determine the femoral neck osteotomy (**A**). Similarly, the pubofemoral arch may be palpated to aid in finding useful landmarks (**B**).

with a reamer in situ and its relationship to the so-called teardrop and other landmarks verified (Fig. 9). Failure to do so can result in poor cup placement or inadvertent reaming through the acetabular floor. We prefer to use an uncemented cup of appropriate size with supplemental screws if required.

Sufficient soft-tissue releases should be performed to adequately prepare the femur. The patient may require an iliopsoas tenotomy or other soft-tissue release if fixed deformity persists or if there is difficulty achieving the desired leg length. The femur is prepared according to the surgeon's usual technique for primary arthroplasty unless a previous femoral osteotomy requires modification of the technique, such as an intraoperative corrective osteotomy.

It is wise to locate the sciatic nerve early, to protect it during the procedure and to ensure it still is mobile after trial reduction of the joint when the knee is in extension. This is particularly important if lengthening the limb is intended. The greater trochanter should be reattached with wires, and if no trochanter is present, the gluteus medius and minimus can be sutured directly to the femur if they are not too retracted. If they are absent or extremely atrophic, the tensor fascia lata may be directly sutured to the greater trochanter.[30] The use of a cup that will capture the femoral head should be considered if there is a high risk of postoperative instability.

Postoperative Management

The patient should remain at partial weight bearing for 6 weeks postoperatively to allow adequate healing of the abductors. Although some authors suggest immobilization in a short, one-leg hip spica, we recommend that physiotherapy should begin immediately postoperatively, but without active abduction for the first 6 weeks. A hip brace is an attractive alternative to a hip spica if relative immobilization is desirable.

Routine antibiotics and thromboembolic prophylaxis should be used, and if the arthrodesis had occurred spontaneously or was associated with marked heterotopic ossification, consideration should be given to the use of radiation therapy or anti-inflammatories to minimize the risk of recurrence.

Outcomes of Conversion of Hip Arthrodesis

Several studies have evaluated the outcomes of converting a hip arthrodesis to a THA.[2,20-22,25,26,28,31-34] The overall follow-up periods ranged from 1 to 16.5 years. Patients generally noticed an improvement in their pain, walking, and overall function.[28] Personal satisfaction ranged from 71.5% to 91%.[20,22] Strathy and Fitzgerald[34] evaluated 80 THAs with a follow-up of 9 to 15 years using the Mayo Clinic hip score and found that 45% of patients (36 of 80) had good to excellent results while an additional 17.5% (14 of 80) were rated as fair.

Back pain is a common complaint several years after hip arthrodesis. Overall, 73% to 92% of patients found that a conversion procedure completely relieved their back discomfort.[2,21,22,26,28] Ipsilateral knee pain was substantially improved in 33% to 100% of patients.[2,21,22,28] Lubahn and associates[2] reviewed 17 patients and found that 70% experienced relief of their contralateral hip pain. Brewster and associates[25] found an overall relief of back, ipsilateral knee, and contralateral hip pain in 31 of 33 patients. Similarly, Perugia and associates[20] found that 85% of their patients (16 of 21) noticed relief of pain in other joints after conversion THA.

As would be expected, the range of motion after conversion of an arthrodesis to a THA is less than with a primary THA. Amstutz and Sakai[28] found a mean of 78° of flexion (range 45° to 125°) with a 54° (range 15° to 95°) arc of rotation and 7.5° flexion deformity. Similarly, Kilgus and associates[22] reported an average of 87° (range 25° to 135°) of flexion with 48° arc of abduction-adduction and a rotational arc of 46°. A persistent fixed flexion deformity was seen postoperatively by Lubahn and associates[2] in 7 of 18 patients with a measured average of 18° (range 5° to 30°). A similar average flexion range has been seen in other studies. The range of movement obtained may be reduced when the original arthrodesis is secondary to hip sepsis. Perugia and associates[20] in their study of 21 hips reported an average range of motion of 80% of normal in their noninfected cases, but this dropped to 55% to 60% of normal in patients who had an original arthrodesis secondary to infection. Similarly, Hardinge and associates[21] found that the least gain in range of motion was seen in patients with spontaneous fusion due to infection.

Postoperatively, a substantial number of patients may continue to limp. In one study[20] 38% of patients (8 of 21) limped while the remainder of patients required no walking aids 1 year postoperatively. Kilgus and associates[22] showed that 5 of 41 patients required more walking support while 12 of 41 required fewer supports after conversion THA. Almost 85% of patients described by Brewster and associates[25] required no walking aids 1 year postoperatively. However, in a recent study, Reikerås and associates[33] demonstrated that while no patient required a walking aid preoperatively, 74% (34 of 46) required some walking support after the conversion procedure. A positive Trendelenburg sign has been found in 34% to 69% of patients.[22,28] When the abductor lever arm is not restored adequately, there is a higher risk of a positive sign.[22,28] However, the strength of the abductors can continue to improve for months to even years after the surgery.[20,22]

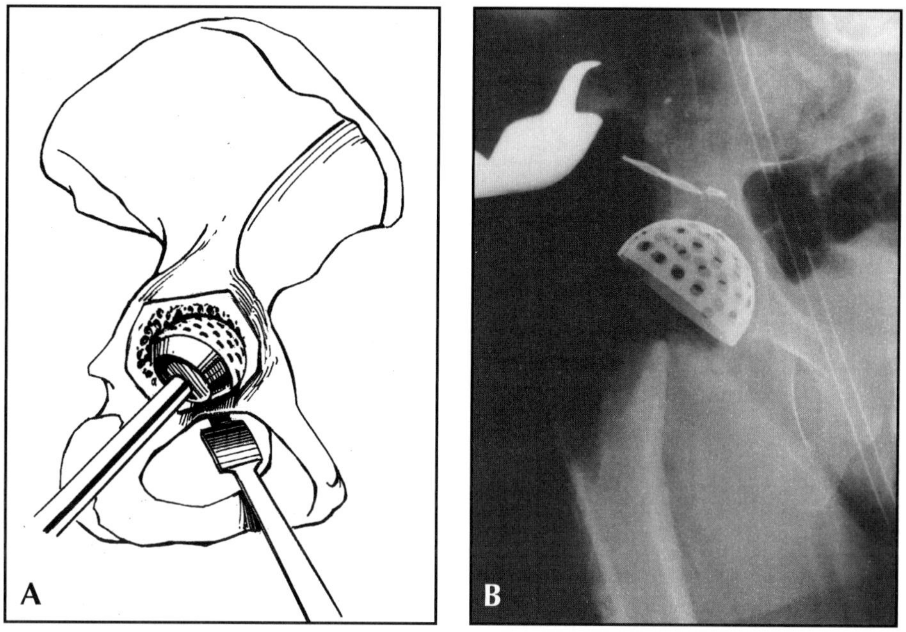

Fig. 9 A, The reaming begins in the inferior portion of the acetabulum at the level of the teardrop. This can be identified by the superior rim of the obturator foramen. **B,** Intraoperatively, a radiograph should be obtained to confirm starting position of the reamer.

After a hip arthrodesis patients usually have a leg-length discrepancy with the side of the fusion generally the shorter of the two. Several studies have shown a substantial improvement in leg-length inequality after conversion to a THA. Kilgus and associates[22] saw an improvement from a mean preoperative leg-length discrepancy of 3.9 cm to 1.4 cm postoperatively. Similarly, Hardinge and associates[21] found an improvement from 2.9 cm to 0.6 cm, and Amstutz and associates[28] reported an improvement in mean leg-length discrepancy of 1.1 cm (3.3 to 2.2 cm). Overall, these studies show a 33% to 79% improvement in leg-length discrepancy.

Although converting a hip arthrodesis to a THA has been shown to improve local pain, function, discomfort in other joints, range of motion, and leg-length discrepancy, there are a number of complications associated with this procedure. There is a higher failure rate of the procedure compared to primary THA. Strathy and associates[34] documented a failure rate of 26% (21 of 80 patients) with a follow-up of 9 to 15 years. These patients included 9 with infection and 12 requiring revision for loosening or dislocation. Twenty of these poor results were seen in patients who had undergone a surgical ankylosis. An increased failure rate was also seen in those undergoing conversion THA when younger than 50 years of age. Overall, conversion THAs in 10 of 26 patients (36%) younger than 50 years old with a surgical ankylosis were successful compared to a 62% (21 of 34) success rate in those older than 50 years. A younger age and prior history of surgical fusion were also found to be risk factors for failure of conversion THA by Kilgus and associates.[22] These authors also concluded that a higher failure rate occurs in patients who have undergone two or more prior operations or in those with a history of injury. Their overall failure rate was 22% (9 of 41). Kreder and associates[32] recently reviewed 40 patients who had undergone a conversion procedure and found substantial morbidity. Within 4 years, there was a 10% revision rate while 5% of patients underwent resection arthroplasty.

As with primary hip replacement, aseptic loosening is the most common mode of failure. The infection rate after conversion to a THA has ranged from 1.8% to 12%.[21,22,25,28,32,34] Other complications have included deep vein thrombosis/pulmonary embolism, dislocation, sciatic nerve palsy, greater trochanter detachment, and heterotopic ossification.

Summary

With the predictably good outcome now found with THA, hip arthrodesis has limited indications today. The procedure still has a role in the case of the young, heavy demand male with an isolated arthritic hip condition, and developments such as the Cobra head plate have considerably improved success rates. However, a long-term hip arthrodesis can have profound effects on a patient's daily function and activities of daily living. In addition, gait pattern is considerably affected as well as other joints such as the lower back, ipsilateral knee, and contralateral hip.

Many patients with a hip arthrodesis will eventually require a takedown of the fused hip and conversion to a THA. The primary indications include fusion in malposition, pseudarthrosis, or severe pain in other joints. The surgeon undertaking such a task must be familiar with the arthrodesis techniques that have been used in the past as well as the equipment that may be required to extract the fixation hardware. Clinical assessment with particular attention to leg-length discrepancy, position of the arthrodesis, and function of the abductors is of paramount importance. The surgeon must carefully review preoperative radiographs to plan the procedure. The surgeon must also be aware of the presence of pathology in other joints.

After takedown of a hip arthrodesis and conversion to a THA, patients cannot expect the result to equal the success rates of primary THA. Patients generally can expect an improvement in function and mobility. Back pain and ipsilateral knee pain are usually improved postoperatively, but the effect on contralateral hip pain is less predictable. Many patients will continue to show a positive Trendelenburg sign, but further improvement in strength of the hip abductors can be expected with time. Leg-length discrepancy is generally improved substantially after THA. However, a substantial number of patients will require a walking aid postoperatively.

Overall, the risk of complications and the rates of revision after converting an arthrodesed hip to a THA are quite high. The procedure can be complex. Consideration should be given to referring these patients to a specialized center under the care of an experienced arthroplasty surgeon if preoperative planning suggests that the conversion will not be straightforward.

References

1. Lipscomb PR, McCaslin FE Jr: Arthrodesis of the hip: Review of 371 cases. *J Bone Joint Surg Am* 1961;43:923-938.
2. Lubahn JD, Evarts CM, Feltner JB: Conversion of ankylosed hips to total hip arthroplasty. *Clin Orthop* 1980;153:146-152.
3. Barmada R, Abraham E, Ray RD: Hip fusion utilizing the cobra head plate. *J Bone Joint Surg Am* 1976;58:541-544.
4. Barnhardt T, Stiehl JB: Hip fusion in young adults. *Orthopedics* 1996;19:303-306.
5. Benaroch TE, Richards BS, Haideri N, Smith C: Intermediate follow-up of a simple method of hip arthrodesis in adolescent patients. *J Pediatr Orthop* 1996;16:30-36.
6. Brien WW, Golz RJ, Kuschner SH, Brien EW, Wiss DA: Hip joint arthrodesis utilizing anterior compression plate fixation. *J Arthroplasty* 1994;9:171-176.
7. Roberts CS, Fetto JF: Functional outcome of hip fusion in the young patient: Follow-up study of 10 patients. *J Arthroplasty* 1990;5:89-96.
8. Schneider R: Hip arthrodesis with the cobra head plate and pelvic osteotomy. *Reconstr Surg Traumatol* 1974;14:1-37.
9. Carter PJ, Wickstrom J: Arthrodesis of the hip: An assessment of results in one hundred patients. *South Med J* 1971;64:451-458.
10. Stewart MJ, Coker TP Jr: Arthrodesis of the hip: A review of 109 patients. *Clin Orthop* 1969;62:136-150.
11. Stinchfield FE, Cavallaro WU: Arthrodesis of the hip joint: A follow-up study. *J Bone Joint Surg Am* 1950;32:48-58.
12. Lam SJ: Arthrodesis of the hip: With special reference to early mobilisation without external splintage. *J Bone Joint Surg Br* 1968;50:14-23.
13. Thompson FR: Combined hip fusion and subtrochanteric osteotomy allowing early ambulation. *J Bone Joint Surg Am* 1956;38:13-22.
14. Watson-Jones R, Robinson WC: Arthrodesis of the osteoarthritic hip joint. *J Bone Joint Surg Br* 1956;38:353-377.
15. Duncan CP, Spangehl M, Beauchamp C, McGraw R: Hip arthrodesis: An important option for advanced disease in the young adult. *Can J Surg* 1995;38(suppl 1):S39-S45.
16. Murrell GA, Fitch RD: Hip fusion in young adults: Using a medial displacement osteotomy and cobra plate. *Clin Orthop* 1994;300:147-154.
17. Callaghan JJ, Brand RA, Pedersen DR: Hip arthrodesis: A long-term follow-up. *J Bone Joint Surg Am* 1985;67:1328-1335.
18. Sofue M, Kono S, Kawaji W, Homma M: Long term results of arthrodesis for severe osteoarthritis of the hip in young adults. *Int Orthop* 1989;13:129-133.
19. Sponseller PD, McBeath AA, Perpich M: Hip arthrodesis in young patients: A long-term follow-up study. *J Bone Joint Surg Am* 1984;66:853-859.
20. Perugia L, Santori FS, Mancini A, Manili M, Falez F: Conversion of the arthrodesed hip to a total hip arthroplasty: Indications and limitations. *Ital J Orthop Traumatol* 1992;18:145-153.
21. Hardinge K, Williams D, Etienne A, MacKenzie D, Charnley J. Conversion of fused hips to low friction arthroplasty. *J Bone Joint Surg Br* 1977;59:385-392.
22. Kilgus DJ, Amstutz HC, Wolgin MA, Dorey FJ: Joint replacement for ankylosed hips. *J Bone Joint Surg Am* 1990;72:45-54.
23. Gore DR, Murray MP, Sepic SB, Gardner GM: Walking patterns of men with unilateral surgical hip fusion. *J Bone Joint Surg Am* 1975;57:759-765.

24. Waters RL, Barnes G, Husserl T, Silver L, Liss R: Comparable energy expenditure after arthrodesis of the hip and ankle. *J Bone Joint Surg Am* 1988;70:1032-1037.

25. Brewster RC, Coventry MB, Johnson EW Jr: Conversion of the arthrodesed hip to a total hip arthroplasty. *J Bone Joint Surg Am* 1975;57:27-30.

26. Hardinge K, Murphy JC, Frenyo S: Conversion of hip fusion to Charnley low-friction arthroplasty. *Clin Orthop* 1986;211:173-179.

27. Spangehl MJ, Younger AS, Masri BA, Duncan CP: Diagnosis of infection following total hip arthroplasty. *J Bone Joint Surg Am* 1997;79:1578-1588.

28. Amstutz HC, Sakai DN: Total joint replacement for ankylosed hips: Indications, technique, and preliminary results. *J Bone Joint Surg Am* 1975;57:619-625.

29. Davis JB: The muscle-pedicle bone graft in hip fusion. *J Bone Joint Surg Am* 1954;36:790-799.

30. Besser MI: A muscle transfer to replace absent abductors in the conversion of a fused hip to a total hip arthroplasty. *Clin Orthop* 1982;162:173-174.

31. Kempf I, Jenny JY: Total prosthesis after ankylosis of the hip joint: Report of 22 cases. *Int Orthop* 1991;15:239-243.

32. Kreder HJ, Williams JI, Jaglal S, Axcell T, Stephen D: A population study in the Province of Ontario of the complications after conversion of hip or knee arthrodesis to total joint replacement. *Can J Surg* 1999;42:433-439.

33. Reikerås O, Bjerkreim I, Gundersson R: Total hip arthroplasty for arthrodesed hips: 5- to 13-year results. *J Arthroplasty* 1995;10:529-531.

34. Strathy GM, Fitzgerald RH Jr: Total hip arthroplasty in the ankylosed hip: A ten-year follow-up. *J Bone Joint Surg Am* 1988;70:963-966.

32

Total Hip Replacement for the Dislocated Hip

Greg Jaroszynski, MD, FRCSC
Ian G. Woodgate, FRACS
Khaled J. Saleh, MD, MSc, FRCSC
Allan E. Gross, MD, FRCSC

Total hip replacement for the patient with a dysplastic hip is difficult. Certain problems that are encountered during total hip replacement are more pronounced when the hip is completely dislocated. The classification that we find most practical is that of Hartofilakidis and associates.[1] Type 1 hips are those with dysplasia, in which the femoral head is still within the true acetabulum (Fig. 1). Type 2 hips are those with low dislocation, in which the femoral head is in a false acetabulum, the inferior lip of which is in contact with or overlaps the true acetabulum (Fig. 2). Type 3 hips are those with high dislocation, in which the false acetabulum has no contact with the true acetabulum (Fig. 3). This classification corresponds with the Crowe classification as follows:[2] type 1 hips (dysplasia) correspond with Crowe type I and II hips, type 2 hips (low dislocation) correspond with Crowe type III hips, and type 3 hips (high dislocation) correspond with Crowe type IV hips. Type 2 hips (low dislocation) and type 3 hips (high dislocation) present the surgeon with certain technical problems that must be addressed during the planning and implementation of total hip replacement. These problems are related to limb-length discrepancy, placement and coverage of the cup, the need for small femoral and acetabular components, and the surgical technique.

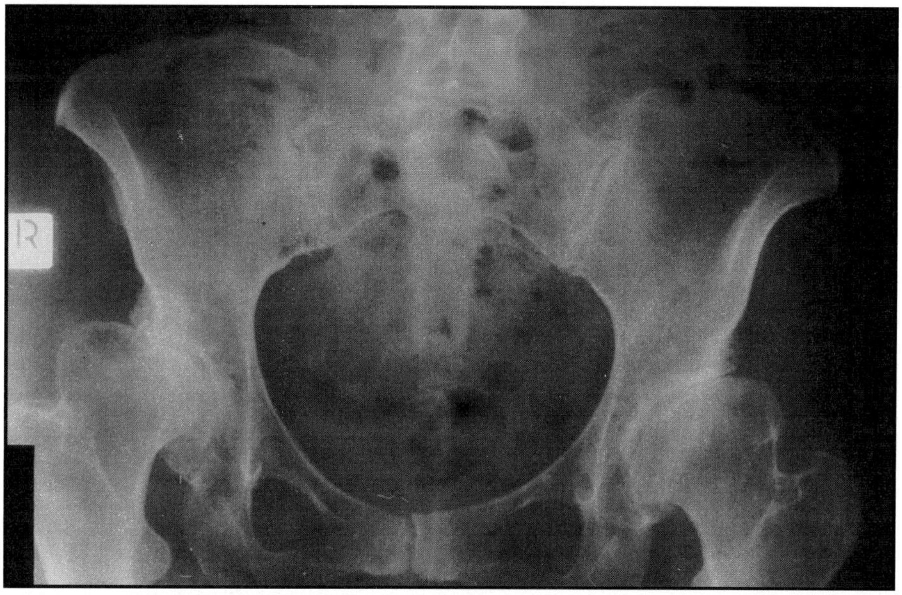

Fig. 1 Anteroposterior (AP) radiograph of the pelvis of a 43-year-old woman who had bilateral dysplasia of the hip (type 1 disease). The acetabula are shallow, and the femoral heads are poorly covered but are still within the true acetabula.

Limb-Length Discrepancy

Dealing with limb-length discrepancy is an important part of the surgical treatment of unilateral type 2 (low) and type 3 (high) dislocation. In comparison with the usual population of patients who are managed with total hip replacement, these patients are younger, tend not to use external walking aids or shoe lifts, and are predominantly female. In the experience of the senior author (A.G.), these patients consider limb-length discrepancy to be one of the reasons for having the surgery, and this aspect of the overall problem should not be minimized by the surgeon. The limb is lengthened by lowering the acetabulum back to or nearer to its anatomic position or by inserting a femoral component that is longer than the length of femoral bone that is removed.

The limb can be lengthened at the time of surgery by as much as 4 cm.[3] The sciatic nerve must be carefully monitored. In all cases in which the limb is to be lengthened by more than 2 cm, we

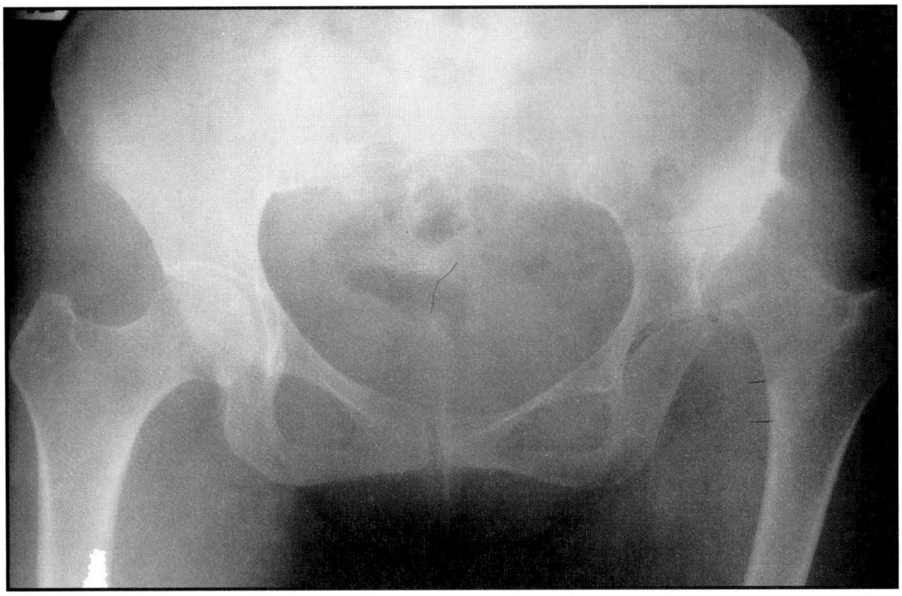

Fig. 2 AP radiograph of the pelvis of a 50-year-old woman who had a low dislocation of the left hip (type 2 disease). The floor of the false acetabulum is in contact with the roof of the true acetabulum.

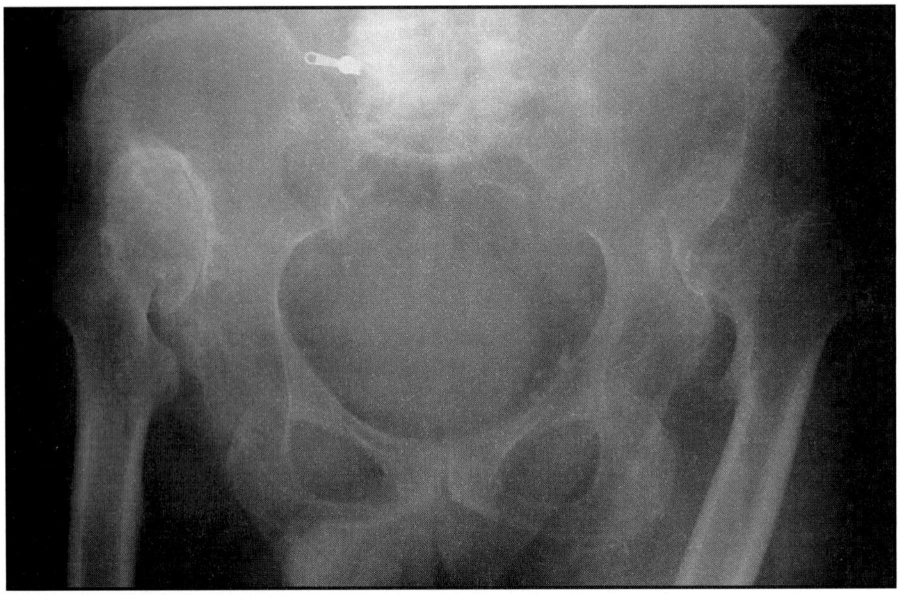

Fig. 3 AP radiograph of the pelvis of a 60-year-old man who had bilateral high dislocation (type 3 disease). There is no contact between the true and false acetabula.

identify the nerve in order to check its tension after reduction of the trial components. Excessive dissection of the nerve should be avoided because of the danger of devascularization, but the nerve must be visualized and palpated. The trial reduction should be carried out with the knee flexed, and the tension in the nerve is then evaluated as the knee is gradually extended. Experience in evaluating nerve tension is invaluable, and a wake-up test is, at least early in one's experience, safer and more reassuring. The senior author performs a wake-up test only when there is some question about the degree of tension in the nerve. If the surgeon anticipates the performance of a wake-up test, both the anesthesiologist and the patient must be informed prior to the induction of anesthesia. During the wake-up test, the patient is instructed to dorsiflex his or her toes on command (dorsiflexion is considered to be more sensitive than plantar flexion). If the patient has been previously instructed to do this, he or she responds with less lightening of the anesthetic. Another method for the evaluation of the sciatic nerve is monitoring of somatosensory-evoked potentials.[4] This method requires additional resources, may be too sensitive, and should be reserved for centers at which a high volume of complex hip operations are performed.

In our experience, the femoral nerve also may be damaged by excessive lengthening. This nerve is not monitored intraoperatively, but it should be evaluated postoperatively along with the sciatic nerve. If there is a femoral nerve palsy, the patient should be positioned in bed with the hip flexed to about 70° in order to relax the femoral nerve. If both the femoral nerve and the sciatic nerve are damaged by stretch, then the patient should be positioned with the hip flexed to relax the femoral nerve and the knee flexed to relax the sciatic nerve.

If there is excessive sciatic nerve tension when a trial reduction is done, the limb has been lengthened too much. It must be shortened by reconstruction of the acetabulum at a higher level or by shortening of the femur. Femoral shortening can be carried out by means of a subtrochanteric osteotomy[5,6] (Fig. 4) or by resection of more bone from the proximal part of the femur.

A subtrochanteric shortening osteotomy is associated with the potential problem of nonunion. A long stem or a modular stem may be necessary to provide stable fixation of the osteotomy site. A step-cut, oblique, or chevron

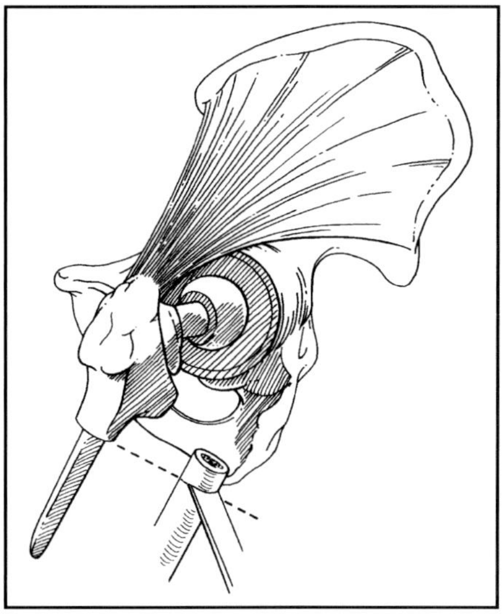

Fig. 4 Illustration of a subtrochanteric osteotomy. A segment of bone can be resected to allow femoral shortening if reduction is difficult or if the nerve is under too much tension, or both. If necessary, the femur can be derotated to neutralize excessive anteversion. The osteotomy site is stabilized by the stem or, if necessary, with a short plate or cortical strut. (© C. Chang, 2000)

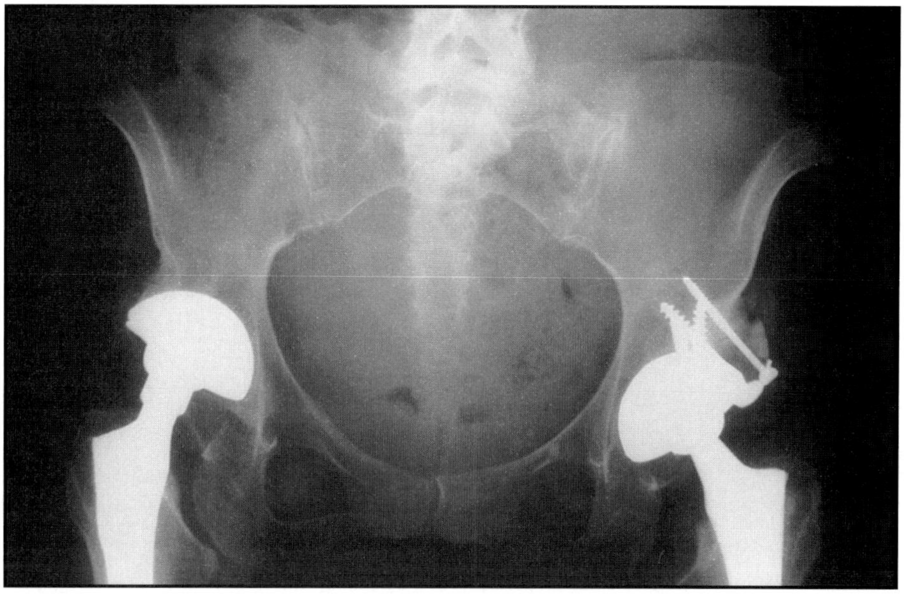

Fig. 5 AP radiograph of the pelvis of a 50-year-old woman, obtained 7 years after replacement of the right hip with use of an uncemented cup in a high position, with restoration of length with use of a long-neck femoral component. The left hip had been reconstructed 3 years previously with an uncemented cup and a shelf autograft at the correct anatomic level. (Figure 1 is the preoperative radiograph of this patient.)

osteotomy can be used to obtain rotational stability, or cortical struts or a plate can be used to stabilize the osteotomy site. Cortical struts or a plate are particularly useful when an uncemented femoral component is used.[5,6] We prefer to use cortical struts or a plate to stabilize the site of a transverse osteotomy because this allows for easier adjustment of the version. A step-cut, oblique, or chevron osteotomy is technically difficult and requires adjusting the version while allowing for the configuration of the osteotomy. Shortening by resection of more proximal femoral bone avoids the problems associated with osteotomy but involves the resection of metaphyseal bone, which is needed for stabilization of the implant and osseous ingrowth.

Placement and Coverage of the Cup

Placement of the cup depends on the amount of available bone stock and the magnitude of the limb-length discrepancy. The cup can be placed at the correct or nearly-correct level with or without a bone graft. The other options are placement of the cup at a high hip center[7,8] and centralization of the cup.[1,9] Both of these techniques avoid the use of a structural graft. The advantage of a high hip center as advocated by Harris is that the surgeon can place a small uncemented cup into live host bone and avoid the disadvantages associated with the use of structural autograft.[7,8] This method is also technically easier. The disadvantages of a high hip center are that there is a higher rate of component loosening,[10,11] there is a potentially higher rate of dislocation because of impingement against the ischium, and a smaller cup with less polyethylene is usually used. Limb-lengthening is possible but must be done on the femoral side. In addition, further surgery may be difficult because bone stock has not been restored. However, a high hip center is indicated when there is adequate bone stock with a minimal-to-moderate limb-length discrepancy of 2 to 3 cm and the cup is not placed so high that lengthening of more than 3 cm is necessary on the femoral side (Fig. 5). Lengthening of more than this amount on the femoral side can cause impingement of the femoral neck against the ischium and potential dislocation.

Centralization of the socket in order to obtain coverage of the cup without a graft may be achieved by reaming to the inner cortex of the ilium and placing a small cup in a protruded position[9] (Fig. 6) or by creating a controlled comminuted fracture of the medial wall (cotyloplasty) in order to allow for medial advancement of the socket.[1] The use of an oblong socket also has been advocated to restore the hip center without the use of structural graft.[12]

The practice of the senior author is to place the cup at the correct or nearly correct anatomic level, and, if it has less than 70% coverage by host bone, to use a shelf autograft (Fig. 7).

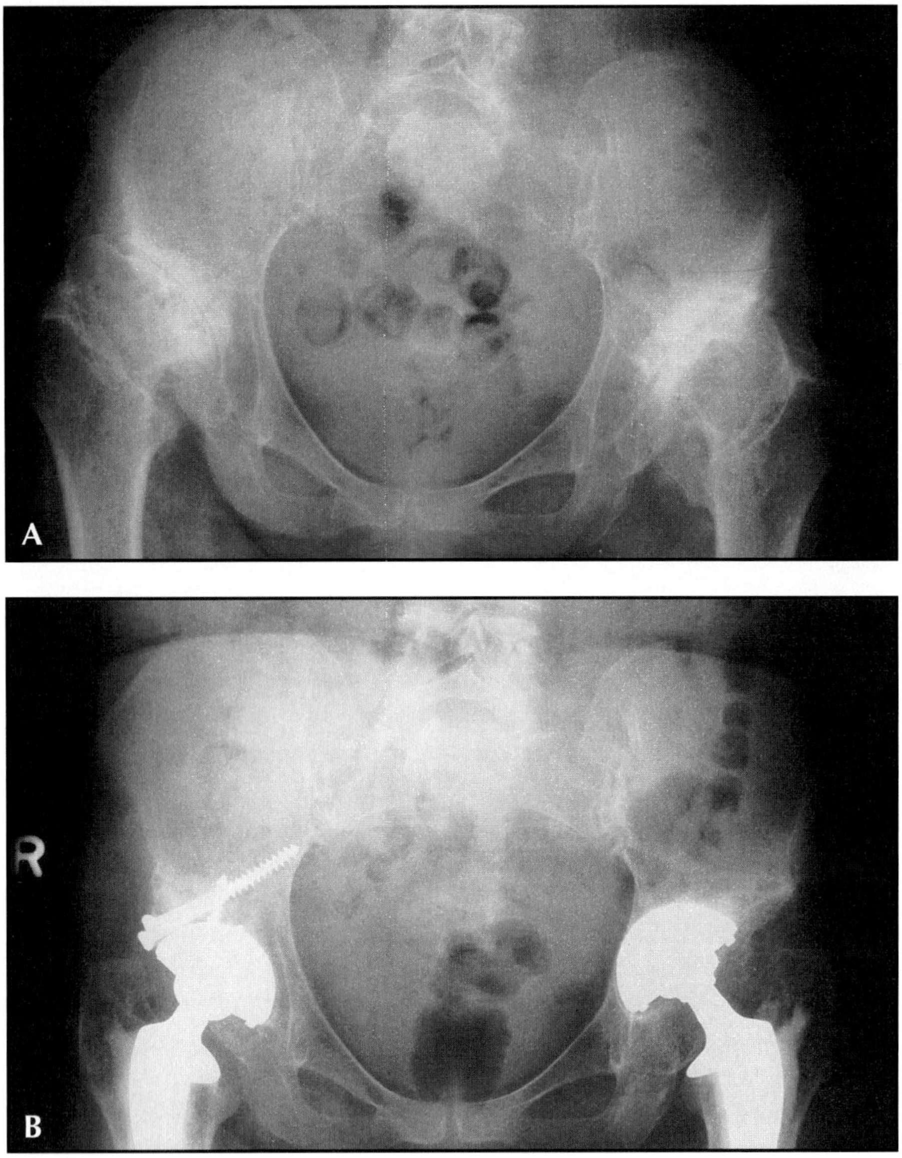

Fig. 6 A, AP radiograph of the pelvis of a 50-year-old woman who had bilateral dysplasia of the hip and secondary osteoarthritis. **B,** AP radiograph of the pelvis, obtained 4 years after reconstruction of the left hip with centralization of an uncemented cup. The cup is in a protruded position. The right hip was reconstructed with an uncemented cup and a shelf autograft.

Components

Special components should be available during the surgical treatment of a dysplastic hip. The cup should have an inner diameter of 22 or 26 mm and can be cemented or uncemented. Cups with an outer diameter of as small as 36 mm should be available; however, the larger the diameter of the cup, the thicker the polyethylene, which is an advantage in these young patients. The surgeon must achieve a balance between cup diameter and cup coverage. The femoral component must be small and should have a straight stem in order to accommodate the anteversion. Stems with a distal diameter of between 5 and 10 mm, or modular stems, should be available.

Surgical Technique

Prior to surgery, an accurate clinical and radiographic measurement of leg length is important. If the patient has a fixed pelvic obliquity, then the apparent leg length (as measured from the umbilicus to the medial malleolus) should be used to determine the amount of lengthening that is necessary. The surgeon should decide on the level of the cup and template it at that level on the radiograph. The surgeon should note how much of the cup is uncovered and anticipate whether or not a bone graft is going to be necessary. The final decision, however, will depend on the intraoperative findings. Templates can be used to determine the level of the neck cut, but the cut usually is made at the level of the lesser trochanter because of the problem of excessive anteversion if the cut is made more proximally.

Surgical Approach

Type 1 hips (dysplasia) can be approached through a conventional posterior[13] or lateral[14] approach without disturbing the greater trochanter, unless the trochanter is riding high due to previous osteonecrosis of the femoral head. Under those circumstances, the surgeon may elect to perform a trochanteric osteotomy in order to advance the greater trochanter distally. Type 2 hips (low dislocation) and type 3 hips (high dislocation) may require a more elaborate approach in order to obtain extensive pelvic exposure and to advance the greater trochanter if indicated. A trochanteric osteotomy provides excellent pelvic exposure. This allows the surgeon to identify the false and true acetabula and, if necessary, to reconstruct the acetabulum with a bone graft. A trochanteric osteotomy also allows for lengthening of the extremity. A transverse osteotomy in which the vastus lateralis is dissected off the greater trochanter offers the best pelvic exposure but carries the risk of nonunion and, even more importantly, of trochanteric

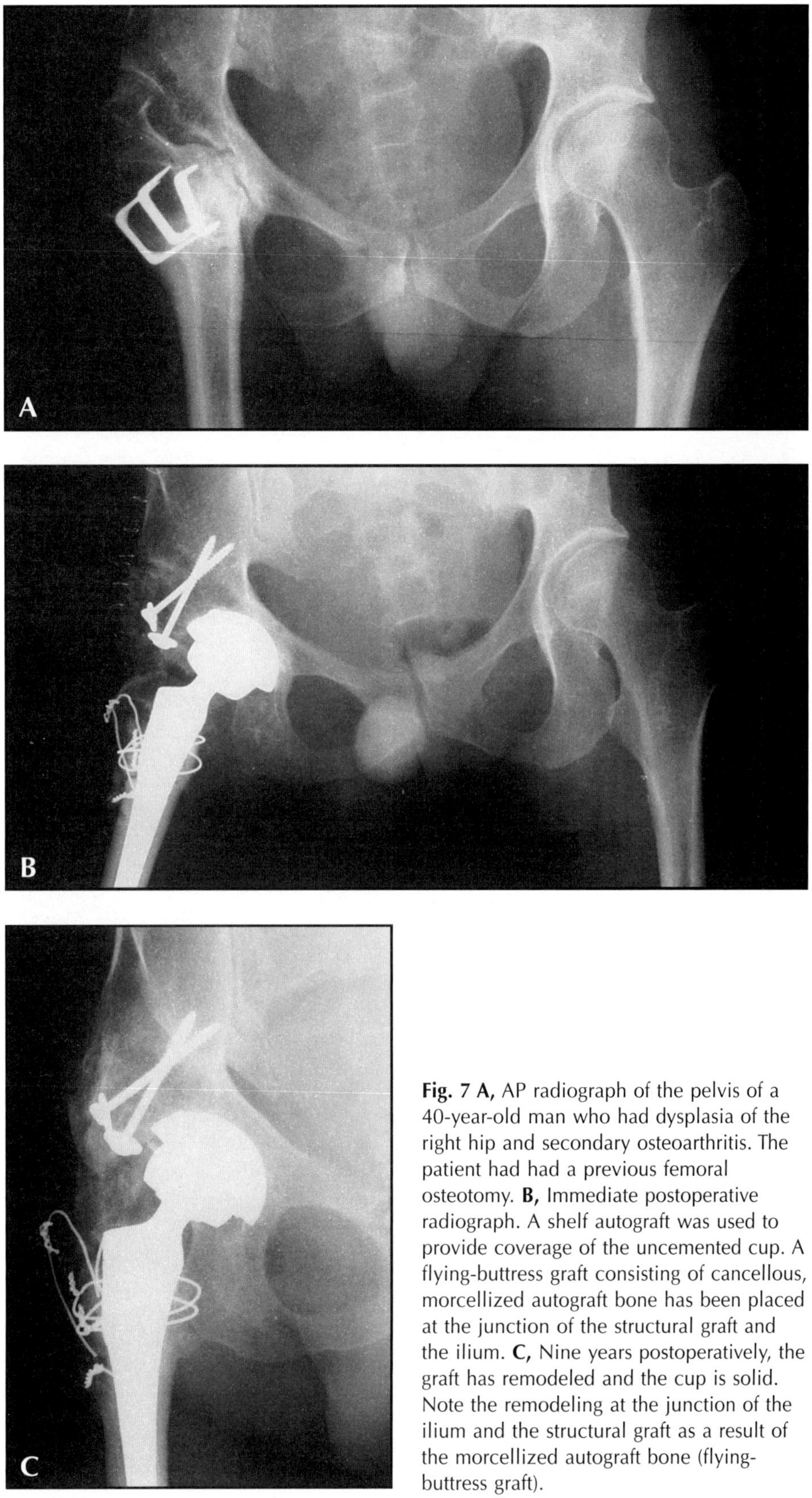

Fig. 7 A, AP radiograph of the pelvis of a 40-year-old man who had dysplasia of the right hip and secondary osteoarthritis. The patient had had a previous femoral osteotomy. **B,** Immediate postoperative radiograph. A shelf autograft was used to provide coverage of the uncemented cup. A flying-buttress graft consisting of cancellous, morcellized autograft bone has been placed at the junction of the structural graft and the ilium. **C,** Nine years postoperatively, the graft has remodeled and the cup is solid. Note the remodeling at the junction of the ilium and the structural graft as a result of the morcellized autograft bone (flying-buttress graft).

migration.[15] A trochanteric slide osteotomy retains the attachment of the vastus lateralis, which protects against trochanteric migration[15,16] (Fig. 8). A trochanteric slide is our preferred approach if a grafting procedure or lengthening of more than 3 cm is anticipated. If the leg is lengthened, it is necessary to keep the trochanteric fragment long in order to ensure bone-to-bone apposition for healing.

A subtrochanteric osteotomy that is performed for femoral shortening and derotation can also be used for exposure, allowing preservation of the greater trochanter while still providing good pelvic exposure for bone-grafting[5,6] (Fig. 4). If a trochanteric osteotomy has already been performed, special care is needed to preserve the blood supply and muscular attachments to the femur proximal to the subtrochanteric osteotomy.

The sciatic nerve is identified after the approach has been completed, the hip has been dislocated, and the level of the true acetabulum has been identified. The nerve is most easily found distal to the true acetabulum in the fat deep to the gluteus maximus, just proximal to the tendon. The nerve is not dissected out because of the danger of devascularization, but it is visualized and not just palpated. If the hip is completely dislocated, identification of the nerve may be difficult because of the redundancy of the false capsule. Under these circumstances, it may be easier to find the nerve when the limb has been brought more out to length when the trial components are in place and the hip is reduced. If this technique is used, it is important to keep the knee flexed so that undue tension is not created in the nerve.

Acetabulum

It is important to identify the desired level for placement of the cup. The level of the true acetabulum can be identified

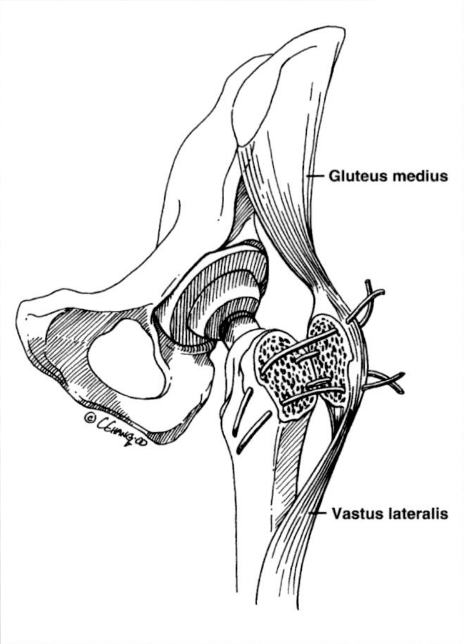

Fig. 8 Illustration of a trochanteric slide osteotomy. The abductors and the vasti are attached to the trochanteric fragment. The trochanter with the attached muscles is retracted anteriorly. Leaving the vastus lateralis attached to the trochanter prevents postoperative trochanteric migration. The traditional trochanteric osteotomy does not leave the vastus lateralis attached; although that method allows intraoperative proximal retraction of the trochanter and better pelvic exposure, it is associated with a higher risk of postoperative trochanteric migration. (© C. Chang, 2000)

with use of the obturator foramen as a landmark. If there is any doubt at all, a radiograph should be made before reaming is started. When reaming is started, the fovea can often be identified. After the level for placement of the cup has been identified, reaming should be started with use of very small reamers, usually 36 mm in diameter. A drill hole is made through the medial part of the acetabulum, and a depth-gauge is used to decide how deep to ream. The senior author stops reaming 0.5 to 1 cm from the inner cortex. A trial cup is then inserted, and, if less than 70% of the cup is covered, bone grafting is performed. The femoral head is used for the bone graft. The cartilage is reamed

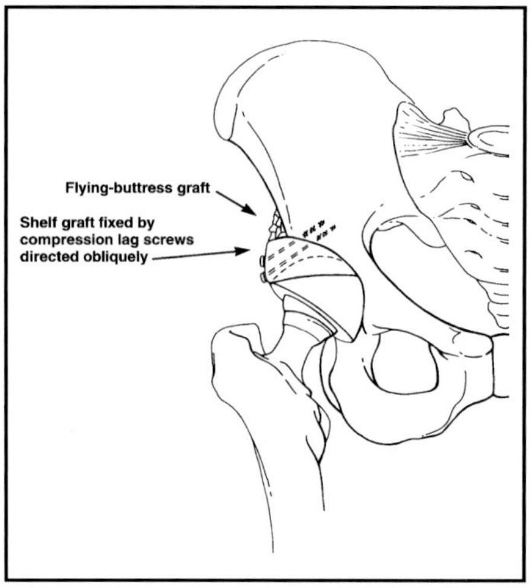

Fig. 9 Illustration of a shelf autograft fixed with two cancellous screws placed in a vertical-to-oblique direction. Note the flying-buttress graft consisting of morcellized autograft bone. (© C.Chang, 2000)

off, but the subchondral bone is kept intact. The graft is placed at the superior edge of the acetabulum or just inside it and is fixed with two cancellous screws, usually 4.5 mm in diameter. The screws are placed in an oblique-to-vertical direction. The cancellous surface of the graft should not be exposed to host soft tissue because this surface is more easily resorbed than the subchondral bone is. The cancellous surface should abut the cup. In addition, we place a flying-buttress graft consisting of cancellous, morcellized, autogenous bone between the top of the shelf graft and the ilium (Fig. 9). The ilium at the junction and just proximal to the shelf graft is roughened or perforated with multiple small drill holes to encourage union and remodeling.

Femur

On the femoral side, the predetermined neck cut is usually made at the level of the lesser trochanter. This is necessary because cutting the neck short decreases the degree of neck anteversion, allowing for easier insertion and fitting of the femoral component. Small reamers and broaches should be used, and the femoral component should have a straight and narrow stem.

Sciatic Nerve

If the limb is to be lengthened by more than 2 cm, the sciatic nerve is identified. Reduction of the hip with the trial components in place is carried out with the knee flexed. The knee is then gradually extended while the tension in the nerve is monitored. If the surgeon is still not sure about whether the nerve is being stretched too much, then a wake-up test must be performed. If the hip is too tight for reduction of the trial components, if the nerve is too tense, or if a wake-up test reveals sciatic nerve weakness, then the femur must be shortened. Proximal shortening of the femur or subtrochanteric osteotomy may be necessary.[5,6] It is our practice to shorten the femur proximally in order to avoid the technical difficulty and potential complications (such as nonunion) associated with a subtrochanteric osteotomy. Proximal shortening, however, should not be performed distal to the lesser trochanter because there will not be enough of a metaphyseal flare left to support the femoral implant. In addition, if a trochanteric approach has been used, trochanteric reattachment may be difficult. Under these circumstances, a subtrochanteric osteotomy should be used.

Results of Treatment

We reviewed the results of 67 total hip replacements that were performed with use of a shelf autograft in 58 patients (48 women and 10 men). The average age of the patients at the time of surgery was 52 years (range, 30 to 65 years), and the average duration of follow-up was 10 years (range, 5 to 17 years). Thirty-nine hips were classified as type 1 (dysplasia); 17 as type 2 (low dislocation); and 11 as type 3 (high dislocation). The acetabular components included 42 metal cups that were inserted without cement, 22 all-polyethylene cups that were inserted with cement, 2 all-polyethylene cups that were inserted without cement, and 1 bipolar prosthesis. On the femoral side, 51 stems were inserted without cement and 16 were inserted with cement. A transgluteal approach was used in 41 hips; a transtrochanteric approach (through a transverse trochanteric osteotomy) in 22; and a Smith-Petersen approach in 4. Fifty-four hips were reconstructed within 1 cm of the true hip center, and 13 were reconstructed more than 1 cm higher than the true hip center.

Four patients had a total of five incomplete nerve palsies (two sciatic and three femoral), all of which resolved completely. Four patients had a hip dislocation, and two of them required revision of the cup. Four patients had a trochanteric nonunion and escape, and one had a fibrous union.

Eleven (16%) of the 67 cups were revised (10 hips) or were awaiting revision (1 hip), and two others were radiographically loose but were asymptomatic. Three of the 10 acetabular revisions were performed because of nonunion at the site of the graft and 7, because of loosening of the cup. Three of the 10 acetabula that were revised required no further grafting, 4 required morcellized graft, and 3 required another structural graft. Four (6%) of the 67 femoral components were revised, and 2 others were radiographically loose but were asymptomatic. Overall, 13 (19%) of the 67 hips were revised (12 hips) or were awaiting revision (1 hip). Two hips had revision of both components.

Kaplan-Meier analysis revealed that the probability of survival at 14 years was 78% for the cups and 85% for the stems. The average duration of survival was 14.2 years (95% confidence interval, 12.6 to 15.9 years) for the cups and 15.3 years (95% confidence interval, 14.0 to 16.0 years) for the stems. Cox regression analysis was used to assess the influence of covariates (gender, age, type of prosthesis, degree of dysplasia, and vertical and horizontal placement of the hip center) on survivorship. Only the degree of dysplasia and the vertical displacement from the so-called true anatomic center had a significant effect on survivorship ($r = 0.29$, $P = 0.0095$). Survivorship was not affected by age, gender, or the use of cement. Seven (18%) of the 39 type 1 hips failed; the average duration of survival in this group was 15 years (95% confidence interval, 13.2 to 16.8 years). Three of the 17 type 2 hips failed; the average duration of survival in this group was 11.5 years (95% confidence interval, 9.4 to 13.5 years). Three of the 11 type 3 hips failed; the average duration of survival in this group was 10.1 years (95% confidence interval, 7.3 to 12.9 years).

Three hips (4%) had a nonunion at the site of the graft. All three required revision of the cup. One of these hips required another structural graft because of severe graft resorption, and the other two healed with screw fixation and placement of morcellized autograft at the site of the nonunion. Seven hips (10%) had resorption of more than one third of the graft; six of these hips had moderate resorption (resorption of one third to one half of the graft), and one had severe resorption (resorption of more than one half of the graft). Of the six hips that had moderate resorption, three had revision of the cup with no need for further structural grafting, one was awaiting revision of a loose cup, one was revised because of a loose femoral component, and one was asymptomatic with no loosening of the cup. The hip with severe resorption required revision of the cup with insertion of a new structural graft, as mentioned above. One other hip required insertion of another structural graft following displacement of the original graft as a result of a dislocation in the early postoperative period.

Discussion

Total hip replacement is more difficult for dislocated (type 2 and type 3) hips than it is for subluxated (type 1) hips. Exposure of the false and true acetabula and identification of the sciatic nerve requires experience and a good surgical approach. In patients with unilateral involvement, the limb-length discrepancy is more severe. Placement of the cup at the correct anatomic level is difficult and may require femoral shortening. This can be accomplished by resecting more femoral bone proximally or by performing a subtrochanteric osteotomy. Coverage of the cup must be achieved to prevent early loosening, and there are various surgical methods that can be used to accomplish this.

Coverage of the cup can be achieved by placing a small cup in a superior[7,8] or protruded[1,9] position or by using an oblong socket.[12] These techniques are advantageous in that they allow the surgeon to avoid the use of a structural autograft, which is associated with certain disadvantages, including technical difficulty, resorption, fragmentation, and loosening of the cup.[7,8]

Advocates of the use of a high hip center have recommended placement of a small socket in a high, but not a lateral, position.[7,8] The advantages of this technique are the avoidance of a structural graft and the ability to place a cementless cup against bleeding host bone. The disadvantages are that the use of a small cup (and therefore thin polyethylene) may be necessary and that there is an increased risk of femoral and acetabular component loosening.[10,11] In addition, this technique does not restore bone stock for subsequent revision surgery. Despite these disadvantages, however, the use of a high hip center is an attractive option if limb length can be restored with use of a long-neck prosthesis, there is adequate bone stock, and the hip is stable. The authors who have advocated this technique have done so on the basis of their own poor results with femoral head autografts.[7,8] Anderson and Harris[17] recently reported on 18 patients (20 hips) who had a primary total hip replacement with use of a cementless cup. All of the hips had either low (type 2) or high (type 3) dislocation. After an average duration of follow-up of 83 months, none of the cups had been revised and none were loose. Although most of the cups were placed in a relatively high position, it was necessary to use a bulk femoral head autograft in four hips. All four grafts united, and none resorbed. In the 20 hips that formed the basis of the study, the center of the hip was placed an average of 28 mm proximal to the interteardrop line. In nine of the hips, the center of the hip was placed at least 35 mm proximal to the interteardrop line; these hips were arbitrarily designated by the authors as having a high hip center. The authors stressed that in these 9 hips, the lateral placement of the cup was normal.

Centralization of the cup by means of cotyloplasty[1] or reaming to the floor of the true acetabular fossa[9] also avoids the use of a structural autograft. We have had no personal experience with cotyloplasty, but this technique has yielded good results and reestablishes the hip center.[1] This technique, which involves the creation of a controlled fracture of the medial wall of the acetabulum, is complicated and should only be undertaken by surgeons who have been specifically trained in this method. Long-term problems of protrusio and cup loosening must be monitored. Hartofilakidis and associates[18] reported on a series of 84 hips (67 patients) that were treated with total hip replacement because of a high dislocation. In 49 of the hips, a cemented cup was inserted at the correct anatomic level with use of the cotyloplasty technique. Those authors reported an overall success rate of 87% after an average duration of follow-up of 6.4 years, with a cumulative rate of survival of the cup of 95% at 5 years and 90% at 10 years.

In 1988, McQueary and Johnston[9] advocated centralization by reaming to the inner cortex and use of cement to provide coverage at the correct anatomic level, but a subsequent review of these patients revealed an unacceptable prevalence of cup loosening.[19] In their 1988 study, the authors reported on a series of 61 hips in 48 patients who had insertion of the cup at the correct anatomic level with use of cement and without bone grafting. After an average duration of follow-up of 8.5 years, no revisions had been performed for aseptic loosening, but six hips (10%) had radiographic evidence of loosening.[9] When this same group of patients was evaluated after an average duration of follow-up of 16 years, survivorship analysis revealed that the rate of survival at 15 years was 85% with revision as the end point but 68% with radiographic loosening as the end point.[19] The authors of the later study expressed concern about the prevalence of acetabular loosening at 15 years. Type 2 and type 3 hips (low and high dislocation) had a higher prevalence of loosening than did type 1 hips (dysplasia).[19]

Dorr and associates[20] reported on 24 hips that were treated with a medial protrusio technique and insertion of an uncemented cup at the correct anatomic level. After an average duration of follow-up of 7 years, no cup had been revised. The authors advocated reaming medially until coverage of 80% of the cup is achieved. Hips with complete dislocation required more medialization than those with subluxation.

Numair and associates[21] presented a series of 182 Charnley total hip replacements in 141 patients with dysplasia. A cemented cup was placed in the true acetabulum without a bone graft. After an average duration of follow-up of 10 years, the rate of acetabular revision was higher in the group of hips that had been reconstructed because of complete dislocation (15%; 7 of 46) than it was in the group of hips that had been reconstructed because of subluxation (9%; 12 of 136). In addition, the rate of definite or possible loosening of the cup was higher in the group of hips with dislocation (11%; 5 of 46) than it was in the group of hips with subluxation (4%; 5 of 136). On the basis of these results, the authors concluded that contemporary grafting techniques should be considered when total hip replacement is performed for the treatment of a completely dislocated hip.[21]

Use of an oblong cup allows the cup to be placed at the anatomic level. The oblong elongated part of the cup fills in the deficient segment and allows further stabilization with screws. This cup has been used mainly for revision arthroplasty of the acetabulum.[12] It has been advocated for primary replacement in hips with low and high dislocation,[12] but we are not aware of any reports on the long-term results of such treatment. The primary disadvantage associated with the use of this device for the treatment of hips with dysplasia is the failure to restore bone stock. Moreover, reaming superior to the true acetabulum in order to seat the elongated part of the cup destroys what valuable bone stock there is.[12]

Our results with the use of structural femoral autografts to provide coverage of the cup have been very encouraging. We advocate the technique outlined above because it restores bone stock for future revision surgery, restores the hip center, and restores limb length in an anatomic way.[22] A cemented or uncemented cup can be used. In our series, only 3 of the 10 hips that had revision of the cup required another structural graft, confirming that this technique restores bone stock for revision surgery. Good long-term results with such structural autografts also have been reported by other authors.[23-25] Garvin and associates[23] reported on 23 hips that were followed for an average of 14 years. Six hips had required structural bone-grafting to support the cup, and all of these reconstructions were still intact with no evidence of loosening of the cup at the time of the latest follow-up. There were only two acetabular revisions in the entire series: one was performed in a type 2 hip (low dislocation), and the other was performed in a type 3 hip (high dislocation). Martí and associates[24] reviewed the results of 63 total hip replacements after an average duration of follow-up of 10 years. All hips required structural grafting of the acetabulum because of congenital dysplasia (53 hips) or traumatic dysplasia (10 hips). The authors advocated the use of two or three small structural grafts fixed with screws and reported no extensive resorption of the grafts at 10 years. Two cups were definitely loose, and two cups were probably loose. The authors stated that the hips with complete dislocation had poorer clinical scores than those with dysplasia but noted that there was no radiographic difference between these groups. Rodriguez and associates[25] reported on 29 hips in 23 patients who required structural grafting during total hip replacement for dysplasia. After an average duration of follow-up of 11 years, three cups (10%) had been revised for loosening and eight cups (28%) were probably loose. Graft resorption was not a problem.

The recent article by Bal and associates[26] also confirms that healed bulk femoral head grafts can provide bone stock for revision arthroplasty with use of an uncemented cup. In that study, nine patients (nine hips) with congenital displacement who had had a previous total hip replacement with use of a cemented cup and a shelf bulk autograft (six hips) or allograft (three hips) had a revision arthroplasty with use of an uncemented cup. After an average duration of follow-up of 76 months, all nine acetabular shells were functioning well. The authors concluded that the previously placed bulk autograft or allograft provided bone stock for revision with an uncemented cup at the correct anatomic level.

Summary

Replacing the dislocated hip is technically more challenging than replacing the subluxated hip. Overall, clinical and radiographic results have not been as good for hips that are completely dislocated.[22,24,26] The surgical approach must allow for identification of the false and true acetabula, identification of the sciatic nerve, and lengthening of the leg.

In patients with a dislocated hip who are managed with total hip replacement, coverage of the cup can be achieved by medialization, creation of a high hip center, or use of a structural graft. Bone grafting allows the cup to be placed in an anatomic position, provides bone stock for additional surgery, and restores leg length. Our results and the results of other authors confirm that these grafts remain intact for at least 10 years and restore bone stock for additional surgery. This is particularly important in this relatively young population.

References

1. Hartofilakidis G, Stamos K, Karachalios T, Ioannidis TT, Zacharakis N: Congenital hip disease in adults. Classification of acetabular deficiencies and operative treatment with acetabuloplasty combined with total hip arthroplasty. *J Bone Joint Surg Am* 1996;78:683-692.
2. Crowe JF, Mani VJ, Ranawat CS: Total hip replacement in congenital dislocation and dysplasia of the hip. *J Bone Joint Surg Am* 1979;61:15-23.
3. Edwards BN, Tullos HS, Noble PC: Contributory factors and etiology of sciatic nerve palsy in total hip arthroplasty. *Clin Orthop* 1987;218:136-141.
4. Black DL, Reckling FW, Porter SS: Somatosensory-evoked potential monitored during total hip arthroplasty. *Clin Orthop* 1991;262:170-177.
5. Becker DA, Gustilo RB: Double-chevron subtrochanteric shortening derotational femoral osteotomy combined with total hip arthroplasty for the treatment of complete congenital dislocation of the hip in the adult: Preliminary report and description of a new surgical technique. *J Arthroplasty* 1995;10:313-318.
6. Yasgur DJ, Stuchin SA, Adler EM, DiCesare PE: Subtrochanteric femoral shortening osteotomy in total hip arthroplasty for high-riding developmental dislocation of the hip. *J Arthroplasty* 1997;12:880-888.
7. Russotti GM, Harris WH: Proximal placement of the acetabular component in total hip arthroplasty: A long-term follow-up study. *J Bone Joint Surg Am* 1991;73:587-592.
8. Jasty M, Anderson MJ, Harris WH: Total hip replacement for developmental dysplasia of the hip. *Clin Orthop* 1995;311:40-45.
9. McQueary FG, Johnston RC: Coxarthrosis after congenital dysplasia: Treatment by total hip arthroplasty without acetabular bone-grafting. *J Bone Joint Surg Am* 1988;70:1140-1144.
10. Kelley SS: High hip center in revision arthroplasty. *J Arthroplasty* 1994;9:503-510.
11. Pagnano MW, Hanssen AD, Lewallen DG, Shaughnessy WJ: The effect of superior placement of the acetabular component on the rate of loosening after total hip arthroplasty: Long-term results in patients who have Crowe type-II congenital dysplasia of the hip. *J Bone Joint Surg Am* 1996;78:1004-1014.
12. DeBoer DK, Christie MJ: Reconstruction of the deficient acetabulum with an oblong prosthesis: Three- to seven-year results. *J Arthroplasty* 1998;13:674-680.
13. Marcy GH, Fletcher RS: Modification of the posterolateral approach to the hip for insertion of femoral head prosthesis. *J Bone Joint Surg Am* 1954;36:142-143.
14. Hardinge K: The direct lateral approach to the hip. *J Bone Joint Surg Br* 1982;64:17-19.
15. McGrory BJ, Bal BS, Harris WH: Trochanteric osteotomy for total hip arthroplasty: six variations and indications for their use. *J Am Acad Orthop Surg* 1996;4:258-267.
16. Glassman AH, Engh CA, Bobyn JD: A technique of extensile exposure for total hip arthroplasty. *J Arthroplasty* 1987;2:11-21.
17. Anderson MJ, Harris WH: Total hip arthroplasty with insertion of the acetabular component without cement in hips with total congenital dislocation or marked congenital dysplasia. *J Bone Joint Surg Am* 1999;81:347-354.
18. Hartofilakidis G, Stamos K, Karachalios T: Treatment of high dislocation of the hip in adults with total hip arthroplasty: Operative technique and long-term clinical results. *J Bone Joint Surg Am* 1998;80:511-517.
19. MacKenzie JR, Kelley SS, Johnston RC: Total hip replacement for coxarthrosis secondary to congenital dysplasia and dislocation of the hip: Long-term results. *J Bone Joint Surg Am* 1996;78:55-61.

20. Dorr LD, Tawakkol S, Moorthy M, Long W, Wan Z: Medial protrusio technique for placement of a porous-coated, hemispherical acetabular component without cement in a total hip arthroplasty in patients who have acetabular dysplasia. *J Bone Joint Surg Am* 1999;81:83-92.

21. Numair J, Joshi AB, Murphy JCM, Porter ML, Hardinge K: Total hip arthroplasty for congenital dysplasia or dislocation of the hip: Survivorship analysis and long-term results. *J Bone Joint Surg Am* 1997;79:1352-1360.

22. Morsi E, Garbuz D, Stockley I, Catre M, Gross AE: Total hip replacement in dysplastic hips using femoral head shelf autografts. *Clin Orthop* 1996;324:164-168.

23. Garvin KL, Bowen MK, Salvati EA, Ranawat CS: Long-term results of total hip arthroplasty in congenital dislocation and dysplasia of the hip: A follow-up note. *J Bone Joint Surg Am* 1991;73:1348-1354.

24. Martí RK, Schüller HM, van Steijn MJ: Superolateral bone grafting for acetabular deficiency in primary total hip replacement and revision. *J Bone Joint Surg Br* 1994;76:728-734.

25. Rodriguez JA, Huk OL, Pellicci PM, Wilson PD Jr: Autogenous bone grafts from the femoral head for the treatment of acetabular deficiency in primary total hip arthroplasty with cement: Long-term results. *J Bone Joint Surg Am* 1995;77:1227-1233.

26. Bal BS, Maurer T, Harris WH: Revision of the acetabular component without cement after a previous acetabular reconstruction with use of a bulk femoral head graft in patients who had congenital dislocation or dysplasia: A follow-up note. *J Bone Joint Surg Am* 1999;81:1703-1706.

33

Primary Total Hip Arthroplasty After Infection

Graham M. Robbins, MD
Bassam A. Masri, MD, FRCSC
Donald S. Garbuz, MD MHSc, FRCSC
Clive P. Duncan, MD, FRCSC

Introduction

Of the more than 200,000 total hip arthroplasties (THAs) performed annually in the United States, only a small number are performed after a proven infection of the hip joint or proximal femur. Although some infections produce severe early destruction of the hip joint, a large proportion of patients, if treated promptly, regain good hip function and seek treatment much later in life only when secondary degenerative changes occur.[1] It is, therefore, always necessary to be aware of the possibility of previous infection and to inquire about it specifically. Previously "cured" bone and joint infections should always be treated with a healthy degree of skepticism because the first recurrence of bone infection may be delayed for many decades. Gallie[2] reported a case of femoral osteomyelitis that first occurred in a 10-year-old girl and first recurred after nearly 80 years. The risk that a previous infection of the hip region poses to a hip arthroplasty is multifactorial. The type of infection (osteomyelitis or septic arthritis), the activity (active or quiescent), the time since infection (recent or historic), the organism (pyogenic, tuberculous, or fungal), and the technique of reconstruction employed will all contribute to the outcome.

One or more of the authors or the departments with which they are affiliated have received something of value from a commercial or other party related directly or indirectly to the subject of this chapter.

Osteomyelitis

In the western world there has been a progressive reduction in the prevalence of osteomyelitis.[3] Craigen and associates[4] found that the incidence in Glasgow had fallen significantly, halving from 87 to 42 per 10,000 population per year between 1970 and 1988 ($P = 0.007$).

In its neonatal form, osteomyelitis differs from that of later childhood or adult life in that metaphyseal infection may readily pass into the femoral head, causing osteonecrosis, septic arthritis, and severe hip destruction. Ever since *Staphylococcus aureus* was first isolated from osteomyelitis by Pasteur[5] in the late 1800s, it has remained the predominant infecting organism, implicated in about 90% of cases (88% [140 of 159] to 95% [392 of 411]) of cases where an organism is isolated.[4,6] The remainder are largely *Staphylococcus epidermidis* and streptococci.

More recently, there has been a shift in the prevalence of certain causative organisms, with fewer cases caused by *S aureus*. There has also been a significant increase (12% [8 of 65] to 42% [8 of 19]; $P < 0.001$) in the proportion of cases that are subacute and that have a greater tendency to relapse.[3,4]

With modern antibiotic management, most recurrences of osteomyelitis are apparent within the first year.[6] Of the 18% (119 of 655) of cases of osteomyelitis that recurred, Gillespie and Mayo[6] found that 66% had occurred by 6 months, 82% by 1 year, and only 6% after more than 5 years. In 50% of these cases there was only one episode of recurrence. Infection was located in the proximal femur in 7% (20 of 275) to 12% (76 of 655) and the pelvis in 3% (20 of 655) to 5% (13 of 275).[4,6] Recurrence rates at both sites were similar at 15% (3 of 20) in the pelvis and 18% (14 of 76) in the proximal femur.

Septic Arthritis

As with osteomyelitis, the predominant infecting organism in septic arthritis is *S aureus*. Of 141 adult hips with septic arthritis, Kelly[7] found *S aureus* in 77%, gram-negative organisms in 16%, and streptococci in 4%. *Haemophilus influenzae* is rare in adults, having a peak incidence at age 2 years, whereas gram-negative organisms, which generally have a worse outcome, have an increased prevalence in adults.[7]

While the clinical picture suggests the diagnosis of septic arthritis in the older child or adult, in infancy the diagnosis is often difficult and delayed. The by-products of leukocytes and bacteria rapidly produce cartilage erosions and may subsequently affect the bone of the femoral head and acetabulum. In addition, increased intracapsular pressure, capsular tension with dislocation, and transphyseal emboli can produce ischemia and osteonecrosis of the epiphysis. The outcome may be anywhere between complete resolution with little damage to the joint, to a coxa magna, a spontaneous bony or fibrous ankylosis, or complete destruction of the proximal femur with dislocation.

Trochanteric overgrowth or acetabular dysplasia may occur; each of them can have an adverse effect on future arthroplasty. The outcomes of septic arthritis managed before the use of antibiotics provide very little insight into how new cases will fare today. Little good data are available because few centers have a large experience with this relatively rare condition. For example, the Mayo Clinic reports treating fewer than four children and eight adults per year between 1958 and 1973, of which only 20% (31 of 156) involved the hip.[7,8]

Of all joints, infection of the hip joint is particularly incapacitating. Morrey and associates[8] found that 85% of their clinically unsatisfactory results after septic arthritis were when the hip had been affected.

Tuberculous Bone and Joint Infections

Although the prevalence of pulmonary tuberculosis has fallen dramatically over the last few decades, the prevalence of extrapulmonary tuberculosis has remained steady, with just under 400 cases of skeletal tuberculosis per year in the United States, of which 13% (90 of 676) involved the hip.[9,10] In the western world, tuberculous arthritis is now very rare in children, mainly affecting people in their fifth and sixth decades. More recently, infection rates in the developed world have been increasing in subgroups of the population due to various host factors (immunosuppression, malnourishment) as well as the development of increasingly resistant strains. Although there does not appear to be an increased risk of contracting tuberculosis in patients who are infected with the human immunodeficiency virus (HIV), increased rates of reactivation have been observed in these patients.[11,12]

Radiographically, tuberculous bone infections normally have a destructive appearance, with adjacent osteopenia and minimal sclerosis. However, they may also simulate pyogenic arthritis with a florid periosteal reaction, sclerosis, and sequestrum formation.

Fungal Bone and Joint Infections

Fungal joint infections differ from pyogenic or tuberculous infections in that there is less joint destruction, and there is evidence that it is not always necessary to irrigate or débride the joint in primary infections.[13-15] Spontaneous infection of the natural hip joint usually is caused by noncandidal fungi, whereas candidal infection at the site of a prosthetic joint is usually associated with immunosuppression, intravenous therapy, drug abuse, or direct inoculation. Candida is the only fungus reported to have caused infections at the site of hip arthroplasties.[16]

Other Organisms

Although a wide variety of other organisms are known to cause bone infections such as brucellosis[17] and syphilis, isolation of these organisms from bone can be difficult, and infections with these organisms at the site of a joint arthroplasty have not yet been described.

Factors Predisposing to Recurrent Sepsis

Intravenous Drug Abuse

The high risk of joint infection is related to the activity of injection and does not appear to be adversely affected by the presence of HIV. Munoz-Fernandez and associates[18] demonstrated an incidence of joint infection in intravenous drug abusers of 5% (25 of 482) if they are positive for HIV and 7% (6 of 85) if they are not. They also found when comparing these 31 joint infections in 567 intravenous drug abusers (irrespective of HIV status) with 21 joint infections in 616 nonintravenous drug abusers that there was a fourfold increase in infection of the hips, sacroiliac joints, and sternocostal joints (64.5% versus 16.6%) in the intravenous drug abusers. It is therefore reasonable to assume that while the active intravenous drug abuser presents an unacceptable risk of further hip infection after THA, the risks with the truly reformed abuser are acceptable.

Hemoglobinopathies

Patients with hemoglobinopathies such as sickle-cell disease have an increased risk of bone and joint infection. Engh and associates[19] reported that 29% of patients (20 of 70) with complete hemoglobinopathies followed for 10 years required treatment for osteomyelitis. All fully documented infections were caused by gram-negative organisms and 80% (8 of 10) were *Salmonella* species. Fifty percent (5 of 10) had femoral involvement, and although 90% (9 of 10) of the infections were limited to the diaphysis and, therefore, did not directly invade the hip joint itself, at THA the femoral stem would have encroached upon this area. In sickle-cell disease with collapse of the femoral head, the radiologic features give little indication whether or not infection is present. Scintigraphy in the form of sequential technetium bone and indium leukocyte scans is therefore recommended in this group to differentiate between infection and infarction as a cause of pain.

Ongoing Sources of Infection

Although treatable sources of ongoing sepsis remote from the hip should obviously be addressed, the actual threat posed to performing a THA is unclear. del Sel and Charnley[20] described primary THA in 31 patients with actively infected hip joints on the opposite side (infections at the site of hip implants, Girdlestone arthroplasties, or septic arthritis), five of which had draining sinuses. Although perioperative antibiotics were rarely used, at mean follow-up of 3.5 years (8 months to 10 years) there were no infections on the clean side. On looking at the risk factors present in 34 of 803 patients with hip replacements in whom a deep infection occurred, Surin and associates[21] found that while the risk increased threefold ($P < 0.05$) in the presence of a remote infection, there was no correlation between the infecting organisms at the two different sites and, therefore, no evidence of a causal relationship.

Occult Infection

Cases have been reported of occult infection in the hip, with a previous historic infection at another site. Coutts and associates[22] reported on a 60-year-old woman who had suffered an osteomyelitis of the left femur and a lumbar vertebra that had been quiescent for 43 years. At the time of a right hip arthroplasty there was no macroscopic evidence of infection, and cultures were negative; however, there were scattered microabscesses representing areas of focal acute and chronic osteomyelitis. At 8-year follow-up there was no evidence of infection.

Tuberculosis can easily be overlooked from the differential diagnosis and should always be considered in cases of hip destruction. Hecht and associates[23] described four cases of reactivation of previously unsuspected tuberculosis in patients who had a normal erythrocyte sedimentation rate (ESR), C-reactive protein (CRP), and leukocyte count preoperatively and for whom no intraoperative cultures had been performed.

Implantation With Active Sepsis

Several historic reviews outline the results of arthroplasty of the hip in the face of gross sepsis. Hunt and Larson[24] reported the outcome of one-stage treatment with aggressive débridement, Vitallium cup arthroplasty, and perioperative antibiotics for the treatment of pyogenic infection in 27 hips.

Of those with signs of active sepsis at surgery, 43% (3 of 7) had no evidence of recurrence, one had a transient recurrence, and 43% (3 of 7) recurred. In the absence of signs of active infection at the time of arthroplasty, the recurrence rate was only 15% (3 of 20).

In 1965, Harris and Aufranc[25] described their experience with the same mold arthroplasty implant in nine patients with active intra-articular infection following internal fixation of femoral neck fractures. The majority (4 of 7) were treated with two-stage reconstruction with 3 to 5 weeks of antibiotics. All healed with no substantial pain or evidence of recurrence of infection at mean follow-up of 3 years (1 to 11 years).

Similarly, Hughes and associates[26] performed hip arthroplasties on three patients in whom hip fractures previously treated with nail-plate devices had become infected, and two patients were converted using a two-stage technique. All patients were free of infection at a minimum follow-up of 6 years, after treating one with a one-stage technique and two with staged procedures.

The Exclusion of Active Infection

History and Examination

While systemic symptoms such as a fever or obvious local symptoms such as a discharging sinus would alert the clinician to the presence of active sepsis, in the vast majority of previously infected hips that come to arthroplasty, any remaining activity of the infection is low and these features are absent. Hardinge and associates[1] emphasized the importance of ensuring that the onset of hip symptoms is slowly progressive. Even after many decades of quiescence, rapidly increasing pain from a joint that has previously been infected raises the suspicion that the infection may have been reactivated, particularly with tuberculosis.

Hematologic Investigations

White Blood Cell Count The white blood cell count (WBC) is usually noncontributory[27] and can often be normal even in actively infected hips. For this reason it cannot reliably exclude infection.

Erythrocyte Sedimentation Rate The ESR is a nonspecific inflammatory marker and can be difficult to interpret because transient elevation may be produced by any concomitant minor illness, and it may be permanently raised in chronic conditions such as connective tissue disorders. In an attempt to exclude chronic infection of the hip joint, the ESR has been extensively investigated in the context of the suspected infection at the site of a THA. A review of these studies shows that a cutoff of 30 mm/h has a diagnostic sensitivity of 60% to 94% and specificity of 65% to 85%.[27-30]

C-Reactive Protein The CRP is an acute phase protein. This has also been studied in detail with respect to revision hip arthroplasty. Sanzén and associates[31] found that unless another probable cause was apparent, a CRP above 20 mg/L indicated that deep sepsis was present.

Improved diagnostic accuracy may be obtained by considering the ESR and CRP results together. Spangehl and associates[27] demonstrated that all 35 of 202 hip replacements that were complicated with deep infection had an ESR at least greater than 30 mL/h or a CRP above 10 mg/L. They suggested that a normal ESR and CRP effectively exclude infection, and an elevation of both indicates an 83% probability of sepsis (Table 1).

Plain Radiographs

The radiologic appearance of bone infection can be confusing. Initially infection is usually more extensive than is radiographically apparent; however, during the early stages of resolution, the

Table 1
The predictive value of investigations in the diagnosis of infection of a hip arthroplasty

Tests	All Negative	All Positive
Erythrocyte sedimentation rate + C-reactive protein	0% [0 to 4%] (0 of 95)	83% [62% to 95%] (20 of 24)
Erythrocyte sedimentation rate + C-reactive protein + aspiration	0% [0 to 4%] (0 of 86)	89% [52% to 100%] (8 of 9)
Erythrocyte sedimentation rate + C-reactive protein + aspiration + histology	0% [0 to 4%] (0 of 84)	100% [40% to 100%] (4 of 4)

(Adapted with permission from Spangehl MJ, Masri BA, O'Connell JX, Duncan CP: Prospective analysis of preoperative and intraoperative investigations for the diagnosis of infection at the sites of two hundred and two revision total hip arthroplasties. *J Bone Joint Surg Am* 1999;81:672-683.)

radiographic bony destruction may appear to progress. Chronic osteomyelitis may appear as sclerosis with adjacent osteoporosis, a fusiform thickening of the cortex, or even an extensive thickened involucrum, but it is very difficult to ascertain the activity of the infection. Osteoarthritis secondary to a healed septic arthritis should evolve slowly with subchondral sclerosis and marginal osteophytes. Conversely in reactivation of infection, there is usually a more sudden clinical deterioration with rapid bone destruction, often associated with local osteoporosis. CT may demonstrate the anatomy better than plain radiographs but again gives little indication of the activity of the infection, unless adjacent soft-tissue changes indicate edema or abscess formation.

Magnetic Resonance Imaging

Active osteomyelitis typically appears dark on T1 images and bright on T2, and with chronicity the bright T2 marrow signal becomes more heterogeneous. Schauwecker[32] in his review of 11 published series on MRI of bone infection found cumulative sensitivities and specificities for MRI of 95% (188 of 197) and 88% (103 of 117).

Tang and associates[33] concluded that MRI was particularly useful for demonstrating the presence of active infection in cases with previous chronic osteomyelitis, with a sensitivity of 100% (10 of 10). Where anatomic distortion was present as a result of longstanding infection, Mason and associates[34] found MRI more sensitive (100% [11 of 11]) than indium-labeled WBC scans (63% [5 of 8]) for demonstrating active infection.

Scintigraphy

Unfortunately, no nuclear medicine scan is specific for infection; the scans simply show different elements of the inflammatory and metabolic response of the bone to infection. None of the scans can be accurately interpreted in isolation.

Technetium Bone Scan The technetium Tc 99m (^{99m}Tc) methylene diphosphonate scan is a very sensitive but nonspecific indicator of osteoblastic activity and remains the so-called work horse of nuclear medicine investigation. Osteomyelitis that has been chronically active for many years continues to produce increased uptake of isotope, and even after effective treatment, the scan may remain positive for over a year. Its specificity for activity of infection is therefore poor. Al-Sheikh and associates[35] looked at 21 patients with subacute or chronic bone infection, found the sensitivity of ^{99m}Tc scanning for active infection to be 100%, and concluded that a negative technetium scan ruled out ongoing infection.

Gallium Citrate Scanning Gallium citrate is taken up by leukocytes and is a better indicator of infection than ^{99m}Tc methylene diphosphonate scanning alone, the two scans often being used sequentially. Its disadvantage is that it is generally less sensitive than a ^{99m}Tc methylene diphosphonate scan and less specific than the indium-labeled WBC scan.[36] It is therefore not routinely used by the authors.

Indium-Labeled WBC Scans In a prospective study of 42 patients, Merkel and associates[36] demonstrated this technique to be superior to sequential technetium-gallium bone scanning in the diagnosis of low-grade musculoskeletal sepsis. Of 30 patients with histologic and bacteriologic proof of the presence or absence of sepsis, the indium-labeled WBC scan was significantly more sensitive (83%) and specific (86%) than the sequential technetium-gallium scan (48% and 57% respectively; $P < 0.01$). Similarly, in 21 patients with subacute or chronic bone infection, Al-Sheikh and associates[35] reported the sensitivity and specificity of technetium scanning to be 100% and 25%, gallium scanning 80% and 83%, and indium-labeled WBC scanning 80% and 75%, respectively.

The method of preparation of the WBC marker affects the population of cells that are labeled. Some authors who have primarily labeled polymorphonuclear cells have criticized the test as being a poor tool for identifying chronic infection. Merkel and associates[36] report better detection of chronic infection with their technique in which a third of the labeled leukocytes were lymphocytes. Datz and Thorne[37] found no difference between the sensitivity of indium-labeled WBC scans in lesions less than 2 weeks old (90% [62 of 69]) and those 2 weeks to 3 months old (86% [74 of 86]).

The identification of active infection is further complicated by any process where remodeling is occurring, as is seen in a degenerated hip. Where radiographs were normal, there was a cumulative sensitivity of 94% (182 of 194) and specificity of 95% (360 of 380) with technetium scanning in cases of suspected osteomyelitis.[32] In the presence of any underlying osteoblastic process, although the sensitivity remained high (95% [250 of 262]), the specificity was poor (33% [110 of 330]). In the same review, the reported sensitivity and specificity for gallium scans were 81% (209 of 257) and 69% (188 of 272) respectively, and for indium-labeled WBC scans, 88% (422 of 480) and 85% (389 of 457), respectively. Schauwecker[32] recommends that if there is underlying bone disease, combined indium-labeled WBC and technetium bone scanning is the investigation of choice. More specifically, around the hip, where there may be degenerative changes and also active bone marrow, he recommends the combination of an indium-labeled WBC scan and a technetium sulfur colloid marrow scan.[32]

Indium-Labeled Polyclonal Antibodies The use of labeled nonspecific antibodies that accumulate in areas of inflammation appears to be better than technetium or gallium citrate scanning.[38] Subsequent developments of this and other techniques, such as polymerase chain reaction amplification of bacterial DNA, may soon provide clinically useful markers of infection.

Aspiration Biopsy

Cherney and Amstutz[39] reported no growth on the preimplantation aspiration of any of the 23% of hips (7 of 31) that had a recurrence of infection after arthroplasty, and the true value of preoperative joint aspiration biopsy has been questioned. In our experience with hip arthroplasties complicated by deep infection, aspiration has proved to be a useful diagnostic tool, with a sensitivity of 86% and a specificity of 94% for 35 infections in 180 hips.[27] Other groups have reported similar results;[29,40] however, we have not yet accumulated sufficient experience with primary arthroplasty of previously infected hips to support a similar statement. If doubt persists, we perform multiple core needle biopsies of the affected bone for both bacteriologic and histologic analysis, to try to distinguish between osteonecrosis and chronic osteomyelitis. We do not, however, have data to support the efficacy of this practice.

Mantoux Test

Shivaram and associates[10] found that the Mantoux test was strongly positive in all of 10 patients with active tuberculous osteomyelitis of the spine. Therefore, it should be performed in all cases of suspected tuberculous infection.

Treatment Options for Painful Hip Degeneration Secondary to Sepsis

After all conservative measures have been exhausted, except for the few patients in which an osteotomy may be of benefit, the surgical options after the onset of painful secondary arthritis in the infected or postinfected hip, other than THA, are a Girdlestone resection arthroplasty or a hip arthrodesis.

Girdlestone Arthroplasty

Girdlestone popularized femoral head and neck resection, which he first performed in 1923.[41] He later reported that his first patient could still walk 10 miles a day at the age of 76 years, 21 years after this operation.[42] However, the reported outcome of Girdlestone resection has been very variable.

Haw and Gray[43] reported patient satisfaction with 77% of hips (31 of 40), at a mean follow-up of 10 years, increasing to 92% (22 of 24 hips) if performed as a secondary or as a salvage procedure. Furthermore, patients younger than 50 years of age were more satisfied (89% [8 of 9 hips]) than those who were older (74% [23 of 31 hips]). Forty-seven percent of hips (19 of 40) were pain free, with pain reduced in 30% (12), unchanged in 18% (7), and worse in only 5% (2 of the 40 hips). The mean limb shortening in this series was 4 cm but it is often reported to be greater, requiring an unacceptably high shoe raise. Other authors have often found a much less satisfactory outcome of the procedure.[44,45] Petty and Goldsmith[45] described moderate to severe pain in 76% (16 of 21), whereas Bittar and Petty[44] described a poor functional outcome with only 42% of patients (14 of 33) satisfied at a mean follow-up of 6 years (3 to 13 years).

This procedure results in a slow lurching gait because of the mechanical disadvantage of the abductors, and the energy efficiency is less than half that of a normal hip.[46] Shepherd[47] made the observation that "many patients achieve no more than a 'fair' result, but 'poor' results are few." Except for use as a salvage procedure, the functional result of a Girdlestone is generally considered unacceptable today. There are, however, cases in which this procedure should be considered, such as with uncontrollable hip infection or in intravenous drug abusers whose repeated bacteremias and even direct inoculation of the hip joint put at considerable risk of further infection. In addition, it may be the procedure of choice in some underdeveloped regions of the world where arthroplasty implants are unaffordable and hip fusion is unacceptable.

Arthrodesis

Following hip arthrodesis, most patients are able to walk at least 1 mile and continue with their occupations.[48,49] Callaghan and associates[48] reported that at over a 17-year follow-up, there was a slight limitation of daily activities in 64% of patients (18 of 28) and moderate or severe limitation in 29% (8 of 28). Similarly, at an over 20-year follow-up, Sponseller and associates[49] found no substantial limitation in 34% of patients (18 of 53). Patient satisfaction at 20 years has been reported in 59% (30 of

Table 2
Correlation between organisms isolated at initial infection and the subsequent prosthetic infection

Author	Hip Arthroplasty	Number of Hips	Same Organism	Different Organism
Carlsson et al[59]	Revision	7	57% (4)	43% (3)
Cherney and Amstutz[39]	Primary & revision	9	67% (6)	33% (3)
McDonald et al[60]	Revision	11	64% (7)	36% (4)

51) to 77% (41 of 53), particularly in those patients undergoing the procedure at a younger age, although this may no longer apply with the increased expectations of today's patients.[49,50]

The long-term deleterious effect of a hip arthrodesis on other joints, particularly the lumbar spine, ipsilateral knee, and contralateral hip, is well recognized.[48-50] In the study by Sponseller and associates,[49] 57% of patients (30 of 53) followed for an average of 38 years experienced low back pain, although in none of these was it considered to be incapacitating. There often is also a substantial limb length inequality, and most patients have a moderate to severe limp, decreased walking speed, and gait efficiency of only 53%.[46,51,52]

Performing a primary hip arthrodesis after joint infection is unusual today. The more common scenario is the conversion to a THA of a hip that was fused following previous infection to provide relief of symptoms from other joints. Hip arthrodesis does, however, retain its role in the treatment of the younger patient after a unilateral hip infection, particularly when the clinical setting indicates that durability is more important than mobility.

The Outcome of Primary Arthroplasty After Infection

In assessing the outcome of THA after sepsis, the following areas should be considered: first, whether there is reactivation of the infection and second, the functional and radiologic outcome of the arthroplasty.

Outcome of Arthroplasty After Pyogenic Infection

Recurrence of Infection In reviewing many of the historic series, it is difficult to determine which cases were true recurrences and which were newly acquired infections. In most cases the isolated organisms are those that are commonly found infecting THA where there is no previous history of sepsis, and therefore, without phage typing of the organisms from both episodes, the true origin of the infection remains uncertain.

The incidence of deep hip sepsis after one-stage primary arthroplasty for the treatment of quiescent hip infection is reported to be from 0 (0 of 27) to 10% (4 of 42).[1,53,54] Hardinge and associates[1] using a cemented Charnley THA, without antibiotics systemically or in the cement, had no recurrence of infection in any of 13 quiescent hips. They suggest several criteria to help exclude active infection before implantation. These include no discharge for 20 years and quiescence for a definite (though unspecified) period. They also recommend that the patient be in good systemic health and have experienced a gradual deterioration of the hip over a number of years. Serial radiographs should have shown slow progression of the degenerative changes with sclerosis and osteophytes, and both the WBC count and ESR should be normal. Jupiter and associates[53] described how in one case, 43 years after multifocal septic arthritis, although there was no evidence of infection at surgery and cultures were normal, on sectioning the femoral head there were areas of acute and chronic osteomyelitis with microabscesses but no bacteria. Laforgia and associates[54] reported deep sepsis occurring in 4 of 42 quiescent hips, of which two were related to poor wound healing. In addition, over half of the patients (20 of 38) were from the preantibiotic era. At the time of arthroplasty they found cultures were positive for *S epidermidis* in 5 of 42 hips and *Pseudomonas* in 1 of 42 hips.

Laforgia and associates[54] found positive intraoperative cultures in 6 of 42 hips, and Hardinge and associates[1] in 1 of 13. None of these hips developed a subsequent deep prosthetic infection despite the erratic use of antibiotics in less than half the cases.

Wilson and associates[55] successfully treated two cases of *S aureus* hip sepsis by débridement and antibiotics, with a second-stage implantation of the prosthesis after 1 and 3 years. In a retrospective review of 43 infections in 3,051 hip replacements, Schmalzried and associates[56] demonstrated a 12-fold increase in the infection rate following a history of previous hematogenous septic arthritis of the hip (8.2%), compared with uninfected osteoarthritic hips (0.7%). In their series of THA after hip infection, Cherney and Amstutz[39] demonstrated a much higher rate of recurrent infection after a hematogenous septic arthritis (44% [4 of 9]) or an infection at the site of a hip replacement (37% [5 of 8]) than for an infection at the site of a hemiarthroplasty (17% [1 of 6]) or internal fixation implant (25% [2 of 8]). Hardinge and associates[57] reported no cases of reactivation of infection (mixed cases of tuberculous and pyogenic sepsis) in 17 fused hips in which there had been sound bony union present for 10 or more years. The risk of recurrence of an infection continues for many years. In their review of recurrence of infection after revision hip replacements complicated by deep infection, using survival analysis, Went and associates[58] demonstrated that of those hips initially thought to be cured of infection (70 of 98 hips), 10% became infected after 3 years and 26% by 10 years.

Reinfecting Organism When infection of a hip arthroplasty occurs after previous hip sepsis, whether as a primary or revision procedure, there is a variable correlation between the original organisms and that of the subsequent infection. Where both the original infecting organism and that subsequently infecting the prosthesis are known, they have generally been found to be the same in approximately two thirds of cases[39,59,60] (Table 2).

In 73% of hips (8 of 11) that became reinfected, McDonald and associates[60] isolated more than one organism. In the staged reconstruction of infected THAs with an antibiotic-loaded interval spacer, Younger and associates[61] found that of the 17% of patients (5 of 30) with positive cultures at the second stage in so-called two-stage exchange arthroplasty, only one of five was with the same organism, and in this case there had been no recurrence of infection. In another study [62] they demonstrated that the same organism recurred in only one of three recurrences in 61 so-called two-stage exchange arthroplasties.

A similar poor correlation is found with the organisms causing infections at the site of total knee arthroplasty.[63] Six of 65 total knee arthroplasties (9%) performed an average of 5 years after septic arthritis had positive cultures at surgery; however, of the four for which the initial infecting organisms were known, the organism was the same in two and different in two. The patients with positive cultures were all treated with 2 weeks of antibiotics, and there were no deep infections in this group. Recurrence, or new infection, did occur in 15% of knees (3 of 20) with a previous history of septic arthritis and osteomyelitis, and 4% of knees (2 of 45) in which only septic arthritis had been present. The overall rate of deep infection in this group was increased at 7.7% (5 of 65) compared with 1.7% of 7,308 knee replacements in the authors' practice. While indicating the lack of consistency of infecting organisms, the fourfold increase in deep infection may indicate the effect of the previous infection on the soft tissues of the knee, and caution should be used in extrapolating such figures to the more deeply sited hip joint. In a smaller study, Farrell and Bryan[64] found no recurrence of infection in 10 knee arthroplasties performed a mean of 13 years after a septic arthritis.

Function After THA in Quiescent Cases Following primary hip arthroplasty for the treatment of hip arthrosis from previous infection, improvement in Charnley hip scores[65] (graded 1 to 6 for each of pain, walking function, and range

Table 3
The success of revision of the infected THA with respect to staging and the use of antibiotic cement

	One Stage	Two Stage
Antibiotics in cement	82% (976 of 1,189)	91% (385 of 423)
Plain cement	58% (35 of 60)	82% (130 of 158)

(Adapted with permission from Garvin KL, Hanssen AD: Infection after total hip arthroplasty: Past, present, and future. *J Bone Joint Surg Am* 1995;77:1576-1588.)

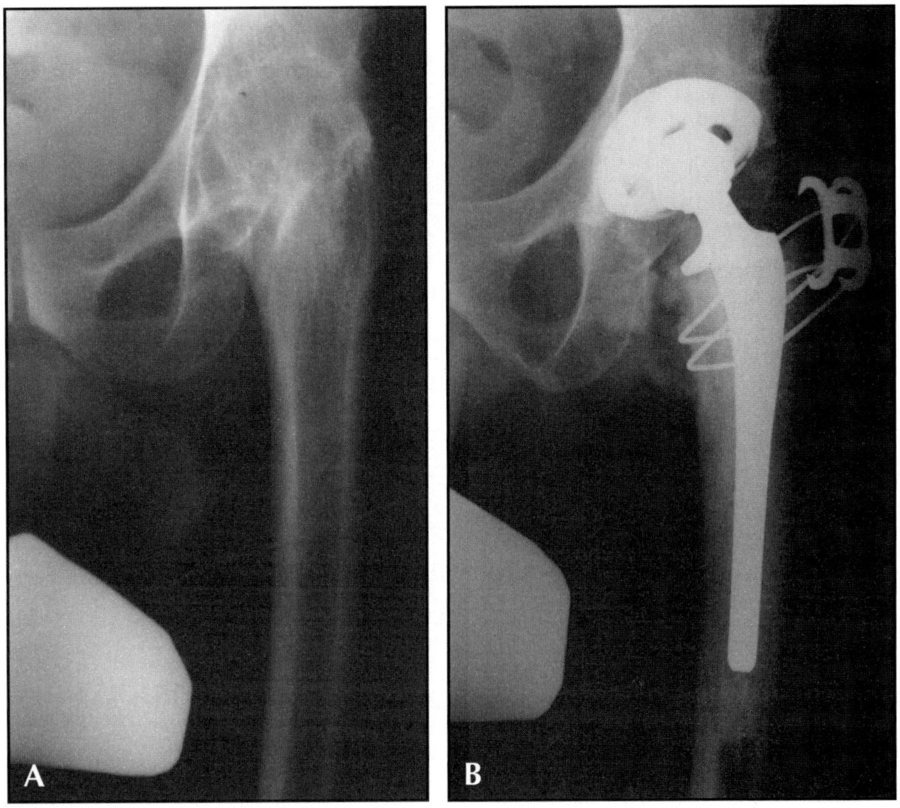

Fig. 1 A and **B,** If spontaneous fusion has occurred after a septic arthritis, there is a high risk of heterotopic bone formation after hip arthroplasty, and prophylactic measures are recommended.

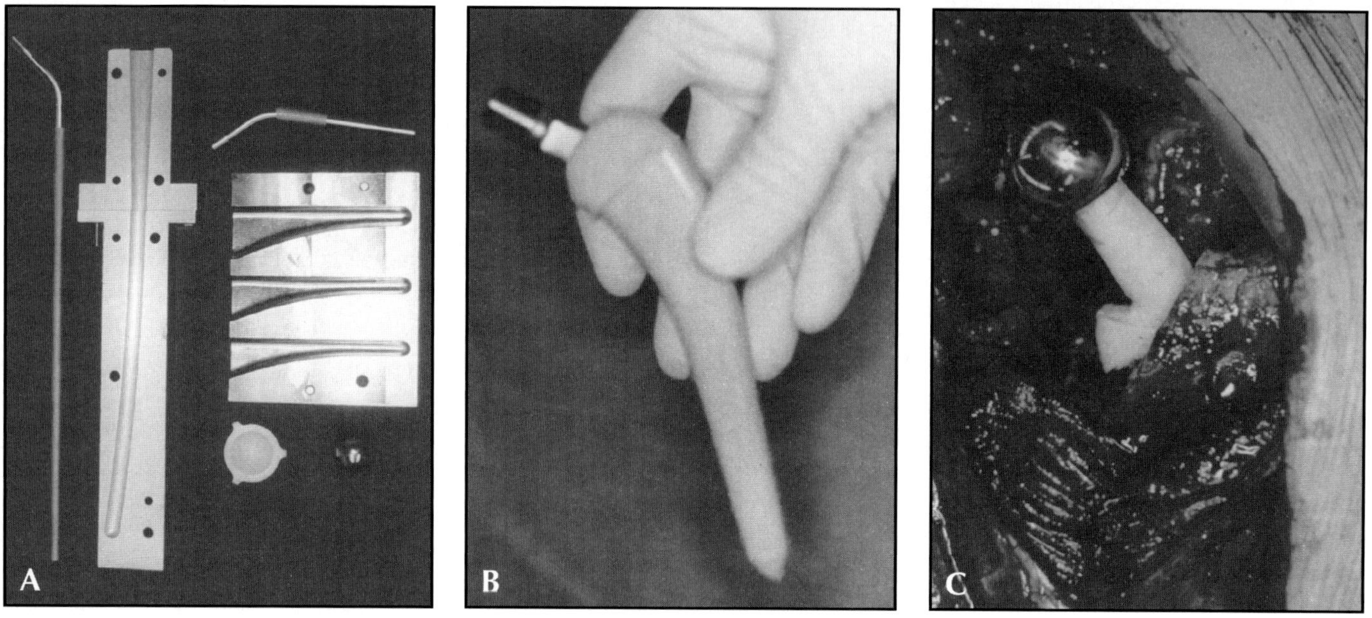

Fig. 2 A, The molds used to make the PROSTALAC femoral component. **B,** The PROSTALAC prior to insertion. **C,** Insertion of the PROSTALAC.

of movement) from 8.3 to 16.0 (in 13 hips) and 9.3 to 15.7 (in 28 hips) has been reported, with a corresponding reduction in cane or crutch requirement from 57% (16 of 28) to 18% (5 of 28).[1,54] In the conversion of 14 hips fused following infection, the improvement in Charnley hip score was from 10.1 to 15.3, with a reduction in cane or crutch requirement from 50% (7 of 14) to 21% (3 of 14) and wheelchair use from 2 of 14 to none. Of 24 hips with quiescence of infection for at least 1 year, Jupiter and associates[53] found that the mean Harris hip score had increased from 36 to 86 out of 100, equating to 75% excellent, 17% good, and 8% fair results. Wilson and associates[55] reported two cases of recent sepsis, treated with so-called staged reconstruction, with one excellent Hospital for Special Surgery hip score (36 of 40) at 3 years' follow-up and one good score (31 of 40) at 30 months.[66] The numbers in these studies are small, and although the functional result does not appear to be as good as those seen in hips without prior sepsis, this may in part reflect the severity of the preexisting hip disease.

In reviewing the radiographs of their series of hip replacements after septic arthritis, Laforgia and associates[54] found that at a mean follow-up of 5 years (2 to 17 years), there were progressive radiolucent lines in 4 of 42 cups, and one cup was loose, comparable to the results of arthroplasty without prior sepsis.

Outcome of Arthroplasty After Tuberculous Infection

Recurrence of Infection Laforgia and associates[54] reported reactivation in 1 of 72 hips undergoing THA a mean of 40 years (17 to 72 years) from the onset of infection. Only 6 of the 68 patients had received antituberculous therapy. Ten had had a chronic sinus, but only one was actively draining at the time of the hip arthroplasty, and it healed without recurrence. Jupiter and associates[53] found no reactivation in any of seven treated and healed tuberculous hips, as did Hardinge and associates[1] in 27 patients and Eskola and associates[67] in 18.

Johnson and associates[68] reported two cases of reactivation of tuberculosis after THA. In both cases, childhood infection had not been treated with antituberculous chemotherapy, and although intraoperative specimens of the capsule, femur, and acetabulum were all negative on culture and histology, tuberculous infection recurred by 1 year, after disease-free intervals of 37 and 42 years. The density of bacilli in infected bone is much less than in infected sputum, making the diagnosis of tuberculous osteomyelitis particularly difficult.[54] Hunt and Larson[24] treated six hips with a cup arthroplasty and perioperative antituberculous therapy, and although one of six had a positive intraoperative culture for tuberculosis, there were no cases of reactivation. Kim and associates[69] reported reactivation of tuberculosis in 1 of 20 patients, where the patient had discontinued antituberculous therapy against medical advice; however, the infection fully resolved on completion of therapy. They noted that although all cultures at surgery were negative, nearly half (9 of 20) showed histologic signs of tuberculosis with lymphocytes, epithelioid cells, and Langerhans giant cells. In 20% (4 of 20), areas of caseous necrosis were visible. The preoperative ESR has not been found to be predictive of the risk of reactivation.[54] The reported incidence of reactivation of tuberculous infection is therefore from 0 (0 of 27) to 5% (1 of 20).[1,24,53,54,67,69] Opinion differs about the use of additional perioperative antituberculous treatment to prevent this small risk of recurrence. Whereas some authors[53,68] recommend a full course of antituberculous therapy only if it has not previously been given, Eskola and associates[67] recommend that antituberculous therapy be given perioperatively in all cases, even those that have been previously treated.

Functional Outcome in THA Following Tuberculous Infection Following primary hip arthroplasty for the treatment of posttuberculous hip arthrosis, improvement in mean Charnley hip scores of 7.1 to 13 (20 hips) and 8.9 to15.8 (38 hips) have been reported, with a corresponding reduction in cane dependence from 42% (16 of 38) to 16% (6 of 38).[54,69] Although there was good relief of pain and improved walking ability, there was a more modest improvement in range of movement.[69] In 34 fused hips, the mean Charnley hip score increased from 10.2 to 14.9, and the use of a cane improved slightly from 21% (8 of 34) to 15% (5 of 34). The complication rate was not unusually high in 72 arthroplasties, but a marked leg length discrepancy persisted in 14% of cases.[54]

Jupiter and associates[53] described how in seven hips (five were ankylosed, one fibrous ankylosis, one very degenerated), the mean Harris hip score increased from 57 to 91 points, representing 71% excellent and 29% good results.

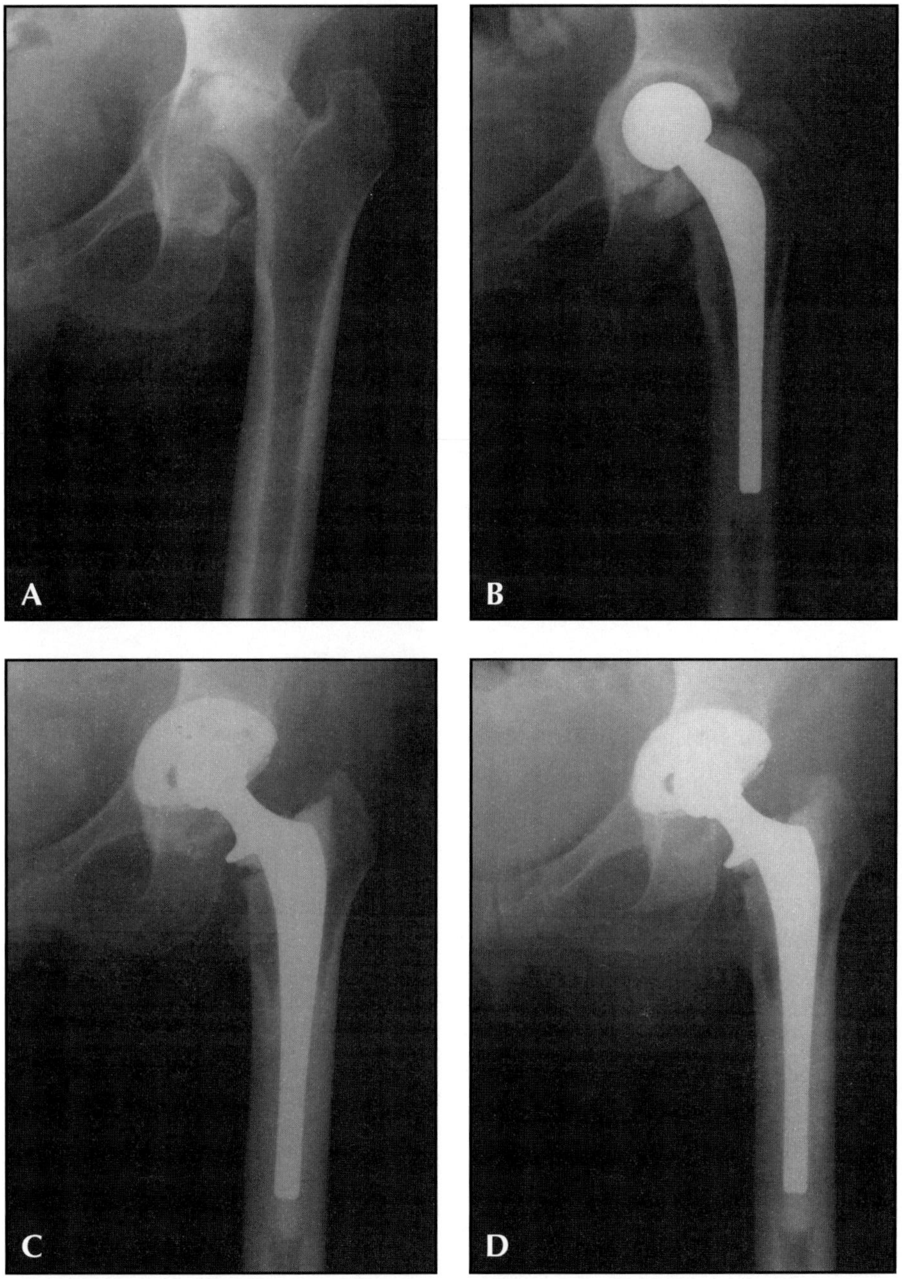

Fig. 3 A, Active septic arthritis (*Staphylococcus aureus*) **B,** Treatment with a PROSTALAC. **C** and **D,** Appearance at 1 and 4 years after arthroplasty, respectively.

Eskola and associates[67] reported an improvement in hip flexion arc from a mean of 40° (0° to 90°) to 86° (55° to 120°). For the 17 of 18 patients whose implants remained (one deep infection was treated with a Girdlestone arthroplasty), they reported good or excellent results in 83% (15 of 18), fair in 11% (2 of 18). Only one was poor, the Girdlestone arthroplasty. Seven hips had persistently marked quadriceps wasting, which improved little with surgery and physical therapy, and the leg-length inequality improved from a mean of 19 mm (0 to 50 mm) to 5 mm (0 to 20 mm). Radiologically, Laforgia and associates[54] found evidence of cup loosening in 7 of 72 hips; however, there was evidence of femoral loosening in 13 of 72 at a mean follow-up of 5 years (2 to 17 years).

Reconstruction Technique

Although the presented data demonstrate generally good results after hip

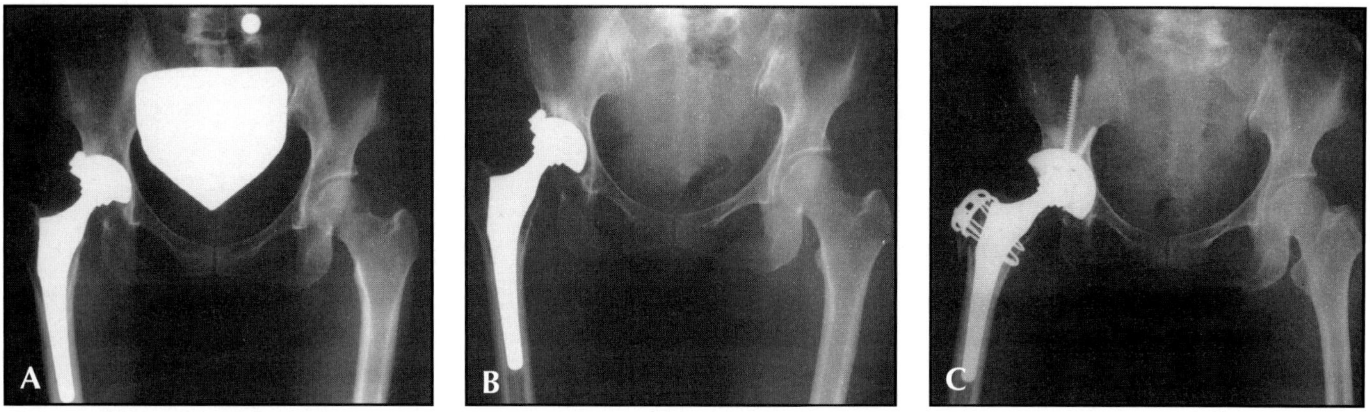

Fig. 4 A, After arthroplasty for tuberculous arthritis (previously treated with a PROSTALAC). **B,** Reactivation of tuberculosis was suspected when osteolysis developed, but this was due to polyethylene wear. **C,** No recurrence after revision of acetabular component.

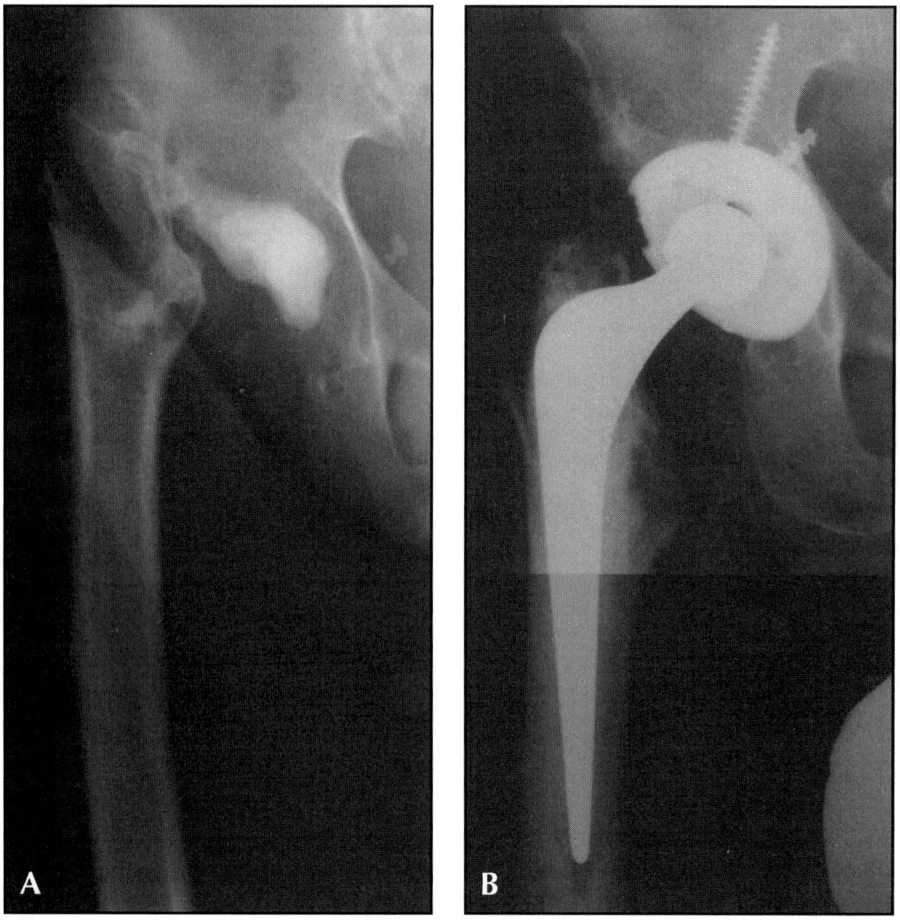

Fig. 5 A, Septic arthritis (*Staphylococcus aureus*) treated with a Girdlestone resection arthroplasty and antibiotic-loaded cement depot in the acetabulum. **B,** After successful eradication of infection and reimplantation.

replacement following infection, with low reinfection rates and good function, the size of these series and the variability of treatment methods preclude their sole use in determining the optimum treatment of these patients. The patient with an infection that was adequately treated many years before, with no episodes of recurrence, and in whom current investigations exclude active sepsis, is clearly suitable for implantation. However, determining the optimal treatment for the patient with a more recent or even current infection is more difficult.

At the time of arthroplasty the decisions must be made between one stage or two and whether to use an uncemented implant or one with antibiotic-loaded cement. Although there is little guidance in the literature to answer these questions specifically with respect to primary hip replacement, the wealth of information on the treatment of infection at the site of hip arthroplasty can provide some guidelines. The management of these cases represents the treatment of an active infection and, therefore, has a considerably higher risk of recurrence than a previously infected natural hip joint. The risk may be similar to that expected with the treatment of a current or recent septic arthritis.

One- or Two-Stage Reconstruction?

In primary THA after previous infection that is quiescent, the rates of deep

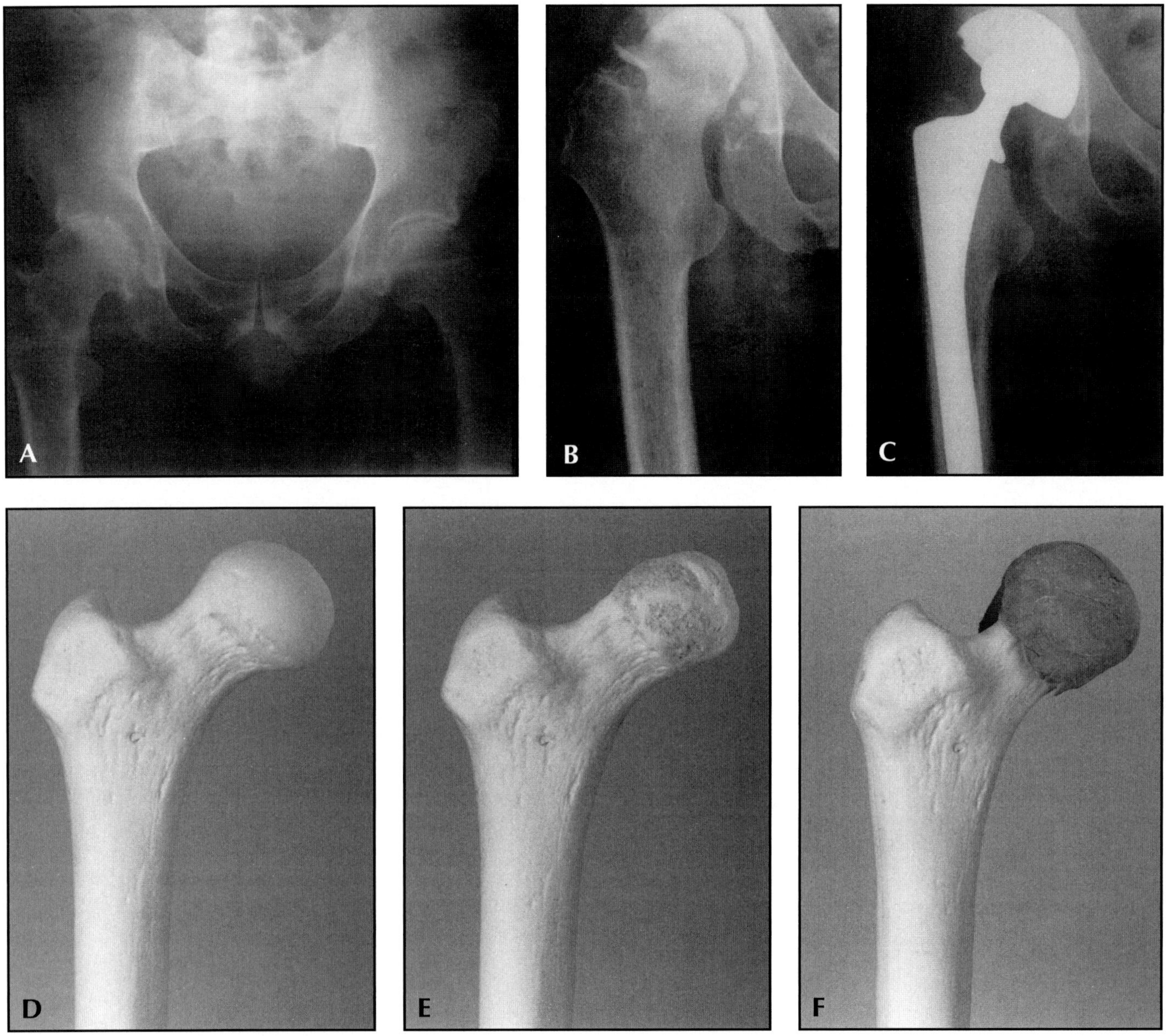

Fig. 6 A, Acute septic arthritis (*Staphylococcus aureus*), treated by **B,** Débridement of the femoral head and resurfacing with antibiotic-loaded cement. **C,** After successful eradication of infection and reimplantation. **D** through **F,** Model to represent débridement and resurfacing with antibiotic-loaded polymethylmethacrylate.

sepsis after single-stage arthroplasty are reported to be between 0 (0 of 27) and 10% (4 of 42).[1,53,54] Hardinge and associates[1] noted that the pain of secondary osteoarthritis is slowly progressive, and a rapid deterioration should raise the suspicion of reactivation of infection, which should be ruled out before proceeding to arthroplasty. Buchholz and associates[70] reported their first 10-year experience with one-stage revision hip arthroplasty using antibiotic-loaded cement, during which they used gentamicin, erythromycin, or antibiotics as directed by preoperative cultures. They successfully eradicated infection in 77% (448 of 583) at the first attempt and 88% after further exchange, if required.

Raut and associates[71] described their experience with 57 so-called one-stage exchange arthroplasties for infection at the site of THA with actively draining sinuses, using gentamicin-loaded cement. At a mean follow-up of 7.5 years (2 to 12.5 years), infection had been controlled in 86% (49 of 57). The authors concluded that even the presence of an actively

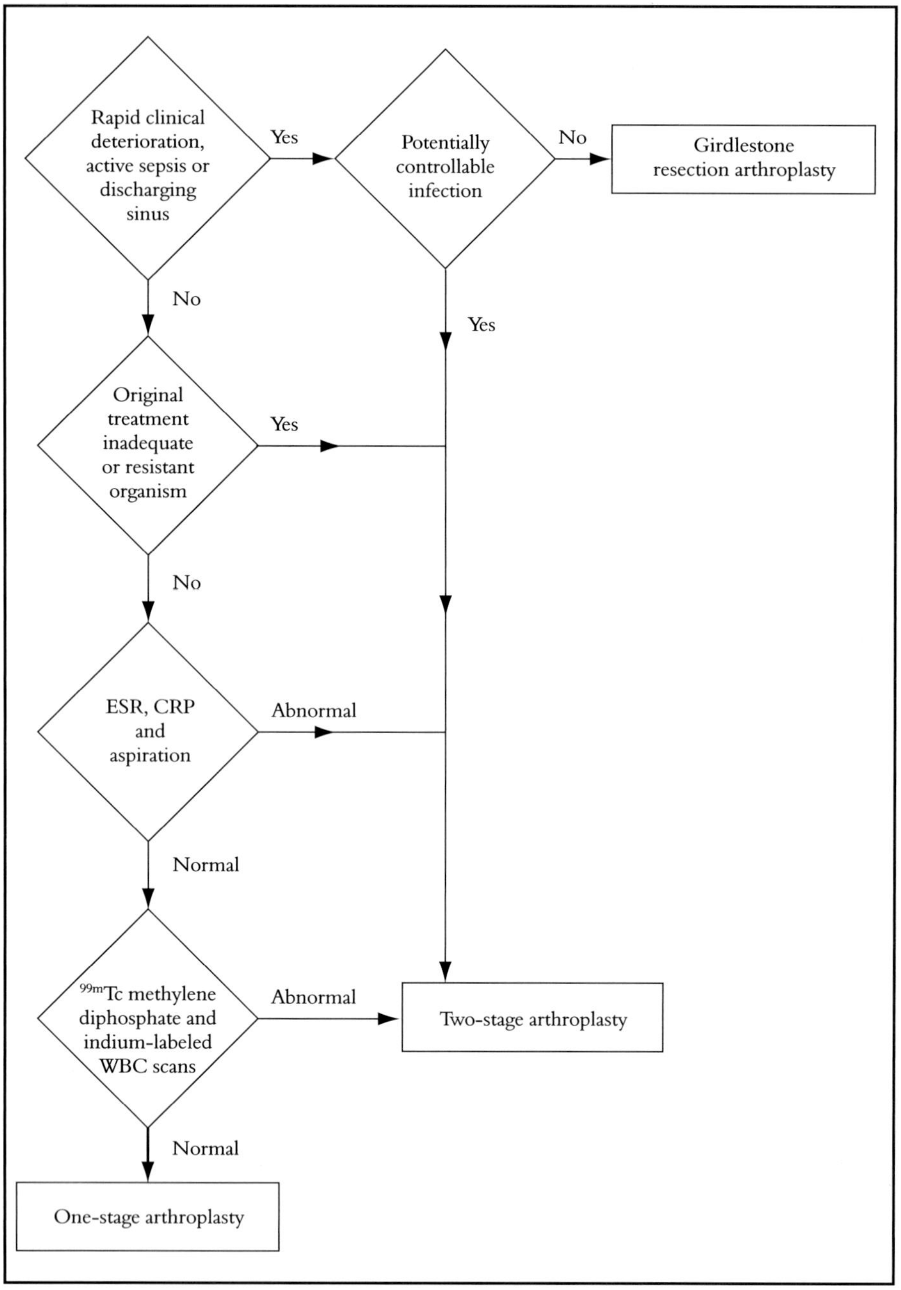

Fig. 7 Treatment algorithm.

Table 4
Surgical requirements for natural and prosthetic hip infections

Infection	Natural Joint	Prosthetic Joint
Pyogenic	Open	Remove implant
Tuberculous	Closed	Retain implant
Fungal	Closed	Remove implant

draining sinus was not in itself a contraindication to a so-called one-stage exchange arthroplasty.

In a prospective multicenter trial of 77 hip replacements with proven infection, Carlsson and associates[59] performed 59 revisions in one stage and 18 in two, with a mean interval of 1 year (2 to 41 months). At follow-up of between 6 months and 6 years, 78% of one-stage reconstructions were considered successful, with recurrence in 8% (5 of 59) and possible recurrence in a further 14% (8 of 59). Similarly 77% of those performed in two stages had succeeded with 17% recurrence (3 of 18) and one doubtful case. Although these failure rates of one- and two-stage techniques appear comparable, the patients with one-stage revisions had been given 6 months of postoperative antibiotics, and follow-up was less than a year in 34% (20 of 59) and 2 years in 61% (36 of 51). Sanzén and associates[31] reported similar cure rates at 2- to 9-year follow-up of 76% (55 of 72) in one-stage revision, 65% (11 of 17) with two-stage revision without gentamicin beads, and 83% (11 of 13) with two stages of revision and beads.

Garvin and Hanssen[72] demonstrated in their review of 29 series that in the absence of antibiotic cement, a one-stage revision had a 58% (35 of 60) cure rate compared to 82% (130 of 158) for a two-stage procedure. Similarly, with antibiotic cement, the one-stage cure rate was 82% (976 of 1,189) compared to 91% (385 of 423) for two-stage. The studies differ greatly in exact management details, which precludes statistical analysis. There is, however, an apparent benefit in using antibiotic-loaded cement in one-stage arthroplasty, whereas for a staged reconstruction, the benefit, if any, is much reduced (Table 3).

In performing staged revision arthroplasty, most authors recommend a delay between stages of 6 weeks to 6 months; however, this remains controversial and some authors have found no correlation between the time interval from débridement to implantation and the recurrence of infection.[39] In revision hip arthroplasty with cement that did not contain antibiotics, McDonald and associates[60] found that at a mean follow-up of 5.5 years (2 to 13.6 years), the reinfection rate was significantly higher when reimplantation was at less than 1 year (27% [7 of 26]) than when it was greater (7% [4 of 56]; $P < 0.001$), suggesting that a longer period may be beneficial in these cases.

The Role of Antibiotic-Loaded Cement

While the addition of antibiotics to cement is unusual in North America, in the United Kingdom over half (57%) of surgeons routinely use antibiotic-loaded cement, even in routine primary cases.[73] Polymethylmethacrylate bone cement has been shown experimentally to decrease leukocyte migration,[74] reduce leukocyte ability to phagocytose, to a lesser extent kill the most common infecting agents (*S aureus* and *S epidermidis*),[75] and detrimentally affect the complement cascade.[76] In addition, the exothermic polymerization may cause local bone injury, promoting bacterial colonization; therefore, a theoretical case can be made against its use. However, as well as a potential bactericidal effect of the polymethylmethacrylate monomer itself, there may be additional bactericidal benefit from the exothermic polymerization process, which produces a surface temperature of up to 70° in vivo and internal temperatures of up to 125°.[77]

The cement also can be used as a vehicle for antibiotic delivery, and while the duration of antibiotic release from cement in vitro is less than suggested in some of the earlier studies,[78-80] several clinical studies have demonstrated the effectiveness of antibiotic-loaded cement in reducing the incidence of deep sepsis in THA.[81,82] Furthermore, in an in vivo study, Masri and associates[83] demonstrated therapeutic levels of tobramycin in the periprosthetic fluid up to 4 months after implantation of antibiotic-loaded spacers. Josefsson and associates,[81] in a prospective trial comparing gentamicin cement with systemic prophylactic antibiotics, found a significant reduction in deep sepsis from 1.6% (13 of 812) to 0.4% (3 of 821; $P < 0.01$) with gentamicin cement. At later follow-up of greater than 5 years, the difference was still significant ($P < 0.05$) at 1.9% (16 of 835) compared to 0.8% (7 of 853), respectively.[82]

In performing primary THA on hips with quiescent sepsis, at a mean follow-up of 5 years (2 to 19 years) Laforgia and associates[54] found that infection or reactivation had occurred in none of nine hips that had gentamicin in the cement but did in 4 of 33 hips without gentamicin. However, the use of systemic antibiotics was erratic, and they were given only to one of the four who developed an infection.

Garvin and Hanssen[72] presented the results of 29 series of revision THAs. They demonstrated a cumulative cure rate for single-stage revision of 58% (35 of 60) without antibiotics and 82% (976 of 1,189) with, supporting the case for antibiotic-loaded cement in single-stage arthroplasty. A similar but less marked benefit was demonstrated for two-stage revisions at 82% eradication (130 of 158) without antibiotic cement and 91% (385 of 423) with its use.

In their studies of patients reimplanted with a prosthesis using cement that does not contain antibiotics in two-stage exchange arthroplasty for infection at the site of THA, McDonald and associates[60] looked at patients infected with what they considered to be more virulent organisms (methicillin-resistant staphylococci, group D streptococci, gram-negative bacilli). Infection recurred in 1 of 13 patients (8%) treated with antibiotics for more than 28 days, and in 3 of 7 (43%) treated for less. Although the numbers were small and not statistically significant ($P = 0.055$), there appears to be a clear beneficial trend of using a prolonged course of systemic antibiotics if antibiotics are not present in the cement.

Concern has been raised about the production of resistant organisms when antibiotic-loaded cement is used. Hope and associates,[84] in their study of 91 patients with coagulase negative staphylococcal infection at the site of THA, demonstrated a significantly higher incidence of gentamicin-resistant organisms when gentamicin had been present in the cement (88% [30 of 34]) than when plain cement was used (16% [9 of 57]; $P < 0.001$).

In addition to using standard antibiotics in cement, we have previously described the use of streptomycin-loaded bone cement as an adjunct to conventional therapy in the management of active tuberculous osteomyelitis,[85] and amphoteracin B-loaded cement for the treatment of fungal infections.[86]

Definitive Reimplantation With Antibiotic-Loaded Cement Versus Cementless Technique

To the best of our knowledge, there are no studies that compare the outcome of primary THA after sepsis with so-called cemented versus cementless implants in sufficient numbers to draw statistical conclusions.

In revision hip arthroplasty, several studies have demonstrated that prostheses inserted without cement at the second stage in two-stage exchange arthroplasty achieve similar results to those implanted with antibiotic-loaded cement. Using an uncemented implant, Nestor and associates[87] report an 82% (28 of 34) cure of infection at mean of 4 years (2 to 6 years), with an 8-month (3 to 19 months) interval in the revision of infected THAs that had originally been implanted with cement. A similar result of an 87% (34 of 39 patients) cure of infection at a mean of 4 years (2.5 to 7 years) was presented by Lai and associates[88] using two-stage revision of uncemented THAs with a 1-year (2 to 25 months) interval. They also demonstrated a marked benefit in using antibiotic-impregnated beads during the interval, with recurrence of infection in 6% (2 of 34) of those with beads and 50% (3 of 6) of those without.

The Influence of the Type of Organism on Infection Eradication After Hip Replacement for Previous Sepsis

There is controversy over which organisms are harder to treat and, therefore, more likely to recur. In their mixed series of 31 hip replacements after hip sepsis, both spontaneous and postoperative, Cherney and Amstutz[39] found a minimum 3-year infection eradication rate of 78% (14 of 18) for gram-positive bacteria, 58% (7 of 12) for gram-negative bacteria, and 66% (2 of 3) for anaerobes, and concluded that their success rate was higher for infections caused by gram-positive organisms than for those caused by gram-negative organisms. The series is too small to draw statistical conclusions. In fact, of the nine cases of spontaneous infection in which no previous implant was present, the opposite trend was shown, with infection eradication rates of 50% (2 of 4) and 60% (3 of 5) for infections caused by gram-positive and gram-negative organisms, respectively.

Buchholz and associates[70] reported greater difficulty eradicating infections caused by gram-negative organisms in one-stage revision for infection at the site of THA. Their success rate was 43% (62 of 145) compared to 72% (197 of 274) for infections caused by *S aureus*. Similarly, Jupiter and associates[53] found that at the site of implant, infections caused by gram-negative organisms were more difficult to eradicate. Many authors, however, have found no real evidence to indicate that gram-negative organisms are any harder to treat than others. Sanzén and associates[31] found no difference in infection eradication rates between different organisms (82% [51 of 62] for gram-positive cocci, 82% [9 of 11] for gram-negatives, and 78% [14 of 18] for anaerobes). Tsukayama and associates[89] reported that all of 13 infections caused by gram-negative organisms in their series were cured with the use of tobramycin-loaded cement beads. While the above data apply to revision THA, there are no data in the literature regarding reimplantation of the hip after an acute infection.

Use of Allografts After Infection

In the reconstruction of the hip damaged by infection, on occasion there will be such extensive bone loss from the acetabulum or proximal femur that augmentation with an allograft may be desirable. There are no reports on the outcome of bulk allografts in primary hip arthroplasty after infection; however, their use in reconstruction of infection at the site of THA with bone loss is well described and can provide some guidance. Wang and Chen[90] reported their experience using allografts in two-stage revision for infection at the site of THA. At a mean follow-up of 4 years (2 to 7 years) they found recurrent infection in 13% (2 of 16) with morcellized grafts, and 0 of 6 where bulk and morcellized graft were used. Both recurrences were with virulent organisms: one was a methicillin-resistant *S aureus* and the other was a *Pseudomonas* organism. Similarly, Berry and associates[91] found 8% of bulk allografts (1 of 13) were complicated by deep infection after a two-stage revision at a mean follow-up of 42 months (24 to 97 months). Alexeeff and associates[92] reported no recurrent infections in 11 hips that were reconstructed with bulk allograft after deep infection at a mean follow-up of 48 months (24 to 72 months), although the latter differed in using an antibiotic-loaded cement spacer in the interval between stages. It can therefore be concluded that the selective use of a bulk allograft is not contraindicated by a history of previous, but no longer active, hip sepsis.

Surgical Technique

Preoperative Assessment

Clinical The presence of any signs of active infection should be sought and excluded. There is often contracture of the flexors or adductors, which should be quantified, and the power of the abductors should be assessed, particularly if they have been violated by a previous operation. Any leg-length inequality is determined and the neurovascular status of the limbs recorded.

Radiologic In addition to the usual radiographs, unless the acetabulum is very well preserved, Judet views should be obtained to assess the available bone stock.

Surgical Details

The technical difficulty of the arthroplasty will depend on the degree of soft-tissue contracture and the extent of bone loss. In many cases where treatment was early and effective such that the patient made a good functional recovery, the anatomy will be well preserved, and the technique will not be substantially different from a routine primary hip replacement. In other cases, particularly those of neonatal sepsis, there may be extensive distortion of the pelvic and femoral anatomy, which may require modified techniques with special components and sometimes bone graft.

Previous incisions should be used if present and appropriate, and any sinuses should be fully excised. Severe contractures may require release of the adductors or iliopsoas. Antibiotics should be withheld until synovial specimens have been taken for culture, which should include studies for tuberculosis and fungi, if suspected.

The original acetabulum may be filled with scar, and in cases with marked bone loss and a proximally displaced greater trochanter, the hip center may be difficult to ascertain. Here, an intraoperative anteroposterior radiograph of the pelvis with the reamer in situ can be very useful for ensuring correct placement of the cup in relation to the so-called tear drop. Following longstanding infection of the hip, the proximal femur may be distorted with a narrow intramedullary canal and an anteverted femoral neck, which may cause difficulty with reaming and an increased risk of femoral fracture. If the previous infection led to a spontaneous fusion, this represents an increased risk of heterotopic ossification, and prophylactic measures of anti-inflammatories or radiotherapy should be considered (Fig.1).

Although the surgery may in some cases be technically demanding, the reported complications rates, with respect to nerve injury and dislocation, while only based on small series, do not appear to be greatly increased.[54,67]

The Authors' Preferred Protocol

In primary hip replacement, we recommend a two-stage reconstruction in cases of resistant organisms at the initial infection, if the primary treatment appears to have been inadequate or if there is a sinus or other evidence of a recent flare-up. Similarly, in the presence of an elevated ESR or CRP; positive hip aspiration; positive bone biopsy, histology, or cultures; or positive sequential technetium-indium scans, which suggest ongoing sepsis, a two-stage procedure is indicated. An MRI may indicate active sepsis but is not routinely used in our assessment.

Since 1986, in staged procedures, we have used the PROSTALAC (Prosthesis of Antibiotic-Loaded Acrylic Cement) concept (Figs. 2 through 4). With the use of a system of molds, a femoral component is fashioned from a narrow stemmed femoral component that is encased in antibiotic-impregnated cement. A constrained acetabular component is also cemented with antibiotic-loaded cement. Because the PROSTALAC is a temporary low-demand implant, the concerns about high antibiotic concentrations weakening the cement can largely be disregarded, and we typically use 2.4 to 3.6 g of tobramycin and 1.0 to 1.5 g of vancomycin per 40 g of cement powder. The actual choice of antibiotic depends on the historic or preoperative cultures; however, the concentrations used are much higher than those used in definitive cementation of an implant. Appropriate parenteral antibiotics are administered for 6 weeks. If a repeat aspiration of the hip 4 weeks after completion of the antibiotics is negative for bacterial growth, and the ESR and CRP have returned to normal, the second stage is performed using hybrid or cementless fixation depending on the patient's age and the surgeon's preference.

Before the PROSTALAC was available, the first stage consisted of either a Girdlestone arthroplasty and antibiotic-loaded cement depot placed in the acetabulum (Fig. 5), or we have also successfully used a technique of forming a surface hemiarthroplasty from antibiotic-loaded cement (Fig. 6). These earlier techniques have the theoretical advantage that they do not violate the femoral canal. However, spread of infection simply as a result of the PROSTALAC stem has not been noted, and ambulation is greatly improved.

We have previously reported a 100% (6 of 6) eradication rate with this two-stage regimen for primary hip replacements in the presence of active pyogenic hip infection and 94% (45 of 48) for revision of infection at the site of THA at a minimum follow-up of 2 years.[62]

If the history of deterioration is slowly progressive, there are no clinical features of active sepsis, and the inflammatory markers, aspiration, and nuclear medicine scans are negative, we would advocate a one-stage arthroplasty using antibiotic-loaded cement for the femoral component and either an all-polyethylene acetabular component inserted with antibiotic-loaded cement or a porous-coated acetabular component inserted without cement (Fig. 7).

The Treatment of Reactivation of Infection: Is Surgery Required?

Once well established, pyogenic infection of a hip arthroplasty warrants treatment with prosthetic exchange. In contrast, tuberculous infections have been treated successfully with antituberculous therapy and retention of the prosthesis in cases where the components are solidly fixed[93] (Table 4). In fungal prosthetic hip infections, to date there have been no reports of successful treatment without implant removal. However, successful irradication of infection has been reported for staged reimplantation.[16,94]

References

1. Hardinge K, Cleary J, Charnley J: Low-friction arthroplasty for healed septic and tuberculous arthritis. *J Bone Joint Surg Br* 1979;61:144-147.
2. Gallie WE: First recurrence of osteomyelitis eighty years after infection. *J Bone Joint Surg Br* 1951;33:110-111.
3. Jones NS, Anderson DJ, Stiles PJ: Osteomyelitis in a general hospital: A five-year study showing an increase in subacute osteomyelitis. *J Bone Joint Surg Br* 1987;69:779-783.
4. Craigen MA, Watters J, Hackett JS: The changing epidemiology of osteomyelitis in children. *J Bone Joint Surg Br* 1992;74:541-545.
5. Pasteur L: De l'extension de la theorie des germes a l'etiologie de quelques maladies communes. *Bull Acad Med* 1880;9:435-447.
6. Gillespie WJ, Mayo KM: The management of acute haematogenous osteomyelitis in the antibiotic era: A study of the outcome. *J Bone Joint Surg Br* 1981;63:126-131.
7. Kelly PJ: Bacterial arthritis in the adult. *Orthop Clin North Am* 1975;6:973-981.
8. Morrey BF, Bianco AJ Jr, Rhodes KH: Septic arthritis in children. *Orthop Clin North Am* 1975;6:923-934.
9. Farer LS, Lowell AM, Meador MP: Extrapulmonary tuberculosis in the United States. *Am J Epidemiol* 1979;109:205-217.
10. Shivaram U, Wollschlager C, Khan F, Khan A: Spinal tuberculosis revisited. *South Med J* 1985;78:681-684.
11. Chaisson RE, Slutkin G: Tuberculosis and human immunodeficiency virus infection. *J Infect Dis* 1989;159:96-100.
12. Watson JM, Gill ON: HIV infection and tuberculosis. *BMJ* 1990;300:63-65.

13. Fitzgerald E, Lloyd-Still J, Gordon SL: Candida arthritis: A case report and review of the literature. *Clin Orthop* 1975;106:143-147.

14. Noyes FR, McCabe JD, Fekety FR Jr: Acute candida arthritis: Report of a case and use of amphotericin B. *J Bone Joint Surg Am* 1973;55:169-176.

15. Svirsky-Fein S, Langer L, Milbauer B, Khermosh O, Rubinstein E: Neonatal osteomyelitis caused by Candida tropicalis: Report of two cases and review of the literature. *J Bone Joint Surg Am* 1979;61:455-459.

16. Evans RP, Nelson CL: Staged reimplantation of a total hip prosthesis after infection with Candida albicans: A report of two cases. *J Bone Joint Surg Am* 1990;72:1551-1553.

17. Samra Y, Hertz M, Shaked Y, Zwas S, Altman G: Brucellosis of the spine: A report of 3 cases. *J Bone Joint Surg Br* 1982;64:429-431.

18. Munoz-Fernandez S, Macia MA, Pantoja L, et al: Osteoarticular infection in intravenous drug abusers: Influence of HIV infection and differences with non drug abusers. *Ann Rheum Dis* 1993;52:570-574.

19. Engh CA, Hughes JL, Abrams RC, Bowerman JW: Osteomyelitis in the patient with sickle-cell disease. *J Bone Joint Surg Am* 1971;53:1-15.

20. del Sel HJ, Charnley J: Total hip replacement following infection in the opposite hip. *Clin Orthop* 1979;141:138-142.

21. Surin VV, Sundholm K, Bäckman L: Infection after total hip replacement: With special reference to a discharge from the wound. *J Bone Joint Surg Br* 1983;65:412-418.

22. Coutts RD, Schiller AL, Harris WH: Subclinical osteomyelitis of the femoral head: Two cases illustrating a special problem in the use of total hip replacement. *Clin Orthop* 1972;86:68-72.

23. Hecht RH, Meyers MH, Thornhill-Joynes M, Montgomerie JZ: Reactivation of tuberculous infection following total joint replacement: A case report. *J Bone Joint Surg Am* 1983;65:1015-1016.

24. Hunt DD, Larson CB: Treatment of the residua of hip infections by mold arthroplasty: An end-result study of thirty-three hips. *J Bone Joint Surg Am* 1966;48:111-125.

25. Harris WH, Aufranc OE: Mold arthroplasty in the treatment of hip fractures complicated by sepsis: A report on nine cases. *J Bone Joint Surg Am* 1965;47:31-42.

26. Hughes PW, Salvati EA, Wilson PD Jr, Blumenfeld EL: Treatment of subacute sepsis of the hip by antibiotics and joint replacement: Criteria for diagnosis with evaluation of twenty-six cases. *Clin Orthop* 1979;141:143-157.

27. Spangehl MJ, Masri BA, O'Connell JX, Duncan CP: Prospective analysis of preoperative and intraoperative investigations for the diagnosis of infection at the sites of two hundred and two revision total hip arthroplasties. *J Bone Joint Surg Am* 1999;81:672-683.

28. Forster IW, Crawford R: Sedimentation rate in infected and uninfected total hip arthroplasty. *Clin Orthop* 1982;168:48-52.

29. Levitsky KA, Hozack WJ, Balderston RA, et al: Evaluation of the painful prosthetic joint: Relative value of bone scan, sedimentation rate, and joint aspiration. *J Arthroplasty* 1991;6:237-244.

30. Magnuson JE, Brown ML, Hauser MF, Berquist TH, Fitzgerald RH Jr, Klee GG: In-111-labeled leukocyte scintigraphy in suspected orthopedic prosthesis infection: Comparison with other imaging modalities. *Radiology* 1988;168:235-239.

31. Sanzén L, Carlsson AS, Josefsson G, Lindberg LT: Revision operations on infected total hip arthroplasties: Two- to nine-year follow-up study. *Clin Orthop* 1988;229:165-172.

32. Schauwecker DS: The scintigraphic diagnosis of osteomyelitis. *AJR Am J Roentgenol* 1992;158:9-18.

33. Tang JS, Gold RH, Bassett LW, Seeger LL: Musculoskeletal infection of the extremities: Evaluation with MR imaging. *Radiology* 1988;166:205-209.

34. Mason MD, Zlatkin MB, Esterhai JL, Dalinka MK, Velchik MG, Kressel HY: Chronic complicated osteomyelitis of the lower extremity: Evaluation with MR imaging. *Radiology* 1989;173:355-359.

35. Al-Sheikh W, Sfakianakis GN, Mnaymneh W, et al: Subacute and chronic bone infections: Diagnosis using In-111, Ga-67 and Tc-99m MDP bone scintigraphy, and radiography. *Radiology* 1985;155:501-506.

36. Merkel KD, Brown ML, Dewanjee MK, Fitzgerald RH Jr: Comparison of indium-labeled leukocyte imaging with sequential technetium-gallium scanning in the diagnosis of low-grade musculoskeletal sepsis: A prospective study. *J Bone Joint Surg Am* 1985;67:465-476.

37. Datz FL, Thorne DA: Effect of chronicity of infection on the sensitivity of the In-111-labeled leukocyte scan. *AJR Am J Roentgenol* 1986;147:809-812.

38. Rubin RH, Fischman AJ, Needleman M, et al: Radiolabeled, nonspecific, polyclonal human immunoglobulin in the detection of focal inflammation by scintigraphy: Comparison with gallium-67 citrate and technetium-99m-labeled albumin. *J Nucl Med* 1989;30:385-389.

39. Cherney DL, Amstutz HC: Total hip replacement in the previously septic hip. *J Bone Joint Surg Am* 1983;65:1256-1265.

40. Lachiewicz PF, Rogers GD, Thomason HC: Aspiration of the hip joint before revision total hip arthroplasty: Clinical and laboratory factors influencing attainment of a positive culture. *J Bone Joint Surg Am* 1996;78:749-754.

41. Taylor RG: Pseudarthrosis of the hip joint. *J Bone Joint Surg Br* 1950;32:161-165.

42. Girdlestone GR: Discussion on treatment of unilateral osteoarthritis of the hip-joint. *Proc R Soc Med* 1945;38:363-368.

43. Haw CS, Gray DH: Excision arthroplasty of the hip. *J Bone Joint Surg Br* 1976;58:44-47.

44. Bittar ES, Petty W: Girdlestone arthroplasty for infected total hip arthroplasty. *Clin Orthop* 1982;170:83-87.

45. Petty W, Goldsmith S: Resection arthroplasty following infected total hip arthroplasty. *J Bone Joint Surg Am* 1980;62:889-896.

46. Waters RL, Perry J, Conaty P, Lunsford B, O'Meara P: The energy cost of walking with arthritis of the hip and knee. *Clin Orthop* 1987;214:278-284.

47. Shepherd MM: A further review of the results of operations on the hip joint. *J Bone Joint Surg Br* 1960;42:177-204.

48. Callaghan JJ, Brand RA, Pedersen DR: Hip arthrodesis: A long-term follow-up. *J Bone Joint Surg Am* 1985:67:1328-1335.

49. Sponseller PD, McBeath AA, Perpich M: Hip arthrodesis in young patients: A long-term follow-up study. *J Bone Joint Surg Am* 1984;66:853-859.

50. Perugia L, Santori FS, Mancini A, Manili M, Falez F: Conversion of the arthrodesed hip to a total hip arthroplasty: Indications and limitations. *Ital J Orthop Traumatol* 1992;18:145-153.

51. Amstutz HC, Sakai DN: Total joint replacement for ankylosed hips: Indications, technique, and preliminary results. *J Bone Joint Surg Am* 1975;57:619-625.

52. Kilgus DJ, Amstutz HC, Wolgin MA, Dorey FJ: Joint replacement for ankylosed hips. *J Bone Joint Surg Am* 1990;72:45-54.

53. Jupiter JB, Karchmer AW, Lowell JD, Harris WH: Total hip arthroplasty in the treatment of adult hips with current or quiescent sepsis. *J Bone Joint Surg Am* 1981;63:194-200.

54. Laforgia R, Murphy JC, Redfern TR: Low friction arthroplasty for old quiescent infection of the hip. *J Bone Joint Surg Br* 1988;70:373-376.

55. Wilson PD Jr, Aglietti P, Salvati EA: Subacute sepsis of the hip treated by antibiotics and cemented prosthesis. *J Bone Joint Surg Am* 1974;56:879-898.

56. Schmalzried TP, Amstutz HC, Au MK, Dorey FJ: Etiology of deep sepsis in total hip arthroplasty: The significance of hematogenous and recurrent infections. *Clin Orthop* 1992;280:200-207.

57. Hardinge K, Williams D, Etienne A, MacKenzie D, Charnley J: Conversion of fused hips to low friction arthroplasty. *J Bone Joint Surg* 1977;59:385-392.

58. Went P, Krismer M, Frischhut B: Recurrence of infection after revision of infected hip arthroplasties. *J Bone Joint Surg Br* 1995;77:307-309.

59. Carlsson AS, Josefsson G, Lindberg L: Revision with gentamicin-impregnated cement for deep infections in total hip arthroplasties. *J Bone Joint Surg Am* 1978;60:1059-1064.

60. McDonald DJ, Fitzgerald RH Jr, Ilstrup DM: Two-stage reconstruction of a total hip arthroplasty because of infection. *J Bone Joint Surg Am* 1989;71:828-834.

61. Younger AS, Duncan CP, Masri BA: Treatment of infection asssociated with segmental bone loss in the proximal part of the femur in two stages with use of an antibiotic-loaded interval prosthesis. *J Bone Joint Surg Am* 1998;80:60-69.
62. Younger AS, Duncan CP, Masri BA, McGraw RW: The outcome of two-stage arthroplasty using a custom-made interval spacer to treat the infected hip. *J Arthroplasty* 1997;12:615-623.
63. Jerry GJ Jr, Rand JA, Ilstrup D: Old sepsis prior to total knee arthroplasty. *Clin Orthop* 1988;236:135-140.
64. Farrell MJ Jr, Bryan RS: Total knee arthroplasty after septic arthritis. *Orthop Clin North Am* 1975;6:1057-1062.
65. Charnley J: The long-term results of low-friction arthroplasty of the hip performed as a primary intervention. *J Bone Joint Surg Br* 1972;54:61-76.
66. Salvati EA, Wilson PD Jr: The long-term results of femoral-head replacement. *J Bone Joint Surg Am* 1973;55:516-524.
67. Eskola A, Santavirta S, Konttinen YT, Tallroth K, Hoikka V, Lindholm ST: Cementless total replacement for old tuberculosis of the hip. *J Bone Joint Surg Br* 1988;70:603-606.
68. Johnson R, Barnes KL, Owen R: Reactivation of tuberculosis after total hip replacement. *J Bone Joint Surg Br* 1979;61:148-150.
69. Kim YY, Ko CU, Lee SW, Kwak BM: Replacement arthroplasty using the Charnley prosthesis in old tuberculosis of the hip. *Int Orthop* 1979;3:81-88.
70. Buchholz HW, Elson RA, Engelbrecht E, Lodenkämper H, Röttger J, Siegel A: Management of deep infection of total hip replacement. *J Bone Joint Surg Br* 1981;63: 342-353.
71. Raut VV, Siney PD, Wroblewski BM: One-stage revision of infected total hip replacements with discharging sinuses. *J Bone Joint Surg Br* 1994;76:721-724.
72. Garvin KL, Hanssen AD: Infection after total hip arthroplasty: Past, present, and future. *J Bone Joint Surg Am* 1995;77:1576-1588.
73. Leach WJ, Wilson NI: Trends in infection prophylaxis in orthopaedics. *J R Coll Surg Edinb* 1992;37:265-266.
74. Petty W: The effect of methylmethacrylate on chemotaxis of polymorphonuclear leukocytes. *J Bone Joint Surg Am* 1978;60:492-498.
75. Petty W: The effect of methylmethacrylate on bacterial phagocytosis and killing by human polymorphonuclear leukocytes. *J Bone Joint Surg Am* 1978;60:752-757.
76. Petty W, Caldwell JR: The effect of methylmethacrylate on complement activity. *Clin Orthop* 1977;128:354-359.
77. Meyer PR Jr, Lautenschlager EP, Moore BK: On the setting properties of acrylic bone cement. *J Bone Joint Surg Am* 1973;55:149-156.
78. Chapman MW, Hadley WK: The effect of polymethylmethacrylate and antibiotic combinations on bacterial viability: An in vitro and preliminary in vivo study. *J Bone Joint Surg Am* 1976;58:76-81.
79. Hill J, Klenerman L, Trustey S, Blowers R: Diffusion of antibiotics from acrylic bone-cement in vitro. *J Bone Joint Surg Br* 1977;59:197-199.
80. Levin PD: The effectiveness of various antibiotics in methyl methacrylate. *J Bone Joint Surg Br* 1975;57:234-237.
81. Josefsson G, Lindberg L, Wiklander B: Systemic antibiotics and gentamicin containing bone cement in the prophylaxis of postoperative infections in total hip arthroplasty. *Clin Orthop* 1981;159:194-200.
82. Josefsson G, Gudmundsson G, Kolmert L, Wijkström S: Prophylaxis with systemic antibiotics versus gentamicin bone cement in total hip arthroplasty: A five-year survey of 1688 hips. *Clin Orthop* 1990;253:173-178.
83. Masri BA, Duncan CP, Beauchamp CP: Long-term elution of antibiotics from bone- cement: An in vivo study using the prosthesis of antibiotic-loaded acrylic cement (PROSTALAC) system. *J Arthroplasty* 1998;13:331-338.
84. Hope PG, Kristinsson KG, Norman P, Elson RA: Deep infection of cemented total hip arthroplasties caused by coagulase-negative staphylococci. *J Bone Joint Surg Br* 1989;71: 851-855.
85. Masri BA, Duncan CP, Jewesson P, Ngui-Yen J, Smith J: Streptomycin-loaded bone cement in the treatment of tuberculous osteomyelitis: An adjunct to conventional therapy. *Can J Surg* 1995;38:64-68.
86. Marra F, Robbins GM, Duncan CP, et al: Amphotericin B-loaded bone cement for the treatment of Candida albicans osteomyelitis. *Can J Surg*, in press.
87. Nestor BJ, Hanssen AD, Ferrer-Gonzalez R, Fitzgerald RH Jr: The use of porous prostheses in delayed reconstruction of total hip replacements that have failed because of infection. *J Bone Joint Surg Am* 1994;76:349-359.
88. Lai K-A, Shen W-J, Yang C-Y, Lin R-M, Lin C-J, Jou I-M: Two-stage cementless revision THR after infection: 5 recurrences in 40 cases followed 2.5-7 years. *Acta Orthop Scand* 1996;67:325-328.
89. Tsukayama DT, Estrada R, Gustilo RB: Infection after total hip arthroplasty: A study of the treatment of one hundred and six infections. *J Bone Joint Surg Am* 1996;78:512-523.
90. Wang J-W, Chen C-E: Reimplantation of infected hip arthroplasties using bone allografts. *Clin Orthop* 1997;335:202-210.
91. Berry DJ, Chandler HP, Reilly DT: The use of bone allografts in two-stage reconstruction after failure of hip replacements due to infection. *J Bone Joint Surg Am* 1991;73:1460-1468.
92. Alexeeff M, Mahomed N, Morsi E, Garbuz D, Gross A: Structural allograft in two-stage revisions for failed septic hip arthroplasty. *J Bone Joint Surg Br* 1996;78:213-216.
93. Spinner RJ, Sexton DJ, Goldner RD, Levin LS: Periprosthetic infections due to Mycobacterium tuberculosis in patients with no prior history of tuberculosis. *J Arthroplasty* 1996;11:217-222.
94. Younkin S, Evarts CM, Steigbigel RT: Candida parapsilosis infection of a total hip-joint replacement: Successful reimplantation after treatment with amphotericin B and 5-fluorocytosine. A case report. *J Bone Joint Surg Am* 1984;66:142-143.

34

Primary Total Hip Arthroplasty After Acetabular Fracture

Dana C. Mears, MD, PhD
John H. Velyvis, MD

After a displaced acetabular fracture, a patient may be predisposed to the development of symptomatic posttraumatic degenerative arthritis of the hip joint or osteonecrosis of the femoral head. In selected patients, a total hip arthroplasty (THA) may eventually be necessary irrespective of the method of initial management.[1-3] On the basis of a review of the results described by Letournel and Judet[2] and Matta[4] and on the basis of our experience, we determined that the likelihood that treatment will culminate in an arthroplasty is related to the initial type of fracture; the magnitude of the provocative force; the age and weight of the patient; and, when the initial management of the fracture was open reduction and internal fixation, the duration of the delay from the injury to the surgical procedure. When the initial acetabular deformity is relatively minor and when the acetabulum unites, especially following nonsurgical treatment, a conventional arthroplasty is likely to lead to an uncomplicated recovery and a satisfactory outcome. Nevertheless, in selected cases, one or more complicating factors may be encountered. Following nonsurgical treatment of an acetabular fracture, residual displacement may hamper a subsequent arthroplasty because of an occult or frank nonunion of the acetabulum or possibly because of a malunion or a malaligned nonunion.[5] When the initial management of an acetabular fracture was surgical, a belated arthroplasty performed to manage posttraumatic arthritis may be impeded by dense scar tissue, heterotopic bone, avascularity of the hip muscles or the acetabulum, obstructive hardware, or occult infection.[6] On the basis of a review of the few prior studies in the literature,[7-10] we found that the overall prognosis for a patient managed with a THA after an acetabular fracture is less favorable than that for one managed with an arthroplasty performed because of primary degenerative arthritis. In the present study, we address the principal concerns regarding management with THA after initial treatment of an acetabular fracture with closed or open reduction.

In view of the principal shortcoming of acute management with THA following an acetabular fracture, namely, the vulnerability to premature failure and the subsequent need for one or more surgical revisions, the potential therapeutic alternatives merit serious consideration. For example, young male laborers or other young, exceptionally active individuals are highly susceptible to premature failure of an arthroplasty.[11] In such patients, one therapeutic alternative is arthrodesis of the hip, which is mainly indicated if there is relative preservation of the osseous architecture of the hip joint. The other criteria for an arthrodesis, namely, a normal contralateral hip, normal knees, and an asymptomatic lower back, also must be met.[12] Currently, most individuals in North America are reluctant to consider arthrodesis. When a patient has osteonecrosis of the femoral head, loss of acetabular bone stock, marked osteoporosis, or a persistent acetabular nonunion that impairs the mechanical stability of a hip fusion and hampers the healing of the bone, the likelihood of achieving a solid fusion is considerably compromised. In such complex cases, the main practical alternative is a resection arthroplasty, with or without the use of a cement spacer.[13]

Certain other symptomatic acetabular fractures may be associated with secondary problems that can be addressed by reconstruction of the hip, thus preserving the hip as a functional joint. Examples of the problems include heterotopic bone leading to hip stiffness; symptoms related to the hardware; a symptomatic nonunion or malunion of the acetabulum and/or hemipelvis; and, occasionally, a localized and indolent infection. In each of these situations, all relevant diagnostic clinical and radiographic methods are used in an attempt to determine whether the hip joint has intact and congruent bearing surfaces. Whenever it is technically possible, and especially in a younger patient, every attempt should be made to salvage a functional hip joint.[14]

Clinical Assessment

The typical presenting symptoms of posttraumatic arthritis or osteonecrosis of the femoral head include local or referred pain, a limp, and a decreased level of activity. If the acetabulum, or another site in the pelvic ring, has a persistent nonunion, the patient may complain of pelvic instability with gross motion of the nonunion site or sites. A marked deformity of the pelvic ring can be an associated complicating factor, but this is rare. After an open reduction of the acetabulum, particularly when an extensile exposure has been used, stiffness may develop secondary to extensive heterotopic bone. Young obese men who sustain a closed head injury in addition to the acetabular fracture are notoriously susceptible to this problem.

During the physical examination, a shortened leg or an antalgic or stiff-hipped gait may be evident. Tenderness about the hip and the presence of a surgical scar, along with a flexion or other type of contracture and stiffness, are commonly observed. The ipsilateral lower extremity is examined carefully for subtle findings of a sciatic nerve palsy, such as hypoesthesia of the foot or motor weakness. When a patient has these findings, even a slight intraoperative injury to the sciatic nerve creates a substantial risk for the development of a postoperative complete footdrop because of the extraordinary susceptibility of a peripheral nerve to a second injury, or "double crush syndrome" as described by Osterman.[15]

When open reduction of the acetabulum culminates in a chronically painful hip, the potential for a deep wound infection needs to be considered. Most such infections are occult, with such subtle clinical findings that hematologic, bacteriologic, and radiographic studies, and even an aspiration arthrogram, may not confirm the diagnosis. In an exceptional case, a frank wound infection with an open sinus tract may complicate the presentation of grossly infected bone. From the time of presentation, the patient should be managed with suitable antibiotic therapy, and surgical planning should include multiple débridements, techniques for plastic coverage of the wound, and consideration of a belated arthroplasty.

Radiographic Assessment

When a minimally displaced acetabular fracture progresses to posttraumatic arthritis, the preparation for a THA may be adequately accomplished by scrutiny of standard anteroposterior pelvic and frog-leg lateral radiographs. In more complex cases, additional pelvic radiographs may be helpful.[2,3] The 45° inlet and outlet radiographs reveal pelvic ring deformities, including central protrusion and vertical or posterior displacement of a hemipelvis. The 45° obturator oblique radiograph highlights deformities of the anterior column and the posterior wall, while the corresponding iliac oblique radiograph depicts the posterior column and the anterior wall. A CT scan may provide the optimal view of an occult nonunion and of incarcerated hardware such as a screw. When a patient has an exceptional deformity that involves the entire pelvic ring, a three-dimensional CT scan may help the surgeon to identify the sites and vectors of the deformity.[16] When there is extensive heterotopic bone formation, a combination of imaging modalities merits consideration in order to fully characterize the magnitude of the problem. A CT scan along with Judet oblique radiographs are crucial to fully ascertain the extent of the anterior and posterior heterotopic ossification.[17]

When an occult deep wound infection is suspected after a prior open acetabular reduction, either an aspiration arthrogram or a technetium Tc 99m bone scan may be helpful. An infection is a causative factor for heterotopic bone formation.[18] Ironically, when a patient has florid heterotopic bone, an aspiration arthrogram may be impossible and a technetium Tc 99m bone scan may lose much of its sensitivity in the detection of infection. In addition to a complete blood cell count with differential and a determination of the erythrocyte sedimentation rate and C-reactive protein level, a gallium Ga 67 citrate scan or an indium white blood cell scan may be valuable, but only in rare cases.[19,20]

Preoperative Planning

When the clinical and radiographic assessments are complete, the specific focal problems of the patient are carefully analyzed to plan the arthroplasty. A discrete acetabular defect may arise from the site of a displaced acetabular fragment following surgical removal of a loose fragment or from an area of marginal or central impaction. The defect may vary widely in size, from minute to structurally important. As a general rule, a defect with a diameter of less than 10 mm is not structurally important, a defect with a diameter of 10 to 25 mm is moderately important, and a defect with a diameter of greater than 25 mm is very important (Fig. 1). Such defects can be characterized by one of the available classification schemes, such as that of D'Antonio and associates[21] and that of Gross and associates[22] (Tables 1 and 2). Most of the available classification schemes distinguish isolated cavitary lesions from segmental defects. The more structurally important segmental group can be subdivided into defects involving a wall or a rim as opposed to a column or, ultimately the most sinister form, a transverse dissociation or nonunion. These types of defects represent progressively more challenging reconstructive problems. Irrespective of its size, such a defect may possess a well-circumscribed boundary or a highly irregular one, and its borders may have well-vascularized or avascular bone. All of these factors have profound implications for the therapeutic plan.

A wide variety of deformities of the acetabulum and the pelvic ring may be encountered. When a late deformity is present, it may involve a limited portion of the acetabulum, such as the anterior or posterior column or the medial wall. This type of deformity may be evident as a linear step-off. Alternatively, after an unreduced fracture of both columns, a

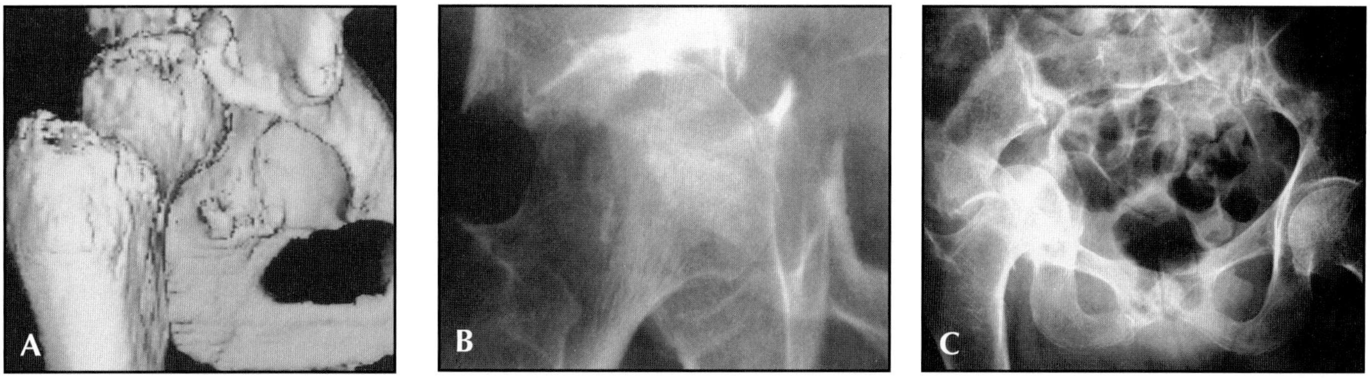

Fig. 1 The structural importance of acetabular defects is related to their size, location, and characterization as a cavitary or segmental lesion. **A,** Oblique three-dimensional CT scan, obtained 1 year after a fracture-dislocation of the posterior wall, showing a large segmental defect of the posterior wall secondary to failed fixation. **B,** Anteroposterior (AP) radiograph of a hip, obtained 2 years after a transtectal transverse fracture that was treated nonsurgically, showing a central segmental defect of moderate size, with a principal axis of more than 10 mm but less than 25 mm. **C,** AP radiograph of a pelvis, obtained 2 years after a transtectal T-type fracture that was treated nonsurgically, showing progression to a large central segmental defect with a principal axis of approximately 50 mm.

"secondary incongruity" may represent a malrotation of each portion of the acetabulum, manifesting as a protrusion of the fragments around the imploded femoral head.[2] Nevertheless, in this situation, while the center of rotation of the femoral head is somewhat altered biomechanically, there is no true focal acetabular defect. This deformity, therefore, is readily addressed with use of a standard cementless cup of a somewhat enlarged size, or a so-called jumbo cup[23] (Fig. 2).

Table 1
Classification of acetabular deficiencies in THA according to the system of D'Antonio and associates[21]

Type	Deficiency
I	Segmental deficiencies
IA	Peripheral
IB	Central (medial wall absent)
II	Cavitary deficiencies
IIA	Peripheral
IIB	Central (medial wall intact)
III	Combined deficiencies
IV	Pelvic discontinuity
V	Arthrodesis

Table 2
Classification of acetabular deficiencies in THA according to the system of Gross and associates[22]

Type	Deficiency
I	Contained cavitary defect (protrusio)
II	Uncontained (structural rim defect)
IIA	Minor column (shelf defect) with > 50% of cup coverage
IIB	Major column (acetabular defect) with > 50% loss of cup contact and loss of one or both columns

At the time of a THA for posttraumatic arthritis following an acetabular fracture, a nonunion is particularly likely to be encountered after a posterior wall or column injury. However, after an injury pattern such as a transverse fracture or a fracture of both columns, a nonunion is an uncommon problem that occurs primarily when florid displacement is uncorrected. Preoperative multiplanar imaging of the acetabulum is particularly helpful to characterize the magnitude, site, and vector of displacement of the nonunion. The degree of malalignment of an acetabular nonunion has considerable therapeutic implications and can be broadly subdivided into three categories that correspond to the magnitude of the acetabular defect. When the nonunion gap is less than 10 mm, it can be readily obliterated by packing it with autograft harvested from the femoral head. Alternatively, the fracture fragments may be sufficiently mobile to approximate the fracture surfaces with use of suitable bone-holding forceps. The fixation of the fragments can be achieved with use of lag screws, a plate, a cup with multiple screws, or a ring. When a nonunion defect is 10 to 25 mm, scar tissue, heterotopic bone, or fracture callus may considerably impede an attempted open reduction. The gap can be obliterated with morcellized or bulk autograft. For structural augmentation, one of several strategies may be considered. Fine stainless-steel or titanium mesh can be used to buttress the acetabulum to facilitate impaction grafting.[24] Alternatively, a cup inserted with multiple screws can be used as a form of a hemispherical plate. For defects that are larger than 25 mm, one of several specialized devices may be used. A cage or ring combined with a cemented cup can be used to immobilize multiple acetabular bone fragments and to obliterate the acetabular defect.[25,26] To fill a superior acetabular defect, a bilobed cup can be used. As an alternative strategy, when the nonunion gap exceeds 25 mm, serious consideration should be given to realignment and reapproximation of the acetabulum.[5] Otherwise, a

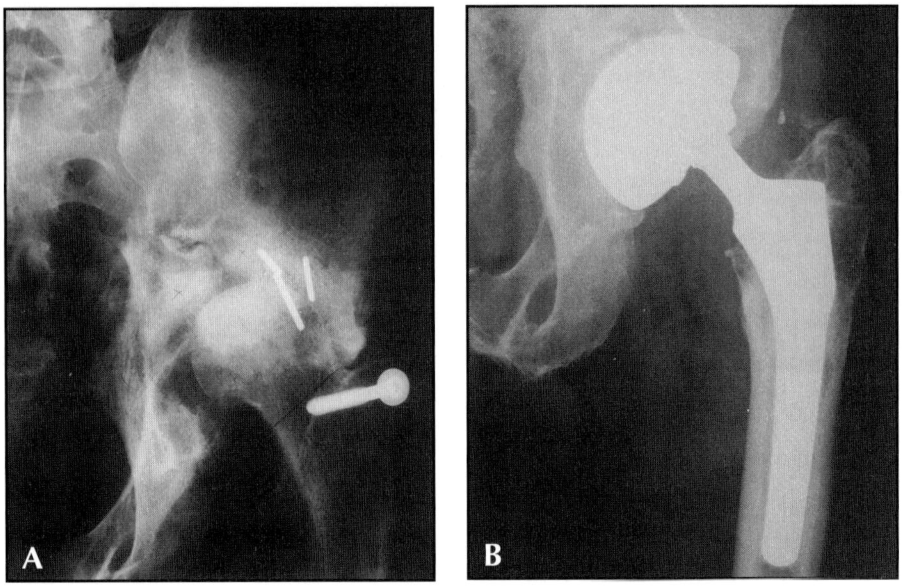

Fig. 2 A 48-year-old man sustained a T-type acetabular fracture, which was managed with limited internal fixation. Subsequent symptomatic posttraumatic arthritis was complicated by an excessively large superocentral acetabular defect and necrotic bone in the roof. Three years after the injury, as part of a THA, the necrotic bone was removed and a structural autograft from the femoral head was used to obliterate the acetabular defect. **A,** AP radiograph of the right hip, obtained 3 years after the injury, showing the large acetabular defect. **B,** AP radiograph obtained after the THA, showing the large defect obliterated by a jumbo cup.

technical failure with a persistent nonunion, premature loosening of the cup, or other complication is likely to ensue. During preoperative preparation for such a case, a three-dimensional CT scan is helpful to optimally characterize the pelvic deformity.

Optimal Timing of the Arthroplasty

After initial management of an acetabular fracture, THA is typically considered when a patient is seen with evidence of secondary degenerative change 1 year or more after the initial injury. By that time, the acetabulum is usually united, even though there may be a defect or a deformity. Occasionally, a serious problem with the hip (for example, an early secondary displacement of the fracture, possibly with failed internal fixation) is recognized within a few days or weeks after the initial injury and following either nonsurgical or surgical treatment.

An unacceptable deformity often is not adequately appreciated radiographically. For instance, when a patient has a displaced transverse or posterior fracture-dislocation and osteopenia, the femoral head typically undergoes rapid abrasive wear that may culminate in the loss of 50% or more of its surface area. Likewise, late recognition of marginal or central acetabular impaction may not be consistent with a realistic capability to achieve a satisfactory belated surgical correction. Unfortunately, both conventional radiography and CT may fail to provide a realistic representation of a hip with an extraordinary amount of loss of surface area of the femoral head or extensive acetabular impaction.

When a THA is indicated, a question may arise about the need to delay the procedure until the acetabular fracture has fully united so that the cup can be inserted into a stable osseous bed. The best solution depends on the severity of the particular acetabular deformity and the experience of the surgeon. There are potential advantages to undertaking a THA as soon as the hip has been shown radiographically to have incongruent articular surfaces and thus an overwhelming potential for a rapid onset of pain. The foremost advantage is minimization of the delay between the acute fracture and the recovery from the arthroplasty. Also, when an unacceptable deformity of the acetabulum is recognized soon after the injury, either as a failure to achieve an acceptable reduction or as a delayed displacement, the defect can typically be adequately minimized or even fully corrected at the time of a promptly executed arthroplasty.

For some hips with a displaced fracture, open reduction and internal fixation needs to be considered when an incongruity has been recognized early.[14] In the absence of marked impaction or abrasion of the articular surfaces, and especially in a young adult who has a simple fracture pattern, delayed open reduction is preferred. In an inactive elderly or otherwise infirm patient in whom comminution and impaction secondary to osteoporosis can be anticipated, acute management with an arthroplasty may be a more realistic endeavor. When it is difficult to predict the extent of irreversible damage radiographically, consent for open reduction with a possible THA is obtained and the appropriate resources are organized for both procedures.

Surgical Approaches

Depending on the focal anatomic and pathologic problem, such as heterotopic ossification, one of several standard surgical approaches may be preferred[26-31] (Fig. 3). Typically, when posttraumatic arthritis develops after an acetabular fracture has healed with minimal deformity, either a conventional anterior Hardinge approach[31] or a posterior approach is highly suitable. When there is a substantial acetabular deformity or heterotopic bone, a modified or alternative exposure may be preferred. If a fractured posterior wall or column requires an extensive surgical field, then a full Kocher-Langenbeck incision[2] is used. For adequate visualization of both the anterior and the posterior aspect of the acetabulum and the adjacent hip joint, a triradiate incision with preservation of the greater trochanter is highly appropriate. When the entire hemipelvis is involved in the deformity and needs a corrective osteotomy as part of the arthroplasty, then an extended iliofemoral approach may be used. In this situation, we prefer a modified or limited extended iliofemoral approach whereby the gluteal tendons and adjacent greater trochanter as well as the piriformis tendons are preserved intact. If the ipsilateral sacroiliac joint is displaced, typically in external rotation, open reduction can be achieved by means of a variety of exposures. With the extended iliofemoral or triradiate approach, a release of the insertions of the external oblique muscle from the iliac crest and the iliacus muscle from the internal iliac fossa provides a suitable access. Alternatively, if the arthroplasty is performed with a conventional anterior or posterior approach to the hip, a second incision along the anterior iliac crest can be used to approach the sacroiliac joint. Whenever a secondary deformity of the pelvic ring culminates in malalignment of the acetabulum by more than 25° in a single plane, initial correction of the pelvic ring is usually indicated prior to the THA. Otherwise, after insertion of the cup, an iatrogenic deformity would ensue as the pelvic ring deformity was corrected. For deformities that involve both hemipelves, the multiple corrective osteotomies and the arthroplasty may be undertaken as a combined sequential procedure (Fig. 4) or as separate procedures at two different times. The relevant determinants include the experience of the surgeon, the magnitude and complexity of the deformities, the presence of heterotopic bone, and the potential comorbidities of the patient. Some of the principal determinants and the corresponding therapeutic strategies are outlined in Table 3.

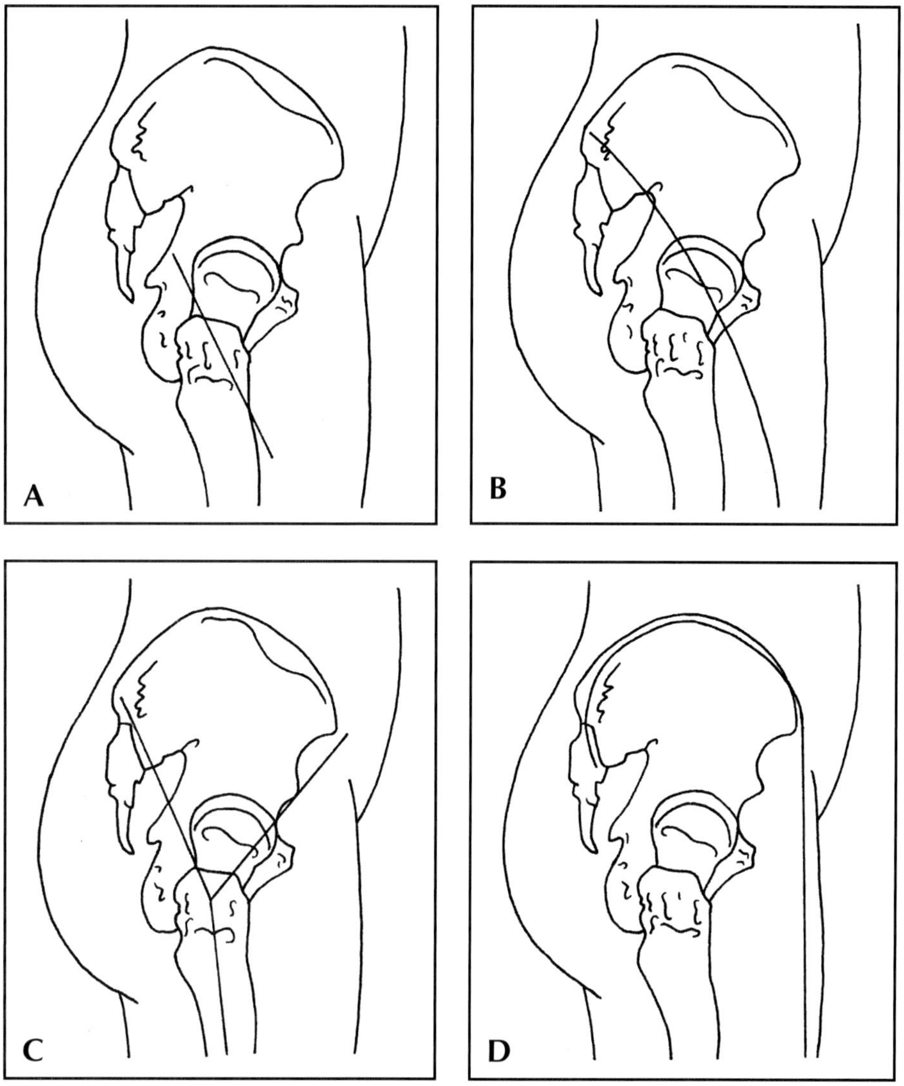

Fig. 3 The surgical approaches commonly used in THA for late reconstruction of acetabula with various defects and accompanying deformities. **A**, The modified Hardinge (anterolateral) incision. Our preferred modification of the approach includes an orientation of 30° from the long axis of the limb so that more direct visualization of the acetabulum is achieved with a shorter incision. **B**, The Kocher-Langenbeck incision. **C**, The modified triradiate incision, with preservation of the greater trochanter. **D**, The limited extended iliofemoral incision.

Preparation of the Acetabulum

After routine resection of the femoral neck and head, the acetabulum is débrided of residual fibrocartilage and granulation tissue. The acetabulum is carefully examined for a defect, deformity, or nonunion. If such a site is identified, its osseous surfaces are meticulously denuded so that the structural problem can be carefully assessed. The subsequent stages depend on the nature of the problem. If the acetabulum displays necrotic bone, then the dead bone is removed until a uniformly bleeding bed is achieved.

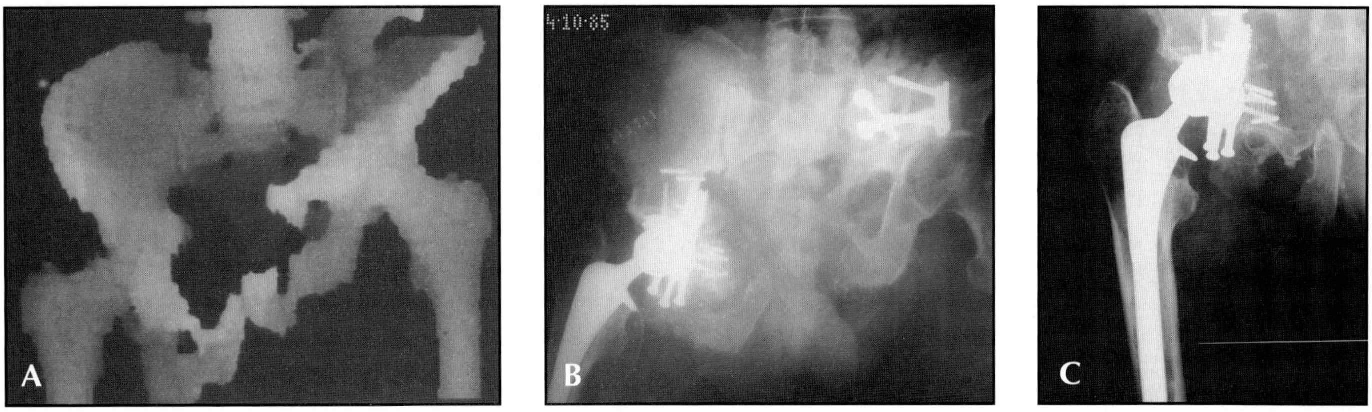

Fig. 4 CT scan and radiographs showing a displaced iliac-wing, or so-called crescent, fracture of the left hip and a T-type acetabular fracture of the right hip. **A,** A three-dimensional CT scan, obtained at the time of presentation, showing a persistent vertical and rotational deformity of the left hemipelvis and a displaced nonunion of the right T-type acetabular fracture with distal displacement of the inferior half of the acetabulum. **B,** Postoperative AP radiograph showing a partial correction of the left pelvic deformity and a right cementless total hip replacement with immobilization of the acetabulum. **C,** AP radiograph of the right hip, obtained 11 years after arthroplasty, showing a successful long-term result. The patient had no pain.

Subsequently, the acetabulum is reamed to restore a hemispherical concavity that is suitable for the insertion of a cementless cup. A large jumbo cup may be needed to obliterate a residual acetabular recess (Fig. 2).

Contained Defects

For a small contained defect, impaction grafting with morcellized bone from the femoral head is preferred.[24,32-35] When a defect is 25 mm or more in its largest dimension, a structural autograft should be considered. In some instances, a femoral head-and-neck autograft can be shaped to fit precisely into the defect (Fig. 5). If it is slightly oversized, it may be impacted to achieve a stable fit. In other instances, fixation with supplementary lag screws or a plate may be necessary. When the cup is placed on a bed of autograft, a cementless cup is the most appropriate choice. When the bed consists of allograft, and especially when it involves the weight-bearing surface, use of a cemented cup is preferred.[36] If the defect greatly exceeds 25 mm in its largest dimension, another useful option is a ring or cage.

Use of a Ring or Cage

Historically, a ring or cage was used in conjunction with a cemented polyethylene cup (Fig. 6). The more recent designs include the availability of a metal-backed polyethylene liner that is mechanically secured to the cage so that the use of bone cement is unnecessary. A wide variety of cages with diverse extension plates are available for special problems[25,26,28] (Fig. 7). The principal advantage of the cage is the potential to use a device with a predictable shape to obliterate a highly irregular defect. Frequently, supplementary bone graft is needed to fill any gaps that remain between the outer surface of the cage and the intact pelvis. The cage may function as a type of fixation plate that immobilizes the site of a transverse nonunion. Nevertheless, despite its current popularity, a cage has certain shortcomings. The foremost problem is a potential for loosening when its anchoring screws are inserted in osteopenic bone. Where there is a nonunion and osteopenic bone, failure to achieve a rapid union of the acetabulum contributes greatly to premature loosening of the cage. A shortcoming that pertains to previous designs in which the cup was attached to the cage with bone cement is late deterioration of this interface, with subsequent loss of fixation of the cup. This problem is not uncommon after a period of 5 to 10 years. An additional shortcoming of the various cages with a superior or inferior flange or hook is the anatomic configuration of such devices. Typically, such a cup does not fit properly in a highly deformed acetabulum. Most cages are too thick to permit realistic contouring with standard bending instrumentation. A review of the indications for the use of a variety of these devices is summarized in Table 4.

Intermediate or Uncontained Defects

The most common site of an intermediate or uncontained defect is the posterior wall (Fig. 8). In this situation, the displaced and ununited fragment of wall typically is maintained, by scar tissue, in a highly displaced location with superior and posterior malalignment. To achieve a nearly anatomic reduction, the surfaces attached by scar tissue must be fully mobilized, which inevitably provokes extensive avascularity. As an alternative technique, we prefer to denude the deep, former articular surface of the displaced fragment so that it contacts the structural graft and provides a potential source of blood supply.

After curettage, whenever feasible, the defect is prepared with conventional acetabular reamers. Likewise, the true acetabulum is reamed in a conventional manner. The resected femoral head is denuded of residual cartilage with use of cup arthroplasty reamers or so-called reverse acetabular reamers and is used as a structural autograft. A v-shaped notch is made in the femoral head so that the notch interlocks into the damaged section of the posterior wall. The autograft is anchored with use of three 3.5- or 4.0-mm fully threaded screws. Then, the acetabulum is reamed again to the optimal diameter. Any persistent small defect at the junction between the graft and the residual acetabulum is filled with morcellized cancellous bone. Then, a metal backing for a cementless cup in an appropriate size is impacted into the acetabular recess and is anchored with two or three cancellous screws.

Table 3
Guidelines for surgical strategies to address pelvic and acetabular deformities as part of a THA

Type of Defect	Treatment
Intrinsic acetabular defects	
Small superior acetabular defect	Morcellized impaction grafting if contained defect, supplementary mesh if uncontained defect, cementless cup
Large superior acetabular defect	Structural or morcellized grafting, cementless cup, jumbo cup, bilobed cup, protrusio cage
Medial acetabular defect	Central mesh, morcellized impaction grafting, cage
Posterior acetabular defect	Structural or morcellized grafting, posterior plate, mesh, standard cup, cage
Associated deformities of pelvic ring	
Iliac defect, nonunion, malalignment	Open reduction and internal fixation of ilium, standard cup
External rotational deformity of ipsilateral or contralateral sacroiliac joint	Open reduction and internal fixation of sacroiliac joint, standard cup
Unstable, windswept pelvis	Open reduction and internal fixation of both sacroiliac joints, standard cup
Vertical defect	
Ipsilateral	Reduction of hemipelvis, long-stemmed component
Contralateral	Reduction of hemipelvis, standard cup

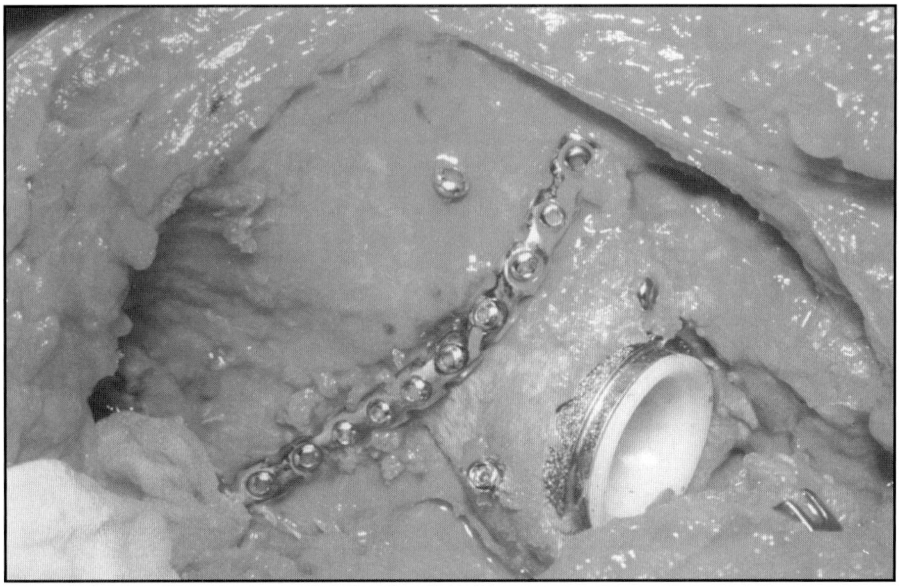

Fig. 5 A T-type fracture of the posterior wall that initially was managed nonsurgically progressed to a nonunion with deformity and degenerative change. Two years later, the posterior column was stabilized through a Kocher-Langenbeck approach with a reconstruction plate, while the defective wall was replaced with a precisely fitting structural autograft and lag screws. This intraoperative photograph was obtained after a metal-backed cup was secured to the pelvis while the autograft was secured with multiple screws.

Large Uncontained Defects

Large uncontained defects present a principal structural problem in the posterior, superior, or central aspect of the acetabulum. Some reconstructive recommendations are described for each type of defect.

When a patient has a large defect in the posterior part of the acetabulum that involves the wall and the adjacent column, perhaps the most formidable mechanical challenge is the transfer of the patient from the bed to a chair. Thus, a highly stable configuration of the reconstruction is essential. Historically, the most popular form of reconstruction has been the application of a posterior plate with the use of a structural autograft (Figs. 5 and 8). Alternative potential solutions include the use of a cage or a mesh, which is anchored around the rim of the defect with screws. Then, impaction grafting of the defect is performed with autologous bone in order to create a suitable bed for the cup.

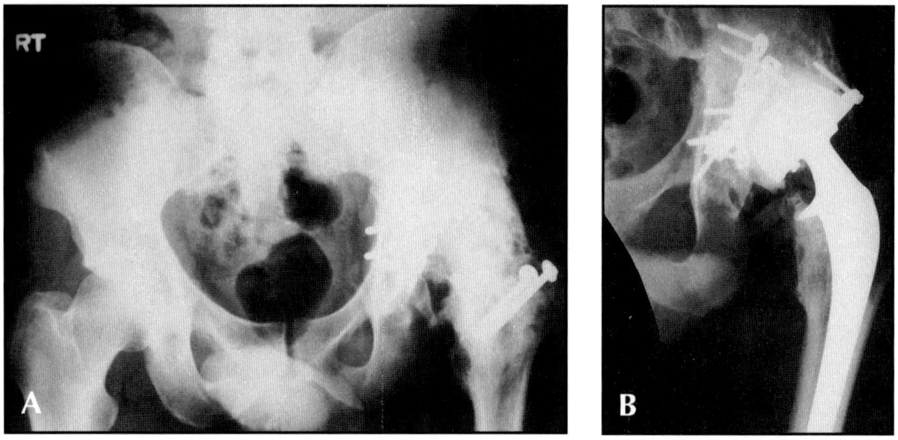

Fig. 6 Radiographs of a 28-year-old man who sustained a transverse fracture of the posterior wall of the left acetabulum. Open reduction and internal fixation was performed with use of a triradiate incision. Within 2 weeks, the posterior wall fragment had displaced; subsequently, the hip progressed to posttraumatic arthritis with grade IV heterotopic bone formation. Two years later, a THA was performed and augmented with a Müller ring to stabilize the wall defect. **A,** AP radiograph, obtained 2 years after the open reduction and internal fixation, showing grade IV heterotopic bone formation and a fusion of the hip. **B,** AP radiograph, obtained 5 years after THA, showing stable fixation of the ring along with a cemented polyethylene cup and a cementless stem.

Table 4
Devices to manage a large defect and indications for their use

Device	Indication
Mesh	Superior or middle central defect or superior posterior wall defect (remaining acetabulum must be intact)
Bilobed cup	Superior wall and dome defect
Müller ring	Central, superior defect
Ganz ring with hook inobturator foramen	Nonunion of transverse fracture

Another option is the fabrication of a custom implant that is designed on the basis of a three-dimensional CT scan or a corresponding model of the hip (Fig. 9). While this method permits the use of an unlimited variety of shapes to address truly unique structural problems, it possesses several shortcomings. Not only is this technique costly, but only a single implant design can be available during the procedure. If an unanticipated defect within an avascular bed is identified during the surgery, so that additional bone has to be excised, then the custom implant no longer fits precisely into the defect. In this situation, structural autograft or, suboptimally, allograft is needed to restore the structural stability of the reconstruction.

A viable solution for a defect in the superior aspect of the acetabulum that includes a corresponding segment of wall is a bilobed or oblong cup.[37] One newer modular model permits the application of a lobe of three different sizes for obliteration of the corresponding defects (Fig. 10). The principal shortcoming of a bilobed cup is the need to orient it so that the lobe is directed superiorly. If a defect is posterosuperior, the lobe cannot be redirected or the articular portion of the cup will be malaligned and provoke instability of the total hip prosthesis.

For repair of a defect in the central aspect of the acetabulum, use of a structural autograft, a cage, or a central mesh should be considered[38] (Fig. 11). For the latter two methods, morcellized autograft initially is placed into the base of the defect prior to insertion of the hardware. If a central mesh is used, a 5- to 10-mm-thick layer of morcellized cancellous bone graft is impacted in place after insertion of the mesh.

If the defect is exceedingly large, a bed of morcellized cancellous bone graft is inserted into the acetabulum to a thickness of approximately 5 mm. A layer of mesh that obliterates the entire defect is placed inside the bone graft and is supported by the adjacent intact acetabulum. Extra-articular screws may be inserted to anchor the periphery of the mesh to the lateral wall of the acetabular rim. Additional bone graft is impacted into the mesh until a continuous layer that is 5 to 10 mm thick has been established. A second layer of mesh is inserted into the acetabulum with two additional extra-articular anchoring screws. An additional layer of impacted bone graft is used to cover the second mesh. Then, a cup is cemented into the bone graft. In this construct, the secondary layer of mesh serves to compartmentalize the bone graft and thereby to inhibit late subsidence.

Nonunion

When a partial union of a displaced acetabular fracture creates a gap of as much as 25 mm, the fracture gap is usually managed with débridement and obliteration with autograft. If a mobile nonunion is encountered, the opposing surfaces are approximated and immobilized with appropriate fixation. Any residual fracture gaps are obliterated with bone graft. The preferred strategies for fixation of a nonunion site include the use of lag screws or the insertion of a cup as a hemispherical plate, both of which avoid exposure of the posterior column, which is the most suitable site for plate fixation. The application of a plate to the posterior column in the setting of a nonunion is likely to result in osteo-

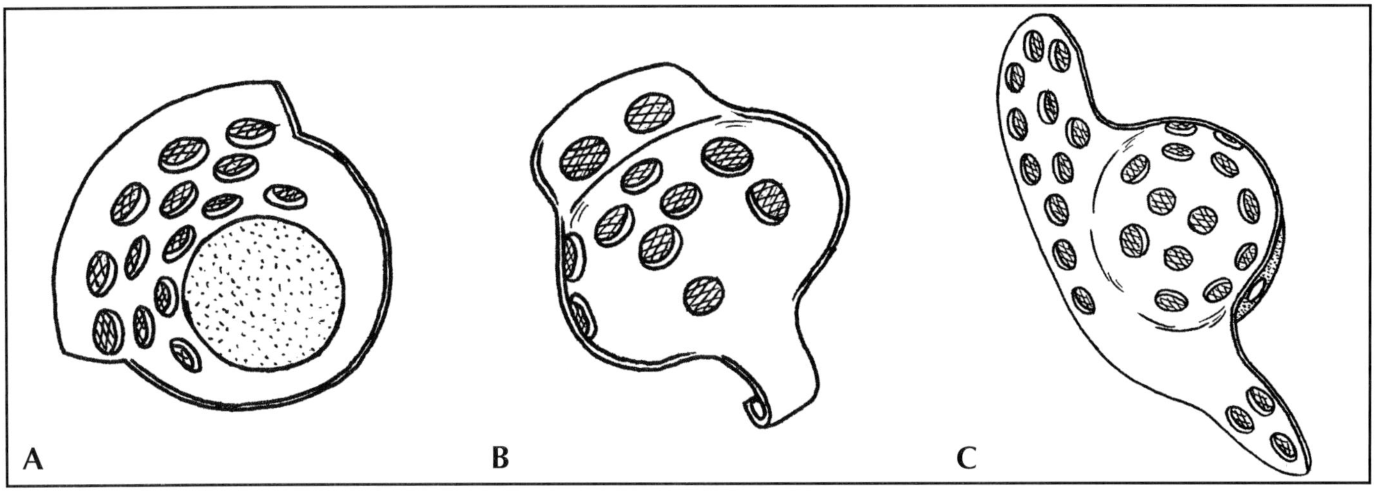

Fig. 7 Drawings showing multiple designs of cages with diverse extension plates that are available for use with a cemented cup. **A,** Müller ring with a smaller posterosuperior flange. **B,** Ganz ring with a superior flange and an inferior hook for anchorage in the obturator foramen. **C,** Burch-Schneider cage with large superior and inferior flanges for anchoring screws.

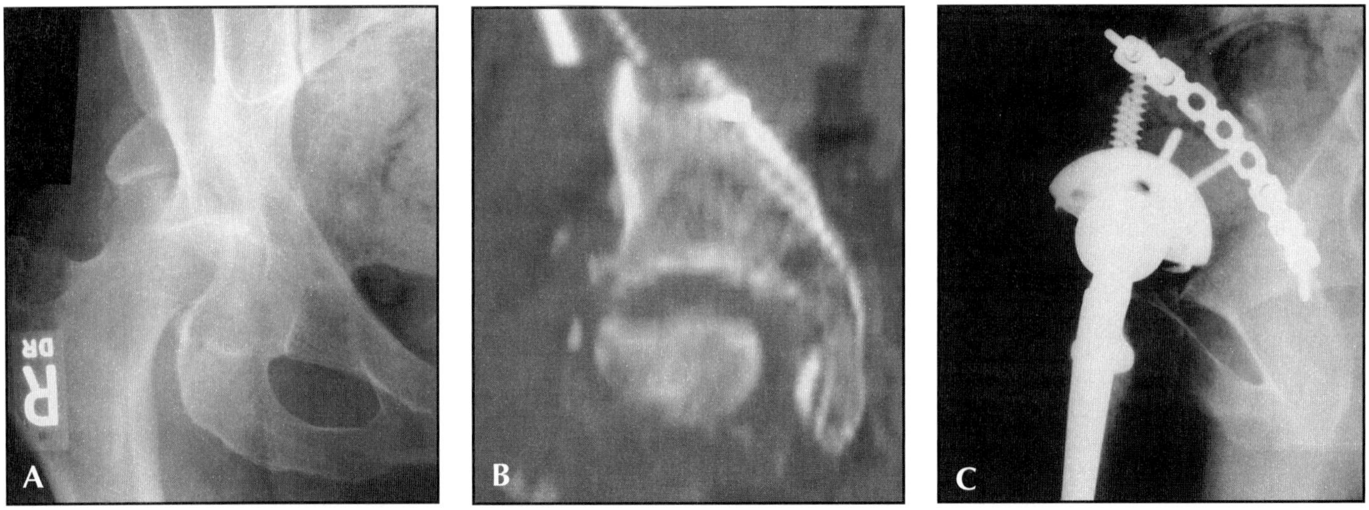

Fig. 8 Radiographs and CT scan from a 53-year-old man who had a fracture of the posterior wall that was managed with an acute open reduction and internal fixation with use of a plate. **A,** AP radiograph of the right hip, obtained at the time of the injury, showing the fracture-dislocation of the posterior wall. **B,** Transaxial CT scan, obtained 4 weeks after the injury, showing erosive damage to more than 30% of the femoral head. This finding was not visualized on plain radiographs made at that time. **C,** Iliac oblique radiograph, obtained after THA, showing the structural autograft secured with two cancellous screws.

necrosis of the acetabulum as the periosteal blood supply is compromised by the elevation of soft tissues and revascularization is impeded by the plate.

Another technique of fixation is the use of cables around the acetabulum[39] (Fig. 12). This method is particularly suitable for a transverse fracture pattern. The cable is passed around the inner pelvic wall with a standard or modified Statinski vascular clamp. We have procured custom-made modified clamps that are stiffer and have jaws designed to rigorously grip the end of a 2-mm cable. The advantages of this method include minimal denuding and devascularizing of the hemipelvis and prolonged integrity of the fixation in osteopenic bone, where screws are vulnerable to a rapid onset of loosening. The principal liability of the cabling technique is the potential for a neurovascular injury during the passage of the cable along the inner pelvic table.

Insertion of the Femoral Stem

Currently, the optimal design of a cemented or cementless femoral stem

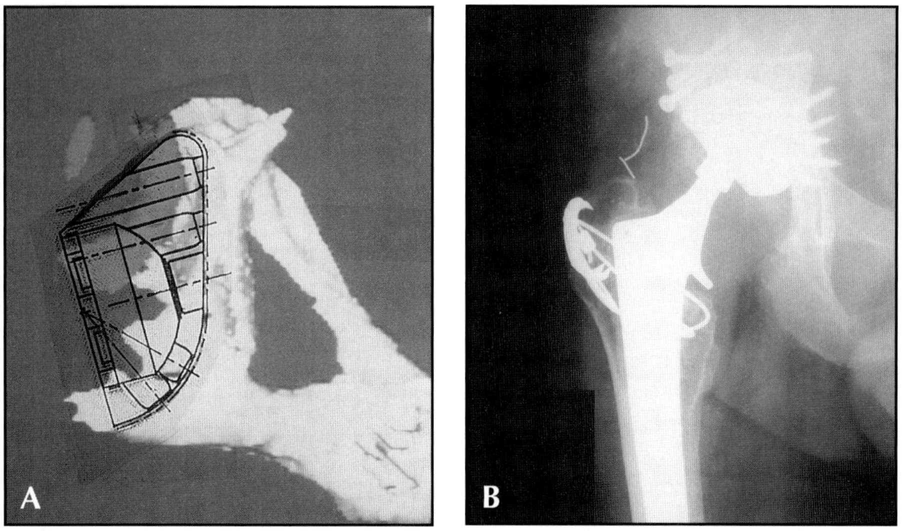

Fig. 9 CT scan and radiograph from a 35-year-old man who sustained a fracture of the posterior wall and posterior column of the right acetabulum and was managed initially with limited internal fixation. **A,** Transaxial three-dimensional CT reconstruction with a template of the custom cup. **B,** AP radiograph of the right hip, obtained 6 years after THA, showing continued stable fixation of the cup in a superior position.

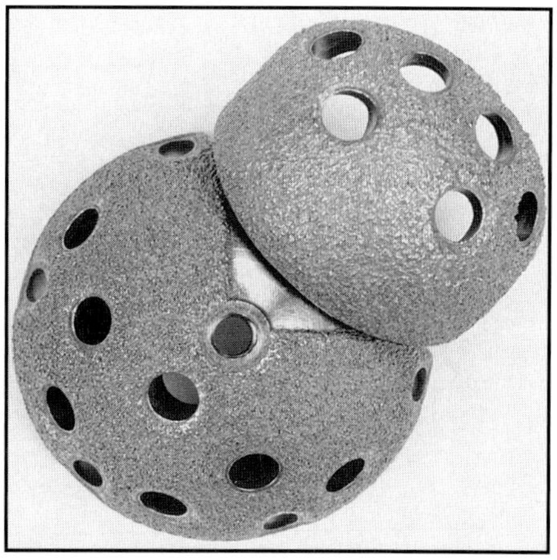

Fig. 10 Photograph showing the modular bilobed cup (Mars, Biomet, Warsaw, IN), which allows application of a lobe of three different sizes to obliterate corresponding acetabular defects. The polyethylene liner is secured mechanically to the bilobed cup, in contrast to the conventional cage.

remains highly controversial.[40] As a general rule, in the United States, a cementless design is favored for use in younger adults. In the few previous reports in the literature on THA performed after an acetabular fracture, some investigators acknowledged an exceptionally high prevalence of premature loosening of cementless stems.[6,7,41,42] They described the development of a relative osteopenia of the proximal part of the femur even in young men. This observation has been interpreted to mean that the period of inactivity and limited weight bearing that immediately follows the acute injury, combined with the additional period of limited weight bearing that accompanies the onset of posttraumatic arthritis of the hip before the THA, culminates in disuse osteoporosis. In such a patient, the application of a cemented stem merits consideration.

Strategies to Address Anticipated Problems

When a THA is performed after an acetabular fracture, problems may arise that need special consideration and an appropriate alteration of the technique. Infrequently, a concomitant fracture of the proximal part of the femoral shaft or an intertrochanteric fracture is an additional problem that may lead to a secondary malunion, retained metal, the development of heterotopic bone, or a nonunion in rare cases.[43-47] The principal factors that are most likely to influence acetabular reconstruction are sciatic nerve injury, obstructive hardware, heterotopic ossification, occult infection, and osteonecrosis.

Sciatic Nerve Injury

After initial surgical management of a posterior fracture-dislocation of the acetabulum, the sciatic nerve usually becomes attached to the site of the posterior fixation with scar tissue. The extent of the scar tissue varies considerably and may progress to its most sinister form, in which supplementary heterotopic bone is encountered. When a THA is performed after a posterior fracture-dislocation has been initially managed with surgery, we prefer to use an anterolateral or a modified Hardinge approach[31] (Fig. 3, *A*). In this way, the need for posterior dissection is minimized. In many cases, some degree of contusion of the sciatic nerve accompanies the initial traumatic injury. At the time of the arthroplasty, the sciatic nerve is particularly vulnerable to a clinically important secondary injury as a manifestation of the "double crush syndrome," which may result from a seemingly trivial retraction.[15] Whenever possible, the principal posterior fixation is left in situ, although not infrequently one or two obstructive screws may need to be entirely or partly removed. In certain cases in which a persistent nonunion or malunion of the posterior column or a retained plate needs to be exposed, a complete exposure of the relevant segment of the sciatic nerve should precede the osseous reconstruction or metal removal. In order to minimize the tension on the nerve, the knee is maintained in a position of more than 90° of flexion during the remainder of the arthroplasty except for the brief period when the hip is being reduced.

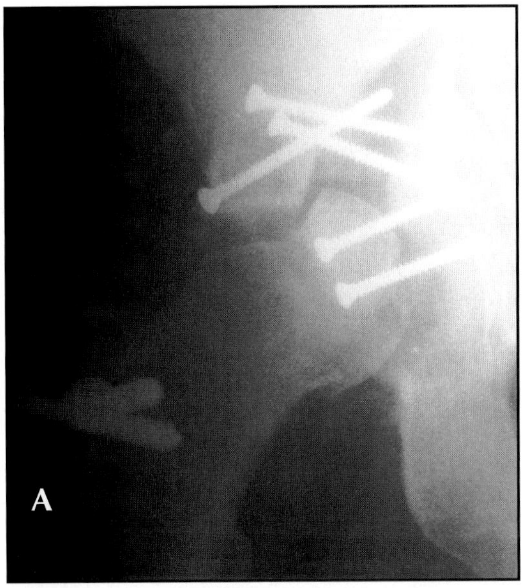

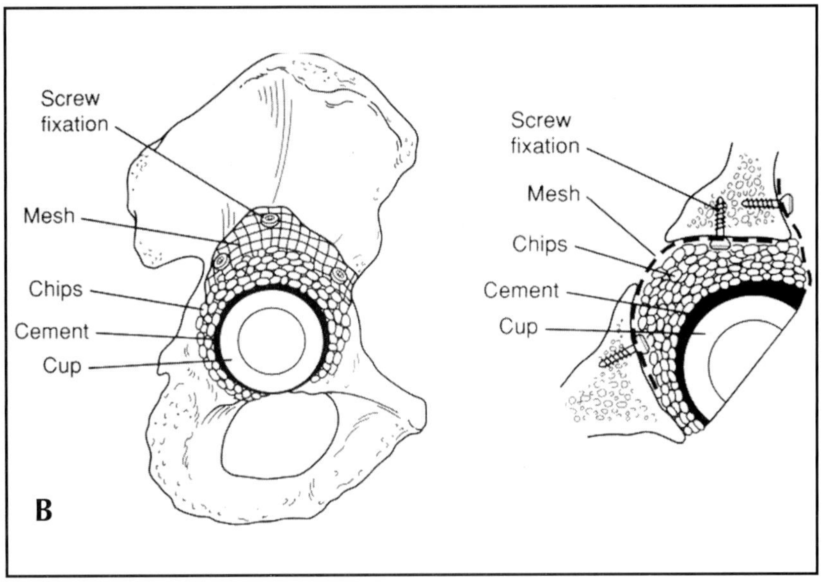

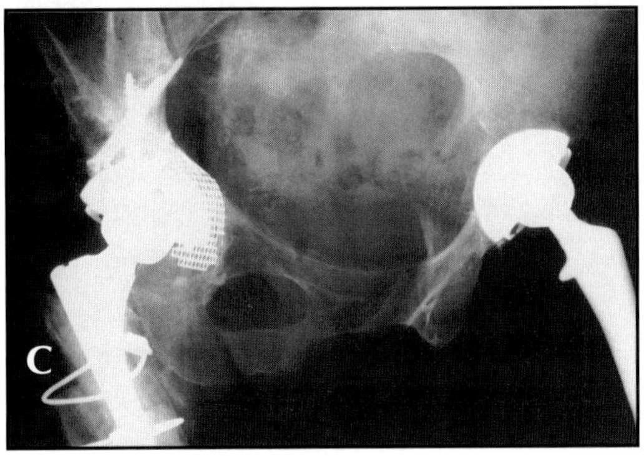

Fig. 11 Radiographs and schematic of the hip of a 56-year-old man who had failure of fixation of a transverse acetabular fracture of the right hip and was managed with a THA with use of central mesh, morcellized bone graft, and lag screws. **A,** AP radiograph, obtained before THA, showing failure of internal fixation solely with lag screws and marked abrasive destruction of the femoral head. **B,** Schematic drawing of the central mesh and morcellized impacted bone chip. **C,** Obturator oblique radiograph, obtained after hybrid THA, showing a central mesh and a metal-backed cup secured with three screws.

In an attempt to monitor the function of the sciatic nerve during a surgical procedure, somatosensory evoked potentials and continuous electromyographic measurements both have been used. Some early reports expressing enthusiasm for measurements of somatosensory evoked potentials have been published.[48-50] Nevertheless, a disturbing trend, which has been documented, has been a prevalence, albeit a low one, of false-positive and false-negative results.[48,51,52] The latter is a particular problem that undermines the confidence of the surgeon in the reliability of this method. Other problems include a substantial latent period, which may be exacerbated by the complexities in the interpretation of the results. Recent evaluations of continuous electromyographic monitoring have indicated that this method has more advantages than the former one.[53,54] Unlike recordings of somatosensory evoked potentials, electromyographic measurements represent virtually instantaneous changes in nerve function. Also, electromyographic measurements are technically less demanding to obtain and require less sophisticated and less costly instrumentation. While the methods can be used in combination, it appears that isolated use of motor-nerve monitoring is the most practical option.

Intraoperative spontaneous electromyographic recordings are obtained with use of sterile needle electrodes from the muscles innervated by the common peroneal nerve (tibialis anterior and peroneus longus muscles) and the posterior tibial nerve (abductor hallucis and flexor hallucis longus muscles). Unlike the situation with somatosensory evoked potential monitoring, a neurotechnologist is not needed to evoke electromyographic activity. The data are continuously recorded from the muscles; any mechanical or thermal irritation of the sciatic nerve results in a burst or train of neuromuscular discharges, which usually persists until the offending stimulus is removed.[54]

Obstructive Hardware

In many patients who have a THA after open reduction and internal fixation of an acetabular fracture, some of the hardware is directly visualized once the

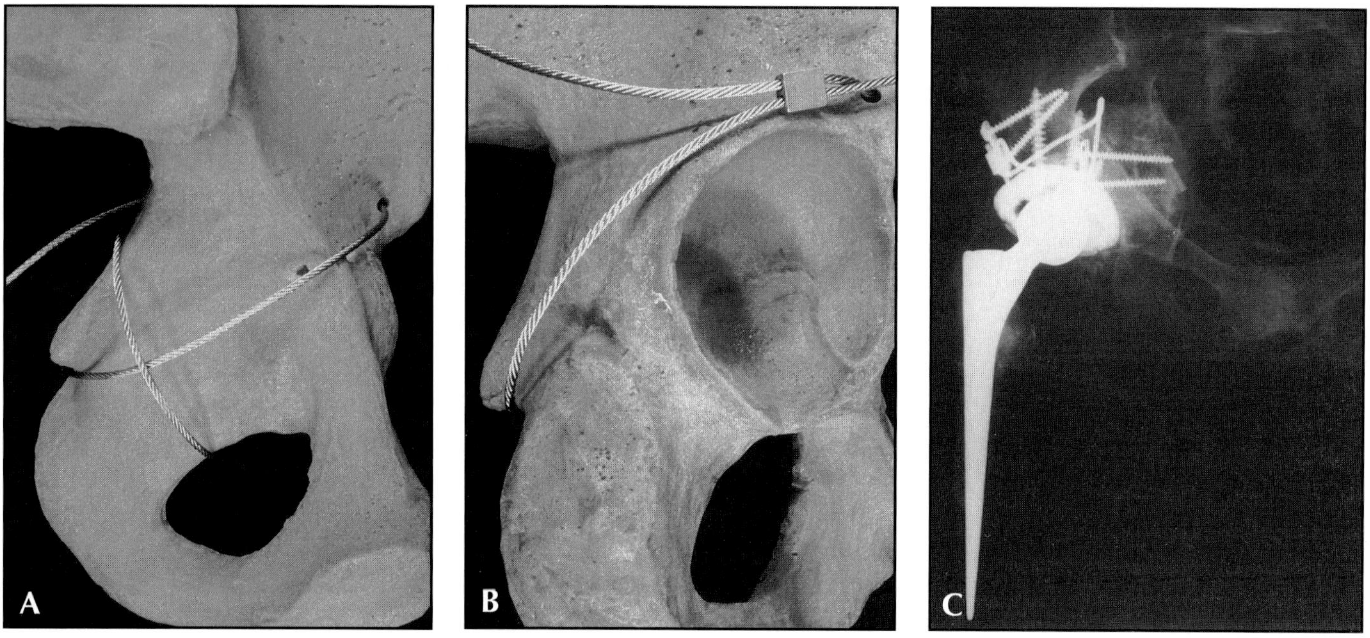

Fig. 12 The use of cables for reconstruction of the inner pelvic table in a so-called geriatric acetabular fracture pattern in which the quadrilateral plate is displaced medially. **A,** Photograph of an intact anatomic pelvic model, showing the position of the cables on the inner pelvic table. **B,** Photograph of an intact anatomic pelvic model, showing the position of a cable on the outer pelvic table. **C,** AP radiograph made after THA with two cables that buttress the crucial quadrilateral surface; the patient is a 62-year-old woman with osteopenic bone who sustained a T-type acetabular fracture with marked displacement of the posterior column, including most of the quadrilateral surface.

articular surface of the acetabulum is exposed. This problem may be indicative of loose or broken hardware that has migrated, or it may be a sequela to an eroded osseous surface or a malpositioned implant. Generally, appropriate preoperative imaging allows this problem to be recognized or at least suspected so that a suitable preoperative plan can be made. When a plate on the posterior column is directly visualized within the acetabulum, or when the plate or its associated screw is struck by an acetabular reamer, the feasibility of leaving the plate in situ needs to be considered. The potential problems that may be encountered during an attempt to remove the entire plate include the risk of an iatrogenically induced injury to the sciatic nerve, the inevitable blood loss, and the extensive surgical time needed to remove the plate. Occasionally, with certain patterns of acetabular malunion in the presence of a thick layer of heterotopic bone, most of the structural integrity of the posterior column is provided by the heterotopic bone. On removal of the heterotopic bone and the underlying plate, the residual acetabulum may be weakened to a substantial degree, even to the point where a fracture occurs through the remaining defective bone.[6] Once this problem arises, a successful arthroplasty necessitates structural replacement of the posterior column, which is a formidable technical challenge. We recommend that, whenever feasible, impaction grafting of the acetabulum with morcellized femoral-head autograft be performed to cover the exposed bottom surface of the plate and to restore a 5- to 10-mm thick osseous supportive layer for the cup. If a segment of a protruding screw or another nonstructural portion of hardware intrudes into the acetabulum, it may be trimmed with a diamond burr without compromising the structural integrity of the posterior column.

Heterotopic Ossification

When a lateral exposure (especially an extended lateral approach) was used for the fixation of an acetabular fracture, some degree of heterotopic bone is typically seen.[5] Occasionally, clinically important heterotopic ossification develops after a Kocher-Langenbeck approach, whereas it rarely develops after an ilioinguinal exposure. While the amount of heterotopic ossification may be limited, an extensive region of dense scar tissue usually surrounds the radiographically demonstrable area. This area may be impregnated with multiple small deposits of bone that are radiographically invisible. Such tissue must be excised to permit dislocation of the hip and subsequent completion of the THA. If the preoperative radiographs display extensive grade III or IV heterotopic bone according to the system of Brooker and associates,[55] a rigorous characterization of the extent of the problem is essential. Both supplementary iliac and obturator oblique radiographs are needed to determine the magnitude of the anterior and posterior extent of the heterotopic ossification.[17] A CT scan is useful to document that the hip capsule and adjacent muscles are intact, which indicates that excision of the heterotopic ossification is feasible. Prior to the removal of the heterotopic ossification, the precise distribution of the bone, the optimal approaches to the sites, and the potential anatomic hazards are reviewed. One typical pattern involves heterotopic ossification that is limited to the site of the hip capsule and does not extend into the adjacent hip muscles or femoral head. In this situation, removal of the heterotopic ossification during the THA may be highly successful (Fig. 6). The opposite extreme involves circumferential heterotopic bone that infiltrates radially from the femoral head and neck to pervade the capsule and the adjacent muscles, with associated osseous bars that anchor the entire proximal part of the femur to the pelvis. Almost all of these more florid cases are encountered in patients who have had a closed head injury, particularly young obese men. Despite the use of postoperative radiation therapy, the likelihood for recurrent formation of massive heterotopic ossification is great.[51] With the loss of the normal tissue planes and mobile interfaces, resection of heterotopic ossification when there is such extensive involvement is a formidable undertaking. Considerable blood loss can be anticipated, and arrangements for transfusion and intraoperative salvage of blood are needed.

Following such an extensive procedure, the risk of a serious deep wound infection is considerable. If such an infection does develop, it has been our experience that, despite the use of multiple surgical débridements, formation of scar tissue usually progresses to a virtual fusion of the hip. Alternatively, a resection arthroplasty may become necessary to control the infection. This measure is reserved solely for infections that culminate in extensive necrosis of the involved bone and neighboring soft tissues. After adequate débridements of bone and soft tissue, a cement spacer is inserted to obliterate the dead space and to provide a temporary reservoir of a suitable antibiotic. It has been our experience that, when the residual viable tissues have been extensively covered with scar tissue in the aftermath of the infection, the late functional outcome of a resection arthroplasty with a cement spacer often is functionally equivalent to that of a secondarily performed THA with regard to pain relief, stability, and mobility. In fact, after a resection arthroplasty with a cement spacer, many patients refuse to consider additional surgery even if a surgeon recommends conversion to a total hip replacement.

Once the amount and the site of distribution of the heterotopic ossification have been characterized, the optimal surgical approach can be selected. Although grade I or II heterotopic ossification does not materially influence the approach, grade III or IV heterotopic ossification has an impact on the surgical plan. If heterotopic ossification is localized solely to the posterior aspect of the hip joint, the use of a Kocher-Langenbeck approach is recommended (Fig. 3, *B*). If heterotopic ossification is both anterior and posterior to the hip joint, we prefer to use a triradiate incision with preservation of the greater trochanter and the adjacent gluteal insertions.[30]

The excision of two patterns of heterotopic ossification is especially challenging. In some patients with mature heterotopic ossification, the extra bone is virtually indistinguishable from the intact pelvis. Furthermore, the soft-tissue boundaries, such as the capsule, may be wholly or substantially lost because they have been replaced by bone. In contrast, progressive removal of heterotopic ossification in a patient who has preservation of the soft-tissue intervals can be documented by visualization of conspicuous osseous landmarks, such as the anterior inferior iliac spine and the junction between the femoral neck and the greater trochanter. The other challenging pattern of heterotopic ossification is ossification that infiltrates deeply into the adjacent soft tissues such as the gluteus minimus. At the time of the initial cutaneous incision, the first hint of this pattern is typified by evidence of bone in the deep fascia. To dislocate the hip, resection of the involved portion of the gluteus minimus may be necessary. Other local muscles that are likely to contain ossified portions include the indirect head of the rectus femoris, the iliopsoas, and the short external rotators.

During resection of heterotopic ossification around the superior portion of the hip joint, the insertions of the gluteal muscles into the trochanteric region must be carefully preserved. The exposure of a fixation plate on the posterior column or an isolated screw is a valuable landmark for identifying the surface of the intact pelvis. As a rule, such hardware is left in situ. In this way, if another approach to the hip subsequently becomes necessary, possibly for a revision arthroplasty, the hardware continues to serve as a marker of the normal pelvic surface, so that overenthusiastic removal of recurrent heterotopic bone does not progress to a catastrophic resection of the acetabulum. In cases with the most extensive heterotopic ossification, the anterior inferior iliac spine is an additional useful anterior landmark. Supplementary image intensification can be used to delineate the position of the acetabular rim. During THA, the femoral neck is provisionally divided in its midportion with a power saw. Sufficient heterotopic ossification is removed so that the proximal part of the femoral shaft can be placed in approximately 90° of external rotation. Afterward, the standard cut at the base of the femoral neck is made with the use of an alignment guide. Once the heterotopic ossification has been completely removed, the remainder of the arthroplasty continues in a conventional fashion.

Often, the most extensive cases of heterotopic bone around the hip are encountered in patients with an acetabular fracture and an associated fracture of the proximal or midpart of the femur who had combined internal fixation performed through contiguous surgical fields. In the most florid cases, the heterotopic bone can extend from the iliac crest to the distal femoral metaphysis so that both the hip and the ipsilateral knee are ankylosed. A suitable release of the hip and knee involves both a resection of the massive amount of bone and a complete quadricepsplasty. Despite the use of postoperative radiation therapy and/or treatment with indomethacin, recurrent heterotopic ossification is almost a certainty.[51,56] Nevertheless, the patient may be grateful for a moderate functional improvement in gait and the ability to transfer.

In some cases of massive heterotopic ossification, the findings on preoperative radiographs are consistent with some degree of posttraumatic degenerative arthritis of the hip. Even with an adequate CT scan, the surgeon may be unable to determine whether complete removal of the heterotopic ossification will permit a functional restoration of a mobile and painless hip joint. The patient's preoperative consent and the corresponding discussion may be directed toward surgical resection of the heterotopic ossification, with a possible supplementary THA, if features of severe degenerative changes in the hip joint are observed during the procedure.

Following a THA that is accompanied by the removal of extensive heterotopic ossification, the use of one or more postoperative prophylactic measures is recommended.[51] Radiation therapy with a dose of 700 cGy on the first postoperative day is a standard recommendation.[57] Alternatively, the use of indomethacin for a period of at least 6 weeks has been advised. In a recent randomized, prospective study to assess the formation of heterotopic ossification after open reduction of acute acetabular fractures, Matta and Siebenrock[56] reported that indomethacin had no therapeutic beneficial effect as prophylaxis against heterotopic ossification. Other surgeons have used a combination of radiation therapy and indomethacin.[58] Despite the use of prophylactic regimens, the formation of clinically important heterotopic ossification or a complete recurrence of it after resection is not unlikely in hips with florid heterotopic ossification following a closed head injury. It has been our experience that this sobering event may transpire even though years of "maturation" of the heterotopic ossification may ensue after the acetabular fracture and prior to the THA.

Occult Infection

An occult infection may be a source of chronic pain in the hip after open reduction and internal fixation of the acetabulum, and it may be the cause of deterioration of the joint surfaces. Certain circumstances should heighten suspicion of an occult infection. The use of an extended lateral approach for the initial treatment of an acetabular fracture is a risk factor, particularly when the dissection is undertaken along both the inner and the outer pelvic table. Another factor is heterotopic ossification, which may be provoked in part by the infection itself. Additional factors include morbid obesity, an immunocompromised patient, and previous radiation therapy to the pelvis.

While clinical, hematologic, radiographic, or other findings may indicate an infection, clear evidence of an infection is typically not available until the arthroplasty is performed. When dense scar tissue or heterotopic bone is anticipated, a preoperative aspiration or even a trephine biopsy of the hip may fail to confirm the infection. At the time of the arthroplasty, specimens of joint fluid should be sent to the laboratory for analysis, including a Gram stain and a histologic scrutiny for white blood cells. A highly reliable method is intraoperative examination of a frozen section obtained from membrane or pericapsular granulation tissue. The presence of 10 white blood cells per high-power field is presumptive evidence of an infection.[59] If the hip is infected, our preferred method is to perform a thorough débridement, including resection of the femoral head and neck and any necrotic acetabular bone. Following pulsatile jet lavage and antibiotic irrigation, a cement spacer that has been impregnated with an antibiotic, typically gentamicin, is inserted into the acetabulum.[60,61] The wound is closed in layers over a suction drain. Postoperatively, after the identification of the pathogen, appropriate intravenous antibiotics are given for at least 6 weeks. Upon the cessation of antibiotic therapy, a trephine biopsy of the hip is performed under image intensification. If the specimen is sterile, insertion of the total hip prosthesis is considered. If the specimen reveals a persistent infection, multiple surgical débridements with replacement of the cement spacer and continued intravenous antibiotic therapy are undertaken until the infection is eradicated.

Osteonecrosis of the Acetabulum

Another potential complicating factor is osteonecrosis of the acetabulum.[62] Following a single extensile approach or two simple approaches for acute reconstruction of an acetabular fracture, the blood supply to the acetabular bone may be heavily compromised for a prolonged period of years. At the time of a belated arthroplasty, necrotic acetabular bone may thwart the insertion of the cup and may predispose the patient to premature acetabular loosening. When a THA is being considered for a patient with posttraumatic arthritis after an extended lateral approach or a two-incision approach, the surgeon is advised to review the prior surgical report to determine whether an extensive intraoperative dissection on the inner and outer pelvic tables was performed. A helpful, although subtle, radiographic sign of acetabular necrosis is an increased radiodensity, especially in the region of the dome (Fig. 13). If the cup is inserted into an avascular bed, a serious potential complication is an insidious protrusion of the cup through the medial acetabular wall. In the most florid case, a transverse dissociation may occur (Fig. 14).

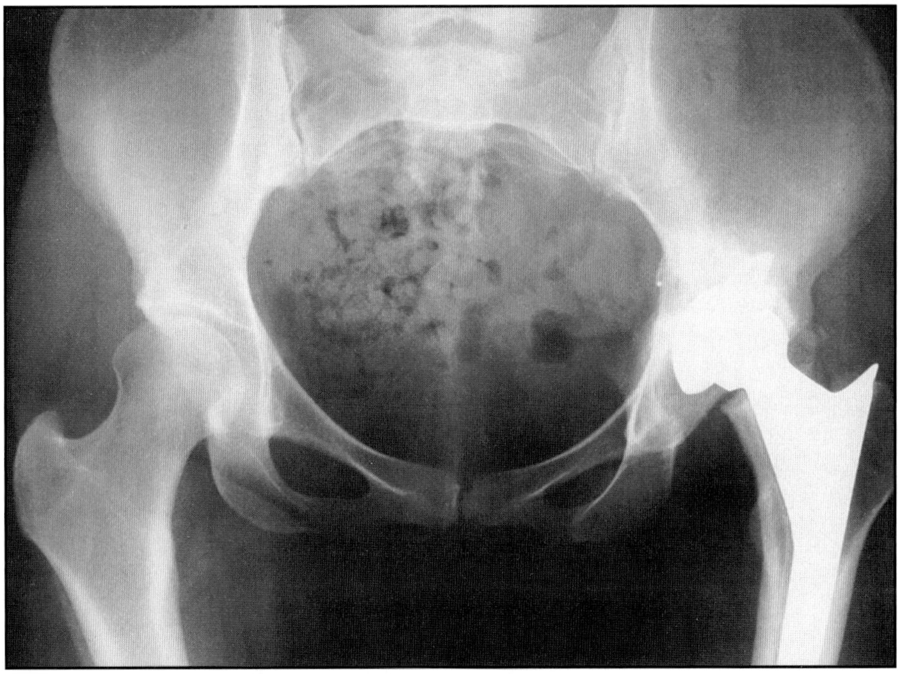

Fig. 13 Increased radiodensity of the acetabular roof on the left side is a subtle but important finding of acetabular osteonecrosis. The radiograph is that of a 28-year-old woman who sustained a transverse fracture that was managed acutely with open reduction and was managed 1 year later with removal of the metal. Three years after the injury, a THA was performed to manage posttraumatic arthritis. Within another 2-year period, the patient complained of recurrent hip pain, and an aspiration arthrogram confirmed an aseptically loose cup. This AP radiograph shows superior migration of the failed cup into the necrotic acetabular roof.

The optimal method of addressing acetabular osteonecrosis is to reduce its potential for development at the time of the initial open reduction; for instance, use of the extended lateral approach should be minimized, and the blood supply to all of the major acetabular fragments should be maintained. At the time of the arthroplasty, if a cementless cup is used, it must be placed on viable bone. Even if a cemented cup is selected, a viable osseous bed markedly improves the longevity of the fixation. When the preoperative radiographs indicate an extensive area of periacetabular osteonecrosis, the feasibility of successfully anchoring the cup on viable bleeding and structurally sound bone must be carefully reviewed. In exceptional cases, a resection arthroplasty may provide a superior and more predictable outcome than a THA.

After a thorough inspection of the preoperative images, the feasibility of reconstructing a stable acetabulum needs to be determined. For a particularly large acetabular defect that is further complicated by a suspicion of extensive avascular bone, a frank discussion with the patient about the magnitude of the problem and the potential need for resection arthroplasty may be advisable before embarking on the procedure. If the potential for acetabular reconstruction remains unclear to the surgeon, a review of the clinical and radiographic features with an orthopaedist who is highly experienced with this problem may be beneficial.

Salvage of Complex Late Cases

A limited spectrum of acetabular fractures, after failure of the initial open reduction and internal fixation, have a heterogeneous mixture of complicating factors. A patient may have a serious deep wound infection, possibly with persistent drainage through a sinus tract. The gluteus medius and minimus muscles may have been damaged by an injury to the superior gluteal nerve, heterotopic bone formation, or osteonecrosis, or they may even have been injured secondary to a life-saving embolic occlusion of a traumatic laceration of the internal iliac artery. Substantial acetabular bone loss may have occurred as a result of avascularity or infection or occasionally other factors. In some of these situations, a THA may be feasible, even if a multistaged reconstruction is necessary. Nevertheless, in certain situations, such as complete loss of the posterior column (Fig. 15), a THA may be technically unrealistic. Furthermore, the functional outcome of a THA with respect to pain relief and durability may not be any better than that of the principal surgical alternative, a resection arthroplasty with or without the insertion of a cement spacer.[63-66]

Acute Management With THA After Acetabular Fracture in Highly Selected Patients

Fractures in elderly individuals represent the most rapidly growing spectrum of

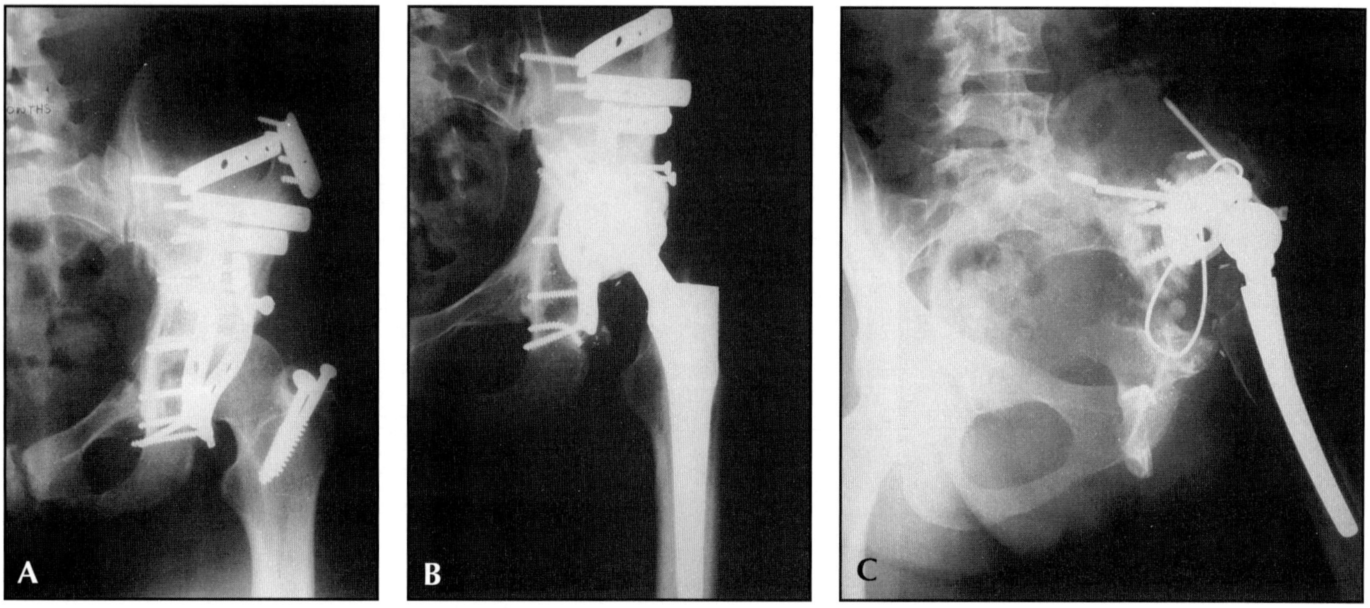

Fig. 14 Radiographs from a 24-year-old woman who sustained a fracture of both columns of the left acetabulum, which was initially treated with open reduction through a triradiate approach and dissection on the outer and inner pelvic tables. **A,** AP radiograph obtained 10 months after open reduction and internal fixation. **B,** AP radiograph made soon after THA and 6 years after the initial injury. **C,** Iliac oblique radiograph, obtained 2 years after THA, showing a completely loose cup and a transverse dissociation secondary to marked osteolysis of the anterior and posterior columns.

acetabular trauma.[67-69] The specific indications for acute management with THA after a displaced acetabular fracture have yet to be clearly defined but may include marked impaction, extensive abrasion or fracture of the femoral head, a completely displaced femoral neck fracture, marginal or central impaction of the acetabulum involving more than 30% of its surface area, and extensive acetabular comminution in the presence of osteopenic bone. Other relative indications include delayed presentation, substantial medical comorbidities, morbid obesity, and advanced age. We have been encouraged by our early experience with THA in the treatment of selected acute fractures.[39]

Postoperative Management

After the THA, a patient is managed with an abduction bolster or split Russell traction for 24 hours to minimize the risk of postoperative dislocation. In general, bed-to-chair transfers are initiated on the first postoperative day, with touch-down or light partial weight bearing beginning on the second day. Substantial partial weight bearing is begun at 4 to 6 weeks after the arthroplasty, with full weight bearing at 6 to 8 weeks. When an elderly patient who has compromised strength, agility, and balance compared with a younger adult is managed with a THA, partial weight bearing or weight bearing as tolerated is almost essential or the risk of a fall becomes excessive. Therefore, the acetabular repair requires sufficient structural integrity so that some degree of immediate weight bearing is feasible.

Whenever practical, vigorous progressive resistance exercises of the hip abductors, quadriceps, and hamstrings, as well as active range-of-motion exercises, including flexion, extension, and abduction of the hip joint, are encouraged.[6,70] A program of continuous passive motion may be used at the discretion of the surgeon. Prophylactic intravenous antibiotics with a second-generation cephalosporin are used routinely for 48 hours. Prophylaxis against thromboembolism includes the application of elastic stockings, sequential compression devices, and an appropriate course of anticoagulation with warfarin or low-molecular-weight heparin.

Patients who have previously had open reduction and internal fixation of an acetabular fracture and who had grade I or II heterotopic ossification and/or an extended lateral approach prior to the belated THA are managed with low-dose radiation (a single dose of 700 cGy). Alternatively, indomethacin can be used in younger female patients in whom radiation exposure should be avoided. When indomethacin and anticoagulation with low-molecular-weight heparin or warfarin are used concomitantly, appropriate medical supervision is needed to minimize the risk of a coagulopathy.

Clinical Outcome of THA After Acetabular Fracture

According to a few prior studies on the late outcome of a belated total hip replacement after closed or open treatment of an acetabular fracture,[7,8,42,71] the clinical outcome is generally less favorable than that after THA performed to manage degenerative arthritis. Undoubtedly, the outcome of belated THA after acetabular fracture is best when the fracture pattern is one of minor displacement with union, especially following nonoperative treatment. In earlier published reports, such as one by Boardman and Charnley,[72] even when open reduction of the acute acetabular fracture had been performed, the indication for the late THA typically was a posterior fracture-dislocation, such as a posterior wall fracture, for which an isolated posterior surgical approach was used to achieve fixation with lag screws or a single plate. In contrast to the simple pattern fractures of the posterior column, posterior wall, and transverse fractures, few of the more complex patterns, such as a fracture of both columns, a T-type fracture, or an anterior column-posterior hemitransverse fracture, were managed surgically until recently. For example, Boardman and Charnley,[72] in a study of the outcomes of 68 Charnley low-friction arthroplasties, reported that 55 of the acute acetabular fractures were managed nonsurgically and the remaining 13 were treated with primary open reduction and internal fixation. After a relatively short period of follow-up (an average of 3.5 years), the patients had good results with respect to pain and function. Waddell and Morton (unpublished data, 1994), in a study of 34 patients, reported that 29 were managed initially with open reduction. Satisfactory rates of success were noted after an average follow-up period of 2 years. Earlier studies by multiple authors have described comparable rates of success over similarly brief follow-up periods, regardless of whether the initial management of the diverse patterns of the acetabular fractures was open or closed.[8,10,73-75]

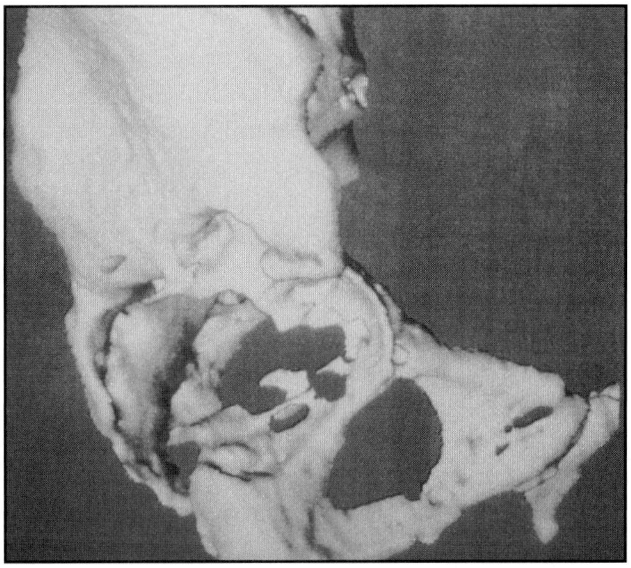

Fig. 15 Three-dimensional CT scan of the hip of a 73-year-old woman who had complete, traumatic loss of the posterior acetabular column. This acetabular defect presents one of the most challenging reconstruction problems because it can be very difficult to achieve a stable acetabular component that will resist the forces that are imposed by sitting and sitting transfers, as well as standing and walking.

Romness and Lewallen,[7] in a longer-term evaluation of 55 belated arthroplasties performed after an acetabular fracture, observed that the rate of radiographic acetabular loosening at an average of 7.5 years postoperatively was 52.9%; the loosening was symptomatic in 27.5%, and it progressed to a revision in 13.7%. In contrast, Stauffer,[9] in a 10-year follow-up study of 231 hips in which a Charnley arthroplasty had been performed for degenerative arthritis, reported that 36.8% had features of radiographic loosening and the rate of revision was 8.2%. The rates of radiographic loosening of the femoral component (29%), symptomatic loosening (16%), and revision (8%) were remarkably similar in the two series. When the two series were compared with respect to the results in patients who were older than age 60 years, the rates of loosening of the femoral component were similar; however, the rate of loosening of the acetabular component was 38.5% in the series described by Romness and Lewallen compared with approximately 4.8% in the series reported by Stauffer. Romness and Lewallen concluded that the fourfold to fivefold increase in the rate of failure of THA after an acetabular fracture was primarily attributable to damage or loss of acetabular bone stock. They recommended an initial open reduction as a way to reconstruct the osseous anatomy, even if that procedure fails to prevent posttraumatic degeneration. In contrast, Carnesale and associates,[71] in a study of 56 hips with an acetabular fracture, including 11 that were treated surgically, discouraged open reduction as the initial choice of treatment for an acetabular fracture because of the corresponding deterioration of the outcome after belated arthroplasty.

More recently, Mears and Ward (unpublished data, 1996) evaluated a series of 36 patients who underwent a THA after previous open reduction and internal fixation of the acetabulum. Most patients (83%) had had a triradiate extended lateral surgical exposure with dissection along the inner and outer pelvic walls. The rate of radiographic loosening was 58%, and the rate of surgical revision was 36% within 2 years after the primary arthroplasty. The high rate of premature technical failure was, in part, a reflection of the use of an unsatisfactory design of a cementless femoral stem. Nevertheless, at the time of the revision arthroplasties, multiple acetabular biopsies confirmed the high likelihood of widespread osteonecrosis in the central aspect of the acetabulum that correlated with the initial dissections along the inner and outer pelvic walls.

Weber and associates[42] reported on 63 patients who were followed for an average of 9.6 years after a primary THA following failed open reduction of an acetabular fracture. The 10-year rate of survival of the components was 78%, and the rate of revision, which was performed mainly because of aseptic loosening of one or both components, was 51%. Notable risk factors for revision included age younger than 50 years, weight greater than 80 kg, and large residual combined segmental and cavitary deficiencies in the osseous acetabulum. Mont and associates[11] also observed a poorer outcome after THAs performed in younger patients, who generally are more active and have an increased body weight compared with older individuals.

For many reasons, the use of extensile or multiple pelvic incisions has diminished greatly during the past decade. Nevertheless, there is currently no convincing documented evidence that acute management with open reduction and internal fixation improves the success of a subsequent THA performed for posttraumatic arthritis. Ironically, it has been our experience that the best late results of THA after acetabular fracture have been documented when the arthroplasties were performed acutely. In a series of 57 patients managed with an acute THA after acetabular fracture, the principal problems were postoperative dislocation in two hips (3.5%), one of which progressed to a revision of the cup, and a symptomatic loose cup in one hip (1.6%), which was revised at 3 years.[76] In one other hip, grade IV heterotopic bone developed after the acute THA. The heterotopic ossification was resected, and there was no recurrence at 20 months after the arthroplasty. There were no deep wound infections and no cases of radiographic or symptomatic femoral loosening. The discussion of these results is not meant to be a recommendation for THA for more than an exceptional acetabular fracture, especially in elderly patients. Nevertheless, an analysis of the results of open reduction and internal fixation of acute acetabular fractures highlights a therapeutic dilemma. Even in the most experienced hands, as Letournel and Judet[2] meticulously documented, certain patterns of acetabular fracture have an abysmal prognosis.

A small group of patterns of displaced acetabular fractures and clinical scenarios have a low likelihood for a favorable outcome after open reduction and internal fixation, and an open reduction of such fractures may compromise the outlook for a successful subsequent THA. These fracture patterns include abrasion, impaction, or fracture of the femoral head; a displaced fracture of the femoral neck; acetabular impaction; certain comminuted fractures; multiple associated fractures; and osteopenic bone. The clinical scenarios include advanced patient age, morbid obesity, substantial medical comorbidities, and a delay between the injury and the surgery. In certain patients who have several of these complicating factors, some alternative method of primary management seems to be preferable. When the primary factor is comminution and impaction with relatively minor displacement, most surgeons may lean toward nonsurgical treatment. When a patient has substantial displacement, especially an elderly patient with osteopenic bone, acute THA merits more careful consideration.

Summary

In most cases, when THA is performed after an acetabular fracture, it is done to manage secondary degenerative change or, possibly, osteonecrosis of the femoral head. Secondary complicating factors may be encountered during the THA. After initial nonsurgical treatment of an acetabular fracture, an occult or frank acetabular nonunion and malunion are not uncommon and may extend to the residual pelvic ring. After surgical treatment, intrusive hardware, heterotopic bone, dense scar tissue, ischemic muscle or bone, and occult infection are additional hazards that may be encountered. When acute sciatic nerve palsy, whether induced traumatically or iatrogenically, accompanies the initial acetabular injury, the palsy is likely to be exacerbated during a subsequent THA. A careful clinical and radiographic evaluation is needed, along with the formulation of a detailed surgical strategy. The need for specialized arthroplasty instruments, fixation devices, and autograft or, occasionally, allograft has to be identified.

When heterotopic bone is evident, an extensile approach may be needed to allow adequate exposure for its complete removal. After a bone defect and/or a nonunion with displacement has been characterized, one or more strategies for obliteration of the defect are considered; these include the use of impaction grafting, a structural graft, a cup inserted with multiple screws, mesh, or a suitable ring or other fixation device.

Evaluation of results has shown that, overall, the late outcome of THA after acetabular fracture is inferior to that of arthroplasty performed because of degenerative arthritis. Although open reduction and internal fixation of an acute acetabular fracture was previously hypothesized as an effective way to improve the anticipated late outcome of THA by the elimination of a large fracture gap or the prevention of a potential nonunion, current observations do not support that hypothesis. An initial open reduction may compromise the outcome of a subsequent THA by compromising the blood supply of the acetabulum and by initiating the formation of scar tissue, heterotopic bone, or an occult or frank infection.

For a highly selected group of especially severe acetabular fractures, particularly those in elderly patients, THA appears to be a promising therapeutic alternative.

References

1. Vail TP, McCollum DE: Complex primary acetabular replacement, in Callaghan JJ, Rosenberg AG, Rubash HE (eds): *The Adult Hip*. Philadelphia, PA, Lippincott-Raven, 1998, vol 2, pp 1183-1200.
2. Letournel E, Judet R: *Fractures of the Acetabulum*, ed 2. Berlin, Germany, Springer-Verlag, 1993, pp 359-386.
3. Tile M (ed): *Fractures of the Pelvis and Acetabulum*, ed 2. Baltimore, MD, Williams & Wilkins, 1995, pp 176-184.
4. Matta JM: Fractures of the acetabulum: Accuracy of reduction and clinical results in patients managed operatively within three weeks after the injury. *J Bone Joint Surg Am* 1996;78:1632-1645.
5. Mears DC, Rubash HE (eds): *Pelvic and Acetabular Fractures*. Thorofare, NJ, Slack, 1986, pp 422-439.
6. Jimenez ML, Tile M, Schenk RS: Total hip replacement after acetabular fracture. *Orthop Clin North Am* 1997;28:435-446.
7. Romness DW, Lewallen DG: Total hip arthroplasty after fracture of the acetabulum: Long-term results. *J Bone Joint Surg Br* 1990;72(suppl 5):761-764.
8. Pritchett JW, Bortel DT: Total hip replacement after central fracture dislocation of the acetabulum. *Orthop Rev* 1991;20:607-610.
9. Stauffer RN: Ten-year follow-up study of total hip replacement. *J Bone Joint Surg Am* 1982;64:983-990.
10. Rogan IM, Weber FA, Solomon L: Abstract: Total hip replacement following fracture dislocation of the acetabulum. *J Bone Joint Surg Br* 1979;61(suppl 2):252.
11. Mont MA, Maar DC, Krackow KA, Jacobs MA, Jones LC, Hungerford DS: Total hip replacement without cement for non-inflammatory osteoarthrosis in patients who are less than forty-five years old. *J Bone Joint Surg Am* 1993;75:740-751.
12. Callaghan JJ, McBeath AA: Arthrodesis in, Callaghan JJ, Rosenberg AG, Rubash HE (eds): *The Adult Hip*. Philadelphia, PA, Lippincott-Raven, 1998, pp 749-759.
13. Carangelo RJ, Schutzer SF: Resection arthroplasty in, Callaghan JJ, Rosenberg AG, Rubash HE (eds): *The Adult Hip*. Philadelphia, PA, Lippincott-Raven, 1998, pp 737-747.
14. Johnson EE, Matta JM, Mast JW, Letournel E: Delayed reconstruction of acetabular fractures 21-120 days following injury. *Clin Orthop* 1994;305:20-30.
15. Osterman AL: The double crush syndrome. *Orthop Clin North Am* 1988;19:147-155.
16. Mears DC, Ward AJ, Wright MS: The radiological assessment of pelvic and acetabular fractures using three-dimensional computed tomography. *Intern J Orthop Trauma* 1992;2:196-209.
17. Moed BR, Smith ST: Three-view radiographic assessment of heterotopic ossification after acetabular fracture surgery. *J Orthop Trauma* 1996;10:93-98.
18. Evans BG: Late complications and their management, in Callaghan JJ, Rosenberg AG, Rubash HE (eds): *The Adult Hip*. Philadelphia, PA, Lippincott-Raven, 1998, pp 1149-1161.
19. Fitzgerald RH Jr, Davis LP, Rajan DK: Radionuclide imaging, in Callaghan JJ, Rosenberg AG, Rubash HE (eds): *The Adult Hip*. Philadelphia, PA, Lippincott-Raven, 1998, pp 373-391.
20. Schauwecker DS: The scintigraphic diagnosis of osteomyelitis. *AJR Am J Roentgenol* 1992;158:9-18.
21. D'Antonio JA, Capello WN, Borden LS, et al: Classification and management of acetabular abnormalities in total hip arthroplasty. *Clin Orthop* 1989;243:126-137.
22. Gross AE, Allan DG, Catre M, Garbuz DS, Stockley I: Bone grafts in hip replacement surgery: The pelvic side. *Orthop Clin North Am* 1993;24:679-695.
23. Emerson RH Jr, Head WC: Dealing with the deficient acetabulum in revision hip arthroplasty: The importance of implant migration and use of the jumbo cup. *Sem Arthroplasty* 1993;4:2-8.
24. Slooff JH, Schreurs BW, Buma P, Gardeniers JWM: Impaction morcellized allografting and cement. *Instr Course Lect* 1999;48:79-89.
25. Müller ME: Acetabular revision, in Salvati EA (ed): *The Hip: Proceedings of the Ninth Open Scientific Meeting of the Hip Society*. St Louis, MO, CV Mosby, 1981, pp 46-56.
26. Peters CL, Curtain M, Samuelson KM: Acetabular revision with the Burch-Schneider antiprotrusio cage and cancellous allograft bone. *J Arthroplasty* 1995;10:307-312.
27. Moed BR: Acetabular fractures: The Kocher-Langenbeck approach, in Wiss DA (ed): *Fractures: Master Techniques in Orthopaedic Surgery*. Philadelphia, PA, Lippincott-Raven, 1998, pp 631-655.
28. Matta JM, Reilly MC: Acetabular fractures: The ilioinguinal approach, in Wiss DA (ed): *Fractures: Master Techniques in Orthopaedic Surgery*. Philadelphia, PA, Lippincott-Raven, 1998, pp 657-673.
29. Helfet DL, Bartlett CS, Malkani AL: Acetabular fractures: The extended iliofemoral approach, in Wiss DA (ed): *Fractures: Master Techniques in Orthopaedic Surgery*. Philadelphia, PA, Lippincott-Raven, 1998, pp 675-695.
30. Mears DC, MacLeod MD: Acetabular fractures: The triradiate and modified triradiate approaches, in Wiss DA (ed): *Fractures: Master Techniques in Orthopaedic Surgery*. Philadelphia, PA, Lippincott-Raven, 1998, pp 697-724.
31. Hardinge K: The direct lateral approach to the hip. *J Bone Joint Surg Br* 1982;64:17-19.
32. Gie GA, Linder L, Ling RS, Simon JP, Slooff TJ, Timperley AJ: Impacted cancellous allografts and cement for revision total hip arthroplasty. *J Bone Joint Surg Br* 1993;75:14-21.
33. Ling RS: Femoral component revision using impacted morsellised cancellous graft. *J Bone Joint Surg Br* 1997;79:874-875.
34. Paprosky WG, Magnus RE: Principles of bone grafting in revision total hip arthroplasty: Acetabular technique. *Clin Orthop* 1994;298:147-155.
35. Slooff TJ, Huiskes R, van Horn J, Lemmens AJ: Bone grafting in total hip replacement for acetabular protrusion. *Acta Orthop Scand* 1984;55:593-596.
36. Capello WN, Hellman EJ, Feinberg JR: Revision of the acetabular component: Use of cement, in Callaghan JJ, Rosenberg AG, Rubash HE (eds): *The Adult Hip*. Philadelphia, PA, Lippincott-Raven, 1998, vol 2, pp 1439-1448.
37. DeBoer DK, Christie MJ: Revision of the acetabular component: Oblong cup, in Callaghan JJ, Rosenberg AG, Rubash HE (eds): *The Adult Hip*. Philadelphia, PA, Lippincott-Raven, 1998, vol 2, pp 1461-1468.
38. Slooff TJ JH, Buma P, Gardeniers JWM, Schreurs BW, Schimmel JW, Huiskes R: Revision of the acetabular component: Bone packing, in Callaghan JJ, Rosenberg AG, Rubash HE (eds): *The Adult Hip*. Philadelphia, PA, Lippincott-Raven, 1998, vol 2, pp 1449-1459.
39. Mears DC, Shirahama M: Stabilization of an acetabular fracture with cables for acute total hip arthroplasty. *J Arthroplasty* 1998;13:104-107.
40. Galante JO: Overview of total hip arthroplasty in, Callaghan JJ, Rosenberg AG, Rubash HE (eds): *The Adult Hip*. Philadelphia, PA, Lippincott-Raven, 1998, vol 2, pp 829-838.
41. Sim FH, Stauffer RN: Management of hip fractures by total hip arthroplasty. *Clin Orthop* 1980;152:191-197.
42. Weber M, Berry DJ, Harmsen WS: Total hip arthroplasty after operative treatment of an acetabular fracture. *J Bone Joint Surg Am* 1998;80:1295-1305.
43. Mehlhoff T, Landon GC, Tullos HS: Total hip arthroplasty following failed internal fixation of hip fractures. *Clin Orthop* 1991;269:32-37.
44. Soballe K, Boll KL, Kofod S, Severinsen B, Kristensen SS: Total hip replacement after medial-displacement osteotomy of the proximal part of the femur. *J Bone Joint Surg Am* 1989;71:692-697.

45. Tabsh I, Waddell JP, Morton J: Total hip arthroplasty for complications of proximal femoral fractures. *J Orthop Trauma* 1997;11:166-169.

46. Patterson BM, Salvati EA, Huo MH: Total hip arthroplasty for complications of intertrochanteric fracture: A technical note. *J Bone Joint Surg Am* 1990;72:776-777.

47. Boos N, Krushell R, Ganz R, Müller ME: Total hip arthroplasty after previous proximal femoral osteotomy. *J Bone Joint Surg Br* 1997;79:247-253.

48. Vrahas M, Gordon RG, Mears DC, Krieger D, Sclabassi RJ: Intraoperative somatosensory evoked potential monitoring of pelvic and acetabular fractures. *J Orthop Trauma* 1992;6:50-58.

49. Helfet DL, Koval KJ, Hissa EA, Patterson S, DiPasquale T, Sanders R: Intraoperative somatosensory evoked potential monitoring during acute pelvic fracture surgery. *J Orthop Trauma* 1995;9:28-34.

50. Helfet DL, Schmeling GJ: Somatosensory evoked potential monitoring in the surgical treatment of acute, displaced acetabular fractures: Results of a prospective study. *Clin Orthop* 1994;301:213-220.

51. Templeman DC, Olson S, Moed BR, Duwelius P, Matta JM: Surgical treatment of acetabular fractures. *Instr Course Lect* 1999;48:481-496.

52. Middlebrooks ES, Sims SH, Kellam JF, Bosse MJ: Incidence of sciatic nerve injury in operatively treated acetabular fractures without somatosensory evoked potential monitoring. *J Orthop Trauma* 1997;11:327-329.

53. Helfet DL, Anand N, Malkani AL, et al: Intraoperative monitoring of motor pathways during operative fixation of acute acetabular fractures. *J Orthop Trauma* 1997;11:2-6.

54. Moed BR, Ahmad BK, Craig JG, Jacobson GP, Anders MJ: Intraoperative monitoring with stimulus-evoked electromyography during placement of iliosacral screws: An initial clinical study. *J Bone Joint Surg Am* 1998;80:537-546.

55. Brooker AF, Bowerman JW, Robinson RA, Riley LH Jr: Ectopic ossification following total hip replacement: Incidence and a method of classification. *J Bone Joint Surg Am* 1973;55:1629-1632.

56. Matta JM, Siebenrock KA: Does indomethacin reduce heterotopic bone formation after operations for acetabular fractures? A prospective randomised study. *J Bone Joint Surg Br* 1997;79:959-963.

57. Lo TC, Healy WL, Covall DJ, et al: Heterotopic bone formation after hip surgery: Prevention with single-dose postoperative hip irradiation. *Radiology* 1988;168:851-854.

58. Moed BR, Letournel E: Low-dose irradiation and indomethacin prevent heterotopic ossification after acetabular fracture surgery. *J Bone Joint Surg Br* 1994;76:895-900.

59. Della Valle CJ, Bogner E, Desai P, et al: Analysis of frozen sections of intraoperative specimens obtained at the time of reoperation after hip or knee resection arthroplasty for the treatment of infection. *J Bone Joint Surg Am* 1999;81:684-689.

60. Spangehl MJ, Masri BA, O'Connell JX, Duncan CP: Prospective analysis of preoperative and intraoperative investigations for the diagnosis of infection at the sites of two hundred and two revision total hip arthroplasties. *J Bone Joint Surg Am* 1999;81:672-683.

61. Hanssen AD, Rand JA: Evaluation and treatment of infection at the site of a total hip or knee arthroplasty. *Instr Course Lect* 1999;48: 111-122.

62. Mears DC: Avascular necrosis of the acetabulum. *Op Tech Orthop* 1997;7:241-249.

63. Younger AS, Duncan CP, Masri BA, McGraw RW: The outcome of two-stage arthroplasty using a custom-made interval spacer to treat the infected hip. *J Arthroplasty* 1997;12:615-623.

64. Haddad FS, Masri BA, Garbuz DS, Duncan CP: The treatment of the infected hip replacement: The complex case. *Clin Orthop* 1999;369:144-156.

65. Pagnano MW, Trousdale RT, Hanssen AD: Outcome after reinfection following reimplantation hip arthroplasty. *Clin Orthop* 1997;338:192-204.

66. Nestor BJ, Hanssen AD, Ferrer-Gonzalez R, Fitzgerald RH Jr: The use of porous prostheses in delayed reconstruction of total hip replacements that have failed because of infection. *J Bone Joint Surg Am* 1994;76: 349-359.

67. Lonner JH, Koval KJ: Polytrauma in the elderly. *Clin Orthop* 1995;318:136-143.

68. DeMaria EJ, Kenney PR, Merriam MA, Casanova LA, Gann DS: Survival after trauma in geriatric patients. *Ann Surg* 1987;206: 738-743.

69. McCoy GF, Johnston RA, Duthie RB: Injury to the elderly in road traffic accidents. *J Trauma* 1989;29:494-497.

70. Joly JM, Mears DC: The role of total hip arthroplasty in acetabular fracture management. *Op Tech Orthop* 1993;3:80-102.

71. Carnesale PG, Stewart MJ, Barnes SN: Acetabular disruption and central fracture-dislocation of the hip: A long-term study. *J Bone Joint Surg Am* 1975;57:1054-1059.

72. Boardman KP, Charnley J: Low-friction arthroplasty after fracture-dislocations of the hip. *J Bone Joint Surg Br* 1978;60:495-497.

73. Coventry MB: The treatment of fracture-dislocation of the hip by total hip arthroplasty. *J Bone Joint Surg Am* 1974;56:1128-1134.

74. Harris WH: Traumatic arthritis of the hip after dislocation and acetabular fractures: Treatment by mold arthroplasty: An end-result study using a new method of result evaluation. *J Bone Joint Surg Am* 1969;51: 737-755.

75. Westerborn A: Central dislocation of the femoral head treated with mold arthroplasty. *J Bone Joint Surg Am* 1954;36:307-314.

76. Mears DC: Surgical treatment of acetabular fractures in elderly patients with osteoporotic bone. *J Am Acad Orthop Surgeons* 1999;7: 128-141.

SECTION

7

Knee: Adult Reconstruction

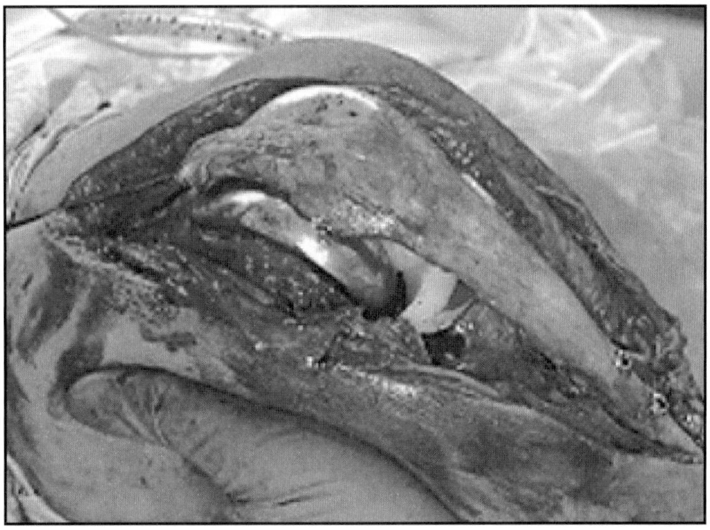

35 Principles of Revision Total Knee Arthroplasty: Overview

36 Revision Total Knee Arthroplasty: Planning, Management, Controversies, and Surgical Approaches

37 Revision Total Knee Arthroplasty: Planning, Controversies, and Management—Infection

38 Periprosthetic Fractures Following Total Knee Arthroplasty

39 Periprosthetic Osteolysis With Total Knee Arthroplasty

40 Ligament Instability in Total Knee Arthroplasty

41 Patellofemoral Complications Following Total Knee Arthroplasty

42 Infection After Total Knee Arthroplasty

43 Thromboembolic Disease in Total Knee Arthroplasty

44 Maximizing Ultra High Molecular Weight Polyethylene Performance in Total Knee Replacement

45 Mobile-Bearing Knee Replacement: Concepts and Results

46 Revision Anterior Cruciate Ligament Reconstruction: Report of 11-Year Experience and Results in 114 Consecutive Patients ***(with video clip on enclosed CD)***

47 Evaluation and Treatment of Recurrent Instability After Anterior Cruciate Ligament Reconstruction ***(with video clip on enclosed CD)***

35

Principles of Revision Total Knee Arthroplasty: Overview

Victor M. Goldberg, MD

Revision total knee arthroplasty (TKA) is technically more difficult, has increased complications, and potentially has a higher rate of failure than primary TKA.[1-7] The causes of failure of a TKA include infection and mechanical problems associated with loosening, wear, instability, and dysfunction of the extensor mechanism. The success of the revision TKA is affected significantly by identifying the specific cause of the failure of the primary procedure. Data suggest that exploratory knee surgery without a stated diagnosis has a very low rate of success.[8] Most important, there must be a high level of suspicion for infection, and although normal preoperative tests may be obtained, the clinical judgment of the surgeon at surgery is critical.

There are a number of important steps in performing a revision TKA.[2,5] These include understanding the cause of the failure; preoperative planning; consideration of prior incisions; prosthetic options; technical planning; adequate exposure; removal of the implant; restoration of stability and kinematics of the knee by restoring anatomy and joint line, balancing the soft tissues, and restoring mechanical alignment; soft-tissue repair; and finally, well-supervised postoperative rehabilitation.

The principles of surgical technique require restoring bony defects, obtaining fixation of the revision components, and restoring stability and kinematics of the knee.[3,5] It is critical to correct and restore mechanical limb alignment and provide anatomic component position to obtain soft-tissue stability and balance with a functional range of motion.

The sequence of surgical steps begins with excellent exposure of the knee, protecting the extensor mechanism and preserving bone.[9] Removal of the failed components requires patience and the availability of appropriate osteotomes, saws, and high-speed power equipment. Clear sight of the implant-bone interface must be obtained, usually by the use of electrocautery to define the margins of each component. Care must be taken when removing the patella to protect as much of the residual bone as possible. When an all-polyethylene patellar component is present without loosening, retention of the implant may be indicated. To determine the type and extent of bone graft needed, the surgeon must assess bone loss by defining whether the defect is contained, noncontained or segmental, or massive.[10,11]

The principles of the revision transcend any individual design. Although some surgeons proceed by reestablishing the tibial platform first, others approach the femur first; both approaches have similar principles.[5,12] The important principles are restoration of the joint line, balancing the flexion and extension space, and restoration of the extensor mechanism and patellofemoral articulation. Restoration of the joint line is a critical step.[3] The usual landmarks to help define the joint line are the head of the fibula, the epicondylar ridge, and the inferior pole of the patella. Finally, reconstruction of the patellofemoral articulation is completed. Intramedullary stems may be useful when prosthetic augmentation or bone grafts are used, when osteoporotic bone is present, or when a periprosthetic fracture is treated.[5,13] It is generally easier for the surgeon to balance and stabilize the flexion gap first before restoring stability of the knee in extension. The inferior pole of the patella should never be below the level of the joint line to ensure appropriate extensor mechanism function and satisfactory flexion of the knee.

The availability of newer, modular components that may be customized intraoperatively has clearly improved the surgical technique and enabled the surgeon to restore the anatomy of the knee.[5,12] Fixation of the components is usually accomplished with polymethylmethacrylate. Supervised rehabilitation, with conservative weight bearing, and the use of stabilizing braces are an adjunct to a successful outcome. However, although primary TKA yields greater than a 90% success rate 10 years after surgery, most studies of revision TKAs report only an 80% satisfactory outcome.[1,2,7]

In summary, the key concepts in accomplishing a successful revision TKA include determining the mode of failure, appropriate preoperative planning, surgical technique, and restoration of knee anatomy. Finally, it is important to select a component with the least constraint possible to accomplish the goals of revision TKA.

References

1. Friedman RJ, Hirst P, Poss R, Kelley K, Sledge CB: Results of revision total knee arthroplasty performed for aseptic loosening. *Clin Orthop* 1990;255:235-241.
2. Insall JN, Dethmers DA: Revision of total knee arthroplasty. *Clin Orthop* 1982;170:123-130.
3. Goldberg VM, Figgie MP, Figgie HE III, Sobel M: The results of revision total knee arthroplasty. *Clin Orthop* 1988;226:86-92.
4. Elia EA, Lotke PA: Results of revision total knee arthroplasty associated with significant bone loss. *Clin Orthop* 1991;271:114-121.
5. Haas SB, Insall JN, Montgomery W III, Windsor RE: Revision total knee arthroplasty with use of modular components with stems inserted without cement. *J Bone Joint Surg Am* 1995;77:1700-1707.
6. Whiteside LA: Cementless revision total knee arthroplasty. *Clin Orthop* 1993; 286:160-167.
7. Jacobs MA, Hungerford DS, Krackow KA, Lennox DW: Revision total knee arthroplasty for aseptic failure. *Clin Orthop* 1988; 226:78-865.
8. Mont MA, Serna FK, Krackow KA, Hungerford DS: Exploration of radiographically normal total knee replacements for unexplained pain. *Clin Orthop* 1996;331:216-220.
9. Rand JA: Preoperative planning and templating, in Rand JA (ed): *Total Knee Arthroplasty*. New York, NY, Raven Press, 1993, pp 93-114.
10. Engh GA: Bone defect classification, in Engh GA, Rorabeck CH(eds*): Revision Total Knee Arthroplasty*. Baltimore, MD, Williams & Wilkins, 1997, pp 63-120.
11. Engh GA, Herzwurm PJ, Parks NL: Treatment of major defects of bone with bulk allografts and stemmed components during total knee arthroplasty. *J Bone Joint Surg Am* 1997;79:1030-1039.
12. Rosenberg, AG, Verner JJ, Galante JO: Clinical results of total knee revision using the Total Condylar III prosthesis. *Clin Orthop* 1991;273:83-90.
13. Kraay MJ, Goldberg VM, Figgie MP, Figgie HE III: Distal femoral replacement with allograft/prosthetic reconstruction for treatment of supracondylar fractures in patients with total knee arthroplasty. *J Arthroplasty* 1992;7: 7-16.

36

Revision Total Knee Arthroplasty: Planning, Management, Controversies, and Surgical Approaches

Henry D. Clarke, MD
Giles R. Scuderi, MD

Introduction

Revision total knee arthroplasty can be a complicated procedure and is fraught with numerous potential complications. Problems including delayed wound healing, extensor mechanism disruption, intraoperative fracture, and infection may result from inadequate surgical exposure or poor soft-tissue handling. In addition, patient-specific factors influence the occurrence of these undesirable results. Careful preoperative evaluation and attention to intraoperative surgical technique may help avoid potentially catastrophic problems.

Preoperative Evaluation

Comorbidities

Patients with systemic conditions and other comorbidities have been reported to be at risk for wound-healing problems. Careful preoperative evaluation and optimization of these conditions may help prevent postoperative complications.

Inadequate nutrition has been shown to delay wound healing and recovery after surgery.[1-4] A total lymphocyte count of less than 1,500/mm^3 or a serum albumin of less than 3.4 g/dL have been defined as indicators of poor nutrition.[2,4] A delay in wound healing has also been noted in patients with underlying malignant disease, likely due to their overall debilitated state.[5] Obesity may also delay wound healing, but rather than due to systemic effects, the delay may be related to technical factors during surgery. Wong and associates[6] have reported a linear relationship between increasing weight and wound problems following total knee replacement. In distinction, Stern and Insall[7] did not identify any increase in wound-related complications.

Increased wound complications and infection also have been noted in patients with rheumatoid arthritis.[6,8-10] The poor wound healing may be related to the atrophic skin, poor nutritional status, and vasculitis encountered in some of these patients.[8] Higher infection rates may be due to inhibited neutrophil function.[10] It is difficult to determine whether these effects are independent of the corticosteroids used in this population.[8,10]

Diabetes mellitus is another systemic condition associated with higher wound complications and infection rates.[1,6,11-14] Hyperglycemia has been shown to impede wound healing by inhibiting collagen synthesis and slowing capillary ingrowth.[13] The increased infection rate appears to be a result of deficiencies in polymorphonuclear neutrophil function.[12-16] Optimal perioperative control of diabetes and hyperglycemia has been shown to reduce the risk of infection and wound complications.[13,17-19]

Patients taking corticosteroids are also at increased risk for wound healing problems and infection.[8,20] Direct effects of these medications include a reduction in collagen synthesis and inhibition of macrophage function, including migration to sites of inflammation and secretion of proteinases and collegenase.[8,21] Duration of corticosteroid administration greater than 3 years appears to be associated with increased wound complications.[8] Patients on other immune modifying chemotherapy agents may also be at increased risk.[16]

Smoking can also produce detrimental effects on soft-tissue healing. Nicotine is known to potentiate cardiovascular effects, including peripheral vasoconstriction, that may result in significant tissue hypoxia.[22,23] Cotinine, which is a metabolite of nicotine, has a long half-life and may be used as an effective marker of abstinence.[22,24] Systemic levels of cotinine should fall to the background levels seen in nonsmokers within 8 days.[24] Cessation of smoking for several weeks prior to surgery should be encouraged, but even abstinence during the perioperative period may be beneficial.[25]

Anemia has been cited as another factor that may contribute to wound complications. However, it appears that wound oxygen tension is the critical variable rather than absolute hemoglobin levels. Both angiogenesis and fibroblast function are inhibited by inadequate oxygen tension.[3] The mild, normovolemic anemia that occurs routinely in postoperative patients may not impede wound healing.[3,17,26] In patients with good cardiac and pulmonary function, a hematocrit as low as 15% to 18% may allow adequate healing.[3] Poor wound oxygen tension is associated with increased infection rates because wound hypoxia also appears to inhibit neutrophil bactericidal activity.[27,28] Thus, it seems advisable to correct factors that contribute to low tissue perfusion, including a low hematocrit, dehydration, and peripheral vasoconstriction.

Peripheral vascular disease should also be evaluated carefully before surgery. Vascular surgery consultation should be sought for any patient with a history of claudication or prior bypass surgery. In addition, physical findings such as poor pedal pulses, venous stasis changes, or significant vascular calcifications noted on routine radiographic examination should prompt a complete evaluation. Furthermore, we avoid the use of an intraoperative tourniquet in any patient with a history of a prior ipsilateral lower extremity bypass or revascularization procedure.

Anatomic Considerations

Patient-specific knee anatomy can make the surgery technically more difficult. Preoperative consideration of these factors allows the surgeon to anticipate how best to facilitate safe and expeditious exposure, rather than making a hasty intraoperative decision. This information is particularly important for surgeons who perform these difficult procedures on an occasional basis. Numerous prior incisions and adherent tissue can complicate the exposure and predispose to postoperative wound problems. Obesity, patella baja, bony abnormalities, restricted motion, ankylosis, and significant malalignment also may contribute to difficult surgical exposure that can result in local soft-tissue trauma, extensor mechanism disruption, and component malposition. A number of prophylactic measures and specific surgical techniques may be used to minimize complications resulting from systemic comorbidities and individual anatomic features.

Skin Incisions

Vascular Anatomy

The skin overlying the anterior knee receives its blood supply from an anastomosis of vessels that run just superficial to the deep fascia. This anastomosis is different than the better known deep anterior anastomosis that provides vascular supply to the patella and integuments of the knee.[29] Vessels that perforate through the deep fascia, including branches of the inferior and superior genicular arteries, the saphenous branch of the descending genicular artery, and recurrent branches of the anterior tibial artery, feed the superficial anastomosis.[30] This network of vessels courses parallel to the surface for a considerable distance in the loose areolar layer that separates the deep fascia from the subcutaneous fat.[30,31] Terminal vessels to the dermis and epidermis pass through the subcutaneous fat, but there is little communication in these more superficial layers.[30] Because the skin relies on this plexus of perforating vessels running just superficial to the deep fascia, undermining of the skin and creation of elevated skin and subcutaneous flaps should be minimized. Furthermore, because the primary vascular supply originates from the medial side, creation of large lateral flaps should be particularly avoided.[30,32-34]

Prior Incisions

A single, longitudinal anterior midline incision provides the most extensile exposure and is preferred for both primary and revision total knee replacement. In patients without significant risk factors, this skin incision usually is well tolerated. When a single prior anterior incision exists, it should be used in subsequent revision procedures. In these circumstances, we limit subcutaneous dissection and maintain full thickness flaps to minimize trauma to the plexus of vessels. If multiple incisions or a single anterior incision located well away from the midline exists, selection of the appropriate skin incision requires more careful consideration. A single, transverse anterior incision may be crossed by a new perpendicular longitudinal incision with little concern. In distinction, creation of parallel longitudinal incisions should be avoided. If the prior incision is considered to be too far from the midline and would necessitate creation of a large laterally based subcutaneous flap, we may consider using a new incision. In these circumstances, adequate skin bridges (~5 cm) should be maintained.[35] In any circumstance in which we consider the patient to be at high risk for developing wound problems because of the number and orientation of prior incisions or because of other patient comorbidities, we do not hesitate to use preoperative techniques to optimize the local soft-tissue environment. These techniques include the sham incision, soft-tissue expansion, and rotational or free soft-tissue flaps.

Sham Incision

The sham incision is mentioned for historic interest because we no longer use this technique. Rather than a prophylaxis against wound problems, the sham incision is simply a predictor of wound healing complications. Approximately 2 weeks before the planned total knee procedure, the intended skin incision is made and extended through the subcutaneous tissue to the level of the extensor mechanism.[36] The incision is then closed in the standard fashion and the wound is observed. If the wound heals without complications, the intended knee procedure is performed. If skin necrosis occurs, a soft-tissue coverage procedure, such as a fasciocutaneous or muscle flap, is performed prior to the arthroplasty. In these circumstances, if full-thickness slough occurs, the risk of deep infection is reduced because no arthrotomy was performed and the prosthesis was not directly exposed. The development of soft-tissue expansion techniques around the knee has superseded the use of the sham incision in our practice.

Tissue Expanders

Soft-tissue expansion has been performed by plastic surgeons throughout the body and recently has been used about the knee before reconstructive surgery. Expandable, saline-filled implants are inserted in the subcutaneous space. Periodically, saline is injected into a separate, subcutaneous access port. The overlying soft tissue is gradually expanded in size according to the concept of stress relaxation.[37] However, the process involves more than a simple stretching of the overlying skin. Although thinning of the dermis and subcutaneous fat does occur, the epidermis hypertrophies.[38] The nature of the tissue also changes, with higher mitotic activity in the epidermis and vascular dilatation in the dermis.[38] A distinct fibrous capsule, which we have found to be quite useful at the time of closure, also develops around the tissue expander. In addition to providing supplemental tissue, expansion acts as a stimulus for angiogenesis, producing increased vascularity in the overlying region, which may be the result of a relative hypoxia that occurs during the expansion process.[39,40]

Insertion of the tissue expanders is performed under local anesthesia. A small incision oriented parallel to the planned incision is made and a subcutaneous pocket is created. The expanders are then inserted and oriented perpendicularly to one another. Typically one to three 200-mL expanders are used. Expansion is begun after 1 week, and approximately 10% of the required value is expanded on a weekly basis. Knee replacement may be performed approximately 2 weeks after the final expansion. The expanders can easily be removed at the time of surgery. At the time of closure surplus tissue often is encountered and should be trimmed. We now routinely use subcutaneous drains in the dead spaces created by each expander pocket to minimize superficial hematoma formation and wound drainage. Drains are removed when the output is less than or equal to 10 cc per shift or 30 cc per 24-hour period.

Successful results of the use of soft-tissue expanders before total knee replacement have been reported but are limited in number.[41-44] The early experience at our institution with the first 10 patients was excellent, with no significant wound complications and early primary healing.[37] In the latest expanded series of 29 knees, minor wound complications, such as erythema or skin blisters, occurred after 21% of the tissue expansion insertions and 18% of the knee replacements. One major complication occurred after soft-tissue expansion and involved full-thickness skin necrosis in a patient whose skin had been extensively irradiated; the planned arthroplasty procedure was subsequently deferred (FD Cushner, personal communication, 1999). Following the knee replacement, three knees developed persistent drainage, and two knees developed subcutaneous hematomas. The persistent drainage resolved with immobilization and local wound compression, whereas the two subcutaneous hematomas required surgical evacuation. In our experience, this technique prevented major wound complications and eliminated the need for more complex soft-tissue procedures.

Fasciocutaneous Flaps and Muscle Flaps

Soft-tissue flaps, including facsiocutaneous flaps, rotational muscle or myocutaneous flaps, and free muscle flaps, represent salvage procedures when soft-tissue necrosis or dehiscence occurs. However, in certain patients with severe soft-tissue scarring, extensive deformities, or irradiated skin, soft-tissue coverage procedures may be performed either prior to total knee replacement or at the time of the arthroplasty. The goals of treatment include avoidance of deep infection and retention of the prosthesis. Wounds smaller than 2 to 4 cm may be left to heal by secondary intent.[45,46] Skin grafting may be considered if the anticipated time for secondary healing exceeds the 5 to 7 days of postoperative immobilization that is required after skin grafting. Fasciocutaneous flaps also have been successfully employed in circumstances of superficial necrosis.[47,48] These vascular flaps rotate skin, subcutaneous tissue, and deep fascia about a pedicle. Hallock[49] has recommended a maximum length-to-width ratio of 2.5 to 1. Infection and an exposed prosthesis are contraindications to the use of this technique.[50]

If extensive or full-thickness necrosis occurs with exposure of the prosthesis, rotational muscle flaps or free flaps are required. Simple closure over an exposed prosthesis has a poor success rate.[51] The medial gastrocnemius rotation flap provides the most reliable results.[47,51-54] A lateral gastrocnemius flap may also be used on the lateral side. If the necrosis is extensive, free flaps such as transfer of the latissimus dorsi muscle, rectus abdominous muscle, or scapular free flap may be required.[55] Despite successful prosthesis retention, the functional outcomes and range of motion seen in these patients after soft-tissue coverage procedures are inferior to the results obtained in patients who do not encounter wound-healing problems.[47,53] Treatment of wound dehiscence that occurs in association with infection is more difficult and has a higher failure rate.[47] However, even in these cases, prosthesis removal, débridement, intravenous antibiotics and rotational muscle flap coverage followed by delayed reimplantation can be successful.[53,56]

Surgical Exposure

Many intraoperative decisions affect the ease of exposure and influence the incidence of complications. In addition to avoiding rough soft-tissue handling and use of mechanical self-retaining

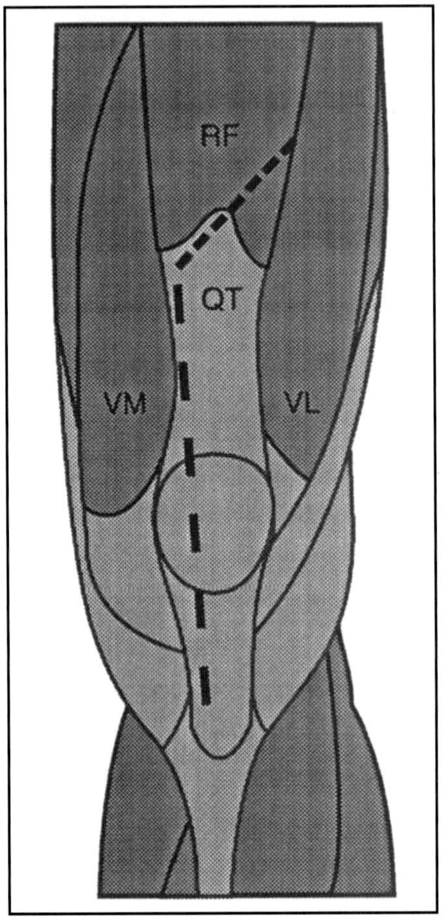

Fig. 1 The quadriceps snip is an oblique proximal and lateral extension of the standard medial parapatellar arthrotomy. The quadriceps snip is extended into the substance of the vastus lateralis as far as required to allow patellar eversion. QT = quadriceps tendon; RF = rectus femoris; VL = vastus lateralis; VM = vastus medialis.

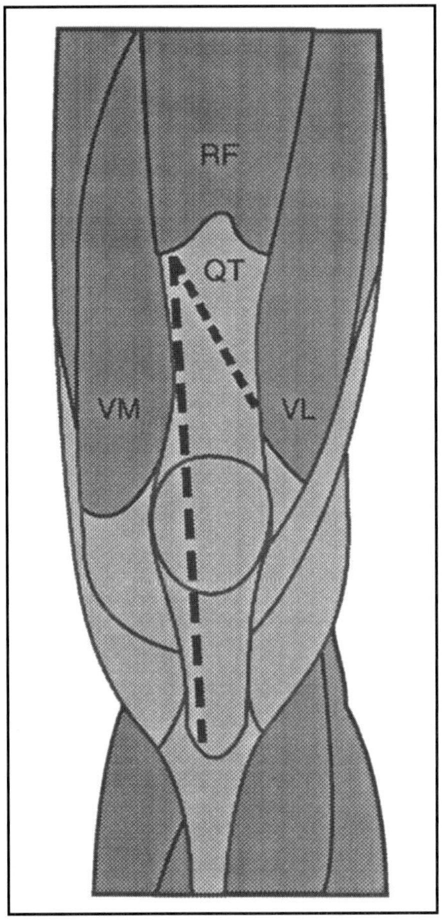

Fig. 2 The modified V-Y quadriceps turndown. Beginning at the apex of the standard medial parapatellar arthrotomy a distal oblique incision is made.

retractors, adequate hydration of the exposed tissue should be maintained with intermittent irrigation. Just as selection of the optimal skin incision is important, choice of the arthrotomy used is also important. Furthermore, the prudent use of additional surgical techniques to provide extensile exposure in these difficult cases is critical.

Arthrotomy

A medial parapatellar arthrotomy is the preferred preliminary step because it is versatile and can be incorporated into more extensile exposures. Proximally, the medial parapatellar arthrotomy can be extended with a quadriceps snip, or it can be incorporated into a modified V-Y turndown or tibial tubercle osteotomy.

Quadriceps Snip

The quadriceps snip represents a proximal and lateral extension of the standard medial parapatellar arthrotomy that helps allow eversion of the patella in obese patients, patients with stiff knees, and patients with patella infera. Beginning at the proximal apex of the quadriceps tendon, the standard arthrotomy is extended proximally and laterally, at an angle of approximately 45°, into the substance of the vastus lateralis (Fig. 1). The length of this extension is variable and may be continued until eversion of the patella is possible. In rare instances, this technique may not allow complete eversion and a tibial tubercle osteotomy can also be performed. At the end of the operation, the quadriceps snip is closed in the same way as the standard arthrotomy. Patients in whom a quadriceps snip is used do not require any modification of their postoperative rehabilitation and may participate in standard physical therapy protocols. Garvin and associates[57] have reported the initial favorable experience with use of the quadriceps snip. In patients with bilateral knee replacements where a quadriceps snip had been performed on one side only, Cybex muscle testing at final follow-up did not show any differences in quadriceps strength between the two sides. Similarly, Barrack and associates[58] compared patients in whom a quadriceps snip had been used with a control group of patients in whom only a standard medial parapatellar arthrotomy had been performed; at final follow-up these two groups were identical in every outcome parameter measured. In our practice, we do not hesitate to use this technique because avoidance of an extensor mechanism disruption is a paramount concern during these procedures.

V-Y Quadriceps Turndown

The V-Y quadriceps turndown was first described by Coonse and Adams[59] in 1943 and was subsequently modified by Aglietti and associates.[60] After a standard medial parapatellar arthrotomy, an additional incision extends distally and laterally at an angle of 45° along the tendinous portion of the vastus lateralis (Fig. 2). This forms an inverted V of tissue that allows eversion and distal displacement of the patella and provides excellent exposure. At the time of closure, the quadriceps tendon may be lengthened, creating the Y. This approach can be helpful in the

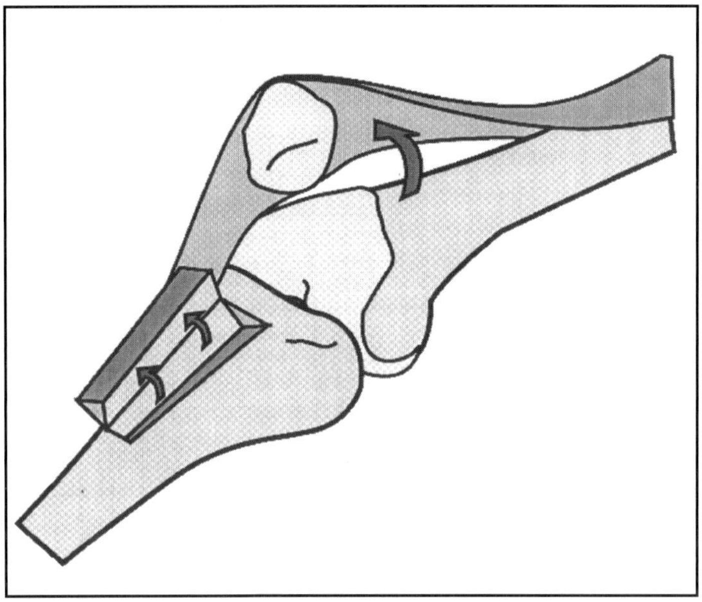

Fig. 3 The tibial tubercle osteotomy allows eversion of the tibial tubercle and extensor mechanism in continuity. The osteotomized tubercle is hinged laterally on the intact periosteal sleeve.

ankylosed knee but does require modifications in the postoperative rehabilitation, including partial weight bearing, bracing, and limited range of motion. Another disadvantage is that some patients develop a persistent extensor lag.

Trousdale and associates[61] have reported their experience with the V-Y quadricepsplasty. Cybex testing did not reveal any statistically significant quadriceps strength differences in patients who had undergone knee replacement with a V-Y quadriceps turndown on one side versus a knee replacement with the routine exposure on the contralateral side. However, 5 of 14 patients had an extensor lag greater than 5°.[61] Barrack and associates[58] have also reported problems with extension lag in patients after this procedure. Because of the excellent success that we have experienced with the use of the quadriceps snip, we do not currently use this technique. In cases where the quadriceps snip does not provide adequate exposure, we prefer to use the tibial tubercle osteotomy.

Tibial Tubercle Osteotomy

The tibial tubercle osteotomy was first described by Dolin[62] in 1983 and has been popularized by Whiteside.[63] This technique may be performed in conjunction with a quadriceps snip if patella eversion is inadequate after maximal extension into the lateralis muscle. It may also be used to allow access to the tibial canal in order to facilitate controlled extraction of well-fixed tibial stems. After the standard arthrotomy is performed, the periosteum is incised 1 cm medial to the tibial tubercle. Next, the cortex of the tibia is cut along the medial edge of the tibial tubercle with an oscillating saw for a distance of 6 cm. The lateral cortex is then osteotomized, while the distal cut is tapered to minimize a stress riser. A bone block measuring approximately 6 cm long, 2 cm wide, and 1 cm thick is thus created. The lateral periosteum and musculature remain attached to the tubercle and act as a soft-tissue hinge, allowing the osteotomized segment to be everted and displaced laterally (Fig. 3). At the time of closure the tubercle is reattached with three stainless steel wires oriented distally in an oblique fashion. Depending on component design, screw fixation is an alternative. If rigid fixation is obtained, the patient is allowed full weight bearing and unrestricted range of motion. Advantages of this technique include lower incidences of extensor lag and quadriceps weakness than with the V-Y quadricepsplasty. Whiteside[63] has reported his experience with the use of this technique in 136 patients; only two patients demonstrated an extensor lag. Barrack and associates[58] have also reported a significantly lower degree of extensor lag in patients who had undergone a tibial tubercle osteotomy than in those who had undergone a V-Y quadricepsplasty. The main disadvantages of this technique are the major complications related to surgical technique that have been reported to occur in up to 23% of cases.[64] Reported complications include tibial shaft fractures, displacement of the osteotomized tubercle, and patellar tendon rupture.[63-66] We use the tibial tubercle osteotomy in selected patients in whom the quadriceps snip fails to provide adequate exposure.

Additional Technical Details

In addition to the major techniques described above, a number of other maneuvers may be used to improve exposure. These may be used in conjunction with the previously described techniques. Sharply transecting the lateral patellofemoral ligaments and sharply releasing the fat pad along the lateral edge of the patellar tendon may facilitate patellar eversion. Furthermore, an early lateral patellar retinacular release may be performed. It is also important to remember that if the patellar component does not need to be revised, eversion of the patella is not necessarily required, and it may be sufficient to simply subluxate the patella laterally. We also raise a few millimeters of periosteum along the medial margin of the patellar tendon to prevent tendon rupture. If excessive tension in the extensor mechanism occurs, we believe this maneuver encourages a controlled peel of the tendon from the bone rather than sudden catastrophic failure. Other techniques to improve exposure in the revision setting or stiff knee include performing an early arthrolysis. During a revision arthroplasty, if a modular tibial component is present, the polyethylene component can be removed from the metal tray. This maneuver will relax the surrounding capsular structures. Abundant fibrous scar tissue is commonly encountered in the suprapatellar pouch and should be sharply excised. Moreover, both sharp and blunt dissection may be used to reestablish the medial and lateral gutters. Finally, a femoral peel may be used and involves circumferential subperiosteal elevation of the soft-tissue sleeve from the distal femur.[67] Each of these maneuvers can help gain adequate exposure and should be used where necessary.

Summary

Revision total knee arthroplasty can be a technically challenging procedure fraught with potential complications. In many cases, obtaining adequate exposure is difficult, and failure to do so can directly cause technical errors and complications. Patient-specific systemic comorbidites and anatomic details can further complicate the procedure. Careful preoperative evaluation can help to facilitate optimal results. Furthermore, specific surgical techniques help to improve the surgical exposure and can minimize complications such as wound healing problems, component malposition, and extensor mechanism disruption. All surgeons undertaking these procedures require a thorough understanding of these principles.

References

1. Cruse PJ, Foord R: A five-year prospective study of 23,649 surgical wounds. *Arch Surg* 1973;107:206-210.
2. Dickhaut SC, DeLee JL, Pase CP: Nutritional statistics. Importance in predicting wound healing after amputation. *J Bone Joint Surg Am* 1984;66:71-75.
3. Hunt TK, Hopf HW: Wound healing and wound infection: What surgeons and anesthesiologists can do. *Surg Clin North Am* 1997;77:587-606.
4. Jensen JE, Jensen TG, Smith TK, Johnston DA, Dudrick SJ: Nutrition in orthopaedic surgery. *J Bone Joint Surg Am* 1982;64:1263-1272.
5. Glenn F, Moore SW: The disruption of abdominal wounds. *Surg Gynec Obstet* 1941;72:1041-1046.
6. Wong RY, Lotke PA, Ecker ML: Factors influencing wound healing after total knee arthroplasty. *Orthop Trans* 1986;10: 497.
7. Stern SH, Insall JN: Total knee arthroplasty in obese patients. *J Bone Joint Surg Am* 1990;72:1400-1404.
8. Garner RW, Mowot AG, Hazleman BL: Wound healing after operations on patients with rheumatoid arthritis. *J Bone Joint Surg Br* 1973;55:134-144.
9. Grogan TJ, Dores F, Rolling J, Amstutz HC: Deep sepsis following total knee arthroplasty. *J Bone Joint Surg Am* 1986;68:226-234.
10. Wilson MG, Kelley K, Thornhill TS: Infection as a complication of total knee replacement arthroplasty: Risk factors and treatment in sixty-seven cases. *J Bone Joint Surg Am* 1990;72:878-883.
11. Ecker ML, Lotke PA: Postoperative care of the total knee patient. *Orthop Clin North Am* 1989;20:55-62.
12. England SP, Stern SH, Insall JN, Windsor RE: Total knee arthroplasty in diabetes mellitus. *Clin Orthop* 1990;260:130-134.
13. McMurray JF Jr: Wound Healing with Diabetes Mellitus. Better glucose control for better wound healing in diabetes. *Surg Clin North Am* 1984;64:769-778.
14. Menon TJ, Thjellesen D, Wroblewski BM: Charnley low-friction arthroplasty in diabetic patients. *J Bone Joint Surg Br* 1983;65:580-581.
15. Delamaire M, Maugendre D, Moreno M, Le Goff MC, Allannic H, Genetet B: Impaired leukocyte functions in diabetic patients. *Diabet Med* 1997;14:29-34.
16. Dennis PA: Wound complications in total knee arthroplasty. *Instr Course Lect* 1997;46:165-169.
17. Heughan C, Chir B, Grislis G, Hunt JK: The effect of anemia on wound healing. *Ann Surg* 1974;179:163-167.
18. Rassias AJ, Marrin CAS, Arruda J, Whalen PK, Beach M, Yeager MP: Insulin infusion improves neutrophil function in diabetic cardiac surgery patients. *Anesth Analg* 1999;88:1011-1016.
19. Zerr KJ, Furnary AP, Grunkemeier GL, Bookin S, Knahere V, Starr A: Glucose control lowers the risk of wound infection in diabetes after open heart operations. *Ann Thorac Surg* 1997;63:356-361.
20. Green JP: Steroid therapy and wound healing in surgical patients. *Br J Surg* 1965;52:523-525.
21. Werb Z.: Biochemical actions of glucocorticoids on macrophages in culture: Specific inhibition of elastase, collagenase, and plasminogen activator secretion and effects on other metabolic functions. *J Exp Med* 1978;147:1695-1712.
22. Benowitz NL, Kuyt F, Jacob P: Influence of nicotine on cardiovascular and hormone effects of cigarette smoking. *Clin. Pharmacol Ther* 1984;36:74-81.
23. Jensen JA, Goodson WH, Hopf HW, Hunt TK: Cigarette smoking decreases tissue oxygen. *Arch Surg* 1991;126:1131-1134.
24. Benowitz NL, Kuyt F, Jacob P, Jones RT, Osman AL: Cotinine disposition and effects. *Clin Pharmacol Ther* 1983;34:604-611.
25. Craig S, Rees TD: The effects of smoking on experimental skin flaps in hamsters. *Plast Reconstr Surg* 1985;75:842-846.
26. Jonsson K, Jensen JA, Goodson WH III, et al: Tissue oxygenation, anemia and perfusion in relation to wound healing in surgical patients. *Ann Surg* 1991;2145:605-613.
27. Allen DB, Maguire JJ, Mahdavian M, et al: Wound hypoxia and acidosis limit neutrophil bacterial mechanisms. *Arch Surg* 1997;132: 991-996.
28. Hopf HW, Hunt TK, West JM, et al: Wound tissue oxygen tension predicts the risk of wound infection in surgical patients. *Arch Surg* 1997;132: 997-1005.
29. Scapinelli R: Blood supply of the human patella: Its relation to ischaemic necrosis after fracture. *J Bone Joint Surg Br* 1967;49:563-570.
30. Younger ASE, Duncan CP, Masri B: Surgical exposures in revision total knee arthroplasty. *J Am Acad Orthop Surg* 1998; 6:55-54.
31. Taylor GI, Palmer JH: The vascular territories (angiosomes) of the body: Experimental study and clinical applications. *Br J Plast Surg* 1987;40:113-141.
32. Colombel M, Mariz Y, Dahhan P, Kenesi C: Arterial and lymphatic supply of the knee integuments. *Surg Radiol Anat* 1998;20:35-40.
33. Johnson, DP: Midline or parapatellar incision for knee arthroplasty: A comparative study of wound viability. *J Bone Joint Surg Br* 1988;70:656-658.
34. Johnson DP, Eastwood DM: Lateral patellar release in knee arthroplasty: Effect on wound healing. *J Arthroplasty* 1992;7(suppl):407-431.
35. Ranawat CS, Flynn WF Jr: Principles of planning and prosthetic selection for revision total knee replacement, in Scott WN (ed): *The Knee.* St. Louis, MO, Mosby-Year Book, 1994, pp 1297-1303.
36. Rothaus KO: Plastic and reconstructive surgery, in Insall JN (ed): *Surgery of the Knee.* New York, NY, Churchill-Livingstone, 1993, pp 1200-1201.
37. Gold DA, Scott SC, Scott WN: Soft tissue expansion prior to arthroplasty in the multiply operated knee - A new method of preventing catastrophic skin problems. *J Arthroplasty* 1996;11:512-521.
38. Pasyk KA, Argenta LC, Austad ED: Histopathology of human expanded tissue. *Clin Plast Surg* 1987;14:435-445.
39. Argenta LC, Marks MW, Pasyk KA: Advances in tissue expansion. *Clin Plast Surg* 1985; 12:159-171.

40. Cherry GW, Austad E, Pasyk K, McClatchey K, Rohrich RJ: Increased survival and vascularity of random-pattern skin flaps elevated in controlled, expanded skin. *Plast Reconstr Surg* 1983;72:680-687.

41. Mahomed N, Mckee N, Solomon P, Lahoda L, Gross AE: Soft tissue expansion before total knee arthroplasty in arthrodesed joints. A report of two cases. *J Bone Joint Surg* 1993;76B:88-90.

42. Namba RS, Diao E: Tissue expansion for staged reimplantation of infected total knee arthroplasty. *J Arthroplasty* 1997;12:471-474.

43. Santore RF, Kaufman D, Robbins AJ, Dabezies EJ: Tissue expansion prior to revision total knee arthroplasty. *J Arthroplasty* 1997;12: 475-478.

44. Weinzweig N, Dowden RV, Stulberg BN: The use of tissue expansion to allow reconstruction of the knee. *J Bone Joint Surg Am* 1987;69: 1238-1240.

45. Hemphill CS, Ebert FR, Muench AG: The medial gastrocnemius muscle flap in the treatment of wound complications following total knee arthroplasty. *Orthopaedics* 1992;15:477-480.

46. Nahabedian MY, Orlando JC, Delanois RE, Mont MA, Hungerford DS: Salvage procedures for complex soft tissue defects of the knee. *Clin Orthop* 1998;356:119-124.

47. Adam RF, Watson SB, Jarratt JW, Noble J, Watson JS: Outcome after flap cover for exposed total knee arthroplasties. A report of 25 cases. *J Bone Joint Surg Br* 1994;76:750-753.

48. Shaw AD, Ghosh SJ, Quaba AA: The island posterior calf fasciocutaneous flap: An alternative to the gastrocnemius muscle for cover of knee and tibial defects. *Plast Reconstr Surg* 1998;101:1529-36.

49. Hallock GG: Salvage of total knee arthroplasty with local fasciocutaneous flaps. *J Bone Joint Surg Br* 1990;76:1236-1239.

50. Lewis VL Jr, Mossie RD, Stulberg DS, Bailey MH, Griffith BH: The fasciocutaneous flap: A conservative approach to the exposed knee joint. *Plast Reconstr Surg* 1990;85:252-257.

51. Bengtson S, Carlsson A, Relander M, Knutson K, Lidgren L: Treatment of the exposed knee prosthesis. *Acta Orthop Scand* 1987;58:662-665.

52. Eckhardt JJ, Lesavoy MA, Dubrow TJ, Wackyum PA: Exposed endo-prosthesis. *Clin Orthop* 1990;251:220-229.

53. Gerwin M, Rothaus KO, Windsor RE, Brause BD, Insall JN: Gastrocnemius muscle flap coverage of exposed or infected knee prosthesis. *Clin Orthop* 1993;286:64-70.

54. Sanders R, O'Neill T: The gastrocnemius myocutaneous flap used as a cover for the exposed knee prosthesis. *J Bone Joint Surg Br* 1981;63:383-386.

55. Craig SM: Soft tissue considerations in the failed total knee arthroplasty, in Scott WN (ed): *The Knee*. St. Louis, MO, Mosby-Yearbook, 1994, pp 1279-1295.

56. McPherson EJ, Patzakis MJ, Gross JE, Holtom PD, Song M, Dorr LD: Infected total knee arthroplasty: Two-stage reimplantation with a gastrocnemius rotational flap. *Clin Orthop* 1997;341:73-81.

57. Garvin KL, Scuderi G, Insall JN: Evolution of the quadriceps snip. *Clin Orthop* 1995;321: 131-137.

58. Barrack RL, Smith P, Munn B, Engh G, Rorabeck C: Comparison of surgical approaches in total knee arthroplasty. *Clin Orthop* 1998;356:16-21.

59. Coonse K, Adams JD: A new operative approach to the knee joint. *Surg Gynecol Obstet* 1943;77:344-347.

60. Aglietti P, Windsor RE, Buzzi R, Insall JN: Arthroplasty for the stiff or ankylosed knee. *J Arthroplasty* 1989;4:1-5.

61. Trousdale RT, Hanssen AD, Rand JA: V-Y quadricepsplasty in total knee arthroplasty. *Clin Orthop* 1993;286:48-55.

62. Dolin MG: Osteotomy of the tibial tubercle in total knee replacement: A technical note. *J Bone Joint Surg Am* 1983;65:704-706.

63. Whiteside LA: Exposure in difficult total knee arthroplasty using tibial tubercle osteotomy. *Clin Orthop* 1995;321:32-35.

64. Wolff AM, Hungerford DS, Krackow KA, Jacobs MA: Osteotomy of the tibial tubercle during total knee replacement. *J Bone Joint Surg Am* 1989;71:848-852.

65. Ries MD, Richman JA: Extended tibial tubercle osteotomy in total knee arthroplasty. *J Arthroplasty* 1996;11:964-967.

66. Ritter MA, Carr K, Keating EM, Faris PM, Meding JB: Tibial shaft fracture following tibial tubercle osteotomy. *J Arthroplasty* 1996;11: 117-119.

67. Windsor RE, Insall JN: Exposure in revision total knee arthroplasty: The femoral peel. *Techniques Orthop* 1988;3:1-4.

37

Revision Total Knee Arthroplasty: Planning, Controversies, and Management—Infection

Sandeep Munjal, MD
Matthew J. Phillips, MD
Kenneth A. Krackow, MD

Deep sepsis of a total knee arthroplasty is a devastating complication. Preventing infection is an integral part of performing the procedure, while early and appropriate treatment of the established infection is of utmost importance. In recent reports, deep infection complicates 1.3% to 2.9% of total knee arthroplasties.[1-7]

Etiology

Infection that occurs in the perioperative period is generally the result of contamination at the time of surgery. Late infection may occur in a previously sterile joint that becomes septic secondary to hematogenous seeding of the arthroplasty.

Multiple factors that increase the risk of infection have been identified. These factors may be exogenous or endogenous. Exogenous factors are generally controlled by the surgeon and therefore must be addressed at the time of surgery. Numerous improvements in surgical techniques during the past 30 years have resulted in a significant decline in infection rate. The routine use of broad-spectrum antibiotics perioperatively,[8-11] laminar flow operating rooms,[12] sterile isolation gowns,[13] limiting the number of operating room personnel,[14,15] and modern total condylar designs have all contributed to a decreased incidence of postarthroplasty infection. Endogenous or host factors that predispose certain patients to septic complications have also been identified. Diabetes mellitus, rheumatoid arthritis and its variants, corticosteroid use, immunosuppressive medications, extreme old age, concurrent infections, prior history of septic arthritis, obesity, and prior knee surgery increase the risk of early and/or late sepsis of the knee.[4,5,7,16-18]

Microbiology

Staphylococcus aureus and *Staphylococcus epidermidis* are the most common organisms isolated in septic arthroplasties. Together, these microbes are identified in more than half of all infected arthroplasties in a wide range of studies.[4,7,19-28]

Gram-negative bacilli can be involved when an arthroplasty infection results from acute wound complications or late hematogenous seeding. Indolent infections that present 3 to 24 months after surgery are often caused by avirulent organisms such as coagulase-negative staphylococci, viridans streptococci, anaerobic gram-positive cocci, and coryneform bacteria. Candida organisms that contaminate the wound perioperatively have caused rare cases of indolent prosthetic joint infections.[29] Hematogenous infections of arthroplasties are typically caused by virulent organisms such as *S aureus*, beta-hemolytic streptococci, and gram-negative bacilli.[30,31]

Diagnosis

Arthroplasties may become infected at any time following implantation of the prosthesis and can present a diagnostic challenge. No test is 100% sensitive and specific; thus, the diagnosis of infection ultimately relies on the surgeon's perception of the clinical presentation, the findings on physical examination, and the interpretation of the laboratory results. The consequences of misdiagnosis are considerable because reimplantation into an infected tissue bed without appropriate débridement is likely to result in persistent infection.

Clinical Presentation

The three-stage classification system described by Coventry[32] and later by Fitzgerald and associates[33] is based on the mode or timing of the presentation of infection and is perhaps the most common system used for classification of infection after arthroplasty. The system was initially described for total hip arthroplasty; however, it can be used for total knee arthroplasty infections as well.

Type I infections occur in the immediate postoperative period. The patient is seen during the first postoperative month, and the diagnosis is often evident on the basis of the medical history and physical examination. Systemic signs of infection, such as fever, chills, and sweating, may be present. Pain is usually continuous, and, on local examination, the wound may be erythematous, swollen, fluctuant, and tender. Wound drainage, if present, is usually purulent. Type I infections are caused by infected hematomas or superficial wound infections that spread contiguously to the periprosthetic space. The diagnostic challenge is to determine whether or not a superficial infection has penetrated deep to fascia.

Because moderate elevation is expected during this time period, laboratory tests such as white blood cell (WBC) count and erythrocyte sedimentation rate (ESR) are of limited use, C-reactive protein (CRP) normalizes within 3 weeks of surgery, much earlier than ESR,[34] and a persistent high level of CRP suggests infection but is not diagnostic.

Clinically, it is difficult to distinguish between sterile and infected hematomas. Culture of drainage fluid has not been reliable.[35] Aspiration is helpful, but if the patient has received antibiotics within the preceding weeks, a false-negative result may be obtained.

Treatment of the wound is the primary consideration. Surgical management of tense effusions or hematomas, whether or not infection is present, is preferred. Infection in this time period is initially treated with surgical débridement, administration of antibiotics, and attempted retention of the components.

Type II infections are also believed to originate at the time of the surgery, but because of a small inoculum or the low virulence of the organism, the onset of symptoms is delayed. The patient is seen between 6 and 24 months after the index procedure. The hallmark of this type of infection is a gradual deterioration in function and an increase in pain. Pain is often present from the time of the original procedure; it may be activity-related or it may occur at night and during rest. Often, the only clue to infection is early loosening of the components. Systemic symptoms may not be a part of the presentation; however, there may be a history of prolonged wound drainage at the time of the index procedure. Persistent swelling and stiffness are often seen and may be difficult to distinguish from reflex sympathetic dystrophy.

Type III infections are the least common and are caused by hematogenous spread to a previously asymptomatic arthroplasty, usually 2 or more years after the arthroplasty. Generally, an acute febrile episode is accompanied by sudden rapid deterioration in the function of the knee. The diagnosis can usually be based on history and physical examination. Seeding can occur at the site of a loose prosthesis, a solidly osseointegrated prosthesis, or a solidly fixed, cemented prosthesis. Patients with a type III infection typically have a significant pain-free interval. A type III infection is likely to occur in patients who are immunosuppressed, such as those who have had a renal transplant or who have been managed with immunosuppressive medications for inflammatory arthropathy; those who have recurrent episodes of bacteremia (such as intravenous drug abusers); and those who need repeat urinary catheterization.[36,37] Other associated factors include recent dental work,[38] respiratory infection, remote periprosthetic infection, open skin lesions, endoscopy, and contamination of surgery sites.

Preoperative Investigations

Plain Radiographs

Plain radiographs should routinely be obtained when evaluating the painful total knee replacement, even though they are unremarkable in most patients, particularly during the early period. Occasionally, the patient will have diagnostic changes such as periostitis, rapidly progressive osteolysis, or endosteal scalloping. A complete radiolucency that develops around a component over a short period of time is highly suggestive of advanced infection.[39] Subchondral bone resorption and patchy osteoporosis are more subtle, earlier findings that present in some infected patients.[40] Periprosthetic osteolysis is the most common finding, but it is nonspecific. Periosteal new bone formation, with or without loosening of a component, has been considered by some authors to be pathognomonic of deep infection.[41]

Laboratory Tests

The WBC count is rarely abnormal in patients with suspected total knee infection. In one series,[25] only 28% of infected knees had a WBC count greater than 11,000/mm^3. When a patient does have an abnormal WBC count, the systemic infection is usually clinically obvious and is either of type I or type III origin.[42]

The ESR and CRP are useful laboratory screening investigations for the diagnosis of a potential infection following total joint replacement. Average ESRs of more than 50 mm/h have been reported in different series of infected total knee arthroplasties,[25,28,43,44] but both false-positive and false-negative results are seen. False-positive results can occur because of other inflammatory conditions such as rheumatoid arthritis. The ESR may remain elevated for months after an uncomplicated joint arthroplasty and during the early postoperative period. The CRP is also an acute phase reactant synthesized by the liver and is found only in trace amounts under normal conditions. The CRP levels increase from trace amounts to maximum values within 48 hours of surgery and then return to trace amounts in approximately 2 to 3 weeks.[45,46]

The ESR and CRP levels must be interpreted carefully before a revision surgery. The physician must determine whether any other factors, such as rheumatoid arthritis, recent surgery, neoplasia, collagen vascular disease, infection, or an inflammatory condition, are present. If no such conditions are prsent, an ESR of more than 30 or 35 mm/h and a CRP level of more than 10 mg/L should be considered abnormal and warrant additional investigation to rule out infection.[42]

Radionuclide Imaging

Scintigraphy can assist in the diagnosis of infection following joint replacement; however, scintigraphy is limited by the cost of scans, the time required, and, most importantly, its inability to yield consistently acceptable levels of sensitivity and specificity. Often, scans are no more accurate than other, less expensive serologic investigations.

Technetium Tc 99m (^{99m}Tc) bone scans are sensitive but not specific. Infection is only one of the many causes of accelerated bone turnover; other causes include loosening, trauma, and tumor. In addition, persistent increased uptake of ^{99m}Tc adjacent to asymptomatic total knee arthroplasties, particularly around the tibial component, is expected for up to 1 year.[40] ^{99m}Tc scintigraphy has a sensitivity of 95% in detecting total knee arthroplasty infection; its specificity is only 20%.[47]

Gallium Ga 67 citrate is a radioisotope that accumulates in areas of inflammation. Upon intravenous injection, gallium binds to serum transferrin and is carried into the extracellular space, including sites of infection. Gallium scan sensitivity is high, and a negative scan can reliably rule out infection; however, because gallium may show increased uptake at uninfected sites of bone remodeling, the positive predictive value is 70% to 75%.[47]

Indium In 111(^{111}In)–labeled WBCs are useful for the diagnosis of increased vascularity and WBC uptake, and ^{111}In–labeled WBC scintigraphy has been used to study periprosthetic infection. An early study demonstrated an accuracy of 84%,[48] and a more recent report on 38 total knee replacements also reported a diagnostic accuracy of 84%.[49]

Other radiolabeled markers, such as radiolabeled immunoglobulin G, have been investigated, and although preliminary results are encouraging,[50] their routine use cannot be advocated until further studies are available. Radionuclide scans can be beneficial in situations in which results from serologic studies may be falsely elevated, and aspirate cultures are unreliable because of the administration of antibiotics.

Aspiration

Aspiration of the knee is the "standard of care for determining whether there is deep joint infection."[39] Laboratory studies of the aspirate can also identify the bacterial species and antibiotic sensitivity. A synovial fluid WBC count of greater than 25,000/mm^3 or a differential with more than 75% polymorphonuclear leukocytes (PMNLs) suggests infection.[51] Also, elevated protein and low glucose are consistent with infections.

False-negative aspirations are not uncommon, and a single negative aspiration does not rule out infection.[40] The most common reason for a false-negative result is the administration of antibiotics before aspiration. If there is any suspicion of infection and the first aspirate is negative, we routinely repeat weekly aspirations for 3 to 4 weeks.

Management of Established Infection

Several options in the management of septic knee arthroplasty are available, including chronic antibiotic suppression, irrigation and débridement with prosthesis retention, arthrodesis, amputation, and débridement with reimplantation. A number of factors must be considered before the treatment option is selected. These factors include the time elapsed from the index procedure, host factors affecting treatment of the infection, soft-tissue condition, implant status in terms of fixation, the type of organism and its sensitivity to antibiotics, and, most importantly, the patient's expectations and functional requirements. The goal of treatment is eradication of the infection with alleviation of symptoms and a functional lower extremity.

Planning for any proposed treatment option will require an accurate history that includes documentation of the index surgery if performed at a different institution, prior cultures and sensitivity, prior radiographs for comparison, and treatment received. High-risk hosts with altered immunity resulting from immunosuppressive medication, systemic illnesses such as diabetes, rheumatoid arthritis, or malnourishment should be identified and conditions optimized. Remote sources of bacteremia should be identified and treated.

Physical examination should include assessment and documentation of neurovascular status, joint motion, and stability. Because it significantly affects the treatment choice, careful assessment of the extensor mechanism is mandatory. The soft tissue around the knee should be evaluated and the incision planned in patients with multiple incisions. The potential need for soft-tissue coverage prior to reconstruction should also be recognized.

Antibiotic Suppression

To sterilize an infected arthroplasty with antibiotics alone is difficult, typically impossible. Long-term suppression with antibiotics alone is rarely indicated. In rare circumstances when a patient's medical condition precludes surgery and removal of well-fixed components and the organism has a low degree of virulence and is susceptible to an oral antibiotic, chronic oral suppression may be justified. Although this treatment method is rarely indicated, it is commonly attempted and only prolongs the presence of infection and complicates subsequent treatment attempts.[52]

Débridement With Prosthetic Retention

Débridement with prosthetic retention involves removal of all intra-articular infected material and retention of the prosthesis. Suggested treatment criteria include short duration of infection (less than 2 to 3 weeks), susceptible gram-positive organisms, absence of prolonged drainage of the sinus tract, and no prosthetic loosening.[53] Results of a multicenter study indicated success with open débridement in less than 20% of 154 knees.[54] However, infections caused by gram-negative organisms or *S aureus*, those occurring in older patients, and those with a longer duration of symptoms appear to be associated with an increased failure rate when such cases are treated with débridement only.

Several authors have suggested using an implantable antibiotic pump to deliver antibiotics locally in combination with surgical débridement and retention of the prosthesis.[55,56] This technique can provide high concentrations of local antibiotics for prolonged periods of time with minimal side effects, as compared to intravenous antibiotics. In one reported series,[56] the duration of antibiotic treatment averaged 18 weeks with reported success in 10 (78%) of 13 knees. We have no personal experience with this technique, although it can be a useful adjunct in the management of selected patients.

Arthrodesis

Removal of components and surgical arthrodesis is rarely performed as a first line of management; however, it is a potentially beneficial means of managing infected arthroplasties with a low risk of reinfection and reliable pain relief and knee stability. Absence of knee motion and its effect on activities of daily living counterbalance some of its advantages.[52]

Generally, we consider an arthrodesis after a failed reimplantation in patients with high functional demand, single-joint disease, or extension mechanism disruption with a poor soft-tissue envelope. Special situations, such as an immunocompromised host, an organism requiring highly toxic antibiotic therapy, and even socioeconomic factors, may dictate the selection of the one procedure that has the best chance for success.

Many factors affect the success of knee fusion. Prior knee implant, extent of bone loss, control of infection, and the surgical technique can affect the outcome of surgery. Time of union ranges from 2.5 months for failed resurfacing implants to 22 months for hinged implants.[57,58] Arthrodesis with biplanar external fixator accomplished union in 66% of patients; uniplanar fixation achieved union in only 33%.[59] Intramedullary nailing appears to be more reliable, with an overall success rate in the literature of 83% of 107 patients who were treated specifically for an infected total knee arthroplasty.[54,60-68]

Complications of arthrodesis include nonunion, reinfection, and ipsilateral limb fracture. Causes of nonunion include bone deficiency, persistent infection, poor bone opposition, malalignment, and inadequate immobilization.[57,64]

Surgical Tips Arthrodesis is the option of choice when satisfactory revision is not expected because of severe bony or ligamentous deficiency. Sometimes, patient factors also may dictate the use of this arthrodesis. Meticulous surgery, adequate débridement and preparation of bone ends, and rigid fixation are key to success.

The scar from the prior surgery should be used whenever possible. Dissection of soft tissue should be limited to preserve bone vascularity, as much bone as possible should be preserved, and a healthy surrounding soft-tissue envelope should be achieved. Most knees require one thorough débridement; however, additional débridement may be necessary for knees with extensive tissue necrosis.[52]

Adequate opposition of vascular bone is probably the most significant factor influencing solid fusion, and every effort should be made to maximize the contact area between the distal femur and proximal tibia. A resurfacing implant may require only a few millimeters of bone resection, whereas hinged components with stems may induce additional bone loss. Bone deficiency should be augmented with cancellous bone grafts placed "peripherally" around the arthrodesis site to allow revascularization from the surrounding tissues.

Because some bone loss and shortening is expected, the optimum position for fusion in most patients will be near full extension. Limb shortening in most patients studied averages 3.0 cm (range, 1 to 6 cm).[63,68] In the absence of bone loss, the optimum position of fusion is 10° to 15° of flexion to allow for foot clearance.

Amputation

Amputation is reserved as a final option in the presence of life-threatening systemic sepsis. The incidence of amputation following failed total knee surgery should decrease with earlier attempts at arthrodesis, when there is adequate bone stock and a viable soft-tissue envelope, rather than with repeated attempts at revision in the presence of infection and decreased use of stemmed hinged implants.[69,70]

Sometimes, amputation may also be warranted for a nonfunctional extremity or nonambulatory patient with severe contractures.

Reimplantation

The most commonly used protocol for the treatment of infected total knee arthroplasty is the two-stage exchange arthroplasty, which involves removal of the prosthesis and cement, with subsequent arthroplasty at a later date and an intervening period of antibiotic administration. One-stage reimplantations have also been reported in the literature.[21,71,72] However, most series contain small numbers of participants, and success has not been corroborated by other groups.[73]

We have no personal experience with one-stage revision and believe, like many authors,[7,23,51,74-82] that two-stage exchange arthroplasty is still the treatment of choice for infected total knee replacements. However, if one-stage revision is chosen for a sensitive gram-positive infection, certain aspects of the protocol of Freeman and associates[71] make sense. These aspects include performing separate surgical preparation and draping for the débridement and reimplantation portions of the procedure, using separate instruments for reimplantation, using antibiotic-loaded cement for fixation, and continued administration of antibiotics for 3 months following the procedure.

Two-stage reimplantation usually implies revision arthroplasty that occurs more than 4 to 6 weeks following prosthetic removal.

Stage 1 Reimplantation This stage involves adequate exposure, component and cement removal, cement spacer/articulation, and closure.

Exposure Adequate exposure is crucial for revision knee surgery. Intra-articular access can be limited by a tight or compromised extensor mechanism, and lateral release or a rectus snip may be required to facilitate exposure and relieve tension on the tibial tubercle. Other more aggressive options include V-Y turndown quadricepsplasty,[51,82-85] tibial tubercle osteotomy,[86-89] or a medial distal femoral peel.[90,91] We usually augment our exposure with a rectus snip and/or tibial tubercle osteotomy.

The previous knee arthroplasty incision is typically used, although other preexisting incisions, which may raise suspicion about skin bridges, future healing, etc, must be considered. Subcutaneous dissection should be minimized, and lateral undermining should always proceed beneath the superficial fascia. Interestingly, wound healing problems associated with the first-stage prosthesis removal or second-stage reimplantation have clearly not been a problem, in our experience, even in the presence of draining sinuses, which we hypothesize is due to the generally increased vascularity of the overall inflammatory state.

A standard medial arthrotomy and distal periosteal incision 1 cm medial to the tibial tubercle is made, preserving the periosteum in continuity with the patellar tendon. Initial lateral patellar release, synovectomy, and excision of thickened subcapsular reactive tissue may help in patellar eversion and with the general exposure. In most patients, these measures, along with subperiosteal dissection around the proximal tibia beneath the superficial medial collateral ligament, allow adequate exposure for débridement and removal of components and cement.

The rectus snip[83,85,87] is a modification of the quadriceps turndown and can provide some measure of increased exposure. The rectus snip maintains both a vastus medialis bridge and a vastus lateralis bridge.[92] The "snip" is the proximal lateral oblique extension across the quadriceps tendon of the standard midline capsular incision. A tibial tubercle osteotomy as described by Whiteside[88] is extremely useful in stiff knees and situations in which more extensile exposure is required. In general, an oscillating saw is used to cut the proximal medial cortex; the bone block is usually 8 to 10 cm long and 2 to 3 cm wide.

We prefer to drill multiple small holes in the lateral cortex prior to completing the osteotomy. This technical point may seem obvious; however, all practitioners of this method do not necessarily use it. Its important function is to define the lateral "cracking" line, which is otherwise difficult to define because most surgeons leave the lateral musculature and fascia intact. This practice provides vascularity and added strength of reattachment.

After making the medial and distal saw cuts for the tubercle osteotomy, curved small and then medium-sized osteotomes are used to approximately or precisely reach the line of preperforation just described. A final technical point is the preservation of a proximal shelf of bone, if possible. The presence of the bone shelf blocks proximal migration of the tubercle fragment so long as the fragment is held down against the substrate bone. In this way, the screws or wires used for reattachment of the tubercle are not solely responsible for blocking the sheer forces created with tension on the quadriceps tendon.[93]

Component and Cement Removal Prosthetic components in the septic knee may be grossly loose or well-fixed. Most recent knee designs include modular tibial inserts, removal of which further facilitates exposure. If the prosthesis to be removed has an all-polyethylene tibial component, the plateau portion may be removed first by using an oscillating saw, cutting the stem off through the cement implant interface.[94] The femoral component should be addressed next. If the component is not loose, thin osteotomes or thin high-speed burrs can be used to loosen it. A Gigli saw can also be used to loosen the anterior cortex and flange.[95] Posterior and condylar interfaces should also be loosened using curved osteotomes or a special intercondylar osteotome before any significant extraction force is applied. Applying any significant extraction force before the prosthesis is loose may result in femoral fracture.[94] Once the fixation has been loosened, the femoral prosthesis can be removed with a simple mallet and impactor or more elaborate femoral extractor devices that attach directly to some prosthetic designs.

The tibial component is removed next. The accessible interface between the implant and bone should be loosened with an oscillating saw and thin osteotomes; the extractor can then be tapped to exert proximal extraction force. If excessive force seems necessary for extraction, further loosening should be performed with thin osteotomes or high-speed burrs before more extraction force is applied. All polyethylene patellar components should be removed by transecting the pegs with the oscillating saw at the cement implant interface. The remaining pegs are removed next with a high-speed burr. It may be safest to leave patellar component removal for last. If the residual patellar bone is quite thin, early inadvertent fracture can be prevented by leaving the entire construct intact.

After the prostheses are out, attention is next directed to cement removal. Fragmentation is facilitated by using special osteotomes, and cement fragments can be retrieved with grasping forceps. Cement removal around stems may require special cement-extraction instruments and techniques similar to cement removal in revision hip surgery. Meticulous removal of all cement particles is mandatory. We follow a rigid protocol of confirming and documenting total removal of cement by obtaining intraoperative radiographs. Multiple radiographs may be necessary on occasion to locate and remove intramedullary cement. In addition, cement is much easier to see after fresh, pulse irrigation. Cement may be retained in the bone holes created by drills or spikes to affix cutting blocks during the primary arthroplasty, and particular attention must be paid to this possibility. During a primary procedure, intrusion of methylmethacrylate under pressure frequently leads to deep tracking of cement into these residual spaces.

Cement Spacer The use of an antibiotic-loaded cement spacer was first reported by Cohen and associates[96] and later by Wilde and Ruth[78] who reported a 90% success rate with the use of these spacers. Booth and Lotke[20] also reported more than 90% success with a two-stage exchange with an interim period using an antibiotic-loaded cement spacer. The authors concluded that reimplantation was facilitated by these spacers.

The hamburger bun-type cement spacer is probably the most common form of spacer. In addition to maintaining joint space and extremity length, these spacers can reduce scarring and decrease the difficulty of reimplantation.[73] However, some caution is necessary. Mixing cement in a bowl permits air to become trapped and leads to expansion of the spacer at terminal curing. Despite careful measuring and planning, the spacer may not fit. Additionally, with irregular bone surfaces, this type of spacer may not be as mechanically secure as it should be and may subsequently become dislocated.

In situations in which a fixed space alone is desired, we currently pack rather doughy cement into the tibiofemoral defect while exerting strong longitudinal traction at the ankle and foot. Such a spacer molded to the existing bone ends is quite stable, diffuses forces more effectively across the residual surfaces, and is not associated with significant bone loss or spacer subluxation.

The most commonly used antibiotics in cement spacers are tobramycin, vancomycin, and gentamicin. Different antibiotics have different elution characteristics. For example, tobramycin elutes in a much higher concentration early on and decays at a much faster rate than vancomycin.[97] The local antibiotic level can also be much higher than parenteral therapy[98,99] and vastly exceed the minimal inhibitory concentration of most susceptible pathogens.

We use 2.4 g of tobramycin and 2 g of vancomycin per one 40-g package of bone cement. As previously described, the spacer is inserted in the doughy stage and pushed into place to mold well to the residual surfaces. We prefer to release the tourniquet as the cement is warming and irrigate the cavity in an attempt to prevent any thermal damage to the surrounding soft tissues. We also prefer to use a thin layer of cement between the femur and patella to prevent scarring of the extensor mechanism.

Although the use of handmade spacers is most prevalent, use of articulating spacers has also been reported. The technique has been described by Scott and associates[100] and by Kane and associates.[101] The knee is thoroughly débrided, components are removed, and after sterilization, the same components are reimplanted with high-concentration, antibiotic-laden cement. The cement is applied with "poor technique" for planned suboptimal fixation. Although achieving component stability is desired, future removal should not be made difficult, especially regarding further bone loss with removal. We have no experience with this technique and are generally concerned about placing foreign material that is not specifically antibiotic eluting.

Another approach involves the use of the commercially prepared prosthesis of antibiotic-loaded acrylic cement (PROSTALAC; Smith & Nephew Richards, Memphis, TN), first reported in 1992 by Duncan and associates.[102] Both of these approaches can be expected to preserve joint movement and elute high levels of antibiotics.

Unlike first-generation PROSTALAC components, which were cement-on-cement articulations, current designs contain small stainless steel runners and polyethylene tibial skids[73] to provide lower friction and allow a better gait as compared to cement-on-cement high-friction articulation. Later PROSTALAC designs also include posterior stabilized options with a transverse bar in the femoral runner and a cement post on the tibial component.

The advantages of these articulated systems include providing mobility for the patient and mobility for the tissues between the stages of removal and permanent implantation; however, certain concerns about this approach must be noted. The patient has undergone two-stage surgery specifically for the purpose of removing foreign material and eliminating its presence in the site of infection. Placement of antibiotic-eluting cement into the infected or contaminated space has proven to be quite successful and has basically become the standard of care. Leaving any additional impregnated metal, or other metal and polyethylene in the case of the sterilized reimplanted components, has not yet been proven to be as safe. Also, with any functioning articulation, during this period when the knee is very likely not optimally "balanced" with less than optimal constraint in the residual "prosthetic components," subluxation may occur.

Wound Closure and Reattachment of the Osteotomy Maximal, reasonable hemostasis is achieved after the tourniquet is released, the cement spacer or spacers are placed, and closed wound suction drains are placed. With the capsular closure, we always avoid using permanent, nonabsorbable suture material. When a rectus snip has been used, we closed it with ordinary figure-of-8 heavy (No. 1 or "0") sutures.

We have had uniform success reattaching the tubercle osteotomy fragment with heavy Vicryl (No. 3) sutures. The sutures are placed through the medial and the lateral cortices of the subjacent tibia and tied over the tubercle fragment itself. We do not use articulating spacers but rather fixed, molded spacers. Our patients have experienced no difficulty with failure of this fixation and are spared any potential downside of retained hardware in the presence of infection or significant contamination. The fascia and subcutaneous tissue are also closed with appropriate absorbable material, and meticulous skin closure is essential.

Interval Period Postoperatively, a bulky Jones dressing or, quite frequently, a cylinder or long leg cast is applied. We usually do not apply the cast at surgery; however, in those instances in which it is applied, routine bivalving in the recovery room to prevent swelling-compression problems should be strongly considered. Drains are removed at 2 days. Infectious disease consultation is obtained in the postoperative period if it was not obtained previously. Consultation is advantageous from the standpoint of selecting the optimally appropriate antibiotic or antibiotics as well as follow-up of antibiotic administration to ensure adequate drug levels. If definitive cultures have been obtained ahead of time, broad-spectrum or organism-specific antibiotics are continued during the immediate postoperative period. Culture and sensitivity results from material obtained at surgery are used by the infectious disease consultant from that point on.

Antibiotic treatment is planned for a minimum of 6 weeks and rarely as long as 10 weeks. The time period may be adjusted depending on the presumed virulence of the organism versus its susceptibility, the clinical appearance of the wound, and the laboratory results, primarily, the CRP level and, secondarily, the ESR.

In patients in whom tibial tubercle osteotomies were performed, extensor mechanism precautions are initiated, which include avoiding active extension from a position of flexion and avoiding passive flexion. For patients who are out of a cast or brace with articulated spacers, active flexion and straight leg raising are permitted. Straight leg raising should be performed with the knee in a brace.

We do not allow full weight bearing with the spacers and recommend toe touch to "medium," or 25%, partial weight bearing as comfortable. At 2 weeks, skin staples are removed, and radiographs to confirm the position of the spacers are obtained. One to 2 weeks after antibiotic administration ends, the patient is seen again in the office for knee aspiration and culture. In the rare instance of a positive culture, the patient is scheduled for another débridement and placement of antibiotic loaded cement spacers.

Stage 2 (Reimplantation) Prosthetic Reconstruction During the second stage (reimplantation), the previous incision is used. We do not use any prophylactic antibiotics until further cultures and specimens are obtained. Any earlier tibial tubercle osteotomy should be well healed, but the site is usually identified, and a second tibial tubercle osteotomy is performed at the same site. If the previous site is not clear, this issue is ignored, and the tubercle is osteotomized as in a virgin situation. Aspirate or joint fluid is obtained and sent for aerobic, anaerobic, and fungal cultures plus an urgent Gram staining. The cement spacer is splintered/fragmented using a sharp osteotome and is relatively easy to remove.

A thorough re-débridement is performed. In many patients, bone defects need to be addressed. Other issues to be addressed include constraint, depending on bone loss, ligament integrity, and the symmetry of the soft-tissue capsular ligamentous sleeve. The details of these choices are beyond the scope of this particular article and are covered elsewhere.

Intraoperative Investigations

A number of intraoperative investigations can be performed to aid in the diagnosis of infection at the initial revision surgery and occasionally to determine the likelihood of persistent infection at the time of the second-stage intervention.

Intraoperative Frozen Sections Intraoperative frozen sections have become a valuable tool for the diagnosis of infection. Mirra and associates[103] reported that more than five PMNLs per high-power field is evidence of probable infection, and a lack of PMNLs is evidence of no infection. Lonner and associates[104] recommended considering 10 PMNLs per high-power field to improve specificity

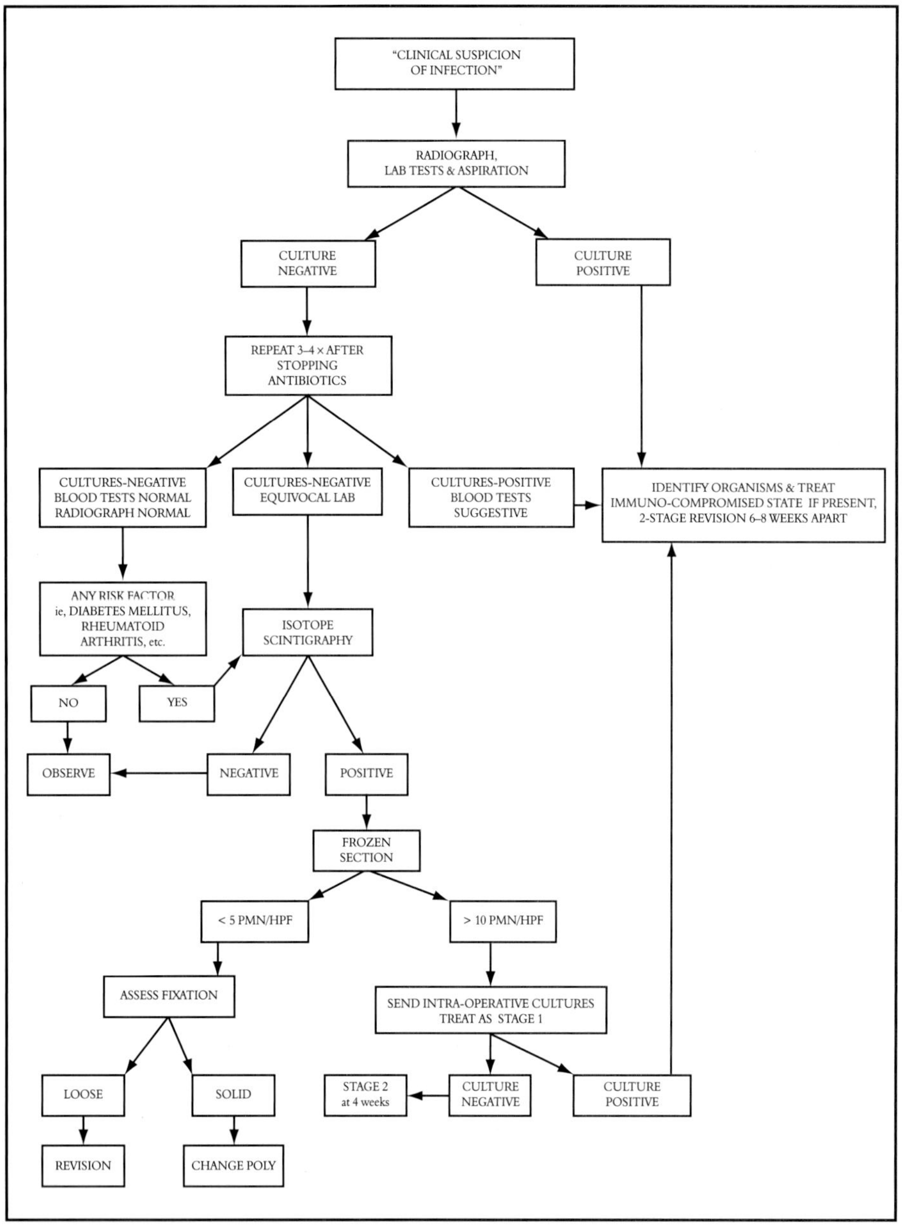

Fig. 1 Protocol for diagnosis and treatment of infection after total knee arthroplasty. PMN/HPF = polymorphonuclear leukocytes per high-power field.

without reducing sensitivity. In their analysis of 175 revision arthroplasties, specificity improved from 96% to 99% when 10 instead of 5 PMNLs per high-power field was used as an index of infection. The sensitivity remained the same at 84%. For the most accurate interpretation, the tissues should be obtained from areas that appear most inflamed and examined by experienced pathologists.

Gram Stain Intraoperative Gram staining produces a high percentage of false-negative results,[105,106] while a positive Gram stain is strong evidence of infection. A negative Gram stain cannot be considered as evidence for absence of infection and thus, in equivocal situations, is not a useful investigation.

Surgeon's "Gut Feeling" In some knees, there may be diffuse synovitis, turbid joint fluid, formation of slime, and areas of granulation tissues, which are all suspicious features of continued infection with equivocal frozen sections and other laboratory tests. We believe that in such circumstances it is safer to obtain additional intraoperative cultures, repeat a débridement, and operate again at a later date after final results of the culture.

Intraoperative Cultures Intraoperative cultures are often used as a standard for the diagnosis of infection and are useful during stage 1 in patients with suspected infection if the organism is not identified before surgery. During stage 2, results of intraoperative cultures do not contribute any decisions made in terms of reimplantation, but they may play a role in postoperative decision-making in terms of antibiotic therapy.

Positive culture results do not represent a standard for the absolute diagnosis of intra-articular infection. Fitzgerald and associates[107] noted positive cultures in 25% of 437 hips that had not been operated on previously, and other authors have reported similar high rates of false-positive results in total hip replacement.[108,109] In more recent reports, the incidence of false-positive results is between 6% and 13% in patients who have undergone revision hip surgery.[110-112]

Molecular Analysis Molecular technology may be used to diagnose the presence of bacterial DNA and RNA. Polymerase chain reaction techniques enable large volumes of identical copies to be obtained from small quantities of starting material. Bacterial DNA and RNA can then be identified.[113,114]

Molecular technology techniques are currently being developed; however, their ability to identify small quantities of bacteria may make them susceptible to false-positive results from contaminants. As with frozen-section and aspiration testing, false-negative results are also possible from sampling error.

Surgical Tips

In the revision setting, every effort should be made to achieve a functionally stable knee. An array of trials should be used to achieve flexion-extension balance. Tissues may stretch during surgery. In most revisions, we use a posterior stabilized implant and try to balance the collaterals. Preserving bone is essential. Oversized components may be needed to restore stability; however, overstuffing should be avoided in patients with stiff knees. Although it is ideal to restore the joint line after revision, occasionally joint line elevation cannot be avoided in revision total knee arthroplasty and satisfactory knee extension takes precedence over joint line restoration.

Summary

Routine blood work that includes ESR, CRP, and glucose levels, and plain radiographs and knee aspirations are obtained from our patients who have clinical suspicion of infection. If the culture result is positive and blood tests suggest infection, the surgical plan is a two-stage revision with an interval period of intravenous antibiotic administration. Risk factors are identified, and the patient's condition optimized. An infectious disease consultant is also involved in the treatment care plan and advises the patient about the best antibiotic, management of proper antibiotic levels, and home care.

If culture results are negative, cultures are repeated every week for 3 to 4 weeks after the patient stops taking antibiotics. If the cultures yield positive results, a two-stage revision protocol is initiated. In patients who have 3 to 4 negative culture results, normal blood tests and radiographs, and no history of any immunocompromised state, such as diabetes or rheumatoid arthritis, diagnoses such as polyethylene wear or synovitis can be considered. If patients have any involved risk factor or blood tests, equivocal or suggestive, isotope scintigraphy is requested. We examine tissue in patients with positive scans and equivocal blood test results with clinical suspicion of infection. We prefer an open arthrotomy, which allows us to take multiple specimens for frozen section, assess fixation of the implant, and look for any other signs of infection. If the frozen section reveals more than 10 PMNLs per high-power field, we proceed to stage 1 revision after obtaining intraoperative cultures. If an organism grows in the cultures, stage 2 protocol is initiated. If no cultures are obtained at 7 to 10 days of incubation, we may consider earlier stage 2 revision at 4 to 6 weeks (Fig. 1).

In patients in whom the frozen section reveals less than 5 PMNLs per high-power field, component fixation should be assessed, and if they are loose, revision of the knee should be initiated. As with a septic revision, use of antibiotic-impregnated cement can be considered for fixation. If the components are well fixed, a polyethylene tibial tray is exchanged. In either circumstance, intraoperative cultures should be obtained, and if they yield positive results, antibiotics should be continued for 6 to 12 weeks.

Conclusion

Although preventing infection is an integral part of performing total joint arthroplasty, early and appropriate management of infection can yield acceptable results. No test is 100% sensitive and specific. A high index of suspicion is the key for early diagnosis.

Blood tests, radiographs, and scans can be helpful in making a diagnosis; however, aspiration is the standard of care for determining deep joint infection. Intraoperative investigations and histologic examination can be valuable in equivocal situations, and molecular analysis may improve the diagnostic ability in the future.

In most infections, a two-stage protocol with an intervening period of antibiotic administration is the most favored option in the literature for healing established infection with predictable success.

References

1. Fitzgerald RH Jr: Infections of hip prostheses and artificial joints. *Infect Dis Clin North Am* 1989;3:329-338.
2. Grogan TJ, Dorey F, Rollins J, Amstutz HC: Deep sepsis following total knee arthroplasty: Ten-year experience at the University of California at Los Angeles Medical Center. *J Bone Joint Surg Am* 1986;68:226-234.
3. Hanssen AD, Rand JA: Evaluation and treatment of infection at the site of a total hip or knee arthroplasty. *J Bone Joint Surg Am* 1998;80:910-922.
4. Poss R, Thornhill TS, Ewald FC, Thomas WH, Batte NJ, Sledge CB: Factors influencing the incidence and outcome of infection following total joint arthroplasty. *Clin Orthop* 1984;182:117-126.
5. Rand JA, Fitzgerald RH Jr: Diagnosis and management of the infected total knee arthroplasty. *Orthop Clin North Am* 1989;20:201-210.
6. Salvati EA, Robinson RP, Zeno SM, Koslin BL, Brause BD, Wilson PD Jr: Infection rates after 3,175 total hip and total knee replacements performed with and without a horizontal unidirectional filtered air-flow system. *J Bone Joint Surg Am* 1982;64:525-535.
7. Wilson MG, Kelley K, Thornhill TS: Infection as a complication of total knee-replacement arthroplasty: Risk factors and treatment in sixty-seven cases. *J Bone Joint Surg Am* 1990;72:878-883.
8. Doyon F, Evrard J, Mazas F: An assessment of published trials on antibiotic prophylaxis in orthopaedic surgery. *French J Orthop Surg* 1989;3:49-53.
9. Heath AF: Antimicrobial prophylaxis for arthroplasty and total joint replacement: Discussion and review of published clinical trials. *Pharmacotherapy* 1991;11:157-163.
10. Hill C, Flamant R, Mazas F, Evrard J: Prophylactic cefazolin versus placebo in total hip replacement: Report of a multicentre double-blind randomised trial. *Lancet* 1981;1:795-796.
11. Norden CW: Antibiotic prophylaxis in orthopedic surgery. *Rev Infect Dis* 1991;13(suppl 10):S842-S846.
12. Lidwell OM, Lowbury EJ, Whyte W, Blowers R, Stanley SJ, Lowe D: Effect of ultraclean air in operating rooms on deep sepsis in the joint after total hip or knee replacement: A randomised study. *Br Med J (Clin Res Ed)* 1982;285:10-14.
13. Ritter MA: Intraoperative controls of bacterial contamination during total knee replacement. *Clin Orthop North Am* 1989;20:49-53.
14. Fitzgerald RH Jr, Kelly PJ: Total joint arthroplasty: Biologic causes of failure. *Mayo Clin Proc* 1979;54:590-596.

15. Nelson CL: Prevention of sepsis. *Clin Orthop* 1987;222:66-72.

16. Gristina AG, Kolkin J: Total joint replacement and sepsis. *J Bone Joint Surg Am* 1983;65: 128-134.

17. Petty W, Bryan RS, Coventry MB, Peterson LFA: Infection after total knee arthroplasty. *Orthop Clin North Am* 1975;6:1005-1014.

18. Jerry GJ Jr, Rand JA, Ilstrup D: Old sepsis prior to total knee arthroplasty. *Clin Orthop* 1988;236:135-140.

19. Bengtson S, Knutson K, Lidgren L: Treatment of infected knee arthroplasty. *Clin Orthop* 1989;245:173-178.

20. Booth RE Jr, Lotke PA: The results of spacer block technique in revision of infected total knee arthroplasty. *Clin Orthop* 1989;248:57-60.

21. Borden LS, Gearen PF: Infected total knee arthroplasty: A protocol for management. *J Arthroplasty* 1987;2:27-36.

22. Bliss DG, McBride GG: Infected total knee arthroplasties. *Clin Orthop* 1985;199:207-214.

23. Jacobs MA, Hungerford DS, Krackow KA, Lennox DW: Revision of septic total knee arthroplasty. *Clin Orthop* 1989;238:159-166.

24. Lettin AW, Neil MJ, Citron ND, August A: Excision arthroplasty for infected constrained total knee replacements. *J Bone Joint Surg Br* 1990;72:220-224.

25. Morrey BF, Westholm F, Schoifet S, Rand JA, Bryan RS: Long-term results of various treatment options for infected total knee arthroplasty. *Clin Orthop* 1989;248:120-128.

26. Rand JA, Bryan RS, Chao EY: Failed total knee arthroplasty treated by arthrodesis of the knee using the Ace-Fischer apparatus. *J Bone Joint Surg Am* 1987;69:39-45.

27. Salvati EA, Small RD, Brause BD, et. al: Infections Associated with orthopedic devices, in Sugarman B, Young EJ (eds): *Infections Associated with Prosthetic Devices.* Boca Raton, FL, CRC Press, 1984, pp 181-218.

28. Windsor RE, Insall JN, Urs WK, Miller DV, Brause BD: Two-stage reimplantation for the salvage of total knee arthroplasty complicated by infection: Further follow-up and refinement of indications. *J Bone Joint Surg Am* 1990;72:272-278.

29. Lambertus M, Thordarson D, Goetz MB: Fungal prosthetic arthritis: Presentation of two cases and review of the literature. *Rev Infect Dis* 1988;10:1038-1043.

30. Brause BD: Infected orthopaedic prosthesis, in Bison AL, Waldvogel FA (eds): *Infections Associated with Indwelling Medical Devices.* Washington DC, American Society for Microbiology, 1989, pp 111-128.

31. Inman RD, Gallegos KV, Brause BD, Redecha PB, Christian CL: Clinical and microbial features of prosthetic joint infection. *Am J Med* 1984;77:47-53.

32. Coventry MB: Treatment of infections occurring in total hip surgery. *Orthop Clin North Am* 1975;6:991-1003.

33. Fitzgerald RH Jr, Nolan DR, Ilstrup DM, Van Scoy RE, Washington JA II, Coventry MB: Deep wound sepsis following total hip arthroplasty. *J Bone Joint Surg Am* 1977;59:847-855.

34. Larsson S, Thelander U, Friberg S: C-reactive protein (CRP) levels after elective orthopedic surgery. *Clin Orthop* 1992;275:237-242.

35. Insall JN: Infection in total knee arthroplasty. *Instr Course Lect* 1982;31:42-48.

36. Hughes PW, Salvati EA, Wilson PD Jr, Blumenfeld EL: Treatment of subacute sepsis of the hip by antibiotics and joint replacement: Criteria for diagnosis with evaluation of twenty-six cases. *Clin Orthop* 1979;141:143-157.

37. Irvine R, Johnson BL Jr, Amstutz HC: The relationship of genitourinary tract procedures and deep sepsis after total hip replacements. *Surg Gynecol Obstet* 1974;139:701-706.

38. Stinchfield FE, Bigliani LU, Neu HC, Goss TP, Foster CR: Late hematogenous infection of total joint replacement. *J Bone Joint Surg Am* 1980;62:1345-1350.

39. Windsor RE, Insall JN: Management of the infected total knee arthroplasty, in Insall JN, Windsor RE, Scott WN, Kelly MA, Aglietti P (eds): *Surgery of the Knee,* ed 2. New York, NY, Churchill Livingstone, 1993, vol 2, pp 959-974.

40. Lotke PA: Treatment of the infected total knee replacement, in Lotke PA (ed): *Postoperative Infections in Orthopaedic Surgery: Prevention and Treatment.* Park Ridge, IL, American Academy of Orthopaedic Surgeons, 1992, pp 47-71.

41. Fitzgerald RH Jr: Total hip arthroplasty sepsis: Prevention and diagnosis. *Orthop Clin North Am* 1992;23:259-264.

42. Spangehl MJ, Younger AS, Masri BA, Duncan CP: Diagnosis of infection following total hip arthroplasty. *J Bone Joint Surg Am* 1997;79: 1578-1588.

43. Levitsky KA, Hozack WJ, Balderston RA, et al: Evaluation of the painful prosthetic joint: Relative value of bone scan, sedimentation rate, and joint aspiration. *J Arthroplasty* 1991;6: 237-244.

44. Rand JA, Brown ML: The value of indium III leukocyte scanning in the evaluation of painful or infected total knee arthroplasties. *Clin Orthop* 1990;259:179-182.

45. Aalto K, Osterman K, Peltola H, Rasanen J: Changes in erythrocyte sedimentation rate and C-reactive protein after total hip arthroplasty. *Clin Orthop* 1984;184:118-120.

46. O'Neill DA, Harris WH: Failed total hip replacement: Assessment by plain radiographs, arthrograms, and aspiration of the hip joint. *J Bone Joint Surg Am* 1984;66:540-546.

47. Davis LP: Nuclear imaging in the diagnosis of the infected total joint arthroplasty. *Semin Arthroplasty.* 1994;5:147-152.

48. Merkel KD, Brown ML, Dewanjee MK, Fitzgerald RH Jr: Comparison of indium-labeled leukocyte imaging with sequential technetium-gallium scanning in the diagnosis of low-grade musculoskeletal sepsis: A prospective study. *J Bone Joint Surg Am* 1985;67: 465-476.

49. Rand JA: Sepsis following total knee arthroplasty, in Rand JA (ed): *Total Knee Arthroplasty.* New York, NY, Raven Press, 1993, pp 349-375.

50. Lind P, Langsteger W, Koltringer P, Dimai HP, Passl R, Eber O: Immunoscintigraphy of inflammatory processes with a technetium–99m labeled monoclonal antigranulocyte antibody (Mab BW 250/183). *J Nucl Med* 1990;31:417-423.

51. Insall JN: Infection of total knee arthroplasty. *Instr Course Lect* 1986;35:319-324.

52. Hanssen AD: Management of the infected total knee arthroplasty, in Engh GA, Rorabeck CH (eds): *Revision Total Knee Arthroplasty.* Baltimore, MD, Williams & Wilkins, 1997, pp 371-393.

53. Burger RR, Basch T, Hopson CN: Implant salvage in infected total knee arthroplasty. *Clin Orthop* 1991;273:105-112.

54. Bengtson S, Knutson K: The infected knee arthroplasty: A 6-year follow-up of 357 cases. *Acta Orthop Scand,* 1991;62:301-311.

55. Davenport K, Traina S, Perry C: Treatment of acutely infected arthroplasty with local antibiotics. *J Arthroplasty* 1991;6:179-183.

56. Perry CR, Hulsey RE, Mann FA, Miller GA, Pearson RL: Treatment of acutely infected arthroplasties with incision, drainage, and local antibiotics delivered via an implantable pump. *Clin Orthop* 1992;281:216-223.

57. Brodersen MP, Fitzgerald RH Jr, Peterson LF, Coventry MB, Bryan RS: Arthrodesis of the knee following failed total knee arthroplasty. *J Bone Joint Surg Am* 1979;61:181-185.

58. Drinker H, Potter TA, Turner RH, Thomas WH: Arthrodesis for failed knee arthroplasty. *Orthop Trans* 1979;3:302.

59. Knutson K, Hovelius L, Lindstrand A, Lidgren L: Arthrodesis after failed knee arthroplasty: A nationwide multicenter investigation of 91 cases. *Clin Orthop* 1984;191:202-211.

60. Behr JT, Chmell SJ, Schwartz CM: Knee arthrodesis for failed total knee arthroplasty. *Arch Surg* 1985;120:350-354.

61. Bengtson S, Knutson K, Lidgren L: Revision of infected knee arthroplasty. *Acta Orthop Scand* 1986;57:489-494.

62. Donley BG, Matthews LS, Kaufer H: Arthrodesis of the knee with an intramedullary nail. *J Bone Joint Surg Am* 1991;73:907-913.

63. Ellingsen DE, Rand JA: Intramedullary arthrodesis of the knee after failed total knee arthroplasty. *J Bone Joint Surg Am* 1994;76:870-877.

64. Figgie HE III, Brody GA, Inglis AE, Sculco TP, Goldberg VM, Figgie MP: Knee arthrodesis following total knee arthroplasty in rheumatoid arthritis. *Clin Orthop* 1987;224:237-243.

65. Goldberg JA, Drummond RP, Bruce WJ, Viglione W, Lennon WP: Huckstep nail arthrodesis of the knee: A salvage for infected total knee replacement. *Aust NZ J Surg* 1989;59:147-150.

66. Stiehl JB, Hanel DP: Knee arthrodesis using combined intramedullary rod and plate fixation. *Clin Orthop* 1993;294:238-241.

67. Wilde AH, Stearns KL: Intramedullary fixation for arthrodesis of the knee after infected total knee arthroplasty. *Clin Orthop* 1989;248:87-92.

68. Bono JV, Windsor RE, Laskin RS, et al: Abstract: Intramedullary arthrodesis following failed septic total knee arthroplasty. *Proceedings of the American Academy of Orthopaedic Surgeons 62nd Annual Meeting.* Orlando, FL. Rosemont, IL, American Academy of Orthopaedic Surgeons, 1995, p 143.

69. Hanssen AD, Trousdale RT, Osmon DR: Patient outcome with reinfection following reimplantation for the infected total knee arthroplasty. *Clin Orthop* 1995;321:55-67.

70. Isiklar ZU, Landon GC, Tullos HS: Amputation after failed total knee arthroplasty. *Clin Orthop* 1994;299:173-178.

71. Freeman MA, Sudlow RA, Casewell MW, Radcliff SS: The management of infected total knee replacements. *J Bone Joint Surg Br* 1985;67:764-768.

72. Goksan SB, Freeman MA: One-stage reimplantation for infected total knee arthroplasty. *J Bone Joint Surg Br* 1992;74:78-82.

73. Masri BA, Duncan CP, Beauchamp CP: The modified two-stage exchange arthroplasty in the treatment of the infected total knee replacement: The PROSTALAC system and other articulated spacers, in Engh GA, CH Rorabeck (eds): *Revision Total Knee Arthroplasty.* Baltimore, MD, Williams & Wilkins, 1997, pp 394-424.

74. Insall JN, Thompson FM, Brause BD: Two-stage reimplantation for the salvage of infected total knee arthroplasty. *J Bone Joint Surg Am* 1983;65:1087-1098.

75. Walker RH, Schurman DJ: Management of infected total knee arthroplasties. *Clin Orthop* 1984;186:81-89.

76. Teeny SM, Dorr L, Murata G, Conaty P: Treatment of infected total knee arthroplasty: Irrigation and debridement versus two-stage reimplantation. *J Arthroplasty* 1990;5:35-39.

77. Hofmann AA, Kane KR, Tkach TK, Plaster RL, Camargo MP: Treatment of the infected total knee arthroplasty using an articulating spacer. *Clin Orthop* 1995;321:45-54.

78. Wilde AH, Ruth JT: Two-stage reimplantation in infected total knee arthroplasty. *Clin Orthop* 1988;236:23-35.

79. Whiteside LA: Treatment of infected total knee arthroplasty. *Clin Orthop* 1994;299:169-172.

80. Hirakawa K, Stulberg BN, Wilde AH, Bauer TW, Secic M: Results of 2-stage reimplantation for infected total knee arthroplasty. *J Arthroplasty* 1998;13:22-28.

81. Goldman RT, Scuderi GR, Insall JN: 2-stage reimplantation for infected total knee replacement. *Clin Orthop* 1996;331:118-124.

82. Trousdale RT, Hanssen AD, Rand JA, Cahalan TD: V-Y quadricepsplasty in total knee arthroplasty. *Clin Orthop* 1993;286 48-55.

83. Insall JN: Total knee arthroplasty, in Insall JN (ed): *Surgery of the Knee.* New York, NY, Churchill Livingstone, 1984.

84. Scott RD, Siliski JM: The use of a modified V-Y quadricepsplasty during total knee replacement to gain exposure and improve flexion in the ankylosed knee. *Orthopedics* 1985;8:45-48.

85. Vince KG: Revision knee arthroplasty, in Chapman MW, Madison M (eds): *Operative Orthopaedics*, ed 2. Philadelphia, PA, JB Lippincott, 1993, vol 3, pp 1981-2010.

86. Dolin MG: Osteotomy of the tibial tubercle in total knee replacement: A technical note. *J Bone Joint Surg Am* 1983;65:704-706.

87. Vince KG: Revision knee arthroplasty technique. *Instr Course Lect* 1993;42:325-339.

88. Whiteside LA: Exposure in difficult total knee arthroplasty using tibial tubercle osteotomy. *Clin Orthop* 1995;321:32-35.

89. Wolff AM, Hungerford DS, Krackow KA, Jacobs MA: Osteotomy of the tibial tubercle during total knee replacement: A report of twenty-six cases. *J Bone Joint Surg Am* 1989;71:848-852.

90. Windsor R, Insall J: Exposure in revision total knee arthroplasty: The femoral peel. *Tech Orthop* 1988;3:1-4.

91. Windsor RE, Scuderi GR, Insall JN: Revision of well-fixed, cemented, porous total knee arthroplasty: Report of six cases. *J Arthroplasty* 1988;3(suppl):S87-S94.

92. Peters PC: Surgical exposure for revision total knee arthroplasty, in Engh GA, Rorabeck CH (eds): *Revision Total Knee Arthroplasty.* Baltimore, MD, Williams & Wilkins, 1997, pp 195-204.

93. Krackow KA (ed): *The Technique of Total Knee Arthroplasty.* St Louis, MO, CV Mosby, 1990.

94. Moreland JR: Techniques for removal of prosthesis and cement in knee revision surgery, in Engh GA, Rorabeck CH (eds): *Revision Total Knee Arthroplasty.* Baltimore, MD, Williams & Wilkins, 1997, pp 224-234.

95. Firestone TP, Krackow KA: Removal of Femoral Components during revision knee arthroplasty. *J Bone Joint Surg Br* 1991;73:514.

96. Cohen JC, Hozack WJ, Cuckler JM, Booth RE Jr: Two-stage reimplantation of septic total knee arthroplasty: Report of three cases using an antibiotic-PMMA spacer block. *J Arthroplasty* 1988;3:369-377.

97. Masri BA, Duncan CP, Beauchamp CP, Paris NJ, Arntrop J: Tobramycin and vancomycin elution from bone cement: An in-vitro and in-vivo study. *Orthop Trans* 1994-1995;18:130.

98. Brien WW, Salvati EA, Klein R, Brause B, Stern S: Antibiotic impregnated bone cement in total hip arthroplasty: An in vivo comparison of the elution properties of tobramycin and vancomycin. *Clin Orthop* 1993;296:242-248.

99. Salvati EA, Callaghan JJ, Brause BD, Klein RF, Small RD: Reimplantation in infection: Elution of gentamicin from cement and beads. *Clin Orthop* 1986;207:83-93.

100. Scott IR, Stockley I, Getty CJ: Exchange arthroplasty for infected knee replacements: A new two-stage method. *J Bone Joint Surg Br* 1993;75:28-31.

101. Kane K, Plaster R, Tkach T, Camargo M, Hoffman A: Treatment of infected total knee replacement arthroplasty using an articulated spacer. *Clin Orthop* 1995;321:44-54.

102. Duncan CP, Beauchamp CP, Masri B, McGraw RW, Paris N, Breault M: Abstract: The antibiotic loaded joint replacement system: A novel approach to the management of the infected knee replacement. *J Bone Joint Surg Br* 1992;74(suppl 3):296.

103. Mirra JM, Amstutz HC, Matos M, Gold R: The pathology of the joint tissues and its clinical relevance in prosthesis failure. *Clin Orthop* 1976;117:221-240.

104. Lonner JH, Desai P, Dicesare PE, Steiner G, Zuckerman JD: The reliability of analysis of intraoperative frozen sections for identifying active infection during revision hip or knee arthroplasty. *J Bone Joint Surg Am* 1996;78 1553-1558.

105. Chimento GF, Finger S, Barrack RL: Gram stain detection of infection during revision arthroplasty. *J Bone Joint Surg Br* 1996;78: 838-839.

106. Athanasou NA, Pandey R, de Steiger R, Crook D, Smith PM: Diagnosis of infection by frozen section during revision arthroplasty. *J Bone Joint Surg Am* 1995;77:28-33.

107. Fitzgerald RH Jr, Peterson LF, Washington JA II, Van Scoy RE, Coventry MB: Bacterial colonization of wounds and sepsis in total hip arthroplasty. *J Bone Joint Surg Am* 1973;55: 1242-1250.

108. Murray WR: Results in patients with total hip replacement arthroplasty. *Clin Orthop* 1973;95:80-90.

109. Tietjen R, Stinchfield FE, Michelsen CB: The significance of intracapsular cultures in total hip operations. *Surg Gynecol Obstet* 1977;144:699-702.

110. Barrack RL, Harris WH: The value of aspiration of the hip joint before revision total hip arthroplasty. *J Bone Joint Surg Am* 1993; 75:66-76.

111. Fehring TK, Cohen B: Aspiration as a guide to sepsis in revision total hip arthroplasty. *J Arthroplasty* 1996;11:543-547.

112. Spangehl MJ, Duncan CP, O'Connell JX, Masri BA: Abstract: Prospective analysis of preoperative and intraoperative studies for the diagnosis of infection in 210 consecutive revision total hip arthroplasties. *Proceedings of the American Academy of Orthopaedic Surgeons 64th Annual Meeting.* San Francisco, CA, Rosemont, IL, American Academy of Orthopaedic Surgeons, 1997, p 197.

113. Rapley R, Theophilus BD, Bevan IS, Walker MR: Fundamentals of the polymerase chain reaction: A future in clinical diagnostics? *Med Lab Sci* 1992;49:119-128.

114. Clarke AM, Mapstone NP, Quirke P: Molecular biology made easy: The polymerase chain reaction. *Histochem J* 1992;24:913-926.

38

Periprosthetic Fractures Following Total Knee Arthroplasty

Douglas A. Dennis, MD

Periprosthetic fractures following total knee arthroplasty (TKA) are a potentially devastating complication to both the patient and the surgeon. Complication rates of treatment reported in the literature range widely, from 25% to 75%, even in the hands of both skilled and experienced surgeons.[1-4] A meta-analysis of 195 fractures in 12 published reports of ipsilateral supracondylar femoral fractures demonstrated complication rates of 30% with both nonsurgical and surgical treatment methods.[5] Various treatment modalities have been used to manage these challenging fractures. The purpose of this review is to analyze the prevalence, pathogenesis, mechanism of injury, risk factors, classification, and treatment of these fractures.

Supracondylar Femoral Fractures

Prevalence and Pathogenesis

The reported prevalence of supracondylar femoral fracture following TKA has ranged from 0.3% to 2.5%.[3,6-12] Various factors have been implicated in the pathogenesis of this fracture. These include stress shielding from the anterior flange of the femoral component, inadequate osseous remodeling due to postoperative hypovascularity, a relative difference in elastic modulus between the implant-covered distal part of the femur and the femoral cortex, endosteal ischemia from metal or bone cement,[13,14] and osteolysis of the distal part of the femur secondary to polyethylene wear debris.[15]

The majority of these fractures result from a combination of axial and torsional loads.[10,16,17] Most occur following minimal falls, whereas others are secondary to motor vehicle accidents, seizures, or closed manipulation of a stiff knee after TKA.[18]

Risk Factors

A review of the literature shows that patients with conditions associated with osteopenia are clearly at greater risk of sustaining a supracondylar femoral fracture after TKA.[4-7,10,19-24] Patients with rheumatoid arthritis,[2,4,7,18,19,24] those being treated with corticosteroids,[4,5,18,22,24] those of advanced age,[4,10] and females[8,10,14,18,19,25,26] are all at greater risk for supracondylar femoral fracture. Additional risk factors include neurologic disorders,[10] a previous revision TKA,[4,27] and rotationally constrained implants that create increased torsional load transfer to bone.[10,28]

Both clinical and biomechanical data strongly suggest that anterior notching of the distal femoral cortex increases the risk of this fracture, with 40% to 52% of reported fractures associated with an anterior notch.[2,3,6,7,10,19,29,30] A theoretical mathematical analysis revealed that a 3-mm notch results in a 30% reduction in torsional bone strength.[10] A biomechanical analysis of cadaveric femora revealed a mean reduction of 18% in bending strength and a mean decrease of 42% in torsional strength when a full-thickness anterior notch was present.[31] Ritter and associates,[13] however, in a review of 670 TKAs, observed that 138 femora (20.6%) exhibited a notch of at least 3 mm, yet a supracondylar fracture developed in only two. This finding emphasizes the potential for osseous remodeling to decrease the risk of fracture should an anterior notch occur.

To reduce the risk of supracondylar femoral fracture after TKA, use of walking aids by patients with substantial osteopenia and an unsteady gait pattern is recommended. Additionally, should an anterior notch of the distal part of the femur be created intraoperatively, the surgeon should consider implantation of a femoral component with an attached diaphysis-engaging stem to support the weakened distal part of the femur.

Classification

Numerous systems of classification of supracondylar femoral fractures after TKA have been developed.[5,32-34] The system found most valuable in my management of these fractures was created by Rorabeck and associates.[34] Their classification takes into account both the status of the prosthesis (that is, whether it is intact or failing) and the displacement of the fracture. Type I is assigned if the fracture is undisplaced and the prosthesis is intact; type II, if the fracture is displaced and the prosthesis is intact; and type III, if the fracture is displaced or undisplaced and the prosthesis is loose or failing (that is, if there is substantial instability or polyethylene wear).[33]

Treatment Options

The goals of treatment are to obtain and maintain good postfracture alignment

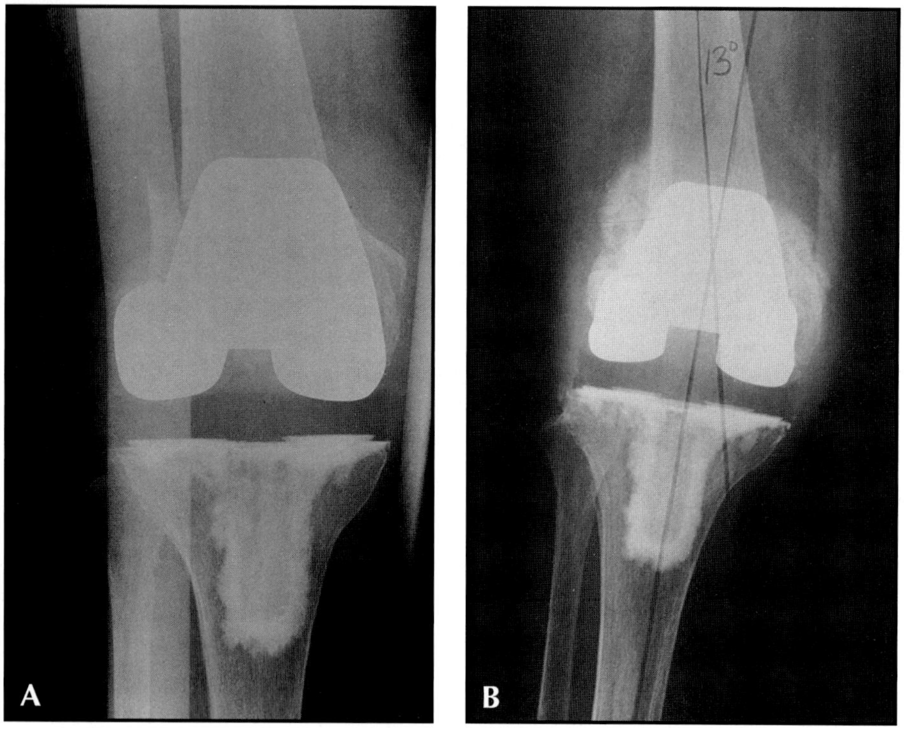

Fig. 1 A, Anteroposterior (AP) radiograph of a minimally displaced supracondylar femoral fracture in a patient with advanced osteopenia. **B,** AP radiograph made 6 months following nonsurgical treatment with cast immobilization. Despite corrective reduction and cast-wedging, a valgus malunion resulted.

and stability to allow early range of motion.[10,33,35,36] There are a myriad of both nonsurgical and surgical treatment options for the management of supracondylar femoral fractures. The nonsurgical options include skeletal traction; application of a cast, pins and plaster; and cast-bracing. The surgical options include use of a condylar plate; intramedullary fixation, either flexible or rigid (interlocking); revision TKA; external fixation; cerclage wiring with strut allograft fixation; and arthrodesis. Determination of clearly superior treatment methods is difficult because of the limited number of cases that have been evaluated in most reports.[5,10] While fracture configuration plays a role in the choice of treatment method, fracture displacement, the degree of osteopenia, and the status of the prosthetic components (intact or failing) are my primary determinants of the fracture management method. Treatment results are closely associated with postfracture alignment and stability.[8,14,22,27,35-37] Fracture displacement, intercondylar extension, and comminution are negative prognostic factors.[27] High malunion rates are common in association with varus, flexion, and internal rotation deformities typically seen as a result of forces exerted by the adductor and gastrocnemius muscle groups.[3] Varus femoral malunion is associated with a risk of premature failure of the TKA. Figgie and associates[3] reported on 12 fractures that had united with varus malposition of the femoral component. Progressive radiolucent lines at the bone-cement interface were seen in 9 of the 12 cases.

The superiority of nonsurgical[4,8,18,19,27,38-40] treatment over surgical[2,3,10,12,14,26,35-37,41-49] treatment has been controversial. Chen and associates[5] performed a review of 12 published studies (195 fractures) and found no significant difference ($P < 0.90$) between the prevalence of successful results in the nonsurgical treatment group (67%) and that in the surgical group (69%). More recently, surgical treatment has been shown to provide better results when used for displaced fractures,[45,48,50] probably because of improvements in surgical techniques and the available fracture fixation devices. Moran and associates[48] reviewed a series of 24 cases of displaced supracondylar fracture after TKA. Nine fractures were managed nonsurgically and all nine had an unsatisfactory result, primarily because of malunion. Fifteen were managed with open reduction and internal fixation, and 10 had a satisfactory result. The choice of treatment method should be based on the patient's health, fracture displacement, comminution, severity of osteopenia, and status of the prosthetic components (loose, unstable, or malaligned).

Nonsurgical Treatment

The advantages of nonsurgical treatment are that it is noninvasive and the infection rate is negligible. Union is likely, particularly in nondisplaced fractures. Nonsurgical treatment is uniformly recommended as the initial management of nondisplaced fractures.[3-5,23,27,29,39] Chen and associates[5] found an 83% rate of successful results in a literature review. Disadvantages include a relatively high malunion rate and functional loss, particularly in patients with a displaced fracture through osteopenic bone, in whom maintenance of reduction is difficult.[3,4,10,14,18,19,23,27,35-37] Additionally, nonsurgical treatment often requires prolonged immobilization, which leads to loss of motion and reduced walking capacity.[2,4,5,10,18] Culp and associates[10] reported the results in 30 patients treated nonsurgically. Fifteen patients (50%) had increased pain or decreased ambulatory status following nonsurgical care, whereas this was true of only 13% of patients treated with surgery. Use of a cast resulted in an average loss of motion of 26°. Harlow and Hofmann[23] performed a literature review that included 142 supracondylar fractures following TKA that were treated nonsurgically. Twenty-nine percent of these fractures eventually required surgical care.

In summary, nonsurgical treatment is best reserved for nondisplaced fractures that do not demonstrate intercondylar extension. Nonsurgical treatment of displaced fractures can be attempted with initial closed reduction and subsequent immobilization, although accurate maintenance of reduction of fractures through osteopenic bone is often difficult, with malunion commonly occurring (Fig. 1). An initial 4- to 6-week period of cast immobilization, followed by a gentle range of motion in a hinged knee brace under the guidance of a physiotherapist is favorable. If nonsurgical management is selected, biweekly radiographs for the first 6 weeks are recommended to closely monitor fracture alignment.

Surgical Treatment

Open reduction and fixation with a condylar plate provides the potential advantages of anatomic reconstruction, rigid fixation, and an early range of motion. Maintenance of reduction can be a problem, particularly when a patient has a comminuted fracture through osteopenic bone, and malunion is commonly observed (Fig. 2). Figgie and associates[3] reviewed 10 cases in which this treatment method was used. Fracture alignment was lost in eight. In cases of substantial osteopenia of the distal femoral fragment, adjunctive use of polymethylmethacrylate to enhance fixation may improve results, as evidenced by the 100% success rate without malunion in the six cases reported on by Zehntner and Ganz.[50] Additionally, Healy and associates[45] advocated packing strips of corticocancellous allograft into the distal femoral fracture to augment condylar plate fixation (Fig. 3).

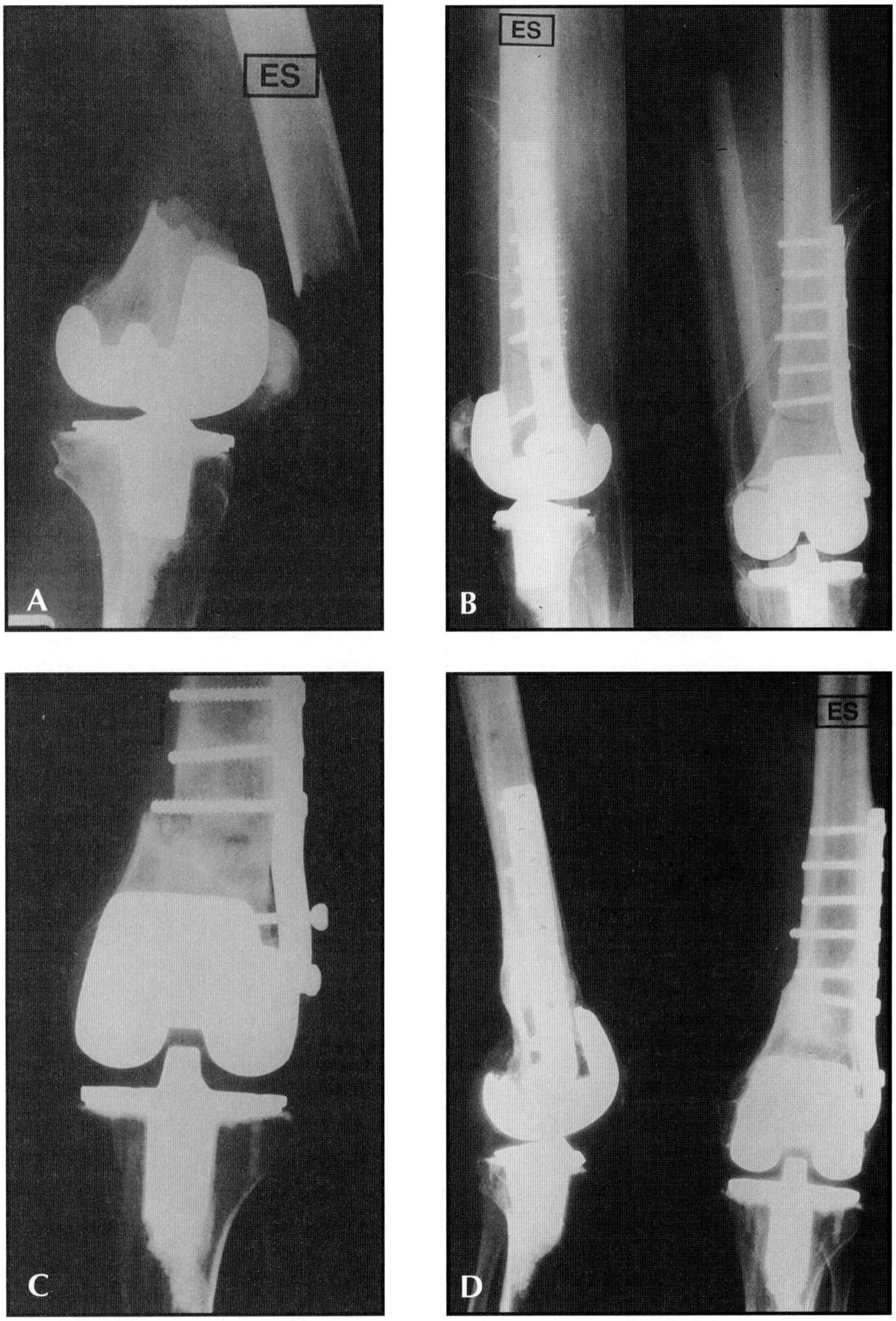

Fig. 2 A, Radiograph of a displaced supracondylar femoral fracture. **B,** Early lateral and AP radiographs made after open reduction and internal fixation (with a condylar plate), demonstrating satisfactory fracture reduction. **C,** Three-month postoperative AP radiograph demonstrating delayed union with slight loss of fracture reduction. **D,** Six-month postoperative lateral and AP radiographs demonstrating fracture malunion with mild varus malalignment.

Others[51] have used intramedullary fibular graft placed in a retrograde fashion to enhance plate-and-screw fixation. Use of a condylar plate is best reserved for less comminuted, displaced fractures with satisfactory bone stock.

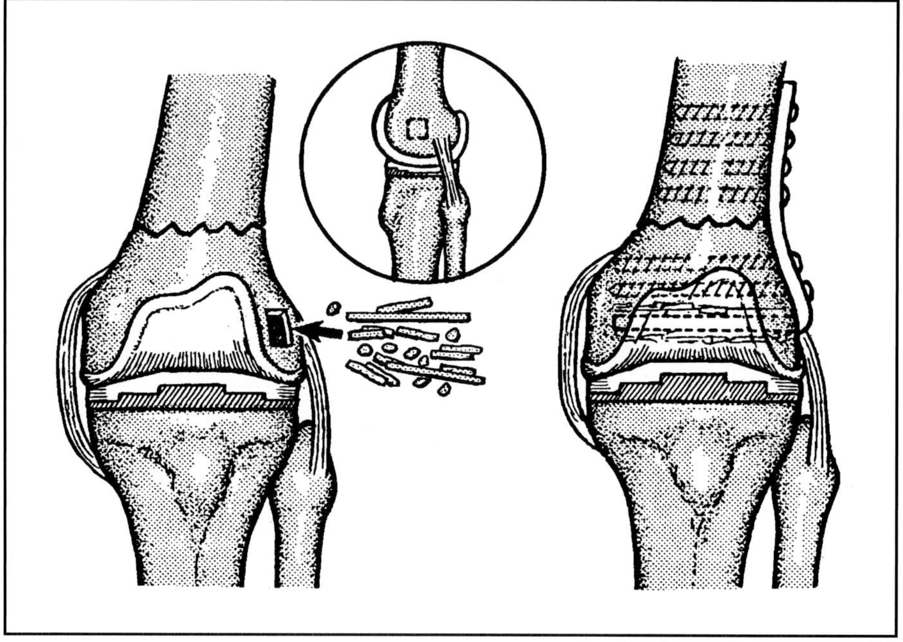

Fig. 3 Polymethylmethacrylate or bone graft may be used to augment the distal fixation of the implant used for treatment of the fracture in patients who have extreme osteopenia of the distal condylar fragment. (Reproduced with permission from Healy WL, Siliski JM, Incavo SJ: Operative treatment of distal femoral fractures proximal to total knee replacements. *J Bone Joint Surg Am* 1993;75:32.)

Use of flexible intramedullary rods is an efficient and less invasive treatment option.[26,52] Shortening and rotational malunion occasionally occur as a result of the reduced axial and rotational stability provided by this technique. Ritter and associates[52] reviewed 22 cases treated with Rush rods and found that union had been obtained in 100% without a major complication. This technique should be considered for mildly displaced fractures in patients in poor health. It is a minimally invasive procedure with limited morbidity.

Rigid supracondylar interlocking rod fixation offers the advantage of being minimally invasive while providing good axial, angular, and rotational stability in most cases.[1,21,24,41,42] It can be performed with use of a minimal patellar-tendon-splitting approach with percutaneous placement of interlocking screws in cases with lesser comminution, with maintenance of the fracture hematoma and osseous blood supply (Fig. 4). Contraindications include a long preexisting total hip intramedullary stem, loose total knee components, severe comminution, and an extremely distal fracture. This method of fixation may also be used for supracondylar femoral fractures proximal to a posterior cruciate-substituting total knee prosthesis. With these designs, access to the medullary canal may be blocked by the intercondylar box of the femoral component. Maniar and associates[53] described a technique of opening an aperture in the intercondylar femoral box with use of a diamond-tip metal-cutting burr (Midas Rex, Fort Worth, TX) to allow passage of the interlocking intramedullary rod. Overall, a review of 19 cases from four published reports revealed union in all cases, no malalignment, and minimal complications.[21,24,41,42]

Revision TKA provides the advantage of stable fixation with a diaphysis-engaging intramedullary femoral stem, allowing early range of motion and weight bearing.[3,5,6,12,22,29,37,54] This technique is selected for extremely distal or comminuted fractures when stable fixation is difficult to secure, or for any fracture associated with loose, unstable, or substantially malaligned total knee components. Additionally, revision TKA is frequently required in cases in which nonsurgical or other methods of surgical treatment have failed. This procedure is often technically demanding, even in the hands of a skilled arthroplasty surgeon, and it is best reserved for surgeons who have considerable skill and experience in revision TKA. Use of constrained total knee components, despite their risk of premature failure, is frequently required. Markedly comminuted fractures in osteopenic bone may require distal fracture-fragment excision with replacement with either structural allograft[3,22] or a distal femoral replacement prosthetic component.[6] In the meta-analysis by Chen and associates,[5] 11 supracondylar fractures proximal to total knee prostheses were treated with revision TKA. A satisfactory result was obtained in 10 cases.

Additional treatment modalities such as external fixation,[12,44] cerclage wiring with strut allograft fixation, and arthrodesis have been less frequently utilized, and there is a lack of adequate reports on them in the literature. A suggested treatment algorithm is provided in Figure 5.

Treatment Summary

Obtaining and maintaining fracture alignment is critical for the success of any treatment method. Rigid fixation allows an early range of motion, resulting in a superior functional result. There is a high probability of success with nonsurgical treatment of minimally displaced fractures. Maintenance of reduction of displaced fractures with nonsurgical measures is often difficult, particularly when there is associated osteopenia and comminution. Review of more recent studies demonstrates a trend toward

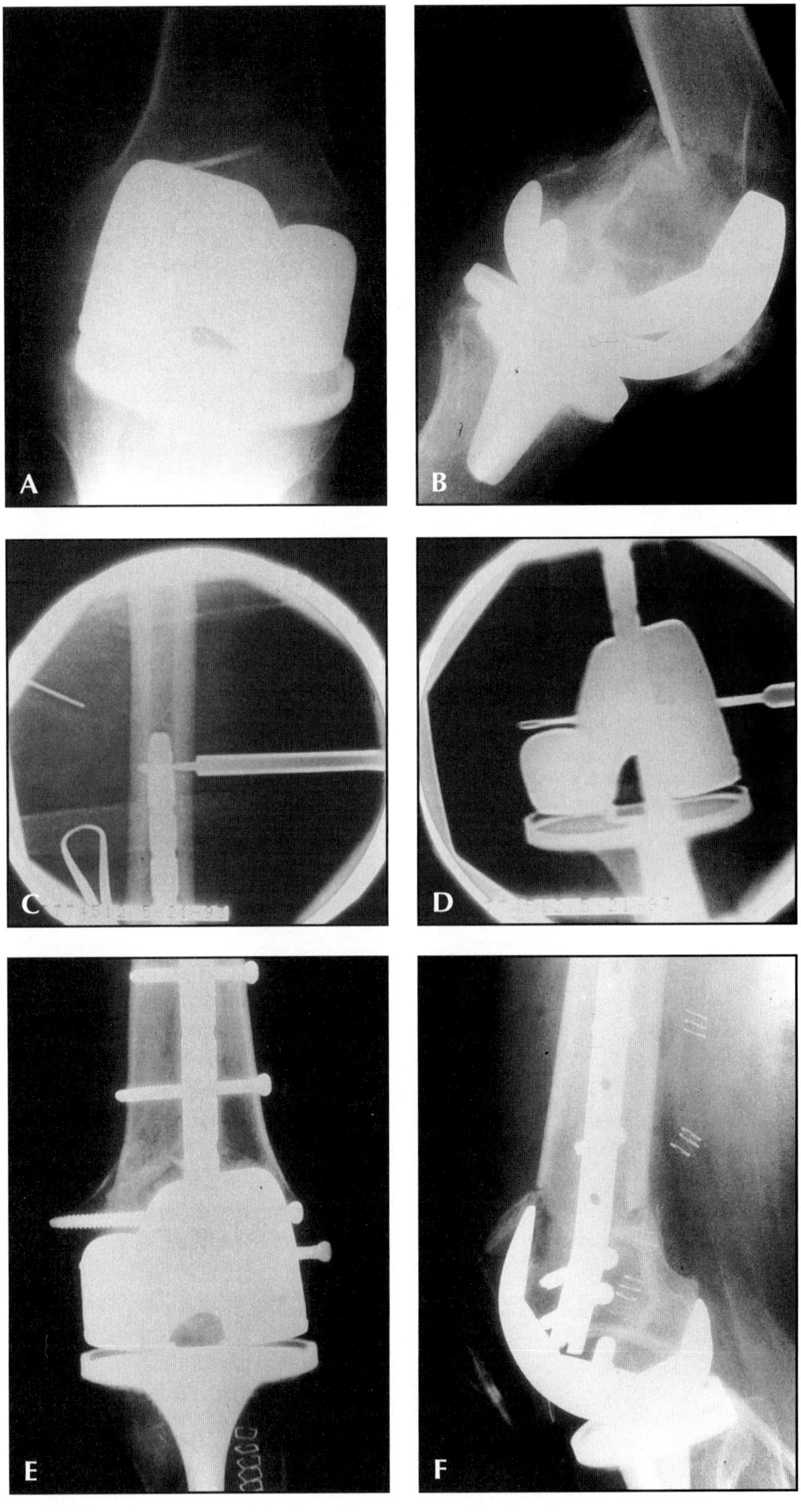

Fig. 4 Preoperative AP (**A**) and lateral (**B**) radiographs of a displaced supracondylar femoral fracture. **C** and **D,** Intraoperative fluoroscopic images showing placement of an interlocking screw into a rigid supracondylar intramedullary nail. Postoperative AP (**E**) and lateral (**F**) radiographs made following treatment with an interlocking supracondylar intramedullary nail inserted with use of a percutaneous technique.

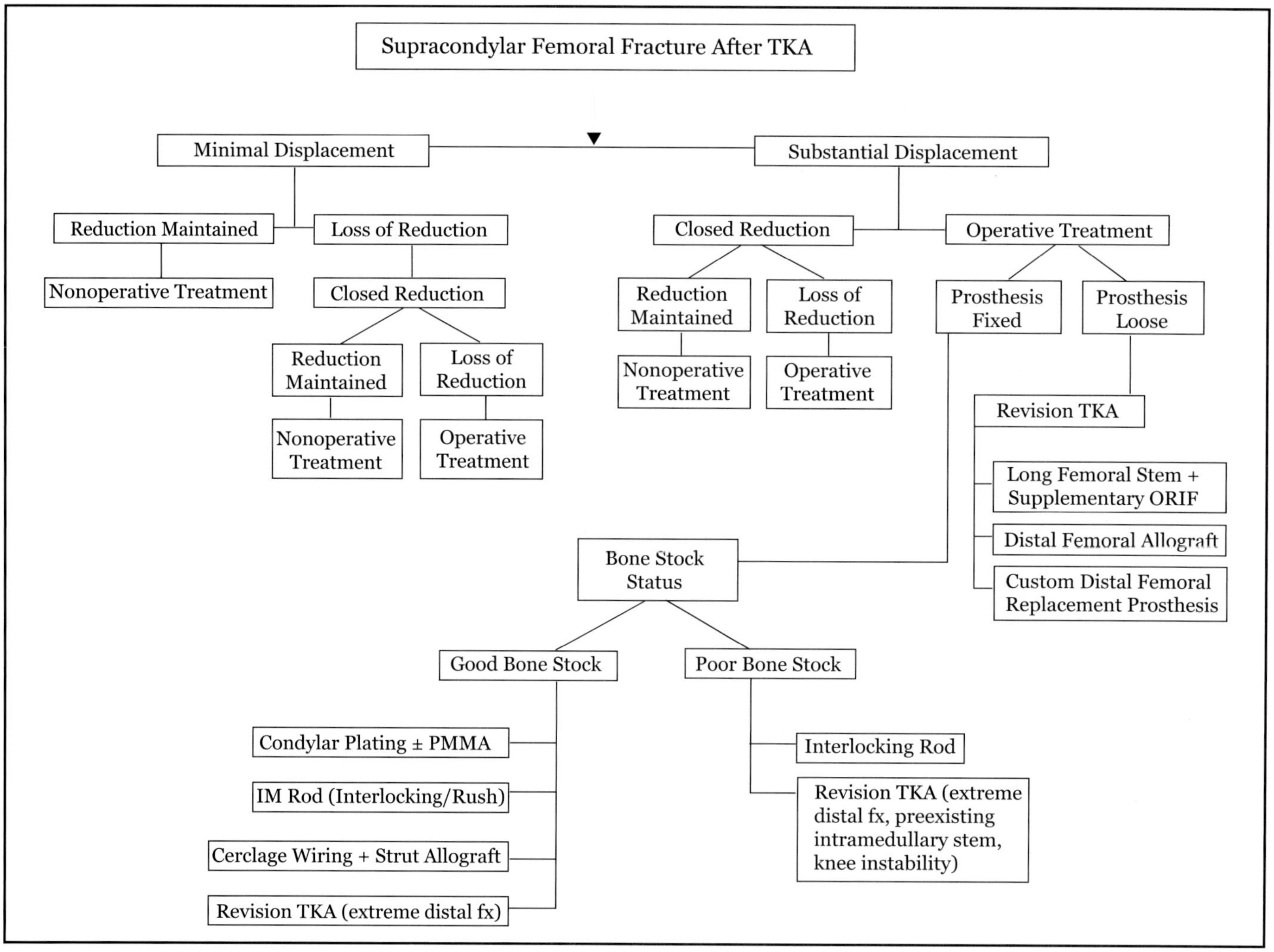

Fig. 5 Schematic of treatment options for supracondylar femoral fracture. TKA = total knee arthroplasty, IM = intramedullary, PMMA = polymethylmethacrylate, fx = fracture, and ORIF = open reduction and internal fixation.

superior results with surgical treatment of displaced fractures.[3,6,22,29,37,48] Use of a condylar plate, which increases the chance of obtaining rigid fixation and allows early range of motion, is best reserved for less comminuted fractures with good bone stock. Revision TKA is recommended for patients with loose, unstable, or substantially malaligned components; severe comminution; an extremely distal fracture; and failure of other treatment methods.

Use of a supracondylar interlocking rod is becoming the treatment of choice for the majority of displaced supracondylar femoral fractures. It provides good axial, angular, and rotational stability. Clinical studies have shown high union rates with minimal complications.[1,21,24,41,42] Contraindications to this treatment method include a long preexisting intramedullary stem from a previous total hip arthroplasty, severe comminution, an extremely distal fracture, and failed TKA components.

Tibial Fractures

Tibial fracture following total knee arthroplasty is an infrequent complication with a reported prevalence of 0.4% to 1.7%.[55-57] These fractures may occur intraoperatively or postoperatively.[57] Intraoperative fractures occur most commonly during component removal, bone retraction, trial reduction, or preparation for insertion of a stemmed tibial component.[58] There are several etiologies for postoperative tibial fractures.[37,56-63] Many occur after traumatic events. Others are associated with malalignment, knee instability, or component loosening. Rand and Coventry[56] observed 15 stress fractures of the tibia after Geomedic and Polycentric TKA (Howmedica, Rutherford, NJ). All cases were associated with axial malalignment and component malposition. Tibial shaft fractures after extended tibial tubercle osteotomy have also been reported.[62,63]

Tibial fractures were classified by Felix and associates[57] on the basis of their anatomic location and the status of the prosthetic fixation (Fig. 6). Type I fractures involve the tibial plateau and the fixation interface of the tibial component. Type II fractures occur adjacent to the stem of the tibial component. Fractures distal to the tibial stem are classified as type III, and those involving the tibial tubercle are classified as type IV. In their review of 102 tibial fractures after TKA, Felix and associates observed 61 type I, 22 type II, 17 type III, and 2 type IV fractures.[57] Eighty-three fractures occurred postoperatively, and 19 occurred during the performance of the TKA. These fractures were observed more commonly in female patients.

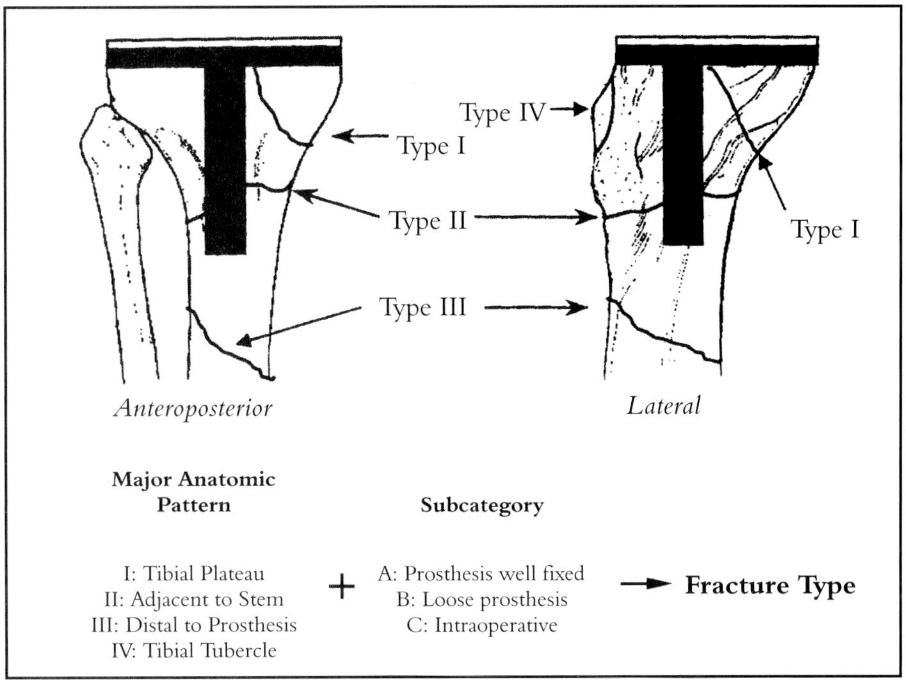

Fig. 6 Mayo classification of periprosthetic tibial fractures. (Reproduced with permission from Stuart MJ, Hanssen AD: Total knee arthroplasty: Periprosthetic tibial fractures. *Orthop Clin North Am* 1999;30:280.)

Treatment of periprosthetic tibial fractures is based on the fracture location and the status of the prosthetic components.[23,55-58] Fractures associated with prosthetic loosening or substantial instability are best managed with component revision, typically with a diaphysis-engaging tibial intramedullary stem, and supplementary open reduction and internal fixation of additional fracture fragments, if possible. In cases with a high degree of comminution, excision of fracture fragments and replacement with prosthetic augmentation or structural bone graft may be required. Cases lacking instability, malalignment, or loosening are treated with use of standard principles of tibial fracture care.

Patellar Fractures

Patellar fracture is an infrequent complication of TKA,[64-66] although a prevalence as high as 21% has been reported.[67] Various etiologies for patellar fracture have been proposed.[65-78] The finding of an increased prevalence of patellar fracture associated with patellofemoral malalignment is supported by biomechanical studies that demonstrated that contact forces substantially increase with patellofemoral malalignment.[79] Both the eccentricity and the magnitude of patellofemoral loads increase with patellar subluxation,[80] increasing the risk of patellar fracture.

Excessive, asymmetrical, or inadequate patellar resection increases the probability of patellar fracture. Excessive patellar resection, especially if the subchondral bone is removed, predisposes to patellar fracture.[81] Reuben and associates[82] demonstrated that a patellar osteotomy resulting in a patellar osseous thickness of less than 15 mm substantially increases anterior patellar strain. Conversely, minimal patellar resection, resulting in a greater thickness of the patella-patellar component composite, increases patellofemoral joint-reaction forces and tension within the quadriceps tendon. Use of a femoral component with an excessive anteroposterior diameter or implantation of a femoral component in a flexed position increases patellofemoral joint-reaction forces and theoretically increases the probability of fracture.[71,83] Asymmetrical patellar resection can also result in impaired mechanical strength of the patella, particularly if the lateral facet is overresected. Finally, it has been shown that, when the patella is prepared for component fixation, the creation of a large central peg-hole increases anterior patellar strain more than smaller peripheral peg designs do, thereby increasing the risk of fracture.[84,85]

Surgical disruption of the patellar blood supply, resulting in osteonecrosis, has been associated with patellar fracture.[66,69,72,84,86] Analyses of patellar blood supply have demonstrated both extraosseous and intraosseous vascular systems[87-90] (Fig. 7). The extraosseous system comprises a peripatellar anastomotic ring supplied by six main arteries. The superior portion of the vascular ring passes anterior to the quadriceps tendon, while the inferior portion passes posterior to the patellar tendon through the fat pad. The intraosseous system comprises the midpatellar, polar,

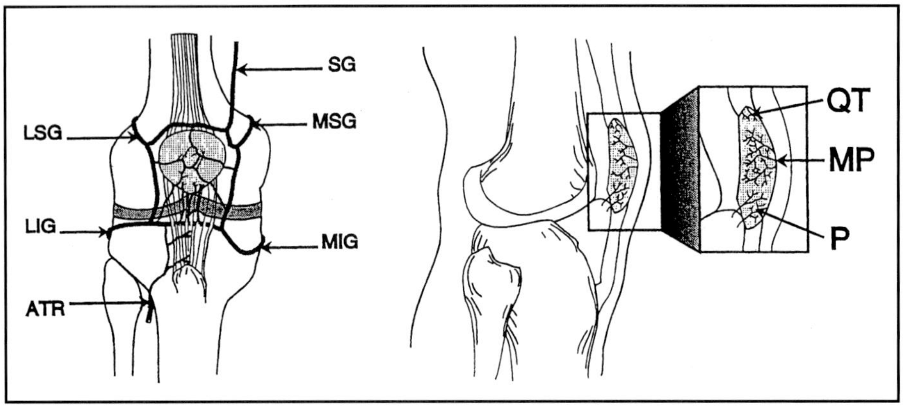

Fig. 7 Diagram demonstrating the extraosseous (left) and intraosseous (right) blood supplies of the patella. LSG = lateral superior genicular artery, LIG = lateral inferior genicular artery, ATR = anterior tibial recurrent artery, SG = supreme genicular artery, MSG = medial superior genicular artery, MIG = medial inferior genicular artery, QT = quadriceps tendon blood supply, MP = midpatellar blood supply, and P = polar blood supply. (Reproduced with permission from Dennis DA: Patellofemoral complications in total knee arthroplasty: A literature review. *Am J Knee Surg* 1992;5:157.)

and quadriceps tendon blood supplies. The midpatellar vessels penetrate anteriorly through the middle third of the patella, branching into both the proximal and the distal pole. The polar vasculature passes through the proximal part of the fat pad, posterior to the patellar tendon, entering the inferior pole of the patella. Scapinelli[89,90] observed minimal vascular penetration into the superior pole and the periphery of the patella, whereas Bjorkstrom and Goldie[87] demonstrated a superior vascular supply via the quadriceps tendon.

Substantial disruption of patellar vascular systems occurs during routine performance of TKA.[65-67,69,70,72,86,88,91-95] The medial superior and inferior genicular arteries are divided during a medial peripatellar arthrotomy. Damage to the lateral inferior genicular artery is common during lateral meniscectomy or fat-pad excision. The lateral superior genicular artery is at risk when a lateral retinacular release is performed. The intraosseous vascular system can be compromised during creation of fixation holes, particularly large central holes. Technetium bone scans following TKA have demonstrated reduced patellar vascularity if a lateral retinacular release had been performed.[94,95] McMahon and associates[93] also found reduced patellar vascularity following lateral retinacular release, but they determined that fat-pad excision has no detrimental effect. Histological evaluations of patellar specimens following patellar fracture have documented the presence of osteonecrosis.[69,91]

Component malposition can affect the prevalence, type, severity, and prognosis of patellar fractures.[65,96] Errors in joint-line position, lower extremity alignment, or patellar coverage by the prosthesis may increase the risk of fracture. Major malalignment has been associated with more complex fracture patterns and a worse prognosis.

Additional risk factors for patellar fracture include increased flexion following TKA, thermal necrosis, and revision TKA. Windsor and associates[97] reported that patients with knee flexion of greater than 95° generate increased patellofemoral compression forces and frequently have higher activity levels. The heat of polymerization of the polymethylmethacrylate (reported to be as high as 80°C to 90°C in TKA) may exceed the coagulation temperature of tissue proteins, causing thermal necrosis of bone.[93,98-101] Grace and Sim[99] reported that the prevalence of patellar fracture following primary TKA (0.12%) was much lower than that after revision TKA (0.61%).

Patellar fractures are best avoided through proper patellar resection (duplication of the original patellar thickness and creation of symmetry of medial and lateral facet thickness), use of a smaller peripheral fixation peg design, assurance of central patellar tracking, and maintenance of the patellar blood supply through fat-pad preservation, avoidance of large central-fixation peg designs, and preservation of the lateral superior genicular artery if a lateral retinacular release is required.

Treatment of patellar fractures is controversial. Some require no treatment as they may go unrecognized by the patient. Additional options include immobilization, open reduction and internal fixation with or without component revision, partial patellectomy with tendon repair, and total patellectomy.[65,66,97,99,102-104] In what I believe is the largest series of patellar fractures presented to date, Ortiguera and Berry (unpublished data, 1999) reported on 78 cases. Fractures were classified according to the status of the patellar component fixation, the integrity of the extensor mechanism, and the quality of the remaining bone stock. Nonsurgical treatment was highly successful for the management of fractures with a stable patellar component and an intact extensor mechanism. Surgical treatment was selected for 31 patients. A complication rate of 39% (12 of 31 patients) was observed, and 16 revision surgeries were required.

Overall, results of surgical treatment of patellar fractures have been suboptimal,[65,66] and nonsurgical treatment is recommended as long as there is no component dislocation or loosening and as long as disruption of the extensor mechanism is not complete. Because of the inferior results reported with surgical treatment, I favor nonsurgical treatment of displaced fractures with substantial associated extensor lag, as long as fixation of the patellar component is maintained. Treatment with immobilization in extension for 4 to 6 weeks frequently results in satisfactory restoration of the function of the extensor mechanism.

References

1. Henry SL, Booth RE Jr: Management of supracondylar fractures above total knee prostheses. *Tech Orthop* 1994;9:243-252.
2. Bogoch E, Hastings D, Gross A, Gschwend N: Supracondylar fractures of the femur adjacent to resurfacing and MacIntosh arthroplasties of the knee in patients with rheumatoid arthritis. *Clin Orthop* 1988;229:213-220.
3. Figgie MP, Goldberg VM, Figgie HE III, Sobel M: The results of treatment of supracondylar fracture above total knee arthroplasty. *J Arthroplasty* 1990;5:267-276.
4. Merkel KD, Johnson EW Jr: Supracondylar fracture of the femur after total knee arthroplasty. *J Bone Joint Surg Am* 1986;68:29-43.
5. Chen F, Mont MA, Bachner RS: Management of ipsilateral supracondylar femur fractures following total knee arthroplasty. *J Arthroplasty* 1994;9:521-526.
6. Madsen F, Kjaersgaard-Andersen P, Juhl M, Sneppen O: A custom-made prosthesis for the treatment of supracondylar femoral fractures after total knee arthroplasty: Report of four cases. *J Orthop Trauma* 1989;3:332-337.
7. Aaron RK, Scott R: Supracondylar fracture of the femur after total knee arthroplasty. *Clin Orthop* 1987;219:136-139.
8. Delport PH, Van Audekercke R, Martens M, Mulier JC: Conservative treatment of ipsilateral supracondylar femoral fracture after total knee arthroplasty. *J Trauma* 1984;24:846-849.
9. Webster DA, Murray DG: Complications of variable axis total knee arthroplasty. *Clin Orthop* 1985;193:160-167.
10. Culp RW, Schmidt RG, Hanks G, Mak A, Esterhai JL Jr, Heppenstall RB: Supracondylar fracture of the femur following prosthetic knee arthroplasty. *Clin Orthop* 1987;222:212-222.
11. Hanks GA, Mathews HH, Routson GW, Loughran TP: Supracondylar fracture of the femur following total knee arthroplasty. *J Arthroplasty* 1989;4:289-292.
12. Rorabeck CH, Taylor JW: Periprosthetic fractures of the femur complicating total knee arthroplasty. *Orthop Clin North Am* 1999;30:265-277.
13. Ritter MA, Faris PM, Keating EM: Anterior femoral notching and ipsilateral supracondylar femur fracture in total knee arthroplasty. *J Arthroplasty* 1988;3:185-187.
14. Short WH, Hootnick DR, Murray DG: Ipsilateral supracondylar femur fractures following knee arthroplasty. *Clin Orthop* 1981;158: 111-116.
15. Rand JA: Supracondylar fracture of the femur associated with polyethylene wear after total knee arthroplasty: A case report. *J Bone Joint Surg Am* 1994;76:1389-1393.
16. Hohl M: Fractures about the knee, in Rockwood CA Jr, Green DP (eds): *Fractures in Adults*, ed 2. Phildelphia, PA, JB Lippincott, 1984, pp 1429-1444.
17. Insall JN: Fractures of the distal femur, in Insall JN (ed): *Surgery of the Knee*. New York, NY, Churchill Livingstone, 1984, pp 413-448.
18. Sisto DJ, Lachiewicz PF, Insall JN: Treatment of supracondylar fractures following prosthetic arthroplasty of the knee. *Clin Orthop* 1985;196:265-272.
19. Hirsh DM, Bhalla S, Roffman M: Supracondylar fracture of the femur following total knee replacement: Report of four cases. *J Bone Joint Surg Am* 1981;63:162-163.
20. Schatzker J, Lambert DC: Supracondylar fractures of the femur. *Clin Orthop* 1979;138:77-83.
21. Jabczenski FF, Crawford M: Retrograde intramedullary nailing of supracondylar femur fractures above total knee arthroplasty: A preliminary report of four cases. *J Arthroplasty* 1995;10:95-101.
22. Kraay MJ, Goldberg VM, Figgie MP, Figgie HE III: Distal femoral replacement with allograft/prosthetic reconstruction for treatment of supracondylar fractures in patients with total knee arthroplasty. *J Arthroplasty* 1992;7:7-16.
23. Harlow ML, Hofmann AA: Periprosthetic fractures, in Scott WN (ed): *The Knee*. St Louis, MO, Mosby Year Book, 1994, vol 2, pp 1405-1417.
24. McLaren AC, Dupont JA, Schroeber DC: Open reduction internal fixation of supracondylar fractures above total knee arthroplasties using the intramedullary supracondylar rod. *Clin Orthop* 1994;302:194-198.
25. Rinecker H, Haibock H: Surgical treatment of peri-prosthetic fractures after total knee replacement. *Arch Orthop Unfallchir* 1977;87: 23-29.
26. Ritter MA, Stiver P: Supracondylar fracture in a patient with total knee arthroplasty: A case report. *Clin Orthop* 1985;193:168-170.
27. Cain PR, Rubash HE, Wissinger HA, McClain EJ: Periprosthetic femoral fractures following total knee arthroplasty. *Clin Orthop* 1986;208:205-214.
28. Roscoe MW, Goodman SB, Schatzker J: Supracondylar fracture of the femur after GUEPAR total knee arthroplasty: A new treatment method. *Clin Orthop* 1989;241:221-223.
29. Booth RE Jr: Management of periprosthetic fractures. *Orthopedics* 1994;17:845-847.
30. Scott RD: Letter: Anterior femoral notching and ipsilateral supracondylar femur fracture in total knee arthroplasty. *J Arthroplasty* 1988;3:381.
31. Lesh ML, Schneider DJ, Pellegrini VD: Abstract: Biomechanical evaluation of the effects of anterior cortical notching of the femur in total knee arthroplasty. *65th Annual Meeting Proceedings*. Rosemont, IL, American Academy of Orthopaedic Surgeons, 1998, p 238.
32. DiGioia AM III, Rubash HE: Periprosthetic fractures of the femur after total knee arthroplasty: A literature review and treatment algorithm. *Clin Orthop* 1991;271:135-142.
33. Rorabeck CH, Taylor JW: Classification of periprosthetic fractures complicating total knee arthroplasty. *Orthop Clin North Am* 1999;30: 209-214.
34. Rorabeck CH, Angliss RD, Lewis PL: Fractures of the femur, tibia, and patella after total knee arthroplasty: Decision making and principles of management. *Instr Course Lect* 1998;47:449-458.
35. Dennis DA: Periprosthetic fractures following total knee arthroplasty. *Tech Orthop* 1999;14: 138-143.
36. Dennis DA: Periprosthetic fractures following total knee arthroplasty: The good, bad, and ugly. *Orthopedics* 1998;21:1048-1050.
37. Cordeiro EN, Costa RC, Carazzato JG, Silva J dos S: Periprosthetic fractures in patients with total knee arthroplasties. *Clin Orthop* 1990;252: 182-189.
38. Oni OO: Supracondylar fracture of the femur following Attenborough stabilized gliding knee arthroplasty. *Injury* 1982;14:250-251.
39. Nielsen BF, Petersen VS, Varmarken JE: Fracture of the femur after knee arthroplasty. *Acta Orthop Scand* 1988;59:155-157.
40. Sochart DH, Hardinge K: Nonsurgical management of supracondylar fracture above total knee arthroplasty: Still the nineties option. *J Arthroplasty* 1997;12:830-834.
41. Rolston LR, Christ DJ, Halpern A, O'Connor PL, Ryan TG, Uggen WM: Treatment of supracondylar fractures of the femur proximal to a total knee arthroplasty: A report of four cases. *J Bone Joint Surg Am* 1995;77:924-931.
42. Murrell GA, Nunley JA: Interlocked supracondylar intramedullary nails for supracondylar fractures after total knee arthroplasty: A new treatment method. *J Arthroplasty* 1995;10:37-42.
43. Ayers DC: Supracondylar fracture of the distal femur proximal to a total knee replacement. *Instr Course Lect* 1997;46:197-203.
44. Biswas SP, Kurer MH, MacKenney RP: External fixation for femoral shaft fracture after Stanmore total knee replacement. *J Bone Joint Surg Br* 1992;74:313-314.
45. Healy WL, Siliski JM, Incavo SJ: Operative treatment of distal femoral fractures proximal to total knee replacements. *J Bone Joint Surg Am* 1993;75:27-34.

46. Howes JP, Sakka SA, Riley TBH: A modified prosthesis with an interlocking nail stem for the treatment of supracondylar femoral fractures after total knee replacement: A report of three cases. *Orthopedics Internat Ed* 1995;3: 303-308.

47. MacEachern AG, Ling RS: Ununited supracondylar fracture of the femur following Attenborough stabilized gliding knee arthroplasty treated by distal femoral replacement. *Injury* 1983;15:214-216.

48. Moran MC, Brick GW, Sledge CB, Dysart SH, Chien EP: Supracondylar femoral fracture following total knee arthroplasty. *Clin Orthop* 1996;324:196-209.

49. Smith WJ, Martin SL, Mabrey JD: Use of a supracondylar nail for treatment of a supracondylar fracture of the femur following total knee arthroplasty. *J Arthroplasty* 1996;11: 201-213.

50. Zehntner MK, Ganz R: Internal fixation of supracondylar fractures after condylar total knee arthroplasty. *Clin Orthop* 1993;293: 219-224.

51. Tani Y, Inoue K, Kancko H, Nishioka J, Hukuda S: Intramedullary fibular graft for supracondylar fracture of the femur following total knee arthroplasty. *Arch Orthop Trauma Surg* 1998;117:103-104.

52. Ritter MA, Keating EM, Faris PM, Meding JB: Rush rod fixation of supracondylar fractures above total knee arthroplasties. *J Arthroplasty* 1995;10:213-216.

53. Maniar RN, Umlas ME, Rodriguez JA, Ranawat CS: Supracondylar femoral fracture above a PFC posterior cruciate-substituting total knee arthroplasty treated with supracondylar nailing: A unique technical problem. *J Arthroplasty* 1996;11:637-639.

54. Engh GA, Ammeen DJ: Periprosthetic fractures adjacent to total knee implants: Treatment and clinical results. *J Bone Joint Surg Am* 1997;79: 1100-1113.

55. Healy WL: Tibial fractures below total knee arthroplasty, in Insall JN, Scott WN, Scuderi GR (eds): *Current Concepts in Primary and Revision Total Knee Arthroplasty*. Philadelphia, PA, Lippincott-Raven, 1996, pp 163-167.

56. Rand JA, Coventry MB: Stress fractures after total knee arthroplasty. *J Bone Joint Surg Am* 1980;62:226-233.

57. Felix NA, Stuart MJ, Hanssen AD: Periprosthetic fractures of the tibia associated with total knee arthroplasty. *Clin Orthop* 1997;345:113-124.

58. Stuart MJ, Hanssen AD: Total knee arthroplasty: Periprosthetic tibial fractures. *Orthop Clin North Am* 1999;30:279-286.

59. Bryan RS, Peterson LF, Combs JJ Jr: Polycentric knee arthroplasty: A preliminary report of postoperative complications in 450 knees. *Clin Orthop* 1973;94:148-152.

60. Chmell MJ, Moran MC, Scott RD: Periarticular fractures after total knee arthroplasty: Principles of management. *J Am Acad Orthop Surg* 1996;4:109-116.

61. Kjaersgaard-Andersen P, Juhl M: Ipsilateral traumatic supracondylar femoral and proximal tibial fractures following total knee replacement: A case report. *J Trauma* 1989;29:398-400.

62. Ritter MA, Carr K, Keating EM, Faris PM, Meding JB: Tibial shaft fracture following tibial tubercle osteotomy. *J Arthroplasty* 1996;11: 117-119.

63. Whiteside LA: Exposure in difficult total knee arthroplasty using tibial tubercle osteotomy. *Clin Orthop* 1995;321:32-35.

64. Tria AJ Jr, Harwood DA, Alicea JA, Cody RP: Patellar fractures in posterior stabilized knee arthroplasties. *Clin Orthop* 1994;299:131-138.

65. Goldberg VM, Figgie HE III, Inglis AE, et al: Patellar fracture type and prognosis in condylar total knee arthroplasty. *Clin Orthop* 1988;236:115-122.

66. Hozack WJ, Goll SR, Lotke PA, Rothman RH, Booth RE Jr: The treatment of patellar fractures after total knee arthroplasty. *Clin Orthop* 1988;236:123-127.

67. Cameron HU, Fedorkow DM: The patella in total knee arthroplasty. *Clin Orthop* 1982;165:197-199.

68. Doolittle KH II, Turner RH: Patellofemoral problems following total knee arthroplasty. *Orthop Rev* 1988;17:696-702.

69. Scott RD, Turoff N, Ewald FC: Stress fracture of the patella following duopatellar total knee arthroplasty with patellar resurfacing. *Clin Orthop* 1982;170:147-151.

70. Clayton ML, Thirupathi R: Patellar complications after total condylar arthroplasty. *Clin Orthop* 1982;170:152-155.

71. Ranawat CS: The patellofemoral joint in total condylar knee arthroplasty: Pros and cons based on five- to ten-year follow-up observations. *Clin Orthop* 1986;205:93-99.

72. Leblanc JM: Patellar complications in total knee arthroplasty: A literature review. *Orthop Rev* 1989;18:296-304.

73. Thompson FM, Hood RW, Insall J: Patellar fractures in total knee arthroplasty. *Orthop Trans* 1981;5:490-491.

74. Lynch AF, Rorabeck CH, Bourne RB: Extensor mechanism complications following total knee arthroplasty. *J Arthroplasty* 1987;2:135-140.

75. Ahmed AM, Burke DL, Hyder A: Force analysis of the patellar mechanism. *J Orthop Res* 1987;5:69-85.

76. Dupont JA, Baker SA: Complications of patellofemoral resurfacing in total knee arthroplasty. *Orthop Trans* 1982;6:369.

77. Rand JA: Patellar resurfacing in total knee arthroplasty. *Clin Orthop* 1990;260:110-117.

78. Roffman M, Hirsh DM, Mendes DG. Fracture of the resurfaced patella in total knee replacement. *Clin Orthop* 1980;148:112-116.

79. Kaufer H: Mechanical function of the patella. *J Bone Joint Surg Am* 1971;53:1551-1560.

80. Huberti HH, Hayes WC: Patellofemoral contact pressures: The influence of q-angle and tendofemoral contact. *J Bone Joint Surg Am* 1984;66:715-724.

81. Josechak RG, Finlay JB, Bourne RB, Rorabeck CH: Cancellous bone support for patellar resurfacing. *Clin Orthop* 1987;220:192-199.

82. Reuben JD, McDonald CL, Woodard PL, Hennington LJ: Effect of patella thickness on patella strain following total knee arthroplasty. *J Arthroplasty* 1991;6:251-258.

83. Stulberg SD, Stulberg BN, Hamati Y, Tsao A: Failure mechanisms of metal-backed patellar components. *Clin Orthop* 1988;236:88-105.

84. Rand JA, Gustilo RB: Technique of patellar resurfacing in total knee arthroplasty. *Tech Orthop* 1988;3:57-66.

85. Goldstein SA, Coale E, Weiss AP, Grossnickle M, Meller B, Matthews LS: Patellar surface strain. *J Orthop Res* 1986;4:372-377.

86. Brick GW, Scott RD: The patellofemoral component of total knee arthroplasty. *Clin Orthop* 1988;231:163-178.

87. Bjorkstrom S, Goldie IF: A study of the arterial supply of the patella in the normal state, in chondromalacia patellae and in osteoarthrosis. *Acta Orthop Scand* 1980;51:63-70.

88. Kayler DE, Lyttle D: Surgical interruption of patellar blood supply by total knee arthroplasty. *Clin Orthop* 1988;229:221-227.

89. Scapinelli R: Blood supply of the human patella: Its relation to ischaemic necrosis after fracture. *J Bone Joint Surg Br* 1967;49:563-570.

90. Scapinelli R: Studies on the vasculature of the human knee joint. *Acta Anat* 1968;70:305-331.

91. Insall J, Scott WN, Ranawat CS: The total condylar knee prosthesis: A report of two hundred and twenty cases. *J Bone Joint Surg Am* 1979;61:173-180.

92. Scott WN, Rubinstein M, Scuderi G: Results after knee replacement with a posterior cruciate-substituting prosthesis. *J Bone Joint Surg Am* 1988;70:1163-1173.

93. McMahon MS, Scuderi GR, Glashow JL, Scharf SC, Meltzer LP, Scott WN: Scintigraphic determination of patellar viability after excision of infrapatellar fat pad and/or lateral retinacular release in total knee arthroplasty. *Clin Orthop* 1990;260:10-16.

94. Scuderi G, Scharf SC, Meltzer LP, Scott WN: The relationship of lateral releases to patella viability in total knee arthroplasty. *J Arthroplasty* 1987;2:209-214.

95. Wetzner SM, Bezreh JS, Scott RD, Bierbaum BE, Newberg AH: Bone scanning in the assessment of patellar viability following knee replacement. *Clin Orthop* 1985;199:215-219.

96. Figgie HE III, Goldberg VM, Figgie MP, Inglis AE, Kelly M, Sobel M: The effect of alignment of the implant on fractures of the patella after condylar total knee arthroplasty. *J Bone Joint Surg Am* 1989;71:1031-1039.

97. Windsor RE, Scuderi GR, Insall JN: Patellar fractures in total knee arthroplasty. *J Arthroplasty* 1989;4(suppl):S63-S67.

98. Berman AT, Reid JS, Yanicko DR Jr, Sih GC, Zimmerman MR: Thermally induced bone necrosis in rabbits: Relation to implant failure in humans. *Clin Orthop* 1984;186:284-292.

99. Grace JN, Sim FH: Fracture of the patella after total knee arthroplasty. *Clin Orthop* 1988;230:168-175.

100. d'Hollander A, Burny F, Monteny E, Donkerwolcke M: Extraosseous variations of temperature during polymerization of acrylic cement in hip arthroplasties. *Acta Orthop Scand* 1976;47:186-188.

101. Willert HG, Ludwig J, Semlitsch M: Reaction of bone to methacrylate after hip arthroplasty: A long-term gross, light microscopic, and scanning electron microscopic study. *J Bone Joint Surg Am* 1974;56:1368-1382.

102. Ritter MA, Campbell ED: Postoperative patellar complications with or without lateral release during total knee arthroplasty. *Clin Orthop* 1987;219:163-168.

103. Ritter MA, Herbst SA, Keating EM, Faris PM, Meding JB: Patellofemoral complications following total knee arthroplasty: Effect of a lateral release and sacrifice of the superior lateral geniculate artery. *J Arthroplasty* 1996;11:368-372.

104. Le AX, Cameron HU, Otsuka NY, Harrington IJ, Bhargava M: Fracture of the patella following total knee arthroplasty. *Orthopedics* 1999;22:395-399.

39

Periprosthetic Osteolysis With Total Knee Arthroplasty

Gerard A. Engh, MD
Deborah J. Ammeen, BS

With early hinged metal knee components, osteolysis occurred only after aseptic loosening. The osteolysis was secondary to cement fragmentation. Although particulate metal debris from the articulating surfaces could have contributed to a histiocytic response, the osteolysis was, most probably, a response to particulate cement.

The earliest reports of osteolysis adjacent to total knee implants were single case studies published in the mid to late 1980s.[1] The first cases reported were from a group of cementless Synatomic total knee implants (DePuy, Warsaw, IN) with osteolysis around the tibial fixation screws.[2] Coincidentally, the Synatomic tibial component was the first widely used modular implant. At that time, no one identified modular implants as a source of wear debris that might cause osteolysis.

Clinical Presentation of Osteolysis

The clinical manifestations of osteolysis rarely occur within the first 5 years after surgery. Quite commonly, the lesions are visible on radiographs before the patient develops symptoms. Occasionally, advanced lesions of osteolysis are present without the patient having significant knee pain or functional limitations. For this reason, it is important that the surgeon emphasize the need for routine follow-up radiographs on all patients with joint replacement.

One or more of the authors or the departments with which they are affiliated have received something of value from a commercial or other party related directly or indirectly to the subject of this chapter.

Joint Effusion

A joint effusion occurs when the synovial membrane is saturated with a large volume of particulate wear debris from a total knee implant. When the joint capsule is intact, synovial fluid pressure is increased. If the path of least resistance is through periprosthetic bone, osteolysis may develop in this location as a response to the particulate debris. However, if the joint capsule is weak, herniation of the capsule into the surrounding soft tissues can create a synovial pseudocyst lined by hyperplastic synovium.[3,4] These extracapsular cysts can be tense and painful and can expand to a pronounced size (Fig. 1). Pseudocysts also can be difficult to aspirate because of detritus that clogs the aspiration needle. The excision of the cyst is rarely successful without full component revision. Also, simple cyst excision may result in the development of a chronic draining sinus and a potential pathway for opportunistic infection (unpublished data).

Synovial pseudocysts commonly are associated with a large joint effusion. Usually, it is not difficult to aspirate the knee joint. The fluid is usually yellow, rarely serosanguinous, and usually nonviscous. Examination under light microscopy with polarization may reveal shards of polyethylene. Particulate metal debris is not visible with light microscopy of these specimens.

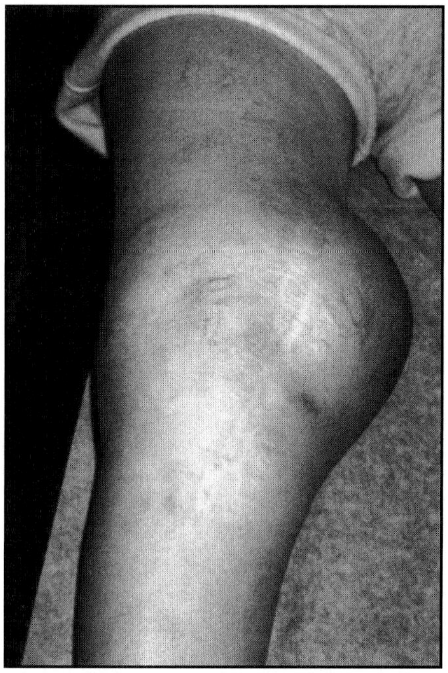

Fig. 1 A large pseudocyst is present on the medial side of this patient's knee.

Loss of Flexion/Knee Pain

Commonly, patients with long-standing particulate synovitis gradually lose knee flexion and have increasing knee pain and stiffness. Patients describe the pain as a deep ache that is aggravated by activity.

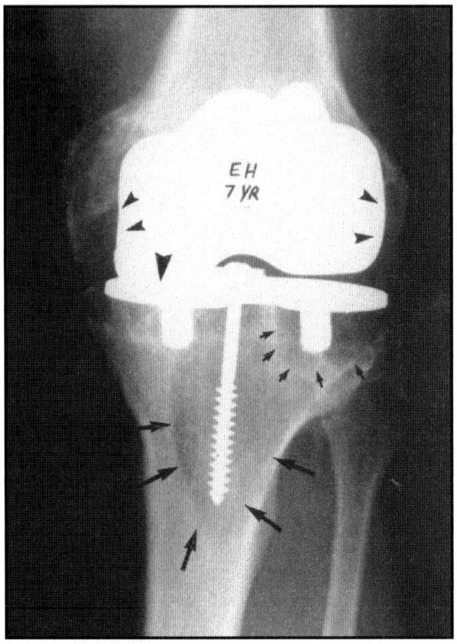

Fig. 2 Osteolysis is outlined (*arrows*) by a rim of reactive new bone.

Patterns of Osteolysis

The location of osteolysis is determined by the presence of an access route to periprosthetic bone. Access routes are created wherever an implant is not bonded rigidly at its fixation interface and components do not cover the resected bone surfaces. An all-polyethylene tibial component rarely covers the entire resected surface of the proximal tibia. Thus, the design deficiencies of an implant and the positioning of the components could be responsible for the development and location of osteolytic lesions.

Many of the early total knee implants with all-polyethylene tibial components were available in only two sizes; hence, the implant poorly covered the tibia. Despite the range of implant sizes available today, cancellous bone might remain exposed and become part of the "available joint space."[5] This bone is less resistant to intra-articular fluid pressure than bone bonded to the implant by cement or bone ingrowth. With increased intra-articular fluid volume and increased pressure secondary to implant wear, synovial fluid laden with wear debris could move into bone in such locations.

Osteolysis With Cementless Components

One characteristic of cementless implants that influences the frequency and location of osteolytic lesions is the amount and location of smooth metal on the underside of the component. A common feature of cementless femoral components is that small sections of the anterior or posterior flanges are not coated with a beaded surface for bone ingrowth. Bone does not bond to the implant in these smooth areas; instead, fibrous tissue forms, making an access channel for synovial fluid and debris.

Osteolytic lesions, often demarcated by a rim of new bone, develop as a result of extraosseous fluid pressure (Fig. 2). Osteolysis also can develop if the femoral component is oversized anteriorly, leaving a recess between the anterior flange of the femoral component and the host bone. In many instances, the bone remodels away from the anterior flange of the femoral component in response to debris.

Often, osteolytic lesions develop adjacent to the posterior condyles. As previously mentioned, some cementless femoral designs have areas of smooth metal on the posterior condyles that provide an access route for fluid and debris. In many instances the resected posterior condylar surfaces are incompletely capped by the component. Posterior condylar lesions often expand from this location into the periprosthetic bone.

Screw holes or other openings in the metal surface of the component also provide a route for debris to access the cancellous bone. The Synatomic total knee implant used large cancellous titanium screws placed through holes in the cobalt-chrome alloy tibial baseplate. In a study by Peters and associates,[2] osteolytic lesions developed in proximity to the screws, and in many cases there was an intact fibrous-tissue membrane surrounding the screw. Particulate polyethylene debris and metal debris were implicated as causes of the lesion. In cases of severe lesions, the osteolysis expanded through the adjacent metaphyseal cortex. Although in some instances the lesions were extensive, implant loosening and component migration rarely were encountered.

The configuration of the porous coating on the undersurface of the tibial component also influences the development of osteolysis. Cementless tibial components with patches of porous coating connected by smooth metal tracks are likely to channel debris from the joint surface to the area surrounding the stem.[6] Whiteside[6] found that 28 of 124 Ortholoc (Wright Medical Technology, Arlington, TN) modular prostheses with patches of porous coating had osteolysis compared to no cases from a group of 675 knees with porous coating that covered the entire undersurface of the tibial tray. Similarly, osteolysis was identified around the smooth pegs of the Ortholoc I (Wright Medical Technology) tibial tray.[7]

Fractures of Cementless Components

Once bone ingrowth is achieved with a cementless device, changes in alignment rarely occur unless the component or bone fractures. A metal-backed tibial component may fracture (Fig. 3), particularly if made of titanium, and the patient may develop an angular deformity of the knee. Although recurrent deformity occurs with baseplate fracture, a broken metal tray is not recognized easily on routine follow-up radiographs because the fractured pieces rarely separate. Radiographs must be inspected carefully to identify a slight sag or angulation of the broken plateau.

Fractured tibial baseplates have been reported with the Press Fit Condylar knee (PFC, Johnson & Johnson, Warsaw, IN).[8] Tibial trays with thin metal, a sintered surface, and design features such as slots, screw holes, and sharp corners have stress concentrations that make the tray more likely to fracture.[9] The Porous Coated Anatomic knee (PCA, Howmedica, Rutherford, NJ) featured slots in the tibial tray adjacent to a central post that allowed the surgeon access to the porous-coated stem if component removal was necessary. Although this tray was made of cobalt-chrome alloy, fractures have been encountered with it.[10]

Cementless femoral components also may fail by component fracture, most commonly at the junction of the posterior chamfer. Thin metal at the region of the posterior chamfer was a design flaw of the Ortholoc II implant (Wright Medical Technology).[11] The loss of bone support from osteolysis and stress concentrations in areas of thin metal have led to cementless component fracture.[12] Campbell and associates[13] reported implant failure due to fracture of the femoral component in 2 of 65 cementless PFC knees. Parks and Topoleski[9] also identified femoral component fractures as a mechanical failure mode of total knee implants.

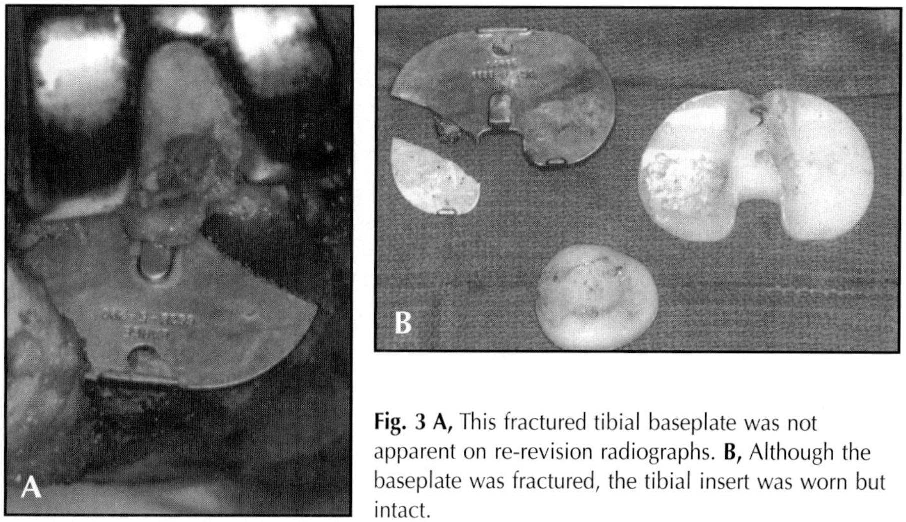

Fig. 3 A, This fractured tibial baseplate was not apparent on re-revision radiographs. **B,** Although the baseplate was fractured, the tibial insert was worn but intact.

Osteolysis in Cemented Components

Osteolysis can develop adjacent to a cemented implant without the components becoming loose. In our experience, a cemented component is more likely to loosen than a bone ingrown cementless implant if exposed to an abnormally large particulate load. This might be related to the poor tensile strength of methylmethacrylate. Lesions associated with cemented components most likely originate in areas where the bone-cement interface is demarcated with fibrous tissue. Voids in the bone-cement interface are a conduit for debris that ultimately can lead to linear osteolysis and fixation failure.

If cement does not penetrate and bond to host bone, a linear radiolucency can be seen on early postoperative radiographs. This is particularly common in revision situations in which the bone is densely sclerotic. If debris filters along the fixation interface, the lucency may progress and ultimately lead to aseptic loosening of the component. This loss of fixation by a biologic process in response to particulate debris was identified as the mechanism of fixation failure with acetabular components of total hip arthroplasty.[14] Cemented knee components might also migrate with loss of fixation. On radiographs, the implant appears to have subsided (Fig. 4) or to be malpositioned because of recurrent angular deformity. Cement fragmentation with implant loosening causes additional debris that contributes to progressive bone destruction.

Angular deformity also occurs when an all-polyethylene tibial component loses bone support because of an osteolytic bone defect. If osteolysis develops adjacent to an all-polyethylene tibial component, the loss of bone support beneath the plateau can lead to polyethylene deformation (Fig. 5). Linear osteolysis rarely progresses around the stem of an all-polyethylene tibial component; thus, the implant sags while the stem of the implant remains fixed. The patient often develops recurrent deformity in the knee. Such osteolytic lesions may not be apparent on weight-bearing radiographs because the lesion is obliterated by implant deformation into the defect. A comparison of weight-bearing and non–weight-bearing radiographs is useful in identifying plastic deformation. With repetitive stress, an all-polyethylene tibial component may fracture from fatigue (Fig. 6).

Radiographs

The anteroposterior (AP) radiograph is often as helpful as the lateral radiograph for identifying osteolysis with both cemented and cementless components. Lesions appear as scalloped defects at the margins of the femoral or tibial components (Fig. 7). In the femur, the lesions often expand into the surrounding metaphysis, and bone loss is seen on radiographs in the part of the condyle not hidden by the metallic prosthesis. The extent of bone loss often is outlined by new bone formation, suggesting an attempt by host bone to contain or heal the lytic process. These new sclerotic lines are usually present on both the AP and lateral radiographs and may be the only evidence of osteolysis.

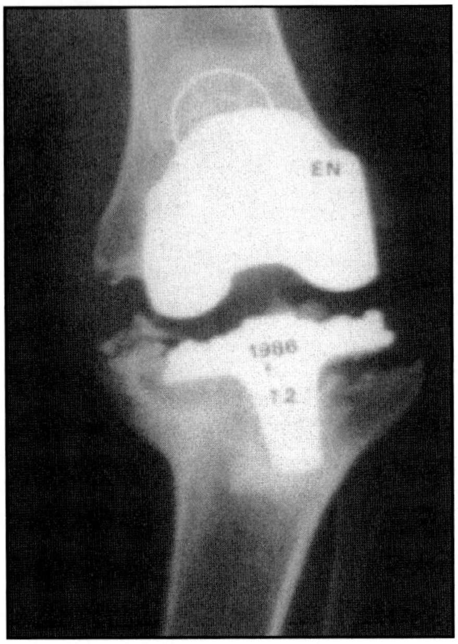

Fig. 4 This tibial component has shifted into varus with loss of bone support secondary to osteolysis.

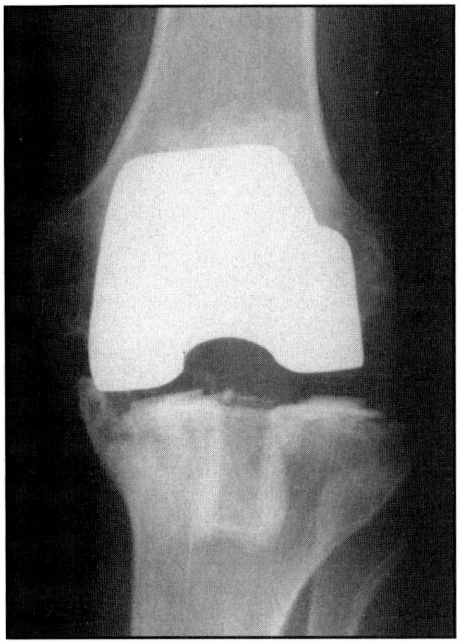

Fig. 5 Although this all-polyethylene tibial component is not loose, the medial plateau has sagged from the loss of bone support.

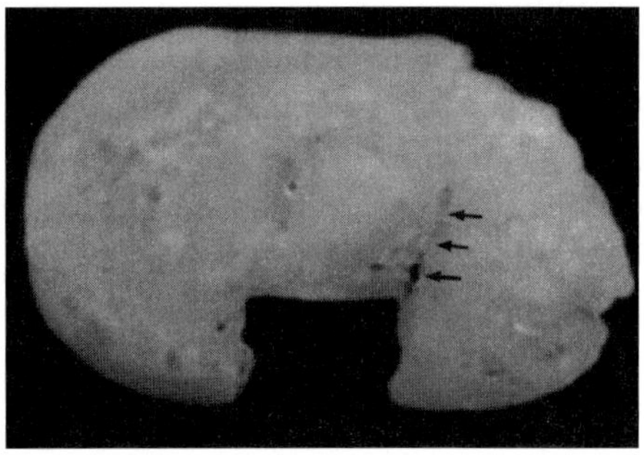

Fig. 6 An all-polyethylene tibial component that has fractured (*arrows*) from loss of bone support with osteolysis.

Intraoperative Inspection of Osteolytic Lesions

At the time of revision surgery, the surgeon must search carefully for the osteolytic lesions. Quite often cortical defects are not apparent, and the osteolytic defects can be overlooked. The margins of the components must be cleared of fibrous tissue and carefully probed for an entry site to the lytic area. An entry channel is always present because the osteolytic defect is an expansion of the available joint space. When the entry channel is located and the defect probed, a clear yellow fluid similar to the patient's joint fluid will exude from the damaged bone segment. The most common entry sites on the femoral side are along the margins of the posterior femoral condyles (Fig. 8). Tibial defects may originate at any area adjacent to the tibial tray.

Management Options

Osteolysis is visible on radiographs before a component becomes aseptically loose. In some instances, full-thickness polyethylene wear has occurred, and the metallic tibial baseplate has articulated with the femoral component. Because full-thickness wear of the polyethylene alone is not painful, the patient might not return for follow-up evaluation. As the articulating metal parts continue to wear, the patient gradually develops an effusion, increasing stiffness, and low-grade pain in the knee.

Observation of the Lesion

It is reasonable to observe and carefully monitor relatively small osteolytic lesions. Serial radiographs are particularly helpful in ascertaining that a lesion is new and does not represent a preoperative bone defect from causes other than debris generation. These radiographs also are useful in determining the rate of progressive bone damage. Some lesions appear to stabilize and become contained by a surrounding border of new bone. Surveillance is recommended with such lesions if the patient is asymptomatic and has no significant risk of fracture from the lesion. It is helpful to establish patient concurrence with a treatment plan while observing the progression of the lesion.

Partial Revision

When the femoral and tibial components are stable, partial revision surgery may be an attractive alternative. Often, the surgeon is reluctant to remove well-fixed components, particularly when extensive bone damage from osteolysis combined with damage from implant removal will lead to a complex revision procedure. Usually, the removal of knee implants with significant periprosthetic osteolysis requires reconstruction with allograft bone and a stemmed revision component or a conversion to a linked revision implant system—two options surgeons would like to avoid.

To determine if component retention is judicious, the surgeon must inspect the articulating surface of the femur. It is reasonable to retain the femoral component if the component has no visible or palpable damage. Often, slight burnishing of the component makes this decision difficult. It is helpful to palpate the burnished area with a probe because this palpation often reveals surface roughness far beyond that identified by digital palpation. It also is important to consider the patient's age and activity level because it may be acceptable to retain a somewhat less pristine component surface in an inactive, elderly individual.

The surgeon also must examine articulating surfaces of the tibia for wear damage. When the articular wear of the components is extensive, with delamination after a relatively short in vivo interval, the surgeon must consider the underlying reasons for this accelerated polyethylene wear. If there is a reasonable explanation, such as a heat-pressed polyethylene insert (Howmedica), a carbon fiber-reinforced insert (Zimmer, Warsaw, IN), or a Hylamer-M insert (DePuy), and the components are correctly aligned, a simple insert exchange is prudent.[15] If the implants are not correctly aligned and malalignment has contributed to asymmetric polyethyelene wear, the surgeon can consider an angled bearing to correct the malalignment.[16]

The polyethylene insert must be examined for wear and signs of impingement, particularly if the patient has a posterior-stabilized implant. Although not a posterior-stabilized device, the Synatomic Knee had a high incidence of osteolysis associated with impingement of the high central eminence of the polyethylene insert against the intercondylar notch of the femoral implant. The impingement resulted in motion of the modular tibial insert and accelerated wear on the backside of the polyethylene and the tibial baseplate. Polyethylene exchange without revising the femoral and tibial components was successful with Synatomic inserts with a customized low central eminence (personal experience).

A similar phenomenon is seen with some of the contemporary posterior-stabilized knee designs. The post of the insert must be inspected carefully because post wear has been identified as an additional source of wear debris (CH Rorabeck, MD, personal communication, 1999). If the post of the insert has significant wear, the surgeon must decide whether the impingement can be corrected without performing a full knee revision.

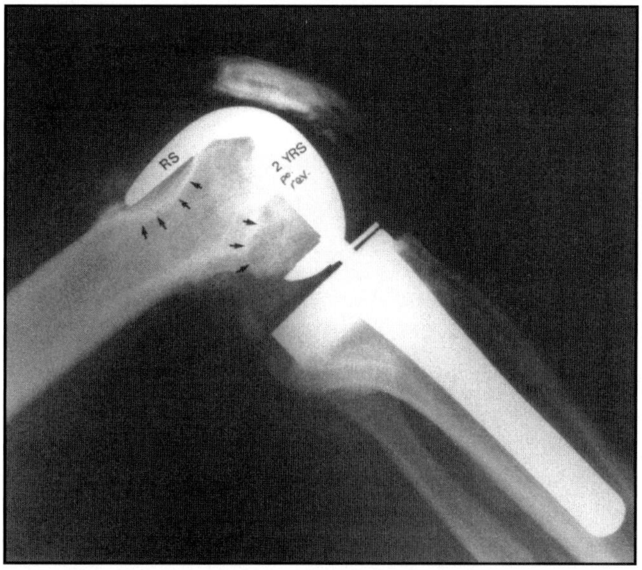

Fig. 7 Osteolytic lesions (*arrows*) at the anterior and posterior margins of this femoral component.

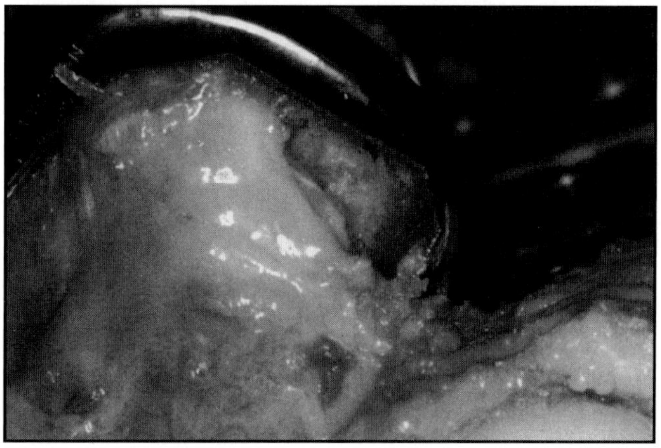

Fig. 8 Femoral osteolysis most commonly is found along the margins of the femoral component and posterior femoral condyles.

When contemplating component retention, the surgeon also must inspect the tibial baseplate and the backside of the modular polyethylene. Tibial baseplate wear was identified in modular tibial components with both snap-fit and tongue-in-groove style locking mechanisms for the modular inserts.[17] Backside wear of the polyethylene is evident by the wearing away of material in all areas except directly over the screw holes. Machine markings imprinted for product identification also can be used to evaluate backside polyethylene wear. The etchings on the back of inserts are inscribed to a depth of at least 0.3 mm. The loss of such markings is evidence of insert micromotion and an inadequate tibial tray locking mechanism.[18] If backside wear of the insert is evident, the modular locking mechanism is poor, and tibial component retention should not be considered.

Visible damage to the tibial baseplate is a sign of a poor modular locking mechanism. Most tibial baseplates are made of titanium alloy, a relatively soft metal that is prone to wear even when articulating against polyethylene. A stippled area, defined as an extensive area of wear in a discrete pattern, has been identified in tibial trays with relatively poor locking mechanisms. Often, this stippled pattern is oriented in a direction that indicates insert rotation. Laboratory examination of worn tibial components recovered at revision surgery and retrieved from well-functioning knees at autopsy has confirmed substantially greater insert micromotion between the insert and the tibial baseplate than with nonimplanted, new, out-of-the-box tibial components. In many instances the slack (insert motion under minimal load) of these recovered inserts ranges from hundreds of microns to more than a thousand microns.[17]

Insert exchange alone is a viable option in a knee with osteolysis if the original insert demonstrated acceptable wear after an in vivo interval of more than 10 years.[15] Both the femoral and tibial baseplate must be stable and undamaged. Screws that were placed for cementless tibial tray fixation should be removed because the screws are a conduit for debris with the revision tibial insert. The osteolytic defects must be located by probing the margins of the components. Once an entry site is identified, the entry portal can be enlarged to evacuate tissue and fluid from the osteolytic cyst. After the osteolytic lesion is thoroughly debrided, the same portal is used to repair the bone defect. Although the benefit of using allograft to restore bone and provide support for the retained components has not been documented, we believe large-chunk allograft should be used to fill the defects created by osteolysis (personal experience). The allograft bone is tightly impacted into the defect with a bone punch to prevent the bone graft from dislodging with patient activities.

When a total knee arthroplasty fails by wear or osteolysis in less than 10 years after implantation, tibial insert exchange is unpredictable and full knee revision usually is indicated. Engh and associates[15] reported a 27% failure rate with tibial insert revision because of accelerated wear of the new insert. If the tibial baseplate is worn and the insert delaminated, isolated insert is contraindicated except with elderly, low-demand patients.

Full Knee Revision

The need and timing of revision surgery has not been defined for patients in whom osteolysis is identified on follow-up radiographs. Whenever fracture occurs through an osteolytic defect or whenever loss of component fixation and subsidence occur, full revision is the only option. Because these patients are symptomatic, the decision to proceed with surgery is easy for both the surgeon and the patient. When dealing with small osteolytic lesions, the decision to perform a partial versus a full revision should be based on the reported results with the implant system in situ, the time interval until the development of osteolysis, and intraoperative inspection of the components. Often the extent of osteolytic defects and implant damage are underestimated on prerevision radiographs; therefore, a full revision knee system should always be available whenever planning a partial revision.

In most cases of full knee revision for osteolysis, it is necessary to use either a modular revision implant system with allografts or a linked (rotating-hinged) implant system. The decision is made on a knee by knee basis. In most instances, rotating hinges should be reserved for revising knees with large osteolytic lesions that cannot be managed with less-constrained devices. Such knees are those with recurvatum instability or marked collateral ligament deficiency. The use of rotating hinges is reasonable in low-demand, elderly individuals, whereas allograft reconstruction with revision components is preferable for younger, active patients. An advantage of composite reconstructions with allograft bone and long-stemmed components is that allograft bone restores a cancellous structure that readily heals to the patient's bone at the base of a large osteolytic defect. Allograft bone also provides a cancellous surface for cement interdigitation.

When fully revising a knee with large osteolytic defects, the surgeon must adhere to the following three principles: (1) When necessary, reconstitute cancellous bone structure in the metaphyseal region of the knee for cement interdigitation and rigid component stability. (2) Use a long-stemmed revision component that engages the diaphyseal segment of the femur or tibia. (3) Use the least amount of implant constraint that is needed for satisfactory knee stability.

Keeping these principles in mind, the decision of how best to proceed with the revision is made after implant removal and curettage of the osteolytic bone defects. The surgeon must decide if adequate knee stability can be achieved without a linked component. Instability resulting purely from bone loss can be corrected by allograft repair of the bone defects; however, a linked device is necessary if the capsular and collateral ligaments are absent. Commonly, ligament imbalance may be present, but adequate stability can be achieved by releasing the contracted structures. Spacer blocks can be used to assess relative knee stability before committing to a hinged device.

Allograft Reconstruction

Using progressively larger rigid reamers, the surgeon opens the intramedullary canals of the femur and tibia until encountering endosteal resistance. The severity of bone deficiency is assessed to determine if augments or bone grafts are necessary. Defects up to 12 mm in depth from the planned resection levels of the distal femur are amenable to distal femoral augments, as long as reasonable cancellous bone is present for cement interdigitation. Defects more than 12 mm in depth are best repaired with allografts. In most instances, the surgeon can use a female reamer to prepare a femoral head allograft that fills a similar but slightly smaller hemispherical-shaped defect in the patient's bone that has been prepared with a male reamer. Kirschner wires (K-wires; Zimmer) can hold the allograft in place temporarily.

With the allografts in place, the surgeon makes a rough bone resection to facilitate the positioning of contemporary knee-revision instruments. If the allograft interferes with insertion of the intramedullary guide, the canal is reopened with a high-speed burr. Bone resections are performed on the allograft and host bone. To permit axial loading of the allograft, the stems of the components are not cemented to the intramedullary canal. Once the allograft is secured between the component and host bone, the K-wires are removed.

If a whole-segment allograft is needed, the allograft is placed in an Allogrip bone-holding device (DePuy), and an arthroplasty is performed on the allograft. A long-stemmed component is implanted with the stem protruding from the intramedullary canal of the allograft. The allograft-revision composite is placed into the patient's prepared intramedullary canal. With the composite in place, the allograft is shortened until the knee can be brought to full extension. Next, the surgeon implants a tibial insert that is of appropriate thickness to provide stability in extension. With the knee at 90° flexion, the femoral epicondyles of the patient are reattached to the allograft to restore stability in flexion.

Clinical Results of Revision Surgery for Osteolysis

At a mean follow-up of 41 months (range, 24 to 72 months), the clinical and radiographic results were excellent in 23 of 25 cases of tibial osteolysis managed at our institute with different surgical options.[19] Both limited revision with insert exchange and full knee revision were successful, although two cases of insert exchange were pending re-revision for progression of osteolytic lesions. Ten patients who underwent tibial component revision and five who underwent full revision have fared well. Structural allografts were used in three tibial revisions and in four full revisions. Neither aseptic loosening nor recurring osteolysis was identified in any of these patients.

Large structural allografts are indicated in revision surgery that involves large osteolytic bone defects. Ghazavi and associates[20] reported successful outcomes in 77% of cases (23 of 30) where a large structural allograft was used in the revision. Both revision and hinged components were used in this study. The seven failures were due to infection (three knees), aseptic loosening of the tibial component (two knees), graft nonunion (one knee), and graft fracture (one knee). In another study, standard long-stemmed revision components were used in conjunction with structural allografts to reconstruct major bone deficiency.[21] Twenty-nine femoral head and six full-segment allografts were used for bone defect reconstruction. At a mean follow-up interval of 4.2 years, there were no revisions or re-operations. Three of four components that were press-fit to the host bone subsided but did not require re-revisions. In these patients, the clinical results were inferior to those of patients with cemented revision components.

Rotating-hinge components are the alternative choice for revision surgery with large osteolytic bone defects. In a review from the Mayo Clinic, Rand and associates[22] reported aseptic loosening and a higher infection rate using rotating hinges in revision surgery. The aseptic loosening rate was 13% and the infection rate was 16% at a mean of 4.2 years after revision arthroplasty. Another author reported progressive radiolucencies in 20% of rotating hinges at 2-year follow-up.[23]

At our institution, the current approach to revision knee surgery with large, progressive osteolytic defects is to repair the bone defects with allograft bone and to use the minimal constraint necessary for a stable, well-functioning arthroplasty. Hinged devices are reserved for unstable knees that cannot reliably be managed with varus-valgus constrained components. Such cases include knees with complete loss of collateral stability, either medially or laterally, or global instability with a compromised extensor apparatus.

References

1. Dannenmaier WC, Haynes DW, Nelson CL: Granulomatous reaction and cystic bony destruction associated with high wear rate in a total knee prosthesis. *Clin Orthop* 1985;198:224-230.
2. Peters PC Jr, Engh GA, Dwyer KA, Vinh TN: Osteolysis after total knee arthroplasty without cement. *J Bone Joint Surg Am* 1992;74:864-876.
3. Chavda DV, Garvin KL: Failure of a polyethylene total knee component presenting as a thigh mass: Report of a rare complication of total knee arthroplasty. *Clin Orthop* 1994; 303: 211-216.
4. Yasuda M, Inoue K, Ikawa T, Yukioka M, Shichikawa K: A giant thigh mass in a patient with total knee arthroplasty for Charcot joint. *Clin Orthop* 1995;317:159-161.
5. Schmalzried TP, Jasty M, Harris WH: Periprosthetic bone loss in total hip arthroplasty: Polyethylene wear debris and the concept of the effective joint space. *J Bone Joint Surg Am* 1992;74:849-863.
6. Whiteside LA: Effect of porous-coating configuration on tibial osteolysis after total knee arthroplasty. *Clin Orthop* 1995;321:92-97.
7. Whiteside LA: Cementless total knee replacement: Nine- to 11-year results and 10-year survivorship analysis. *Clin Orthop* 1994;309: 185-192.
8. Cook SD, Thomas KA: Fatigue failure of noncemented porous-coated implants: A retrieval study. *J Bone Joint Surg Br* 1991;73:20-24.
9. Parks NL, Topoleski LDT: Revision total knee implants: Materials and design considerations, in Engh GA, Rorabeck CH (eds): *Revision Total Knee Arthroplasty*. Baltimore, MD, Williams & Wilkins, 1997, pp 121-136.
10. Morrey BF, Chao EY: Fracture of the porous-coated metal tray of a biologically fixed knee prosthesis: Report of a case. *Clin Orthop* 1988; 228:182-189.
11. Whiteside LA, Fosco DR, Brooks JG Jr: Fracture of the femoral component in cementless total knee arthroplasty. *Clin Orthop* 1993; 286:71-77.

12. Huang CH, Yang CY, Cheng CK: Fracture of the femoral component associated with polyethylene wear and osteolysis after total knee arthroplasty. *J Arthroplasty* 1999;14:375-379.

13. Campbell MD, Duffy GP, Trousdale RT: Femoral component failure in hybrid total knee arthroplasty. *Clin Orthop* 1998;356:58-65.

14. Schmalzried TP, Guttmann D, Grecula M, Amstutz HC: The relationship between the design, position, and articular wear of acetabular components inserted without cement and the development of pelvic osteolysis. *J Bone Joint Surg Am* 1994;76:677-688.

15. Engh GA, Koralewicz LM, Pereles TR: Clinical results of modular polyethylene insert exchange with retention of total knee arthroplasty components. *J Bone Joint Surg Am* 2000;82:516-523.

16. Shaw JA: Angled bearing inserts in total knee arthroplasty: A brief technical note. *J Arthroplasty* 1992;7:211-216.

17. Engh GA, Rao A, Ammeen DJ, Sychterz CJ: Abstract: Tibial baseplate wear: A major source of wear debris with contemporary modular knee implants. *Proceedings of the American Academy of Orthopaedic Surgeons 67th Annual Meeting*, Orlando, FL. Rosemont, IL, American Academy of Orthopaedic Surgeons, 2000, p 283.

18. Furman BD, Schmieg JJ, Bhattacharyya S, Li S: Assessment of backside polyethylene wear in three different metal backed total knee designs. *Trans Orthop Res Soc* 1999;24:149.

19. Engh GA, Parks NL, Ammeen DJ: Tibial osteolysis in cementless total knee arthroplasty: A review of 25 cases treated with and without tibial component revision. *Clin Orthop* 1994; 309:33-43.

20. Ghazavi MT, Stockley I, Yee G, Davis A, Gross AE: Reconstruction of massive bone defects with allograft in revision total knee arthroplasty. *J Bone Joint Surg Am* 1997;79:17-25.

21. Engh GA, Herzwurm PJ, Parks NL: Treatment of major defects of bone with bulk allografts and stemmed components during total knee arthroplasty. *J Bone Joint Surg Am* 1997;79: 1030-1039.

22. Rand JA, Chao EY, Stauffer RN: Kinematic rotating-hinge total knee arthroplasty. *J Bone Joint Surg Am* 1987;69:489-497.

23. Shaw JA, Balcom W, Greer RB III: Total knee arthroplasty using the kinematic rotating hinge prosthesis. *Orthopedics* 1989;12:647-654.

40

Ligament Instability in Total Knee Arthroplasty

Michael A. Kelly, MD

Satisfactory stability of soft tissue is critical to the clinical success of a total knee arthroplasty (TKA). Instability in TKA may be broadly classified into extension and flexion instabilities; the incidence varies in recent reports[1-5] (Fig. 1). Clinical presentation of the unstable TKA may vary accordingly and may be influenced by the design of the individual prosthesis. With this is mind, it should be noted that a posterior cruciate ligament (PCL) substituting prosthesis may provide some stability to the knee in flexion, but would provide no prosthetic stability to varus/valgus ligament laxity. A constrained condylar-type implant will provide both flexion as well as varus/valgus stabilizing effects.

Extension instability following TKA can be classified into symmetric and asymmetric extension instability.[3,6] Symmetric instability occurs when the size of the extension gap exceeds the thickness of prosthetic components. An excessive tibial resection will affect both flexion and extension gaps and can be successfully managed with a thicker tibial polyethylene. Excessive femoral bone resection is a more serious problem to correct. The proper solution is to use distal femoral augments to restore bone loss, maintain the correct joint line position, and fill the extension space. Modular knee systems provide such augments as well as a variety of intramedullary stems to augment femoral fixation in this situation. Knees with excessive ligament length, which makes soft-tissue balance difficult, may present infrequently. If this condition is suspected preoperatively, for example, as in genu recurvatum, initial underresection of the distal femur may assist in ligament balancing. The preferred solution intraoperatively is to augment the distal femur when possible. Although a thicker tibial polyethylene may resolve the instability, it will lead to the deleterious effects of proximal migration of the joint line, and possibly patella baja.[7]

The author or the departments with which he is affiliated have received something of value from a commercial or other party related directly or indirectly to the subject of this chapter.

Asymmetric extension instability, which is much more common than symmetric extension instability, is associated with soft-tissue release that is insufficient to correct the associated angular deformity in the arthritic knee.[3] Valgus deformity may require lateral soft-tissue release to restore proper alignment and stability to the TKA.[6] Various soft-tissue release patterns are described in the literature, and most surgeons accept very little medial laxity for stabilization of these knees.[6,8] Varus deformity requires a medial release, and most surgeons will accept a small amount of lateral laxity and anticipate some lateral tightening over time.[9] Excessive ligament releases leading to instability may occur but fortunately have been rare. There may be occasional situations associated with severe angular deformity, particularly valgus deformity, whereby soft-tissue balance cannot be achieved. Suitable solutions are to consider a prosthesis with greater constraint or possibly ligament tightening techniques as described by Krackow.[10]

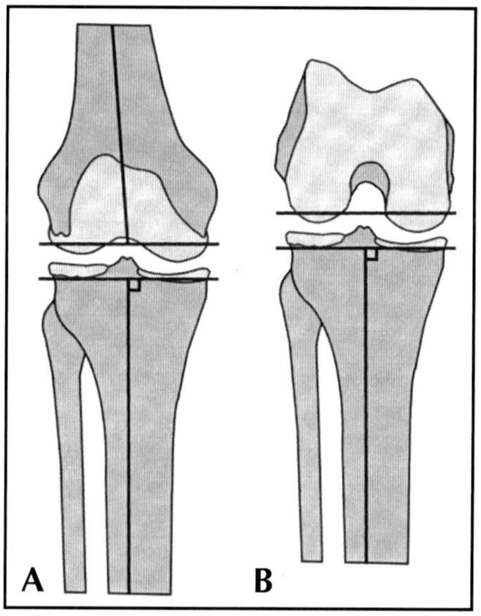

Fig. 1 A, Extension gap. Distal femoral and proximal tibial resection. **B,** Flexion gap. Posterior femoral and proximal tibial resection.

Bone loss associated with angular deformity should not lead to ligament instability. The bone defect may be managed with cement, bone graft, or prosthetic substitution. The ligament balancing principles of TKA remain the same. A unique situation that may occur, intraoperatively and lead to asymmetric instability is iatrogenic injury to the superficial medial collateral ligament (MCL). Repair of the MCL is rarely successful, and a constrained condylar knee is often indicated. Intramedullary stems

Table 1
Factors leading to flexion instability of TKA

Undersized femoral component
Mismanagement of flexion contracture
Malrotation of the femoral component
PCL laxity in cruciate-retaining TKA
Rheumatoid arthritis
PCL recession
Polyethylene wear
PCL substituting designs
Cam-spine interaction (in posterior stabilized TKA design)

should be used on both the femoral and tibial sides whenever a constrained condylar knee is selected.

Flexion instability of TKA is more common than extension instability and an increased incidence over the past decade has been noted.[1-4] This condition occurs when the flexion space is too large for the tibial component. There are a number of factors that may lead to this condition, and the etiology may be multifactorial (Table 1). An undersized femoral component may lead to an excessive flexion gap. Using an anterior femoral referencing surgical technique in this situation will lead to excessive posterior femoral condylar bone resection and an enlarged flexion gap. This result was not uncommon with the size limitations of early TKA designs and was managed with additional distal femoral bone resection to equalize the extension gap. The preferred solution today is to use a posterior referencing system, avoiding excessive posterior femur resection and inclining the distal femoral cut to 3° of flexion to avoid anterior femoral notching when between sizes.

Mismanagement of a flexion contracture may lead to an unstable TKA in flexion. It is tempting to resolve an existing flexion contracture at the time of prosthetic trial components by switching to a thinner tibial polyethylene. Although this action will eliminate the flexion contracture, it may lead to instability of the TKA in flexion. The solution is the correct management of the flexion contracture to create equal flexion and extension gaps. Any posterior femoral osteophytes should be removed and the posterior capsule released carefully off the femur. If a flexion contracture persists, additional distal femoral bone should be resected to balance the gaps.

Malrotation of the femoral component may lead to an asymmetric flexion gap and result in flexion stability.[11] Proper femoral component rotation may be achieved using the transepicondylar axis or the anteroposterior axis of the femur, as described by Anouchi and associates,[11] as a surgical reference. Secondary anatomic landmarks and ligament tension may be used to ensure symmetric ligament stability in flexion and proper femoral component rotation.[3]

Overrelease of the valgus knee may lead to excessive lateral laxity in flexion with subsequent flexion instability. This has been reported to lead to occasional cases of posterior dislocation of PCL-substituting knees, especially in patients who regain excellent knee flexion.[6] A titrated lateral soft-tissue release that achieves proper ligament balance laterally and medially in flexion and extension should be used. There is no consensus in the literature regarding lateral soft-tissue release to correct a valgus deformity.[6,8] The posterolateral capsule and iliotibial band can be released using a "pie crusting" surgical technique. Further release of the lateral collateral ligament may be needed if the deformity is significant. The popliteus tendon is preserved, when possible, to assist in posterolateral flexion stability. This is particularly important with PCL-substituting knees.

Recently, PCL release or recession has been recommended in PCL-retaining knee designs to properly balance the tension of PCL. Some surgeons have recommended this release at the tibial insertion of the PCL, while authors advocate selective PCL release from the femur. This is to avoid excessive tightness of the PCL, which may lead to a stiff, painful TKA and the early onset of articular polyethylene wear. Excessive release may lead to increased flexion laxity in these knees. Additionally, late rupture of the PCL may occur, leading to flexion instability. Posterior articular polyethylene wear associated with flat-on-flat cruciate tibial designs may lead to subtle flexion instability, as well.

Waslewski and associates[12] reported on early PCL deficiency leading to flexion instability. Patients typically presented with persistent effusions, anterior knee pain, and instability episodes with activities of daily living. Examination revealed an effusion, posterior sag, positive quadriceps active test, and a visible anterior translation of the tibia on the femur while extending the leg from a seated 90° flexed position. Laskin and O'Flynn[13] noted an increased incidence of posterior instability and recurvatum in patients with rheumatoid arthritis in using a PCL-retaining TKA design. Typically, nonsurgical treatment has been unsuccessful in these cases.[14] Revision TKA using a thicker tibial polyethylene may be used. However, Pagnano and associates[5] reported a revision operation that focuses on balancing the flexion/extension spaces in conjunction with a posterior stabilized knee design. They noted marked improvement in 19 of 22 revision TKAs using these principles.

PCL-substituting designs may provide some flexion stability in TKA. However, different prosthetic designs have different spine and cam mechanisms producing such stability. These mechanisms provide different degrees of "jump distances" in flexion to assist in stabilizing the TKA, and surgeons should be aware of these variations as they balance these knees in flexion.

The clinical manifestations of flexion instability in substituting designs may be dramatic and present with a posterior dislocation.[3,15,16] Early dislocation may be successfully managed with closed reduction and a period of bracing. Activity precautions limiting deep flexion or figure-of-4 positions are recommended. Recurrent prosthetic dislocation will require revision to a thicker tibial component or to a constrained condylar knee.

In summary, soft-tissue balance is critical to a successful total knee arthroplasty. The flexion and extension gaps should be symmetrically balanced. In the setting of angular deformity, soft-tissue releases to create a rectangular soft-tissue gap in flexion and extension rather than a trapezoidal, poorly balanced gap may be necessary. A PCL-substituting TKA may provide some knee stability in flexion but provides no medial-lateral stabilizing effects. A constrained condylar design may be necessary to provide such stability in rare occasions.

References

1. Dejour D, Deschamps G, Garotta L, Dejour H: Laxity in posterior cruciate sparing and posterior stabilized total knee protheses. *Clin Orthop* 1999;364:182-204.
2. Dorr LD, Scrocki JH: Mechanisms of failure of total knee arthroplasty, in Scott WN (ed): *The Knee*. St. Louis, MO, Mosby Yearbook, 1994.
3. Insall JN: Complications in total knee arthroplasty, in Insall JN, Windsor RE, Scott WN, Kelly MA, Aglietti P (eds): *Surgery of the Knee*, ed 2. New York, NY, Churchill Livingstone, 1993, pp 891-934.
4. Lonner JH, Siliski JM, Scott RD: Prodromes of failure in total knee arthroplasty. *J Arthroplasty* 1999;14:488-492.
5. Pagnano MW, Hanssen AD, Lewallen DG, Stuart MJ: Flexion instability after primary posterior cruciate retaining total knee arthroplasty. *Clin Orthop* 1998;356:39-46.
6. Insall JN: Surgical techniques and instrumentation in total knee arthroplasty, in Insall JN, Windsor RE, Scott WN, Kelly MA, Aglietti P (eds): *Surgery of the Knee*, ed 2. New York, NY, Churchill Livingstone, 1993, pp 739-804.
7. Martin JW, Whiteside LA: The influence of joint line position on knee stability after condylar knee arthroplasty. *Clin Orthop* 1990; 259:146-156.
8. Buechel FF: A sequential three-step lateral release for correcting fixed valgus knee deformities during total knee arthroplasty. *Clin Orthop* 1990;260:170-175.
9. Laskin RS, Schob CJ: Medial capsular recession for severe varus deformities. *J Arthroplasty* 1987;2:313-316.
10. Krackow KA: Deformity, in *The Technique of Total Knee Arthroplasty*. Baltimore, MD, CV Mosby, 1990.
11. Anouchi YS, Whiteside LA, Kaiser AD, Milliano MT: The effects of axial rotational alignment of the femoral component on knee stability and patellar tracking in total knee arthroplasty demonstrated on autopsy specimens. *Clin Orthop* 1993;287:170-177.
12. Waslewski GL, Marson BM, Benjamin JB: Early, incapacitating instability of posterior cruciate ligament-retaining total knee arthroplasty. *J Arthroplasty* 1998;13:763-767.
13. Laskin RS, O'Flynn HM: Total knee replacement with posterior cruciate ligament retention in rheumatoid arthritis: Problems and complications. *Clin Orthop* 1997;345:24-28.
14. Peters CL, Hennessey R, Barden R, Galante JO, Rosenberg AG: Revision TKA with cemented posterior stabilized or constrained condylar prostheses: A minimum 3 year and average 5 year follow-up. *J Arthroplasty* 1997;12:896-903.
15. Galiant BJ, Vernace JV, Booth RE Jr, Rothman RH: Dislocation of the posterior stabilized total knee arthroplasty: A report of two cases. *J Arthroplasty* 1988;3:363-367.
16. Gebhard JS, Kilgus DJ: Dislocation of a posterior stabilized total knee prosthesis: A report of two cases. *Clin Orthop* 1990;254:225-229.

41

Patellofemoral Complications Following Total Knee Arthroplasty

Michael A. Kelly, MD

Introduction

The incidence of patellofemoral complications following total knee arthroplasty (TKA) has been reported as being between 2% and 10%.[1-4] Lynch and associates[3] evaluated 281 patients with TKAs at 6 years' follow-up, noting a 10% incidence of extensor mechanism complications. Complications included quadriceps and patellar-tendon rupture, patellar fracture, patellar subluxation, patellar pain, and malrotated patella. Brick and Scott[1] reported in 1988 that more than 50% of revision TKAs were attributed to patellofemoral complications. This report led to reevaluation of routine patellar resurfacing with TKA. The literature remains divided regarding this issue, with several authors suggesting selected patellar resurfacing to avoid the associated complications.[5-7]

Early TKA designs did not include patellofemoral resurfacing. Residual patellofemoral symptoms were noted in up to 30% of patients, prompting design modifications.[8] Scuderi and associates[8] noted an improved quality of arthroplasty with TKA designs allowing for patellofemoral resurfacing. However, associated with this improved clinical success was a variety of extensor mechanism complications. Most of these complications were related to errors in surgical technique and component design issues. Recent improvements in surgical technique and instrumentation as well as in patellofemoral component design have led to an overall decreased incidence of extensor mechanism complications. This chapter will review patellar fractures, patellofemoral instability, extensor mechanism rupture, patellar component failure, and soft tissue impingement syndromes.

The author or the departments with which he is affiliated have received something of value from a commercial or other party related directly or indirectly to the subject of this chapter.

Patellar Fractures

The incidence of patellar fractures following TKA varies from 0 to 21%. Various causative factors have been attributed to these fractures (Table 1). Excessively thin or thick patellae have been associated with patellar fractures. Reuben and associates[9] reported increased patellar strains with residual patellar bone less than 15 mm thick, suggesting a possible risk of fracture. However, this has not been reported clinically, with good clinical success noted by Greenfield and associates[10] with bony patellar remnants typically 12- to 13-mm thick. Excessively large femoral components may overstuff the patellofemoral compartment, increasing the risk of patellar fracture (Table 1).

The patella has a complex extraosseous and intraosseous blood supply.[11] Avascularity of the patella may occur during a routine paramedian surgical approach combined with a lateral release, contributing to an increased incidence of patellar fracture. Correct patellar tracking is critical to a successful TKA, with maltracking of the patella possibly leading to a shear-type patellar fracture (Fig. 1). The importance of preserving the superior lateral geniculate artery during the lateral release remains controversial,[4,12] although I continue to preserve this vessel when possible.

Table 1
Patellar Fractures

Mechanical compromise secondary in improper patellar resection, peg fixation, and cementation
Patellar maltracking
Avascularity of the patella
Prosthetic design
Obesity
Increased knee flexion
Excessive patient activity
Trauma

Large central patellar component fixation lugs have been associated with an increased incidence of patellar fracture. Most recent designs have used three smaller, peripheral fixation lugs to minimize this risk.

Goldberg and associates[13] have reported on patellar fracture patterns and their influence on clinical outcome. Patellar fractures that do not involve loose patellar components, disruption of the extensor mechanism, or major

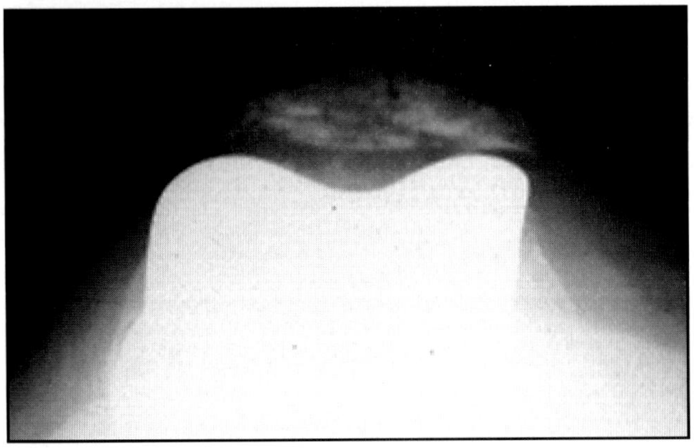

Fig. 1 Horizontal shear-type patellar fracture secondary to maltracking of the patella.

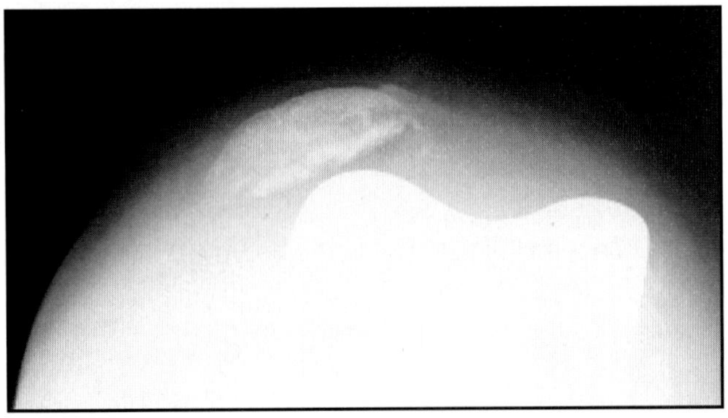

Fig. 2 Dislocating patella following TKA.

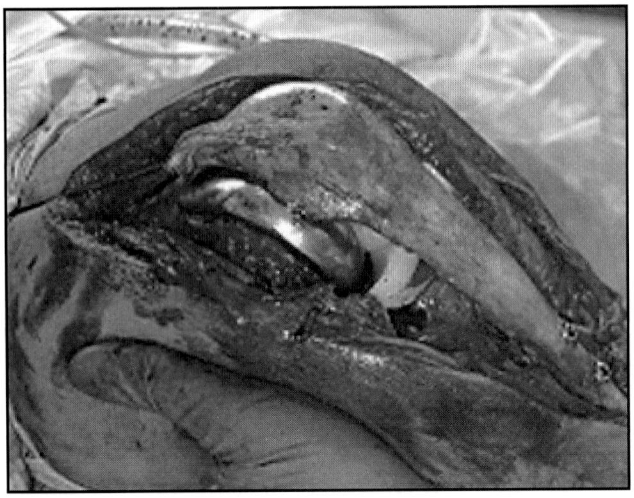

Fig. 3 Rupture of the patellar tendon following TKA with patella alta.

component malalignment may be treated nonsurgically with good clinical success.[13-15] Surgical treatment of patellar fractures is associated with poor results and a high complication rate.[8,13,14] Surgery typically is reserved for fractures associated with implant loosening or displaced patellar fractures with significant extensor lag.[8] Elaborate open reduction and internal fixation techniques should be avoided. Simple patellar cerclage or a possible partial patellectomy with extensor mechanism repair may be more successful alternatives. A loose component may be removed and the patella resurfaced if 10 to 12 mm of bone remains. If not, a patelloplasty is preferred.

Patellofemoral Instability

The incidence of symptomatic patellar instability after TKA has been reported to range from 1% to 20%[3,16-18] (Fig. 2). Most instances are secondary to errors in surgical technique and largely avoidable. Less frequent causes include trauma and specific prosthetic design issues. Patellofemoral subluxation is more common than frank dislocation, and nonsurgical treatment typically is unsuccessful.

Reoperation for patellar instability is reported to be 1%, and it is critical to ascertain the specific etiology of maltracking in determining the surgical treatment. Radiographic evaluation should include patellofemoral axial views. A modified Merchant view with 30° of knee flexion is preferred. CT may be useful in determining possible malrotation of the femoral component using the transepicondylar axis as the anatomic landmark for proper rotation.

In the case of symptomatic patellar subluxation with normally aligned prosthetic components, a lateral retinacular release may be sufficient. A proximal patellar realignment for recurrent patellar subluxation-dislocation secondary to quadriceps imbalance is preferred.[8] Others have favored a distal realignment to correct maltracking of the patella.[19] Whiteside[19] advocates a distal realignment with a medial transfer of the medial portion of the patellar tendon. An increased incidence of wound complications and patellar tendon rupture has been reported with distal realignment procedures.[20] If significant prosthetic component malalignment is determined to be the etiology of the patellofemoral instability, revision of the components is the preferred solution. Internal malrotation of the femoral or tibial component is the more common surgical error.

Extensor Mechanism Rupture

Extensor mechanism rupture is a devastating complication of TKA. Fortunately this occurs infrequently, with rupture of the patellar tendon more common than rupture of the quadriceps[3] (Fig. 3). The etiology of failure is multifactorial, often including surgical technique. Although nonsurgical treatment has been reported, most ruptures require surgery.

Regardless of surgical technique, repair of patellar tendon ruptures often is associated with poor clinical results and persistent extensor lag. Clinical results of acute repairs are superior to those of chronic repairs, with Cadambi and Engh[21] demonstrating the benefits of augmenting the surgical repair with the semitendinosus tendon. Chronic patellar tendon rupture with significant extensor lag may be managed with extensor mechanism allograft[22] (Fig. 4). This technique is quite useful in restoring effective extensor strength. However, this surgery is complex, and the patient should be counseled regarding the limited goals of such a procedure. Perhaps nowhere in the surgical technique of TKA is prevention more critical than in preserving the integrity of the patellar tendon.

Patellar Component Failure

Most present-day TKA designs incorporate an all-polyethylene patellar component with several peripheral lugs for cement fixation. These components have performed quite well, with infrequent loosening (less than 2%).[2] Virtually all of these patellar components demonstrate some cold flow polyethylene deformation. However, no significant clinical consequences have been observed with available long-term follow-up.[8]

Multiple factors have been associated with patellar component failure, including oversizing the femoral component, increased thickness of the patellar implant composite, increased knee flexion, and patient activity as well as patient obesity. Metal-backed patellar designs were introduced in the 1980s. Theoretically the advantage of these designs was to minimize polyethylene deformity, allowing for more uniform load distribution and cementless fixation. However, the failure rate of these designs far exceeded that of the cemented all-polyethylene patellar components.[1,23-26]

Failure modes of metal-backed patellar components include poor ingrowth into porous designs with subsequent loosening, polyethylene wear and fracture, peg failure secondary to high shear forces, dissociation of both the polyethylene and the metal, and component fracture.[23-26] Often these modes of failure expose the femoral component to the metal of the patellar component with secondary metal-on-metal wear and rapid global joint failure. In these situations, revision of all knee components may be necessary.

Berry and Rand[27] have reported the difficulties associated with isolated patellar revision surgery, noting a significant complication rate. Management options vary from observation to surgical intervention. Revision of a loose patellar component may be performed if adequate bone stock remains. If the remaining patellar bone is inadequate for resurfacing (less than 10-mm thick), either a patelloplasty preserving the existing bone or a formal patellectomy may be performed.[8]

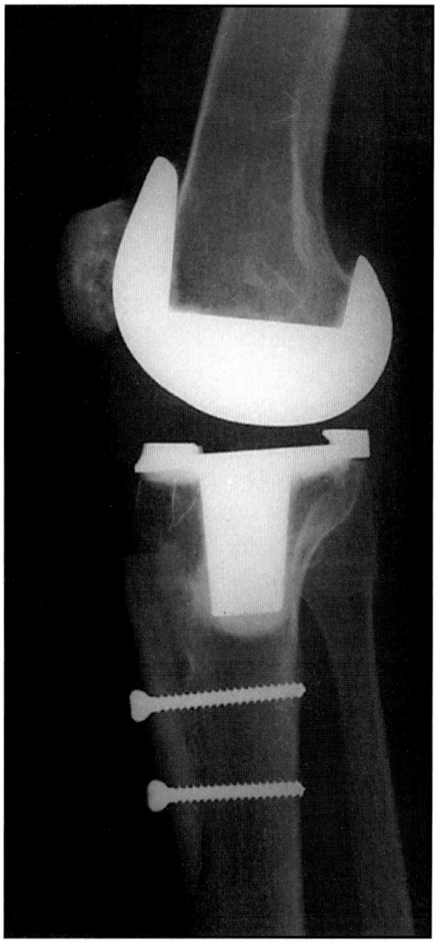

Fig. 4 Extensor mechanism allograft used in a patient with chronic patellar tendon rupture and extensor lag.

Soft-Tissue Impingement

A variety of soft-tissue impingement syndromes occurring after TKA has been reported. The patellar clunk is the most significant of these syndromes, causing a painful clunking sensation in the patellofemoral compartment with active knee extension from 60° to 30°.[8] The pathology involves the formation of a fibrous nodule on the undersurface of the distal quadriceps. This nodule becomes entrapped between the patellar component and the underlying femoral component, causing pain. The patellar clunk has been more frequent in posterior cruciate ligament–substituting designs. However, recent femoral design changes, with deepening and elongation of the femoral trochlea as well as excision of the synovium on the undersurface of the quadriceps at the initial surgery, have markedly reduced the incidence of this problem.[2]

If the soft-tissue impingement is diagnosed early, an exercise program with repetitive knee flexion, such as riding a stationary bicycle, may resolve the problem. Persistent symptoms may be managed successfully with arthroscopic debridement, as reported by Diduch and associates.[28] Superior arthroscopic portals and prophylactic perioperative antibiotics should be used. Recurrence of the soft-tissue nodule is uncommon.

Summary

Patellofemoral complications following TKA are largely avoided with proper surgical technique. A variety of surgical exposures, including the midvastus and subvastus approach, has resulted in good clinical success. It is critical to maintain the integrity of the extensor mechanism. The surgeon should be prepared to use specific surgical techniques to assist in exposing the stiff knee and to avoid injury to the patellar tendon. These techniques may include the quadriceps snip, modified V-Y quadriceps turndown, and tibial tubercle osteotomy. When tibial tubercle osteotomy is necessary, the technique of Whiteside,[19] using wire fixation of the osteotomy, is preferred.

Selection of the proper femoral component size is important. In general, the surgeon should avoid selecting an excessively large femoral component and overstuffing the patellofemoral compartment. Similarly, the surgeon should restore the patella-implant composite to the original patellar thickness or slightly less when possible. Femoral component positioning is critical to proper patellofemoral tracking. The femoral component rotation should be aligned with the transepicondylar axis of the femur.[29] The anteroposterior axis of the femur as described by Whiteside and Arima[30] is a useful secondary landmark to ensure proper femoral component placement. A slightly lateral femoral component position is favored when possible to further facilitate proper patellar tracking.

Proper rotation of the tibial component is important. A variety of surgical techniques and anatomic landmarks may be used to establish proper tibial component rotation. The surgeon must avoid internal rotation of the tibial component leading to an increased quadriceps angle and lateral maltracking of the patella.

The patellar osteotomy may be performed using either a calibrated cutting system or an eyeball technique. The surgeon should avoid an oblique osteotomy placing the patellar component on the lateral facet. A cemented all-polyethylene component placed in a medialized position to improve patellar tacking is preferred.[31] Proper soft-tissue tension may require a lateral retinacular release in a small percentage of cases. The superior lateral genicular artery is preserved when possible with the release. Proper patellofemoral tracking must be obtained at the time of the primary TKA.

The diagnosis and treatment of the more frequent complications of the extensor mechanism following TKA have been discussed. Although these complications may be successfully treated, most may be largely avoided with proper surgical technique and prosthetic component design.

References

1. Brick GW, Scott RD: The patellofemoral component of total knee arthroplasty. *Clin Orthop* 1988;231:163-178.
2. Healy WL, Wasilewski SA, Takei R, Oberlander M: Patellofemoral complications following total knee arthroplasty: Correlation with implant design and patient risk factors. *J Arthroplasty* 1995;10:197-201.
3. Lynch AF, Rorabeck CH, Bourne RB: Extensor mechanism complications following total knee arthroplasty. *J Arthroplasty* 1987;2:135-140.
4. Scuderi G, Scharf SC, Meltzer LP, Scott WN: The relationship of lateral releases to patella viability in total knee arthroplasty. *J Arthroplasty* 1987;2:209-214.
5. Barrack RL, Wolfe MW, Waldman DA, Milicic M, Bertot AJ, Myers L: Resurfacing of the patella in total knee arthroplasty: A prospective, randomized, double-blind study. *J Bone Joint Surg Am* 1997:79:1121-1131.
6. Boyd AD Jr, Ewald FC, Thomas WH, Poss R, Sledge CB: Long-term complications after yotal knee arthroplasty with or without resurfacing of the patella. *J Bone Joint Surg Am* 1993;75:674-681.
7. Picetti GD III, McGann WA, Welch RB: The patellofemoral joint after total knee arthroplasty without patellar resurfacing. *J Bone Joint Surg Am* 1990;72:1379-1382.
8. Scuderi GR, Insall JN, Scott WN: Patellofemoral pain after total knee arthroplasty. *J Am Acad Orthop Surg* 1994;2:239-246.
9. Reuben JD, McDonald CL, Woodard PL, Hennington LJ: Effect of patella thickness on patella strain following total knee arthroplasty. *J Arthroplasty* 1991;6:251-258.
10. Greenfield MA, Insall JN, Case GC, Kelly MA: Instrumentation of the patellar osteotomy in total knee arthroplasty: The relationship of patellar thickness and lateral retinacular release. *Am J Knee Surg* 1996;9:129-132.
11. Brick GW, Scott RD: Blood supply to the patella: Significance in total knee arthroplasty. *J Arthroplasty* 1988;4(suppl):S75-S79.
12. Ritter MA, Herbst SA, Keating EM, Faris PM, Meding JB: Patellofemoral complications following total knee arthroplasty: Effect of a lateral release and sacrifice of the superior lateral geniculate artery. *J Arthroplasty* 1996;11: 368-372.
13. Goldberg VM, Figgie HE III, Inglis AE; et al: Patellar fracture type and prognosis in condylar total knee arthroplasty. *Clin Orthop* 1988;236:115-122.
14. Hozack WJ, Goll SR, Lotke PA, Rothman RH, Booth RE Jr: The treatment of patellar fractures after total knee arthroplasty. *Clin Orthop* 1988;236:123-127.
15. Tria AJ Jr, Harwood DA, Alicea JA, Cody RP: Patellar fractures in posterior stabilized knee arthroplasties. *Clin Orthop* 1994;299:131-138.
16. Grace JN, Rand JA: Patellar instability after total knee arthroplasty. *Clin Orthop* 1988;237:184-189.
17. Kirk P, Rorabeck CH, Bourne RB, Burkart B, Nott L: Management of recurrent dislocation of the patella following total knee arthroplasty. *J Arthroplasty* 1992;7:229-233.
18. Merkow RL, Soudry M, Insall JN: Patellar dislocation following total knee replacement. *J Bone Joint Surg Am* 1985;67:1321-1327.
19. Whiteside LA: Distal realignment of the patellar tendon to correct abnormal patellar tracking. *Clin Orthop* 1997;344:284-289.
20. Rand JA, Morrey BF, Bryan RS: Patellar tendon rupture after total knee arthroplasty. *Clin Orthop* 1989;244:233-238.
21. Cadambi A, Engh GA: Use of a semitendinosus tendon antogenous graft for rupture of the patellar ligament after total knee arthroplasty: A report of seven cases. *J Bone Joint Surg Am* 1992;74:974-979.
22. Emerson RH Jr, Head WC, Malinin TI: Reconstruction of patellar tendon rupture after total knee arthroplasty with an extensor mechanism allograft. *Clin Orthop* 1990;260:154-161.
23. Bayley JC, Scott RD, Ewald FC, Holmes GB Jr: Failure of the metal-backed patellar component after total knee replacement. *J Bone Joint Surg Am* 1988;70:668-674.
24. Dennis DA: Removal of well-fixed cementless metal-backed patellar components. *J Arthroplasty* 1992;7:217-220.
25. Rosenberg AG, Andriacchi TP, Barden R, Galante JO: Patellar component failure in cementless total knee arthroplasty. *Clin Orthop* 1988;236:106-114.

26. Stulberg SD, Stulberg BN, Hamati Y, Tsao A: Failure mechanisms of metal-backed patellar components. *Clin Orthop* 1988;236:88-105.

27. Berry DJ, Rand JA: Isolated patellar component revision of total knee arthroplasty. *Clin Orthop* 1993;286:110-115.

28. Diduch DR, Scuderi GR, Scott WN, Insall JN, Kelly MA: The efficacy of arthroscopy following total knee replacement. *Arthroscopy* 1997;13:166-171.

29. Poilvache PL, Insall JN, Scuderi GR, Font-Rodriguez DE: Rotational landmarks and sizing of the distal femur in total knee arthroplasty. *Clin Orthop* 1996;331:35-46.

30. Whiteside LA, Arima J: The anteroposterior axis for femoral rotational alignment in valgus total knee arthroplasty. *Clin Orthop* 1995; 321:168-172.

31. Hofmann AA, Tkach TK, Evanich CJ, Camargo MP, Zhang, Y: Patellar component medialization in total knee arthroplasty. *J Arthroplasty* 1997;12:155-160.

42

Infection After Total Knee Arthroplasty

Robert T. Trousdale, MD
Arlen D. Hanssen, MD

Introduction

Over the past 25 years, total knee arthroplasty (TKA) has become an accepted and successful means to treat end-stage knee arthritis. The majority of the implants remain intact and function well for many years. Of all the complications that can occur after a TKA, infection remains one of the most dreaded and difficult to manage.[1-3] Fortunately, with improved patient selection and surgical techniques and proper medical management, infections after TKA are relatively rare.[4-6] The outcome of an infected TKA is more optimistic now than in the 1970s.[7]

Treatment goals of the infected TKA include alleviation of pain, maintenance of a functional extremity, and in most cases, elimination of the infection. In general, there are six basic management options for treatment of an infected TKA: (1) antibiotic suppression; (2) surgical débridement with prosthesis retention; (3) resection arthroplasty: (4) arthrodesis; (5) reinsertion of another prosthesis (immediate exchange or delayed); and (6) amputation.[8]

This chapter will describe our current approach to the management of a patient with an infected knee prosthesis, first discussing the decision variables that determine selection of the various treatment options.

Table 1
Decision variables

Is the infection superficial or deep?
How long has the infection been present?
What are the host factors that may affect treatment outcome?
What is the status of the extensor mechanism and soft tissues about the knees?
Is the implant loose?
What is the infecting organism?
What are the patient's expectations?
What are the surgeon's expectations and available resources to treat the infection?

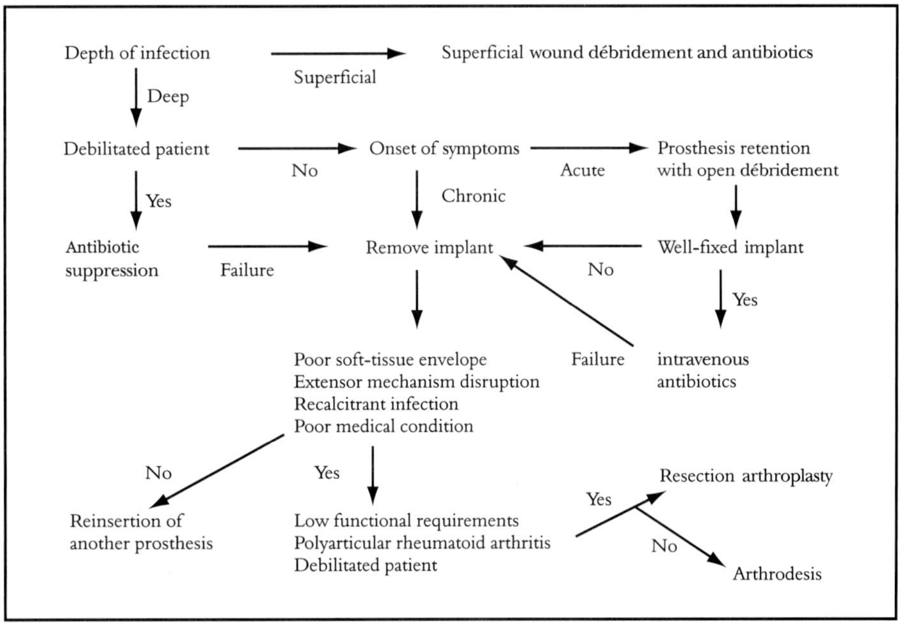

Fig. 1 Treatment algorithm for infection after TKA. (Reproduced with permission from Hanssen AD: Management of the infected total knee arthroplasty, in Engh GA, Rorabeck CH (eds): *Revision Total Knee Arthroplasty.* Baltimore, MD, Williams & Wilkins, 1997, pp 372-393.)

Decision Variables and Treatment Options

Once the diagnosis of a deep periprosthetic infection has been made, there are several questions that must be asked before treatment is begun.[9-22] These questions are outlined in Table 1. Considering these variables, the suggested treatment algorithm is shown in Figure 1.

Antibiotic Suppression

Antibiotics alone will never completely eliminate a deep periprosthetic infection but can occasionally suppress the infection in selected circumstances. For antibiotic suppression to be successful, the following criteria should be met: the organism must be of low virulence and susceptible to a well-tolerated oral antibiotic, and the prosthesis must be well fixed.

Patients who are potentially good candidates for suppression meet these criteria and have an implant in place that will be difficult to remove (such as a hinged implant or long cemented stems), and/or their medical condition precludes multiple surgeries. Absolute contraindications to antibiotic suppression include the presence of a draining sinus and a loose implant with the presence of a resistant organism. Combined results from several series reveal success in only 21% (63 of 299) of these patients. Many of these series do not comment on the exact inclusion criteria, so it is difficult to state the true success rate of antibiotic suppression if all of the appropriate selection criteria were used.

Débridement and Prosthesis Retention

Débridement may be indicated for the patient who presents either in the early postoperative period or for an acute presentation of an infection around a securely fixed and well-functioning implant.[23] For the patient to be considered a reasonable candidate for débridement and prosthetic retention, the infection should be present for less than 2 to 3 weeks (based on clinical symptoms), the implant well fixed and with no marked bony defects, and the organism susceptible to a well-tolerated antibiotic.[24] The soft-tissue envelope about the knee should also be intact, with no history of prolonged drainage or a sinus tract. Although results of débridement and prosthesis retention are difficult to compare in light of the differing inclusion criteria, combining results from multiple series, overall success has been reported in 29.8% (143 of 480 knees). Timing of the débridement appears to be critical to the success of this technique. Early postoperative infections are more successfully treated with débridement than those that occur by late hematogenous spread. Schoifet and Morrey[25] reported results of débridement and prosthesis retention in 37 infected total knee arthroplasties. All were treated with open débridement and temporary intravenous antibiotics. At an average follow-up of 8.8 years, the overall success rate was extremely poor at 23%. The duration of infection averaged 21 days in successfully treated knees, compared to 36 days in the failures. It was interesting to note that when all the above-described favorable criteria were present, the long-term success rate exceeded 50%. *Staphylococcus aureus* portended a lower success rate in this series, as it was present in only 29% of the successfully treated knees compared with 58% of the failures. Unconstrained knees were also slightly more likely to have a successful outcome than hinged constrained components. The role of arthroscopy, antibiotic pumps, duration of intravenous antibiotic therapy, and number of débridements that are optimal is unknown. Presently we favor open surgical débridement with polyethylene exchange if the tibial tray is modular. Intravenous antibiotics currently are administered for 4 weeks, and the decision whether chronic antibiotic suppression is desirable is made based on the status of the host and virulence of the infecting organism.

Definitive Resection Arthroplasty

Definitive resection arthroplasty involves implant removal without the intention of subsequent reconstruction. This procedure is best reserved for those patients who have minimal ambulatory demands (such as patients with severe polyarticular rheumatoid arthritis) and those with poor tissues and/or insufficient bone stock that preclude reconstruction. Nonambulators find resection arthroplasty tolerable because it allows the patient to sit more readily than does an arthrodesis. Although resection arthroplasty usually achieves successful eradication of the infection, all patients have limited ambulatory capacity and knee instability, and most have some discomfort and require some form of ambulatory aid.

Arthrodesis

Arthodesis remains a viable option for a small subset of patients with an infected TKA. Arthrodesis provides reliable pain relief and excellent stability and has a low risk of reinfection. These advantages are counterbalanced by a leg that is restricted to near-full extension, with the obvious difficulties with certain daily activities. Arthrodesis is reserved for young patients who have high functional demands, isolated single-joint disease, extensor mechanism disruption, poor soft-tissue envelope around the knee requiring soft-tissue reconstruction, and systemic immunocompromised and infecting organisms that are highly resistant to conventional antibiotics. Patients for whom knee fusion is contraindicated include those with ipsilateral ankle or hip disease, bilateral knee disease, contralateral amputation, and severe unreconstructible bone defects.

The ability to obtain a solid fusion is dependent on the type of prior implant that was present, severity of bone deficiency, adequate control of infection, and fusion technique. Union occurs more reliably after a resurfacing TKA than a hinged prosthesis (86% versus 51%). Union also occurs more readily if the infection is eliminated (62% versus 19%). Fusion with an intramedullary rod is more reliable than with external fixation (83% versus 71%) and occurs more commonly with biplanar external fixation than uniplanar external fixation (66% versus 33%).

Potential problems with knee arthrodesis include gait disturbances, limb shortening, nonunion, reinfection, ipsilateral hip fracture, neurovascular injury, pin site problems, and nail breakage or migration. Although intramedullary nails have a more reliable union rate than external fixators, the complication rate is also high, up to 56% of cases in some series.

Amputation

Amputation is an unfortunate possibility for any patient whose TKA becomes infected. However, this procedure is rarely required because alternative salvage techniques are usually successful. The factors that most commonly lead to amputation include multiple revision attempts for chronic infection, use of a hinged prosthesis, severe bone loss, intractable pain, and occasionally life-threatening uncontrollable sepsis. Amputation as a salvage for most patients with an infected TKA is a debilitating procedure. In one series of 23 patients treated with above-knee amputation for a failed TKA, only 7 were ambulatory. Twenty of the 23 patients used a wheelchair part of the day and 55% were confined to the wheelchair.

Reimplantation

The preferred treatment method for most patients with an infected TKA is reimplantation after a thorough débridement and administration of appropriate antibiotics.[26-28] Reimplantation provides the best opportunity for improved functional outcome, but it is also complicated by a higher reinfection rate than those of some other salvage procedures (arthrodesis, resection, or amputation). Contraindications for reimplantation include persistent infection, medical conditions preventing multiple reconstructive procedures, and a severely immunocompromised host. Relative contraindications for reimplantation include extensor mechanism disruption, poor bone stock, and a poor soft-tissue envelope about the knee.

Controversial treatment variables include the optimal time delay from removal of the infected implant to reimplantation; the duration and route of antibiotic therapy; the ideal role of antibiotic delivery systems; the efficacy of antibiotic impregnated bone cement used at the time of revision surgery; optimal fixation of the reimplanted knee (cement, uncemented, or hybrid); role of spacers or antibiotic-loaded prostheses to improve functional outcome; and optimal use of bone graft in the face of previous infection.

These treatment variables are extremely difficult to assess in view of the literature because of the relatively small number of patients with multiple treatment variables present.

The optimal delay between resection to reimplantation remains controversial. Reinsertion of a new prosthesis can be performed as a direct exchange or after a variable time delay. Direct exchange is attractive because morbidity is limited, thus possibly improving the overall functional result. Success with direct exchange seems to be dependent on the presence of a gram-positive infection, use of antibiotic-impregnated cement for fixation of the new prosthesis, and prolonged use of intravenous antibiotics after reimplantation. Unfortunately, direct exchange is not as successful in eradicating infection as delayed reimplantation. Furthermore, the salvage of a knee in which reimplantation has failed secondary to reinfection is extremely difficult. For that reason, most surgeons favor the two-stage protocol initially described by Insall and associates.[29] This protocol involves complete soft-tissue débridement with removal of all foreign material, including the prosthesis and cement; 4 to 6 weeks of appropriate dosed intravenous antibiotics; and then reimplantation of a new prosthesis in a delayed fashion.

The delivery of antibiotics can be done by intravenous routes, orally, or locally with antibiotic-impregnated cement, biodegradable antibiotic delivery systems, or antibiotic pumps. The efficacy of oral antibiotics alone has not been formally evaluated in the treatment of an infected TKA. Although the administration of intravenous antibiotics for 3 to 6 weeks prior to the insertion of a new implant has proved to be very successful, no studies have been done allowing comparison of various time courses of intravenous antibiotics. Local antibiotics can be delivered in the form of antibiotic-impregnated cement in the form of beads, spacer blocks, or in the shape of a prosthesis. Although local antibiotic delivery is an attractive concept, their efficacy has not been conclusively demonstrated. Most reports have used antibiotic ratios of only 1 g of antibiotic per batch of bone cement; currently, most surgeons are using much higher dosage ratios (4 to 6 g of antibiotics for a 40-g batch of cement). The efficacy of these dosages has not yet been determined.

The use of antibiotic-impregnated cement for prosthesis fixation at the time of reimplantation does appear to be effective. Antibiotic ratios at the time of reinsertion should be 1 g per patch of cement so as not to compromise the cement's integrity. Some interesting trends are noted when reviewing the available literature concerning the effect of antibiotic cement and delayed reimplantation on reinfection rates (Fig. 2). It appears early reimplantation without antibiotic cement is less successful than direct exchange with antibiotic cement, which is less effective than any technique performed with a two-stage technique. The most successful way to alleviate infection appears to be a two-stage technique with antibiotic spacers, with antibiotic

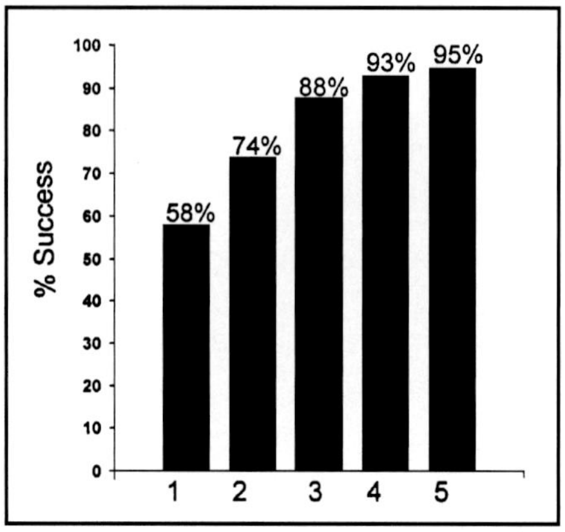

Fig. 2 Bar graph illustrating the effect of antibiotic-impregnated cement and timing of reconstruction for the treatment of the infected TKA. 1 = early reimplantation and no antibiotic-impregnated polymethylmethacrylate (Ab-PMMA); 2 = direct-exchange technique with Ab-PMMA; 3 = two-stage exchange technique and no Ab-PMMA; 4 = two-stage exchange technique with Ab-PMMA only for prosthesis fixation; 5 = two-stage exchange technique with Ab-PMMA for prosthesis fixation and for local antibiotic delivery with beads or spacers.

cement used at the time of component reinsertion.

The effects of delay between insertion and reimplantation on optimal functional outcome has not been clearly established. Periarticular scarring progressively worsens with the increased time delay between resection and reimplantation. The use of spacer blocks to maintain an appropriate space in the ligament tension certainly facilitates the ease of revision and may improve the functional outcome. Disadvantages of spacer blocks include the potential for subluxation of the block and inability to allow motion. Both these disadvantages are addressed by the PROSTALAC (prosthesis of antibiotic-loaded acrylic cement) implants, which provide local antibiotic delivery as well as allowing motion of the knee during the interval between the resection and reimplantation. Using this system, successful elimination of infection in 92% of patients has been reported. Patients are allowed to bear weight and attempt knee range of motion during the interval between resection and reimplantation. Others have used "articulating spacers" made from the removed femoral component. This component is sterilized and a new polyethylene insert is used during the resection phase of treatment. The PROSTALAC and articulating spacers may certainly provide for motion during the resection and may potentially improve the functional outcome of these patients.

Prosthesis selection at the time of reimplantation remains controversial. Ligament insufficiency and bone deficiency often necessitate the use of posterior stabilized or constrained pros thetic designs as well as stemmed components to obtain reasonable prosthetic fixation. If possible, hinged constrained prostheses should be avoided.

Whether the stems should be cemented or press-fit remains controversial. Cement allows the use of an increased load of antibiotic delivery as well as improved immediate fixation. But the management of these prostheses should reinfection occur is difficult. It appears that allograft bone may be used in the face of prior infection, but there are no comparative studies documenting the incidence of recurrent infection in this subgroup.[30]

All decisions that are made in the treatment of a patient with an infected prosthesis should be done with the knowledge that salvage of a reinfection after reimplantation is extremely difficult. Our experience with 24 patients (24 knees) who had another infection following reimplantation is humbling.[31] The average number of surgical procedures for each infected knee was 9.3 (range, 5 to 23). The final outcome of the knee joints included 10 knees (42%) with a successful fusion, 5 (21%) with infected implants on suppressive oral antibiotics, 4 (17%) with an above-knee amputation, 3 (13%) persistent pseudoarthroses, 1 (4%) resection arthroplasty, and 1 uninfected TKA. The difficulties encountered in obtaining a healed wound, obtaining the successful knee arthrodesis, and the successful eradication of infection with nonprosthetic salvage procedures after a failed reimplantation are considerable.

Authors' Preferred Treatment Approach

Acute deep infections in the first few weeks postoperatively, or acute hematogenous infections in a well-functioning and well-fixed prosthesis are aggressively managed with open débridement and intravenous antibiotics for 4 weeks. Occasionally, elderly patients with a well-fixed prosthesis, absence of drainage, and minimal pain are treated with aspiration and chronic oral antibiotic suppression if the microorganism is sensitive to a nontoxic antibiotic. For chronic infections, the treatment methods depend on functional requirements, soft-tissue envelope status, extent of bone loss, and integrity of the extensor mechanism. Definitive resection arthroplasty or above-knee amputation are rarely required. Disruption of the extensor mechanism or a poor soft-tissue envelope may mandate a knee arthrodesis. For adequate bone apposition, an external fixation technique is preferred, but with more severe bone deficiency, a two-stage long intramedullary nailing is performed.

If the patient is a candidate for reinsertion of another prosthesis, a two-stage technique is preferred. After removal of the infected prosthesis, the knee is closed over antibiotic-impregnated beads or spacers. Most commonly a combination of vancomycin and tobramycin is used. The ratio of antibiotic powder per 40-g batch of cement is 3 to 4 g of vancomycin or 3.6 g of tobramycin. The capsule is closed with a running absorbable monofilament suture. Braided subcutaneous sutures are avoided because of bacterial adherence. The skin is closed with a nonabsorable monofilament suture. Postoperatively, the patient is placed in a knee immobilizer or a long leg cast. Most patients are treated with a 4-week course of intravenous antibiotics under the supervision of infectious disease consultants.

Reimplantation of another prosthesis is performed as soon as convenient after the conclusion of the intravenous antibiotics regimen. If there is concern about persistent deep infection, aspiration or débridement for retrieval of tissue culture, with delayed implantation until the culture results are available, can be performed.[32-39] Most patients are empirically reimplanted based on the appearance of tissues at revision surgery, visualization of serologic markers for infection, and histologic analysis of fresh-frozen tissue samples.[40-43] Tissue for culture is obtained at the reimplantation.[44-46] We prefer the use of antibiotic-impregnated bone cement for prosthesis fixation and choose the antibiotic based on sensitivity tests from the original offending organism or organisms. Vancomycin and tobramycin are most commonly used in a ratio of 1 to 2 g per batch of bone cement, as higher dosages weaken the mechanical strength of the cement. Currently, most prostheses used for reimplantation are posterior stabilized or constrained condylar designs. Bone graft is avoided if possible. The patella with severely compromised bone stock is often left unresurfaced. Postoperatively, the patient is continued on prophylactic antibiotics until the results from the intraoperative cultures are available. If these cultures are negative, all antibiotics are discontinued. If these cultures are positive and the organism is the same as the original offending organism, a 4-week course of intravenous antibiotics is administered and then additional chronic oral antibiotics are considered. If the culture results are considered to be a laboratory contaminant, additional antibiotics are not recommended.

References

1. Glynn MK, Sheehan JM: An analysis of the causes of deep infection after hip and knee arthroplasties. *Clin Orthop* 1983;178:202-206.
2. Katz MM, Hungerford DS, Krackow KA, Lennox DW: Reflex sympathetic dystrophy as a cause of poor results after total knee arthroplasty. *J Arthroplasty* 1986;1:117-124.
3. Stern SH, Insall JN: Total knee arthroplasty in obese patients. *J Bone Joint Surg Am* 1990;72:1400-1404.
4. England SP, Stern SH, Insall JN, Windsor RE: Total knee arthroplasty in diabetes mellitus. *Clin Orthop* 1990;260:130-134.
5. Gordon SM, Culver DH, Simmons BP, Jarvis WR: Risk factors for wound infections after total knee arthroplasty. *Am J Epidemiol* 1990;131:905-916.
6. Greene KA, Wilde AH, Stulberg BN: Preoperative nutritional status of total joint patients: Relationship to postoperative wound complications. *J Arthroplasty* 1991;6:321-325.
7. Hanssen AD, Osmon DR, Nelson CL: Prevention of deep periprosthetic joint infection. *Instr Course Lect* 1997;46:555-567.
8. Hanssen AD, Rand JA: Evaluation and treatment of infection at the site of a total hip or knee arthroplasty. *J Bone Joint Surg Am* 1998;80:910-922.
9. Athanasou NA, Pandey R, de Steiger R, Crook D, Smith PM: Diagnosis of infection by frozen section during revision arthroplasty. *J Bone Joint Surg Br* 1995;77:28-33.
10. Barrack RL, Jennings RW, Wolfe MW, Bertot AJ: The value of preoperative aspiration before total knee revision. *Clin Orthop* 1997;345:8-16.
11. Chimento GF, Finger S, Barrack RL: Gram stain detection of infection during revision arthroplasty. *J Bone Joint Surg Br* 1996;78:838-839.
12. Choudhry RR, Rice RP, Triffitt PD, Harper WM, Gregg PJ: Plasma viscosity and C-reactive protein after total hip and knee arthroplasty. *J Bone Joint Surg Br* 1992;74:523-524.
13. Demirkol MO, Adalet I, Unal SN, Tozun R, Cantez S: 99Tc(m)-polyclonal IgG scintigraphy in the detection of infected hip and knee prosteses. *Nucl Med Commun* 1997;18:543-548.
14. Duff GP, Lachiewicz PF, Kelley SS: Aspiration of the knee joint before revision arthroplasty. *Clin Orthop* 1996;331:132-139.
15. Duus BR, Boeckstyns M, Stadeager C: The natural course of radionuclide bone scanning in the evaluation of total knee replacement: A 2 year prospective study. *Clin Radiol* 1990;41: 341-343.
16. Fehring TK, McAlister JA Jr: Frozen histologic section as a guide to sepsis in revision joint arthroplasty. *Clin Orthop* 1994;304:229-237.
17. Fehring TK, McAvoy G: Fluoroscopic evaluation of the painful total knee arthroplasty. *Clin Orthop* 1996;331:226-233.
18. Feldman DS, Lonner JH, Desai P, Zuckerman JD: The role of intraoperative frozen sections in revision total joint arthroplasty. *J Bone Joint Surg Am* 1995;77:1807-1813.
19. Glithero PR, Grigoris P, Harding LK, Hesslewood SR, McMinn DJ: White cell scans and infected joint replacements: Failure to detect chronic infection. *J Bone Joint Surg Br* 1993;75:371-374.
20. Levitsky KA, Hozack WJ, Balderston RA, et al: Evaluation of the painful prosthetic joint: Relative value of bone scan, sedimentation rate, and joint aspiration. *J Arthroplasty* 1991;6: 237-244.
21. Lian G, Cracchiolo A III, Lesavoy M: Treatment of major wound necrosis following total knee arthroplasty. *J Arthroplasty* 1989;(suppl 4):S23-S32.
22. Weiss AP, Krackow KA: Persistent wound drainage after primary total knee arthroplasty. *J Arthroplasty* 1993;8:285-289.
23. Hartman MB, Fehring TK, Jordan L, Norton HJ: Periprosthetic knee sepsis: The role of irrigation and débridement. *Clin Orthop* 1991;273:113-118.
24. Teeny SM, Dorr L, Murata G, Conaty P: Treatment of infected total knee arthroplasty: Irrigation and débridementversus two-stage reimplantation. *J Arthroplasty* 1990;5:35-39.
25. Schoifet SD, Morrey BF: Treatment of infection after total knee arthroplasy by débridementwith retention of the components. *J Bone Joint Surg Am* 1990;72:1383-1390.
26. Grogan TJ, Dorey F, Rollins J, Amstutz HC: Deep sepsis following total knee arthroplasty: Ten-year experience at the University of California at Los Angeles Medical Center. *J Bone Joint Surg Am* 1986;68:226-234.
27. Tsukayama DT, Estrada R, Gustilo RB: Infection after total hip arthroplasty: A total study of the treatment of one hundred and six infections. *J Bone Joint Surg Am* 1996;78: 512-523.
28. Wymenga AB, van Horn JR, Theeuwes A, Muytjens HS, Sloof TJ: Perioperative factors associated with septic arthritis after arthroplasty: Prospective multicenter study of 362 knee and 2,651 hip operations. *Acta Orthop Scand* 1992;63:665-671.
29. Insall JN, Thompson FM, Brause BD: Two-stage reimplantation for the salvage of infected total knee arthroplasty. *J Bone Joint Surg Am* 1983;65:1087-1098.
30. Gabrielsen TA, Trousdale RT: Use of allograft bone in revision total knee arthroplasty in previously septic knees: Short term results. *The Knee* 1995;2:165-170.
31. Hanssen AD, Trousdale RT, Osmon DR: Patient outcome with reinfection following reimplantation for the infected total knee arthroplasty. *Clin Orthop* 1995;321:55-67.
32. Hofmann AA, Wyatt RW, Daniels AU, Armstrong L, Alazraki N, Taylor A Jr: Bone scans after total knee arthroplasty in asymptomatic patients: Cemented versus cementless. *Clin Orthop* 1990;251:183-188.

33. Kantor SG, Schneider R, Insall JN, Becker MW: Radionuclide imaging of asympotmatic versus symptomatic total knee arthroplasties. *Clin Orthop* 1990;260:118-123.

34. Kennedy JG, Rodgers WB, Zurakowski D, et al: Pyrexia after total knee replacement: A cause for concern? *Am J Orthop* 1997;26:549-552.

35. Nijhof MW, Oyen WJ, van Kampen A, Claessens RA, van der Meer JW, Corstens FH: Hip and knee arthroplasty infection: In-111-IgG scintigraphy in 102 cases. *Acta Orthop Scand* 1997;68:332-336.

36. Owen RJ, Harper WM, Finlay DB, Belton IP: Isotope bone scans in patients with painful knee replacements: Do they alter management? *Br J Radiol* 1995;68:1204-1207.

37. Palestri CJ, Swyer AJ, Kim CK, Goldsmith SJ: Infected knee prosthesis: Diagnosis with In-111 Leukocyte, Tc-99m sulfur colloid, and Tc-99m MDP imaging. *Radiology* 1991;179: 645-648.

38. Rand JA, Brown ML: The value of indium-111 leukocyte scanning in the evaluation of painful or infected total knee arthroplasties. *Clin Orthop* 1990;259:179-182.

39. Waldman BJ, Mont MA, Yoon TR, Hungerford DS: Abstract: The value of cell count and differential after aspiration in predicting infection of total knee arthroplasty. *65th Annual Meeting Proceedings*. Rosemont, IL, American Academy of Orthopaedic Surgeons, 1998, p 169.

40. Kolstad K, Levander H: Inflammatory laboratory tests after joint replacement surgery. *Ups J Med Sci* 1995;100:243-248.

41. Larsson S, Thelander U, Friberg S: C-reactive protein (CRP) levels after elective orthopedic surgery. *Clin Orthop* 1992;275:237-242.

42. Mariani BD, Martin DS, Levine MJ, Booth RE Jr, Tuan RS: Polymerase chain reaction detection of bacterial infection in total knee arthroplasty. *Clin Orthop* 1996;331:11-22.

43. Levine MJ, Mariani BA, Tuan RS, Booth RE Jr: Molecular genetic diagnosis of infection total joint arthroplasty. *J Arthroplasty* 1995;10:93-94.

44. Lonner JH, Desai P, Dicesare PE, Steiner G, Zuckerman JD: The reliability of analysis of intraoperative frozen sections for identifying active infection during revision hip or knee arthroplasty. *J Bone Joint Surg Am* 1996;78: 1553-1558.

45. Mirra JM, Marder RA, Amstutz HC: The pathology of failed total joint arthroplasty. *Clin Orthop* 1982;170:175-183.

46. Pace TB, Jeray KJ, Latham JT Jr: Synovial tissue examination by frozen section as an indicator of infection in hip and knee arthroplasty in community hospitals. *J Arthroplasty* 1997;12: 64-69.

43

Thromboembolic Disease in Total Knee Arthroplasty

Miguel A. Jimenez, MD
Robert T. Trousdale, MD

Thromboembolic disease remains a major cause of morbidity and mortality in patients who undergo total knee arthroplasty (TKA). Controversy still exists about the ideal methods of prevention and treatment of thromboembolic disease. This chapter will attempt to answer some of the most commonly asked questions about thromboembolic disease and TKA.

Prophylaxis

The definition of a prophylactic versus a therapeutic regimen has varied over the past 25 years and has often been interchanged in the literature. Prophylaxis should always be considered as a preventive agent given perioperatively. It is used to prevent the morbidity, mortality, and potential legal consequence of thromboembolic disease occurring after TKA.

Thromboembolic disease is not an uncommon occurrence after TKA. According to venographic data, the incidence of deep vein thrombosis (DVT) ranges from 50% to 70%.[1] Asymptomatic pulmonary embolism may occur in up to 10% to 18% of patients.[1] Symptomatic and fatal pulmonary embolism occur much less frequently (1% to 1.9% and 0.2% to 0.7%, respectively).[1,2]

Several national consensus panels have proposed recommendations for preventing thromboembolic disease after TKA, and they all recommend some form of prophylaxis.[3] The high prevalence of thromboembolic disease, combined with the potential of significant morbidity and mortality, prompts surgeons to use some form of prophylaxis in all patients undergoing total hip arthroplasty.

Predisposing Factors for Thromboembolic Disease

Several medical conditions have been shown to increase the risk of thromboembolic disease. Obesity, coronary artery disease, congestive heart failure, trauma, pelvic or limb surgery, extremity immobility for any reason, malignancy, myeloproliferative disorders, nephrotic syndrome, oral contraceptive use, presence of lupus anticoagulant/anticardiolipin antibody, inflammatory bowel disease, history of previous thromboembolic disease, and deficiencies in plasminogen, antithrombin III, protein C, and protein S may all increase the risk of thromboembolic disease after TKA.[4]

It is prudent to attempt to diminish any risk factor present prior to TKA. Encouraging patients to lose weight, maximize treatment of their medical conditions, and avoid the use of birth control pills are certainly reasonable recommendations to minimize the risk of DVT. However, many risk factors cannot be diminished, which is yet another reason why prophylaxis for thromboembolic disease is reasonable.

Pathogenesis

In 1856, Virchow described three predisposing factors for thromboembolic disease: hypercoagulability, venous stasis, and endothelial wall injury (Virchow's Triad). Hypercoagulability is thought to be brought about by tissue debris that is generated during TKA. There may be a secondary effect via stasis or endothelial wall injury. The exact etiology and mechanism of hypercoagulability remain uncertain. Intraoperative venous stasis can occur with tourniquet use, hypotension, and excessive knee flexion while preparing the tibia for surgery. In addition, intraoperative limb immobilization may also contribute to venous stasis. Venous endothelial wall injury may occur intraoperatively from both manipulation and placement of retractors.

Diagnosis of Thromboembolic Disease

In order to make an accurate diagnosis of thromboembolic disease, it must be recognized that the condition can represent a spectrum of diseases ranging from superficial thrombophlebitis, distal calf DVT, proximal thigh or pelvic DVT, nonfatal pulmonary embolism (symptomatic or asymptomatic), and fatal pulmonary embolism.

The clinical examination and diagnostic studies are both instrumental in confirming the diagnosis of thromboembolic disease. Clinical examination is not very predictive of disease. Homan's sign (calf pain with foot dorsiflexion) has a poor predictive value for thromboembolic disease and can occur equally in patients with and without DVT.[5] The location of a thrombus will influence the presence or severity of clinical symptoms. The more proximal the thrombus is located the more likely the patient will be symptomatic, and the more likely that clots will become emboli.[6] Proximal thrombi tend to be associated with distal clots and more commonly lead to diffuse disease.[4] Rarely, extensive venous thrombosis in the femoral and iliac veins will lead to phlegmasia cerulea dolens, characterized by a swollen, tense, painful, blue-tinged limb, that is at risk of venous gangrene. The most common clinical signs of a pulmonary embolus are respiratory rate greater than 25/min, tachycardia (rate greater than 100/min), and increased pulmonic second sound noted on cardiac auscultation.[7] The most common symptoms of a pulmonary embolus are dyspnea and chest pain.[7] A pulmonary embolism will become symptomatic when more than 50% of the pulmonary vascular outflow tract is obstructed.[4] Less obstruction is necessary in patients with underlying cardiopulmonary disease. Less than 55% of patients with fatal pulmonary embolism have any clinical signs of DVT prior to death.[4] Therefore, a high clinical suspicion is essential to make the diagnosis using clinical criteria alone.

Diagnostic studies presently being used to detect DVT include duplex ultrasound, venography, and plethysmography. A duplex scan consists of a real-time B mode ultrasonography and Doppler flow detection. In addition, it is noninvasive, relatively inexpensive, and reproducible. Duplex ultrasound has a high sensitivity and specificity for distal and proximal DVT.[8] However, it has a poor sensitivity for iliac vein clots. Venography is considered the gold standard and is effective in diagnosing thrombi in all locations. However, it is expensive, invasive, and can be associated with chemical phlebitis secondary to contrast dye use.[4] Plethysmography is not very sensitive for partial venous occlusion and it is rarely used as the sole diagnostic tool for the diagnosis of DVT.[4]

Diagnostic studies presently being used for the diagnosis of pulmonary embolism include ventilation/perfusion scans, angiography, and ultrafast CT. A normal perfusion scan can effectively rule out a pulmonary embolism. Unfortunately, an abnormal scan does not necessarily confirm the diagnosis. An abnormal perfusion scan combined with a physician's clinical suspicion of a pulmonary embolism will be confirmed in less than 50% of patients. Abnormal perfusion can occur from atelectasis, pneumothorax, emphysema, and chronic pulmonary disease. A ventilation scan can differentiate abnormal perfusion scans secondary to a pulmonary embolism and other causes. A normal ventilation scan and an abnormal perfusion scan (or V/Q mismatch) suggest a high probability of a pulmonary embolism. Combining a perfusion with a ventilation scan will increase their predictive value. The absence of a V/Q mismatch and low clinical suspicion yields a low probability scan, with a 2% to 9% likelihood of a pulmonary embolism.[9] A documented V/Q mismatch and high clinical suspicion yields a high probability scan with a 96% likelihood of a pulmonary embolism.[9] Pulmonary angiography is considered the gold standard for the diagnosis of pulmonary embolism. However, it is invasive, risky, and expensive. Ultrafast CT, which is both sensitive and specific, is becoming more widely used and may become the predominant diagnostic tool in the future.[4]

Minimizing the Patient's Risk of DVT

Preventive measures can be implemented perioperatively to counteract Virchow's triad. Careful limb manipulation and placement of retractors during surgery can help minimize endothelial wall injury. Ninomiya and associates[10] performed intraoperative angiograms while perfoming TKAs in four cadaver knees. They found that the artery was located posterolaterally and the vein was more centrally located. Placement of retractors in the central and posterolateral tibial plateau regions during the procedure may place the vein and artery at risk. In addition, intraoperative angiograms demonstrated how hyperextension could lead to neurovascular traction injuries. Moreover, the artery and nearby vein are located very close to the posterior tibial plateau cortex. Farrington and associates[11] found that the mean movement of the neurovascular bundle from the posterior tibia cortex was only 3.15 mm when the knee is flexed from zero to 90°. The distance of the neurovascular structures to the posterior tibial cortex was maximal when the knee was flexed from 60° to 90°.

Minimizing tourniquet use may also decrease the duration of venous stasis. Although no studies have shown tourniquet inflation to be a definitive risk factor for DVT; however, thrombogenic factors are released with tourniquet release.[12] It would seem prudent that minimizing tourniquet time may potentially decrease both stasis and the incidence of DVT. Use of intraoperative intermittent pneumatic compression devices may actively decrease stasis that occurs during surgery.

Nonpharmacologic Prophylaxis

Nonpharmacologic prophylactic methods include early mobilization, lower extremity exercises, elastic stockings, continuous passive motion of the knee, and intermittent pneumatic compression. The efficacy of some of these modalities is questionable.[13] However, all are reasonable to use because they are noninvasive, relatively inexpensive, and usually easily tolerated.

Intermittent pneumatic compression can be performed using devices that include the foot, calf, foot and calf combinations, or calf and thigh combinations (Table 1). Westrich and associates[14] examined the venous hemodynamics at the saphenous-femoral junction with various intermittent pneumatic compression pumps as well as with active foot motion. They found that all intermittent pneumatic compression pumps augment peak venous velocity and volume flow.[14] The greatest effects were observed below the great saphenous-femoral vein junction. In addition, they found that active foot flexion increased venous velocity.[14] A single calf contraction can increase peak volume by 8.5 mL/contraction.[14] The precise role of venous velocity and flow volume on the development of thromboembolic disease remains unclear. Optimizing venous flow during the postoperative period would only be helpful in minimizing the patient's risk of developing a DVT when the patient is relatively immobile.

Clagett and associates[3] pooled data from four clinical trials (366 total hip arthroplasty patients) to examine the role of intermittent pneumatic compression in preventing DVT in TKA patients. They found that the relative risk reduction (compared with no treatment) for developing DVT was 82% with the use of intermittent pneumatic compressions. Intermittent pneumatic compression is an effective prophylactic agent if used continuously as soon as it is feasible. Side effects are minimal, but are limited by a patient's intolerance/compliance and difficulties in continued use after hospital discharge.

Pharmacologic Prophylaxis

There are a vast number of pharmacologic agents available to help prevent thromboembolic disease. Some of the most commonly recognized agents include dextran, aspirin, warfarin, and various heparin preparations.

Dextran is a branched polysaccharide that has demonstrated limited efficacy in other surgical patients, but has not been formally studied in TKA patients. It must be administered intravenously and has been associated with serious complications including volume overload, bleeding complications, and anaphylactic reactions.[15] Because of the lack of clinical data, its route of administration, and potential complications, dextran is rarely used as a prophylactic agent in TKA patients.

Aspirin has been a popular method of prophylaxis in TKA patients because it is easy to use and is relatively well tolerated. Despite its common use in the past there is a paucity of well-designed, large, randomized studies. Available data has shown conflicting efficacy. Aspirin can be associated with gastrointestinal upset and bleeding complications. Moreover, intermittent pneumatic compression appears to be more effective than aspirin.[16] Given the clinical uncertainty of aspirin and proven available alternatives, it seems prudent not to use aspirin alone as a prophylactic agent. There are some data that in total hip arthroplasty, aspirin combined with hypotensive anesthesia and intermittent pneumatic compressions may be an effective prophylactic regimen.[17] This has yet to be studied in TKA.

Warfarin has become an extremely popular prophylactic agent in TKA patients. It is used in various dosing regimens (adjusted dose, low dose, or minidose). Adjusted dose warfarin is commonly used and involves giving the patient a 5- to 10-mg dose perioperatively and titrating to an international normalized ratio (INR) of 2 to 3. Warfarin has many attractive features. It is an oral agent that can be continued after discharge from the hospital, the risk of bleeding is relatively low if adequately monitored. The disadvantages include the extremely variable dose response and the careful monitoring required to achieve appropriate anticoagulation. Clagett and associates[3] pooled patient data from seven clinical trials (1,108 TKA patients). They found that the total prevalence of DVT was 49% and the relative risk reduction was 20%, compared to no treatment.

Heparin and heparin derivatives have gained significant popularity as prophylactic agents. Traditional heparin, an extract from pig intestines, has been supplanted by low molecular weight heparins, which are an extract from traditional heparin. The advantages of low molecular weight heparin include their efficacy and potentially fewer side effects than traditional heparins.[4] The most commonly used low molecular weight heparins are enoxaparin and ardaperin. Ardaperin is presently approved by the Food and Drug Administration (FDA) for TKA patients, whereas enoxaparin is approved for both THA and TKA patients. Enoxaparin is administered in a standard dose, ardaperin is administered based on the patient's weight. Multiple studies have suggested that low molecular weight heparins maybe slightly more effective than warfarin in decreasing the risk of thromboembolic disease.[3,18] But low molecular weight heparins have disadvantages, which include subcutaneous administration, and a real potential for bleeding. Clagett and associates[3] combined nine clinical trials (1,409 TKA patients). The total DVT prevalence was 31% and with a relative risk reduction for DVT of 49%, which is more than double the relative risk reduction of warfarin. Many surgeons have chosen either warfarin or low molecular weight heparins as their prophylactic agent of choice. There are no studies comparing warfarin and low molecular weight heparin in TKA patients in which symptomatic thromboembolism was the primary end point. There is a trend in the literature that low molecular weight

Table 1
Intermittent pneumatic compressive devices used by Westrich and associates[14]

Foot Pumps	
	Arteriovenous Impulse Pump
	PlexiPulse Foot Pump
Calf Pump	
	VenaFlow Pump
Foot/Calf Pump	
	PlexiPulse Foot/Calf Pump
Calf/Thigh Pumps	
	Sequential Compression Device (SCD)
	Flowtron
	Jobst Automatic

heparins may be more efficacious than warfarin for DVT prevention, but it may have a slightly higher rate of bleeding complications. A recent study by Stern and associates[19] evaluated the safety of warfarin versus enoxaparin. Two hundred sixty-three patients were studied, with 122 receiving low-dose warfarin for 4 to 6 weeks and 141 receiving enoxaparin for 2 weeks after TKA. The rate of ultrasound-detectable deep vein thrombosis was no different in the two groups (three patients each). The number of bleeding complications was two times higher in the low molecular weight heparin group versus the warfarin group.

One of the advantages of low molecular weight heparins is that monitoring is not required. Prophylaxis with warfarin requires careful monitoring. Bleeding complications seen with warfarin appear to be related to INR levels. Closely monitoring INR levels can reduce bleeding complications and help maintain therapeutic levels. However, because of the extremely variable dose response to warfarin, some bleeding complications may be unavoidable[20] and may be as high as 16%.

Mechanical Prophylaxis

Inferior vena caval filters are used to prevent pulmonary embolism in high-risk patients. Patients with a history of thromboembolic disease should be considered candidates for an inferior vena caval filter. Patients with contraindications to routine prophylactic measures, for example, patients with a history of a cerebral bleed, recent brain, eye, or spinal surgery, or active gastrointestinal bleeding, should also be considered for inferior vena caval filters. Filters are also indicated in patients with a history of a pulmonary embolism who are hemodynamically unstable and to prevent recurrent pulmonary embolism postembolectomy. These filters may also be indicated in high-risk patients with a poor cardiopulmonary tolerance.[4] Emerson and associates[21] described the use of prophylactic Greenfield filters in 49 high-risk total joint arthroplasty patients. Thirty-eight patients received filters preoperatively without anticoagulation. Eleven patients were treated with filters and received postoperative anticoagulation. No clinical embolic episodes were observed and the caval patency remained intact in 96% of the patients. An orthopaedic patient requiring a filter has a time limited risk of a pulmonary embolism and may be best treated with a temporary filter. New technology may produce these innovations in the near future. There is a catheter device now available that is used to introduce fibrinolytic agents, in which the tip opens into a temporary filter to prevent loose clots from embolizing. A similar device may be available in the future. At the present time, there are no FDA-approved temporary filters.

Optimal Duration of Prophylaxis/Surveillance

The optimal duration of prophylaxis in TKA patients is unknown. Several studies suggest that the risk of DVT can persist up to 2 months after surgery.[3] Most surgeons would agree that the highest risk for clot formation occurs perioperatively and would continue prophylaxis for at least the first 5 to 7 days after surgery.[4] Whether it is prudent to continue prophylaxis for longer periods of time remains controversial. The duration of prophylaxis can probably be modified according to the patient's risk of developing thromboembolic disease, as well as the agent being used.

Surveillance is defined as the use of diagnostic tests, either a duplex ultrasound or venography, to confirm the diagnosis of DVT in asymptomatic patients postoperatively. Surveillance would be most effective in the early postoperative period because most DVTs occur in the first 24 to 48 hours.[22] Cost-effectiveness in asymptomatic patients is questionable. Surveillance may be cost effective in high-risk patients, but there is little data to support its routine use.

Summary

Good data exist to support the use of low molecular weight heparins, warfarin, or intermittent pneumatic compression to prevent thromboembolic disease in TKA patients. Emerging data suggest that low molecular weight heparins may be more efficacious than warfarin, but are probably associated with slightly higher bleeding complications. There is little data to support the efficacy of aspirin alone as a prophylactic agent in TKA patients. Routine screening in asymptomatic low risk patients is probably not cost-effective. Prophylactic inferior vena caval filters are recommended in high-risk patients in whom other forms of anticoagulation are not feasible.

References

1. Insall JN, Haas SB: Complications of total knee arthroplasty, in Insall JN, Windsor RE, Scott WN, Kelly MA, Aglietti P (eds): *Surgery of the Knee,* ed 2. New York, NY, Churchill Livingstone, 1993, vol 2, pp 891-934.
2. Stulberg BN, Insall JN, Williams GW, Ghelman B: Deep-vein thrombosis following total knee replacement: An analysis of six hundred and thirty-eight arthroplasties. *J Bone Joint Surg Am* 1984;66:194-201.
3. Clagett GP, Anderson FA Jr, Geerts W, et al: Prevention of venous thromboembolism. *Chest* 1998;114(suppl 5):531S-560S.
4. Gloviczki P, Yao JST (eds): *Handbook of Venous Disorders: Guidelines of the American Venous Forum.* London, England, Chapman & Hall Medical, 1996.
5. Cranley JJ, Canos AJ, Sull WJ: The diagnosis of deep vein thrombosis: Fallibility of clinical symptoms and signs. *Arch Surg* 1976;111:34-36.
6. Lotke PA, Ecker ML, Alavi A, Berkowitz H: Indications for the treatment of deep venous thrombosis following total knee replacement. *J Bone Joint Surg Am* 1984;66:202-208.
7. Manganell D, Palla A, Donnamaria V, Giantini C: Clincal features of pulmonary embolism: Doubts and certainties. *Chest* 1995;107(suppl 1):255-325.
8. Woolson ST, Pottorff G: Venous ultrasonography in the detection of proximal vein thrombosis after total knee arthroplasty. *Clin Orthop* 1991;273:131-135.

9. PIOPED Investigators: Value of the ventilation/perfusion scan in acute pulmonary embolism: Results of the prospective investigation of pulmonary embolism diagnosis (PIOPED). *JAMA* 1990;263:2753-2759.

10. Ninomiya JT, Dean JC, Goldberg VM: Injury to the popliteal artery and its anatomic location in total knee arthroplasty. *J Arthroplasty* 1999;14:803-809.

11. Farrington WJ, Charnley GJ, Harries SR, Fox BM, Sharp R, Huges PM: The position of the popliteal artery in the arthritic knee. *J Arthroplasty* 1999;14:800-802.

12. Sharrock NE, Go G, Sculco TP, Ranawat CS, Maynard MJ, Harpel PC: Changes in circulatory indices of thrombosis and fibrinolysis during total knee arthroplasty performed under tourniquet. *J Arthroplasty* 1995;10:523-528.

13. Pellegrini VD Jr: Thromboembolic disease. *Instr Course Lect* 1997;46:185-189.

14. Westrich GH, Specht LM, Sharrock NE, et al: Venous haemodynamics after total knee arthroplasty: Evaluation of active dorsel to plantar flexion and several mechanical compression devices. *J Bone Joint Surg Br* 1998;80:1057-1066.

15. Hull RD, Raskob GE: Prophylaxis of venous thromboembolic disease following hip and knee surgery. *J Bone Joint Surg Am* 1986;68: 146-150.

16. Haas SB, Insall JN, Scuderi GR, Windsor RE, Ghelman B: Pneumatic sequential-compression boots compared with aspirin prophylaxis of deep-vein thrombosis after total knee arthroplasty. *J Bone Joint Surg Am* 1990;72:27-31.

17. Westrich GH, Farrell C, Bono JV, Ranawat CS, Salvati EA, Sculco TP: The incidence of venous thromboembolism after total hip arthroplasty: A specific hypotensive epidural anesthesia protocol. *J Arthroplasty* 1999;14: 456-463.

18. Hull R, Raskob G, Pineo G, et al: A comparison of subcutaneous low-molecular-weight heparin with warfarin sodium for prophylaxis against deep-vein thrombosis after hip or knee implantation. *N Eng J Med* 1993;329: 1370-1376.

19. Stern SH, Wixson RL, O'Connor D: Evaluation of the safety and efficacy of enoxaparin and warfarin for prevention of deep vein thrombosis after total knee arthroplasty. *J Arthroplasty* 2000;15:153-158.

20. Sutherland CJ, Schurman JR: Complications associated with warfarin prophylaxis in total knee arthroplasty. *Clin Orthop* 1987;219: 158-162.

21. Emerson RH Jr, Cross R, Head WC: Prophylactic and early therapeutic use of the Greenfield filter in hip and knee joint arthroplasty. *J Arthroplasty* 1991;6:129-135.

22. Maynard MJ, Sculco TP, Ghelman B: Progression and regression of deep vein thrombosis after total knee arthroplasty. *Clin Orthop* 1991;273:125-130.

44

Maximizing Ultra High Molecular Weight Polyethylene Performance in Total Knee Replacement

David C. Ayers, MD

Introduction

Total knee replacement (TKR) is the treatment of choice for patients with debilitating arthritis of the knee because of the pain relief and improved function the patient experiences postoperatively. A successful result following TKR is dependent on proper patient selection, surgical technique, implant design, and the avoidance of complications. However, polyethylene wear is inevitable following TKR. New information reveals that polyethylene wear occurs both at the articular surface as well as on the undersurface of the polyethylene insert between the insert and the tibial base plate. Polyethylene wear following TKR has a multifactorial etiology. This chapter will examine ways to maximize the performance of ultra high molecular weight polyethylene (UHMWPE) following TKR with an emphasis on the role of the surgeon in minimizing polyethylene wear.

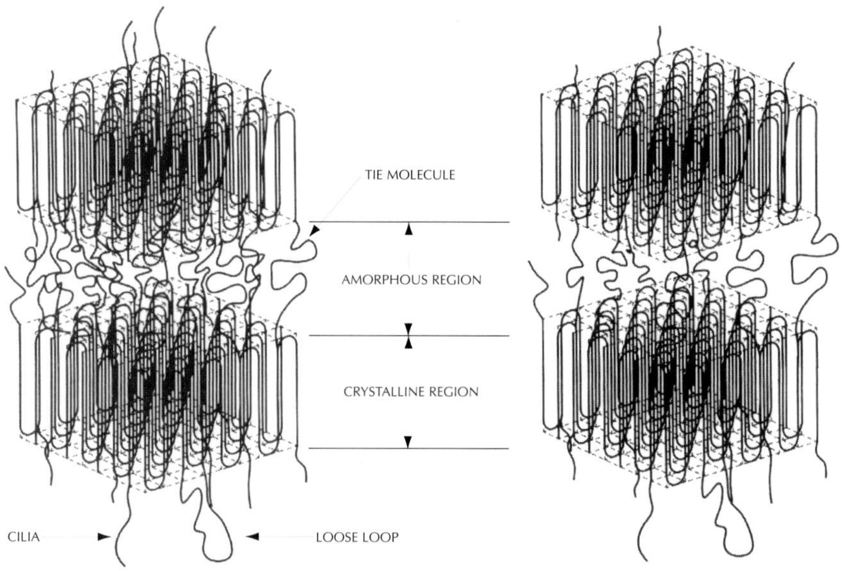

Fig. 1 Molecular structure of UHMWPE (*left*). Molecular structure of high-density polyethylene (*right*). (Reproduced with permission from *Overview and Fundamentals of UHMWPE.* Rutherford, NJ, Howmedica, 1994, p 3).

Polyethylene Structure and Fabrication

The linear structure of polyethylene is a long-chain polymer composed of a carbon backbone chain with hydrogen subgroups. Polyethylene grades differ primarily on the basis of molecular weight and the number of branches that occur along the polymer chain. Medical grade UHMWPE accounts for approximately 0.1% of the annual production of polyethylene and has a molecular weight between 3 and 6 million. As is typical of semicrystalline polymers, UHMWPE has a microstructure consisting of crystalline regions that are highly ordered, as well as amorphous or disordered regions (Fig. 1). Surrounding and connecting the crystalline regions are the bridging tie molecules. One major difference between the morphology of UHMWPE and regular high density polyethylene is the large number of tie molecules in the UHMWPE that act as cross-links between the crystalline regions and provide improved load bearing, stress transfer, and chemical and physical strength. Despite current concerns regarding wear, UHMWPE, when used properly, remains the best polymer available for use in TKR today because of its unique material properties, including high impact resistance, high toughness, high abrasion resistance, and good chemical resistance and biocompatibility.[1]

One of two processes is currently used to make medical grade UHMWPE devices. Components may be compression-molded into the geometry of the prosthetic component directly from the polyethylene powder or be machined

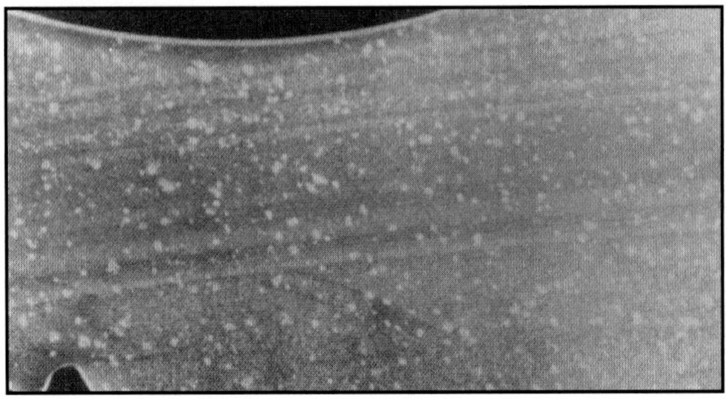

Fig. 2 Inclusion defects within the UHMWPE. (Reproduced with permission from Li S, Burstein AH: UHMWPE: The material and its use in total joint implants. *J Bone Joint Surg Am* 1994;76:1080-1090.)

from either polyethylene bar or sheet stock. In the fabrication of sheet stock, the polyethylene powder is press molded into sheets 1 to 6 inches thick from which the components are machined. Polyethylene bar stock is formed by ram extrusion. The polyethylene powder is placed into a cylinder of a ram extruder and the material is forced through the die by the reciprocating ram. The compacted material passes through a heated zone that must be long enough to allow complete fusion of the material. Bars that are typically supplied to the implant manufacturers are from 2 to 4 inches in diameter. In direct compression molding, polyethylene powder is placed into a mold of the desired component geometry that is then heated under pressure to compress it into the final shape of the device. Devices made in this manner have no external machining lines. This process can be carried out in an inert environment to reduce the oxygen available for oxidation of the material.

There is growing evidence that the manufacturing method of the polyethylene insert may affect its clinical performance. Ritter and associates[2] reported on the results of 2,001 AGC TKAs (AGC; Biomet, Warsaw, IN) evaluated after more than 10 years' follow-up. There was a 98% survival rate at 10 years in this flat-on-flat posterior cruciate ligament (PCL) retaining knee design. The authors concluded that the primary reason for the success of this design was the compression-molded polyethylene. Won and associates[3] studied the effect of UHMWPE resin type and manufacturing method on wear of polyethylene inserts following TKR. Thirteen Miller-Galante I and 10 Miller-Galante II tibial inserts were retrieved at revision surgery. The Miller-Galante I tibial components were made by direct compression molding of Hi-fax 1900 resin and the Miller-Galante II components were made by machining from ram extruded rods of GUR 415 resin. Both groups of inserts were sterilized by gamma radiation in air. The Miller-Galante I retrievals had significantly more wear damage in the form of scratching and embedded metallic debris, whereas the Miller-Galante II retrievals had significantly more wear damage in the form of delamination, complete breakup of material in plates; and particles. In implants that had been in use for 5 years or more, the Miller-Galante II polyethylene had a significantly greater maximum density value than the Miller-Galante I polyethylene. Miller-Galante II components, when sectioned, exhibited a subsurface region of oxidative degradation through which the delamination occurred. No such subsurface degraded region was observed for the Miller-Galante I components. This study suggests that delamination of polyethylene tibial components that have been gamma sterilized in air is influenced by manufacturing method, resin type,[3] or both.

In both bar stock formation and direct compression molding, control of the consolidation parameters is necessary to ensure a homogeneous and defect-free polyethylene. The quality of the consolidation process affects the wear characteristics of a UHMWPE component. Defects have been observed in UHMWPE tibial components. These defects have been observed with the unaided eye, x-ray defraction, and optical analyses[4-9] (Fig. 2). Impurities, or inclusions, within the UHMWPE have been found. Fusion defects are areas within the UHMWPE component where there are areas of polyethylene powder that incompletely consolidate during the manufacturing process. Fusion defect areas have been hypothesized to be highly susceptible to damage after implantation when the UHMWPE is subjected to stress. Wrona and associates[9] showed a statistically significant correlation between fusion defects and UHMWPE component total wear, delamination, and cracking in an implant retrieval study. This study did not control for oxidation of the components, and thus the effect of fusion defects could not be seperated from that of subsurface oxidation.

Factors That Affect Polyethylene Wear

Surgical technique can influence the rate of polyethylene wear following TKR (Fig. 3). Restoration of the mechanical axis of the limb is the single most important factor influencing mechanical complications following TKR. A line from the center of the femoral head to the center of the talus should pass through the center of the knee. Malalignment of the mechanical axis can result in increased forces applied over a smaller area of polyethylene and increased polyethylene wear. Similarly, malposition of the tibial component in the coronal plane is consistently associated with polyethylene radiolucencies at the bone-cement interface and late loosening of the prosthesis. Matsuda and associates[10] reported the results of 20 TKRs that changed alignment at a mean follow-up of 87 months due to wear of the polyethylene insert. Seventeen of the 20 knees were in a varus position on the initial postoperative radiographs. The thickness of the polyethylene significantly decreased in the medial compartment, resulting in increasing varus alignment of the limb. The polyethylene wear rate had a positive correlation with the initial postoperative alignment. The authors concluded that correction of the mechanical axis of the limb is important in order to minimize polyethylene wear. The level of the proximal tibial resection determines the thickness of the polyethylene insert that is used during TKR. The thickness of the polyethylene determines the ability of the polyethylene insert to function as a weight-bearing material. A minimum polyethylene thickness of 8 mm is recommended for a conforming tibial insert. An additional 2 mm of proximal tibial bone must be removed if a modular tibial component is being used, to allow for the metallic base plate. This dictates that a minimum of 10 mm be resected from the uninvolved tibial plateau to use a tibial insert containing 8 mm of true polyethylene. The choice of the knee prosthesis also affects polyethylene wear. An implant should maximize polyethylene contact areas and minimize peak contact stresses. The UHMWPE-tibial base plate locking mechanism should be secure and minimize wear at this interface. Finally, the mechanical properties of the polyethylene should be maintained during the manufacturing and sterilization processes.

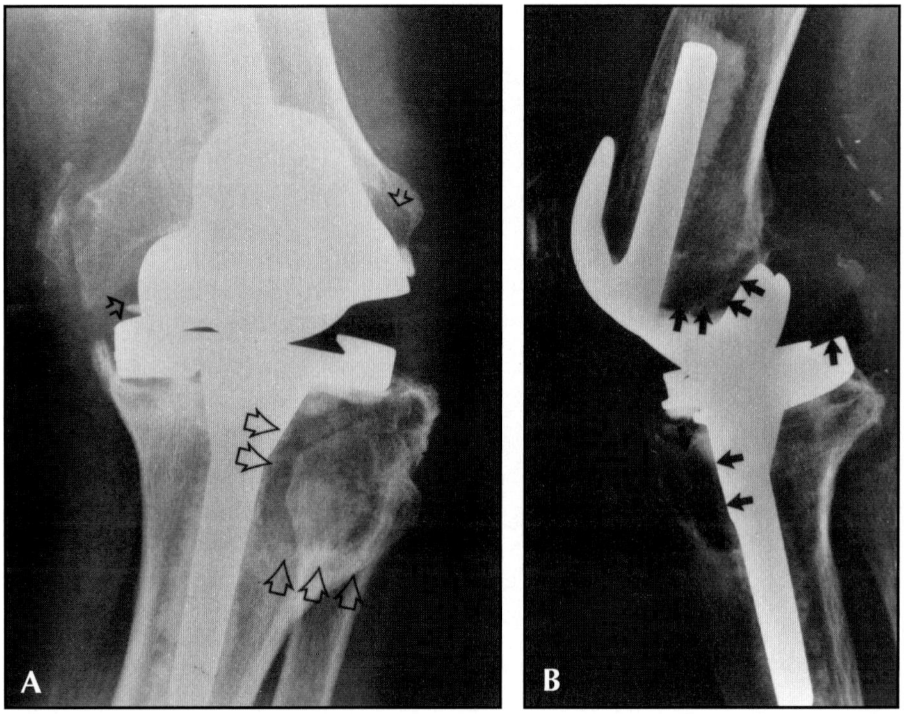

Fig. 3 A, Anteroposterior, and **B,** lateral radiographs of variable axis knee replacement with extensive polyethlene wear. There is a fractured polyethylene insert and base plate. Note the extensive osteolysis in the lateral tibial plateau and the distal femur.

Method of Sterilization

Sterilization of UHMWPE devices may lead to oxidation of the polyethylene and structural changes that alter the mechanical properties of the device and lead to rapid wear and early failure of the implant. The majority of UHMWPE implants historically have been sterilized by gamma radiation, typically with 2.5 Mrad. Gamma radiation in air results in oxidation of the UHMWPE and alters the physical structure of the material by scission of individual polymer chains.[4] Chain scission produces free radicals that in an air environment combine with oxygen to cause oxidative degradation. Oxidative degradation increases mobility of the shortened polyethylene chains, which allows for a change in orientation and an increased percentage of the material that is crystalline.[11,12] Free radicals formed by radiation may exist for years within the polyethylene and react with oxygen over time. Oxidative degradation of the UHMWPE therefore continues during the shelf life of the implant.[4] Shelf life is defined as the time elapsed between sterilization and implantation. The loss of mechanical strength over time as a result of gamma sterilization in air has been shown to strongly influence the development of fatigue wear modes of delamination and cracking. Since 1995, most UHMWPE has been sterilized either by gamma radiation in an inert, oxygen-free environment, or by ethylene oxide.

Wrona and associates[9] demonstrated that the method of sterilization of polyethylene directly affects its mechanical properties and its ability to function as a weight-bearing material. They reported that 40% of all tibial components retrieved had cracking or delamination damage upon close inspection. In tibial components sterilized by gamma radiation in air, 65% had cracking or delamination. When components with delamination are microtomed into thin sections, 91% exhibited a subsurface white band. The white band is an area where there is oxidation of the polyethylene and a resulting loss of mechanical strength and ductility that occurs as a result of gamma sterilization in an oxygen environment. Thus, method of sterilization may play a key role in the long-term success of polyethylene as a weight-bearing material; gamma radiation in an oxygen environment is to be avoided.

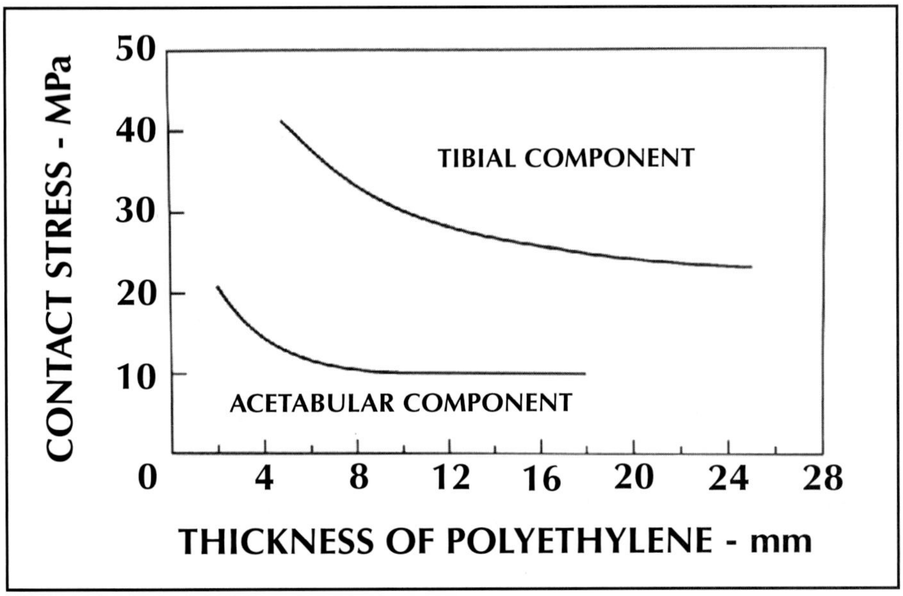

Fig. 4 This graph illustrates that as the thickness of a polyethylene component decreases the contact stress perpendicular to the surface increases. Because the surface is less conforming, the stresses are greater for the tibial component of a TKR at all thicknesses of polyethylene than they are for an acetabular component. A minimum thickness of 8 mm of true polyethylene should be chosen for tibial components. (Reproduced with permission from Bartel DL, Rimnac CM, Wright TM: Evaluation and design of the articular surface, in Goldberg VM (ed): *Controversies of Total Knee Arthroplasty.* New York, NY, Raven Press, 1991, pp 61-73.)

Thickness of the Tibial Polyethylene Insert

As stated earlier, the thickness of the polyethylene insert is an important factor in maximizing the performance of polyethylene as a weight-bearing material in TKR. The thickness of the tibial insert is directly linked to the level of the tibial bone resection. Polyethylene thickness is an important determinant of contact stress distribution within a UHMWPE component and associated UHMWPE damage. Bartel and associates[13] in 1985 delineated the relationship between polyethylene thickness and contact stress in metal-backed UHMWPE implants. The authors showed that the contact stresses increase exponentially when the thickness of the UHMWPE decreases (Fig. 4). They recommended a minimum UHMWPE thickness of 8 mm in knee replacements, based on their study that used a relatively conforming or dished articular geometry.

Widespread use of metal-backed tibial components in knee replacement surgery has resulted in a potential dilemma for surgeons; resect more bone from the proximal tibia to accommodate the metal backing, or use a thinner polyethylene component. Advantages of metal-backed tibial components are that the metal backing stiffens the overall structure and allows more even distribution of load transfer to the supporting bone. Metal backing also prevents gross deformation of the UHMWPE. The disadvantage of the metal-backed tibial component is that the metal backing is added at the potential expense of the UHMWPE because its thickness is often decreased. Manufacturers often include the thickness of the metal backing with the thickness of the UHMWPE when labeling a polyethylene insert. Should the true thickness of the UHMWPE fall below the 8 mm recommended by Bartel and associates,[13] the device becomes more susceptible to surface damage, deformation, and catastrophic failure.

Surgeons may incorrectly emphasize preserving proximal tibial bone by minimizing resection of the proximal tibia during TKR. Goldstein and associates[14] demonstrated that the mechanical strength of the proximal tibia bone diminishes with increasing distance from the articular surface. Fixation of the tibial component in weaker bone could theoretically result in increased potential for implant loosening. This study overemphasizes the role of the subchondral bone plate, and the difference in strength is much less after the subchondral plate is removed. The surgeon often desires to preserve as much bone in the proximal tibia as possible, but a tibial resection level that necessitates the use of a polyethylene insert less than 8 mm thick increases the risk of catastrophic tibial polyethylene wear. The mechanical performance of UHMWPE as a weight-bearing material is directly dependent on the thickness of the UHMWPE insert. It is recommended that the tibial resection level be determined by a measured resection technique that removes the amount of proximal tibia necessary to allow use of a tibial insert at least 8 mm thick in addition to the metal backing, typically 10 mm.

Polyethylene Damage Following TKR

Wear at the articular surface of polyethylene components following TKR is inevitable. The large contact stresses to which the polyethylene is subjected are sufficient to cause wear damage even in highly conforming prosthetic designs. Delamination and pitting are two wear-damage modes commonly seen in TKRs that are caused by fatigue. These damage modes can generate a large amount of debris of relatively large particle size in comparison to that of total hip replacement. During loading of the knee, the contact area moves over the tibial surface, creating large cyclic stresses in the polyethylene that cause cracks to initiate and grow on and below the component surface.

Polyethylene damage of tibial components in TKR has been extensively studied.[5-8,15,16] Retrieval studies have correlated the duration of implantation and patient body weight with the extent of UHMWPE damage. In one study, the three most common modes of damage were found to be delamination, abrasive wear, and adhesive wear.[8] Landy and Walker,[7] in an implant retrieval study, found a high incidence of three-body wear resulting from the entrapment of a third body, such as a bone or polymethylmethacrylate fragment, between the femoral condyle and the UHMWPE. Delamination was also observed and appeared to be initiated by fusion defects within the UHMWPE propagated by the subsurface shear stresses beneath the contact zone. Maximum shear stresses in the UHMWPE occur at a depth of 1 to 2 mm beneath the articular surface. In vivo testing to 10 million cycles demonstrated that if the location of contact between the prosthetic femoral condyles and the UHMWPE remained constant, some surface deformation was observed but surface damage was minimal.[17] However, if sliding was allowed in the sagittal plane, severe delamination and numerous subsurface cracks developed. Blunn and associates[17] have concluded that minimizing sliding and maintaining relatively localized contact area minimizes UHMWPE wear.

The PCL-retaining designs typically have a less conforming or flatter UHMWPE tibial sagittal geometry to permit rollback and function of the PCL. Several studies now suggest that well functioning PCL-retaining prostheses may have a paradoxical anterior translation of the tibia on the femur rather than the anticipated rollback. Dennis and associates[18] have studied in vivo anteroposterior femorotibial translation of TKR in a multicenter analysis. This study compared the femorotibial contact patterns for subjects having a PCL-retaining or PCL-substituting TKR. Femorotibial contact of 72 patients implanted with a TKR performed by one of five surgeons was analyzed using video fluoroscopy. Thirty-one patients were implanted with a PCL-retaining TKR with a flat polyethylene posterior lipped insert, 12 with a PCL-retaining curved polyethylene insert, and 29 with a PCL-substituting TKR. Each subject performed successive deep knee bends to maximum flexion during which video fluoroscopy was used to determine femorotibial contact patterns. The results show a lack of customary posterior femoral rollback in both PCL-retaining designs, and conversely an average anterior femoral translation with knee flexion was observed in both PCL-retaining TKRs. Posterior femoral rollback, less than in normal knees, routinely was observed in PCL-substituting TKRs. This factor was attributed to engagement of the femoral component cam with the tibial post. The abnormal anterior femoral translation observed in PCL-retaining TKRs in this multicenter series was remarkably similar to previous single surgeon series, and may be a factor in the premature polyethylene wear observed in retrieval studies.[19] Studies have been conducted that compare the surface contact areas and areas of maximum contact stresses between various PCL-retaining knee implants and between various PCL-sacrificing implants.[20] More conforming surfaces have been associated with a lower incidence of UHMWPE wear in clinical use.[21]

Hirakawa and associates[22] have suggested that the size and concentration of debris particles might reflect, in part, different dominant wear mechanisms among implants of different designs. They studied tissues from 75 failed primary total knee prostheses from which polyethylene particles were isolated. Implants were divided into four groups: group I; PCL-retaining, flat-on-flat design, heat-pressed polyethylene; group II; PCL-retaining, flat-on-flat design, non–heat-pressed polyethylene; group III; PCL-retaining, congruent design, and group IV; PCL-substituting, congruent design. Polyethylene particles were evaluated for particle size and concentration and implants were compared as to the extent and distribution of wear on the superior and inferior polyethylene surfaces. The more conforming designs (groups III and IV) had fewer and smaller particles and less surface damage than groups I and II. Groups I and II had more rotationally asymmetric wear patterns than groups III and IV. Implants with third-body wear had relatively small debris particles. Implants with thinner polyethylene had more severe surface delamination and more wear between the liner and metal base plate.[22]

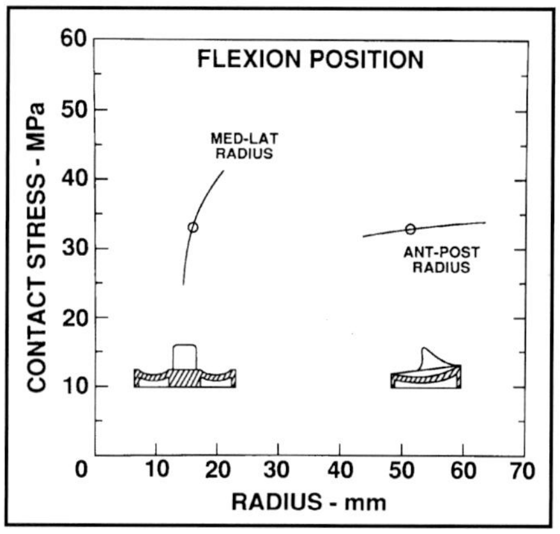

Fig. 5 Compressive contact stress on the tibial component polyethylene as a function of the geometry of the contact surfaces. The conformity in the coronal plane has a greater effect on contact stress than conformity in the sagittal plane. (Reproduced with permission from Bartel DL, Rimnac CM, Wright TM: Evaluation and design of the articular surface, in Goldberg VM (ed): *Controversies of Total Knee Arthroplasty*. New York, NY, Raven Press, 1991, pp 61-73.)

Compressive and tensile stresses that exceed the endurance of the UHMWPE have been demonstrated to exist in tibial components of TKRs by in vitro testing and finite element analysis.[23,24] The yield stress of UHMWPE is approximately 15 MPa. Contact stresses in conforming total knee designs have been shown to vary from 25 MPa compression to 15 MPa tension. These stresses are significantly higher than the contact stresses that are present in hip replacements where the articular surface is more conforming. This is consistent with implant retrieval studies that show that the less conforming tibial components from TKRs experienced greater surface UHMWPE damage than did acetabular components from total hip replacements. Conformity is an important consideration in TKR prosthetic design. Conformity in the coronal plane has been shown to have a greater effect on contact stresses than conformity in the sagittal plane[23] (Fig. 5). The effects of large compressive and tensile maximum stresses are compounded in TKRs because the contact area size and location change during flexion and extension. The tibial component UHMWPE is thus subjected to cyclic stresses that vary an order of magnitude greater than those to which an acetabular component is subjected. Currier and associates[25] have studied the in vitro simulation of fatigue loading of UHMWPE knee components in a knee simulator and on a rolling and sliding wear tester. Tibial components for the knee simulator were gamma-sterilized, implantable components taken from manufacturing inventory. The rolling/sliding disks were machined from bar stock and either gamma sterilized in air and age-accelerated, or left as nonsterilized controls. Cracking and delamination of samples that had been gamma sterilized in air and aged were observed in both types of tests. Contact fatigue damage was visible in as few as 150,000 cycles using the knee simulator at loads of 122 N (275 lb). The rolling/sliding samples showed signs of damage in as few as 130,000 cycles with an estimated stress of 15 MPa. However, cracking and delamination were not seen in the never-sterilized or recently sterilized controls. UHMWPE that has been gamma sterilized in air and aged is shown to be susceptible to contact fatigue damage. These results are important when interpreting in vitro TKR simulations used to assess the performance of tibial inserts.[25]

Incidence of Polyethylene Wear Following TKR

Lonner and associates[26] studied the prodromes of failure in TKR. They studied 102 revision TKRs to determine the prodromal symptoms and radiographic findings associated with failure. Presenting symptoms included pain (84%); swelling (76%); progressive varus or valgus deformity (19%); instability (17%); stiffness (17%); clicking or grinding (7%); patellar pain, or subluxation (4%). Radiographs were diagnostic in 91% of failures, demonstrating complete radiolucencies (80%); polyethylene wear (43%); component breakage (5%); and osteolysis (4%). Gross intraoperative findings included polyethylene wear in 72% of cases. The authors recommended an annual follow-up examination and weight-bearing radiographs be used to ensure adequate surveillance of TKR patients and avoid the complications associated with delay in the diagnosis of polyethylene wear or implant loosening.

A high incidence of accelerated polyethylene wear was first reported by Kilgus and associates[15] in 1991. A series of 176 Porous Coated Anatomic (PCA, Howmedica, Rutherford, NJ) TKRs performed between 1981 and 1987 with a mean follow-up of 60 months was evaluated retrospectively. The average postoperative mechanical axis of the limb in this series was neutral. More than 30% of the patients showed radiographic evidence of polyethylene wear; 10% of the patients underwent revision surgery because of severe polyethylene wear or fracture of the polyethylene insert.

Tsao and associates[27] reviewed 487 PCA total knee replacements performed by a single surgeon between 1982 and 1989. There were 32 clinical failures (7%) due to severe wear of the surfaces of the tibial and patellar polyethylene components. Thirty of these patients underwent revision and the average time to failure was 4.5 years. Significant predictors of an increased risk of failure were thin polyethylene tibial inserts, increased patient weight, and younger patient age. Examination of the retrieved tibial components revealed extensive delamination caused by fracture of the polyethylene at a depth of about 1 mm below the articular surface. The accelerated rate of polyethylene wear in this series and the series of Kilgus and associates[15] may be attributed to heat treatment of the polyethylene, thin polyethylene tibial components, relatively low femoral-tibial contact areas, and high maximal contact stresses.

Wasielewski and associates[28] examined 55 tibial polyethylene components retrieved at revision TKR for evidence of wear after a mean implantation of 34.2 months. Twenty tibial components retrieved were UHMWPE and 35 were carbon-reinforced polyethylene. Severe generalized articular wear was seen in inserts with three-body wear from metal and cement debris. Severe localized delamination wear was seen in inserts with rotational-subluxation patterns of wear. Preoperative varus was found to be related to the occurrence of posteromedial cold flow of polyethylene into tibial tray screw holes. Increasing tibial insert posterior slope was associated with increased posterior wear track location. Articular wear and cold flow into screw holes tended to be greater in the tightest prearthroplasty compartment; medial in varus knees and lateral in valgus knees. The authors concluded that wear patterns and the severity of UHMWPE wear in unconstrained tibial components may be associated with clinical and mechanical factors under the surgeon's control, including component size and position, and knee alignment and ligament balance.[28]

Six hundred sixty-five patients underwent revision TKR at the Mayo Clinic from July 1983 to November 1990.[29] In 24 of these 665 patients (3.6%) surgery was performed due to gross failure of the UHMWPE insert. Although there were multiple styles of knee replacements in this series of 24 polyethylene failures, there are three features common to this group of patients. In all 24 patients the tibial component was positioned in varus, resulting in varus postoperative alignment of the limb. In addition, in all 24 patients the tibial component UHMWPE thickness was equal to or less than 9 mm. As this measurement typically included the metal backing of the tibial component, the actual thickness of the UHMWPE itself varied between 4 to 7 mm in the thinnest area of the insert. Twelve of these 24 patients (50%) exceeded their ideal body weight by more than 20%.[29]

Plante-Bordeneuve and Freeman[30] studied UHMWPE wear following TKR in 27 patients with up to 9 years follow-up. The design of the components gave a nominal contact area of 320 mm^2 on each condyle. The tibial component was UHMWPE at least 6 mm thick, and not heat-treated. The average wear rate was 0.025 mm/yr. The relative wear in the medial and lateral compartments was related to the axis of the leg. None of the retrieved components showed any severe disruption of their surface. The authors concluded that the rate of wear of UHMWPE in a conforming tibiofemoral bearing with a fixed tibial component was slow enough to be safe for use in clinical practice.[30]

Undersurface Wear of the Polyethylene Insert

Wasielewski and associates[31] studied the undersurface of the tibial insert as a contributing source of polyethylene wear debris in TKR patients. Sixty-seven tibial inserts from cementless TKRs were retrieved at autopsy and revision surgery and analyzed for evidence of articular and nonarticular surface wear after a mean implantation time of 62.8 months (range 4 to 131 months). Polyethylene cold flow and abrasive wear on the nonarticular insert surface (undersurface) were assigned a wear severity score. The severity of the articular wear was assessed quantitatively and graded. Corresponding prerevision radiographs were evaluated for evidence of tibial osteolysis and osteolysis around tibial fixation screws. The authors found that severe grade 4 wear of the tibial insert undersurface was associated with tibial osteolysis or osteolysis around screws. Time in situ statistically was related to grade 4 undersurface wear and tibial osteolysis. The occurrence of osteolysis was not statistically related to the severity of wear at the main articular surface. The main articulation between the femoral implant and polyethylene insert has been assumed to be the primary source of polyethylene debris contributing to osteolysis and TKR implant failure. The undersurface of the insert is an additional source of polyethylene debris contributing to osteolysis in the tibia. To lessen polyethylene debris, the authors recommended improving the tibial implant locking mechanism to firmly fix the polyethylene to the metal and decrease relative micromotion. Because motion between the insert and metal tray may be inevitable, the wear characteristics of the inner tray surface should be optimized to minimize wear debris production at this interface.

A mobile-bearing TKR contains a tibial insert that is intended to rotate or rotate and translate in relation to the tibial base plate. One rationale for the use of a mobile-bearing knee prosthesis is that the undersurface wear is better controlled than it is with many modular tibial designs in which no motion is intended. In addition, many believe that the articulation surfaces are more congruent in mobile-bearing knee prostheses, which would decrease the peak stresses in the polyethylene insert during weight-bearing loading cycles. However, Matsuda and associates[32] showed that there are fixed-bearing knees that have better contact stresses and reduced contact forces at 60° and 90° of flexion compared to the Low Contact Stress (LCS, DePuy, Warsaw, IN) knee replacement. In addition, Parks and associates[33] found that the difference between fixed-bearing and mobile-bearing knees with respect to the average and peak stresses on the articular surface of the polyethylene is only 2 to 3 MPa. They also found that the stress on the undersurface of the mobile-bearing knee against the base plate was 40% of the upper surface stress. At present, there are no studies that show that mobile-bearing TKRs have less polyethylene wear or a different rate of osteolysis than a fixed-bearing prosthesis.[34]

Treatment of Polyethylene Wear

One treatment option for patients with polyethylene wear of the tibial insert is exchange of the modular insert with retention of the total knee components. Engh and associates[35] reported on the results of 63 knees (56 patients) treated with revision of the tibial polyethylene insert and retention of well aligned and stable femoral and tibial components. The implants had been in situ for an average of 59 months (2 to 108 months) at the time of the insert exchange. The inserts that were removed were examined and the severity of the articular wear and the undersurface wear was graded. They found that 7 of the 48 exchanges failed at an average of 54 months because of accelerated wear of the new insert. All seven knees required complete revision of all components. Of the 22 exchanges that were performed because of severe wear of the primary insert, 6 failed at an average of less than 5 years. The author concluded that knees in which the insert exchange was performed for advanced wear were more likely to fail again ($P < 0.05$). In addition, primary inserts that were removed from knees that failed after

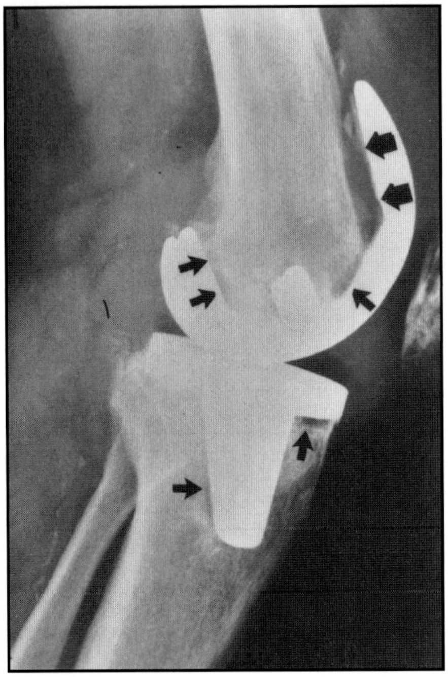

Fig. 6 Lateral radiograph of a patient with extensive polyethylene wear and resultant osteolysis due to three-body wear of the polyethylene.

exchange of the insert had higher delamination scores than those that were removed from knees in which the exchange was successful ($P < 0.05$). Most of the primary inserts had marked undersurface wear at the time of the exchange procedure. Engh and associates[35] concluded that an isolated revision of the tibial polyethylene insert should not be performed when there is accelerated wear of the insert with severe delamination and grade 3 or 4 undersurface wear within 10 years of the primary procedure. Because of the variety of patient-related, implant-related, and technical factors that influence polyethylene wear, the orthopaedist must consider multiple variables whenever contemplating a limited revision or tibial insert exchange.

Ayers and Carr (unpublished data, 1997) reported the results of 26 patients who had undergone an exchange of the tibial insert following a variable axis TKR. All of the patients were more than 10 years from their index operation and each had severe wear of the polyethylene insert. Osteolysis was graded by the Lewis method. Twenty of these 26 patients required TKR within 8 years of the insert exchange. Ayers and Carr concluded that contraindications for insert exchange included loose femoral or tibial component; scratching of the femoral component, osteolysis of grade 1 or more at the time of insert exchange; and if a mal-alignment of the limb could not be corrected by insert exchange alone. Isolated insert exchange was rarely indicated. The indications for isolated tibial insert exchange were well-fixed components; properly aligned components; less than grade 1 osteolysis; and if the etiology of the polyethylene wear could be corrected at the time of insert exchange. This correction typically required the fabrication of an angled tibial insert and ligamentous balancing techniques to achieve equal and symmetric flexion and extension gaps at the time of insert exchange.

Pathophysiology of Osteolysis

Polyethylene wear may lead to osteolysis. Osteolysis has been observed in patients with cemented and cementless TKR around well-fixed and loose components (Fig. 6). The pathophysiology of osteolysis centers on the role of the macrophage and its response to particulate debris, such as polyethylene. Particulate debris may gain access to the bone-cement or the bone-prosthesis interface and elicit formation of a fibrous tissue membrane that contains macrophage and foreign body giant cells.[36] The foreign body debris is phagocytosed by the macrophage. In response, the macrophage produces inflammatory mediators, such as cytokines (interleukins-1 and -6, tumor necrosis factor) and prostinoids (prostaglandins E_2 and F_{2a}), that result in the stimulation of osteoclasts to effect bone resorption. In order for this complex biologic cascade to proceed, the particulate debris must have access to the interface. The bone-cement interface, or alternatively the prosthesis-bone interface in cementless implants, are included as part of the effective joint space.[37] The pressure generated within the joint is sufficient to act as a hydraulic pump to circulate the particulate debris throughout the effective joint space.

A number of factors influence the biologic response to particulate debris: the number of particles present, the size of the particles, the surface chemistry of the particles, and the type of particulate material. Studies have demonstrated that the size distribution of the particles obtained from the inflammatory membrane retrieved from TKR patients with osteolytic defects differs from the size of particulate debris from TKR patients with osteolytic defects.[38] Particulate polyethylene debris retrieved from TKR patients have a higher percentage of particulate material that is larger in size than the debris obtained from total hip replacement patients.[38] Conversely, particulate debris retrieved from TKR patients with osteolysis have a higher percentage of particles in the submicron range. It has been hypothesized that the small, submicron particles may be a greater stimulus to the macrophage to produce inflammatory mediators that result in osteolysis.[38]

Summary

The etiology of polyethylene wear following TKR is multifactorial. Factors such as surgical technique, patient selection, and choice of implant design directly impact the polyethylene wear rate. Surgical technique is directly associated with polyethylene wear; particularly the thickness of the polyethylene insert, the post-operative mechanical axis of the limb, and the alignment of the tibial component in the coronal plane. Patient selection is an important determinant of polyethylene wear, as patient body weight and activity level have been shown to correlate with wear rate. Prosthetic design plays a role in polyethylene wear as femoral-tibial contact areas, peak contact forces, and surface topography of the polyethylene are important considerations. The method by which the polyethylene is manufactured and the method of sterilization are also important determinants of polyethylene wear. Wear of polyethylene is one source of particulate debris following TKR. Phagocytosis of the particulate debris by macrophage occurs at the prosthesis-bone interface. The macrophage produces inflammatory mediators in response to the particulate debris. Inflammatory mediators act at the failed interface to effect bone resorption and produce osteolysis. In summary, the surgeon can play a major role in maximizing polyethylene performance in TKR by understanding the multiple factors that contribute to polyethylene wear and taking steps to lessen their effect.

References

1. Li S, Burstein AH: Current concepts Review: Ultra-high molecular weight polyethylene. *J Bone Joint Surg Am* 1994;76:1080-1090.
2. Ritter MA, Worland R, Saliski J, et al: Flat-on-flat, nonconstrained, compression molded polyethylene total knee replacement. *Clin Orthop* 1995;321:79-85.
3. Won CH, Rohatgi S, Kraay MJ, Goldberg VM, Rimnac CM: Effect of resin type and manufacturing method on wear of polyethylene tibial components. *Clin Orthop* 2000;376:161-171.
4. Streecher RM: Localizing irradiation for sterilization and modification of high molecular weight polyethylenes. *Plas Rubber Process Appl* 1988;10:221-229.
5. Collier JP, Mayor MB, McNamara JL: Analysis of the failure of 122 polyethylene inserts from uncemented tibial knee components. *Clin Orthop* 1991;273:232.
6. Hood RW, Wright TM, Burstein AH: Retrieval analysis of total knee prostheses. *J Biomed Mater* 1983;17:829-842.
7. Landy MM, Walker PS: Wear of UHMWPE components of 90 retrieved knee prostheses. *J Arthroplasty* 1988;(suppl):S73-S84.
8. Wright TM, Bartel DL: The problem of surface damage in polyethylene total knee components. *Clin Orthop* 1986;205:607.
9. Wrona M, Major MB, Collier TP, Jensen RE: The correlation between fusion defects and damage in tibial polyethylene bearings. *Clin Orthop* 1994;229:92-103.
10. Matsuda S, Miura H, Nagamine R, Urabe K, Harimaya K, Matsunobu T, Iwamoto Y: Changes in knee alignment after total knee arthroplasty. *J Arthroplasty* 1999;14:566-570.
11. Rimnac CM, Klein RW, Betts F, Wright TM: Post-irradiation aging of ultra-high molecular weight polyethylene. *J Bone Joint Surg Am* 1994;76:1052-1056.
12. Rose RM, Crugnola A, Ries M, Cimino WR, Paul I, Radin EL: On the origin of high in vivo wear rates in polyethylene components of total joint prostheses. *Clin Orthop* 1979;145:277.
13. Bartel DL, Burstein AH, Toda MD, Edwards DL: The effect of conformity and plastic thickness on contact stresses in metal-backed plastic implants. *T Biotech Eng* 1985;107:193-199.
14. Goldstein SA, Wilson DL, Sonstegard DA: The mechanical properties of human tibial bone as a function of metaphyseal location. *J Biomech* 1983;16:965-969.
15. Kilgus DJ, Moreland JR, Finerman GA, Funahashi TT, Tipon JS: Catastrophic wear of tibial polyethylene inserts. *Clin Orthop* 1991;273:223.
16. Landy MM, Walker PS: Wear in condylar replacement knees: A ten year follow-up. *Trans Orthop Res Soc* 1985;10:96.
17. Blunn GW, Walker PS, Joshi A, Hardinge K: The dominance of cyclic sliding in producing wear in total knee replacements. *Clin Orthop* 1991;273:253-260.
18. Dennis DA, Komistek RD, Colwell CE Jr., Ranawat CS, Scott RD, Thornhill TS, Lapp MA: In vivo anteroposterior femorotibial translation of total knee arthroplasty: a multicenter analysis. *Clin Orthop* 1998;356:47-57.
19. Dennis DA, Komistek RD, Cheal EJ, Stiehl JB, Walker SA: In vivo Femoral condylar lift-off in total knee arthroplasty. *Orthop Trans* 1997;21:1112.
20. Werner FW, Ayers DC, Statler KD, Murray DG: Contact surface areas in cruciate sparing knee replacements. *Trans Ortho Res Soc* 1992;17:331.
21. Colizza WA, Insall JN, Scuderi GR: The posterior stabilized total knee prosthesis. Assessment of polyethylene damage and osteolysis after a ten year minimum follow-up. *J Bone Joint Surg Am* 1995;77:1713-1720.
22. Hirakawa K, Bauer TW, Yamaguchi M, Stulberg BN, Wilde AH: Relationship between wear debris particles and polyethylene surface damage in primary total knee arthroplasty. *J Arthroplasty* 1999;14:165-171.
23. Bartel DL, Bicknell MS: The effect of conformity, thickness and material on stresses in UHMW components for total joint replacement. *J Bone Joint Surg Am* 1986;68:1041-1051.
24. Bartel DL, Rimnac CM, Wright TM: Evaluation and design of the articular surface, in Goldberg VM (ed): *Controversies of Total Knee Arthroplasty*. New York, NY, Raven Press, 1991, pp 61-73.
25. Currier JH, Duda JL, Sperline DK, Collier JP, Currier BH, Kennedy FE: In vitro simulation of contact fatigue damage found in ultrahigh molecular weight polyethylene components of knee prostheses. *Proc Inst Mech Eng [H]* 1998;212:293-302.
26. Lonner JH, Siliski JM, Scott RD: Prodromes of failure in total knee arthroplasty. *J Arthroplasty* 1999;14:488-492.
27. Tsao A, Mintz L, McRae CR, Stulberg SD, Wright T: Failure of the porous-coated anatomic prosthesis in total knee arthroplasty due to severe polyethylene wear. *J Bone Joint Surg Am* 1993;75:19-26.
28. Wasielewski RC, Galante JO, Leighty RM, Nartaradam RN, Rosenberg AG: Wear patterns on retrieved polyethylene tibial inserts and their relationship to technical considerations during total knee arthroplasty. *Clin Orthop* 1994;299:31-43.
29. Rand, JA: Revision total knee arthroplasty, in Morrey (ed): *Total Joint Arthroplasty*. New York, NY, Raven Press, 1993.
30. Plante-Bordeneuve P, Freeman MA: Tibial high density polyethylene wear in conforming tibiofemoral prostheses. *J Bone Joint Surg Br* 1993;75:630-636.
31. Wasielewski RC, Parks N, Williams I, Surprenant H, Collier JP, Engh G: Tibial insert undersurface as a contributing source of polyethylene wear debris. *Clin Orthop* 1997;345: 53-59.
32. Matsuda S, White SE, Williams VG II, McCarthy DS, Whiteside LA: Contact stress analysis in meniscal bearing total knee arthroplasty. *J Arthroplasty* 1998;13:699-706.
33. Parks NL, Engh GA, Topoleski LD, Emperado J: Modular tibial insert micromotion. A concern with contemporary knee implants. *Clin Orthop* 1998;356:10-15.
34. Callaghan JJ, Insall JN, Greenwald AS, Dennis DA, Komistek RD, Murray DW, Bourne RB, Rorabeck CH, Dorr LD: Mobile-bearing knee replacement. *J Bone Joint Surg Am* 2000; 82:1020-1041.
35. Engh GA, Koralewicz LM, Pereles TR: Clinical results of modular polyethylene insert exchange with retention of total knee arthroplasty components. *J Bone Joint Surg Am* 2000;82:516-523.
36. Mirra JM, Marder RA, Amstutz HC: The pathology of failed total joint arthroplasty. *Clin Orthop* 1982;170:175.
37. Schmalzried TP, Jasty M, Harris WH: Periprosthetic bone loss in total hip arthroplasty, polyethylene wear debris and the concept of the effective joint space. *J Bone Joint Surg Am* 1992;74:849-863.
38. Chiba T, Schwenderman CJ, Booth RE, Crossett LS, Rubash HE: A biomechanical, histologic and immunohistology analysis of membranes obtained from failed cemented and cementless TKA. *Clin Orthop* 1994;299: 114-125.

45

Mobile-Bearing Knee Replacement: Concepts and Results

John J. Callaghan, MD
John N. Insall, MD
A. Seth Greenwald, DPhil (Oxon)
Douglas A. Dennis, MD
Richard D. Komistek, PhD
David W. Murray, MD, FRCS
Robert B. Bourne, MD, FRCSC
Cecil H. Rorabeck, MD
Lawrence D. Dorr, MD

Durable long-term fixation has been documented for many designs of fixed-bearing total knee replacement (TKR).[1-4] However, in the late 1970s and the early 1980s, implant fixation and polyethylene wear became recognized as long-term causes of late failure. Mobile-bearing knee replacements, with a polyethylene insert that articulates with a metallic femoral component and a metallic tibial tray, were designed to create a dual-surface articulation. This feature was intended to reduce the surface and subsurface stress states at the bearing surfaces and at the bone-implant surfaces by maximizing the conformity of the tibial and femoral components and allowing mobility of the bearing surface. We reserve the description "meniscal-bearing" is reserved for implants in which the femoral condyle is spherical and the bearing can function like its analogue in nature. These design features were developed to decrease the fatigue wear associated with failure of the polyethylene in knee arthroplasty. Currently, there are few intermediate-term follow-up reports and no long-term follow-up reports, as far as we know, on the use of these devices, but almost every manufacturer of TKR components is developing a product that they hope to introduce to the market. In this chapter, the rationale for the use of mobile-bearing knee devices is explored and the clinical follow-up of these devices is updated. The clinical results of use of the Oxford unicompartmental replacement (Biomet, Warsaw, IN), the Low-Contact Stress knee replacement (LCS; DePuy, Warsaw, IN), and the Self-Aligning knee replacement (SAL; Sulzer, Austin, TX) are highlighted, because these devices have been followed for at least 5 years.

One or more of the authors or the departments with which they are affiliated have received something of value from a commercial party related directly or indirectly to the subject of this chapter.

Why the Clinical Interest in Mobile-Bearing Knees?

Conventional fixed-bearing knee prostheses have proved to be clinically successful but with some reservations. In a study of 101 knees with such a prosthesis,[5] 96% had good-to-excellent clinical results, and the rate of survival of the prosthesis, with revision as the end point, was 96.4% after 10 to 15 years of follow-up.

However, there is an important caveat. Most of the patients involved in these follow-up studies have been elderly individuals with low activity levels, and thus low demands have been placed on the prosthesis. With a few exceptions,[1] there is little evidence that the same results could be duplicated in more active people. Also, even allowing for the preceding reservation, polyethylene wear and osteolysis remain important problems with current fixed-bearing knee prostheses.

Polyethylene Wear

There are two types of polyethylene wear. The first is articular wear, which was observed as a clinical problem in the 1980s and occurred in the so-called round-on-flat designs, which were popular then because they duplicated the normal motions of the knee. Round-on-flat designs, by definition, produce high contact stresses in the polyethylene.[6] When combined with sliding and skidding movements encouraged by an unconstrained articulation, these stresses lead to polyethylene damage and delamination, the particles from which can lead to osteolysis.[7,8]

The solution to this type of polyethylene wear is to design more conformity into the articulation (the so-called round-on-round type of prosthesis). Because there is always a compromise between conformity and freedom of motion within the knee as articular contact stresses are reduced, a kinematic penalty is paid. The increased contact area reduces rotation. While lack of rotation may not be important for elderly patients, it is probably a drawback for younger, more active patients.[9-15]

The second type of polyethylene wear that has been recognized recently is undersurface wear,[16] which occurs between the polyethylene bearing and the tibial baseplate. Initially, tibial components had a monoblock construction; that is, the polyethylene was molded onto the tibial baseplate during manufacture. This type of design has yielded successful and durable long-term results. Unfortunately, increased sizing options have made modularity a virtual necessity so that at present, in most cases, the polyethylene is no longer attached to the tibial baseplate by the manufacturer but is fixed to the baseplate with some kind of locking mechanism by the surgeon during the surgery. No currently used locking mechanism is entirely reliable, and varying degrees of motion occur between the polyethylene and the baseplate. This motion can, of course, result in undersurface wear and the production of polyethylene particles. The problem is compounded because, for manufacturing reasons, the baseplate often is made of titanium and the surface is usually unpolished.

Mobile-Bearing Prostheses

On the basis of all of this information, it would appear that we are at a crossroad. There is little likelihood that additional refinement in the design of fixed-bearing knee prostheses can improve the current results and even less likelihood that it would resolve the aforementioned problems. It is impossible to envision a return to monoblock tibial components, given the desire to closely match the implant size to the dimensions of the knee and to maintain the intraoperative flexibility provided by modularity. To date, implant manufacturers have failed to produce a completely reliable locking mechanism for attaching the polyethylene to the tibial baseplate. The kinematic conflict between low-stress articulations and free rotation cannot be solved by any fixed-bearing knee design.

Therefore, there are two possible options to pursue. One is the development of a new polyethylene or polyethylene alternative that is impervious to wear. The other is to further explore the possibilities of a mobile polyethylene bearing.

Biomechanical Concepts of Mobile Bearings

The success of total knee arthroplasty (TKA) is influenced by a complex interaction between the geometry of an implant design and the active and passive soft-tissue structures that surround the articulation.[17] This interaction, in turn, determines the stability, range of motion, and interface stresses that develop.

Dual-surface articulation between a polyethylene insert and the metallic femoral and tibial tray components is a consequence of mobile-bearing knee designs. These designs offer the advantage of conformal geometry with diminished surface and subsurface stress distributions, while the mobility of the bearings serves to minimize the development of interfacial bone stresses.

One of the principal features of mobile-bearing knee designs is the promotion of load sharing through the relative displacement between the tibial and femoral components. Simply stated, these designs allow the torques and shear forces of gait to be transferred by way of displacements to the soft tissues in a fashion similar to that of the normal knee. Load sharing has many potential advantages. It reduces the loosening stresses that are transferred to the implant-bone interface, and it also promotes soft-tissue strengthening. These tissues, unlike the inert prosthesis, have the capacity to respond and remodel to the challenges of the expanding activities performed as the pain-free knee is rehabilitated. Finally, load sharing may contribute to the reduction of articular wear of these devices by decreasing the joint loads. Thus, in general, soft-tissue involvement should be encouraged in order to decrease the dependency on the intrinsic constraints afforded by condylar geometry. Contemporary mobile-bearing knee designs achieve this involvement, and they can be described in terms of the plateau mobility, which can be (1) pure rotation, (2) rotation with anterior-posterior translation, and (3) unconstrained.[18] With regard to the knee replacements described in the present investigation, the Oxford unicompartmental replacement allows only anterior-posterior translation; the LCS rotating-platform knee, pure rotation; and the LCS meniscal-bearing and SAL knee replacements, rotation and anterior-posterior translation.

Long-term evaluation of the LCS meniscal-bearing total knee system with use of a wear simulator that approximated 10 years of in vivo service life demonstrated low volumetric loss of ultra-high molecular weight polyethylene (UHMWPE) compared with that associated with fixed-plateau designs.[18] Specifically, a 160-mg weight loss over 10 million stance-phase cycles, from a bearing plateau that initially weighed 16,000 mg, has been verified by more than 15 years of clinical success associated with this particular design.[18,19] A reason for this result is the substantial reduction in the proximal and distal contact stress levels suggested by finite element computation analysis.[20,21] The low contact stresses on both articulating surfaces greatly attenuate any effect that increased sliding distances may have on abrasive wear-debris generation.[22,23]

An evolution is occurring in total knee design that will lead to increasing use of mobile-bearing knee systems. Although these systems are regulated by the Food and Drug Administration (FDA) in the United States, the growing use of these systems in other countries is continuing unabated. Mobile-bearing knee designs offer orthopaedic surgeons a unique option for restoring normal, pain-free activity. Because of the mobility that they provide, slight positional malalignment of the components should not substantially affect the expected in vivo service life of the device as long as that malalignment corresponds with the defined mobility of that design. The individual clinical performance of the devices is strongly influenced by the particular design kinematics of both the proximal and the distal surface as well as the distribution of contact stresses. In addition, the volume and size of UHMWPE particles produced by dual-surface articulation are affected by the quality of the polyethylene and the finish of the articulating metallic components. With regard to these parameters, not all mobile-bearing knee systems perform the same.

Design Features of Mobile-Bearing Knee Prostheses

Mobile-bearing knee prostheses are not new. The first to be used was the Oxford device[24] (Biomet, Bridgend, South Wales), which was designed almost 25 years ago, and the second was the LCS prosthesis,[22] which was based on similar concepts and appeared shortly thereafter. Other designs have followed, but, to date, all have enjoyed only limited popularity. The concept of a mobile-bearing knee prosthesis is intellectually attractive and can potentially solve the three problems that have been discussed.

First, if the need to allow rotation at the femorotibial articulation is eliminated and rotation of the tibial polyethylene-tibial tray interface is allowed instead, the contact area of the articular surface can be greatly increased, from approximately 200 square mm^2 in a good fixed bearing to 1,000 mm^2 or more, and there can be a consequent reduction in contact stresses, from approximately 25 MPa in a fixed bearing to 5 MPa or less. The former stresses theoretically result in polyethylene breakdown, whereas the latter should not damage the polyethylene even in active use. The difference is analogous to the indentations left by a high-heeled shoe compared with those caused by a boot.

Second, the problem of wear between the polyethylene bearing and the tibial baseplate also can be resolved. There are insurmountable difficulties with regard to the manufacture of a chromium-cobalt tibial baseplate with a suitable intraoperative locking mechanism for the polyethylene because the material must be cast and not machined. It is relatively easy to make a chromium-cobalt baseplate to accommodate a mobile bearing, and it is also feasible to provide a smooth, highly polished surface on which the mobile bearing can move. It is well known that, however well finished, titanium does not provide a good articulating surface for polyethylene.[25]

Third, a mobile bearing also solves the kinematic conflict of a fixed-bearing knee prosthesis because a highly conforming articular surface can now coexist with free rotation.

The mobile-bearing concept is therefore attractive, but many questions remain to be answered and details need to be dealt with in pursuit of the best mobile-bearing knee design.

Fully Conforming Articulation

A fully conforming articulation has a contact area that remains the same throughout the range of motion, which appears to be the most desirable configuration.

Full Flexion

It has been postulated that the knee flexes about an axis running through the femoral epicondyles,[19] and a femoral component with a constant sagittal radius would therefore be not only possible but desirable. Such a design should allow 120° of flexion but perhaps not more because of posterior impingement of the tibial component. Until now, this degree of flexion has been considered sufficient for a knee prosthesis, but should future knee designs allow full flexion?

A knee design that allows full flexion must have two essential features: it must be posterior stabilized to direct predictable femoral rollback, and the femoral component must have a decreasing sagittal radius. These requirements suggest the need for a hybrid type of mobile-bearing knee prosthesis. If rotation is not required, the conformity of a conventional fixed-bearing knee can be improved and the contact area can be approximately doubled even in flexed positions. Therefore, a hybrid knee would allow a large contact area for the first 20° of flexion (the motion that occurs during the gait cycle) and an improved contact area throughout the rest of knee flexion. Rotation of course would occur at the undersurface.

Axis of Rotation

The proper axis of rotation at the undersurface also remains debatable. For a fully conforming meniscal-bearing knee, both rotation and anterior-posterior translation seem desirable to mimic the motion of the natural knee. Hybrid posterior stabilized mobile-bearing knees do not demand anterior-posterior translation and therefore may be well suited to some type of rotating platform; however, a central axis of rotation is not physiologic because backward movement on one side is accompanied by forward movement on the other.

Prevention of Dislocation of the Bearing

A potential complication associated with mobile-bearing knee prostheses is dislocation of the bearing. To prevent dislocation, some type of restraint on bearing movement seems desirable. This restraint could be provided by a "cylinder in a cylinder" or a "cone within a cone," with the cylinder or cone an extension of the polyethylene insert, which mates with a recess in the baseplate. Alternatively, a post or "mushroom" sprouting from the tibial baseplate could be used to anchor the polyethylene. An anterior or posterior metal stop that projects from the tibial tray may be used to limit unwanted movements.

Mobile-bearing knee designs should follow the tradition of fixed-bearing knee prostheses and have posterior cruciate-retaining (PCR) and posterior-stabilized variants. The former would be a rotating-gliding type, and the latter would most probably be a hybrid type. Although it is possible to envisage a fully conforming posterior-stabilized knee with motion driven by a tibial post fixed to the baseplate, the engineering complexities probably preclude the manufacture of such a design.

Fluoroscopic Evaluation of In Vivo Kinematics of Mobile-Bearing TKA

Previous in vivo kinematic studies with use of fluoroscopy have been conducted on patients with normal knee joints and on those who had implantation of a fixed-bearing PCR or posterior- stabilized TKR of multiple designs[26-30] to determine anteroposterior (AP) femorotibial contact patterns. Those studies have shown that, during a deep knee bend, patients with normal knees exhibited posterior femoral rollback with progressive flexion. In contrast, those who had a fixed-bearing prosthesis often had paradoxical anterior femoral translation (the femoral condyle shifting anteriorly on the tibia) with increasing knee flexion,[26,27] which was the reverse of the situation in the normal knees. Patients who had a posterior-stabilized TKR routinely demonstrated posterior femoral rollback during knee flexion, although it was lesser in magnitude than that in the normal knees.[26,27] When tested during gait, patients who had a PCR or a posterior-stabilized TKR exhibited paradoxical anterior femoral translation, which was attributed to a lack of engagement of the cam and post of the posterior-stabilized TKR in activities that require less flexion, such as gait.[31]

Additional studies involving fluoroscopic evaluation of fixed-bearing TKRs have documented reduced amounts of axial femorotibial rotation[32] and the presence of unicondylar separation of the femoral and tibial condyles (femoral condylar lift-off).[33] We present the following report to summarize the findings of our in vivo kinematic analyses of multiple groups of patients who had been managed with various designs of mobile-bearing TKAs and to compare the in vivo knee kinematics in our patients with those reported in studies involving patients who had had a fixed-bearing TKA.

Materials and Methods

The in vivo kinematics of the knee (anterior-posterior translation, axial rotation, femoral condylar lift-off, and range of motion) have been determined in many studies of meniscal-bearing, posterior-cruciate-sacrificing (PCS) rotating-platform, and posterior-stabilized rotating-platform mobile-bearing TKA designs (LCS).[34-36] All of the TKAs in those studies were judged to have been clinically successful (an excellent result according to The Hospital for Special Surgery knee score[2]) without substantial ligamentous laxity or pain. The knees were analyzed with use of high-frequency, pulsated videofluoroscopy (Radiographic and Data Solutions, Minneapolis, MN) while the patient performed a weight-bearing deep knee bend or normal gait activity. While performing the deep knee bend, each patient placed the foot of the involved lower limb on a designated marker. For this activity, the initial fluoroscopic examination was performed with the knee in full extension. During gait analysis, the involved knee was tracked by the fluoroscopy unit, which was moved manually to capture the knee throughout the stance phase of gait.

The fluoroscopic images were stored on videotape for subsequent redigitization with use of a frame grabber. The contact positions between the femur and the tibia were determined with use of a three-dimensional (3-D) model-fitting technique.[37] The fluoroscopic images were initially captured onto a workstation computer. The 3-D solid models of the femoral and tibial components, made with computer-aided design, were overlaid onto the two-dimensional fluoroscopic perspective images (Fig. 1). Once the 3-D components were precisely fit, the femorotibial contact positions of the medial and lateral condyles were determined with respect to the midline of the tibia in the sagittal plane with use of a sophisticated computer algorithm.[37] A contact position anterior to the midline was denoted as positive, and a position posterior to the midline was denoted as negative. During the deep knee bend, fluoroscopic images were analyzed at 0°, 30°, 60°, and 90° of flexion. Analysis of gait was performed at heel-strike (0%), at 33% and 66% of stance phase, and at toe-off (100%).

Results

Anterior-Posterior Translation Previous analysis of normal knee kinematics with use of videofluoroscopy as the subject performed a weight-bearing deep knee bend has demonstrated that the lateral femoral condyle contacts the tibia anterior to the midline of the tibia in the sagittal plane (an average of +6.5 mm) at full extension.[33] With progressive knee flexion, there is posterior translation of this condyle (posterior femoral rollback) to an average final position of –7.7 mm (an average of 14.2 mm of posterior femoral rollback)[26] (Fig. 2). In contrast, patients with a meniscal-bearing TKR exhibited a posterior contact position at full extension. A small amount of posterior femoral rollback (an average of 4.8

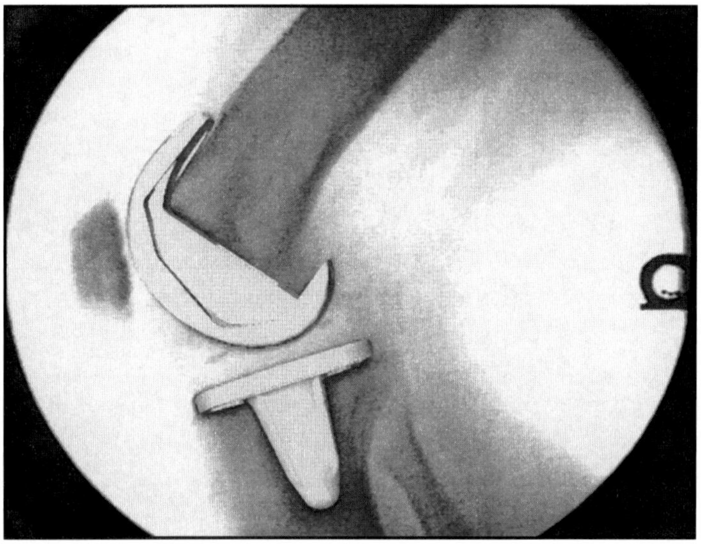

Fig. 1 Three-dimensional solid models of femoral and tibial components, made with computer-aided design, precisely fit over a two-dimensional fluoroscopic image.

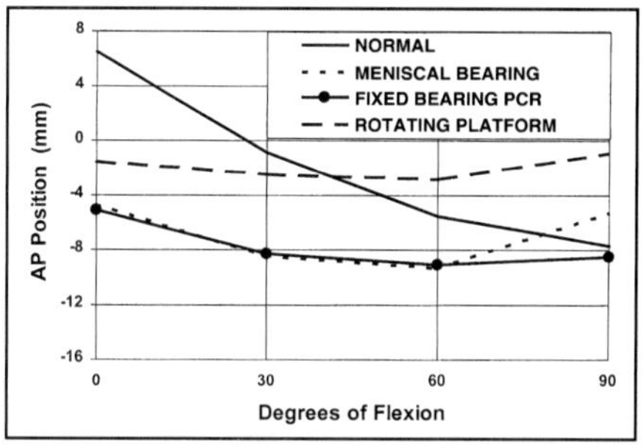

Fig. 2 Graph showing the average AP contact positions of the lateral condyle during a deep knee-bend activity in subjects with normal knees and in those with fixed-bearing PCR, meniscal-bearing, and rotating-platform TKRs.

mm) occurred during the first 60° of flexion, followed by anterior femoral translation as the knee flexed from 60° to 90°.[34,36] Contact pathways in patients who had a meniscal-bearing TKR proved to be quite similar to those in patients with a fixed-bearing PCR TKR.[32,33] Hence, the meniscal-bearing implant may not provide any advantage with regard to the contact pathway.

Patients with a rotating-platform TKR experienced, on the average, minimal anterior-posterior femorotibial translation during a deep knee bend, with femorotibial contact remaining near the middle of the articulating surface of the tibial component[36] (Fig. 2). Substantial variability of contact patterns among subjects managed with either a meniscal-bearing or a rotating-platform design (Fig. 3) was common.

A later analysis was performed to compare the PCS and posterior-stabilized rotating-platform designs (LCS) with regard to AP contact pathways of both the medial and the lateral condyle during a deep knee bend and during normal gait (B Haas, RD Komistek, DA Dennis, unpublished data, Rocky Mountain Musculoskeletal Research Laboratory, Denver, CO). During a deep knee bend, patients managed with a PCS rotating-platform TKR had posterior femoral rollback of the lateral condyle (an average of 3.3 mm) from full extension to 90° of flexion, but they actually experienced anterior translation from 60° to 90° of flexion. The contact position of the medial condyle remained approximately the same (an average of –2.3 mm at 0° and –2.2 mm at 90°) during the deep knee bend (Fig. 4). Patients who had a posterior-stabilized rotating-platform TKR exhibited more substantial posterior femoral rollback of the lateral condyle (an average of 5.9 mm) during the deep knee-bend maneuver. A minimal change in the contact position of the medial condyle was observed throughout the range of flexion (Fig. 5). Again, a high variability in contact positions among individual patients was observed in both design groups, particularly in deep flexion. This variability was attributed, at least in part, to variances in the amount of axial rotation of the bearing among the individual patients. Continual posterior femoral rollback of the lateral condyle throughout the range of flexion (an average of –0.6 mm at 0°, –4.1 mm at 30°, –4.8 mm at 60°, and –6.5 mm at 90°) was observed in all patients managed with a posterior-stabilized rotating-platform design (Fig. 5); this finding was attributed to engagement of the cam-and-post mechanism. In contrast, paradoxical anterior femoral translation of the lateral condyle was observed at some point in the range of flexion in 40% of the patients managed with a PCS rotating-platform TKA.

During gait, patients managed with a PCS rotating-platform TKA experienced minimal change in the AP contact position of the lateral condyle (an average of 2.2 mm) and the medial condyle (an average of 0.2 mm) from heel-strike to toe-off (Fig. 6). Patients managed with a posterior-stabilized rotating-platform TKA also demonstrated minimal change in the AP contact position of the lateral condyle (an average of 1.2 mm) and the medial condyle (an average of 1.1 mm) from heel-strike to toe-off (Fig. 7). In contrast to testing during a deep knee-bend maneuver, testing during gait demonstrated minimal variance (less than 3.0 mm) in contact patterns either medially or laterally among individual patients in both groups.

Axial Femorotibial Rotation During a deep knee bend, patients managed with a PCS rotating-platform or posterior-stabilized rotating-platform TKA generally demonstrated a normal axial femorotibial

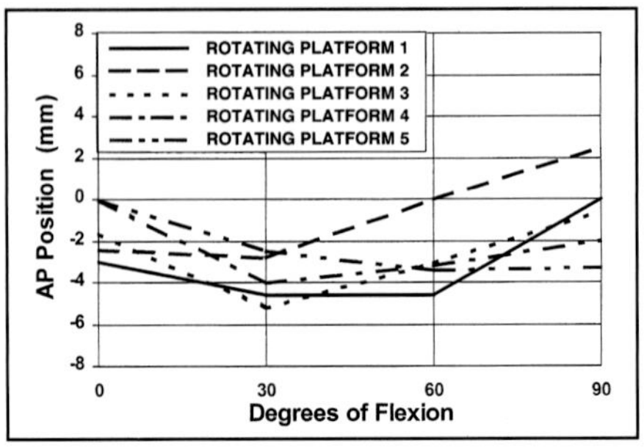

Fig. 3 Graph showing the average AP contact positions of the lateral condyle during a deep knee-bend activity for five randomly selected patients who had a PCS rotating-platform TKR. There is a high variance in contact positions among the individual subjects.

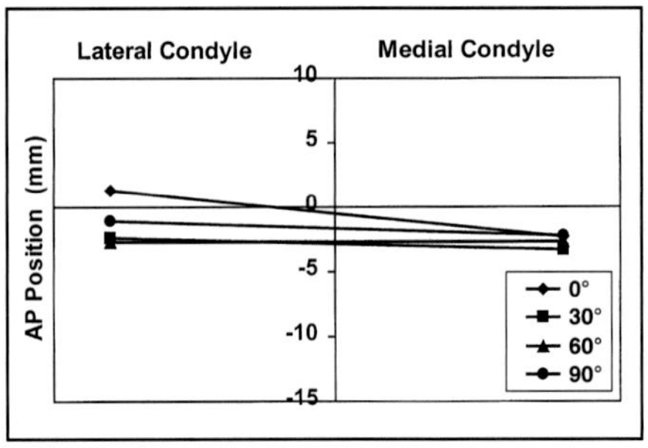

Fig. 4 Graph showing the average AP contact positions of the medial and lateral condyles during a deep knee-bend activity in patients who had a PCS rotating-platform TKR.

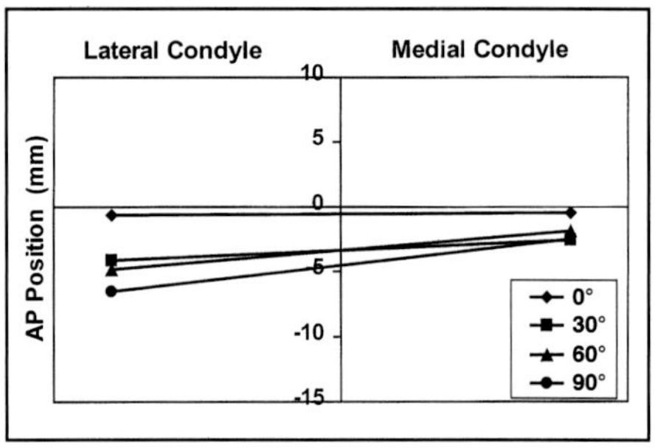

Fig. 5 Graph showing the average AP contact positions of the medial and lateral condyles during a deep knee-bend activity in patients who had a posterior stabilized rotating-platform TKR.

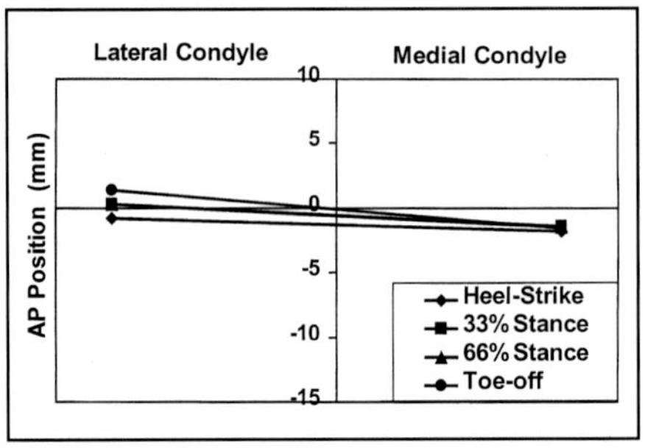

Fig. 6 Graph showing the average AP contact positions of the medial and lateral condyles during gait in patients with a PCS rotating-platform TKR.

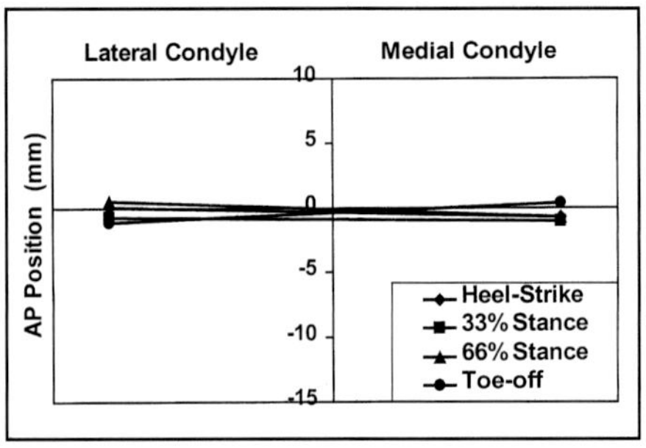

Fig. 7 Graph showing the average AP contact positions of the medial and lateral condyles during gait in patients with a posterior stabilized rotating-platform TKR.

rotational pattern (that is, internal rotation of the tibia with progressive flexion), although it was typically less in magnitude than that reported for normal knees[38] (Table 1). During gait, patients who had been managed with a posterior-stabilized rotating-platform TKR demonstrated, on the average, a normal axial femorotibial rotational pattern whereas those managed with a PCS rotating-platform TKR had an abnormal, reverse rotational pattern (external rotation of the tibia with progressive flexion).

A review of average axial rotational values can be misleading because of the high variability observed among individual subjects. In a separate fluoroscopic study of the gait of 20 patients who had a PCS rotating-platform TKR (LCS), a normal axial rotational pattern was seen in only seven patients, with an abnormal, reverse rotational pattern observed in eight patients and negligible rotation (average, 0.5°) noted in five patients.[35]

Femoral Condylar Lift-Off The occurrence of femoral condylar lift-off at some point in the flexion cycle was common, with a rate of more than 90% with both the PCS and the posterior-stabilized rotating-platform designs.[32,36] This high rate of lift-off was observed during both gait and the deep knee bend maneuver. Femoral condylar lift-off was seen more commonly on the lateral side of the joint, which was attributed to the adduction moment that occurs during the midstance phase of the gait cycle.[33] The magnitude of condylar separation is reported in Table 2. As in previous fluoroscopic evaluations of femoral condylar lift-off in patients managed with a fixed-bearing TKA,[33] lift-off was most commonly observed between 60° and 90° of flexion during a deep knee bend and during the midstance phase of the gait cycle.

Range of Motion The range of motion following meniscal-bearing and PCS rotating-platform TKA has been assessed under passive, non-weight-bearing and active, weight-bearing conditions and compared with previously published data obtained after fixed-bearing PCR and PCS TKAs.[39] Flexion was reduced when it was tested under weight-bearing conditions in all groups (Table 3). The greatest average range of motion was observed in patients who had had a fixed-bearing posterior-stabilized TKA.

Summary of In Vivo Kinematic Studies

In vivo fluoroscopic analyses of various designs of mobile-bearing TKRs during weight-bearing activities have demonstrated that numerous kinematic abnormalities (paradoxical anterior femoral translation, reverse axial rotational patterns, and femoral condylar lift-off) are common (B Haas, RD Komistek, DA Dennis, unpublished data Rocky Mountain Musculoskeletal Research Laboratory,

Denver, CO).[34-36] These kinematic abnormalities are not unlike those reported in similar fluoroscopic evaluations of fixed-bearing TKRs.[26-33]

Typically, patients who have had a mobile-bearing PCS rotating-platform or posterior-stabilized rotating-platform TKA have less anterior-posterior femorotibial translation during gait, with less variability among individual patients, than those who have had a fixed-bearing TKA. This finding is likely related to the increased AP femorotibial conformity allowed in the mobile-bearing designs. This reduction in anterior-posterior translation and intersubject variability was not observed during a deep knee bend activity, however. Posterior femoral rollback after posterior-cruciate-substituting TKAs (those involving implantation of either a mobile-bearing or a fixed-bearing design) is superior to that after PCR arthroplasties.

Axial femorotibial rotation is reduced following implantation of both fixed-bearing and mobile-bearing designs. Reverse axial rotational patterns, which can adversely affect both the range of motion and the patellar stability, are common. Substantial variability in both the magnitude and the pattern of axial rotation among patients is common with both fixed-bearing and mobile-bearing designs.

Femoral condylar lift-off is common after all types of TKAs and does not appear to be affected by bearing mobility. It occurs most commonly on the lateral side of the joint during the deep flexion portion of a deep knee bend activity and during the midstance phase of gait.

When tested under weight-bearing conditions, the amount of flexion obtained following a TKA appears to depend more on condylar geometry than on bearing mobility. The greatest range of flexion in our analyses was observed in patients with a fixed-bearing posterior-stabilized TKR, in which posterior femoral rollback routinely occurs because of engagement of the cam-and-post mechanism, allowing improved knee flexion.[39] In contrast, the least amount of flexion during weight bearing was observed in patients managed with a PCS rotating-platform design, in which anterior femoral translation was often observed during deep flexion, moving the axis of flexion anteriorly and reducing the range of motion. Additionally, the sagittal dwell point (the point where the polyethylene is thinnest) of the PCS rotating-platform TKR evaluated in this report is positioned more anteriorly than it is in most fixed-bearing TKA designs.[39] This, again, may position the axis of flexion anteriorly and limit maximum flexion.

Table 1
Axial femorotibial rotation in the PCS rotating-platform and posterior stabilized rotating-platform TKRs

Type of TKA*	Activity	Rotation (degrees) Average	Maximum	Minimum
PCS-RP	Deep knee-bend	3.4	9.6	0.5†
PS-RP	Deep knee-bend	5.2	13.9	0.1†
PCS-RP	Gait	2.5†	13.2†	0.1†
PS-RP	Gait	3.0	10.9	0.1

*PCS-RP = posterior cruciate-sacrificing rotating platform, and PS-RP = posterior stabilized rotating platform
†Abnormal, reverse rotational pattern

Table 2
Magnitude of femoral condylar lift-off in the PCS rotating-platform and posterior stabilized rotating-platform TKRs

Type of TKA*	Activity	Lift-Off (mm) Average	Maximum	Minimum
PCS-RP	Deep knee-bend	1.4	2.2	1.0
PS-RP	Deep knee-bend	1.9	3.5	1.0
PCS-RP	Gait	1.5	2.2	0.8
PS-RP	Gait	1.5	2.1	0.8

*PCS-RP = posterior cruciate sacrificing rotating platform, and PS-RP = posterior stabilized rotating platform

Table 3
Range of motion associated with different types of TKRs

Type of TKA*	Testing Condition	Average Range of Motion (degrees)
Meniscal-bearing[17]	Non-weight-bearing	121°
Meniscal-bearing[17]	Weight-bearing	100°
PCS-RP	Non-weight-bearing	108°
PCS-RP	Weight-bearing	99°
FB-PCR	Non-weight-bearing	123°
FB-PCR	Weight-bearing	103°
FB-PS	Non-weight-bearing	127°
FB-PS	Weight-bearing	113°

*PCS-RP = posterior cruciate-sacrificing rotating platform, FB-PCR = fixed-bearing posterior cruciate-retaining, and FB-PS = fixed-bearing posterior stabilized

The Oxford Unicompartmental Knee Replacement

Background

In 1978, Goodfellow and O'Connor[40] introduced the concept of the mobile bearing, which is intended to mimic the

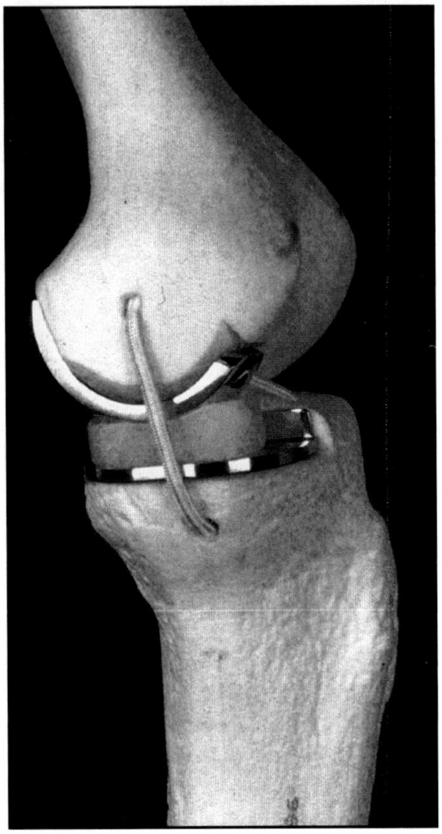

Fig. 8 Photograph of the Oxford unicompartmental knee replacement.

function of the human meniscus. The natural meniscus makes the dissimilar surfaces of the femoral and tibial condyles congruous, doubling the area of their contact and thereby reducing by half the pressure at which loads are transmitted across the joint.[41] The natural meniscus is mobile so that it can follow the rolling and sliding movements of the femoral condyle on the tibial plateau, and it is compliant so that its shape can change to accommodate the varying curvatures that the polyradial femoral condyle presents during flexion and extension.[42]

A mobile polyethylene bearing can mimic the mobility of the natural meniscus, but it is rigid and cannot change shape. The only rigid shapes that can be congruous in all relative positions are a sphere in a spherical socket; therefore, if the surfaces of the prosthesis are to be congruous, the femoral condyle has to be spherical. Some designs of prostheses have a mobile bearing that articulates with a polyradial femoral condyle. These implants exhibit incongruous articulation except in the one position of the joint in which the condyle presents the same curvature as that of the bearing. As already stated, we use the description "meniscal bearing" for implants in which the condyle is spherical and the bearing can function like its analogue in nature. Not all mobile-bearing knee prostheses are meniscal-bearing knee prostheses.

Of the several advantages that might be expected from a meniscal-bearing knee replacement, reduced polyethylene wear is the most obvious. Among the potential disadvantages are the risk of dislocation and the increased dependence on the preserved ligaments to provide stability.

The Prosthesis

The Oxford meniscal-bearing prosthesis has three components (Fig. 8). The metal femoral condyle has a spherical articular surface, and the metal tibial component is flat. In between, there is a mobile polyethylene bearing, which has a spherically concave upper surface and a flat lower surface. The unconstrained bearing is entrapped by the reciprocal shapes of the metal surfaces and by the tension in the soft tissues. Both to avoid dislocation and to confer stability, it is essential that the flexion and extension gaps, defined by the tension in the ligaments, are exactly the same. With the initial design (phase 1), in which the femur was prepared with a saw, such precise ligament balance was difficult to achieve. In 1985, the phase-2 instrumentation was introduced with a spherically concave rotary mill to prepare the femoral condyle. The flexion gap is first defined by excision of thin slices of bone from the tibial plateau and from the posterior surface of the femoral condyle. The distal part of the femur is then milled, in 1-mm increments, until the gap in extension has the same measurement as the gap in flexion. A polyethylene bearing of the appropriate thickness to fill the gap is inserted, and it maintains the ligaments at a constant tension throughout the range of movement. In 1998, the instruments were further modified (phase 3) to simplify their use and to facilitate implantation through a short parapatellar-tendon incision.

Why Unicompartmental?

Between 1977 and 1982, the Oxford implant was used bicompartmentally, with one prosthesis in each compartment of the knee. It soon became apparent that a good result depended on the presence of all of the ligaments, including, in particular, the anterior cruciate ligament (ACL). If the ACL was absent or seriously damaged, the failure rate was about six times higher.[43] Because a majority of osteoarthritic knees that need replacement lack a functional ACL, the usefulness of the implant seemed doubtful. However, during those years we observed that if osteoarthritic joints had an intact ACL, the disease was usually limited to the medial compartment of the joint. The Oxford knee has been used unicompartmentally for such knees since 1982. For knees with an absent ACL, we have preferred fixed-bearing TKRs.

One consequence of the failure of the prosthesis in knees with a deficient ACL was that we collected many used bearings and were able to measure their average wear rate. The Oxford knee provides about 6 cm^2 of congruous contact at both of its surfaces, and little polyethylene wear was expected. The retrieved bearings, in fact, became thinner at an average rate of only 0.03 mm/yr (a rate of 1 mm in 30 years).[44,45]

When possible, we use unicompartmental replacements because they have many advantages over total knee replacements.[46-48] They are less invasive, and because they preserve the cruciate ligaments they result in nearly normal kinematics. The surgery has a lower morbidity rate, blood transfusion is not required, and the implant is less expensive. The postoperative recovery is more rapid, and a better range of movement and more physiologic function are achieved. The concern with unicompartmental replacements is that in general they have had a higher failure rate than TKRs. However, these failures are commonly due to polyethylene wear, which is not a problem with the Oxford meniscal-bearing knee replacement.

A Prosthesis in Search of a Disease

The criteria for use of the Oxford unicompartmental knee are now clearly defined and are all met by the clinicopathologic syndrome of anteromedial osteoarthritis.[49] In this condition, the ACL is intact and the cartilage and bone erosions are limited to the anterior part of the medial compartment. This combination of a functioning ACL and healthy cartilage at the back of the joint has an important consequence. The varus deformity, which is typical of the disease, is present only when the knee is extended—that is, when the eroded anterior articular surfaces are in contact. In flexion, the femur rolls back and presents its intact posterior articular surface to the intact cartilage at the back of the tibial plateau. As a result, the varus deformity corrects every time the knee flexes, and structural shortening of the medial collateral ligament cannot occur. Rupture of the ACL leads to disorderly movement of the femur on the tibia and extension of the cartilage and bone erosions to the back of the joint. Thereafter, the knee is in varus in all positions, secondary shortening of the medial collateral ligament ensues, and the cartilage and bone erosions begin to involve the other joint compartments. This scenario suggests that anteromedial osteoarthritis is not the early manifestation of a global disease of the joint but a focal disorder of the knee and that timely replacement of the eroded medial plateau, before the ACL has stretched or ruptured, could protect both that structure and the lateral compartment from degeneration. In a recent clinical and radiographic study by Weale and associates,[50] 29 knees that had been followed for at least 10 years after an Oxford unicompartmental arthroplasty demonstrated no deterioration of function or progression of arthritis in their retained compartments during that decade.

Anteromedial osteoarthritis, therefore, presents with pathology that is limited to the articular surfaces of one compartment, and all of the ligaments are still normal. In theory, such a knee can be restored to normal function by a unicompartmental surface replacement. For this purpose, a meniscal prosthesis might have two advantages over a fixed-bearing implant: it would be less likely to fail because of polyethylene wear, and its freedom from constraint might allow the intact ligaments to perform more normally.

Indications

Use of an Oxford unicompartmental knee replacement is indicated when there is full-thickness cartilage loss in the medial compartment with or without bone loss. Superficial damage to the ACL, usually caused by osteophyte impingement, is not a contraindication provided that the ligament is functionally intact. A fixed flexion deformity should be less than 15°. The varus deformity should be passively correctable; this is best demonstrated by a valgus-stress radiograph made with the knee in 20° of flexion. The cartilage of the lateral compartment should be full-thickness, which would also be demonstrated by the same radiograph. At surgery, a full-thickness erosion is often found on the medial margin of the lateral condyle, presumably as a result of impingement on the tibial spine, but this is not a contraindication to use of the prosthesis. If the described indications are used, this operation is suitable for about one in four osteoarthritic knees that require replacement.

Many of the contraindications proposed by others are, we believe, unnecessary. In our practice, no knee is excluded because of patellofemoral erosions. Extensive fibrillation and erosion are commonly found on the medial patellar facet and the medial flange of the patellar groove on the femur. The operation corrects the varus deformity and unloads the damaged areas of the patellofemoral joint. We have not had to revise a knee because of patellofemoral pain. The age and weight of the patient and the presence of chondrocalcinosis are not contraindications.

Results

In 1998, Murray and associates,[51] the designers of the Oxford prosthesis, reported the rate of survival of the prostheses in a series of 144 knees that had a medial unicompartmental replacement (phase 1 and phase 2). One knee was lost to follow-up, one phase-1 knee had dislocation of the bearing that was reduced by closed manipulation, and there were no dislocations in the phase 2 knees. The patients ranged in age from 35 to 90 years. The 10-year rate of survival was 98% (95% confidence limits, 93% to 100%). The worst-case rate of survival, derived by assuming that the knee lost to follow-up was a failure, was 97% at 10 years.

The designers' results after the use of the implants need to be regarded with caution as they are susceptible to bias. However, Price and Svard[52] reported on an independent series of patients treated by three surgeons at a nonteaching hospital in Sweden. The study involved 378 medial unicompartmental replacements in knees with anteromedial osteoarthritis, and no patient was lost to follow-up. The 10-year survival rate was 95% (95% confidence limits, 93% to 98%). The worst-case rate of survival was also 95%. Three phase 1 knees had a dislocation of the bearing, and none of the phase 2 knees had a dislocation.

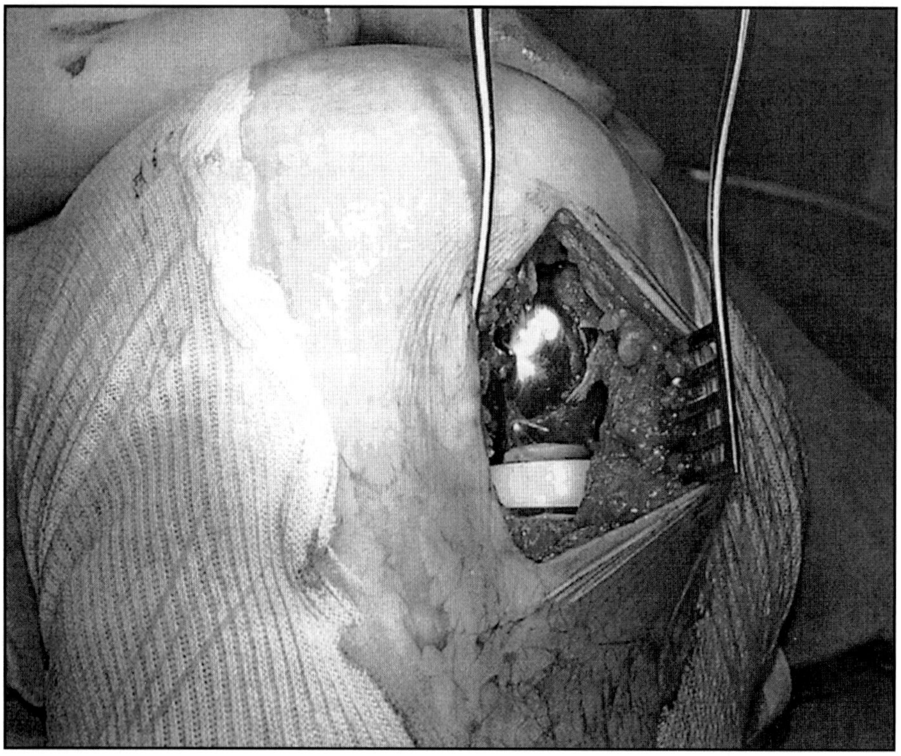

Fig. 9 Intraoperative photograph of the Oxford unicompartmental knee replacement implanted through a short incision.

In contrast, Lewold and associates[53] reported a 5-year rate of survival of only 90% after 699 phase 1 and phase 2 Oxford unicompartmental medial and lateral replacements in the National Arthroplasty Study performed at 19 centers in Sweden. Thirty-seven of the 50 failures occurred less than 2 years after surgery, and the most common cause of early failure was dislocation of the bearing, a complication that occurred only once in the first 2 years in the 522 cases in the series of Murray and associates[51] and Price and Svard.[52] We were able to obtain data from 13 of the 19 centers and found 944 Oxford unicompartmental implants, suggesting that the Swedish register failed to identify more than 25% of the patients. The failure rate from center to center ranged from 0% to as high as 30%. The results reported by Lewold and associates[53] reflect the learning curves associated with a novel technique at 19 centers. The investigators exerted no control over, and collected no information about, the indications that were used. The report by Larsson and associates,[54] who performed a unicompartmental arthroplasty in 71% (102) of all knees that had an arthroplasty for the treatment of osteoarthritis, and the report by Christensen,[55] who performed the procedure in 90% (575) of all such knees, suggest that the indications for the procedure in Sweden may have been wide.

Minimally Invasive Surgery

Since 1998, we have performed the surgical procedure through a short incision from the medial pole of the patella to the tibial tuberosity with use of phase 3 instruments (Fig. 9). With the limited approach, there is minimal damage to the extensor mechanism because the patella is not dislocated and the suprapatellar synovial pouch remains intact. As a result, patients recover much more rapidly.[56] Webb and associates[57] showed that patients achieve straight-leg raising, knee flexion, and independent stair-climbing about three times faster after this procedure than they do after TKR. Furthermore, a comparison of the postoperative radiographs has shown that the operation can be done as reliably through the limited approach with use of the phase 3 instruments as it can be done through a wide incision with use of the phase 2 instruments.

Overview

The Oxford unicompartmental prosthesis has a fully congruent, unconstrained mobile bearing. Retrieval studies have shown that the average wear rate of the polyethylene bearings is very slow (approximately 0.03 mm/yr).[44,45] The indications for use of the implant for the treatment of medial compartment osteo- arthritis are clearly defined and are satisfied in approximately one in four osteoarthritic knees that need replacement.

The 10-year rate of survival of the prosthesis was 98% (95% confidence limits, 93% to 100%) in the designers' series of 144 knees[51] and 95% (95% confidence limits, 93% to 98%) in an independent series of 378 knees.[52] Recent modifications to the instrumentation allow the device to be implanted through a small parapatellar-tendon incision without disturbing the patellofemoral mechanism. This further reduces the perioperative morbidity and allows even more rapid recovery.

When appropriate expertise is available, one fourth of patients who need a knee arthroplasty can enjoy the advantages of unicompartmental rather than tricompartmental replacement without incurring an increased risk of failure in the first 10 years.

Rationale for and Results of the Self-Aligning TKR

In the mid 1980s, a rotating-platform TKR, which provided a congruous articulation from 5° of hyperextension to 90° of flexion and allowed unconstrained rotation as well as anterior-posterior translation limited only by the soft tissues of the knee, was developed at our center (Fig.10). This report describes the results of 172 SAL TKAs performed, between 1990 and 1994, in 141 patients with osteoarthritis of the knee. Twenty-three knees had undergone a prior high tibial valgus osteotomy. All surgery was performed in a laminar airflow theater, with the surgical teams wearing body-exhaust suits. Cefazolin was administered in the perioperative period for antibiotic prophylaxis. All patients were managed with Coumadin (warfarin) as prophylaxis against deep vein thrombosis.

Preoperatively, all patients were assessed by a single observer with use of the Knee Society clinical rating scale,[58] the Western Ontario and McMaster University Osteoarthritis Index,[59] and the Short Form-36 survey.[60] Preoperative evaluation included standing long-leg radiographs, standard AP standing radiographs, and a lateral and axial patellar radiograph of the affected knee. Postoperatively, the same independent observer examined the patient clinically and radiographically at 3 months, 6 months, and yearly thereafter. All radiographs were reviewed by the two senior authors (RBB and CHR).

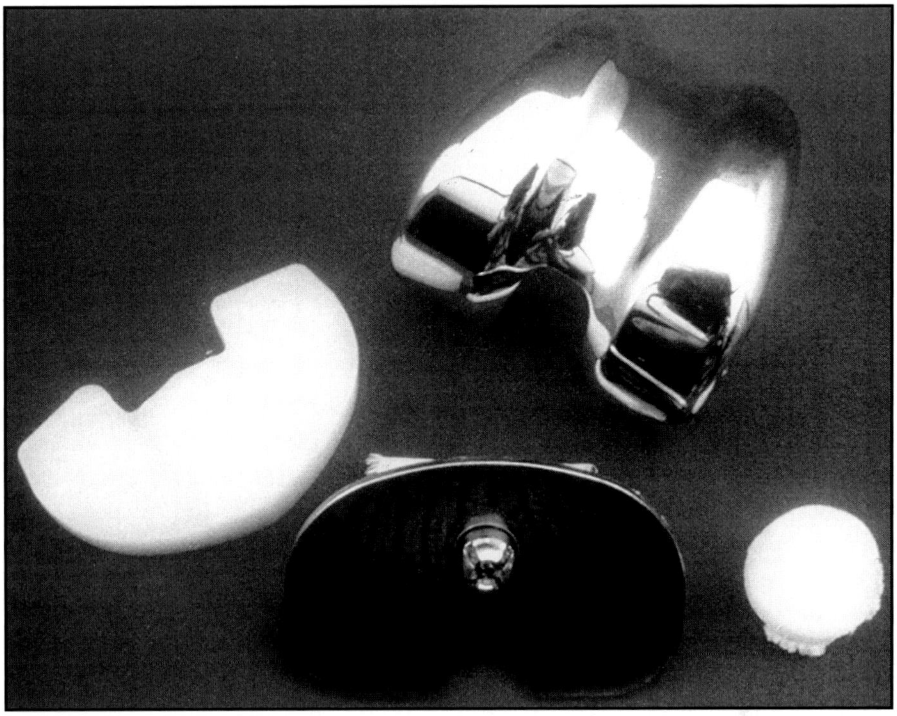

Fig. 10 Photograph of the components of the Self-Aligning-I TKA system, showing a chromium-cobalt femoral component, a nitrite-coated titanium tibial baseplate, a mobile-bearing polyethylene tibial insert, and an all-polyethylene patellar component.

Results

Ninety-five knees were in men and 75 were in women. The patients had an average age of 71 years (range, 47 to 90 years). The average height was 169 cm (range, 147 to 200 cm), and the average weight was 83 kg (range, 50 to 109 kg). All femoral and tibial components were fixed with cement, with the exception of 61 femoral components that were press-fit. Of this group of 61 knees, four were revised because of aseptic loosening of the femoral component. None of the cemented femoral components were revised. An all-polyethylene patellar component was press-fit in 48 knees and cemented in the remaining 124 knees.

At the time of the most recent follow-up, 42 patients had died of causes unrelated to their knee replacement (Table 4). The SAL knee replacements had been functioning well in all of these patients at the time of death. No other patients were lost to follow-up. Eight patients had a revision. Two knees were revised because of polyethylene wear and four, because the press-fit, non porous-coated femoral component had become loose. One patient underwent a revision because of persistent pain, and aseptic loosening of a cemented patellar component was noted intraoperatively. One patient had a revision to exchange a tibial polyethylene insert because of postoperative stiffness.

Fourteen patients needed a reoperation (Table 5). In addition to the eight revisions, a reoperation was performed in four patients because of a deep infection. Three of these patients were treated with a two-stage revision arthroplasty, and the fourth was treated with irrigation, débridement, retention of the components, and suppressive antibiotics. Three traumatic patellar fractures were noted, but only one required revision surgery. One patient had a periprosthetic fracture 6 years postoperatively. The fracture was treated surgically, with a satisfactory outcome. Three patients required manipulation under anesthesia because of postoperative arthrofibrosis.

After 5 to 8 years (average, 5.6 years) of follow-up, 115 knees were available for review. The Knee Society clinical rating had improved from an average of 81 points preoperatively to an average of 155 points at the time of the latest follow-up. The average preoperative range of motion was from 6° ± 7° of extension to 110° ± 15° of flexion. Postoperatively, the average range of motion was from 0° ± 1° to 111° ± 7° (Table 6). Postoperative alignment was neutral in 98 knees, 0° to 5° of

Table 4
Outcomes after TKA with the Self-Aligning-I prosthesis

Clinical Outcome	No. of Knees
Patients who had died*	
< 5 years of follow-up	38
< 5 years of follow-up	4
Patients excluded because of reoperation	14
Patients excluded because of other medical reasons	1†
Patients followed for minimum of 5 years	115

*These patients all had a successful outcome at the time of the last follow-up examination

†This patient had a satisfactory outcome at the time of the last follow-up examination, 3 years after the surgery

Table 5
Reoperations after TKA with the Self-Aligning-I prosthesis*

Indications for Reoperation	No. of Knees
Infection	4
Aseptic loosening of press-fit	4
Femoral component	4
Polyethylene wear	2
Fracture	2
Stiffness	1
Pain	1

*All of these knees were excluded from the present study group

Table 6
Clinical scores according to the system of the Knee Society[58] and range of motion for all Self-Aligning-I TKAs*

	Clinical Score (points)			Range of Motion (degrees)	
	Pain	Function	Total Score	Extension	Flexion
Preoperative	35 ± 15	46 ± 16	81 ± 24	6 ± 7	110 ± 15
Postoperative†	84 ± 7	71 ± 23	155 ± 19	0 ± 1	111 ± 7

*Data are given for the 115 knees that had at least 5 years of follow-up, and the values are given as the average and the standard deviation

†Data are from the latest follow-up examination, which was an average of 5.6 years after the surgery

varus in 72 knees, and 10° to 15° of valgus in 2 knees. No gross instability was noted in any knee. No rotating-bearing polyethylene insert had dislocated at the time of writing. Radiographic review revealed no evidence of osteolysis or implant loosening at the time of the latest follow-up. No additional cases of asymptomatic polyethylene wear were noted. Patellar tracking was noted to be central in 154 knees, and 18 knees required lateral retinacular release to improve patellofemoral tracking. Nine patients required anticoagulant therapy for deep vein thrombosis, and no patient had a clinical pulmonary embolus.

After 5 to 8 years of follow-up, 94% of the patients were satisfied (a good or very good outcome) with the function of the knee and the outcome of the surgery. The remaining 6% rated the outcome as fair.

The results of the SAL total knee replacements in the present investigation are similar to those reported for other rotating-platform TKRs, notably the LCS TKR.[25,61,62] These studies demonstrated a reduction in polyethylene wear.

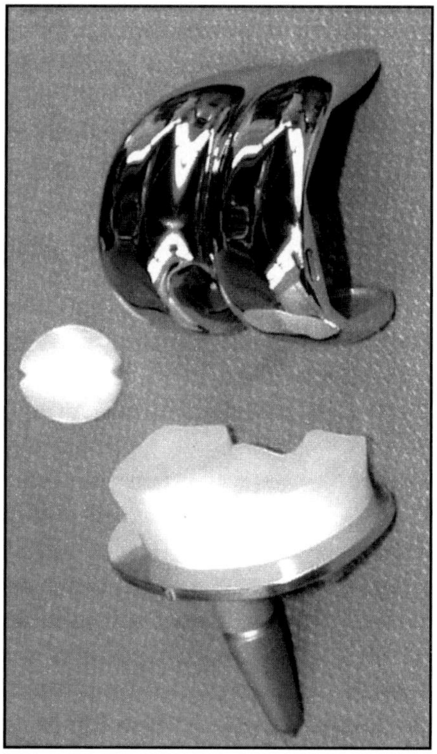

Fig. 11 Photograph of the Self-Aligning-II total knee prosthesis. Note the maintenance of the single axis of curvature for the J-curve of the femoral component, the newer rounded femoral condyles in the mediolateral plane designed to avoid edge-loading, and the change to a chromium-cobalt tibial baseplate from a titanium tibial baseplate.

None of the SAL TKRs had a bearing dislocation, and only four (9.3%) of 43 LCS rotating-platform devices had a bearing dislocation in another study.[63] The present series of SAL TKRs represents the initial learning curve with this device. The encouraging results in this prototype series led to the development of the current SAL TKR with improved instrumentation, a dedicated femoral component, a lower-contact-stress tibial component, and sterilization of the polyethylene in an inert environment (Fig. 11). On the basis of the results with this prosthesis, we concluded that rotating-platform TKRs have the potential to extend the indications for and the longevity of TKR.

The LCS Mobile-Bearing Knee
Design Rationale

The rationale for the design of the LCS mobile-bearing knee was to allow mobility with congruity[7,62,64,65] (Fig. 12). Along these lines, the femoral and tibial components are conforming, in the sagittal plane, from full extension to 30° of flexion to optimize the contact areas and are less conforming from 30° of flexion to full flexion to allow better mobility. The surface geometry of the femoral component in the sagittal plane is demonstrated in Figure 13. The tibial component includes a medial and lateral meniscal-bearing design with a tray cutout to preserve one or both of the cruciate ligaments (hence allowing rotation and anterior-posterior translation) and a rotating-platform design (allowing only rotation) with a relatively deep sagittal-plane conformity for PCS procedures (Fig. 14). The tibial polyethylene insert has a center post that mates with the hollowed-out tibial tray post to allow rotation but no translation. The patellar component is metal-backed and mobile-bearing, with a surface congruent with the patellar groove articulation of the femoral component. All metal backings are porous-coated to allow fixation without cement. The bicruciate-retaining, rotating-platform, and revision knee-device configurations were approved by the FDA and indicated for use with cement in 1985, the PCR device was approved by the FDA for cementless fixation in 1990, and the rotating platform was approved for cementless fixation in 1994.

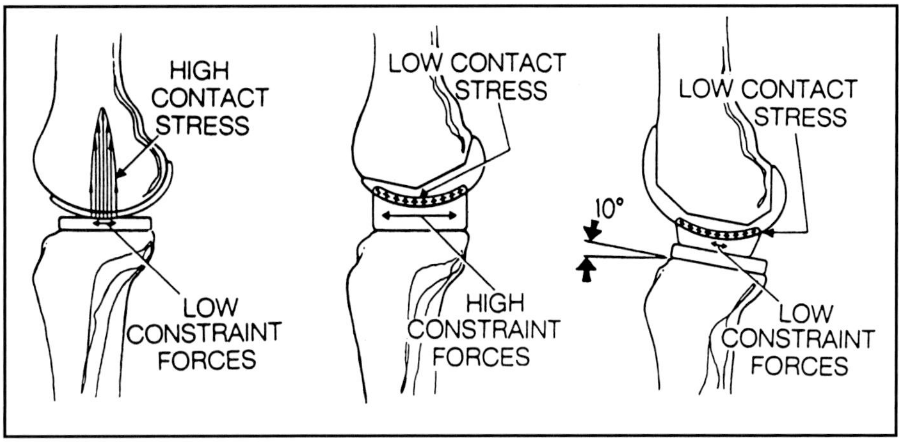

Fig. 12 Illustrations of the three types of knee bearing configurations, showing a point or line-contact device with poor congruity (*left*), a congruent-contact device without inherent axial rotation (*middle*), and a meniscal-bearing congruent-contact device with good mobility (*right*). (Reproduced with permission from Buechel FF, Pappas MJ: New Jersey Low Contact Stress knee replacement system: Ten-year evaluation of meniscal bearings. *Orthop Clin North Am* 1989;20:148.)

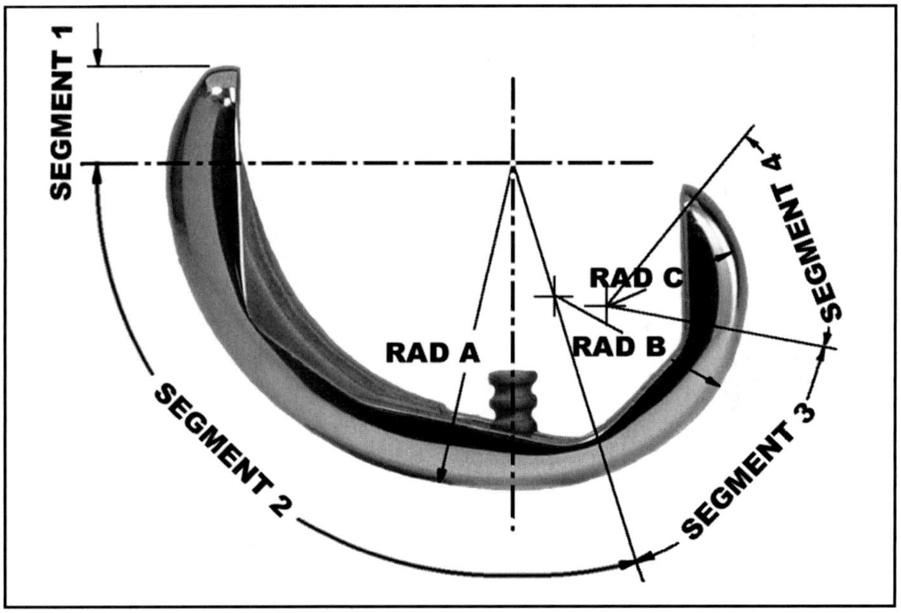

Fig. 13 The geometry of the lateral surface of the New Jersey LCS femoral component. segment 1 represents the patellofemoral bearing surface in full extension, segment 2 is the primary load-bearing surface of the femoral component for both patellar and tibial articulation, and segment 3 and segment 4 are the posterior bearing surfaces used during full flexion. (Reproduced with permission from Buechel FF, Pappas MJ: New Jersey Low Contact Stress knee replacement system: Ten-year evaluation of meniscal bearings. *Orthop Clin North Am* 1989;20:153.)

Summary of Surgical Procedure

The surgical procedure is based on the principle of creating equal flexion and extension gaps while providing a posterior slope to the tibia to prevent shear at the tibial interface. The flexion gap is initially created by resecting the proximal part of the tibial bone (a cut is made perpendicular to the tibial shaft in the coronal plane and is tilted 7° to 10° posteriorly in the sagittal plane). The AP dimension of the femoral component is then sized, and the posterior femoral condyle resection is performed. The flexion gap is checked with a spacer block. Finally, the extension gap is created by removing the amount of the distal aspect of the femur that is necessary to allow the extension gap to equal the flexion gap. The gaps

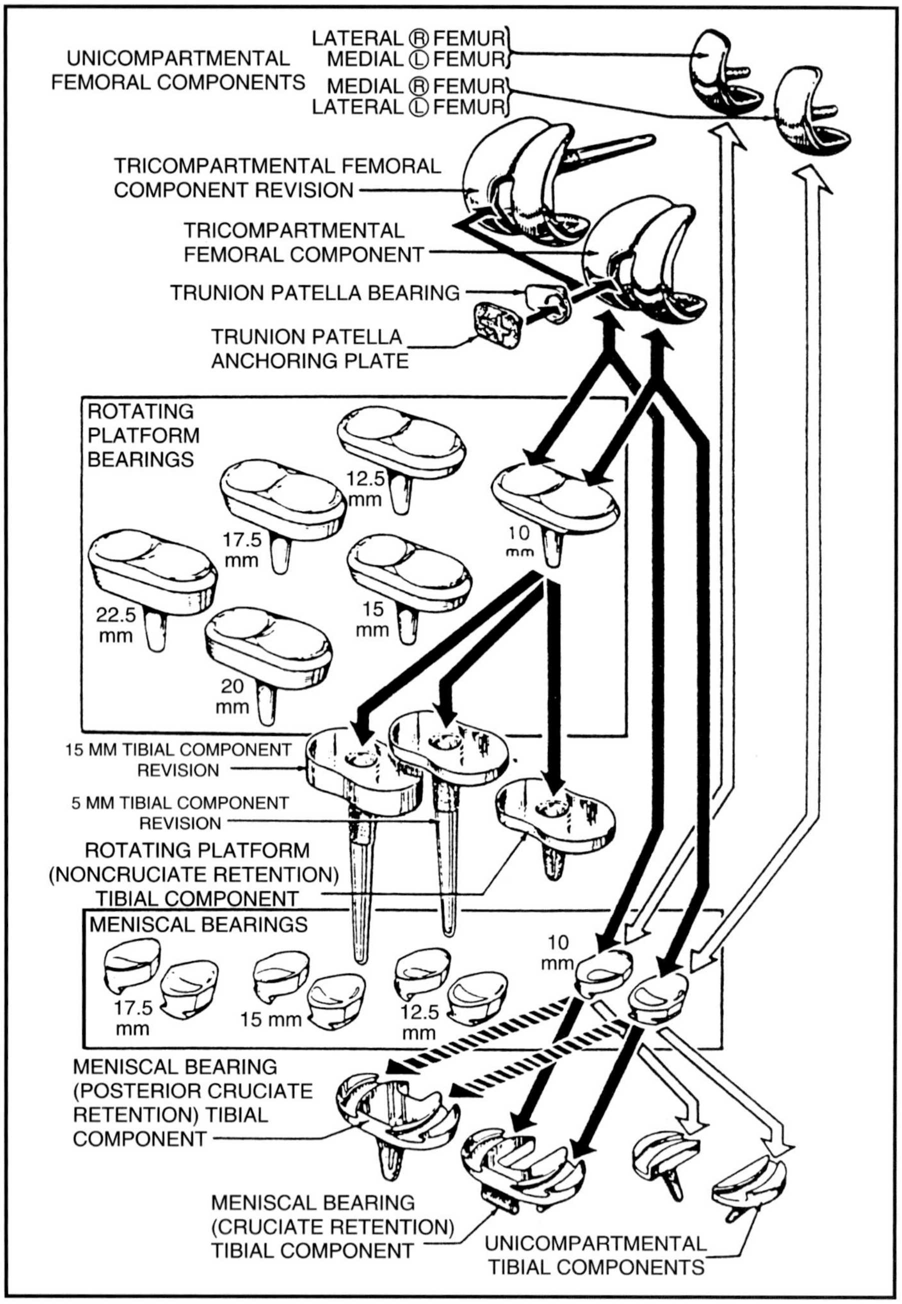

Fig. 14 Drawing of the components of the New Jersey LCS knee replacement system. (Reproduced with permission from Buechel FF, Pappas MJ: New Jersey Low Contact Stress knee replacement system: Ten-year evaluation of meniscal bearings. *Orthop Clin North Am* 1989;20:153.)

are checked for symmetry with use of spacer blocks. To accommodate a deep patellofemoral groove in the femoral implant, the distal part of the femur is cut in a 17° anterior-to-posterior slope. This cut is accommodated by the posterior slope in the tibia (Fig. 15).

Results

Buechel and Pappas[19] followed 46 knees that had a bicruciate-retaining LCS prosthesis for up to 12 years, 57 knees that had a PCR prosthesis for up to 6 years, and 108 knees that had a rotating-platform prosthesis for up to 10 years. Sixty-four knees were fixed with cement, and 147 were fixed without cement. The 12-year rate of survival (with revision as the end point) of the 21 knees with a cemented bicruciate-retaining prosthesis was 90.9%, and the 6-year rate of survival (with revision as the end point) of the 25 knees with a cementless bicruciate-retaining prosthesis was 100%. The 6-year rate of survival of the 57 knees with a cementless PCR meniscal-bearing implant was 97.9%. The 10-year rate of survival of the 43 knees with a cemented rotating-platform design was 97.5%, and the 6-year rate of survival of the 65 knees with a cementless rotating-platform implant was 98.1%.

Sorrells[66] evaluated the results of 665 cementless rotating-platform LCS knee arthroplasties performed between September 1984 and August 1995. Survivorship analysis demonstrated that 94.7% of the components had survived at 11 years, with 13 (2%) revised. Jordan and associates[62] evaluated the results of 473 cementless meniscal-bearing LCS knee arthroplasties performed between May 1985 and February 1991. Seventeen (3.6%) were revised because of mechanical failure. The survival rate of the implant, with revision because of mechanical failure as the end point, was 94.6% at 8 years.

The results of 119 arthroplasties with a cemented LCS rotating-platform TKR and a cemented all-polyethylene patellar component after 9 to 12 years of follow-up were reveiwed.[65] There were no mechanical failures, and none of the components had been revised. The average Hospital for Special Surgery knee rating was 84 points. Knee flexion averaged 102°.

Complications associated with the LCS mobile-bearing knee have included dislocation of the bearings; meniscal, rotating-platform, and patellar dislocations have all been reported.[62,66,67] In the previously discussed series, dislocation occurred in less than 0.5% of cases;

however, Bert[63] reported a prevalence of dislocation of 9.3% (4) of 43 knees. Breakage or wear of the bearings has been reported in less than 2% of cases.[19,62] Even with use of cementless fixation, rates of loosening have been less than 2% in all of the reported series.[19,62,66]

In summary, the LCS mobile-bearing knee prosthesis has been used for 15 years. Although there are few long-term studies, the results reported in the literature are comparable with the best results reported with fixed-bearing devices.

Why Should We Question the Enthusiasm for Mobile-Bearing Knees?

In order to fully endorse a technological design, one must have data that overwhelmingly supports its superiority to its temporal peers. To date, even those who choose to accept the risks associated with use of a prosthesis that has additional moving parts do not have evidence that the mobile-bearing knee design has demonstrated any superiority over fixed-bearing designs. Moving parts always require a mechanical link for attachment, which could fail and result in excessive motion or dislocation of the part and in increased debris within the joint. This complication has occurred with mobile-bearing knees. Weaver and associates[68] and Bert[63] reported that revision was necessary because of failure of the mobile tibial components in the LCS TKR.

Why would a surgeon choose to use a mobile-bearing design? One reason would be an improved functional performance of the knee. However, we know of no reports that have demonstrated that the functional performance of a mobile-bearing knee is better than that of a fixed-bearing knee. Stiehl and associates[29] used fluoroscopy to evaluate the functional kinematics of both fixed-bearing and mobile-bearing knees. They observed that the same paradoxical anterior slide in flexion that occurs with fixed-bearing knees occurs with mobile-bearing knees. Furthermore, Dennis and associates[39] reported an average arc of flexion of 105° with the LCS knee replacement. This flexion range is less than the 110° to 120° that has been reported with some fixed-bearing knees.[69] With flexion averaging only 105°, patients can have some difficulty in descending stairs. None of these clinical series[29,39,69] suggested that the mobile-bearing design is superior to the

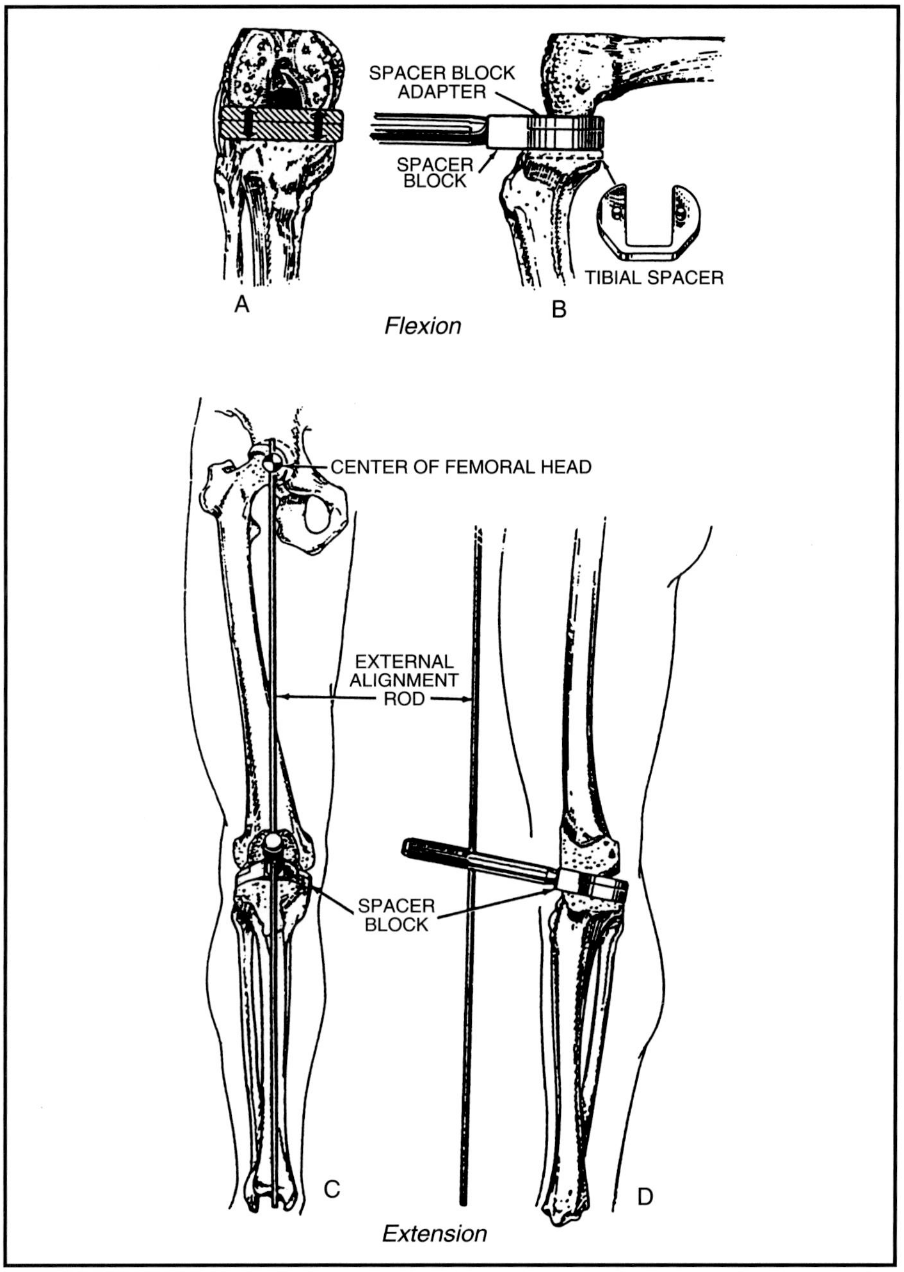

Fig. 15 Illustration showing use of a spacer block to check resection gaps during flexion and extension. **A,** AP view of flexion gap, **B,** lateral view of flexion gap, **C,** AP view of extension gap, and **D,** lateral view of extension gap. (Reproduced with permission from Buechel FF, Pappas MJ: New Jersey Low Contact Stress knee replacement system: Ten-year evaluation of meniscal bearings. *Orthop Clin North Am* 1989;20:160.)

Table 7
Results after arthroplasty with mobile-bearing knee designs

Study	Design*	Intended Motion of Mobile Bearing	No. of Knees	Average Duration of Follow-up (Years)	Rate of Survival (%)
Murray et al[51]	Oxford unicompartmental	Anterior-posterior translation	144	10	98
Lewold et al[53]	Oxford unicompartmental	Anterior-posterior translation	699	5	90
Price and Svard[52]	Oxford unicompartmental	Anterior-posterior translation	378	10	95
Kaper et al[76]	SAL	Anterior-posterior translation, rotation	61	5.6	95
Buechel and Pappas[19]	LCS posterior-cruciate-retaining meniscal-bearing	Anterior-posterior translation, rotation	57	6	98
Jordan et al[62]	LCS posterior-cruciate-retaining meniscal-bearing	Anterior-posterior translation, rotation	473	8	95
Sorrells[66]	LCS rotating-platform	Rotation	665	11	95
Callaghan et al[65]	LCS rotating-platform	Rotation	119	9	100

*LCS = Low-Contact Stress, and SAL = Self-Aligning

fixed-bearing design with regard to providing ligamentous stability and soft-tissue balance of the TKR. Therefore, no functional superiority has been demonstrated with this design concept.

A second reason for choosing a mobile-bearing knee design would be a reduction in the number of mechanical failures and in the rate of revision. To our knowledge, no reports have indicated that the rate of mechanical failure of mobile-bearing knee replacements is superior to that of good fixed-bearing designs. Scuderi and Insall[70] reported that the rate of survival of the metal-backed Insall-Burstein design (Zimmer, Warsaw, IN) was 98.7% at 14 years. Ritter[3] reported that the rate of survival of the AGC knee design (Biomet, Warsaw, IN) was 98% at 15 years. Buechel and Pappas[19] reported that the rate of survival of the rotating-platform design of the LCS knee was 97.5% at 12 years. Jordan and associates[62] reported that 3.6% of 473 LCS knees had been revised at the time of the 8-year follow-up. Clearly, the mobile-bearing design is not superior with regard to the prevention of mechanical failure and revision.

One commonly stated reason for using a mobile-bearing design is that it allows younger patients to be more active. However, this is a theoretical argument because there are no data in the literature that supports this concept, as far as we know. The patients in the series reported by Buechel and Pappas[19] were an average of 64 years old, and those in the study by Jordan and associates[62] were an average of 68 years old. The mobile-bearing design was used in a typical TKR population in both studies. Therefore, no conclusion can be drawn with regard to the superiority of the device for patients who have a high activity level. Furthermore, Ranawat (unpublished data, 1998) reported that a high percentage of patients with a fixed-bearing knee were very active. Eighty-six percent of the 96 patients walked for exercise. These patients also participated in many other sporting activities, including golf, tennis, and gymnasium activities. Fixed-bearing knees provide almost all patients with the ability to participate in their desired activities.

Perhaps the most common argument for the use of a mobile-bearing design is that wear is reduced because the articulation surfaces are more congruent.[71] To date, this improved congruency has been seen only in full extension and perhaps between full extension and 30° of flexion.[25] This large extension contact arc cannot be maintained in flexion because a curvature mismatch of the articulation occurs. Matsuda and associates[72] showed that there are fixed-bearing knees that have better contact stresses and reduced contact forces at 60° and 90° of flexion compared with LCS knee replacements.[73] A study of the Tricon-II mobile-bearing knee (Smith & Nephew Richards, Memphis, TN), by Parks and associates,[16] indicated that the difference between fixed-bearing and mobile-bearing knees with respect to the average and peak stresses on the upper surface is only 2 to 3 MPa. Parks and associates[16] found that there was undersurface stress between the mobile-bearing undersurface of the polyethylene and the metal tray that was 40% of the upper surface stress. We know of no implant-retrieval studies that have shown that the mobile-bearing concept does in fact reduce wear. Long-term studies of fixed-bearing and mobile-bearing knees have shown no difference in the rate of osteolysis.[19,62,70,74] The concept that a mobile-bearing design is associated with less wear than is a well-designed fixed-bearing knee has not been proved and remains a theoretical argument. Perhaps the best argument in favor of the mobile-bearing design is that the undersurface wear is better controlled than it is with some modular tibial designs, which were shown by Parks and associates[16] to be associated with particle formation. Maybe the best knee replacement is a fixed-bearing knee with an all-polyethylene tibial component cemented into the tibial bone.

The increased attention on mobile-bearing knee replacements might be best confined to investigators who desire to do controlled studies in an attempt to prove the superiority of the design. Certainly, a mobile-bearing knee design can be selected by surgeons who prefer it, even though the results will not be different from those with a good fixed-bearing design. However, these surgeons must be willing to accept a 1% to 2% rate of mechanical failure associated with use of a mobile tibial insert.[62,75] It is also important that surgeons do not select the mobile-bearing design because of the expectation that placement of the tibial component does not need to be as accurate as that with a fixed-bearing design and that the mobile insert will correct for malrotation of the tibial component. Again, we know of no data that support this argument, and it is incumbent on the surgeon to perform a good operation no matter what the design because bad surgery always has a much greater chance of leading to a bad result. Furthermore, the findings of Parks and associates[16] suggest that undersurface wear increases with malrotation of a mobile-bearing design.

Summary

In summary, if TKRs are to be performed in patients who are younger and more active than those who had the initial procedures in the 1970s and 1980s, better wear performance is imperative for long-term durability, especially if surgeons continue to consider the versatility associated with modular knee-replacement systems to be a necessity. At least with some designs, including the Oxford knee and the LCS knee, the results after a minimum follow-up of 10 years are comparable with the best results after arthroplasty with fixed-bearing designs in terms of wear, loosening, and osteolysis[4,19,51-53,62,65,66,76] (Table 7). As with fixed-bearing designs, there are additional challenges in terms of optimizing bearing-surface conformity and improving kinematics. Improvements in future designs of mobile-bearing total knee replacements should include better control of bearing mobility patterns to reduce the prevalence of the abnormal kinematic motions that have been observed in fluoroscopic evaluations.

References

1. Diduch DR, Insall JN, Scott WN, Scuderi GR, Font-Rodriguez D: Total knee replacement in young, active patients: Long-term follow-up and functional outcome. *J Bone Joint Surg Am* 1997;79:575-582.
2. Insall JN, Hood RW, Flawn LB, Sullivan DJ: The total condylar knee prosthesis in gonarthrosis: A five to nine-year follow-up of the first one hundred consecutive replacements. *J Bone Joint Surg Am* 1983;65:619-628.
3. Ritter M: 15 year results with the AGC knee. *65th Annual Meeting Proceedings*. Rosemont, IL, American Academy of Orthopaedic Surgeons, 1998.
4. Stern SH, Insall JN: Posterior stabilized prosthesis: Results after follow-up of nine to twelve years. *J Bone Joint Surg Am* 1992;74:980-986.
5. Colizza WA, Insall JN, Scuderi GR: The posterior stabilized total knee prosthesis: Assessment of polyethylene damage and osteolysis after a 10-year-minimum follow-up. *J Bone Joint Surg Am* 1995;77:1713-1720.
6. Szivek JA, Anderson PL, Benjamin JB: Average and peak contact stress distribution evaluation of total knee arthroplasties. *J Arthroplasty* 1996;11:952-963.
7. Bartel DL, Bicknell VL, Wright TM: The effect of conformity, thickness, and material on stresses in ultra-high-molecular weight components for total joint replacement. *J Bone Joint Surg Am* 1986;68:1041-1051.
8. Blunn GW, Walker PS, Joshi A, Hardinge K: The dominance of cyclic sliding in producing wear in total knee replacements. *Clin Orthop* 1991;273:253-260.
9. Hollister AM, Jatana S, Singh AK, Sullivan WW, Lupichuk AG: The axes of rotation of the knee. *Clin Orthop* 1993;290:259-268.
10. Kapandji IA: The knee, in Kapandji IA (ed): *The Physiology of the Joints: Annotated Diagrams of the Mechanics of the Human Joints*, ed 2. Edinburgh, Scotland, Churchill Livingstone, 1970, pp 72-91.
11. Kurosawa H, Walker PS, Abe S, Garg A, Hunter T: Geometry and motion of the knee for implant and orthotic design. *J Biomech* 1985;18:487-499.
12. Markolf KL, Mensch JS, Amstutz HC: Stiffness and laxity of the knee: The contributions of the supporting structures. *J Bone Joint Surg Am* 1976;58:583-593.
13. Mensch JS, Amstutz HC: Knee morphology as a guide to knee replacement. *Clin Orthop* 1975;112:231-241.
14. Piziali RL, Seering WP, Nagel DA, Schurman DJ: The function of the primary ligaments of the knee in anterior-posterior and medial-lateral motions. *J Biomech* 1980;13:777-784.
15. Seering WP, Piziali RL, Nagel DA, Schurman DJ: The function of the primary ligaments of the knee in varus-valgus and axial rotation. *J Biomech* 1980;13:785-794.
16. Parks NL, Engh GA, Topoleski LD, Emperado J: Modular tibial insert micromotion: A concern with contemporary knee implants. *Clin Orthop* 1998;356:10-15.
17. Elias SG, Freeman MA, Gokcay EI: A correlative study of the geometry and anatomy of the distal femur. *Clin Orthop* 1990;260:98-1030.
18. Food and Drug Administration Premarket Application LCS Meniscal Bearing Knee Simulator Studies, July 1984.
19. Buechel FF, Pappas MJ: Long-term survivorship analysis of cruciate-sparing versus cruciate-sacrificing knee prostheses using meniscal bearings. *Clin Orthop* 1990;260:162-169.
20. Morra EA, Postak PD, Greenwald AS: The influence of mobile bearing knee geometry on the wear of UHMWPE tibial Inserts: A finite element study. *Orthop Trans* 1998;22:148.
21. Morra E, Postak PD, Greenwald AS: Abstract: The influence of mobile bearing knee geometry on the wear of ultra-high molecular weight polyethylene tibial inserts: A finite element sudy. *66th Annual Meeting Proceedings*. Rosemont, IL, American Academy of Orthopaedic Surgeons, 1998, p 235.
22. Rose RM, Goldfarb HV: On the pressure dependence of the wear of ultra-high molecular weight polyethylene. *Wear* 1983;92:99-111.
23. Rostoker W, Galante JO: Contact pressure dependence of wear rates of ultra high molecular weight polyethylene. *J Biomed Mater Res* 1979;13:957-964.
24. Goodfellow J, O'Connor J: Abstract: Kinematics of the knee and the prosthetic design. *J Bone Joint Surg Br* 1977;59:119.
25. Buechel FF, Pappas MJ: The New Jersey Low-Contact-Stress knee replacement system:

Biomechanical rationale and review of the first 123 cemented cases. *Arch Orthop Traumatic Surg* 1986;105:197-204.

26. Dennis DA, Komistek RD, Hoff WA, Gabriel SM: In vivo knee kinematics derived using an inverse perspective technique. *Clin Orthop* 1996;331:107-117.

27. Dennis DA, Komistek RD, Colwell CE Jr, et al: In vivo anteroposterior femorotibial translation of total knee arthroplasty: A multicenter analysis. *Clin Orthop* 1998;356:47-57.

28. Hoff WA, Komistek RD, Dennis DA, Gabriel SA, Walker SA: A three dimensional determination of femorotibial contact positions under in vivo conditions using fluoroscopy. *J Clin Biomech* 1998;13:455-470.

29. Stiehl JB, Komistek RD, Dennis DA, Paxson RD, Hoff WA: Fluoroscopic analysis of kinematics after posterior-cruciate-retaining knee arthroplasty. *J Bone Joint Surg Br* 1995;77: 884-889.

30. Stiehl JB, Komistek RD, Paxson RD: Functional kinematic analysis of total knee arthroplasty using dynamic fluoroscopy. *Orthop Trans* 1995;19:462.

31. Dennis DA, Komistek RD, Stiehl JB, Anderson DT, Shoureshi RA: In vivo determination of TKA kinematics during treadmill gait. *Trans Orthop Res Soc* 1999;24:951.

32. Dennis DA, Komistek RD, Northcut EJ, Anderson DT: In vivo analysis of tibiofemoral rotation: Does screwhome rotation occur after total knee arthroplasty? *65th Annual Meeting Proceedings.* Rosemont, IL, American Academy of Orthopaedic Surgeons, 1998.

33. Dennis DA, Komistek RD, Cheal EJ, Walker SA, Stiehl JB: In vivo femoral condylar lift-off in total knee arthroplasty, in press.

34. Stiehl JB, Dennis DA, Komistek RD, Keblish PA: In vivo kinematic analysis of a mobile bearing total knee prosthesis. *Clin Orthop* 1997;345:60-66.

35. Stiehl JB, Dennis DA, Komistek RD, Crane HS: In vivo determination of condylar lift-off and screw-home in a mobile-bearing total knee arthroplasty. *J Arthroplasty* 1999;14:293-299.

36. Stiehl JB, Dennis DA, Komistek RD, Keblish P: In vivo comparison of posterior cruciate retaining and sacrificing mobile bearing total knee arthroplasty. *Am J Knee Surg*, in press.

37. Sarojak ME, Hoff WA, Komistek RD, Dennis DA: Utilization of an automated model fitting process to determine kinematics of TKA. *Trans Orthop Res Soc* 1999;24:953.

38. Jonsson H, Karrholm J, Elmqvist LG: Kinematics of active knee extension after tear of the anterior cruciate ligament. *Am J Sports Med* 1989;17:796-802.

39. Dennis DA, Komistek RD, Stiehl JB, Walker SA, Dennis KN: Range of motion after total knee arthroplasty: The effect of implant design and weight-bearing conditions. *J Arthroplasty* 1998;13:748-752.

40. Goodfellow J, O'Connor J: The mechanics of the knee and prosthesis design. *J Bone Joint Surg Br* 1978;60:358-369.

41. Shrive NG, O'Connor JJ, Goodfellow JW: Load-bearing in the knee joint. *Clin Orthop* 1978;131:279-287.

42. Warren PJ, Olanlokun TK, Cobb AG, Bentley G: Proprioception after knee arthroplasty: The influence of prosthetic design. *Clin Orthop* 1993;297:182-187.

43. Goodfellow J, O'Connor J: The anterior cruciate ligament in knee arthroplasty: A risk- factor with unconstrained meniscal prostheses. *Clin Orthop* 1992;276:245-252.

44 Argenson JN, O'Connor JJ: Polyethylene wear in meniscal knee replacement: A one to nine-year retrieval analysis of the Oxford knee. *J Bone Joint Surg Br* 1992;74:228-232.

45. Psychoyios V, Crawford RW, O'Connor JJ, Murray DW: Wear of congruent meniscal bearings in unicompartmental knee arthroplasty: A retrieval study of 16 specimens. *J Bone Joint Surg Br* 1998;80:976-982.

46. Laurencin CT, Zelicof SB, Scott RD, Ewald FC: Unicompartmental versus total knee arthroplasty in the same patient: A comparative study. *Clin Orthop* 1991;273:151-156.

47. Newman JH, Ackroyd CE, Shah NA: Unicompartmental or total knee replacement? Five-year results of a prospective randomised trial of 102 osteoarthritic knees with unicompartmental arthritis. *J Bone Joint Surg Br* 1998;80:862-865.

48. Rougraff BT, Heck DA, Gibson AE: A comparison of tricompartmental and unicompartmental arthroplasty for the treatment of gonarthrosis. *Clin Orthop* 1991;273:157-164.

49. White SH, Ludkowski PF, Goodfellow JW: Anteromedial osteoarthritis of the knee. *J Bone Joint Surg Br* 1991;73:582-586.

50. Weale AE, Murray DW, Crawford R, et al: Does arthritis progress in the retained compartments after "Oxford" medial unicompartmental arthroplasty? A clinical and radiological study with a minimum ten-year follow-up. *J Bone Joint Surg Br* 1999;81:783-789.

51. Murray DW, Goodfellow JW, O'Connor JJ: The Oxford medial unicompartmental arthroplasty: A ten-year survival study. *J Bone Joint Surg Br* 1998;80:983-989.

52. Price A, Svard U: An independent survival analysis of the Oxford unicompartmental meniscal bearing knee replacement. *67th Annual Meeting Proceedings.* Rosemont, IL, American Academy of Orthopaedic Surgeons, 2000, p 322.

53. Lewold S, Goodman S, Knutson K, Robertsson O, Lidgren L: Oxford meniscal bearing knee versus the Marmor knee in unicompartmental arthroplasty for arthrosis: A Swedish multicenter survival study. *J Arthroplasty* 1995;10: 722-731.

54. Larsson SE, Larsson S, Lundkvist S: Unicompartmental knee arthroplasty: A prospective consecutive series followed for six to 11 years. *Clin Orthop* 1988;232:174-181.

55. Christensen NO: Unicompartmental prosthesis for gonarthrosis: A nine-year series of 575 knees from a Swedish hospital. *Clin Orthop* 1991;273:165-169.

56. Keys G: Reduced invasive approach for Oxford II medial unicompartmental knee replacement: A preliminary study. *Knee*, in press.

57. Webb JM, Topf H, Haikel S, Dodd CA, Goodfellow JW, Murray DW: Abstract: Minimally invasive Oxford unicompartmental knee replacement. *J Bone Joint Surg Br* 1999;81(suppl III):295.

58. Insall JN, Dorr LD, Scott RD, Scott WN: Rationale of the Knee Society clinical rating system. *Clin Orthop* 1989;248:13-14.

59. Bellamy N, Buchanan WW, Goldsmith CH, Campbell J, Stitt LW: Validation study of WOMAC: A health status instrument for measuring clinically important patient relevant outcomes to antirheumatic drug therapy in patients with osteoarthritis of the hip or knee. *J Rheumatol* 1988;15:1833-1840.

60. Ware JE Jr, Kosinski M, Keller SD: *SF-36 Physical and Mental Health Summary Scales: A User's Manual*. Boston, MA, The Health Institute, New England Medical Center, 1994.

61. Buechel FF, Pappas MJ: New Jersey Low Contact Stress knee replacement system: Ten-year evaluation of meniscal bearings. *Orthop Clin North Am* 1989;20:147-177.

62. Jordan LR, Olivo JL, Voorhorst PE: Survivorship analysis of cementless meniscal bearing total knee arthroplasty. *Clin Orthop* 1997;338:119-123.

63. Bert JM: Dislocation/subluxation of meniscal bearing elements after New Jersey Low-Contact Stress total knee arthroplasty. *Clin Orthop* 1990;254:211-215.

64. Barrett DS, Cobb AG, Bentley G: Joint proprioception in normal, osteoarthritic and replaced knees. *J Bone Joint Surg Br* 1991;73:53-56.

65. Callaghan J, Squire M, Goetz D, Sullivan P, Johnston R: Cemented rotating-platform total knee replacement: A nine to twelve-year follow-up study. *J Bone Joint Surg Am*, in press.

66. Sorrells RB: The rotating platform mobile bearing TKA. *Orthopedics* 1996;19:793-796.

67. Buechel FF, Rosa RA, Pappas MJ: A metal-backed, rotating-bearing patellar prosthesis to lower contact stress. An 11-year clinical study. *Clin Orthop* 1989;248:34-49.

68. Weaver JK, Derkash RS, Greenwald AS: Difficulties with bearing dislocation and breakage using a movable bearing total knee replacement system. *Clin Orthop* 1993;290:244-252.

69. Kumar PJ, McPherson EJ, Dorr LD, Wan Z, Baldwin K: Rehabilitation after total knee arthroplasty: A comparison of 2 rehabilitation techniques. *Clin Orthop* 1996;331:93-101.

70. Scuderi GR, Insall JN: Total knee arthroplasty: Current clinical perspectives. *Clin Orthop* 1992;276:26-32.

71. Sathasivam S, Walker PS: Optimization of the bearing surface geometry of total knees. *J Biomech* 1994;27:255-264.

72. Matsuda S, White SE, Williams VG II, McCarthy DS, Whiteside LA: Contact stress analysis in meniscal bearing total knee arthroplasty. *J Arthroplasty* 1998;13:699-706.

73. Heim CS, Postak PD, Greenwald AS: Abstract: Stability characteristics of mobile bearing total knee designs. *66th Annual Meeting Proceedings*. Rosemont, IL, Amercan Academy of Orthopaedic Surgeons, 1999, pp 256-257.

74. Ritter MA, Campbell E, Faris PM, Keating EM: Long-term survival analysis of the posterior cruciate condylar total knee arthroplasty: A 10-year evaluation. *J Arthroplasty* 1989;4: 293-296.

75. Keblish PA, Schmei C, Ward M: Evaluation of 275 Low Contact Stress (LCS) total knee replacements with 2-8 year follow-up. *Orthopedics* 1993;1:168-174.

76. Kaper BP, Smith PN, Bourne RB, Rorabeck CH, Robertson D: Medium-term results of a mobile bearing total knee replacement. *Clin Orthop* 1999;367:201-209.

46

Revision Anterior Cruciate Ligament Reconstruction: Report of 11-Year Experience and Results in 114 Consecutive Patients

Frank R. Noyes, MD
Sue D. Barber-Westin, BS

Introduction

Anterior cruciate ligament (ACL) reconstruction is a popular procedure, performed on an estimated 102,000 patients in the United States each year.[1] Failure of this procedure, resulting in symptomatic instability, occurs in 3% to 10% of knees.[2-11] Therefore, each year, between 3,000 and 10,000 patients are potential candidates for a revision procedure. Because patients are maintaining an active lifestyle for longer periods during the course of their lives, it is believed that this problem of symptomatic instability will only continue to grow and that the number of both primary and revision ACL reconstructions will increase each year.

Although surgical techniques, graft substitutes, and rehabilitation programs continue to improve, ACL reconstructions fail for many reasons. The reasons for failure include, but are not limited to, use of a graft that is biomechanically inadequate,[12] improper intra-articular placement of the graft,[13,14] impingement of the graft in the femoral notch because of inadequate notchplasty or placement,[15,16] improper tensioning of the graft,[17,18] inadequate fixation of the graft because of the fixation device or inadequate bone stock of the host bone,[19,20] failure to correct associated ligament instabilities,[21] failure to correct varus osseous lower limb alignment,[22] and traumatic reinjury. Several authors have defined in detail the etiology of failure of ACL reconstructions.[23-29] This chapter will define important technical issues to be addressed preoperatively and during the procedure and present the results of 11 years of experience with ACL revision reconstruction in 114 consecutive knees.

Preoperative Evaluation and Planning

The first step in planning a revision of a failed ACL reconstruction is a careful assessment of the factors that might have been related to or directly caused the failure so that these problems can be addressed before or during the revision procedure. A meticulous physical examination must be performed to detect any associated ligament deficiencies, excessive valgus or varus lower limb alignment, or gait abnormalities.

Unrecognized lateral collateral ligament (LCL) and posterolateral ligament deficiency or medial collateral ligament deficiency can cause excessive loading on the ACL graft, leading to failure.[21] The important elements of the clinical examination required to detect varus recurvatum, lateral joint opening, and excessive external tibial rotation have been described.[30] During arthroscopy, we perform a lateral joint opening gap test and measure the amount of joint opening with a calibrated nerve hook[31] (Fig. 1). In knees that have insufficient posterolateral structures, 12 mm or more of joint opening will occur at the periphery of the lateral tibiofemoral compartment,[31] indicating that surgical correction should be performed concurrently with the ACL revision reconstruction.

Problems incurred with varus-aligned ACL-deficient knees, and the importance of correcting lower limb malalignment with a high tibial osteotomy (HTO) before ACL reconstruction, have been discussed.[32-34] Problems with varus alignment are especially a concern in patients with a high knee adduction moment measured on gait analysis,[35] or in patients with an abnormal knee hyperextension gait pattern. The hyperextension occurs during the stance phase of gait and can place healing soft tissues and grafts at risk for stretching out postoperatively. This gait abnormality should be corrected before the ACL revision reconstruction by a program that trains patients to walk with the knee slightly flexed throughout stance, to maintain ankle dorsiflexion in early stance, and to maintain an erect trunk-hip attitude during stance.[36]

Lateral radiographs are taken with the knee in full extension to evaluate the location and size of the tibial tunnel.

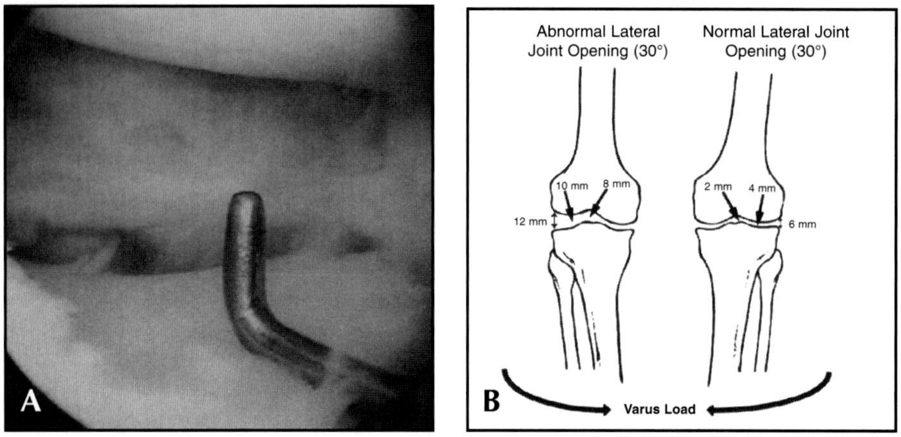

Fig. 1 The arthroscopic gap test for determining the amount of lateral joint opening. **A,** A calibrated nerve hook is used to measure the millimeters of joint space. **B,** In knees that have insufficient posterolateral structures, 8 mm of lateral joint opening will be measured at the intercondylar notch, and 12 mm or more will be measured at the periphery of the lateral tibiofemoral compartment. (Reproduced with permission from Noyes FR, Barber-Westin SD, Hewett TE: High tibial osteotomy and ligament reconstruction for varus angulated anterior cruciate ligament-deficient knees. *Am J Sports Med* 2000;28:282-296.)

Weight-bearing radiographs and posteroanterior 45° knee flexion[37] views to detect osseous alignment and tibiofemoral joint narrowing also are required. MRI is performed when additional preoperative evaluation of tunnel size, position, or associated abnormalities is required.

Other abnormalities or potential problems also must be addressed preoperatively, including patient expectation issues, muscular weakness, painful neuromatous complex regional pain syndromes, and anterior knee pain secondary to patellofemoral cartilage damage. A loss of full knee extension poses special problems. In general, it is important to obtain full knee motion before revision surgery. Exceptions are grafts placed too far anteriorly or cyclops lesions, both of which can produce a mechanical block to full extension. During the revision procedure, the anterior intercondylar blockage might be eliminated by correct graft placement, débridement, and notchplasty. In these knees, there might also be associated tightness to the posterior capsular structures that have shortened, requiring a vigorous postoperative program. If the lack of extension is greater than 5°, we routinely stage the procedure by first performing an arthroscopic débridement and cyclops lesion excision, followed by rigorous rehabilitation to regain full motion, and then proceed with the ACL revision reconstruction.

Considerable counseling and patient education are required on the expected results and outcomes from the revision procedure. This is especially important for patients with knees with preexisting arthrosis or meniscal loss or that require additional major surgical procedures. In nearly one half of revision knees, a major concomitant procedure will be required in addition to the ACL procedure. Patients need to understand the technical difficulties inherent in the procedure and that the results are uniformly not as reliable as those with primary ACL reconstruction. A surgeon-physical therapist team approach is required to provide instruction on rehabilitation to help ensure that the patient will successfully follow the postoperative exercise program.

Graft Options

Currently, no standard procedure exists for revision of failed ACL reconstructions. Graft choices that have been described in the literature include bone–patellar ligament–bone or Achilles tendon allografts[28,38-40] or various autogenous substitutes, including bone–patellar tendon–bone,[40-43] semitendinosus-gracilis tendon,[42] and quadriceps tendon.[43] A few authors have reharvested the ipsilateral patellar tendon several months after the original reconstruction in which this tendon was used.[41,44,45] Results from these graft options are discussed below.

Technical Problems and Solutions at Surgery

Removal of Previously Placed Hardware and Prosthetic Grafts

Preoperatively, a careful examination of radiographs and surgical records will provide information on the type of hardware previously used to ensure that the proper equipment is available for removal of the hardware during the revision procedure. If the existing hardware does not interfere with new tunnel creation, it should be left alone. However, in many cases it must be removed, which can be problematic. Removal of femoral interference screws placed endoscopically during a previous procedure can be difficult, especially if the screw was placed too far posteriorly. Débridement of bone and soft tissue with a curette is usually required. The knee flexion angle that was used to insert the interference screw must be recreated so that the screw can be removed with an endoscopic screwdriver.

Previously placed prosthetic grafts should be removed en bloc to avoid leaving particulate debris, which can promote a marked inflammatory response leading to bone tunnel and articular cartilage deterioration.[46,47] Bone gauges can be used to loosen the bony attachments first, making graft removal easier. Knees with excessive bone loss and osteolysis might require a staged procedure with an autogenous bone graft of the tunnel performed first, followed by revision ACL reconstruction, which must be delayed for at least 6 months to allow osseous healing.

Notchplasty Revision

In many cases, the original ACL reconstruction will have failed because of graft impingement from an inadequate notchplasty. The majority of knees that undergo revision require a careful notchplasty, removing only enough bone to allow adequate visualization and motion of the graft as the knee is moved through a full range of motion without impingement. **(CD-46.1)**

Misplaced or Excessively Wide Tunnels

Several methods can be used to correct for widely misplaced or excessively wide femoral or tibial graft tunnels.[39] There are two options to correct for misplaced femoral tunnels. In some knees, a new femoral tunnel can be created through an outside-in approach, providing an adequate bony bridge between the previous tunnel and the newly created tunnel. If possible, the previously placed interference screw is not removed so that it can act as a buttress to prevent fracture and loss of fixation of the newly placed graft. Care must be taken during the surgical procedure to drill the tunnel in a stepwise manner, starting with an initial 6-mm tunnel that is then overdrilled to the correct diameter.

In other knees, the previous femoral tunnel might be in an excessively abnormal anterior location, making it impossible to locate a new tunnel at the ACL isometric site without breaking into the previous tunnel. A posterior notchplasty of the lateral femoral condyle into the ACL insertion site is created through a limited lateral approach. This allows the graft to be inserted in a posterior position within the anatomic ACL attachment site, maintaining a bony bridge from the previous osseous tunnel. Internal graft fixation with two small-fragment cancellous screws and a back-up suture post provides secure osseous fixation.

An enlarged graft tunnel from a previously failed ACL reconstruction possesses unique problems. One option is to place two stacked cancellous screws to obtain interference graft fixation (Fig. 2). In some cases, excessive widening might be noted at the tibial insertion site as the graft enters the knee joint. When the tibial tunnel extends posteriorly past the normal ACL insertion site, a more vertically oriented posterior graft position occurs. This is viewed as an indication for autogenous bone grafting of the tibial tunnel. In these cases, allografts offer an advantage of having increased osseous size that can accommodate enlarged tunnels, potentially avoiding the need for autogenous bone grafting.

Overly wide or misplaced tibial tunnels also pose special problems in patients with disuse osteopenia and diminished cancellous bone mass of the tibia. In these cases, two stacked interference screws will not provide adequate fixation. Secondary fixation with No. 2 nonabsorbable sutures, passed through the bone end of the graft and tied to a screw or staple post, are required in addition to fixation with interference screws.

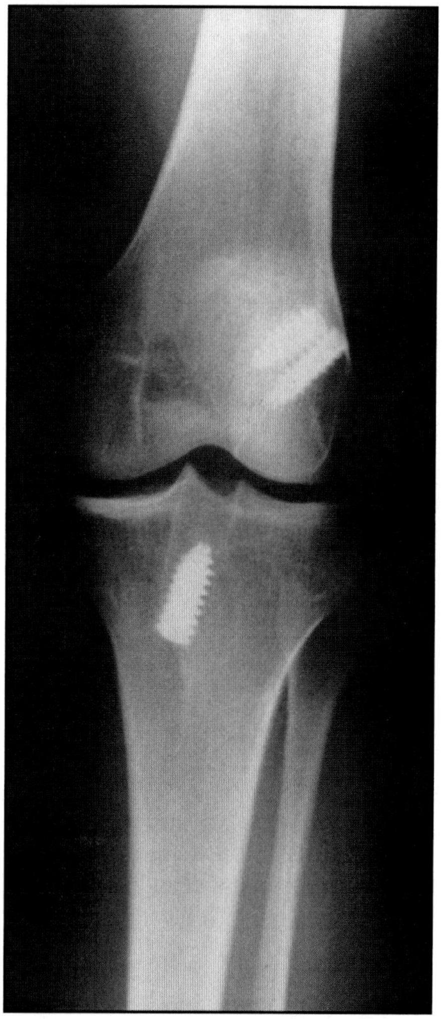

Fig. 2 Two stacked interference screws used in an ACL revision avoided the requirement for an autogenous bone grafting procedure.

Graft Tensioning

Several factors affect graft tensioning during ACL reconstruction, including the type of graft material, tunnel placement, knee flexion angle used during tensioning, the direction of the tensioning force (proximal or distal), and the amount of tension to be applied during graft fixation. Excessive or insufficient tension placed on the graft during ACL reconstruction can lead to failure.[17,18,48-50] Excessive tension can result in overconstraint of the graft, leading to decreased motion or delayed revascularization. Insufficient tension will not correct the abnormal anterior-posterior translation and can result in an incompetent graft that can fail early postoperatively.

During the revision procedure, we directly observe the motion of the graft arthroscopically as the knee is moved through 0° to 120° of flexion to ensure that impingement in the femoral intercondylar notch does not occur. We advocate fixation of the graft in 10° of flexion under a small load (44 N). After graft tensioning and fixation, the joint should not be overconstrained. The goal is to restore the amount of anterior-posterior

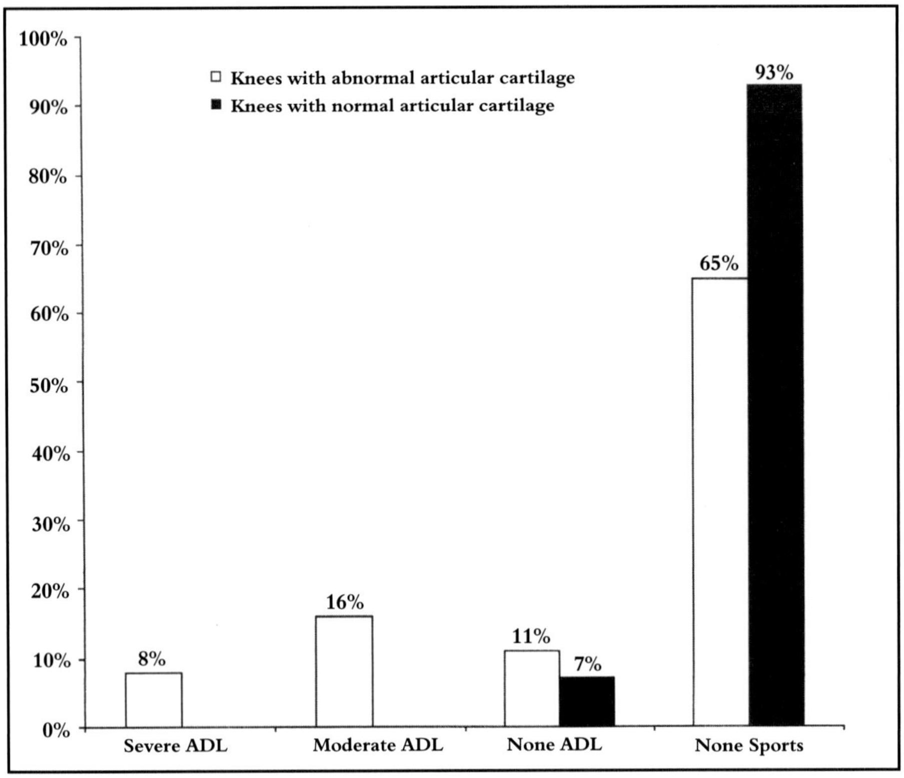

Fig. 3 Comparison of the pain scores at follow-up of 28 knees with normal articular cartilage with scores for 37 knees with abnormal articular cartilage. The difference between the groups was significant ($P < 0.05$). Severe activites of daily living (ADL) = severe pain (constant, not relieved) with activities of daily living. Moderate ADL = moderate pain (frequent, limiting) with activities of daily living. None ADL = no pain with activities of daily living but pain with any sports activity. None Sports = no pain with sports activity. (Reproduced with permission from Noyes FR, Barber-Westin SD: Use of allografts after failed treatment of rupture of the anterior cruciate ligament. *J Bone Joint Surg Am* 1994;76:1019-1031.)

displacement that is present in the normal, contralateral knee.

Results and Outcomes of ACL Revision Procedures

Allografts

Allograft tissue has been used by several authors for ACL revision reconstruction.[38,39,42,47,51,52] In 1995, Johnson and associates[52] reported the results in 14 patients who had had fresh-frozen bone–patellar tendon–bone or Achilles tendon allografts and were followed for between 18 and 30 months postoperatively. Four patients (29%) had failed grafts according to KT-1000 arthrometer (Medmetric, San Diego, CA) testing. Compared with a matched group of primary ACL reconstructions, the allograft group had lower subjective knee scores, International Knee Documentation Committee (IKDC) scores, modified Cincinnati Knee Rating System scores, and stability results. One year later, Johnson and associates[38] reported the results of 25 consecutive patients who had received fresh-frozen allograft revision ACL reconstructions. All patients were followed for between 24 and 36 months postoperatively. Nine patients (36%) had failed grafts with more than 5 mm of increased translation on KT-1000 testing. Seventeen patients (68%) could perform at least light sports activities without pain, swelling, or giving way. Nineteen patients (76%) were satisfied with their results.

Two investigations have compared the results of allograft and autograft ACL revision reconstructions. Getelman and associates[51] compared the results of 14 patients who had fresh-frozen bone–patellar tendon–bone allografts with those of 12 patients who had ipsilateral bone–patellar tendon–bone autogenous grafts. The patients were followed for between 20 and 34 months postoperatively. The allograft group had poorer IKDC rating scores (normal or nearly normal, 29% allografts and 67% autografts; $P < 0.05$), which were related to patellofemoral crepitus and radiographic evidence of joint narrowing. There were five failures in the study; however, the authors did not identify how many were from each subgroup, allograft or autograft.

Uribe and associates[42] followed 54 patients for between 2 and 6.5 years postoperatively. Nineteen received bone–patellar tendon–bone allografts and 35, autogenous grafts (ipsilateral or contralateral patellar tendon or semitendinosus-gracilis tendons). The allograft group had a significantly greater mean increase in KT-1000 test scores than did the autograft group (mean ± SD, 3.3 ± 1.5 mm and 2.2 ± 1.3 mm, respectively; $P < 0.005$). Three knees (6%) had a soft end point; however, the authors did not indicate which type of graft these knees had received. Twenty-nine patients (54%) returned to their preinjury level of activity. All patients felt they had benefited from the surgery and none reported recurrent instability postoperatively.

Clinical Study on Allograft ACL Revision Reconstruction

The results and clinical outcome of a series of 66 consecutive patients (66 knees) who received bone–patellar ligament–bone allograft ACL revision reconstruction have been reported in detail.[39] The results are summarized here.

Sixty-five patients (98%) returned for follow-up an average of 42 months (range, 23 to 78 months) postoperatively. All had received the same graft by the same surgeon, and all followed a similar program of rehabilitation that included immediate knee motion, partial weight bearing for the first 8 to 12 postoperative weeks, and a delay in return to full sports activities for at least 12 postoperative months. Concomitant procedures were common and included meniscus repairs (19 knees), meniscus allografts (10 knees), reconstruction of the LCL (7 knees), advancement of the posterolateral complex (11 knees), reconstruction of the medial collateral ligament (4 knees), and reconstruction of the posterior cruciate ligament (2 knees). The results were assessed using the Cincinnati Knee Rating System.[53]

The overall failure rate was calculated using data derived from both pivot shift and KT-2000 arthrometer testing and included 10 additional knees in which the revision reconstruction had failed early postoperatively. We found that 33% of the reconstructions (25 of 75 knees) failed. However, significant improvements were found for the symptoms of pain, swelling, and giving way ($P < 0.0001$); the functions of walking, stair climbing, and kneeling ($P < 0.001$); and the functions of running, jumping, and twisting/turning ($P < 0.0001$). Forty-two patients (65%) had returned to mostly light sports activities without problems.

Thirty-seven knees (56%) had abnormal articular cartilage surfaces seen during the ACL revision procedure. At follow-up, significant differences were found between these knees and those with normal cartilage surfaces for the variables of pain (Fig. 3), stair climbing, kneeling, running, jumping, twisting/turning, sports activity level, and the overall rating score (Table 1; $P < 0.05$).

Table 1
Effect of the condition of the articular cartilage at the ACL allograft revision reconstruction on the subjective scores and overall rating at follow-up

Variable	Point Scale	Patients With Normal Articular Cartilage*	Patients With Abnormal† Articular Cartilage*	*P* Value‡
Pain	0 to 6	5.9 ± 0.5	4.6 ± 2.1	0.03
Swelling	0 to 6	5.8 ± 0.6	5.2 ± 1.4	0.11‡
Partial giving away	0 to 6	5.9 ± 0.4	5.2 ± 1.5	0.06‡
Full giving away	0 to 6	6.0	5.5 ± 1.4	0.25‡
Walking	0 to 40	38 ± 4	34 ± 8	0.22‡
Stair climbing	0 to 40	36 ± 5	29 ± 11	0.01
Kneeling	0 to 40	28 ± 14	21 ± 14	0.01
Running	40 to 100	84 ± 18	61 ± 21	0.001
Jumping	40 to 100	78 ± 21	57 ± 22	0.01
Twisting and turning	40 to 100	73 ± 21	55 ± 20	0.01
Overall rating	0 to 100			
Follow-up		85 ± 9	71 ± 12	0.0001
Improvement from before surgery		26 ± 10	21 ± 11	0.07

*Values given as mean score ± standard deviation

†Abnormal was defined as fissuring and fragmentation of 15 mm or more in diameter that extended into more than one half of the involved surface or any exposed subchondral bone

‡Contingency table analyses were used for all except the overall rating scores; an unpaired *t* test was used for the analyses of the follow-up scores and the improvement from the preoperative score

NS = not significant

(Adapted with permission from Noyes FR, Barber-Westin SD, Roberts CS: Use of allografts after failed treatment of rupture of the anterior cruciate ligament. *J Bone Joint Surg Am* 1994;76:1019-1031.)

The preoperative overall knee rating score for all 65 knees of 54 ± 10 points significantly improved to 77 ± 13 points at follow-up ($P < 0.0001$). All patients except one had an improvement in this score; the average increase was 23 ± 11 points.

It is concluded that the high failure rate, cost of allograft tissue, and risk of disease transmission brought concerns with this surgical procedure and recommended the use of an autogenous graft for ACL revision reconstruction. Allografts were reserved for knees that did not have suitable autogenous tissues or for knees that required multiple ligament reconstructive procedures. Of note, we found in a previous investigation that the failure rate for ACL allograft reconstructions for chronic ruptures was only 3% (1 of 40 knees) when the procedure was combined with a lateral iliotibial band extra-articular reconstruction.[54] This concept bears further study because allografts, with their delay in remodeling and maturation,[55-57] might require a lateral extra-articular procedure for postoperative graft protection.

Autografts

Different autogenous tissues have been used for ACL revision reconstruction, including the patellar tendon,[40-43,58,59] semitendinosus-gracilis tendons,[58,60] and quadriceps tendon.[43] Only one series has reported on the use of the quadriceps tendon for ACL revision reconstruction. Wirth and Kohn[43] used this tendon in 30 knees followed for between 2 and 18 years postoperatively. In the same investigation, 57 knees underwent autogenous bone–patellar tendon–bone revision reconstruction. The results of the two different graft types were not sorted, nor were failure rates provided. Of all 87 knees, 75% had problems with pain, swelling, or giving way at follow-up. Fifty-two patients (60%) were satisfied with their results.

Uribe and associates[42] used the contralateral patellar tendon in 16 knees and the ipsilateral patellar tendon in 17 knees in their series, which also included

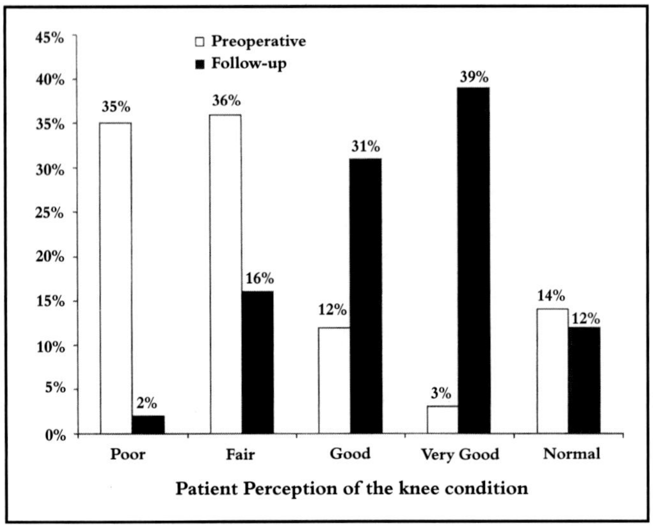

Fig. 4 Patient responses on the rating scale for perception of the overall knee condition before and after bone–patellar tendon–bone autograft ACL revision reconstruction. The difference between evaluations was significant (*P* = 0.0001).

allograft (19 knees) and semitendinosus-gracilis tendon (2 knees) ACL revision reconstructions. At an average of 32 months postoperatively, knees with autogenous grafts had improved stability compared with those that had received allografts. Failure rates were not provided according to graft type. Subjectively and functionally, no significant differences were found between the graft subgroups.

Kartus and associates[41] compared the results of 12 knees in which the ipsilateral patellar tendon was reharvested with results in 12 knees that received contralateral patellar tendon grafts for ACL revision reconstruction. Two years postoperatively, no differences were found between the subgroups on MRI for patellar ligament length, width, thickness, or donor site gap measurements. However, the knees that received the reharvested grafts had lower functional scores and a higher rate of complications, including one postoperative patellar fracture and one postoperative patellar ligament rupture. No failure rates were provided for either subgroup.

Clinical Study on Autograft ACL Revision Reconstruction

The preliminary results of a group of 20 knees that received autogenous bone–patellar tendon–bone grafts for ACL revision reconstruction were reported.[40] In that series, the overall failure rate was 27% at a postoperative average of 27 months. We now present the results of this surgery in 57 consecutive cases (56 knees, including the 20 knees in our preliminary report). In six knees, the revision reconstruction failed before the 2-year follow-up examination. We included these six knees in the calculation of the overall failure rate but not in the other analyses in this study. The study population therefore consisted of 51 knees in 50 patients. All patients were contacted and 48 (49 knees, 96%) returned for an examination at a mean of 34 months (range, 24 to 74 months) postoperatively.

There were 31 men and 17 women whose mean age at the time of surgery was 27 years (range, 14 to 48 years). Most patients were athletically active; 40 (83%) had injured the knee during a sports activity. The mean time from the original knee injury to the revision procedure was 80 months (range, 6 to 218 months).

A total of 218 previous surgical procedures had been done in these knees, including 53 ACL procedures. The failed ACL procedures included primary repairs (11 knees), extra-articular iliotibial band procedures (8 knees), bone–patellar tendon–bone autogenous grafts (14 knees), other autogenous grafts (3 knees), allografts (16 knees), and synthetic grafts (1 knee). Eight patients required HTO, and 9 required reconstruction of the LCL and posterolateral complex.

The results were assessed using the Cincinnati Knee Rating System,[53] KT-2000 arthrometer testing (134 N total anterior-posterior force), comprehensive knee examination, and patient satisfaction questions.

A bone–patellar tendon–bone autograft was used in all knees. In 36 knees (73%), the ipsilateral patellar tendon had not been used previously and was harvested. In 13 knees, the patellar tendon had been used previously for the ACL reconstructions that subsequently failed. Because of patellar tendinitis and pain, the contralateral patellar tendon was used for the revision procedure in five knees. In the remaining eight knees, the ipsilateral patellar ligament was reharvested after careful observation demonstrated that adequate healing in the previous donor site had occurred. The mean time between the original harvest of the patellar tendon and the reharvest for the revision procedure was 48 months (range, 13 to 168 months).

Concurrent surgical procedures were common and included 21 meniscus repairs and 14 reconstructive procedures for lateral or medial ligamentous deficiency. During the revision surgery, 28 knees (57%) had noteworthy damage of the articular cartilage of either fissuring and fragmentation or exposure of subchondral bone.

Results Anterior-posterior displacements significantly decreased from the preoperative arthrometer test (mean, 11.6 ± 3.9 mm) to the follow-up test (mean, 1.2 ± 4.0 mm; *P* = 0.0001). Preoperatively, all knees had a grade 2 or 3 pivot shift. At follow-up, 41 knees (84%) had a grade 0 or 1; 6 (12%), grade 2; and

Table 2
Effect of concomitant surgical procedures on outcome of ACL bone–patellar tendon–bone autograft revision reconstructions

	Pain			Patient Perception of Overall Knee Condition			AP Displacement (mm)			Overall Rating Score		
	Preoperative	Follow-up	*P*	Preoperative	Follow-up	*P*	Preoperative	Follow-up	*P*	Preoperative	Follow-up	*P*
Revision, no other major procedures (N = 30)	4.1	5.7	0.0001	3.8	7.1	0.0001	11.1	0.2	0.0001	64	91	0.0001
Revision and previous HTO (N = 8)	2.2	5.3	0.0007	6.2	4.5*	NS	11.2	4.1*	0.06	51	82*	0.0001
Revision and other ligament reconstruction (N = 11)	3.6	4.9	NS	3.7	6.0	0.03	13.1	2.1	0.0001	58	86	0.0001

*Significantly different from the revision, no other major procedures subgroup, $P < 0.05$

HTO = high tibial osteotomy; AP = anteroposterior; NS = not significant

2 (4%), grade 3. Of the 49 knees followed for at least 2 years, 33 (67%) had a functional reconstruction, 9 (18%) had partial function, and 7 (14%) failed. When the 6 knees that had had early postoperative graft failure were included, 33 knees (60%) were classified as functional, 9 (16%) had partial function, and 13 (24%) failed.

There were significant improvements in pain ($P = 0.0001$), functions of activities of daily living ($P < 0.05$) and sports ($P < 0.001$), patient perception of the overall knee condition ($P = 0.0001$), and the overall rating score ($P = 0.0001$). Preoperatively, 19 of 48 patients (39%) participated in sports activities, all with symptoms or limitations. At follow-up, 30 patients (63%) had returned to athletics without symptoms. Seven other patients with symptoms were participating in sporting activities against our advice.

All patients had at least 135° of knee flexion, and all patients except one had at least 0° of extension. One patient lacked 5° of full extension.

The preoperative mean overall rating score of 61 ± 10 points (range, 43 to 79 points of a possible 100 points total significantly improved to 89 ± 10 points (range, 62 to 100 points) at follow-up ($P = 0.0001$). All knees had an improvement in the overall rating score; the mean improvement was 28 points (range, 4 to 46 points).

The mean preoperative patient perception score of 4.2 ± 2.8 points significantly improved to 6.4 ± 2.0 points (possible total: 10 points) at follow-up ($P = 0.0001$). Patients indicated that the overall condition of 46 knees (94%) had improved by circling at least 1 point higher on the scale at follow-up compared with the preoperative questionnaire (Fig. 4). Two patients rated the overall condition as the same, and one rated the knee condition as worse at follow-up.

When the population was sorted according to concurrent surgical procedures performed with the ACL revision reconstruction, we found that 5 (16%) of the 32 knees that had only the ACL revision reconstruction failed, 2 (22%) of the 9 knees that had an HTO before the revision procedure failed, and 6 (43%) of the 14 knees that had additional ligament procedures performed with the revision reconstruction failed. There was a statistically significant difference between the knees that had only the revision reconstruction and those that had HTO before the revision procedure in the mean patient perception scores, overall rating scores, and anterior-posterior displacement values at follow-up ($P < 0.05$; Table 2).

Additional surgeries were performed in seven knees after the revision reconstruction. Two knees had arthroscopy and removal of painful distal cancellous bone screws. One knee had a twisting reinjury and had a successful repair of a new meniscus tear. One knee had an arthroscopy and partial meniscectomy after a meniscal repair for a tear located in the outer one-third region failed to heal. Three knees had early postoperative increases in anterior-posterior displacement detected on arthrometer testing presumed to be caused by a partial loss of graft fixation. Diagnostic arthroscopy performed between the fourth and sixth postoperative weeks demonstrated that the grafts were intact, and these were treated by distal tibial refixation with an interference screw and a post. At follow-up, one knee had a partially functional graft and two had failed.

Discussion The findings from this study and others[38,39,41-43] regarding ACL revision reconstruction all lead to a similar conclusion, results obtainable from revision surgeries are generally less favorable than those derived from primary ACL reconstructions. The majority of

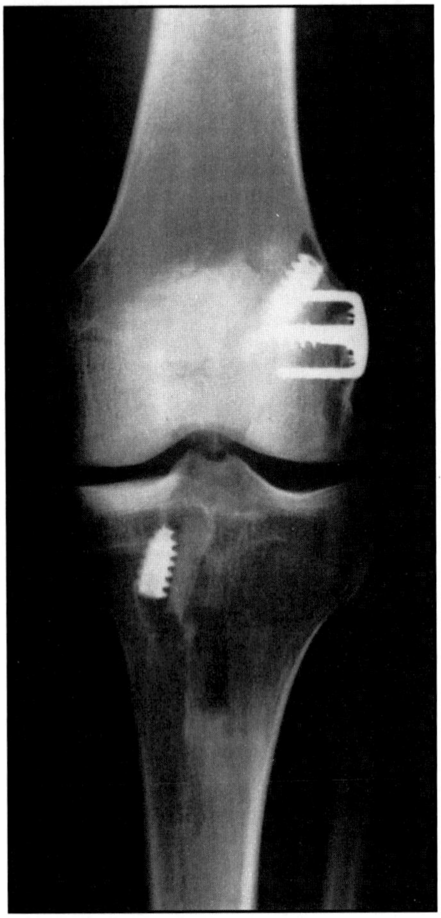

Fig. 5 Osseous fixation of the posterolateral complex proximal advancement procedure performed with an ACL bone–patellar tendon–bone autograft revision reconstruction.

knees requiring revision reconstruction have additional problems, including articular cartilage damage, previous meniscectomy, loss of secondary ligament restraints, varus malalignment, and the necessity for concomitant ligament reconstructions or meniscal repairs. Still, we were encouraged that many patients in our series benefited from the surgery. An improvement in the pain score was reported in 80% of the autograft population and 61% of the allograft population. In the autograft group, 94% (46 knees) rated their overall knee condition as improved compared to the preoperative condition. The overall rating score was improved in 100% of the autograft patients and in all but one of the allograft patients. Finally, 61% of the autograft population and 65% of the allograft population returned to light athletics without symptoms.

Overall Graft Failure Rate The overall failure rate of 24% for the autograft population represented a threefold increase compared with the 7% failure rate we reported[9] in 90 knees that had primary ACL patellar tendon autograft reconstructions. Failure rates obtained by objective instrumented testing of ACL revision reconstructions in which patellar tendon autogenous grafts were used have not been reported by other investigators.[41-43] Failure rates of revision ACL allograft reconstructions remain even higher than those found for patellar tendon autograft reconstructions. Our failure rate of 33% (25 of 75 knees)[39] is similar to the rate of 36% (9 of 25 knees) reported by Johnson and associates.[38]

We found an increased failure rate in our autograft revision series in knees that required a concomitant LCL or posterolateral structure reconstruction compared with knees that did not require such a procedure (27% and 11%, respectively). The reasons for this difference are unclear at the present time. However, one important finding of this series was the amount of time that had elapsed between the failed ACL primary reconstruction and the revision reconstruction (average, 63 months). We hypothesize that, during this time period, the knees suffered deterioration to important structures, including the meniscus, articular cartilage, and secondary restraints. We recommend that the revision procedure be performed earlier to avoid further joint damage and believe that earlier reconstruction might reduce the failure rate.

Effect of the Condition of the Articular Cartilage on Results The condition of the articular cartilage had a statistically significant effect on the outcome in both the allograft and autograft investigations. In the allograft population, significant differences were found between knees with abnormal cartilage surfaces and those with normal cartilage surfaces for pain, stair climbing, kneeling, running, jumping, twisting/turning, sports activity level, and the overall rating score ($P < 0.05$). For the autograft population, one of the 28 patients (4%) that had abnormal articular cartilage surfaces returned to strenuous sports activities compared with 8 of the 21 patients (38%) that had normal articular cartilage surfaces ($P < 0.05$). One half of the patients with abnormal articular cartilage surfaces returned to light recreational activities involving only swimming or bicycling based on our recommendations to avoid strenuous, high-impact activities.

Unrecognized Varus Osseous Alignment and Associated Ligament Deficiencies In the 114 consecutive knees in our two series, 14% required an HTO to correct varus osseous malalignment before the ACL revision surgery. We have discussed the problems incurred in varus-aligned ACL-deficient knees and the importance of correcting lower limb malalignment before ligament reconstruction.[32,33,61] The severity of the condition of these knees was reflected in the poorer outcome compared with other knees in this study in patient perception and the overall rating score at follow-up. Patients who require osteotomy and ACL revision procedures should be counseled regarding realistic outcomes, with an understanding that the goals of the procedure are to decrease or alleviate symptoms with regular activities of daily living and not to return to sports activities.

Twenty-five percent of the knees in our investigations had unrecognized or untreated lateral, posterolateral, or medial ligament deficiencies that most likely were a factor in the failure of the primary ACL reconstructions. Excessive loading can occur on an ACL graft when associated lateral or medial collateral ligament insufficiency is present[21] because of the abnormal amount of medial or lateral joint opening that occurs with activity. Therefore, we routinely correct all associated ligament ruptures during an ACL procedure.

To obtain a successful outcome in a lateral and posterolateral reconstructive procedure, the surgeon must understand the indications for different surgical techniques.[31,62,63] There are three possible procedures: proximal advancement of the entire posterolateral complex, allograft augmentation of the LCL and posterolateral complex, and double-graft substitution using autografts to reconstruct the LCL (bone–patellar tendon–bone) and popliteus tendon and ligament structures (semitendinosus-gracilis tendons). The surgeon must carefully inspect the lateral structures, noting the presence of scar tissue replacement, attachment site integrity, and width and size of the lateral and posterolateral structures to determine which procedure is warranted. In knees with interstitial failure of the posterolateral tissues (without acute traumatic disruption) caused by lax but intact attachment sites, the more simplified proximal advancement can be done (Fig. 5). This procedure is relatively easy to perform without the added surgical complexity and potential morbidity that occurs with major graft reconstructive procedures.[31] When more extensive damage to the posterolateral structures exists, such as after traumatic disruption, a major graft reconstruction is required.[62] In the most severe cases of disruption of all the lateral and posterolateral tissues, in which inadequate collagenous tissues exist, we prefer an autogenous graft replacement of the LCL and posterolateral structures.[63] If autogenous grafts are not available, allografts can be used.

Reharvest of the Patellar Tendon In eight knees (16%) in our autograft revision series, the patellar tendon was reharvested for the reconstruction. In seven of these patients, at least 2 years had elapsed between the original harvest of the patellar tendon and the revision reconstruction. Although the grafts failed in three knees, the small sample size precludes conclusions concerning the efficacy of patellar tendon graft reharvest. Nixon and associates,[64] Benedetto and associates,[65] and Coupens and associates[66] all believed that a patellar tendon graft reharvest was feasible because the tendon resumed a normal appearance on either MRI or ultrasonography between 18 and 24 months postoperatively. Alternatively, Liu and associates[67] reported that persistent morphologic changes lasted up to 7 years postoperatively that could adversely affect the biomechanical properties of the healed donor site. Patellar tendon defects were found in 10 of 12 knees 12 months postoperatively on MRI by Bernicker and associates,[68] who concluded that the graft site cannot be assumed to be completely healed 1 year after harvest. Kartus and associates[41] published the only ACL revision study to date that compares the results of patients who had reharvested patellar tendon grafts (12 knees) and those of patients who had patellar tendon grafts taken from the contralateral knee (12 knees). Two years postoperatively, no differences were found between the subgroups on MRI for patellar tendon length, width, thickness, or donor site gap measurements. However, the knees that received the reharvested grafts had lower functional scores and more complications, including one patellar fracture and one patellar tendon rupture. In our study, no major complications occurred from the reharvesting procedure. We prefer to use the contralateral patellar tendon, the ipsilateral quadriceps tendon–patellar bone graft or semitendinosus-gracilis tendons, instead of a reharvested patellar ligament, for ACL revision reconstruction.

Meniscus Repairs During Revision Procedure One interesting finding from our investigations was that 32% of the knees required meniscal repair during the ACL revision procedure. We could not determine in all cases whether the meniscal tears represented old tears that were not surgically treated, new tears of relatively recent onset, or failed previous repairs. At follow-up, only one of these repairs had required partial resection, and the remainder were asymptomatic for tibiofemoral symptoms. Clinicians should realize, therefore, that meniscal repair is a valid and often successful procedure in knees undergoing ACL revision reconstruction. Repair can be performed for either peripheral tears or more extensive tears extending into the central one-third avascular zone. The meticulous suture method and rehabilitation program required for successful repair of complex meniscal tears has been discussed in detail.[69,70]

Conclusion

From our studies, we conclude that ACL revision reconstruction improves the majority of patients in regard to improved pain scores, improved overall knee rating scores, and allowance of return to light recreational activity. However, in some knees, residual problems exist because of underlying articular cartilage deterioration and previous meniscal loss. We found that, in our patients, an average of 63 months had elapsed between the primary and revision ACL reconstructions. During this time, the majority of knees suffered from multiple giving-way reinjuries and had functional limitations with sports activities, resulting in continued deterioration of the joint. Therefore, earlier consideration is warranted for ACL revision reconstruction before multiple reinjuries and chronic pain and swelling.

One of four knees in our studies had other unrecognized ligament deficiencies that required surgical correction along with the ACL revision procedure. Additionally, one of eight knees was in varus alignment and required an HTO before the ACL revision. We recommend that these procedures be staged to ensure that adequate osseous correction has been achieved and maintained and to reduce the risk of complications.

Meniscus repairs were performed in one of every three knees, and all but one were successful in terms of an absence of joint line pain and additional surgery. These included repairs for tears that extended into the central one-third avascular region.

We found a higher than expected rate of failure after ACL revision in both of our studies that requires further investigation. Our current preferred graft choices are (1) autogenous bone–patellar tendon–bone, with consideration of using the contralateral patellar tendon if the ipsilateral tendon was previously harvested; (2) quadriceps tendon–bone autogenous graft; (3) semitendinosus-gracilis tendon four-strand autogenous graft, provided normal tunnel widths exist; and (4) allografts, with consideration of incorporating an iliotibial band extra-articular procedure for additional graft protection.

References

1. Owings MF, Kozak LJ: Ambulatory and inpatient procedures in the United States, 1996. *Vital Health Stat* 1998;139:1-119.
2. Bach BR Jr, Levy ME, Bojchuk J, Tradonsky S, Bush-Joseph CA, Khan NH: Single-incision endoscopic anterior cruciate ligament reconstruction using patellar tendon autograft: Minimum two-year follow-up evaluation. *Am J Sports Med* 1998;26:30-40.
3. Corry IS, Webb JM, Clingeleffer AJ, Pinczewski LA: Arthroscopic reconstruction of the anterior cruciate ligament: A comparison of patellar tendon autograft and four-strand hamstring tendon autograft. *Am J Sports Med* 1999;27:444-454.
4. Howell SM, Deutsch ML: Comparison of endoscopic and two-incision techniques for reconstructing a torn anterior cruciate ligament using hamstring tendons. *Arthroscopy* 1999;15:594-606.
5. Marcacci M, Zaffagnini S, Iacono F, Neri MP, Loreti I, Petitto A: Arthroscopic intra- and extra-articular anterior cruciate ligament reconstruction with gracilis and semitendinosus tendons. *Knee Surg Sports Traumatol Arthrosc* 1998;6:68-75.
6. Meystre JL, Vallotton J, Benvenuti JF: Double semitendinosus anterior cruciate ligament reconstruction: 10-year results. *Knee Surg Sports Traumatol Arthrosc* 1998;6:76-81.
7. Muneta T, Sekiya I, Yagishita K, Ogiuchi T, Yamamoto H, Shinomiya K: Two-bundle reconstruction of the anterior cruciate ligament using semitendinosus tendon with endobuttons: Operative technique and preliminary results. *Arthroscopy* 1999;15:618-624.
8. Noyes FR, Barber-Westin SD: Reconstruction of the anterior cruciate ligament with human allograft: Comparison of early and later results. *J Bone Joint Surg Am* 1996;78:524-537.
9. Noyes FR, Barber-Westin SD: A comparison of results in acute and chronic anterior cruciate ligament ruptures of arthroscopically assisted autogenous patellar tendon reconstruction. *Am J Sports Med* 1997;25:460-471.
10. Shelbourne KD, Davis TJ: Evaluation of knee stability before and after participation in a functional sports agility program during rehabilitation after anterior cruciate ligament reconstruction. *Am J Sports Med* 1999;27:156-161.
11. Webb JM, Corry IS, Clingeleffer AJ, Pinczewski LA: Endoscopic reconstruction for isolated anterior cruciate ligament rupture. *J Bone Joint Surg Br* 1998;80:288-294.
12. Noyes FR, Butler DL, Grood ES, Zernicke RF, Hefzy MS: Biomechanical analysis of human ligament grafts used in knee-ligament repairs and reconstructions. *J Bone Joint Surg* 1984;66:344-352.
13. Graf B, Uhr F: Complications of intra-articular anterior cruciate reconstruction. *Clin Sports Med* 1988;7:835-848.
14. Hefzy MS, Grood ES, Noyes FR: Factors affecting the region of most isometric femoral attachments: The anterior cruciate ligament. *Am J Sports Med* 1989;17:208-216.
15. Howell SM, Taylor MA: Failure of reconstruction of the anterior cruciate ligament due to impingement by the intercondylar roof. *J Bone Joint Surg* 1993;75:1044-1055.
16. Tanzer M, Lenczner E: The relationship of intercondylar notch size and content to notchplasty requirement in anterior cruciate ligament surgery. *Arthroscopy* 1990;6:89-93.
17. Noyes FR, Butler DL, Paulos LE, Grood ES: Intra-articular cruciate reconstruction: Perspectives on graft strength, vascularization, and immediate motion after replacement. *Clin Orthop* 1983;172:71-77.
18. Yoshiya S, Andrish JT, Manley MT, Bauer TW: Graft tension in anterior cruciate ligament reconstruction: An in vivo study in dogs. *Am J Sports Med* 1987;15:464-470.
19. Kurosaka M, Yoshiya S, Andrish JT: A biomechanical comparison of different surgical techniques of graft fixation in anterior cruciate ligament reconstruction. *Am J Sports Med* 1987;15:225-229.
20. Matthews LS, Soffer SR: Pitfalls in the use of interference screws for anterior cruciate ligament reconstruction: Brief report. *Arthroscopy* 1989;5:225-226.
21. Wascher DC, Markolf KL, Shapiro MS, Finerman GA: Direct in vitro measurement of forces in the cruciate ligaments: The effect of multiplane loading in the intact knee. *J Bone Joint Surg Am* 1993;75:377-386.
22. Noyes FR, Munns SW, Andriacchi TP, et al: The double-varus and triple varus anterior cruciate insufficient knee: Gait analysis and surgical correction. *Tran Am Orthoc Soc Sports Med* 1985;11:41.
23. Carson EW, Simonian PT, Wickiewicz TL, Warren RF: Revision anterior cruciate ligament reconstruction. *Instr Course Lect* 1998;47: 361-368.
24. Getelman MH, Friedman MJ: Revision anterior cruciate ligament reconstruction surgery. *J Am Acad Orthop Surg* 1999;7:189-198.
25. Greis PE, Johnson DL, Fu FH: Revision anterior cruciate ligament surgery: Causes of graft failure and technical considerations of revision surgery. *Clin Sports Med* 1993;12:839-852.
26. Johnson KL, Fu FH: Anterior cruciate ligament reconstruction: Why do failures occur? *Instr Course Lect* 1995;44:391-406.
27. Maday MG, Harner CD, Fu FH: Revision ACL surgery: Evaluation and treatment, in Feagin JA Jr (ed): *The Crucial Ligaments: Diagnosis and Treatment of Ligamentous Injuries About the Knee*, ed 2. New York, NY, Churchill Livingstone, 1994, pp 711-723.
28. Safran MR, Harner CD: Revision ACL surgery: Technique and results utilizing allografts. *Instr Course Lect* 1995;44:407-415.
29. Steadman JR, Seemann MD, Hutton KS: Revision ligament reconstruction of failed prosthetic anterior cruciate ligaments. *Instr Course Lect* 1995;44:417-429.
30. Noyes FR, Stowers SF, Grood ES, Cummings J, VanGinkel LA: Posterior subluxations of the medial and lateral tibiofemoral compartments: An in vitro ligament sectioning study in cadaveric knees. *Am J Sports Med* 1993;21:407-414.
31. Noyes FR, Barber-Westin SD: Surgical restoration to treat chronic deficiency of the posterolateral complex and cruciate ligaments of the knee joint. *Am J Sports Med* 1996;24:415-426.
32. Noyes FR, Simon R: The role of high tibial osteotomy in the anterior cruciate ligament-deficient knee with varus alignment, in DeLee JC, Drez D Jr (eds): *Orthopaedic Sports Medicine: Principles and Practice*. Philadelphia, PA, WB Saunders, 1994, vol 2, pp 1401-1443.
33. Noyes FR, Barber SD, Simon R: High tibial osteotomy and ligament reconstruction in varus angulated, anterior cruciate ligament-deficient knees: A two-to seven-year follow-up study. *Am J Sports Med* 1993;21:2-12.
34. Noyes FR, Roberts CS: High tibial osteotomy in knees with associated chronic ligament deficiencies, in Jackson DW (ed): *Master Techniques in Orthopaedic Surgery: Reconstructive Knee Surgery*. New York, NY, Raven Press, 1995, pp 185-210.
35. Noyes FR, Schipplein OD, Andriacchi TP, Saddemi SR, Weise M: The anterior cruciate ligament-deficient knee with varus alignment: An analysis of gait adaptations and dynamic joint loadings. *Am J Sports Med* 1992;20: 707-716.
36. Noyes FR, Dunworth LA, Andriacchi TP, Andrews M, Hewett TE: Knee hyperextension

gait abnormalities in unstable knees: Recognition and preoperative gait retraining. *Am J Sports Med* 1996;24:35-45.

37. Rosenberg TD, Paulos LE, Parker RD, Coward DB, Scott SM: The forty-five-degree posteroanterior flexion weight-bearing radiograph of the knee. *J Bone Joint Surg Am* 1988;70: 1479-1483.
38. Johnson DL, Swenson TM, Irrgang JJ, Fu FH, Harner CD: Revision anterior cruciate ligament surgery: Experience from Pittsburgh. *Clin Orthop* 1996;325:100-109.
39. Noyes FR, Barber-Westin SD, Roberts CS: Use of allografts after failed treatment of rupture of the anterior cruciate ligament. *J Bone Joint Surg Am* 1994;76:1019-1031.
40. Noyes FR, Barber-Westin SD: Revision anterior cruciate ligament surgery: Experience from Cincinnati. *Clin Orthop* 1996;325:116-129.
41. Kartus J, Stener S, Lindahl S, Eriksson BI, Karlsson J: Ipsi- or contralateral patellar tendon graft in anterior cruciate ligament revision surgery: A comparison of two methods. *Am J Sports Med* 1998;26:499-504.
42. Uribe JW, Hechtman KS, Zvijac JE, Tjin A, Tsoi EW: Revision anterior cruciate ligament surgery: Experience from Miami. *Clin Orthop* 1996;325:91-99.
43. Wirth CJ, Kohn D: Revision anterior cruciate ligament surgery: Experience from Germany. *Clin Orthop* 1996;325:110-115.
44. Karns DJ, Heidt RS Jr, Holladay BR, Colosimo AJ: Case report: Revision anterior cruciate ligament reconstruction. *Arthroscopy* 1994;10: 148-157.
45. Ritchie JR, Parker RD: Graft selection in anterior cruciate ligament revision surgery. *Clin Orthop* 1996;325:65-77.
46. Seemann MD, Steadman JR: Tibial osteolysis associated with Gore-Tex grafts. *Am J Knee Surg* 1993;6:31-38.
47. Sisto DJ, Cook DL: Abstract: Revision of failed synthetic ACL reconstructions. *Arthroscopy* 1996;12:351.
48. Bylski-Austrow DI, Grood ES, Hefzy MS, Holden JP, Butler DL: Anterior cruciate ligament replacements: A mechanical study of femoral attachment location, flexion angle at tensioning, and initial tension. *J Orthop Res* 1990;8:522-531.
49. Gertel TH, Lew WD, Lewis JL, Stewart NJ, Hunter RE: Effect of anterior cruciate ligament graft tensioning direction, magnitude, and flexion angle on knee biomechanics. *Am J Sports Med* 1993;21:572-581.
50. Grood ES, Hefzy MS, Butler DL, Suntay WJ, Siegel MG, Noyes FR: On the placement and initial tension of anterior cruciate ligament substitutes. *Trans Orthop Res Soc* 1983;8:92.
51. Getelman MH, Schepsis AA, Zimmer J: Abstract: Revision ACL reconstruction: Autograft versus allograft. *Arthroscopy* 1995; 11:378.
52. Johnson DL, Irrgang JJ, Caldwell GL Jr, Harner CD, Fu FH : Primary versus revision ACL reconstruction using fresh frozen allograft tissue: A clinical outcome analysis. *Orthop Trans* 1995;19:13.
53. Barber-Westin SD, Noyes FR, McCloskey JW: Rigorous statistical reliability, validity, and responsiveness testing of the Cincinnati Knee Rating System in 350 subjects with uninjured, injured, or anterior cruciate ligament-reconstructed knees. *Am J Sports Med* 1999;27: 402-416.
54. Noyes FR, Barber SD: The effect of an extra-articular procedure on allograft reconstructions for chronic ruptures of the anterior cruciate ligament. *J Bone Joint Surg Am* 1991;73:882-892.
55. Defrere J, Franckart A: Freeze-dried fascia lata allografts in the reconstruction of anterior cruciate ligament defects: A two- to seven-year follow-up study. *Clin Orthop* 1994;303:56-66.
56. Indelicato PA, Bittar ES, Prevot TJ, Woods GA, Branch TP, Huegel M: Clinical comparison of freeze-dried and fresh frozen patellar tendon allografts for anterior cruciate ligament reconstruction of the knee. *Am J Sports Med* 1990;18:335-342.
57. Jackson DW, Grood ES, Arnoczky SP, Butler DL, Simon TM: Freeze dried anterior cruciate ligament allografts: Preliminary studies in a goat model. *Am J Sports Med* 1987;15:295-303.
58. Cross MJ, Purnell MB: Revision reconstruction of the anterior cruciate ligament. *Orthop Trans* 1993;17:931-932.
59. Rubinstein RA, Shelbourne KD, McCarroll JR, Rettig AC, VanMeter CD: The results of a second autogenous bone-patellar tendon-bone anterior cruciate ligament reconstruction after failure of the first reconstruction. *Orthop Trans* 1994;18:742-743.
60. Day B: Abstract: Revision anterior cruciate ligament (ACL) reconstruction after failed bone patella tendon bone reconstruction (BPTB). *Arthroscopy* 1996;12:381-382.
61. Noyes FR, Barber-Westin SD, Hewett TE: High tibial osteotomy and ligament reconstruction for varus angulated anterior cruciate ligament-deficient knees. *Am J Sports Med* 2000;28:282-296.
62. Noyes FR, Barber-Westin SD: Surgical reconstruction of severe chronic posterolateral complex injuries of the knee using allograft tissues. *Am J Sports Med* 1995;23:2-12.
63. Noyes FR, Barber-Westin SD: Treatment of complex injuries involving the posterior cruciate and posterolateral ligaments of the knee. *Am J Knee Surg* 1996;9:200-214.
64. Nixon RG, SeGall GK, Sax SL, Cain TE, Tullos HS: Reconstitution of the patellar tendon donor site after graft harvest. *Clin Orthop* 1995;317:162-171.
65. Benedetto KP, Sperner G, Gloetzer W, Fritschy D, Gautard R: Abstract: Ultrasonographic followup of patellar tendon following graft dissection for ACL-replacement. *Am J Sports Med* 1989;17:709.
66. Coupens SD, Yates CK, Sheldon C, Ward C: Magnetic resonance imaging evaluation of the patellar tendon after use of its central one-third for anterior cruciate ligament reconstruction. *Am J Sports Med* 1992;20:332-335.
67. Liu SH, Hang DW, Gentili A, Finerman GA: MRI and morphology of the insertion of the patellar tendon after graft harvesting. *J Bone Joint Surg Br* 1996;78:823-826.
68. Bernicker JP, Haddad JL, Lintner DM, DiLiberti TC, Bocell JR: Patellar tendon defect during the first year after anterior cruciate ligament reconstruction: Appearance on serial magnetic resonance imaging. *Arthroscopy* 1998;14:804-809.
69. McLaughlin JR, Noyes FR: Arthroscopic meniscus repair: Recommended surgical techniques for complex meniscal tears. *Tech Orthop* 1993;8:129-136.
70. Rubman MH, Noyes FR, Barber-Westin SD: Arthroscopic repair of meniscal tears that extend into the avascular zone: A review of 198 single and complex tears. *Am J Sports Med* 1998;26:87-95.

Reference to Video

Noyes FR: *Revision ACL Reconstruction: Graft Harvest and Preparation (Knee).* Cincinnati, OH, 2000.

47

Evaluation and Treatment of Recurrent Instability After Anterior Cruciate Ligament Reconstruction

Christopher D. Harner, MD
J. Robert Giffin, MD, FRCSC
Roger C. Dunteman, MD
Christopher C. Annunziata, MD
Marc J. Friedman, MD

The annual incidence of anterior cruciate ligament (ACL) injuries in the United States has been estimated to be 1 in 3,000 Americans.[1] Reconstruction is now widely accepted as the treatment of choice for the patient with a functionally unstable ACL deficient knee. By current estimates, more than 100,000 ACL reconstructions are performed annually in the United States.[2] The long-term rates of good and excellent results, in terms of functional stability, relief of symptoms, and return to preinjury level of activity, have been reported to be between 75% and 90%.[3-9] This, however, leaves a substantial group of patients who have an unsatisfactory result from the procedure because of a number of different causes. This chapter will discuss the potential mechanisms of failure of primary intra-articular ACL reconstruction and will provide the treating orthopaedist with a systematic approach for the evaluation of these difficult cases.

Etiology of Failed ACL Reconstruction

Many factors influence the overall success or failure of ACL reconstruction, including the integrity of the secondary restraints, the preoperative laxity of the knee, the status of the articular and meniscal cartilage, the selection of the graft material, the surgical technique, the postoperative rehabilitation, and the motivation and expectations of the patient.[10] Failure may be due to one or more factors, and it may be associated with both graft and non-graft-related conditions. However, there is no universally accepted definition of what qualifies as an unsatisfactory outcome following ACL surgery.[11,12] In addition, there is often a low correlation between the physician's evaluation and the patient's perception of knee stability and function.[4]

Classification of Failure

Failure of an ACL reconstruction can be due to a broad spectrum of potential etiologies ranging from general sources to intra-articular graft failure (Fig. 1). Physicians at the University of Pittsburgh developed a classification system for intra-articular graft failure. Even though failure is based on multiple factors and it is difficult to assign a single causal mechanism, the classification represents an attempt to better identify the cause of failure and to improve the outcomes of revision surgery. It also represents an attempt to be more specific in guiding the surgical management of these complex problems. In all cases, a primary cause is assigned and, when possible, a secondary cause is assigned as well (Fig. 2). The cause can usually be classified into one of the following categories: loss of motion or arthrofibrosis,[13-16] arthritis or recurrent pain,[17,18] extensor mechanism dysfunction,[19-22] or recurrent instability.[4-7] It has been estimated that 0.7% to 8.0% of recurrent instability following primary ACL reconstruction is caused by graft failure.[4-6] In these patients, revision ACL surgery should be considered, as it may be helpful in alleviating symptoms of instability and may improve the functional result.

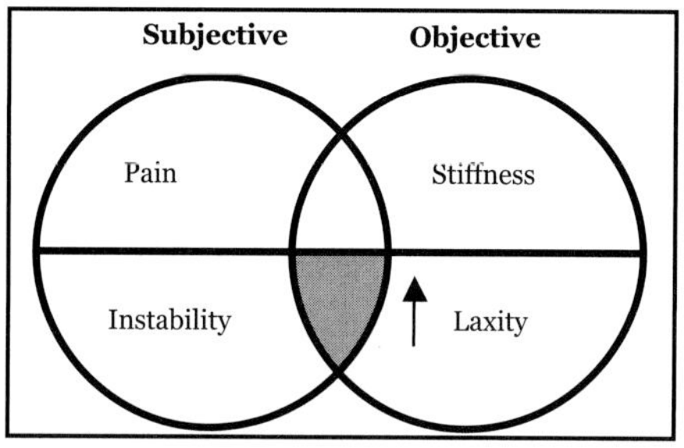

Fig. 1 Illustration showing that failure of ACL reconstruction is due to a broad spectrum of potential causes ranging from subjective patient complaints to objective clinical findings. Intra-articular graft failure (shaded area) commonly results in both recurrent functional instability and increased laxity. (Adapted with permission from Harner CD: Editorial comment. *Clin Orthop* 1996;325:3.)

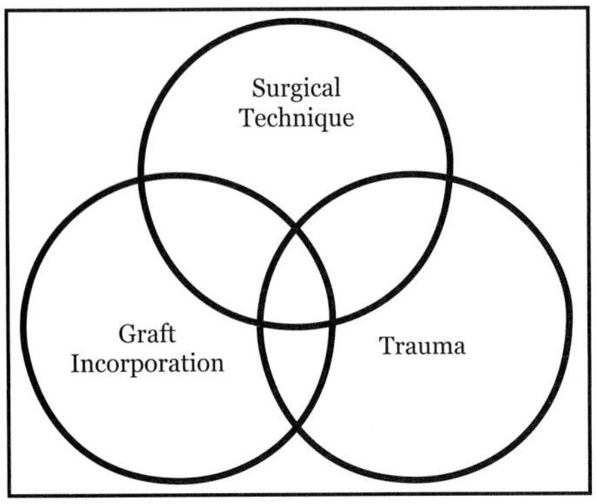

Fig. 2 Illustration showing that the causes of graft failure include surgical error, failure of graft incorporation, and trauma, either alone or in conjunction with one another. (Adapted with permission from Maday MG, Harner CD, Fu FH: Revision ACL surgery: Evaluation and treatment, in Feagin JA Jr (ed): *The Crucial Ligaments: Diagnosis and Treatment of Ligamentous Injuries About the Knee,* ed 2. New York, NY, Churchill Livingstone, 1994, p 712.)

Table 1
Nonanatomic position of bone tunnels causing increased graft tension and subsequent failure

Tunnel Position	Cause of Graft Failure
Femoral	
Anterior	Excessive strain (lengthening) in flexion/laxity in extension
Posterior	Excessive strain in extension/laxity in flexion
Tibial	
Anterior	Excessive strain in flexion/roof impingement in extension
Posterior	Excessive strain in extension/posterior cruciate ligament impingement
Medial/lateral	Impingement on ipsilateral femoral condyle

Often, the cause of failure can be determined by excluding certain factors as well as by noting the time to failure after surgery. Early failure occurs within the first 6 months and is often the result of poor surgical technique, failure of graft incorporation, or possibly excessively aggressive rehabilitation. For example, if the patient complains of persistent functional instability in the early postoperative period and an inappropriate position of the femoral tunnel is seen on radiographs, surgical technique would be assigned as the primary cause of failure. Poor graft incorporation, if found, would be the secondary cause. If review of the surgical records and the radiographs verify that the procedure was technically successful, then the most likely primary cause of failure would be inadequate graft incorporation.

Failure occurring late (more than 1 year after surgery) is most commonly due to trauma. In these cases, technical failure and failure of graft incorporation are ruled out if the knee was functionally stable (with intact secondary restraints) on prior examination and if there is no radiographic evidence of surgical error. The cause of failure could be a major single reinjury (a contact or noncontact mechanism), or it could be repetitive traumatic events (for example, aggressive rehabilitation).

Successful revision surgery requires a methodical and organized approach to identify the potential source (or sources) of failure. A thorough preoperative evaluation, including a detailed history, physical examination, and radiographic evaluation, is of paramount importance before surgery is planned, in order to avoid a repetition of errors.

Failure Caused by Surgical Technique

Technical Errors

Errors in surgical technique are the most common cause of graft failure in patients presenting with recurrent instability after ACL reconstruction.[11,22-28] Technical shortcomings resulting in graft failure after primary reconstruction include nonanatomic tunnel placement, graft impingement, improper tensioning of the graft, and inadequate fixation of the graft in the osseous tunnels.

Tunnel Placement

The consequences of nonanatomic tunnel placement have been described in the literature.[29-36] Inappropriate positioning of either the tibial or the femoral tunnel results in excessive changes in graft length as the knee moves through a range of motion (Table 1). Because biologic ACL grafts can accommodate only small changes in length before undergoing plastic deformation, a malpositioned graft results in either capturing of the knee with subsequent loss of motion or lengthening of the graft over time with subsequent recurrent instability.

In order to achieve stability and to retain a full range of motion, near-anatomic placement of the tunnels is important. Anterior placement of the femoral tunnel is the most common surgical error when a one-incision endoscopic technique is used[10-12,26] (Fig. 3). Improper femoral tunnel placement is most often caused by a failure to visualize the most posterior aspect of the notch adequately. Because the femoral attachment of the ACL is closer to the center of rotation of the knee, small errors in femoral tunnel placement can have deleterious effects on knee kinematics. Ideal femoral tunnel placement is as posterior in the notch as possible without violation of the posterior cortical wall.

Tibial tunnel placement, originally thought to be a less important factor in the outcome of ACL reconstruction, is now known to have a profound effect on the postoperative result.[31-34] Early techniques stressed a relatively anteromedial position, whereas current techniques emphasize a posterior placement of the tibial tunnel, with the ideal position being in the posteromedial portion of the ACL footprint. The tunnel is parallel and posterior to Blumensaat's line when the knee is in full extension[31-34] (Fig. 4). The more posterior position of the tibial tunnel eliminates graft impingement. In patients with major recurvatum or a vertical intercondylar roof, either the tibial tunnel must be placed in a more posterior position or some bone must be removed from the roof of the notch in order to avoid graft impingement with the knee in extension.[2,31] **(CD-47.1)**

Graft Impingement

Graft impingement may be avoided by properly positioning the tunnels and ensuring that an adequate notchplasty has been created.[37-39] Failure to assess the notch architecture for stenosis or intercondylar osteophytes can lead to impingement and secondary graft failure from repetitive trauma and ligament attrition.[33] Notch impingement can also compromise the biologic incorporation of the graft.[40] In addition to a loss of extension, a "cyclops" lesion[41] may form if there is substantial graft impingement. Plain radiographs, CT, or MRI can be helpful in the preoperative assessment of the notch architecture and the subsequent need for a notchplasty. Notchplasty is not without risk, and there has been a recent trend toward decreasing the amount of bone removed during this procedure in order to avoid distorting the anatomic position of the femoral tunnel, which can produce incongruence at the patellofemoral and tibiofemoral articulations.[42]

Graft Tensioning

Improper tensioning of the graft is a potential cause of graft failure. The optimal intraoperative tension remains unknown.[43,44] Factors that affect graft tension include the graft material and length, the tunnel placement, the physiologic joint laxity, the method of graft fixation, and the knee flexion angle at the time of fixation. Of these variables, the knee flexion angle at the time of fixation and graft placement appear to be the most critical.[44] Overzealous tensioning has been associated with decreased motion, delayed vascularization, myxoid degeneration, and resultant graft failure.[45,46] Furthermore, overconstraining the joint may lead to increased joint contact pressures and osteoarthritis.[47] Inadequate tensioning, on the other hand, may lead to persistent instability and a nonfunctioning graft.

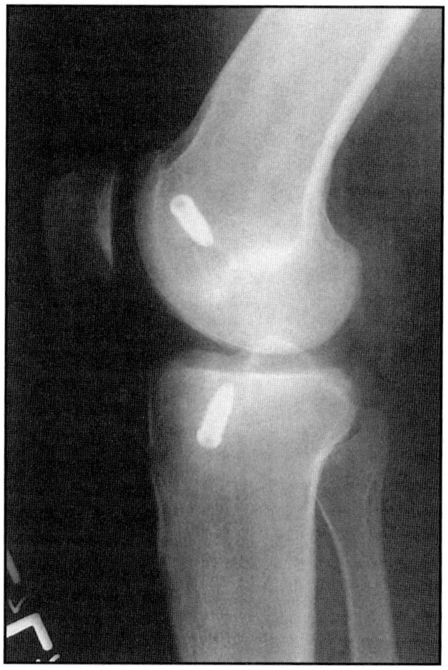

Fig. 3 Lateral radiograph showing anterior placement of the femoral tunnel resulting in graft lengthening and subsequent failure.

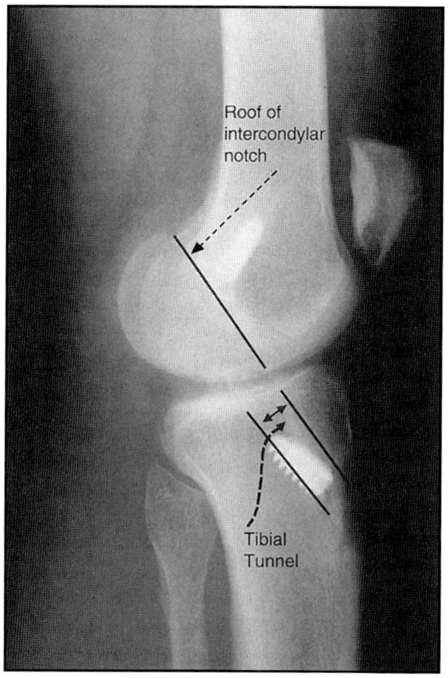

Fig. 4 Lateral radiograph, made with the knee in full extension, demonstrating ideal placement of the tibial tunnel inclined posterior to Blumensaat's line (the line indicating the roof of the intercondylar notch) to avoid graft impingement. The double arrow indicates the width of the tunnel.

Graft Fixation

The stability of the initial graft fixation is critical to the success of ACL reconstruction. The fixation must be secure enough to prevent changes in graft position before healing occurs in the tunnels.[48,49] Advanced rehabilitation protocols require stable fixation that permits immediate knee motion without compromising graft position or tension. Fixation strength depends on the type of graft, the type of fixation device, and the bone quality at the fixation sites.[48] Regardless of the type of graft and the method of fixation, proper surgical technique is critical to avoid pitfalls during insertion of the fixation device.

Graft Material

The structural and material properties of the graft that is selected play a role in the possible failure of the newly reconstructed ACL. Carelessness during graft harvest and preparation may damage the graft substance, thereby affecting its structural and material properties. Although a bone-patellar tendon-bone autograft remains the graft of choice for many surgeons, the doubled semitendinosus and gracilis tendons have recently gained popularity.

The use of allograft material in primary ACL reconstruction has increased in recent years. Basic science and clinical research has provided a greater understanding of the effects of sterilization on the mechanical properties of the graft, its rate of incorporation, and the possibility of an immunologic response.[50-57] The biologic behavior of the different autografts and allografts during incorporation must be understood in order to individualize the rehabilitation program.

The use of synthetic ligaments is not currently recommended for primary or revision ACL reconstruction because of the high complication and failure rates associated with their use.[58,59] The high prevalence of breakage over time, along with reports of effusion, synovitis, and osteolysis, make synthetic grafts undesirable. The value of ligament augmentation devices in improving clinical outcomes has not been proven conclusively, and concerns have been raised regarding the stress-shielding effect of synthetic devices on biologic grafts and their role in delaying graft incorporation.[51,60,61]

Secondary Stabilizers

A surgeon's failure to recognize and treat a combined instability pattern that involves damaged secondary restraints (that is, the medial collateral ligament [MCL], the posterior horn of the medial meniscus, and the posterior aspect of the capsule) to anterior tibial translation may result in the eventual failure of the reconstructed graft. Missed ligamentous and capsular injuries, resulting in combined rotatory instability patterns, place increased loads on the ACL graft.[62] Partial or complete meniscectomy of an irreparable meniscal tear alters the knee-joint kinematics and leads to increased forces on the graft. These forces may have a detrimental effect on graft incorporation and may increase the likelihood of eventual graft failure.

The knee must be carefully examined preoperatively to assess the integrity of the secondary restraints. These findings are confirmed by reexamining the patient while he or she is under anesthesia before proceeding with revision surgery. Close attention must be paid to varus and valgus motion and rotational laxity that are excessive compared with those in the contralateral extremity. Previous surgical reports, imaging studies, and arthroscopic examination are helpful in determining the status of the menisci and the articular cartilage and their possible role in graft failure.

Unrecognized or untreated laxity of the MCL or the posterior oblique ligament, or both, may play a role in the failure of the primary reconstruction. At the time of the revision surgery, it may be necessary to reef these lax tissues and occasionally to perform an advancement of the MCL. If substantial anteromedial rotatory instability is present in the setting of a previous medial meniscectomy, concomitant medial meniscal transplantation should be considered. Meniscal reconstruction with allograft tissue helps to restore the "break-stop" mechanism of the posterior horn of the medial meniscus.

Posterolateral instability is probably the most commonly unrecognized and untreated associated laxity pattern. Surgical options include primary repair, advancement or recession, and augmentation or reconstruction of the popliteus tendon and the popliteofibular and lateral collateral ligaments. If the patient has varus knee alignment and a lateral thrust during the stance phase of gait, a valgus proximal tibial osteotomy should be done to correct the alignment. Persistent lateral thrust after an ACL reconstruction will lead to failure because of chronic repetitive stretching.[63] A medial opening or lateral closing-wedge osteotomy may be performed as a staged procedure or in combination with the reconstruction.

Failure of Graft Incorporation

Failure of incorporation of the ACL graft into the host tissue may be a cause of recurrent instability. The causes of graft failure, which have been studied extensively in a variety of animal models, include inadequate vascularity, immunologic reaction, and stress-shielding associated with use of an augmentation device.[51,54,61,64-67]

Biologic failure should be suspected in patients presenting with recurrent instability without a history of trauma or an identifiable technical error.[12] The process of successful incorporation of both autografts and allografts includes graft necrosis, revascularization, cellular repopulation, collagen deposition, and matrix remodeling.[40,64] This ligamentization process is influenced by the graft source, the host response, and the biomechanical loads affecting the graft during rehabilitation. Furthermore, the rate of incorporation has been shown to depend on both the type of graft material and the method of fixation. This universal biologic healing response should be respected in the design of the early rehabilitation program and in the decision as to when the patient can return to normal activities.

Failure Caused by Trauma

Graft failure due to trauma occurs infrequently and takes one of two forms: early failure secondary to trauma before complete graft incorporation and completion of rehabilitation, and late failure occurring after resumption of full activity. Overaggressive rehabilitation or a premature return to athletics before adequate graft incorporation and return of neuromuscular control of the lower extremity may play a role in early failure. During the first year after reconstruction, the graft strength and stiffness are 30% to 50% of normal and excessive loads can lead to plastic deformation and elongation.[65,66]

As accelerated rehabilitation protocols have gained wider acceptance because of the belief that they improve the functional result and decrease the prevalence of postoperative stiffness associated with ACL reconstruction, the risk of injury to a partially revascularized graft has increased. Furthermore, it is important that the surgeon understand the limitations and parameters of the initial graft fixation and the time course of biologic incorporation. Poorly fixed grafts that require more than 8 to 12 weeks to incorporate do not tolerate early aggressive rehabilitation.

Patients may sustain major trauma to the knee after the graft has matured. Usually these reinjuries occur more than 6 months (late) after the patient has returned to full activity. The prevalence of traumatic reinjury has been reported to be approximately 5% to 10% in the athletic population.[10] These patients present with a new hemarthrosis following an injury and have increased laxity compared with that seen on the previous postoperative examination. In the absence of an identifiable cause of graft failure, it is assumed that the graft had incorporated and was functioning at the time of the new injury.

Preoperative Evaluation of Failed ACL Reconstruction

A comprehensive preoperative evaluation must be performed for all patients being considered for revision ACL surgery. A detailed history, physical examination, and radiographic assessment are essential to determine the etiology of failure, to classify its primary and secondary causes, and to decide whether the patient is an appropriate candidate for revision surgery.

Patients presenting with pathologic anterior laxity on clinical examination that reproduces their symptoms of instability during activities of daily living or athletic activities should be considered candidates for revision surgery. The goals of the surgery are to stabilize the knee, to prevent further injury to the articular cartilage and menisci, and to maximize function. The surgeon must take the time to evaluate the patient as an individual and must be alert to the potential "knee abuser," who will undoubtedly have failure of the revision surgery as well.

The patient must be given realistic goals with regard to the expected outcome and must understand that motivation and compliance are critical to success. These cases are technically demanding and complex, so care must be taken when discussing the long-term prognosis. It has proven difficult (if not impossible) to achieve results similar to those of primary ACL reconstruction; therefore, results should not be compared between the two procedures.[24,56] False expectations on the part of the patient will certainly lead to subjective failure despite an otherwise technically successful procedure.

History

A detailed history should include the chief presenting symptom or symptoms and should elicit the sequence of events that transpired from the time of the initial injury. It is important to determine the nature of the original injury, the preoperative symptoms, the timing of the surgery, the postoperative rehabilitation, the ability to return to preinjury activity, any history of major reinjury, and the time at which the patient realized that he or she was no longer improving. Review of the previous records, including the surgical note, is helpful in determining the extent of the primary surgery. Information about the type of graft used, the status of the menisci, the condition of the articular surfaces, and associated ligamentous injuries at the time of the original procedure can serve as a guide in planning the revision surgery and in making the prognosis.

Pain must be clearly differentiated from instability. The patient who has pain with activities of daily living is different from the patient who has recurrent instability while participating in vigorous sports activity. Potential causes of increasing pain include instability and possibly early arthrosis from a previous meniscectomy or osteochondral injury. If the revision surgery is to be successful, the pain arising from these causes must be addressed separately or simultaneously.[5]

Infection should be considered as a potential cause of pain. Although this is an uncommon complication of ACL reconstruction, the patient must be asked whether there has been purulent drainage, cellulitis, fever, or chills at any time since the original operation. This is especially important if the failed primary reconstruction had been performed with a prosthetic graft.

Physical Examination

A comprehensive physical examination of the patient, including the entire lower extremity, must be performed. The examination usually begins with an observation of gait and lower extremity alignment while the patient is standing. The presence of a lateral thrust during stance phase and/or varus alignment is important to recognize because each can be a source of graft failure due to excessive strain on the reconstructed ACL. In these cases, a valgus high tibial osteotomy should be performed before or in conjunction with the revision ACL surgery.

The presence and extent of an effusion (acute or chronic) are important, as effusion may indicate a variety of abnormalities ranging from recurrent trauma to intra-articular pathology. The range of motion of the knee is carefully assessed to determine whether there is any residual loss due to the original injury and the surgery or whether acute changes from recurrent trauma have led to reduced motion. Differences in heel height and heel-to-buttock distance are useful in measuring loss of extension and flexion.[2,21] Decreased range of motion, extensor mechanism dysfunction, and/or the presence of a bent-knee gait pattern must be addressed before the revision surgery is done. In most cases, a staged surgical procedure should be done; the intent of the initial surgical intervention should be to decrease the loss of motion, and the revision should be performed after an adequate range of motion has been obtained.

The status of the primary ACL reconstruction is evaluated with use of

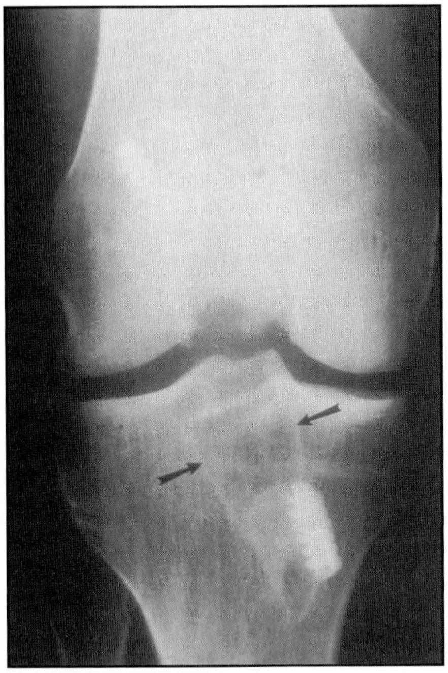

Fig. 5 AP radiograph of a tibial tunnel enlargement (arrows) 6 months after ACL reconstruction with use of a 10-mm-wide bone–patellar tendon–bone autograft.

the Lachman, pivot-shift, and anterior drawer tests. Other provocative tests should also be performed to assess the integrity of the secondary restraints. Particular attention must be paid to excessive varus and valgus motion and rotational laxity. Failure to identify and treat associated ligamentous laxity and combined instability patterns will result in recurrent surgical failure.

Radiographic Evaluation

Radiographic evaluation should include anteroposterior (AP), lateral, 45° posteroanterior (PA) flexion weight bearing, and Merchant views. The AP and lateral radiographs are used to assess the position and size of the femoral and tibial tunnels as well as the type of material used for graft fixation. Assessment of the size of the tunnels is critical in formulating a surgical plan. Expansion of the bone tunnels, seen radiographically, has been well described following ACL reconstruction with use of both autografts (Fig. 5) and allografts.[68-71] Despite appropriate positioning of the tunnels, bone-grafting may be required.

A standing lateral radiograph with the knee in full extension should be made to look for graft impingement. The 45° PA flexion radiograph provides a view of the femoral condylar notch, allowing assessment of its architecture and the degree of articular cartilage narrowing and other associated degenerative changes. A standing long-cassette radiograph should be made to determine the mechanical axis of the lower extremity.

Other imaging modalities that may be used include bone scintigraphy,[72] for the evaluation of potential early degenerative changes; CT, for the definition of bone defects; and MRI. In selected cases, MRI can be helpful in evaluating graft integrity as well as in determining the presence of any associated meniscal, ligamentous, or chondral pathology.

Treatment of Failed ACL Reconstruction

Preoperative Planning

Preoperative discussions should alert the patient to the possible need for a staged procedure if there is major bone-tunnel expansion or arthrofibrosis. If osteolysis or cystic expansion has occurred at the tunnel sites, consideration must be given to removal of hardware and to bone-grafting of lesions, with later revision surgery to occur at 6 to 12 weeks after incorporation of the graft. In selected cases of cystic widening, nonanatomic femoral tunnel placement, or difficult hardware removal, it has been our preference to use the over-the-top position for the reconstructed ACL. An extension loss of more than 5° or a flexion loss of more than 20° should be addressed separately in a staged fashion in an attempt to regain motion before ACL revision is considered.

Skin incisions around the knee should be carefully planned to avoid skin compromise and infection. Surgical technique and handling of the soft tissues must be meticulous to avoid complications in the revision setting. Previous skin incisions should be used or extended if they allow for hardware removal, graft harvesting, and proper placement and fixation of the new graft. Skin bridges of less than 7 cm in width should be avoided.

Graft Selection

The surgeon has numerous options when selecting a graft for revision ACL surgery. Currently, autograft and allograft are the tissues of choice. In the past, synthetic grafts have been used; however, unacceptably high complication and failure rates led to their abandonment in both primary and revision ACL reconstruction.[58,59,73] Many factors must be taken into consideration when a graft is chosen for revision surgery. These include the graft source used in the primary surgery, the incisions used for harvesting the previous graft, the bone-tunnel size (enlargement), and associated ligamentous laxity.[2]

If the surgeon elects to use autogenous tissue, many sources are available, including patellar tendon (contralateral or ipsilateral), hamstring tendon, and quadriceps tendon. Use of autogenous grafts eliminates the potential of disease transmission or immunologic reaction associated with allografts while allowing faster incorporation. However, they pose potential problems. Donor site morbidity and lack of availability are major concerns.

Ipsilateral patellar tendon is often the preferred graft when it is available;[74,75] however, due to its popularity as a graft source during primary ACL reconstruction, it is often not available. This preference for patellar tendon autograft leads to reharvesting of the ipsilateral patellar tendon.[76] An MRI study supported reharvesting of this tendon by demonstrating high signal intensity consistent with edema and scar in the early postoperative period with a subsequent decrease in signal intensity at progressive follow-up intervals.[77] At 18 months, the donor site appeared normal. The authors of that study believed that these findings showed the ability of the patellar tendon to remodel and regenerate.[77] More recently, however, two animal studies demonstrated inferior biomechanical properties of these tendons after harvest. Using a canine model, LaPrade and associates[78] found a substantially lower load to failure in the reharvested patellar tendon compared with that in the contralateral tendon at 1 year postoperatively. Proctor and associates,[79] in a goat model, demonstrated histologic characteristics consistent with reparative scar rather than ligament. Biomechanical testing at 21 months revealed that the tensile strength was inferior to that of the contralateral tendon.[79] These results led the authors of both studies to recommend the use of other graft sources. A recent clinical study by Kartus and associates[80] also argues against the use of reharvested patellar tendon. In that study, 20 patients who had revision ACL surgery were divided into two groups of 10 each. One group had revision surgery with use of reharvested patellar tendon as the graft, and the other group had revision with use of graft harvested from the contralateral patellar tendon. The Lysholm score, International Knee Documentation Committee (IKDC) rating, and Tegner activity score all were lower in the group treated with reharvested patellar tendon. There were also two major complications in that group: a patellar tendon rupture and a patellar fracture. Consequently, Kartus and associates[80] did not recommend use of the ipsilateral patellar tendon for revision ACL reconstruction.

The role of harvest of the contralateral patellar tendon has also been examined. Rubinstein and associates[81] found no major complications in 26 patients in whom a graft from the contralateral patellar tendon was used for primary ACL reconstruction. All patients regained a full range of motion at 3 weeks, and quadriceps strength returned to 93% at 1 year. Even though no patient complained of patellofemoral pain, half experienced patellar tendinitis; most of these cases resolved during the first year. The authors of this study recommended the contralateral patellar tendon as an acceptable graft choice, believing that patellar tendinitis at the donor site resolves quickly, with no long-term effects. However, the possibility of extensor mechanism disruption and patellar fracture in overzealous patients during the postoperative period has been noted as a potential complication.[82] Consideration should be given to use of a graft source other than patellar tendon autograft in the presence of substantial degenerative changes at the patellofemoral joint.

The remaining sources of autogenous tissue are the hamstring and quadriceps tendons. Quadrupled hamstring tendons offer the advantage of being readily available, with decreased donor-site morbidity; however, their size can be a disadvantage in the revision setting.[83] Because hamstring grafts are generally several millimeters smaller in diameter than patellar tendon grafts, which typically have a diameter of 10 mm, their use in revision of a primary reconstruction that had been performed with patellar tendon is limited. In the presence of femoral tunnel enlargement, bone defects, or prior reconstruction with patellar tendon, the hamstring tendons' small size and the lack of a bone block often provide an inadequate fill of the tunne.[12] Bone graft can be used in the enlarged tunnel, and a two-stage procedure can be performed. On the other hand, if new tunnels or an over-the-top position can be used, hamstring tendons make excellent grafts. Another source of autogenous tissue is the quadriceps tendon, which provides both a large cross-sectional area and a single bone block. This graft is helpful when dealing with enlarged tunnels.

The allograft tissue most commonly used in primary and revision ACL reconstruction is the Achilles tendon or the patellar tendon. When an allograft is used, there is no donor-site morbidity, the incisions are smaller, the surgical time is shorter, and there are no size limitations. Disadvantages include longer incorporation time, the possibility of an immunologic reaction, the risk of disease transmission, and higher cost. Jackson and associates[53] demonstrated, in a goat model, slower biologic incorporation of patellar tendon allograft compared with patellar tendon autograft. Even though there have been no reported cases of viral transmission from frozen allogeneic connective tissues when current American Association of Tissue Banks guidelines have been used, infection is still a concern.[50] Attempts to eradicate viruses from tissue with use of radiation have been made, but the dose required to kill a virus (more than 3 Mrad [30,000 gray]) weakens the strength of the allograft tissue by altering its collagen structure.[84] In an attempt to avoid many of these complications, the current techniques used to sterilize grafts include aseptic harvest, multiple antibiotic soaks, multiple cultures, and low-dose irradiation (less than 3 Mrad).[85] Despite these problems, allograft tissue is commonly used in both primary and revision ACL reconstruction. In the revision setting, where larger tunnel diameters are often encountered, the larger size of the allograft bone blocks is extremely useful.

Several studies comparing allograft with autograft for revision ACL reconstruction demonstrated no significant difference between the two groups from either a functional or an objective standpoint.[25,86,87] Uribe and associates[25] reported greater objective stability with autograft than with allograft tissue, with average KT-1000 arthrometer (Medmetric, San Diego, CA) scores of 2.2

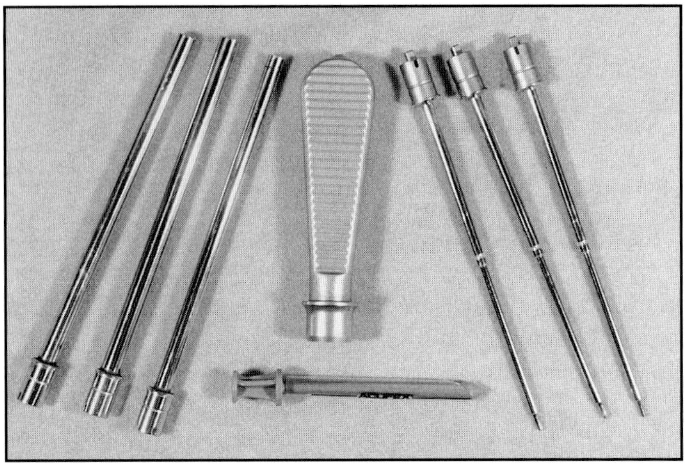

Fig. 6 Photograph showing coring reamers, clear plastic sheaths, and a revision screwdriver set. These instruments are extremely useful during revision surgery.

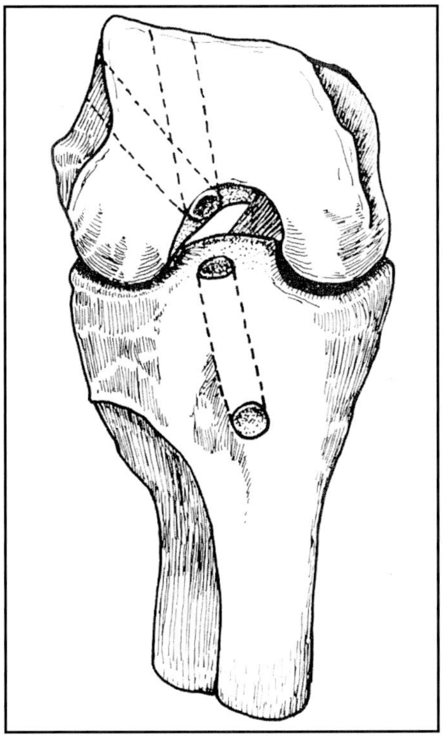

Fig. 7 Drawing showing the tunnel from a two-incision technique entering the femur at a more acute angle than the tunnel from a one-incision technique. This is very useful during revision surgery, especially when posterior cortical wall blowout is encountered.

and 3.3 points, respectively, but these results, as well as the Tegner and Lysholm scores, were not significantly different. Noyes and Barber-Westin[86] found less than 3 mm of displacement on KT-2000 arthrometer testing in 30 of 57 patients in the allograft group and in 12 of 18 in the autograft group. When failures during the first postoperative year were included, 32 of 75 patients in the allograft group and 13 of 22 in the autograft group had a functional reconstruction at an average of 27 months. However, the difference between the groups with regard to the objective and functional results was not significant.

Because each revision ACL reconstruction presents a unique problem, graft selection must be individualized. When the appropriate graft is selected, the surgeon should be able to restore stability to the knee. Because autografts and allografts yield similar results, the potential advantages and disadvantages of each must be considered. The final decision is between the patient and the physician.

Femoral Tunnel

Instruments designed specifically for ACL revision are helpful and should be obtained preoperatively. These instruments include coring reamers and 10-mm plastic sheaths for screw removal (Fig. 6).

As mentioned previously, the surgical error encountered most commonly during ACL reconstruction is anterior positioning of the femoral tunnel[2] (Fig. 3). The surgeon has many options when revising the femoral tunnel. The simplest scenario is when the tunnel has been properly placed. In this case, simply redrilling the previous tunnel is adequate, and hardware can be retained if it does not interfere with proper tunnel placement. The surgeon must be aware of the difficulty with extraction of the screw as well as the large osseous defect created next to the revised tunnel if hardware (that is, the interference screw) is removed. In order to avoid any compromise of the fixation, the screw can be retained and a portion of it can actually be drilled without any adverse effects.[88] The threads can be smoothed with the drill to eliminate graft abrasion, and a soft-tissue graft can be passed into the tunnel and secured on the posterior cortex. If the previous tunnel is more than one tunnel diameter anterior to the anatomic site, a new tunnel can simply be drilled posterior to it. However, if the tunnel is only slightly anterior, possible overlap of the two tunnels can be a problem because of the enlarged tunnel diameter. One choice is to use a smaller graft such as a hamstring tendon graft, as its typical diameter of 7 to 9 mm may allow posterior placement of the graft without tunnel overlap. The hamstring tendon graft can be fixed on the lateral femoral condyle with either an Endobutton (Smith & Nephew, Mansfield, MA) or a two-incision technique, thereby allowing the surgeon to drill the tunnel posteriorly and to effectively eliminate the difficulties encountered with posterior cortical-wall blowout[59] (Fig. 7). Another option is to enlarge the slightly anterior tunnel and to use an allograft with a large bone block. Conversely, when the femoral tunnel is too posterior and there is posterior cortical-wall blowout, a two-incision, over-the-top, or Endobutton technique permits stable fixation on the lateral femoral condyle.

An enlarged femoral tunnel is often encountered during revision of an allograft or synthetic ligament reconstruction.[58,89] The extent of tunnel enlargement can be evaluated on a preoperative radiograph (Fig. 8) or MRI. If the tunnel is more than 15 mm wide, a staged reconstruction with bone-grafting should be considered. An over-the-top technique has also been shown to yield results comparable with those of the standard technique of drilling a femoral tunnel.[90] Other technical options include use of stacked interference screws or a large bone-block allograft to fill the defect. This large bone-block allograft can be rotated either anteriorly or posteriorly, thereby filling the defect and allowing proper positioning of the allograft. Finally, bone-grafting of the enlarged tunnel and an ACL reconstruction can be performed simultaneously or the reconstruction can be done following incorporation of the bone graft.

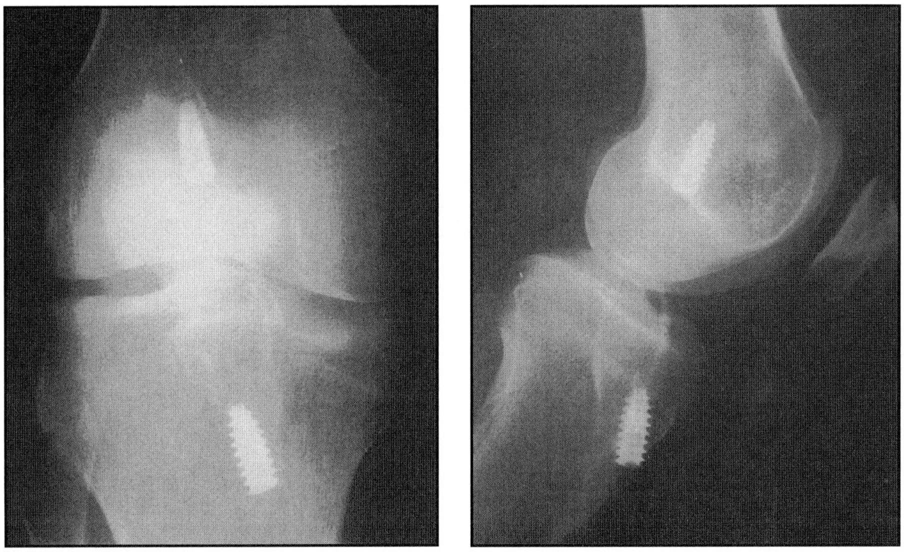

Fig. 8 AP and lateral radiographs of an ACL reconstruction with use of patellar tendon autograft, demonstrating substantial expansion (more than 15 mm) of both the tibial and the femoral tunnel. A staged procedure consisting of bone grafting followed by ACL reconstruction with a hamstring tendon graft was used for revision.

Tibial Tunnel

Even though technical error associated with femoral tunnel placement is a more common reason for failure of ACL reconstruction, correct positioning of the tibial tunnel is also important for a successful outcome. Many of the same techniques used for revising the femoral tunnel apply to the tibial tunnel. However, locating the tibial interference screw can be more difficult. Two techniques are extremely useful for locating the tibial screw: an arthroscope can be inserted up the tibial tunnel to visualize the screw directly, or a radiograph can be used to find the screw and to place a guide-wire into the cannulated screw-hole.

Predictable situations commonly arise when an attempt is made to correct a malpositioned tibial tunnel. If the existing tunnel and hardware are more than one tunnel diameter anterior to the correct position, they can be ignored and a new tunnel can be drilled in a more posterior location. If the tunnel is less than one tunnel diameter anterior to its correct location (slightly anterior), then options similar to those used for the femoral tunnel can be applied. Coring reamers can be used, and the core of bone from the tibia can be placed in the anterior defect, or the tunnel can be expanded and the large bone block from an allograft can be inserted. If the defect is extremely large, bone grafting of the enlarged tunnel with autogenous iliac crest, followed by either simultaneous or delayed ACL reconstruction, can be performed. Brown and Carson[2] described another technique, consisting of identification of the optimal intra-articular location for the tibial tunnel and drilling of a new tunnel divergent to the existing one by varying the external starting point.

Posterior positioning of the tibial tunnel is less frequently encountered, and similar techniques can be used. If the tibial tunnel is grossly (more than one tunnel diameter) posterior, a new tunnel can be drilled anterior to the existing one. If it is only slightly posterior, techniques similar to those used for a slightly anterior tunnel are applicable. Coring reamers, large bone-block allografts, and bone grafting are all acceptable alternatives.

Summary

Revision ACL surgery has become increasingly common. Successful revision surgery requires a thorough preoperative evaluation, including a detailed history and a physical and radiographic examination. Preoperative planning is imperative for a successful outcome, as it limits the potential for repeating the errors that led to the failure of the primary procedure. This begins with a determination of the mechanism of failure. Often, a primary as well as a secondary cause of failure can be identified. Determination of the etiology of failure is the first step in a carefully constructed treatment plan, which includes the type of revision and skin incision, graft and hardware removal, tunnel placement, graft selection and fixation, and the rehabilitation protocol. The preoperative plan should have enough flexibility to accommodate unanticipated findings in the operating room.

Finally, the importance of counseling the patient preoperatively regarding potential results must be emphasized. Given the complexity of revision ACL reconstruction, the patient's expectations must be adjusted to realistically match the potential for success. The goal of successful revision surgery may be only to return the patient to activities of daily living or work, especially if there is evidence of degenerative joint disease. With proper planning and attention to detail, revision ACL surgery can provide a satisfying solution to difficult cases of knee instability.

References

1. Miyasaka KC, Daniel DM, Stone ML, Hirshman P: The incidence of knee ligament injuries in the general population. *Am J Knee Surg* 1991;4:43-48.
2. Brown CH Jr, Carson EW: Revision anterior cruciate ligament surgery. *Clin Sports Med* 1999;18:109-171.
3. Bach BR Jr, Tradonsky S, Bojchuk J, Levy ME, Bush-Joseph CA, Khan NH: Arthroscopically assisted anterior cruciate ligament reconstruction using patellar tendon autograft: Five- to nine-year follow-up evaluation. *Am J Sports Med* 1998;26:20-29.
4. Harter RA; Osternig LR, Singer KM, James SL, Larson RL, Jones DC: Long-term evaluation of knee stability and function following surgical reconstruction for anterior cruciate ligament insufficiency. *Am J Sports Med* 1988;16:434-443.
5. Holmes PF, James SL, Larson RL, Singer KM, Jones DC: Retrospective direct comparison of three intraarticular anterior cruciate ligament reconstructions. *Am J Sports Med* 1991;19:596-600.
6. Howe JG, Johnson RJ, Kaplan MJ, Fleming B, Jarvinen M: Anterior cruciate ligament reconstruction using quadriceps patellar tendon graft: Part I. Long-term followup. *Am J Sports Med* 1991;19:447-457.
7. Kaplan MJ, Howe JG, Fleming B, Johnson RJ, Jarvinen M: Anterior cruciate ligament reconstruction using quadriceps patellar tendon graft: Part II. A specific sport review. *Am J Sports Med* 1991;19:458-462.
8. Kornblatt I, Warren RF, Wickiewicz TL: Long-term follow-up of anterior cruciate ligament reconstruction using the quadriceps tendon substitution for chronic anterior cruciate ligament insufficiency. *Am J Sports Med* 1988;16:444-448.
9. Shelbourne KD, Gray T: Anterior cruciate ligament reconstruction with autogenous patellar tendon graft followed by accelerated rehabilitation: A two- to nine-year followup. *Am J Sports Med* 1997;25:786-795.
10. Johnson DL, Harner CD, Maday MG, Fu FH: Revision anterior cruciate ligament surgery, in Fu FH, Harner CD, Vince KG, Miller KD (eds): *Knee Surgery.* Baltimore, MD, Williams & Wilkins, 1994, pp 877-895.
11. Johnson DL, Fu FH: Anterior cruciate ligament reconstruction: Why do failures occur? *Instr Course Lect* 1995;44:391-406.
12. Maday MG, Harner CD, Fu FH: Revision ACL surgery: Evaluation and treatment, in Feagin JA Jr (ed): *The Crucial Ligaments: Diagnosis and Treatment of Ligamentous Injuries About the Knee*, ed 2. New York, Churchill Livingstone, 1994, pp 711-723.
13. Bach BR Jr, Wojtys EM, Lindenfeld TN: Reflex sympathetic dystrophy, patella infera contracture syndrome, and loss of motion following anterior cruciate ligament surgery. *Instr Course Lect* 1997;46:251-260.
14. Harner CD, Irrgang JJ, Paul J, Dearwater S, Fu FH: Loss of motion after anterior cruciate ligament reconstruction. *Am J Sports Med* 1992:20:499-506.
15. Paulos LE, Rosenberg TD, Drawbert J, Manning J, Abbott P: Infrapatellar contracture syndrome: An unrecognized cause of knee stiffness with patella entrapment and patella infera. *Am J Sports Med* 1987:15:331-341.
16. Shelbourne KD, Wilckens JH, Mollabashy A, DeCarlo M: Arthrofibrosis in acute anterior cruciate ligament reconstruction: The effect of timing of reconstruction and rehabilitation. *Am J Sports Med* 1991;19:332-336.
17. Daniel DM, Stone ML, Dobson BE, Fithian DC, Rossman DJ, Kaufman KR: Fate of the ACL-injured patient: A prospective outcome study. *Am J Sports Med* 1994;22:632-644.
18. Dye SF, Chew MH: Restoration of osseous homeostasis after anterior cruciate ligament reconstruction. *Am J Sports Med* 1993;21:748-750.
19. Aglietti P, Buzzi R, D'Andria S, Zaccherotti G: Patellofemoral problems after intraarticular anterior cruciate ligament reconstruction. *Clin Orthop* 288:195-204.
20. Graf B, Uhr F: Complications of intra-articular anterior cruciate reconstruction. *Clin Sports Med* 1988;7:835-848.
21. Sachs RA, Daniel DM, Stone ML, Garfein RF: Patellofemoral problems after anterior cruciate ligament reconstruction. *Am J Sports Med* 1989;17:760-765.
22. Jaureguito JW, Paulos LE: Why grafts fail. *Clin Orthop* 1996;325:25-41.
23. Johnson DL, Swenson TM, Irrgang JJ, Fu FH, Harner CD: Revision anterior cruciate ligament surgery: Experience from Pittsburgh. *Clin Orthop* 1996;325:100-109.
24. Safran MR, Harner CD: Technical considerations of revision anterior cruciate ligament surgery. *Clin Orthop* 1996;325:50-64.
25. Uribe JW, Hechtman KS, Zvijac JE, Tjin-A-Tsoi EW: Revision anterior cruciate ligament surgery: Experience from Miami. *Clin Orthop* 1996;325:91-99.
26. Wetzler MJ, Bartolozzi AR, Gillespie MJ, Rubenstein DL, Ciccotti MG, Miller LS: Revision anterior cruciate ligament reconstruction. *Op Tech Orthop* 1996;6:181-189.
27. Wirth CJ, Kohn D: Revision anterior cruciate ligament surgery: Experience from Germany. *Clin Orthop* 1996;325:110-115.
28. Greis PE, Johnson DL, Fu FH: Revision anterior cruciate ligament surgery: Causes of graft failure and technical considerations of revision surgery. *Clin Sports Med* 1993;12:839-852.
29. Graf B: Isometric placement of substitutes for the anterior cruciate ligament, in Jackson DW, Drez D Jr (eds): *The Anterior Cruciate Deficient Knee: New Concepts in Ligament Repair*. St. Louis, MO, CV Mosby, 1987, pp 102-113.
30. Hoogland T, Hillen B: Intra-articular reconstruction of the anterior cruciate ligament: An experimental study of length changes in different ligament reconstructions. *Clin Orthop* 1984;185:197-202.
31. Howell SM, Barad SJ: Knee extension and its relationship to the slope of the intercondylar roof: Implications for positioning the tibial tunnel in anterior cruciate ligament reconstructions. *Am J Sports Med* 1995;23:288-294.
32. Howell SM, Clark JA: Tibial tunnel placement in anterior cruciate ligament reconstructions and graft impingement. *Clin Orthop* 1992;283:187-195.
33. Howell SM, Taylor MA: Failure of reconstruction of the anterior cruciate ligament due to impingement by the intercondylar roof. *J Bone Joint Surg Am* 1993;75:1044-1055.
34. Jackson DW, Gasser SI: Tibial tunnel placement in ACL reconstruction. *Arthroscopy* 1994;10:124-131.
35. Romano VM, Graf BK, Keene JS, Lange RH: Anterior cruciate ligament reconstruction: The effect of tibial tunnel placement on range of motion. *Am J Sports Med* 1993;21:415-418.
36. Vergis A, Gillquist J: Graft failure in intra-articular anterior cruciate ligament reconstructions: A review of the literature. *Arthroscopy* 1995;11:312-321.
37. Howell SM, Clark JA, Farley TE: A rationale for predicting anterior cruciate graft impingement by the intercondylar roof: A magnetic resonance imaging study. *Am J Sports Med* 1991;19:276-282.
38. Howell SM, Clark JA, Farley TE: Serial magnetic resonance study assessing the effects of impingement on the MR image of the patellar tendon graft. *Arthroscopy* 1992:8:350-358.
39. Tanzer M, Lenczner E: The relationship of intercondylar notch size and content to notchplasty requirement in anterior cruciate ligament surgery. *Arthroscopy* 1990;6:89-93.
40. Corsetti JR, Jackson DW: Failure of anterior cruciate ligament reconstruction: The biologic basis. *Clin Orthop* 1996;325:42-49.
41. Jackson DW, Schaefer RK: Cyclops syndrome: Loss of extension following intra-articular anterior cruciate ligament reconstruction. *Arthroscopy* 1990:6:171-178.

42. Johnson DL, Miller MD, Fu FH: The arthroscopic "impingement test" during anterior cruciate ligament reconstruction. *Arthroscopy* 1993;9:714-717.

43. Burks RT, Leland R: Determination of graft tension before fixation in anterior cruciate ligament reconstruction. *Arthroscopy* 1988;4:260-266.

44. Bylski-Austrow DI, Grood ES, Hefzy MS, Holden JP, Butler DL: Anterior cruciate ligament replacements: A mechanical study of femoral attachment location, flexion angle at tensioning, and initial tension. *J Orthop Res* 1990;8:522-531.

45. Gertel TH, Lew WD, Lewis JL, Stewart NJ, Hunter RE: Effect of anterior cruciate ligament graft tensioning direction, magnitude, and flexion angle on knee biomechanics. *Am J Sports Med* 1993;21:572-581.

46. Yoshiya S, Andrish JT, Manley MT, Bauer TW: Graft tension in anterior cruciate ligament reconstruction: An in vivo study in dogs. *Am J Sports Med* 1987;15:464-470.

47. Schabus R, Fuchs M, Kwasny O: The effect of ACL-graft preload on the static pressure distribution in the knee-joint. *Orthop Trans* 1989;13:431-432.

48. Butler DL: Evaluation of fixation methods in cruciate ligament replacement. *Instr Course Lect* 1987;36:173-178.

49. Kurosaka M, Yoshiya S, Andrish JT: A biomechanical comparison of different surgical techniques of graft fixation in anterior cruciate ligament reconstruction. *Am J Sports Med* 1987;15:225-229.

50. Ritchie JR, Parker RD: Graft selection in anterior cruciate ligament revision surgery. *Clin Orthop* 1996;325:65-77.

51. Amendola A, Fowler P: Allograft anterior cruciate ligament reconstruction in a sheep model: The effect of synthetic augmentation. *Am J Sports Med* 1992;20:336-346.

52. Harner CD, Fu FH: Editorial: The immune response to allograft ACL reconstruction. *Am J Knee Surg* 1993;6:45-46.

53. Jackson DW, Grood ES, Goldstein JD, Rosen MA, Kurzweil PR, Cummings JF, Simon TM: A comparison of patellar tendon autograft and allograft used for anterior cruciate ligament reconstruction in the goat model. *Am J Sports Med* 1993;21:176-185.

54. Noyes FR, Barber-Westin SD, Roberts CS: Use of allografts after failed treatment of rupture of the anterior cruciate ligament. *J Bone Joint Surg Am* 1994;76:1019-1031.

55. Noyes FR, Barber SD: The effect of a ligament-augmentation device on allograft reconstructions for chronic ruptures of the anterior cruciate ligament. *J Bone Joint Surg Am* 1992;74:960-973.

56. Safran MR, Harner CD: Revision ACL surgery: technique and results utilizing allografts. *Instr Course Lect* 1995;44:407-415.

57. Thompson WO, Harner CD, Jamison JP, Saidman SL, Whiteside-Nimick TE: The immunologic response to fresh frozen bone-patellar tendon-bone allograft ACL reconstruction. *Trans Orthop Res Soc* 1994;19:624.

58. Greis PE, Steadman JR: Revision of failed prosthetic anterior cruciate ligament reconstruction. *Clin Orthop* 1996;325:78-90.

59. Paulos LE, Rosenberg TD, Grewe SR, Tearse DS, Beck CL: The GORE-TEX anterior cruciate ligament prosthesis: A long-term followup. *Am J Sports Med* 1992;20:246-252.

60. Fowler PJ: Semitendinosus tendon and the Kennedy ligament augmentation device in anterior cruciate ligament reconstruction. *Op Tech Orthop* 1992;2:117-124.

61. Jackson DW, Grood ES, Arnoczky SP, Butler DL, Simon TM: Cruciate reconstruction using freeze dried anterior cruciate ligament allograft and a ligament augmentation device (LAD): An experimental study in a goat model. *Am J Sports Med* 1987;15:528-538.

62. Müller WW (ed): *The Knee: Form, Function, and Ligament Reconstruction*. New York, NY, Springer, 1983, pp 63-66, 179.

63. Noyes FR, Barber SD, Simon R: High tibial osteotomy and ligament reconstruction in varus angulated, anterior cruciate ligament-deficient knees: A two- to seven-year follow-up study. *Am J Sports Med* 1993;21:2-12.

64. Arnoczky SP: Biology of ACL reconstructions: What happens to the graft? *Instr Course Lect* 1996;45:229-233.

65. Clancy WG Jr, Narechania RG, Rosenberg TD, Gmeiner JG, Wisnefske DD, Lange TA: Anterior and posterior cruciate ligament reconstruction in Rhesus monkeys: A histological, microangiographic, and biomechanical analysis. *J Bone Joint Surg Am* 1981;63:1270-1284.

66. Drez DJ Jr, DeLee J, Holden JP, Arnoczky S, Noyes FR, Roberts TS: Anterior cruciate ligament reconstruction using bone-patellar tendon-bone allografts: A biological and biomechanical evaluation in goats. *Am J Sports Med* 1991;19:256-263.

67. Rodeo SA, Arnoczky SP, Torzilli PA, Hidaka C, Warren RF: Tendon-healing in a bone tunnel: A biomechanical and histological study in the dog. *J Bone Joint Surg Am* 1993;75:1795-1803.

68. Höher J, Möller HD, Fu FH: Bone tunnel enlargement after anterior cruciate ligament reconstruction: fact or fiction? *Knee Surg Sports Traumatol Arthrosc* 1998;6:231-240.

69. L'Insalata JC, Klatt B, Fu FH, Harner CD: Tunnel expansion following anterior cruciate ligament reconstruction: A comparison of hamstring and patellar tendon autografts. *Knee Surg Sports Traumatol Arthrosc* 1997;5:234-238.

70. Peyrache MD, Djian P, Christel P, Witvoet J: Tibial tunnel enlargement after anterior cruciate ligament reconstruction by autogenous bone-patellar tendon-bone graft. *Knee Surg Sports Traumatol Arthrosc* 1996;4:2-8.

71. Schulte K, Majewski M, Irrgang JJ, Fu FH, Harner CD: Abstract: Radiographic tunnel changes following arthroscopic ACL reconstruction: Autograft versus allograft. *Arthroscopy* 1995;11:372-373.

72. Dye SF, Chew MH: The use of scintigraphy to detect increased osseous metabolic activity about the knee. *Instr Course Lect* 1994;43:453-469.

73. Sledge SL, Steadman JR, Silliman JF, Peloza J, Fullstone AH: Five-year results with the Gore-Tex anterior cruciate ligament prosthesis. *Am J Knee Surg* 1992;5:65-70.

74. Williams RJ, Warren RF, Carson EW, Wickiewicz TL: Revision anterior cruciate ligament reconstruction: The Hospital for Special Surgery experience. *Tech Orthop* 1998;13:375-383.

75. Clancy WG, Pietropaoli MP: Revision anterior ligament reconstruction using the "anatomic endoscopic" method. *Tech Orthop* 1998;13:391-410.

76. Karns DJ, Heidt RS Jr, Holladay BR, Colosimo AJ: Case report: Revision anterior cruciate ligament reconstruction. *Arthroscopy* 1994;10:148-157.

77. Coupens SD, Yates CK, Sheldon C, Ward C: Magnetic resonance imaging evaluation of the patellar tendon after use of its central one-third for anterior cruciate ligament reconstruction. *Am J Sports Med* 1992;20:332-335.

78. LaPrade RF, Hamilton CD, Montgomery RD, Wentorf F, Hawkins HD: The reharvested central third of the patellar tendon: A histologic and biomechanical analysis. *Am J Sports Med* 1997;25:779-785.

79. Proctor CS, Jackson DW, Simon TM: Characterization of the repair tissue after removal of the central one-third of the patellar ligament: An experimental study in a goat model. *J Bone Joint Surg Am* 1997;79:997-1006.

80. Kartus J, Stener S, Lindahl S, Eriksson BI, Karlsson J: Ipsi- or contralateral patellar tendon graft in anterior cruciate ligament revision surgery: A comparison of two methods. *Am J Sports Med* 1998;26:499-504.

81. Rubinstein RA Jr, Shelbourne KD, VanMeter CD, McCarroll JC, Rettig AC: Isolated autogenous bone-patellar tendon-bone graft site morbidity. *Am J Sports Med* 1994;22:324-327.

82. Steadman JR, Saterbak AM: Revision anterior cruciate ligament reconstruction: Techniques and tips — the Vail experience. *Tech Orthop* 1998;13:384-390.

83. Yasuda K, Tsujino J, Ohkoshi Y, Tanabe Y, Kaneda K: Graft site morbidity with autogenous semitendinosus and gracilis tendons. *Am J Sports Med* 1995;23:706-714.

84. Gibbons MJ, Butler DL, Grood ES, Bylski-Austrow DI, Levy MS, Noyes FR: Effects of gamma irradiation on the initial mechanical and material properties of goat bone-patellar tendon-bone allografts. *J Orthop Res* 1991;9:209-218.

85. Shelton WR, Treacy SH, Dukes AD, Bomboy AL: Use of allografts in knee reconstruction: Basic science aspects and current status. *J Am Acad Orthop Surg* 1998;6:165-168.

86. Noyes FR, Barber-Westin SD: Revision anterior cruciate ligament surgery: Experience from Cincinnati. *Clin Orthop* 1996;325:116-129.

87. Getelman MH, Schepsis AA, Zimmer J: Revision ACL reconstruction: Autograft versus allograft. *Arthroscopy* 1995;11:378.

88. Miller MD: Revision cruciate ligament surgery with retention of femoral interference screws. *Arthroscopy* 1998;14:111-114.

89. Fahey M, Indelicato PA: Bone tunnel enlargement after anterior cruciate ligament replacement. *Am J Sports Med* 1994;22:410-414.

90. Karlson JA, Steiner ME, Brown CH, Johnston J: Anterior cruciate ligament reconstruction using gracilis and semitendinosus tendons: Comparisons of the through-the-condyle and over-the-top graft placements. *Am J Sports Med* 1994;22:659-666.

Reference to Video

Friedman M: Revision ACL reconstruction using autogenous hamstring tendon. *ACL Revision Surgery: Technical Concepts.* Van Nuys, CA, 1998.

SECTION

8

Knee: Adult Reconstruction—Osteonecrosis

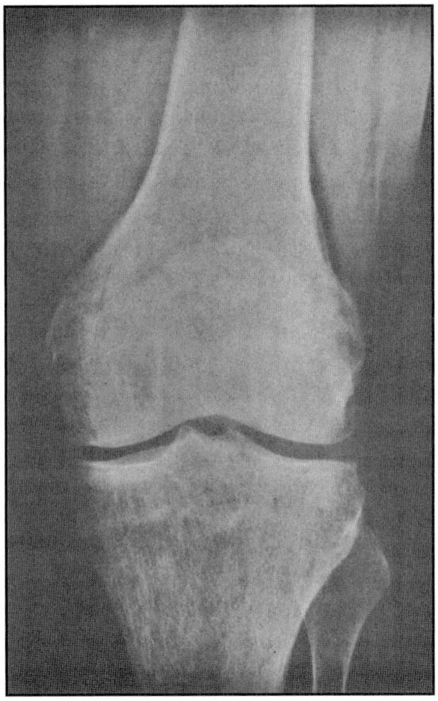

48 Tibial Osteonecrosis

49 Treatment of Osteonecrosis of the Knee

50 Steroid-Associated Osteonecrosis of the Knee: A Comprehensive Review

51 Spontaneous Osteonecrosis of the Distal Femur

52 Surgical Options for the Middle-Aged Patient With Osteoarthritis of the Knee Joint

48

Tibial Osteonecrosis

Jess H. Lonner, MD
Paul A. Lotke, MD

Introduction

Spontaneous osteonecrosis of the medial tibial plateau was first described in 1976 in the French literature by D'Angelejan and associates[1] and later in the English literature by Houpt and associates,[2] nearly 2 decades after Ahlbäck and associates[3] described an analogous lesion in the medial femoral condyle. Since then, osteonecrosis of the medial tibial plateau has been addressed as part of a continuum of change observed in the subchondral bone and metaphysis in patients with varying stages of osteoarthritis.[4-7] Its true incidence is unknown, in part because the condition tends to be recognized less frequently, or misdiagnosed more commonly, than osteonecrosis of the medial femoral condyle.[5-7] These patients, who are usually women age 60 or older, often erroneously undergo arthroscopic surgery for presumed meniscal tears, based on changes observed on MRI studies that are so common in this age group, without symptomatic relief.

Clinical Presentation

As with spontaneous osteonecrosis of the medial femoral condyle, most persons affected with tibial osteonecrosis are women, age 60 years or older. Presenting symptoms often include the acute onset or exacerbation of pain on the medial side of the knee, with or without associated minor trauma or increased activity.[4-6,8] Patients often have a history of insidious knee pain, commonly experienced in the early and mid stages of osteoarthritis. Mechanical symptoms, such as catching, locking, and buckling, are not widespread.

Physical examination reveals a well localized area of tenderness over the medial side of the tibia, usually close to the joint line, and on the posterior aspect of the plateau. Careful and precise palpation will help to distinguish this clinical entity from osteoarthritis, meniscal derangement, or bursitis. Mild effusion and/or synovitis may be observed. Motion is commonly preserved, but may be painful, particularly when the knee undergoes axial loading.

One or more of the authors or the departments with which they are affiliated have received something of value from a commercial or other party related directly or indirectly to the subject of this chapter.

Differential Diagnosis

Meniscal Tears

The interpretation of a degenerative meniscal tear observed on MRI as the cause of symptoms must be done with caution because degenerative tears and signal changes of the medial meniscus are common in this afflicted age group.[6,9,10] Interpreting intrasubstance meniscal degeneration as a clinically relevant or significant finding is particularly problematic if the MRI is obtained early after the onset of symptoms, before MRI changes of osteonecrosis have had the chance to develop.

Bursitis

Pes anserinus bursitis is a common cause of pain in the anteromedial aspect of the knee in this patient group.[11] Bursitis of the semimembranosus bursa, however, is not diagnosed as often, but may be a rare source of posteromedial knee pain. The diagnosis can be established with careful physical examination. MRI can be useful in clarifying the diagnosis.

Insufficiency Fractures

Osteoporosis can lead to a stress fracture on the overloaded aspect of the knee (commonly medial in varus aligned limb). The fracture will usually develop just distal to the flare of the medial tibial plateau. Although careful examination can often confirm the diagnosis, it is difficult to differentiate an insufficiency fracture from pes anserinus bursitis or osteonecrosis. The pain initially may be poorly localized and the radiographs negative for the first 7 to 10 days after injury. Therefore, this diagnosis may be overlooked. MRI or bone scan can assist in establishing the diagnosis, although the latter is nonspecific and will not differentiate well between osteonecrosis and insufficiency fracture.

Etiology

Like spontaneous idiopathic osteonecrosis of the femur, the etiology of tibial osteonecrosis is unknown. Prevailing theories include a vascular ischemic event or localized stress reaction, intraosseous hypertension, and perhaps microfracture.

In osteonecrosis of the knee, a subtle traumatic etiology is the more plausible mechanism.[12] The traumatic theory takes into account that most patients are elderly women in whom osteoporosis is common and in whom a minor traumatic event might cause a microfracture in the weakened subcondylar bone. Once the subcondylar plate has been violated, fluid may enter the marrow space, resulting in an increase in the pressure and causing ischemia and pain. Unfortunately, there is no confirming histologic evidence to support this theory.

The vascular theory is most likely in osteonecrosis of the hip.[13] In a recent study,[14] 74% of patients with osteorecrosis of the hip have been shown to have some underlying coagulopathy or thrombophilia. Glueck and associates[14] noted that in patients with osteonecrosis, an associated finding was a coagulation disorder such as hypofibrinolysis or thrombophilia, including resistance to activated protein C, low protein C, and low stimulated tissue plasminogen activator activity. They speculated that these coagulopathies cause thrombotic venous occlusion in the head of the femur, leading to venous hypertension and hypoxic death of bone. This series of events is less likely involved in the development of spontaneous osteonecrosis of the knee.

Intraosseous compartment pressure measurements have not provided consistent evidence that hypertension exists within the rigid osseous compartment.[15] However, the edema commonly observed within the nonexpandable compartment should intuitively increase the local pressure with the bone marrow, further compromising venous outflow and resulting in localized ischemia.

Pathology

Gross and histologic findings of tibial osteonecrosis are similar to those observed in spontaneous osteonecrosis of the medial femoral condyle.[16] In the early stages of osteonecrosis, slight flattening or discoloration in the articular cartilage may be observed. At the edge of the lesion there may be an irregular line of demarcation on the surface, with a ridge of cartilage of altered color. In the presence of early osteoarthritis, varying degrees of chondromalacia are anticipated.

In the later stages of osteonecrosis, the demarcation can become more pronounced, and chondral delamination may develop. The involved fragment of cartilage, with a thin layer of subchondral bone, can be peeled from its base. It is usually hinged on a normal cartilage segment. For far advanced cases, diffuse chondral fragmentation and degeneration are common. A crater with necrotic detritus and regenerated fibrocartilage may be found.

If subchondral bone of the gross specimen harvested at the time of arthroplasty is studied, a thin layer of whitish yellow necrotic subchondral bone will be noted, sometimes in a fragmented state. A vacant space corresponding to a subchondral fracture, which has begun at the margins and propagated parallel to the surface, is usually present deep in the subchondral bone. In the bed of the crater, above the fractured cleft, necrotic detritus and necrotic trabeculae can be seen. The bone around the necrotic area acquires normal growth characteristics with signs of intense perifocal reparative reaction and sometimes sclerosis. In more advanced cases, in which degenerative changes have already begun, it might be difficult to find a pathology section of a typical necrotic lesion. Sometimes only after close scrutiny can the pathologist find the remnants of a worn crater and fragment. Many believe that osteonecrosis of the knee, as in the hip, is an important and underestimated cause of osteoarthritis.

The histologic appearance of the articular cartilage may be normal or almost normal in the early stages of tibial osteonecrosis. The chondrocytes are grouped in familiar patterns with normal-staining matrix around them. Later, if the process has persisted for a relatively long time, there might be cloning of the chondrocytes and early fibrillation or erosion in the layer of the tidemark, which might become wavy and thicker. The subchondral bone has the typical characteristics of necrosis: the marrow exhibits cell lysis, destruction of fat cells, blood vessels in the stroma, and empty lacunae, or lacunae with pyknotic nuclei. The marrow in more advanced cases has a typical dusty or smoky appearance. There are no signs of reaction. At the base of the crater, in the more superficial layers, some necrotic trabeculae and intense fibrovascular granulation tissue with histocytes and osteoclasts reabsorbing the necrotic tissues can be found. Islands of fibrocartilage may be present as well. The appearance is very similar to that of fractured callus. Proceeding toward the depth of the condyle, the perifocal reaction gradually shifts to new bone formation and deposition of new, immature bone around dead trabeculae or thickening of trabeculae and sclerosis can be seen. This type of reparative reaction can occur very deep in the condyle.

Imaging

Applied imaging studies are similar to those used in the diagnosis and evaluation of osteonecrosis of the medial femoral condyle. The plain radiograph may initially be normal. In more than half of the cases the initial radiographs will show minor preexisting degenerative changes, so common in elderly patients. In some patients, a typical lesion with subchondral lucency surrounded by sclerosis develops. In more advanced cases, collapse of the lesion may result in secondary degenerative changes.

Technetium-99m scans had been used before the advent of MRI. The radionuclide bone scan shows a focal area of increased uptake localized in the tibial plateau. So-called "kissing lesions," with both tibial and femoral uptake, are more indicative of advanced osteoarthritis than osteonecrosis. The radionuclide scan must be positive to confirm the diagnosis of osteonecrosis.[17-19] The static phase image demonstrates a focally intense area of uptake over the affected bone. Al-Rowaih and associates[17] found that the pool phase of a three-phase study did not contribute useful diagnostic or prognostic information, but the presence of a high flow phase and static uptake phase persisting for 6 to 12 months correlated directly with a poor clinical and radiologic outcome.

MRI is undoubtedly the most useful technique for diagnosing early tibial osteonecrosis, providing a vehicle for classification, and a plan for clinical course.[6] However, in some patients the diagnosis may be missed by MRI. Pollack and associates[20] found that in 2 of 10 knees with classic symptoms of osteonecrosis and confirmed with a radionuclide bone scan, the diagnosis was missed using MRI. The authors theorized that the initial small lesions might have been missed because of the thickness of the MRI sections. Subsequently, Nakamura and associates,[21] using a canine model, found a delay in histologic and MRI changes after surgically induced osteonecrosis in the hip. They found that minimal histologic changes could be seen as early as 3 days, but that MRI changes did not manifest until fibrous tissue developed an interface with normal bone. At 2 weeks, four of seven animals showed MRI changes, but it was not until 4 weeks that all animals demonstrated both histologic and MRI evidence of necrosis. It is not unreasonable to suggest that an analogous event may occur in the knee.

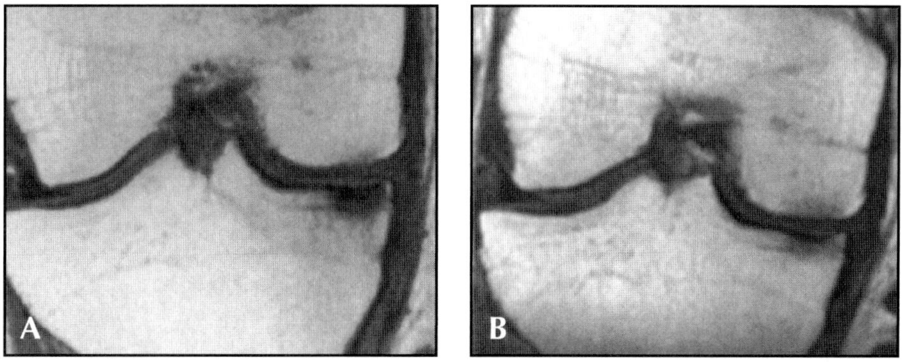

Fig. 1 A, Type A lesion observed on T1-weighted image. Note the localized low signal area in the medial tibial plateau. **B,** Follow-up T1-weighted MRI 1 year after presentation. Symptoms have resolved. Note nearly complete resolution of lesion. (Reproduced with permission from Lotke PA, Ecker ML, Barth P, Lonner JH: Subchondral magnetic resonance imaging changes in early osteoarthrosis associated with tibial osteonecrosis. *Arthroscopy* 2000;16:76-81.)

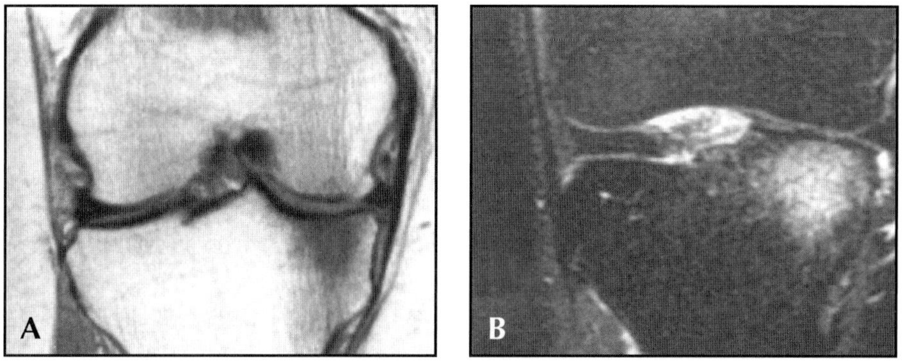

Fig. 2 A, Type B lesion observed on T1-weighted MRI. There is a large area of low signal intensity that extends distal to the physeal scar into the metaphysis. (Reproduced with permission from Lotke PA, Ecker ML, Barth P, Lonner JH: Subchondral MRI changes in early osteoarthrosis associated with tibial osteonecrosis. *Arthroscopy* 2000;16:76-18.) **B,** Type B lesion on fat suppression T2-weighted image highlighting the extent of involvement.

There have been several reports of knees that developed lesions typical of osteonecrosis after undergoing arthroscopic surgery, despite initial MRI examinations that did not show osteonecrosis. In its simplest form, osteonecrosis may result from thermal necrosis induced by the use of lasers during arthroscopic surgery.[22] Brahme and associates[23] reported on seven cases in which there was no evidence of osteonecrosis of the knee on the initial MRI, prior to arthroscopic menisectomy. Repeat MRI performed because of persistent or recurrent pain showed an area of low signal intensity with a T1-weighted image. None of the patients had undergone radionuclide studies prior to the arthroscopic procedures. The authors theorized that the diminished load-bearing capacity of the injured meniscus resulted in microfracture or vascular insufficiency in the contiguous condyle. They did not consider the possibility that the MRI study may have been normal in very early osteonecrosis, and the meniscal tear as seen on MRI may not have been the cause of the presenting symptoms. Bjorkengren and associates,[24] in a study of 16 patients with spontaneous osteonecrosis, reported a 12.5% incidence of false-negative MRIs, despite positive

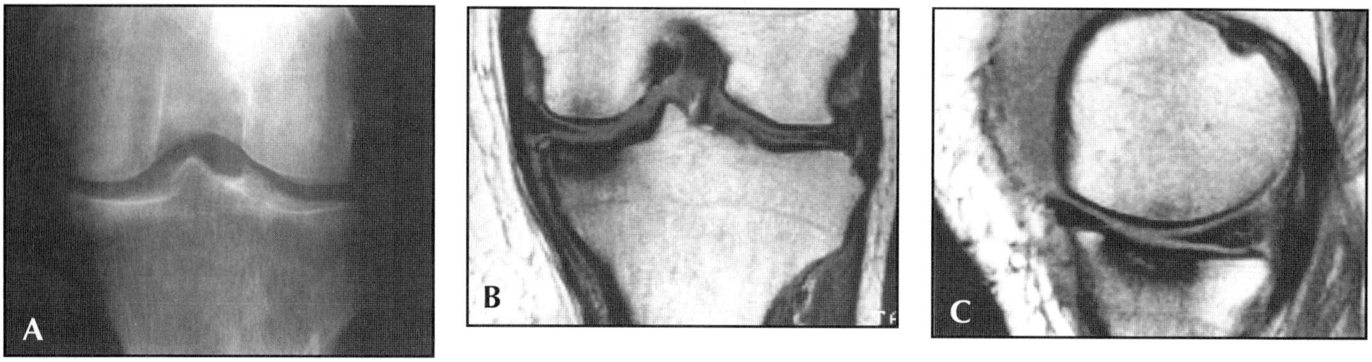

Fig. 3 A, Plain radiograph of a patient with a type C osteonecrotic lesion of the medial tibial plateau. Note mild narrowing of the medial joint space and minimal subchondral sclerosis. **B** and **C,** Coronal and sagittal views, respectively, of type C lesions on T1-weighted MRIs. Note the serpiginous line demarcating an osteonecrotic segment. Note that there is a tear of the posterior horn and body of the medial meniscus. (Reproduced with permission from Lotke PA, Ecker ML, Barth P, Lonner JH: Subchondral magnetic resonance imaging changes in early osteoarthrosis associated with tibial osteonecrosis. *Arthroscopy* 2000;16:76-81.)

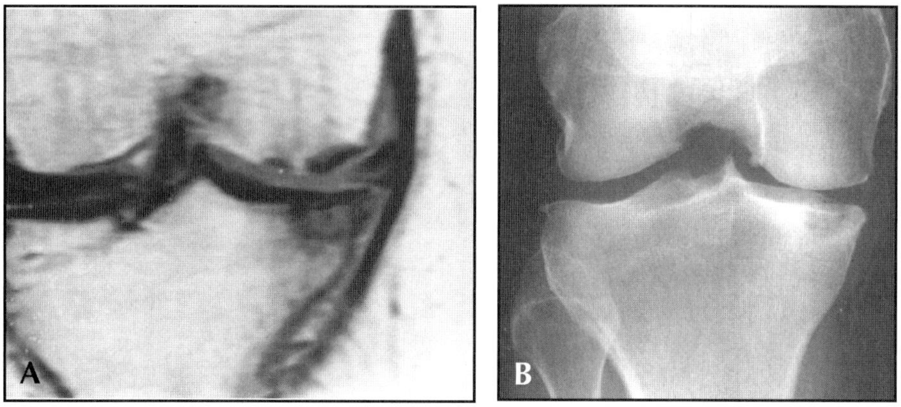

Fig. 4 A and **B,** Type D lesion with collapse of the joint.

bone scans, again calling into question the issue of timing of MRI in the evaluation of spontaneous osteonecrosis of the knee. Fat suppression T2-weighted images may improve the sensitivity of early scans.

Classification

It is useful to classify lesions of tibial osteonecrosis into four types, based on the spectrum of subchondral changes that are observed on MRI.[6]

Type A lesions are relatively small, well localized, low signal areas in the subchondral zone best seen on spin echo T1-weighted images (Fig. 1).

Type B lesions are low signal areas also occurring in the subchondral bone, but extending down into the tibial metaphysis below the epiphyseal line (Fig. 2). They are less focal with a more diffuse area of signal change. They are best appreciated in the spin echo T1- and T2-weighted images, as well as fat suppression images. Type A and B lesions probably represent "preosteonecrotic" lesions that may or may not progress.

Type C lesions have well localized changes in the subchondral bone as well as widespread change into the metaphysis. The pathognomonic characteristic is a well-circumscribed low signal area surrounded by a serpiginous rim of low signal representing reactive bone (Fig. 3). There may be a small area of subchondral collapse that is not visible on standard radiographs. This type C pattern and its serpiginous line is a classic characteristic of true osteonecrosis in bone.

Type D is an extension of the type C pattern. The subchondral collapse is large enough to create secondary changes in bone, and therefore is evident on standard radiographs (Fig. 4).

Clinical Course

The MRI classification can be correlated with the prognosis for an individual lesion. Type A and B lesions, without clearly defined osteonecrotic central segments, generally resolve without surgical intervention, although symptoms may be present for 9 to 12 months. The patient's symptoms may intermittently recur, depending on the extent and severity of associated arthritis. Type C and D lesions may be more likely to require surgery.

In a series of 41 patients with tibial osteonecrosis associated with early osteoarthritis, the type of MRI lesion seen initially was predictive of prognosis.[6] Follow-up MRIs after 1 year routinely showed reduction or absence of lesions when the initial lesion was type A or B. Type C lesions were often reduced in size. At a 2- to 10-year follow-up, 19% of the patients with types A and B lesions had severe symptoms or required surgery, compared with 66% of those patients with type C lesions. Symptomatic relief tended to deteriorate with time. At the end of 1 year, 33 patients (80%) had no or mild symptoms, and 8 (20%) had persistent moderate pain. At 4.5-year follow-up, consistent with progressive osteoarthritis, 12 patients had severe symptoms (29%), 17 (41%) had mild or moderate symptoms, and only 12 (29%) were asymptomatic or had minimal symptoms. The size and depth of the MRI changes noted at the metaphyseal area did not appear to offer prognostic information.[6]

In an earlier study,[7] patients with type D lesions (those with radiographic changes) predictably had the worst prognosis. In that report, 84% of patients with type D lesions eventually required either a total knee or a unicompartmental arthroplasty.

Summary

Spontaneous osteonecrosis of the tibial plateau involves a continuum of change observed in the subchondral zone that is commonly associated with early and mid stages of osteoarthritis. The typical patient is an elderly woman who experiences a sudden onset of pain in the medial aspect of the knee. The diagnosis of this under-appreciated clinical entity may be difficult, but careful examination and judicious use of imaging studies, as well as a high index of suspicion, may facilitate the accurate diagnosis. Although the radiographs may initially be normal (with the exception of mild arthrosis), radionuclide scans and MRI can be of great value. The MRI studies usually show a decreased signal intensity on a T1-weighted image, but may be normal in the early course of the disease. The T2-weighted images and fat suppression views are helpful in establishing a diagnosis and determining the extent of involvement. Recognition of this problem may help to avoid unnecessary intra-articular surgery. Many of these patients have complete or partial resolution of symptoms by 1 year, after a period of protected weight bearing. Nonetheless, surgery may be necessary for more advanced lesions and in those patients with progressive arthrosis.

References

1. D'Anglejan G, Ryckewaert A, Glimet A: Osteonecrose du plateau tibial intern. *Extr Rheum* 1976;8:253-255.
2. Houpt JB, Alpert B, Lotem M, et al: Spontaneous osteonecrosis of the medial tibial plateau. *J Rheumatol* 1982;9:81-90.
3. Ahlbäck S, Bauer GC, Bohne WH: Spontaneous osteonecrosis of the knee. *Arthritis Rheum* 1968;11:705-733.
4. Ecker ML, Lotke PA: Osteonecrosis of the medial part of the tibial plateau. *J Bone Joint Surg Am* 1995;77:596-601.
5. Lotke PA, Ecker ML: Osteonecrosis-like syndrome of the medial tibial plateau. *Clin Orthop* 1983;176:148-153.
6. Lotke PA, Ecker ML, Barth P, Lonner JH: Subchondral magnetic resonance imaging changes in early osteoarthrosis associated with tibial osteonecrosis. *Arthroscopy* 2000;16:76-81.
7. Marmor L: Fracture as a complication of osteonecrosis of the tibial plateau: A case report. *J Bone Joint Surg Am* 1988;70:454-457.
8. Lotke PA, Ecker ML: Osteonecrosis of the knee. *J Bone Joint Surg Am* 1988;70:470-473.
9. Negendank WG, Fernandez-Madrid FR, Heilbrun LK, Teitge RA: Magnetic resonance imaging of meniscal degeneration in asymptomatic knees. *J Orthop Res* 1990;8:311-320.
10. Noble J, Hamblen DL: The pathology of the degenerate meniscus lesion. *J Bone Joint Surg Br* 1975;57:180-186.
11. Moschcowitz E: Bursitis of sartorius bursa: An undescribed malady simulating chronic arthritis. *JAMA* 1937;109:1362.
12. Lotke PA, Abend JA, Ecker ML: The treatment of osteonecrosis of the medial femoral condyle. *Clin Orthop* 1982;171:109-116.
13. Jones JP Jr: Risk factors potentially activating intravascular coagulation and causing nontraumatic osteonecrosis, in Urbaniak JR, Jones JP Jr (eds): *Osteonecrosis: Etiology, Diagnosis, and Treatment*. Rosemont, IL, American Academy of Orthopaedic Surgeons, 1997, pp 89-96.
14. Glueck CJ, Freiberg R, Tracy T, Stroop D, Wang P: Thrombophilia and hypofibrinolysis: Pathophysiologies of osteonecrosis. *Clin Orthop* 1997;334:43-56.
15. Arnoldi CC, Lemperg RK, Linderholm H: Intraosseous hypertension and pain in the knee. *J Bone Joint Surg Br* 1975;57:360-363.
16. Ahuja SC, Bullough PG: Osteonecrosis of the knee: A clinicopathological study in twenty-eight patients. *J Bone Joint Surg Am* 1978;60:191-197.
17. al-Rowaih A, Wingstrand H, Lindstrand A, Bjorkengren A, Thorngren KG, Gustafson T: Three-phase scintimetry in osteonecrosis of the knee. *Acta Orthop Scand* 1990;61:120-127.
18. Lotke PA, Ecker ML, Alavi A: Painful knees in older patients: Radionuclide diagnosis of possible osteonecrosis with spontaneous resolution. *J Bone Joint Surg Am* 1977;59:617-621.
19. Rozing PM, Insall J, Bohne WH: Spontaneous osteonecrosis of the knee. *J Bone Joint Surg Am* 1980;62:2-7.
20. Pollack MS, Dalinka MK, Kressel HY, Lotke PA, Spritzer CE: Magnetic resonance imaging in the evaluation of suspected osteonecrosis of the knee. *Skeletal Radiol* 1987;16:121-127.
21. Nakamura T, Matsumoto T, Nishino M, Tomita K, Kadoya M: Early magnetic resonance imaging and histologic findings in a model of femoral head necrosis. *Clin Orthop* 1997;334:68-72.
22. Janzen DL, Kosarek FJ, Helms CA, Cannon WD Jr, Wright JC: Osteonecrosis after contact neodymium: Yttrium aluminum garnet arthroscopic laser meniscectomy. *AJR Am J Roentgenol* 1997;169:855-858.
23. Brahme SK, Fox JM, Ferkel RD, Friedman MJ, Flannigan BD, Resnick DL: Osteonecrosis of the knee after arthroscopic surgery: Diagnosis with MR imaging. *Radiology* 1991;178:851-853.
24. Bjorkengren AG, AlRowaih A, Lindstrand A, Wingstrand H, Thorngren KG, Pettersson H: Spontaneous osteonecrosis of the knee: Value of MR imaging in determining prognosis. *AJR Am J Roentgenol* 1990;154:331-336.

49

Treatment of Osteonecrosis of the Knee

Paul A. Lotke, MD
Raman Battish, BS
Charles L. Nelson, MD

Introduction

The treatment of osteonecrosis about the knee is divided into the treatment of three principal disorders: (1) spontaneous osteonecrosis of the femoral condyle, (2) tibial osteonecrosis, and (3) steroid-induced osteonecrosis. Although there are several options for treatment regimens, with the exception of conservative therapy for small lesions and total knee arthroplasty for large lesions, the indications and results of other surgical procedures are poorly defined and have not been appropriately stratified for age, size of lesion, and etiology. In general, there are five basic options for the treatment of osteonecrosis: (1) conservative care, (2) core decompression of the distal femur, (3) arthroscopic débridement, (4) proximal tibial osteotomy, and (5) total knee replacement or unicompartmental arthroplasty. These options will be discussed in relationship to the clinical entity. In addition, osteochondral allografts offer an interim response for localized loss of articular cartilage.

Medial Femoral Condyle: Spontaneous Osteonecrosis of the Knee

Conservative Therapy

Conservative treatment generally consists of analgesia as needed, protected weight bearing, and activities to tolerance. Initially the pain is very acute and patients exhibit diminished activity levels. However, as the acute symptoms begin to resolve, patients return to a more normal lifestyle. Excellent to good results can be obtained with conservative means if the lesions are relatively small, that is, less than 40% of the width of the condyle.[1-3] Over time, depending on the size of the lesion, degenerative changes will manifest.[4] Patients with small lesions will continue to function normally with minimal symptoms. However, osteoarthritis will gradually progress depending on the size of the lesion.

Core Decompression

The concept of releasing intraosseous pressure to prevent further necrosis in bone is an extension of the experience that authors have had with decompression of the femoral head for early stages of osteonecrosis of the hip.[5] Jacobs and associates[6] first reported the use of core decompression for the distal femur. They performed core decompression of the distal femur and pathologically confirmed osteonecrosis in 28 knees. Seven knees with stage I and II lesions yielded good results. Furthermore, approximately half of the stage III lesions had good results from the procedure. Recently, Forst and associates[7,8] reported on 16 patients (average age of 64 years) with spontaneous osteonecrosis of the femoral condyle, verified by MRI. Fifteen of these lesions were stage I, with one knee having radiologic signs of femoral condyle flattening. All patients were treated with surgical extra-articular drilling into the affected condyle to achieve core decompression. The acute pain disappeared immediately after surgery for all patients. Successful healing was confirmed by normalization of the bone marrow signal by MRI at a 3-year follow-up. Notably, if femoral condyle flattening was already apparent, the progression of the disease could not always be avoided. Forst and associates[7,8] concluded that core decompression, by extra-articular drilling of the femoral condyle, should be considered an effective treatment for osteonecrosis of the knee prior to collapse. However, the absence of a control group in this study limits any conclusions. It is not possible to know how these patients would have done without core decompression because successful outcomes have been reported for most patients with stage I lesions and minimal femoral flattening.

Core decompression is really an effective treatment for steroid-induced osteonecrosis because steroid-induced osteonecrosis is an entirely different entity with different anatomic involvement in the distal femur. The central factor is that steroid-induced osteonecrosis does not necessarily involve the subchondral plate; the principal involvement is metaphyseal with possible extensions to the subchondral plate. Therefore, it has different structural and mechanical ramifications for the joint surface.

At this time, it appears that core decompression can relieve the initial acute pain that occurs with the onset of spontaneous osteonecrosis of the knee. However, it is still undetermined whether the disease process itself is altered or its progression retarded by early decompression.

Arthroscopic Débridement

Considering the intraosseous focus of osteonecrosis, it appears that arthroscopic débridement and chondroplasty will not delay or alter the natural course and progression of the disease. Miller and associates[9] reviewed a series of five patients with idiopathic osteonecrosis who underwent arthroscopic débridement and abrasion arthroplasty. Although a good postoperative result was reported in four of the five patients after 2.5 years, the progression of osteonecrosis had not been halted.

Arthroscopy may be effective in débriding unstable or delaminating chondral fragments, particularly to resolve mechanical symptoms such as locking or catching. Retrograde drilling through overlying intact cartilage may theoretically stimulate revascularization of the osteonecrotic focus, as in the treatment of osteochondritis dissecans. However, no evidence supports arthroscopy as an effective treatment of spontaneous osteonecrosis in an elderly population. In fact, it may be more advisable to drill in an antegrade, nonarticular direction, thereby avoiding potential articular cartilage damage caused by retrograde drilling. Arthroscopic débridement often is used to diagnose the osteonecrosis and remove fragments of articular cartilage. Still, the results of arthroscopic interventions are neither well defined nor well controlled.[10] In a few reports, osteonecrosis has been noted after arthroscopic treatment for meniscal or degenerative lesions.[11,12] Whether these lesions are new and induced by the arthroscopic treatment or initially overlooked is still undetermined.

Osteochondral Allografts

There have been scattered reports in the literature regarding the use of osteochondral allografts for osteonecrosis of the femoral condyle.[9,13-17] The use of fresh osteochondral allografts has been conceived as an interim response to a localized loss of articular cartilage when there are no other reasonable alternatives.

Fresh osteochondral allografts have been successful in the treatment of posttraumatic defects in the knee. Little has been written regarding the use of these grafts for the treatment of osteonecrosis. Bayne and associates[13] reported on six knees with stage IV spontaneous osteonecrosis of the knee requiring bipolar allografts (needing femoral and tibial articular surfaces); average patient age was 67 years. Five of the six patients had unsatisfactory results with early graft subsidence or fragmentations. We also reviewed three patients with steroid-induced osteonecrosis, each having unsatisfactory results. Overall the results are superior in those patients who underwent treatment for posttraumatic injuries and were in a much younger population. The success rate in this group was 76% in the traumatic patients, 57% in the steroid-induced osteonecrosis group, and only 46% in the spontaneous osteonecrosis group.

Meyers and associates[17] reported on 59 osteochondral allograft transplants, 5 of which were transplanted for osteonecrosis of the medial femoral condyle. Only three of these patients were available for follow-up. Each of these was considered an excellent clinical result. However, there was no mention of the size of the lesion or age of the patients treated.

Flynn and associates[18] reviewed a series of 17 fresh-frozen osteochondral articular allografts used to treat distal femoral osteonecrosis. Seven patients had received corticosteroids, and the remainder were either posttraumatic or spontaneously induced. The average age was only 29.6 years, with an average follow-up of 4 years. Results were considered good or excellent in 12 cases. Of note, 75% of the patients with steroid-induced osteonecrosis had a good or excellent result compared with 67% of the patients with trauma-induced or spontaneous osteonecrosis. A fair result was achieved in the patients with spontaneous osteonecrosis, although the authors stated that one of their failures was in a patient limited by disease in the contralateral knee.

Osteochondral allografts may be an option for younger patients with localized osteonecrosis or with osteochondritis dissecans. However, in the elderly patient with collapse of the subchondral bone, more predictable results may be achieved with an arthroplasty. It is possible that the success of osteochondral allografts may be enhanced with simultaneous unloading procedures, such as proximal tibial osteotomies, or distal femoral osteotomies, if there is an associated malalignment of the mechanical axis. The results of total knee arthroplasty are so good in the older age groups that fresh osteochondral allografts do not seem to be indicated for this population because of the technical difficulties and potential immunogenic responses.

High Proximal Tibial Osteotomy

Proximal tibial osteotomy may be considered for younger, active patients with osteonecrosis of the medial femoral condyle either in the presence of a mechanical axis that has displaced medially or associated with early collapse of the medial compartment. The procedure may also be performed without arthroscopy or arthrotomy if no osteochondral loose bodies or chondral delamination is present. Soucacos and associates[19] have described their approach in stage III and IV osteonecrosis with irreversible destruction in the subchondral bone and cartilage of the medial femoral condyle. Although the authors do not specifically detail the results of treatment, they report that the results were better in stage III osteonecrosis where less than 50% of the condyle was involved and in patients younger than

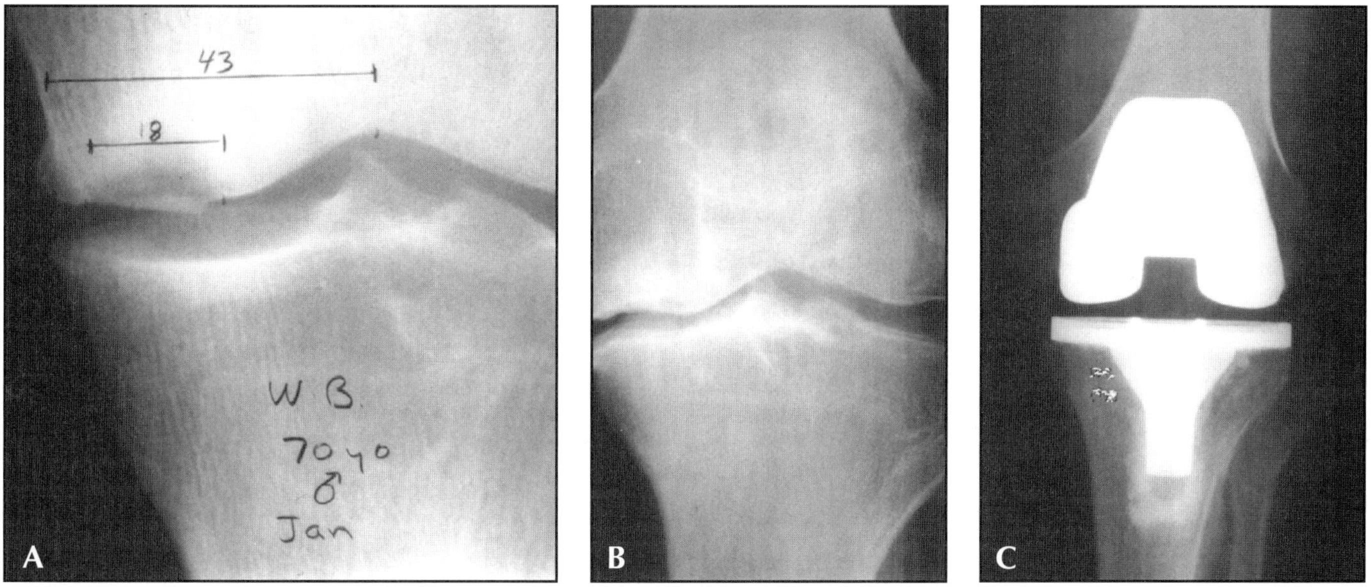

Fig. 1 Radiographs of a 70-year-old man who had sudden onset of pain and a relatively large (41%) lesion in the medial femoral condyle (**A**). Acute symptoms resolved with conservative treatment and the patient did well for 10 years. **B,** Ten years later, the patient has progressive osteoarthritis, increasing pain, and varus deformity. Note the saddle deformity indicative of old collapsing osteonecrosis. **C,** Patient has total knee replacement more than 10 years after original onset of symptoms and diagnosis of osteonecrosis.

65 years of age. Larger lesions and older patients tend to do better with unicompartmental arthroplasty.

Koshino[20] reported on 37 knees treated with proximal tibial osteotomy. Concomitant retrograde drilling or bone grafting behind the lesions was performed in 23 of these patients. At an average follow-up of 67 months and a minimum of 2 years, results were best when the proximal tibial osteotomy was combined with core decompression and bone grafting or with overcorrection of the femoral tibial axis greater than 10° of valgus. The necrotic lesion disappeared radiographically in 13 patients and improved in 17 patients. The results of proximal tibial osteotomy for osteonecrosis in which the preoperative malalignment was corrected were comparable to results obtained after proximal tibial osteotomy for primary arthritis. In the series by Koshino,[20] only one patient subsequently required prosthetic replacement at the follow-up period.

Prosthetic Replacement

Osteonecrosis with debilitating symptoms after failure of conservative therapy or other surgical efforts may be successfully treated with a prosthetic resurfacing arthroplasty (Fig. 1). It is also a viable option in elderly patients who show significant subchondral structural collapse and are significantly disabled by their symptoms.

Proponents of unicompartmental arthroplasty effectively argue that there is a role for unicompartmental replacement of spontaneous osteonecrosis involving one condyle or one tibial plateau. Marmor[21] reported 88% good or excellent results in 34 knees treated with a unicompartmental arthroplasty. Two of his four failures occurred because of subsequent development of symptomatic osteonecrosis in the untreated compartment. Two other failures occurred because of subsidence into compromised bone stock. Clearly, in the setting of osteonecrosis, the possibility of subsequent osteonecrosis of the opposite compartment is a critical concern. Another possibility is that the medial compartment was overstuffed and so increased the pressure on the lateral compartment. Preoperative MRI should be performed to carefully assess the contralateral compartment of the knee when considering a unicompartmental arthroplasty. Any changes involving the epiphysis of metaphyseal bone should be considered as compromised osseous structures that may predispose the subsidence and compromise the long-term survivorship.

Total knee arthroplasty has also produced good and excellent results in well over 94% of patients. Careful review of the literature of these results of total knee arthroplasty for spontaneous osteonecrosis suggests that while satisfactory results are obtainable, there is need to remain guarded in the final results.[22] Ritter and associates[23] reported on 32 knees with spontaneous osteonecrosis of the medial femoral condyle. Using Kaplan-Meier survivorship analyses, the authors reported inferior results compared with

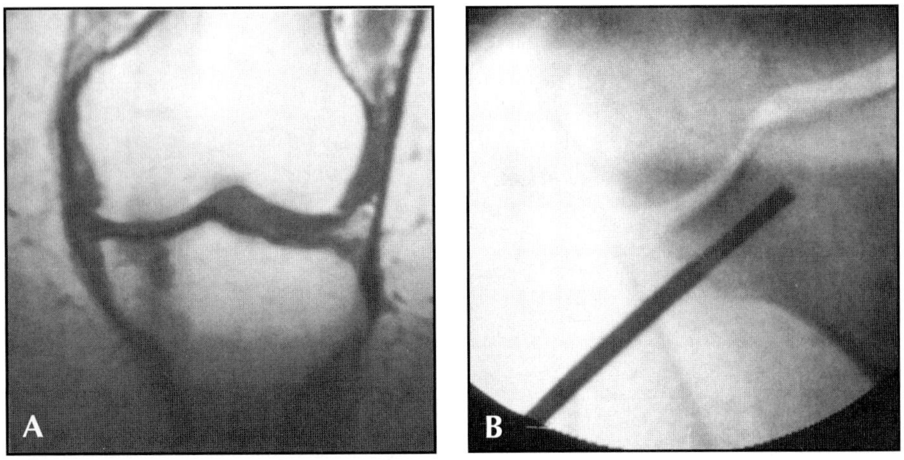

Fig. 2 A and **B**, Radiographs of a 58-year-old woman with medial tibial pain and type B signal changes in the tibial metaphysis from osteonecrosis (**A**). Core decompression of the tibial lesion with fluoroscopically guided trocar is shown (**B**).

matched groups of patients with osteoarthritis. This result is with the posterior cruciate retaining prosthesis. Using pain relief as an end point, the 5-year postoperative success rate was 82% for osteonecrosis and 90% for their osteoarthritic population. Although there was not a statistically significant difference, the authors noted the small sample size prevented attainment of ample statistical power to illustrate a difference between these two groups. At 7 years, 17% of patients with osteonecrosis required revision compared with 0% in the group with osteoarthritis.

Results for total knee arthroplasty in a group of 36 patients with osteonecrosis of the femoral condyles reported by Bergman and Rand,[24] at a mean follow-up of 4 years, were good or excellent in 87% of the patients. Implant survivorship at 5 years was predicted to be 85% using the end point of revision arthroplasty. However, there was only a 68% survivorship when moderate or severe pain was used as a criterion for failure. Although the authors did not find any clinical radiographic evidence of loosening, it is possible that the significant pain resulted when subchondral metaphyseal bone support was compromised by the focus of osteonecrosis.

Tibial Osteonecrosis

Proper recognition of the syndrome is fundamental to appropriate treatment.[25] Typically, elderly patients complain of severe pain in the medial side of the knee, and MRI images show a degenerative meniscal tear in most of these patients. Therefore, if the clinical indications are severe enough, a radionuclide scan should be considered before proceeding with arthroscopic intervention. This scan is particularly important if the MRI was obtained within the first 6 weeks of onset of symptoms, because MRI changes indicative of osteonecrosis may develop weeks after the onset of symptoms.[26]

The treatment for smaller lesions, confined in the metaphysis without evidence of collapse or osteonecrotic serpiginous lines, is generally conservative.[27] They almost always improve, although it may take a long period of time (6 to 9 months). If the patients are very symptomatic and there appears to be well-localized lesion in the tibial metaphysis, best visualized in MRI T2 fat-suppression images, an extra-articular decompression may be considered for relief of pain. Otherwise, conservative management includes the use of nonsteroidal anti-inflammatory medications, analgesia, and activities to tolerance. A cane or crutches may offer some relief during the early onset of symptoms.

In large lesions, where there is definite evidence of osteonecrosis as shown by a low-signal serpiginous line extending into the subchondral zone with or without collapse, the treatment will depend on the temporal recognition of the lesion. If the lesion is still early and without collapse, and the symptoms are very intense, a core decompression may be considered (Fig. 2). There are no firm data at this time to determine if the decompression will prevent collapse of the lesion, but it will reduce the acute symptoms. If the lesion has already collapsed into the subchondral zone, and particularly if it can be visualized on standard radiographs, the prognosis is generally much poorer and most of these patients will need a unicompartmental arthroplasty or total knee arthroplasty. The choice between unicompartmental or total knee replacement depends on the status of the rest of the joint and the surgeon's preference.

Conservative treatment should always be attempted in patients with tibial osteonecrosis. These patients are characterized by advanced age, frequently have other associated degenerative changes in the joint, and almost universally have some meniscal degenerative or signal changes. Indeed, accurate recognition that the symptoms may be coming from the subchondral zone and not the meniscus may save the patients from unnecessary surgery. In addition, if the MRI lesions typical of osteonecrosis develop later, conservative therapy would delay an arthroscopic intervention and may save the surgeon embarrassment if the subchondral lesion proceeds to collapse.

In summary, tibial osteonecrosis occurs on the tibial side of the knee. Patients with tibial osteonecrosis initially have findings similar to those of patients with osteonecrosis of the femoral condyle.

There is sudden pain in the medial side of the knee associated with a spectrum of MRI changes into the subchondral bone. The small lesions will resolve, and minimal residual scar remains in the subchondral bone on MRI. If the lesion is large, it can collapse and show MRI changes of true osteonecrosis. Recognition of this problem may avoid unnecessary surgical intervention. Once collapse has occurred, an arthroplasty is generally the treatment of choice.

Steroid-Induced Osteonecrosis

Steroid-induced osteonecrosis of the knee is a relatively uncommon but debilitating clinical problem that frequently occurs in younger patients and is associated with a variety of disease states. Location and progression of the necrosis may lead to subchondral bone collapse, joint incongruity, and subsequent articular cartilage destruction and may require an arthroplasty. Steroid-induced osteonecrosis of the knee produces a more diffuse pattern of bone necrosis in the distal femur and proximal tibia than does idiopathic osteonecrosis of the knee. The treatment of steroid-induced osteonecrosis will depend on whether the osteonecrotic defect affects the subchondral bone and allows for intra-articular joint collapse. If there is no evidence of joint collapse and pain is intense, core decompression may be considered as a treatment alternative. On the other hand, once the joint surface has been compromised with structural collapse, a knee arthroplasty will be required.

As noted above, if the pain is very intense and the area of principal involvement of necrosis can be identified, then a core decompression may offer relief of symptoms and possibly slow the progression of the disease process. A gadolinium-enhanced MRI scan will be helpful in identifying the location of the symptomatic lesion. Mont and associates[28] reported a series of 79 knees with steroid-induced osteonecrosis. Thirty-two of these knees were treated with conservative modalities, including protected weight bearing, rest, and analgesia. Of these patients, 82% failed and went on to undergo a total knee arthroplasty. A matched group of patients with 47 knees were drilled with good relief of the initial acute symptoms, and only 27% of them failed and went on to total knee arthroplasty. This relatively long-term follow-up study suggested that core decompression might slow the rate of symptomatic progression of steroid-induced osteonecrosis of the knee. In addition, core decompression may extend the symptom-free interval in certain patients with extensive involvement and may delay the need for a knee arthroplasty.

Once there is collapse of the subchondral bone with loss of the joint congruity and subsequent destruction, the need for total knee replacement is evident. However, the structural integrity of large areas of necrotic bone in the knee may adversely effect the fixation and support of total knee arthroplasty. There are only a few series of outcome studies on total knee arthroplasties for steroid-induced osteonecrosis, and these have only had a few cases or anecdotal reports. The largest series is by Seldes and associates.[29] This study reports on 31 knees that had total knee arthroplasties with steroid-induced osteonecrosis. Their average follow-up was 64 months, and they noted an 84% survivorship, with 16% requiring revision. There were an increased number of complications; 19% of the patients had complications. The higher complication rate was attributed, at least in part, to the severity of the patient's underlying disease processes. The authors believe that total knee arthroplasty can be a successful procedure for the chronically ill patient with steroid-induced osteonecrosis.

Summary

There are several options for the treatment of patients with osteonecrosis about the knee. Three appear to be the most effective and include conservative treatment for small lesions without evidence of structural collapse, core decompression for relief of pain and possible delay in structural collapse in the patients with steroid-induced osteonecrosis, and either unicompartmental or total knee arthroplasty. Although other modalities have been reported, these three remain the most widely reported and generally offer the greatest success. With better recognition of these problems, longer duration follow-up, and larger patient series, the answers to the best treatment regimen will become better defined.

References

1. al-Rowaih A, Bjorkengren A, Egund N, Lindstrand A, Wingstrand H, Thorngren KG: Size of osteonecrosis of the knee. *Clin Orthop* 1993;287:68-75.
2. Lotke PA, Abend JA, Ecker ML: The treatment of osteonecrosis of the medial femoral condyle. *Clin Orthop* 1982;171:109-116.
3. Motohashi M, Morii T, Koshino T: Clinical course and roentgenographic changes of osteonecrosis in the femoral condyle under conservative treatment. *Clin Orthop* 1991;266:156-161.
4. Insall JN, Aglietti P, Bullough PG, Windsor RE: Osteonecrosis, in Insall JN, Windsor RE, Scott WN, Kelly MA, Aglietti P (eds): *Surgery of the Knee*, ed 2. New York, NY, Churchill Livingstone, 1993, vol 2, pp 609-633.
5. Steinberg ME, Hayken GD, Steinberg DR: Classification and staging of osteonecrosis, in Urbaniak JR, Jones JP Jr (eds): *Osteonecrosis: Etiology, Diagnosis, and Treatment*. Rosemont, IL, American Academy of Orthopaedic Surgeons, 1997, pp 277-284.
6. Jacobs MA, Loeb PE, Hungerford DS: Core decompression of the distal femur for avascular necrosis of the knee. *J Bone Joint Surg Br* 1989;71:583-587.
7. Forst J, Forst R, Heller KD, Adam G: Spontaneous osteonecrosis of the femoral condyle: Causal treatment by early core decompression. *Arch Orthop Trauma Surg* 1998;117:18-22.
8. Forst J, Forst R, Heller KD, Adam GB: Core decompression in Ahlback's disease: Follow-up and therapy control using MR tomography. *Rofo Fortschr Geb Rontgenstr Neuen Bildgeb Verfahr* 1994;161:142-146.
9. Miller GK, Maylahn DJ, Drennan DB: The treatment of idiopathic osteonecrosis of the medial femoral condyle with arthroscopic debridement. *Arthroscopy* 1986;2:21-29.
10. Koshino T, Okamoto R, Takamura K, Tsuchiya K: Arthroscopy in spontaneous osteonecrosis of the knee. *Orthop Clin North Am* 1979; 10:609-618.

11. Brahme SK, Fox JM, Ferkel RD, Friedman MJ, Flannigan BD, Resnick DL: Osteonecrosis of the knee after arthroscopic surgery: Diagnosis with MR imaging. *Radiology* 1991;178:851-853.

12. Santori N, Condello V, Adriani E, Mariani PP: Osteonecrosis after arthroscopic medial meniscectomy. *Arthroscopy* 1995;11:220-224.

13. Bayne O, Langer F, Pritzker KP, Houpt J, Gross AE: Osteochondral allografts in the treatment of osteonecrosis of the knee. *Orthop Clin North Am* 1985;16:727-740.

14. Convery FR, Meyers MH, Akeson WH: Fresh osteochondral allografting of the femoral condyle. *Clin Orthop* 1991;273:139-145.

15. de la Caffinière JY: Autologous osteochondral graft: A method for resurfacing osteonecrosis of the medial femoral condyle in the elderly. *Rev Chir Orthop* 1978;64:653-660.

16. Marco F, Lopez-Oliva F, Fernandez Fernandez-Arroyo JM, et al: Osteochondral allografts for osteochondritis dissecans and osteonecrosis of the femoral condyles. *Int Orthop* 1993;17: 104-108.

17. Meyers MH, Akeson W, Convery FR: Resurfacing of the knee with fresh osteochondral allograft. *J Bone Joint Surg Am* 1989;71:704-713.

18. Flynn JM, Springfield DS, Mankin HJ: Osteoarticular allografts to treat distal femoral osteonecrosis. *Clin Orthop* 1994;303:38-43.

19. Soucacos PN, Xenakis TH, Beris AE, Soucacos PK, Georgoulis A: Idiopathic osteonecrosis of the medial femoral condyle: Classification and treatment. *Clin Orthop* 1997;341:82-89.

20. Koshino T: The treatment of spontaneous osteonecrosis of the knee by high tibial osteotomy with and without bone-grafting or drilling of the lesion. *J Bone Joint Surg Am* 1982;64:47-58.

21. Marmor L: Unicompartmental arthroplasty for osteonecrosis of the knee joint. *Clin Orthop* 1993;294:247-253.

22. Stern SH, Insall JI, Windsor RW: Total knee arthroplasty in osteonecrotic knees. *Orthop Trans* 1988;12:722-723.

23. Ritter MA, Eizember LE, Keating EM, Faris PM: The survival of total knee arthroplasty in patients with osteonecrosis of the medial condyle. *Clin Orthop* 1991;267:108-114.

24. Bergman NR, Rand JA: Total knee arthroplasty in osteonecrosis. *Clin Orthop* 1991;273:77-82.

25. Lotke PA, Ecker ML, Barth P, Lonner JH: Subchondral magnetic resonance imaging changes in early osteoarthrosis associated with tibial osteonecrosis. *Arthroscopy* 2000;16:76-81.

26. Nakamura T, Matsumoto T, Nishino M, Tomita K, Kadoya M: Early magnetic resonance imaging and histologic findings in a model of femoral head necrosis. *Clin Orthop* 1997; 334:68-72.

27. Lotke PA: Tibial osteonecrosis, in Urbaniak JR, Jones JP Jr (eds): *Osteonecrosis: Etiology, Diagnosis, and Treatment.* Rosemont, IL, American Academy of Orthopaedic Surgeons, 1997, pp 425-428.

28. Mont MA, Tomek IM, Hungerford DS: Core decompression for avascular necrosis of the distal femur: Long-term follow-up. *Clin Orthop* 1997;334:124-130.

29. Seldes RM, Tan V, Duffy G, Rand JA, Lotke PA: Total knee arthroplasty for steroid-induced osteonecrosis. *J Arthroplasty* 1999;14:533-537.

50

Steroid-Associated Osteonecrosis of the Knee: A Comprehensive Review

Kyle Low, MD
Michael A. Mont, MD
David S. Hungerford, MD

Introduction

The knee is second to the hip as the most common area affected by osteonecrosis. Osteonecrosis of the knee occurs in approximately 10% of patients with osteonecrosis of the hip. The disease was first described by Ahlbäck and associates[1] in 1968 and was initially believed to be a single entity. Osteonecrosis of the knee represents two distinct entities, spontaneous osteonecrosis of the knee and steroid-associated osteonecrosis, that share a common pathology. This chapter will focus on the evaluation, pathophysiology, and treatment of steroid-associated osteonecrosis.

Clinical Issues

Steroid-associated osteonecrosis occurs primarily in patients younger than 45 years of age. Women are three to four times more likely to be affected by the disease than men. Patients commonly have an immunocompromising disorder such as systemic lupus erythematosus. Patients have a gradual onset of pain that is localized over the medial or lateral condyle, with the knee examination otherwise unremarkable. The process is bilateral approximately 80% of the time and about 90% of patients have associated hip osteonecrosis involvement. The lesions are typically found on both tibial and femoral condyles and are larger relative to the areas observed in spontaneous osteonecrosis of the knee. A corticosteroid association is common, but is not the only risk factor. Patients with a history of alcoholism,[2,3] Caisson's decompression disease,[4] Gaucher's disease,[5] trauma, arthroscopic meniscectomy (especially with lasers) and those who have undergone anterior cruciate ligament reconstruction are at increased risk of the disease.

Pathogenesis/Pathophysiology

It is still unclear what role corticosteroids play in causing osteonecrosis. Much of what is known about steroid-associated osteonecrosis of the knee is derived from the current understanding of osteonecrosis in the hip. Based on that knowledge, many theories have developed regarding the pathogenesis of steroid-associated osteonecrosis of the knee.

Direct cellular toxicity has been proposed as a mechanism in which steroids can cause osteonecrosis. In animals exposed to steroids, fat has been seen in higher amounts in osteocytes and marrow and this is thought to be toxic to the cells. Unfortunately, no animal models have developed with the same severity of collapse seen in humans.[6,7] Further investigation is needed in this area.

The accumulation of fat in the marrow and osteocytes not only may cause direct cell toxicity, but may also cause an increase in bone marrow pressure. Because cortical bone encloses the cancellous bone, along with marrow, any additional fat can easily increase the intramedullary pressure. The increase in pressure can then cause collapse of the nutrient vessels onto the bone, leading to decreased blood flow, ischemia, and resulting osteonecrosis. It is well documented that areas of osteonecrosis are associated with elevated bone marrow pressure,[8] but it is not known if the increased pressure is the cause or the result of the necrosis. This cellular hypertrophy can be a result of corticosteroid therapy, as well as Caisson's disease, leukemia, or Gaucher's disease.

Lipid emboli of intravascular fat have been proposed as a possible cause of steroid-associated osteonecrosis of the knee.[6,7] It is believed that corticosteroids, as well as gout and alcohol, cause hyperlipidemia. The hyperlipidemia may then cause formation of lipid emboli, which can disrupt circulation.

Steroids may interact with other etiologies, making osteonecrosis a multifactorial disease process.[9] The steroids may be part of a cascade of events. For instance, the steroids may be cytotoxic, which causes cell death, resulting in bone marrow edema and vessel compression. Another example is that the steroids may cause hyperlipidemia that causes lipid emboli to be lodged in the microvasculature. The steroids may also exacerbate a mild condition. For example, a patient may have a subtle hypercoagulable state that may be made worse with the steroids, leading to infarcts in the bone.

Many other mechanisms have been proposed to explain the pathophysiology of this disease. It is well known that osteonecrosis of the femoral head can occur after femoral neck fractures. It is therefore reasonable to believe that osteonecrosis of the knee can occur after trauma. Blunt trauma may disrupt the microvasculature of the knee, resulting in osteonecrosis.

Osteonecrosis may occur following surgery as well. Osteonecrosis of the knee following arthroscopy and meniscectomy with[10,11] and without YAG-lasers[12-14] has been reported. Prues-Latour and associates[13] described nine instances of osteonecrosis of the knee that developed after knee arthroscopy. The patients' average age was 69 years (range, 58 to 82 years). The osteonecrotic lesions were not present on MRI prior to surgery, but lesions were identified by MRI 6 to 48 weeks after surgery. It is believed that the osteonecrosis may be a result of the fluid pressures used during arthroscopy. During arthroscopy, the knee is filled with sterile saline. This process causes an increase in intra-articular pressure that may occlude vessels, resulting in ischemia and eventual osteonecrosis.

Hypofibrinolysis and thrombophilia are coagulation disorders that have both been studied as possible causes of osteonecrosis.[15-18] Thrombophilia is a condition that predisposes patients to forming intravascular thrombi, and hypofibrinolysis is a state in which dissolution of clots takes longer than normal. More than 70% of patients with osteonecrosis have been found to have abnormal levels of certain coagulation factors. Theoretically, these patients may be treated with anticoagulants that may prevent or partially reverse the disease process.

Intravascular coagulation secondary to an autoimmune phenomenon has been studied as well. It is possible that immune complexes are deposited into the vasculature, which may cause venous or arterial damage and eventual osteonecrosis. Animal models with this condition have been found. After corticosteroids were given, osteonecrosis-like lesions developed, although these lesions were metaphyseal and diaphyseal. This pattern is different from that of epiphyseal human lesions, which eventually collapse. The relevance of the animal model studies to the human condition is unclear.

Pathology

The cascade of pathologic events after exposure to the etiology, regardless of the mechanism, is similar in all cases. The causative factor leads to decreased oxygen in the bone. Electrolytes pass through the cell membrane as permeability increases secondary to the hypoxic state. Fluids then enter the cell and lysosomes release degradation enzymes. The action of these enzymes, in addition to the fluid swelling, causes cell lysis. Cell death leads to an inflammatory state with associated edema.

On a larger scale, the center of the region of osteonecrosis usually remains avascular, but sometimes may revascularize. There is more vascularity at the periphery and healing can begin in that area. The osteoclasts and macrophages remove dead bone and tissue. Granulation tissue, followed by fibrous tissue, is then laid down. Osteoblasts then start to form new bone over the dead areas. The resulting bone is much thicker than normal. If the lesion is small it may heal completely. Alternatively, the bone may heal with the center composed of dead bone. Both of these scenarios would result in a painless knee. Larger lesions do not heal well, especially in weight-bearing areas. Unfortunately, bone resorption occurs more quickly than the bone formation. Cancellous bone starts to disappear with continued cell death. Fluid begins to fill the space devoid of bone, leading to the classic crescent sign that is associated with osteonecrosis. As more bone dies, the articular surface starts to flatten and collapse. Even with collapse and bone death, the articular cartilage continues to survive with the help of nutrients supplied by the synovial fluid. Because of the changing mechanics of the knee, more stresses are placed on the articular cartilage, eventually leading to chondrocyte death. Secondary degenerative changes (joint space narrowing, sclerosis, cyst formation, osteophytes) then occur.

Radiographic Evaluation

Anteroposterior (AP), lateral, and sunrise plain radiographic views should be obtained in patients suspected of having osteonecrosis of the knee. In the early stage of the disease process, the radiographic findings may be negative. As the disease worsens, there will be a radiolucent area that develops in the subchondral bone surrounded by a sclerotic ring. Subtle collapse of the surface may be seen. As more bone is lost, the subchondral bone further collapses and the sclerotic ring becomes thicker. Toward the end of the process, there is total bone destruction with associated secondary changes such as joint space narrowing, osteophytes, involvement of the opposite side of the joint, and squaring of the condyles.

MRI is much more sensitive than plain films for detecting osteonecrosis.[19,20] T1-weighted images show an area of low signal intensity surrounded by an area of intermediate signal intensity in the zone of osteonecrosis. On the T2-weighted images, the areas of necrosis appear as an area of low signal intensity surrounded by high signal intensity. The high signal intensity is most likely from associated edema. MRI is the preferred diagnostic test because it is 99% sensitive.

Bone scans have been used as a diagnostic test for osteonecrosis. A recent study compared MRI to bone scans for sensitivity of diagnosing osteo-

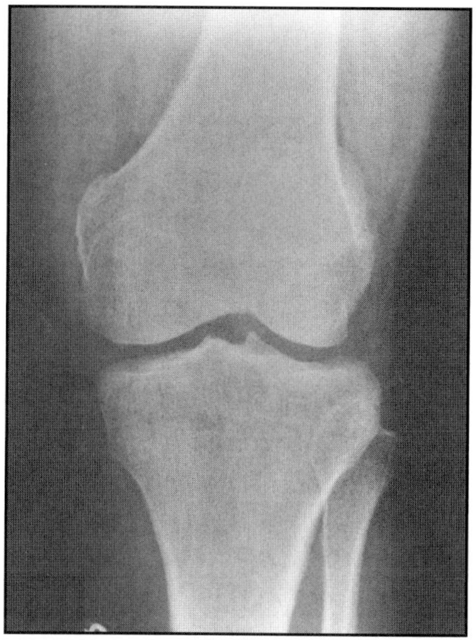

Fig. 1 AP plain radiographic view of a knee with stage I osteonecrosis. No lesions are seen.

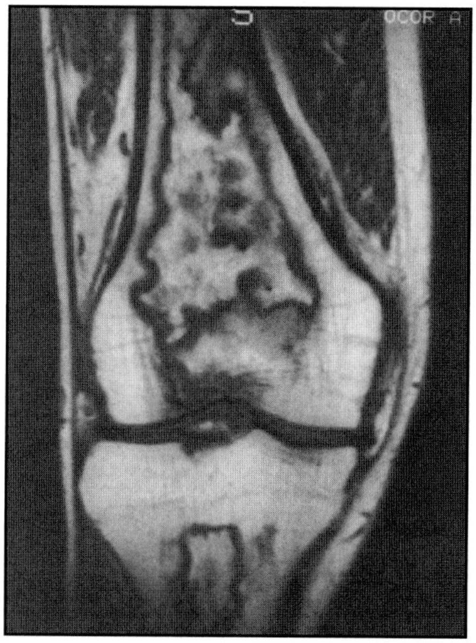

Fig. 2 T1-weighted MRI study of the same knee as in Figure 1. Areas of low signal intensity are surrounded by areas of intermediate signal intensity.

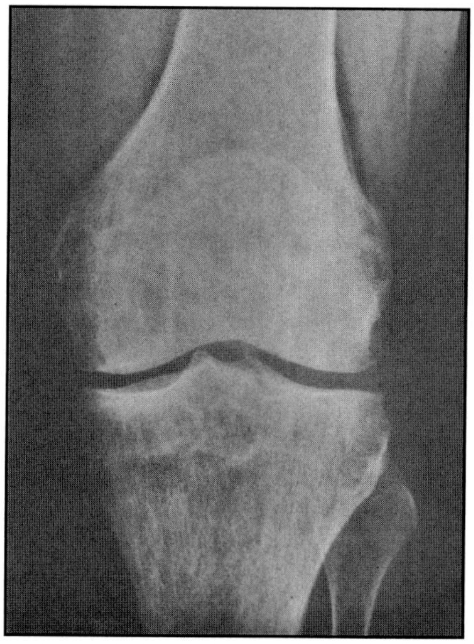

Fig. 3 AP plain radiographic view of a knee with stage II osteonecrosis. Sclerotic and cystic changes are forming.

necrosis. Twenty-four patients were found to have 89 lesions by MRI and histology. Bone scans were only able to detect 55% of the lesions.

Staging

There are many staging systems used for classification of steroid-associated osteonecrosis of the knee. One staging system is based on the Ficat and Arlet system[21] for staging osteonecrosis of the hip. Stage I disease consists of positive changes on MRI, despite negative radiographic findings (Figs. 1 and 2). In stage II, sclerotic and cystic changes are seen on radiographs (Fig. 3). Stage III is associated with subchondral collapse (Fig. 4), and stage IV denotes arthritic changes on both sides of the joint (Fig. 5).

Differential Diagnosis

Prior to establishing a diagnosis of osteonecrosis, various disease processes should be ruled out. These include osteochondritis dissecans, meniscal tears, transient osteonecrosis of the knee, bone bruise, and pes anserine bursitis.

Osteochondritis dissecans of the knee is a disease common in young patients (age 15 to 20 years). Males are affected two to three times more often than females. A history of trauma is given in 50% of cases and the symptoms are gradual in onset. The pain is vague, diffuse, and associated with exercise. Patients may experience acute pain and locking if there is detachment of an osteochondral fragment. It is believed that osteochondritis dissecans of the knee is caused by repetitive overloading of the knee that leads to focal bone damage. The posterolateral aspect of the medial femoral condyle near the intercondylar notch is the most commonly involved area (80% of cases). Diagnosis can be made by plain films, but MRI of the knee can be obtained if the diagnosis is still questionable.

Meniscal tears can mimic osteonecrosis of the knee. The tears can be traumatic (as in valgus–external rotation or varus–internal rotation movements) or degenerative. Patients of all ages may present with meniscal tears. The medial meniscus is more commonly involved than the lateral meniscus. Patients usually present with acute onset of pain and intermittent swelling, and they may also experience popping and locking of the joint. Joint line tenderness and effusion are common findings. The diagnosis is usually confirmed with MRI. Physicians treating a meniscal tear in the setting of osteonecrosis of the knee must be aware that the condition of some patients actually worsens following debridement of the meniscus under arthroscopy.

Bone bruise and transient osteopenia of the knee can be confused with osteonecrosis of the knee. This processes are self-limited and the diagnosis is made primarily by MRI of the knee.

Pes anserine bursitis may be associated with pain over the medial side of the knee. The pain is localized over the proximal medial tibia below the joint line. Swelling and thickening of the bursae can be palpated over the area of tenderness. The diagnosis can be confirmed with an injection of lidocaine into the affected area or by MRI.

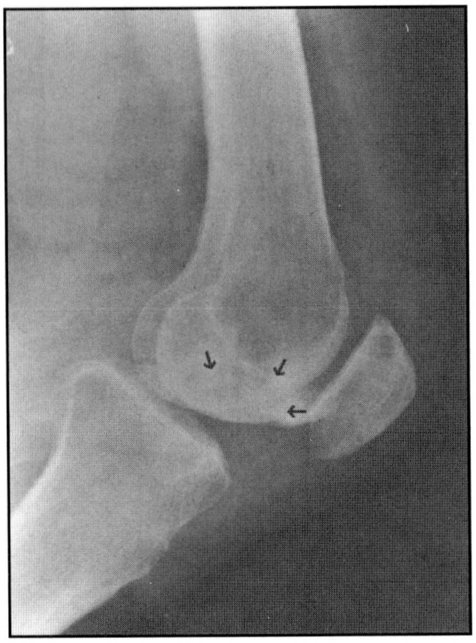

Fig. 4 Lateral plain radiographic view of a knee with stage III osteonecrosis. Subchondral collapse can be seen (arrows).

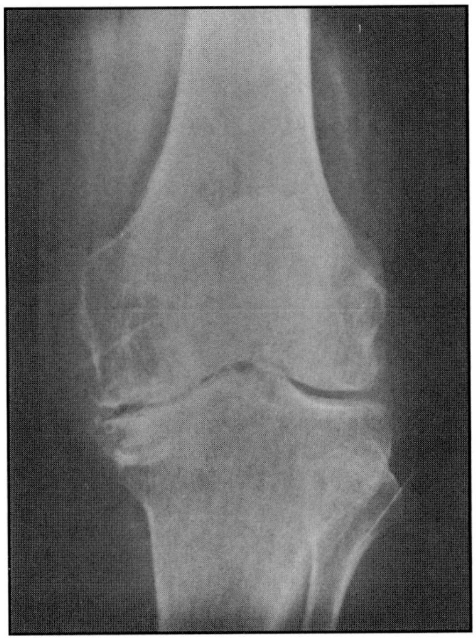

Fig. 5 AP plain radiographic view of a knee with stage IV osteonecrosis. Secondary arthritic changes (joint space narrowing, osteophytes) can be seen on the tibial and femoral surfaces.

Treatment

Several surgical and nonsurgical treatments for steroid-associated osteonecrosis are available; however, nonsurgical treatments have not been as successful as surgery. This factor may be directly related to the large size of most lesions. Mont and associates[22] reported on follow-up results of 32 knees treated nonsurgically. Only 59% had good or excellent results at 2 years, and only 18% of the knees were doing well at 6 years without the need for total knee arthroplasty. Therefore, surgery is currently the treatment of choice.

Arthroscopic débridement has been used to treat steroid-associated osteonecrosis. The results have been mixed.[23,24] Miller and associates[23] treated five knees with arthroscopic débridement and at 31 months' follow-up, results were good in four. They believed that arthroscopy did not change the course of the disease. Wiedel[24] reported results on the study of 10 patients with steroid-associated osteonecrosis of the knees treated by arthroscopic débridement. The author believed that the results were good and that arthroscopy was an effective treatment.

Osteochondral allografts have been used in a few studies as a treatment for knee osteonecrosis.[25,26] Bayne and associates[25] reported on a series of 21 knees treated with fresh nonfrozen allografts. Three of the knees had steroid-associated osteonecrosis, and treatment in all three knees was unsuccessful. This failure was thought to be the result of continued steroid use that caused poor graft incorporation. Flynn and associates[26] reported on a series of 17 knees treated with fresh frozen allograft. At mean follow up of 4.2 years (range, 2 to 9 years), 70% had a good outcome. Perez-Carro and associates[27] published a case report describing arthroscopic placement of bone graft following core decompression for osteonecrosis of the knee and reported a successful outcome. Thus, the information from these studies concerning osteochondral allografts for treating steroid-associated osteonecrosis is limited.

The results of core decompression have been reported by Mont and associates[22] in a series of 47 knees. Eighty-one percent of the knees (34 of 42 knees) had good or excellent results. Patients reported immediate relief that was often sustained (74% success at 10.4 years). Forst and associates[28] also published a report on the use of core decompression in 16 patients with steroid-associated osteonecrosis of the knee. All of these patients experienced immediate relief and did well clinically following the procedure. Core decompression has been very successful in delaying the need for total knee arthroplasty in a large portion of the patient population.

Core decompression is a relatively minor procedure that can be performed on an outpatient basis. Areas of pain are first determined by physical examination. MRI can delineate the extent and location of the disease. The areas to be cored can then be determined. For tibial cores, a small incision is made slightly medial to the tibial tubercle, being careful to avoid the medial saphenous nerve. With the use of fluoroscopy, a 3- to 6-mm Michel trephine is positioned and guided into the medial and lateral plateaus within a few millimeters of the subchondral bone. For femoral cores, a small lateral or medial incision is made just above the flare of the condyle. The 3- to 6-mm Michel trephine is again used and placed into the metaphyseal flare and maneuvered into the medial and lateral femoral condyles within a few millimeters of subchondral bone.

Total knee arthroplasty is the only popular treatment for knees with severe condylar collapse. Mont and Hungerford[29] reported the results of 31 total knee replacements in patients with steroid-associated osteonecrosis of the knee. Fifty-five percent of patients showed good or excellent results at mean 8.2-year follow-up. When the patients with systemic lupus erythematosus were factored out, the remaining patients had excellent results. In the systemic lupus erythematosus patients, results were good in 44%. Seldes and associates[6] studied 31 total knee replacements, with similar results. At 64-month follow-up, 92% of the patients had clinical improvement, although 16% required revision. The 5-year survival rate of the revisions was 84%. Total knee arthroplasty is the only option for treating stage III and IV steroid-associated osteonecrosis of the knee or conditions in which other more conservative treatments have failed. Hopefully, reported results will improve with the use of later-generation prostheses.

Summary

Steroid-associated osteonecrosis of the knee is a disease of young patients (generally younger than 45 years old) who often have underlying immunocompromising disorders. Although many theories have been postulated, the exact pathophysiology of the disorder is still unknown. Precollapse lesions can be treated with core decompression for prolonged symptomatic relief. Later-stage lesions are treated with total knee replacements, which have less than optimal results reported to date.

References

1. Ahlbäck S, Bauer GC, Bohne WH: Spontaneous osteonecrosis of the knee. *Arthritis Rheum* 1968;11:705-733.
2. Hirota Y, Hirohata T, Fukuda K, et al: Association of alcohol intake, cigarette smoking, and occupational status with the risk of idiopathic osteonecrosis of the femoral head. *Am J Epidemiol* 1993;137:530-538.
3. Hungerford DS, Zizic TM: Alcoholism associated ischemic necrosis of the femoral head: Early diagnosis and treatment. *Clin Orthop* 1978;130:144-153.
4. Amstutz HC, Noordin S, Campbell PA, Schmalzried TP: Precision fit surface hemiarthroplasty for femoral head osteonecrosis, in Urbaniak JR, Jones JP Jr (eds): *Osteonecrosis: Etiology, Diagnosis, and Treatment*. Rosemont, IL, American Academy of Orthopaedic Surgeons, 1997, pp 373-383.
5. Jones JP Jr: Etiology and pathogenesis of osteonecrosis. *Semin Arthroplasty* 1991;2: 160-168.
6. Seldes RM, Tan V, Duffy G, Rand JA, Lotke PA: Total knee arthroplasty for steroid-induced osteonecrosis. *J Arthroplasty* 1999;14:533-537.
7. Wang GJ, Moga DB, Richemer WG, Sweet DE, Reger SI, Thompson RC: Cortisone induced bone changes and its response to lipid clearing agents. *Clin Orthop* 1978;130:81-85.
8. Cornell CN, Salvati EA, Pellicci PM: Long-term follow-up of total hip replacement in patients with osteonecrosis. *Orthop Clin North Am* 1985;16:757-769.
9. Amstutz HC, Thomas BJ, Jinnah R, Kim W, Grogan T, Yale C: Treatment of primary osteoarthritis of the hip: A comparison of total joint and surface replacement arthroplasty. *J Bone Joint Surg Am* 1984;66:228-241.
10. Fink B, Schneider T, Braunstein S, Schmielau G, Ruther W: Holmium: YAG laser-induced aseptic bone necroses of the femoral condyle. *Arthroscopy* 1996;12:217-223.
11. Rozbruch SR, Wickiewicz TL, DiCarlo EF, Potter HG: Osteonecrosis of the knee following arthroscopic laser meniscectomy. *Arthroscopy* 1996;12:245-250.
12. Muscolo DL, Costa-Paz M, Makino A, Ayerza MA: Osteonecrosis of the knee following arthroscopic meniscectomy in patients over 50-years old. *Arthroscopy* 1996;12:273-279.
13. Prues-Latour V, Bonvin JC, Fritschy D: Nine cases of osteonecrosis in elderly patients following arthroscopic meniscectomy. *Knee Surg Sports Traumatol Arthrosc* 1998;6:142-147.
14. Santori N, Condello V, Adriani E, Mariani PP: Osteonecrosis after arthroscopic medial meniscectomy. *Arthroscopy* 1995;11:220-224.
15. Glueck CJ, Freiberg R, Tracy T, Stroop D, Wang P: Thrombophilia and hypofibrinolysis: Pathophysiologies of osteonecrosis. *Clin Orthop* 1997;334:43-56.
16. Hungerford DS: Pathogenetic considerations in ischemic necrosis of bone. *Can J Surg* 1981;24:583-587,590.
17. Hungerford DS: Core decompression for the treatment of avascular necrosis of the femoral head. *Semin Arthroplasty* 1991;2:182-188.
18. Hungerford DS, Lennox DW: The importance of increased intraosseous pressure in the development of osteonecrosis of the femoral head: Implications for treatment. *Orthop Clin North Am* 1985;16:635-654.
19. Bjorkengren AG, Al-Rowaih A, Lindstrand A, Wingstrand H, Thorngren KG, Pettersson H: Spontaneous osteonecrosis of the knee: Value of MR imaging in determining prognosis. *AJR Am J Roentgenol* 1990;154:331-336.
20. Healy WL: Osteonecrosis of the knee detected only by magnetic resonance imaging. *Orthopedics* 1991;14:703-704.
21. Ficat RP, Arlet J: Functional investigation of bone under normal conditions, in Ficat P, Arlet J, Hungerford DS (eds): *Ischemia and Necroses of Bone*. Baltimore, MD, Williams & Wilkins, 1980, pp 29-52.
22. Mont MA, Tomek IM, Hungerford DS: Core decompression for steroid-associated avascular necrosis of the femur. *Clin Orthop,* in press.
23. Miller GK, Maylahn DJ, Drennan DB: The treatment of idiopathic osteonecrosis of the medial femoral condyle with arthroscopic debridement. *Arthroscopy* 1986;2:21-29.
24. Wiedel JD: Arthroscopy in steroid-induced osteonecrosis of the knee. *Arthroscopy* 1985;1: 68-72.
25. Bayne O, Langer F, Pritzker KP, Houpt J, Gross AE: Osteochondral allografts in the treatment of osteonecrosis of the knee. *Orthop Clin North Am* 1985;16:727-740.
26. Flynn JM, Springfield DS, Mankin HJ: Osteoarticular allografts to treat distal femoral osteonecrosis. *Clin Orthop* 1994;303:38-43.
27. Perez-Carro L, Gomez-Cimiano FJ, Gomez del Alamo G, Garcia-Suarez G: Core decompression and arthroscopic bone grafting for avascular necrosis of the knee. *Arthroscopy* 1996;12:323-326.
28. Forst J, Forst R, Heller KD, Adam G: Spontaneous osteonecrosis of the femoral condyle: Causal treatment by early core decompression. *Arch Orthop Trauma Surg* 1998;117:18-22.
29. Mont MA, Hungerford DS: Osteonecrosis of the shoulder, knee, and ankle, in Urbaniak JR, Jones JP Jr (eds): *Osteonecrosis: Etiology, Diagnosis, and Treatment.* Rosemont, IL, American Academy of Orthopaedic Surgeons, 1997, pp 429-436.

51

Spontaneous Osteonecrosis of the Distal Femur

Malcolm L. Ecker, MD

Introduction

Spontaneous osteonecrosis of the knee was first reported as a distinct entity by Ahlbäck and associates[1] in 1968. Their series included 40 knees, all of which developed typical lesions in the medial femoral condyle, although the radiographs were initially normal in 12. The condition is also called idiopathic or primary osteonecrosis to distinguish it from secondary osteonecrosis, which is associated with corticosteroid therapy, blood dyscrasias, Gaucher's disease, Caisson's disease, systemic lupus erythematosus, and other rare conditions. Secondary osteonecrosis is more frequently bilateral, usually involves multiple joints, and has a different radiographic appearance.

Clinical Presentation

The usual complaint is the sudden onset of pain on the medial aspect of the knee that may or may not have been precipitated by a specific activity or minor injury. The condition is three times more common in women than men and most of the patients are older than age 60. During the acute phase, which may last 6 to 8 weeks, the pain is frequently worse at night. Depending on the size and stage of the lesion, the pain may either resolve or become a lower grade chronic pain.

Physical examination reveals a well localized area of tenderness over the affected condyle, just proximal to the joint line. In one series, the medial condyle was affected in 102 of 109 knees with spontaneous osteonecrosis of the femoral condyle.[2] The range of motion may be restricted in the acute phase from the pain and muscle spasm. Mild synovitis with a small effusion is common, but a large effusion is unusual. Ligamentous stability is normal.

Imaging Studies

Plain radiographs are obtained first. Radiographs categorize the disease process into five sequential stages. The process can be arrested at any stage, and only the most severe cases reach stage 5.[3] In stage 1, the radiograph is normal and the diagnosis is made using a radionuclide bone scan or MRI. In some patients, the symptoms resolve completely and a radiographic lesion never appears.[4] In stage 2 (Fig. 1, *A*), there is subtle flattening of the weight-bearing portion of the affected condyle that may easily be missed.

The typical lesion of osteonecrosis is seen in stage 3 (Fig. 1, *B*) and consists of a radiolucent area of variable size located in the subchondral bone and bordered proximally and laterally by a sclerotic halo. The lesion may be quantified by the ratio of the width of the lesion to the width of the condyle on the anteroposterior view. This measurement is unaffected by any magnification errors and has been shown to be as accurate a guide to prognosis as more complex measurements of area. Almost all knees with a ratio less than 0.45 have a better prognosis than those knees with a ratio greater than 0.50. MRI may allow further refinement of the prognosis in the early stages.

In stage 4 (Fig. 1, *C*), the sclerotic halo thickens and the subchondral bone begins to collapse. Stage 5 (Fig. 1, *D*) shows further collapse from stage 4 accompanied by secondary changes in the femoral condyle of osteophyte formation, joint space narrowing, and sclerosis. Secondary degenerative changes begin to appear on the tibial side of the joint.

In a series of 40 patients followed for 1 to 7 years, al-Rowaith and associates[5] found that the typical stage 3 lesion was present on the initial radiograph in 19 knees. In 14 of the remaining 21 knees, the typical lesion developed later, at a mean of 28 weeks. The radiograph remained normal in seven knees in which the diagnosis was made with a radionuclide bone scan, and symptoms resolved in all seven. Radionuclide bone scan or scintigraphy is now generally done using technetium-99m because of its short half life (6 hours) and because it is rapidly cleared from the bloodstream. The static-phase image demonstrates a focally intense area of uptake over the affected condyle. The localization of the increased uptake to only the femoral side of the joint is best seen on the lateral view. Increased uptake near the joint line in both the femur and tibia is more indicative of osteoarthritis. al-Rowaith and associates[6] found that the pool phase of a three-phase study did not add useful diagnostic information, but a persistent high-flow phase and static uptake for 6 to 12 months correlated directly with a poor clinical and radiologic outcome.

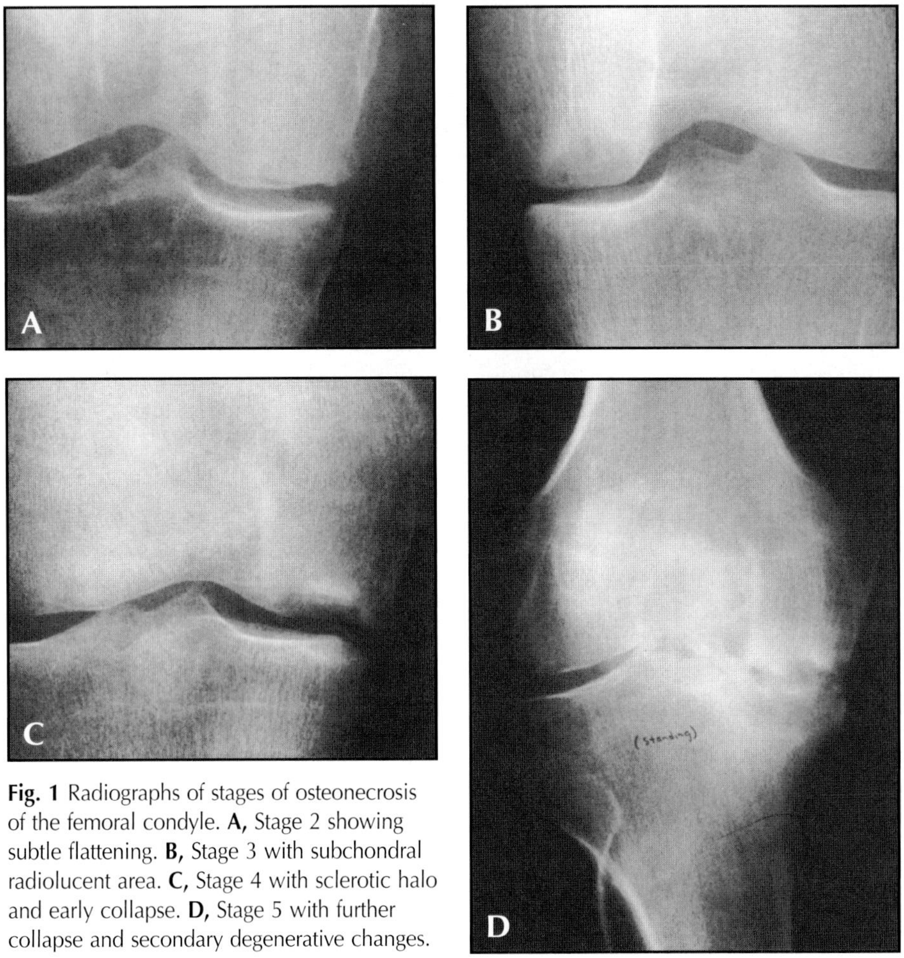

Fig. 1 Radiographs of stages of osteonecrosis of the femoral condyle. **A,** Stage 2 showing subtle flattening. **B,** Stage 3 with subchondral radiolucent area. **C,** Stage 4 with sclerotic halo and early collapse. **D,** Stage 5 with further collapse and secondary degenerative changes.

MRI has shown that the involvement of the condyles is more extensive than can be appreciated on plain radiographs. On the T1-weighted image, the high-intensity image usually produced by the fat in the marrow is replaced by a discrete subchondral area of low signal, sometimes surrounded by an area of intermediate signal intensity. On the T2-weighted images, an area of low signal intensity is surrounded by a variable high-intensity signal, which is thought to be caused by edema surrounding the lesion. Fat suppression images, which normally have low signal in the marrow, show high-intensity signal suggestive of edema that may extend deeply into the marrow (Fig. 2).

In a report by Pollack and associates[7] of 10 knees with classic symptoms of osteonecrosis with positive radionuclide bone scans and normal radiographs, 2 were normal on MRI. The authors theorized that the initial small lesion might have been missed on MRI because of the thickness of the slice.[7] Alternatively, the positive bone scan may have been caused by a condition other than osteonecrosis. Brahme and associates[8] reported on the results of seven patients in whom the initial MRI showed no suggestion of osteonecrosis and who underwent arthroscopic partial meniscectomy. Repeat MRI because of persistent or recurrent pain showed an area of low-intensity subchondral image on the T1-weighted image compatible with osteonecrosis. None of the patients had had a preoperative radionuclide bone scan. The authors theorized that the partial meniscectomy resulted in increased subchondral stress and microfractures but they did not consider that the MRI may have been done too early to detect osteonecrosis.[8] MRI evidence of degenerative meniscal tears is common in the elderly and may not be related to the patient's symptoms. In an analogous study in the canine hip, Nakamura and associates[9] found a delay in histologic and MRI changes after osteonecrosis was induced surgically. Minimal histologic change could be seen in as early as 3 days, but the MRI changes did not appear until an interface developed between the fibrous tissue and bone. At 2 weeks, only four of the seven animals had MRI changes, while all had MRI changes at 4 weeks.

Laboratory Studies

There are no specific abnormal laboratory findings related to spontaneous osteonecrosis.

Pathology

The term osteonecrosis implies that the death of the bone is the primary problem and that the subsequent collapse and overlying articular problems are secondary. With the more frequent use of arthroscopy, physicians are better able to correlate imaging findings with the appearance of the articular cartilage. Ahlbäck and associates[1] obtained core biopsy samples from six knees, all in the later stages of the disease process. The bone in the subchondral area was replaced with fibrous tissue in which there was some bone trabeculae, a few of which were necrotic.

In the early stages, the articular cartilage may show slight flattening and discoloration. As the disease process progresses, a line of demarcation and eventually the articular cartilage may fracture, producing a flap. Eventually the cartilage defect is filled with necrotic debris and the surrounding joint develops the characteristic pathology of osteoarthritis.

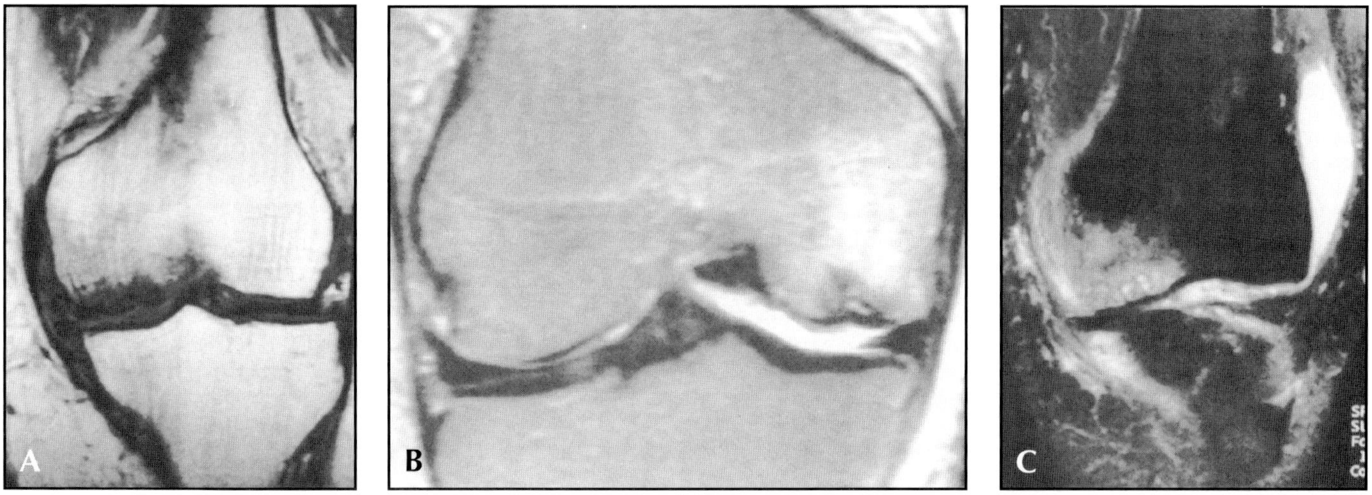

Fig. 2 MRI studies of osteonecrosis of the femoral condyle. **A,** T1-weighted image with discrete subchondral area of low signal. **B,** T2-weighted image with low signal area surrounded by variable high-intensity signal. **C,** Fat-suppression image with high-intensity signal suggestive of edema.

Microscopic analysis reveals dead bone associated with subchondral fracture and collapse. The dead bone in the center has empty lacunae and fatty degeneration. The surrounding area shows reparative bone formation, osteoblastic activity, cartilage formation, and bands of fibrovascular granulation tissue.[10] Pathology early in the course of the process, particularly before radiographic changes are evident, is difficult to obtain. Interestingly, in a series of five patients who were given technetium-99m just prior to undergoing arthroplasty for osteonecrosis, there was a high uptake in the center of the necrotic bone as well as in the surrounding bone.[11]

Etiology

The etiology of spontaneous osteonecrosis of the knee is unknown. Either a vascular or traumatic etiology has been theorized. Because the condition has yet to be experimentally produced and histology is lacking in the early stages of the problem, the discussions are suppositions, drawing on analogies with osteonecrosis of the femoral head. Various coagulopathies have been proposed and found to be more common in osteonecrosis of the hip, supposedly predisposing to thrombotic venous occlusion producing increasing compartment pressure and hypoxic bone death. This predisposition has not been demonstrated in patients with osteonecrosis of the femoral condyle.

The vascular theory proposes that interference with the microcirculation from unknown causes produces edema in the nonexpandable marrow compartment. The increased pressure further diminishes the circulation, producing osseous ischemia. This stage would correspond to the low signal intensity on T1-weighted images seen on the MRI study. If the dead bone collapses, the typical radiographic lesion is produced. If revascularization occurs before collapse, the lesion may heal and the symptoms resolve.

The traumatic theory notes that most of the patients with osteonecrosis of the femoral condyle are elderly women who are more likely to have some degree of osteoporosis. A minor injury might cause a microfracture in the more susceptible subchondral bone. At this stage the radionuclide study would be positive but the MRI could still be normal. Fluid may enter the marrow space through the fracture, increasing the pressure and causing the ischemia. At this point decreased signal would be seen on the MRI study. The lesion may then either progress or resolve.

Prognosis and Clinical Course

The clinical course and the eventual prognosis of spontaneous osteonecrosis of the femoral condyle depend on the extent of the involvement. Early in the disease process, even with normal radiographs, the extent can be evaluated from the radionuclide bone scan or the MRI study. The acute pain is usually intense for 6 to 8 weeks. If the radiograph is normal, a radionuclide bone scan should be done and must be positive to make the diagnosis of osteonecrosis. The MRI study may or may not show decreased signal early, the size of the lesion being a predictor of prognosis. The low-grade pain persists for 6 to 8 months. The process may then resolve with the smaller lesions in 12 to 15 months with no radiographic changes. The radionuclide scan becomes normal and the MRI changes resolve. If the lesion is larger, the symptoms persist and the typical radiographic changes appear and the course is as below.

If the radiographic lesion is less than 45% of the condylar width, the pain pattern is the same as that of patients with no radiographic changes. The mild pain may persist for 6 to 8 months and then gradually resolve. The radiographic lesion stabilizes and does not collapse further. Over the long term, the patient may eventually develop degenerative changes. If the lesion is greater than 50% of the condylar width, the pain becomes progressively severe. Radiographs show further collapse and rapid destruction within 12 months. The MRI study may similarly be useful in determining prognosis earlier in the process.[12]

Treatment

The major issue is to recognize the possibility of osteonecrosis in the patient with acute pain. The trap of ordering an MRI study and performing arthroscopy for the degenerative meniscal tears common in this age group should be avoided. A radionuclide bone scan should be considered if the radiograph and the MRI study are normal or only show degenerative meniscal tears, particularly if the tenderness is over the condyle rather than the joint line.

Conservative treatment is indicated in the early stages of the disease until the size of the lesion and its progression have been defined. It may take 6 months or longer to define the size of the lesion and its progression. Management consists of analgesics as needed and protected weight bearing, usually with a cane. Anti-inflammatory medications are often prescribed but there is no evidence of a significant inflammatory component. These medications may be of minor benefit if there is some secondary synovitis. Conservative management probably does not change the natural history of osteonecrosis. As the acute symptoms resolve, many patients return to their normal lifestyle. As noted previously, good or excellent results will be obtained with conservative management if the lesion is small (less than 45% of the condylar width). If secondary degenerative changes develop later, appropriate treatment can be recommended.[13] Surgical options are discussed in chapter 49 of this volume.

References

1. Ahlbäck S, Bauer GC, Bohne WH: Spontaneous osteonecrosis of the knee. *Arthritis Rheum* 1968;11:705-733.
2. al-Rowaih A, Björkengren A, Egund N, Lindstrand A; Wingstrand H, Thorngren KG: Size of osteonecrosis of the knee. *Clin Orthop* 1993:287:68-75.
3. Aglietti P, Insall JN, Buzzi R, Deschamps G: Idiopathic osteonecrosis of the knee: Aetiology, prognosis and treatment. *J Bone Joint Surg Br* 1983;65:588-597.
4. Lotke PA, Ecker ML, Alavi A; Painful knees in older patients: Radionuclide diagnosis of possible osteonecrosis with spontaneous resolution. *J Bone Joint Surg Am* 1977;59:617-621.
5. al-Rowaith A, Linstrand A, Bjorkengren A, Windstrand H, Thorngren KG: Osteonecrosis of the knee: Diagnosis and outcome in 40 patients. *Acta Orthop Scand* 1991;62:19-23.
6. al-Rowaith A, Wingstrand H, Lindstrand A, Bjorkengren A, Thorngren KG, Gustafson T: Three-phase scintimetry in osteonecrosis of the knee. *Acta Orthop Scand* 1990;61:120-127.
7. Pollack MS, Dalinka MK, Kresssel HY, Lotke PA, Spritzer CE: Magnetic resonance imaging in the evaluation of suspected osteonecrosis of the knee. *Skeletal Radiol* 1987; 16:121-127.
8. Brahme SK, Fox JM, Ferkel RD, Friedman MJ, Flannigan BD, Resnick DL: Osteonecrosis of the knee after arthroscopic surgery: Diagnosis with MR imaging. *Radiology* 1991;178:851-853.
9. Nakamura T, Matsumoto T, Nishino M, Tomita K, Kadoya M: Early magnetic resonance imaging and histologic findings in a model of femoral head necrosis. *Clin Orthop* 1977;334:68-72.
10. Ahuja SC, Bullough PG: Osteonecrosis of the knee: A clinicopathological study in twenty-eight patients. *J Bone Joint Surg Am* 1978; 60:191-197.
11. al-Rowaih A, Björkengren A, Willén H, et al: Primary osteonecrosis in the knee evaluated by histopathology and specimen scintimetry related to clinical radiography, scintimetry and MR. *Chir Organi Mov* 1992;77:257-269.
12. Bjorkengren AG, al-Rowaith A, Lindstrand A, Wingstrand H, Thorngren KG: Spontaneous osteonecrosis of the knee: Value of MR imaging in determining prognosis. *AJR Am J Roentgenol* 1990;154:331-336.
13. Lotke PA, Abend JA, Ecker ML: The treatment of osteonecrosis of the medial femoral condyle. *Clin Orthop* 1982;171:109-116.

52

Surgical Options for the Middle-Aged Patient With Osteoarthritis of the Knee Joint

Arlen D. Hanssen, MD
Michael J. Stuart, MD
Richard D. Scott, MD
Giles R. Scuderi, MD

Arthritic disease of the knee joint hindering lifestyle choices in an active aging population has become increasingly frequent. The pathology within the knee joint can vary from localized unicompartmental arthritis to end-stage tricompartmental arthritis. Associated conditions include extensive meniscal degeneration, ligamentous instability, localized articular cartilage defects, limb malalignment, and joint-line obliquity. Nonsurgical treatments to reduce the pain associated with joint inflammation include activity modification, weight loss, anti-inflammatory or analgesic medications, intra-articular injections, periarticular muscle-strengthening, and stress-offloading with braces or heel wedges. However, when the pain and associated impairment do not resolve satisfactorily with nonsurgical modalities, surgical intervention may be considered.

Surgical options include arthroscopic débridement, ligamentous reconstruction, realignment osteotomy, unicompartmental arthroplasty, and total knee arthroplasty (TKA). In the absence of infection or extensor mechanism disruption, arthrodesis of the knee is an extremely rare option for the active middle-aged patient. For the purposes of this discussion, the middle-aged patient will be defined in chronological terms as being between 40 and 60 years of age. The decision process leading to good patient selection is often complex and depends upon many variables (Table 1). Because most middle-aged patients with arthritis of the knee joint eventually have a TKA, analysis and comparison of several parameters are integral to selecting the best surgical option. These parameters include (1) the clinical results or survivorship associated with a given procedure, (2) the morbidity and attendant complications of the procedure, (3) the difficulty of eventual conversion to a TKA, and (4) the effect of a given procedure on the outcome of an eventual TKA.[1]

The goal of patient selection for a surgical procedure in this young and active population should be extension of the lifetime of the natural knee joint when possible, but the effect on the outcome of eventual prosthetic arthroplasty also should be carefully considered. Although the principle of avoiding TKA for as long as possible in the middle-aged patient is appropriate, performing an alternative procedure that has a limited chance of success or one that has negative implications for the outcome of a subsequent TKA has no logical basis.

Therefore, both patient variables and the capabilities of the surgeon with a specific surgical procedure must be considered. Many reports of clinical results underscore the importance of proper

Table 1
Variables used for selection of the surgical procedure

Historical
Age (chronological, physiological)
Activity level
Pain (severity, location, character)
Mechanical symptoms
Systemic inflammatory disease
Prior joint infection
Prior meniscectomy
Physical examination
Range of motion (total arc, flexion contracture)
Ligamentous deficiencies
Gait (adductor thrust)
Malalignment (magnitude, direction)
Body habitus
Patellofemoral findings (pain, stability)
Radiographic
Alignment (mechanical, anatomical)
Arthritic involvement (location, severity)
Joint-line obliquity
Periarticular deformity
Miscellaneous
Durability of results
Patient expectations
Surgeon capabilities
Potential complications
Postoperative recovery
Effect on subsequent TKA

One or more of the authors or the departments with which they are affiliated have received something of value from a commercial or other party related directly or indirectly to the subject of this chapter.

surgical technique, and many of the difficulties encountered with eventual TKA are due to suboptimal technical performance of the prior procedure. The underlying principle for a successful outcome for all of these surgical options is careful patient selection combined with good surgical technique.

Arthroscopy and Ligament Reconstruction

Although arthroscopic débridement of the knee joint cannot be directly compared with osteotomy, unicompartmental knee arthroplasty, or TKA according to the criteria outlined above, this procedure is often a potential alternative for some middle-aged patients with osteoarthritis of the knee joint. When appropriate, arthroscopic débridement may lengthen the useful lifetime of a knee joint; however, this procedure may have negative effects on the outcome of subsequent surgical procedures if it is used indiscriminately.

The role of arthroscopy in the management of degenerative knee arthritis in the middle-aged yet active patient remains controversial.[2,3] In well selected middle-aged patients with knee arthritis, arthroscopic débridement may be a valuable method for providing transient relief of symptoms.[3,4] Although arthroscopic techniques are continuing to evolve, the natural history of the arthritic process is probably not altered by isolated arthroscopic débridement and lavage. Patients with less extensive arthritis as seen radiographically, less severe involvement of articular cartilage, and a younger age at the time of the operation have more worthwhile improvement.[5] A short duration of pain and mechanical symptoms, and mild-to-moderate radiographic stages of arthritis, correlate with a better result.[6,7] The true outcomes of most of these arthroscopic procedures are difficult to determine, as most investigators have used nebulous inclusion criteria, inadequate study designs, short-term follow-up, as well as limited outcome-based analyses.

The success of an arthroscopic procedure is often enhanced by the concomitant use of other surgical procedures such as ligament reconstruction and osteotomy. Ligament reconstruction can eliminate subluxation episodes and can decrease pain. Restoration of the mechanical axis, alone or in combination with ligament reconstruction, unloads the degenerated compartment. Marrow stimulation techniques, including subchondral bone microfracture and osteochondral transplantation, are recommended for the treatment of focal chondral defects in normally aligned knees of patients younger than 45 years of age. Meniscal transplantation is also indicated for patients younger than 45 years and is not considered in the treatment algorithms for knee arthritis in older middle-aged patients.[8,9]

Surgical débridement of the knee with degenerative changes involves lavage, partial meniscectomy, limited synovectomy, excision of osteophytes, loose body removal, and cartilage-shaving or thermal chondroplasty.[3,10] A carefully recorded history, physical examination, and standing radiographs remain the most important diagnostic tools. One should treat the patient's symptoms and not the MRI study. The primary indications include a discrete chief complaint of well localized joint-line pain with an acute onset, persistent effusion, and catching or locking in a patient who has been treated unsuccessfully with a nonsurgical program.

Excision of symptomatic degenerative meniscal tears or loose bodies can effectively relieve mechanical symptoms and may provide additional pain relief by removing the irritating products of joint degeneration. Occasionally, patients with advanced arthritis are candidates for arthroscopy for the relief of mechanical symptoms caused by meniscal tears, loose chondral flaps, or osteophytes, which appear to cause painful impingement or to block knee motion. It is important to emphasize the importance of axial limb alignment (Fig. 1). If the mechanical axis passes through the lesion, arthroscopy will be unsuccessful.[11,12] There should be normal or nearly normal limb alignment, with only mild to moderate radiographic degenerative changes.[13] Patients with a history of surgery or with arthroscopic evidence of severe (grade 4) chondromalacia are at risk for a poor outcome.[11,14]

Patient satisfaction and a decrease in symptoms following arthroscopic débridement can be marked but also unpredictable.[15] Patients must be counseled about the underlying disease process, the limited goals of the arthroscopic procedure, the potential complications, and the possible need for future reconstructive surgery. Arthroscopic treatment of degenerative arthritis is associated with low morbidity, and serious complications are uncommon. Although the complications of arthroscopy are infrequent and minor, their prevalence appears to be increasing as these procedures become more technically demanding.[12,16] Complication rates have ranged from 7% to 31%,[16] but they are minimized by careful patient selection combined with meticulous attention to detail. Patients older than 50 years of age are at higher risk for complications following arthroscopy.[16,17]

The mechanism of pain relief following arthroscopic treatment of osteoarthritis is obscure, and several prospective, randomized studies have been conducted to address this issue. In one study, the results of arthroscopic débridement were compared, with use of The Hospital for Special Surgery knee scores, with those in a control group that had been treated nonsurgically.[13] Arthroscopic treatment was deemed to have been useful, at a mean duration of follow-up of 2 years. Its main benefit was that it could be used to treat problems that coexisted with osteoarthritis, such as meniscal lesions and loose bodies. In another study, 73 knees were randomized to nonsurgical treatment or arthroscopic débridement.[13] The group treated with débridement had substantially better results at the 1-year and 5-year follow-up evaluations. In another study comparing the results of lavage only with those of arthroscopic débridement, some improvement in quadriceps isokinetic torque was noted after lavage, but neither procedure led to a marked decrease in symptoms.[18] Finally, a prospective, placebo-controlled, blinded, randomized pilot study of 10 patients with symptomatic osteoarthritis was performed.[19] Five patients had skin-puncture wounds only, three underwent arthroscopic lavage and débridement, and two had standard arthroscopic débridement. All five patients with only puncture wounds reported a decrease in pain at 6 months postoperatively; four of the five judged the procedure to have been worthwhile and stated that they would recommend it to family and friends. The three patients who had had lavage and débridement had similar results. Clearly, larger studies with a similar design are required before a more definitive statement on the placebo effect of arthroscopy can be made. Randomized, controlled trials with defined entry criteria, sufficient numbers of patients, and valid, reproducible outcome measures will allow the most unbiased assessment of the risks and benefits of arthroscopic procedures for the treatment of unicompartmental disease of the knee.

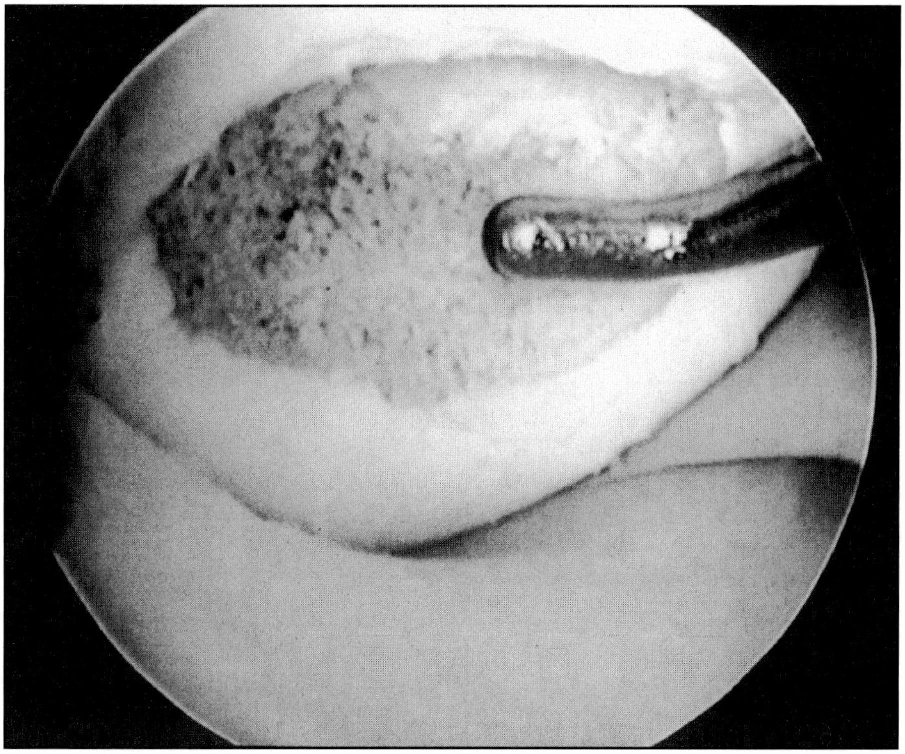

Fig. 1 Arthroscopic view of a focal articular lesion of the medial condyle of the distal part of the femur. The axial limb alignment as seen on a full-length standing radiograph indicated that the weight-bearing line passed directly through the lesion. In addition to arthroscopic débridement or adjunctive surgical techniques such as osteochondral grafting or chondrocyte implantation, a realignment osteotomy is necessary to transfer the weight-bearing forces away from the lesion.

In summary, arthroscopic excision of torn, unstable, degenerative meniscal fragments that are causing joint-line pain, recurrent effusions, and mechanical symptoms is an effective procedure with limited goals. Carefully selected patients with normal or nearly normal limb alignment and mild or moderate unicompartmental degenerative disease can be considered for arthroscopic treatment if a nonsurgical program has been unsuccessful. Treatment of chronic chondral injuries with arthroscopic débridement and chondroplasty provides unpredictable, incomplete, and transient relief of symptoms. Correction of the mechanical axis and elimination of pathological laxity are fundamental issues that must be recognized and addressed. Additional basic science research and well designed clinical trials are necessary to determine whether arthroscopic débridement can relieve symptoms and delay further joint-surface deterioration.

Abrasion arthroplasty is an arthroscopic modification of the Magnuson "housecleaning" arthroplasty, designed to remove dead bone and to expose a vascularized surface and a tissue bed for clot attachment and subsequent fibrocartilage formation.[20,21] In a retrospective study of 126 patients treated for unicompartmental arthritis who were followed for an average of 60 months, those who had had arthroscopic débridement alone had done as well as or better than those who had had abrasion arthroplasty and arthroscopic débridement.[22] An important observation was that 18% of the patients had worsening of the arthritis after the arthroscopic procedure. In another comparative, retrospective study of 110 patients treated with arthroscopic débridement, those in whom the operation included abrasion arthroplasty had a better outcome than those treated with arthroscopic débridement alone; the results were best in patients younger than 40 years of age.[23] In the largest study, 131 patients treated with arthroscopic débridement (Group I) were compared with 28 patients treated with débridement and abrasion arthroplasty (Group II).[24] In Group II, half of the patients had conversion to a TKA within 3 years after the abrasion arthroplasty. The prevalence of patients with worsening of the arthritis was higher after abrasion arthroplasty than it was after arthroscopic débridement alone, and it was concluded that the results of abrasion arthroplasty are unpredictable.

Chronological age is a consideration but not a contraindication in patient selection for reconstruction of the anterior cruciate ligament (ACL). Mild to moderate arthritis does not preclude reconstruction of the ACL. Intra-articular ligament reconstruction has evolved into a reliable procedure with low morbidity. Reconstruction of the ACL can improve stability and decrease pain in the arthritic knee. Endoscopic reconstruction of the ACL with use of patellar tendon allograft provides acceptable clinical results with less pain and less morbidity after graft harvest in this lower-demand patient population. Occasionally, carefully selected patients with normal or nearly normal limb alignment and mild or moderate unicompartmental degenerative disease can be considered for reconstruction of the ACL.[25-27] In a study of 53 patients with chronic deficiency of the ACL, articular cartilage fissuring or exposure of subchondral bone, and normal alignment who were treated with reconstruction of the ACL with use of patellar tendon autograft, there was a decrease in pain in 37 knees and elimination of giving-way episodes in 47 knees; 42 patients were able to return to recreational activities.[28]

The indications for reconstruction of the ACL include recurrent episodes of symptomatic giving-way, despite a comprehensive nonsurgical treatment program, and an unwillingness to modify activities. The goals of surgical intervention include pain relief, restoration of knee stability, and functional improvement in activities of daily living. Although reconstruction of the ACL in the arthritic knee can improve stability both objectively and subjectively, can decrease pain, and can increase the patient's activity level, patients should be counseled that this is a salvage procedure and that it is not intended to facilitate a return to high-demand sports or repetitive impact-loading. These patients need to be cognizant of the limited goals of surgical treatment as well as the progressive nature of the arthritic disease process. The middle-aged patient with an anterior cruciate-deficient knee in the presence of a previous partial meniscectomy or early posttraumatic degenerative arthritis is not an ideal surgical candidate. Reconstruction of the ACL is contraindicated in knees with full-thickness cartilage loss on opposing articular surfaces and in those with secondary bone changes resulting in joint instability.[28]

In young patients with insufficiency of the ACL, cartilaginous lesions in the medial compartment, and varus knee malalignment, a combined procedure consisting of valgus tibial osteotomy and reconstruction of the ACL can be considered. This combined procedure has been performed occasionally in patients during the fourth and fifth decades of life, with encouraging results.[28-34] The techniques have been performed either simultaneously or in stages, with ligamentous reconstruction done after healing of the osteotomy site.[32,35] Again, it must be emphasized that this is a salvage operation; it is not intended to return athletes to competition.[35]

Indications for a valgus-producing proximal tibial osteotomy include medial knee pain, degenerative arthritis involving the medial compartment, and a varus mechanical axis. Biplanar correction techniques address both limb alignment and pathologic laxity. A posteromedial opening or anterolateral closing-wedge osteotomy reduces the tibial slope in the sagittal plane and increases stability in the anterior cruciate-deficient knee. In contrast, an anteromedial opening or posterolateral closing-wedge osteotomy increases the tibial slope in the sagittal plane and increases stability in the posterior cruciate-deficient knee. Contraindications to a lateral closing-wedge osteotomy include intra-articular erosion, primary femoral deformity, and laxity of the medial collateral ligament.[31] The upper age-limit for combined osteotomy and ligamentous reconstruction in the presence of knee arthritis has not been definitively established. The decision process for this procedure is complex and requires careful synthesis of the pattern of ligamentous insufficiency, the location and extent of the arthritis, and the activity level and age of the patient.

Realignment Osteotomy

The goals of osteotomy include pain relief, functional improvement, and allowance of heavy functional demands that would otherwise be precluded by prosthetic replacement. The objective is to transfer the weight-bearing forces from the arthritic portion of the knee to a healthier location of the joint.[36] This principle of force redistribution to increase the life span of the knee joint distinguishes osteotomy from other treatment modalities and is based on the concept that certain high-impact and loading activities are not sanctioned with prosthetic arthroplasty. Functional analysis of young patients following osteotomy has revealed that many patients are able to participate in running and jumping activities that would likely lead to damage of a knee prosthesis.[37-39] Many patients recognize the potential for technological advances during the expected survival period of a knee treated with osteotomy and understand that "buying time" is a viable concept.

The surgeon should discuss all treatment alternatives with the patient and should convey that neither osteotomy nor arthroplasty will result in a "normal" joint. A longer postoperative recovery period with less pain relief after rehabilitation is expected following osteotomy. Prosthetic arthroplasty provides more complete pain relief and a shorter rehabilitation period, and it is more reliable than osteotomy in most patients older than the age of 60 years.[40] These considerations must be balanced against the possible catastrophic complications of infection or prosthetic failure associated with arthroplasty in the young and active patient. It is important to recognize that both physiologic status and lifestyle require careful consideration, as some younger sedentary patients may be better suited to treatment with arthroplasty. The key to success is careful patient selection combined with skillful surgical technique.

The ideal candidate for osteotomy is a thin active individual in the fifth or sixth decade of life who has localized, activity-related, unicompartmental knee pain; no patellofemoral symptoms; a stable knee; and full knee extension with flexion of at least 90°.[9] The location and character of the pain, the desired activity level, and appropriate patient expectations are particularly important. Diffuse or nonspecific knee pain reduces the chance of a successful outcome. Patellofemoral symptoms or meniscal pathology should not be the primary cause of the pain. Substantial retropatellar pain should be a cautionary factor, but mild retropatellar pain does not preclude osteotomy if the primary indication for the osteotomy is unicompartmental tibiofemoral pain.

Symptoms related to knee instability will not be alleviated by osteotomy alone. Moderate or severe instability should not be present, but insufficiency of the ACL does not adversely affect the outcome if the preoperative symptoms can be specifically attributed to an overloading of the degenerated joint compartment. TKA is the treatment of choice for elderly patients with degenerative arthritis and instability.[41]

Posttraumatic arthritis, osteochondritis dissecans, or a prior medial meniscectomy do not adversely affect the outcome, whereas prior combined medial and lateral meniscectomies predict a disappointing outcome.[42,43] Tibiofemoral subluxation, excessive osseous erosion, and diffuse arthritic involvement are also associated with poorer outcomes. Obesity has been associated with lower success rates following high tibial osteotomy, as the surgical technique and the postoperative immobilization are more difficult in these individuals.[44,45] The activity level of these patients should be carefully assessed, as sedentary overweight individuals may be better served by prosthetic replacement (Fig. 2).

The importance of patient selection is underscored by the results of 39 high tibial osteotomies, many of which were performed without precise indications.[46] There were 10 poor results in 9 knees, 4 of which had a preoperative diagnosis of diffuse degenerative arthritis; 2, inflammatory disease; 1, prior septic arthritis; and 1, posttraumatic arthritis with severe deformity. By current standards of patient selection, these patients would be considered poor candidates for realignment osteotomy.

Equally important for a successful clinical outcome is the quality of the surgical technique. In a series of 30 knees treated with tibial osteotomy, in which rigid patient-selection criteria were used, 13 knees had a satisfactory outcome and 17, a poor outcome, at the 51-month follow-up evaluation.[47] There were no technical errors in any knee with a good result, and all had good correction of malalignment. Of the 17 poor results, 10 were in knees in which there had been a technical error: 5 of these knees had undercorrection, 3 had overcorrection, and 2 had joint penetration during the osteotomy. There were 11 complications. These results emphasize the adverse impact of a suboptimal surgical technique on the outcome of corrective osteotomy even when there has been good patient selection.

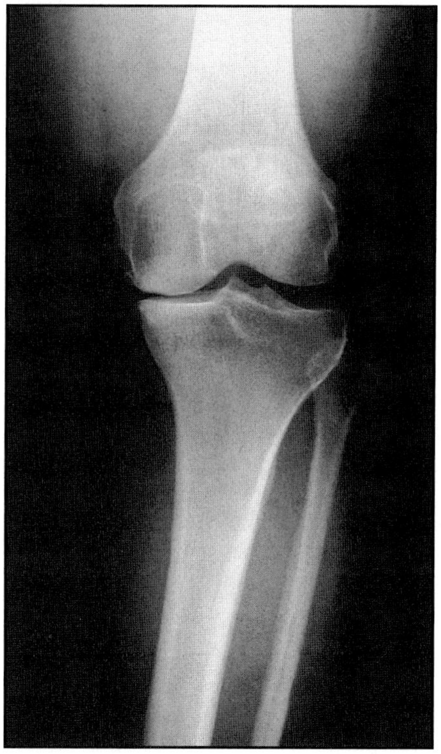

Fig. 2 Anteroposterior standing radiograph of the knee joint in a heavy 52-year-old woman with progressive pain in the medial compartment. The symptoms are typical of degenerative arthritis, and mechanical symptoms of catching or locking are absent. Because of the advanced degenerative changes and the varus limb alignment, this patient is not a good candidate for arthroscopic débridement. Her body habitus is a relative contraindication to realignment osteotomy. TKA or unicompartmental knee arthroplasty is the best surgical option.

One reason for premature failure following osteotomy is undercorrection or overcorrection of the deformity. Like patient selection, the accuracy of postoperative alignment is a primary predictor of success. The difficulty lies in determining the so-called appropriate postoperative alignment, as recommendations have varied widely. Hernigou and associates[48] recommended 3° to 6° of valgus; Cass and Bryan,[49] 10° to 12° of valgus; and Rudan and Simurda,[50] 6° to 14° of anatomic valgus.

Currently, the goal of postoperative alignment is to place the weight-bearing

Table 2
Survival rates in selected series of high tibial osteotomies

Study	No. of Patients	Rate of Survival At 2 Yrs. (%)	At 5 Yrs. (%)	At 7 Yrs. (%)	At 10 Yrs. (%)	At 15 Yrs. (%)
Berman et al[46]	39	87	—	—	—	57*
Cass and Bryan[49]	86	94	87	—	69	—
Coventry et al[44]	87	—	87	—	66	—
			(96)†		(91)†	
			(94)‡		(94)‡	
Healy and Riley[57]	31	92	88	91	80§	—
Hernigou et al[48]	93	—	90	—	45#	—
			(100)#		(100)†	
Matthews et al[45]	40	86**	50	—	28§	—
Ritter and Fechtman[58]	78	95	80	58	58	58*
Rudan and Simurda[50]	128	—	—	—	80	70
Yasuda et al[59]	86	—	88	—	63	—

*The average duration of follow-up was 12 to 13 years

†Value for patients with a relative body weight of less than 1.17

‡Value for patients with postoperative alignment of at least 8° of valgus

§The average duration of follow-up was 9 years

#Value for 20 patients with appropriate postoperative alignment

**The average duration of follow-up was 1 year

line of the extremity within the middle to outer third of the lateral compartment of the knee. This method of measurement of the mechanical axis alignment does not always correlate with the specific ranges of measurement methods based on the anatomic axis because of differences in joint-line obliquity and femoral or tibial bowing. In general, when the goals of mechanical axis translation are achieved, the postoperative anatomical axis measures between 8° and 12° of valgus.

In a series of 93 osteotomies, the fact that the overall 5-year survival rate of 90% diminished to 45% at 10 years obscures results in patients with good postoperative alignment.[48] The 20 patients with good postoperative alignment had no failures after 11.5 years of follow-up. Coventry and associates[44] reported that, for knees with at least 8° of postoperative valgus, the survival rate was 94% at the 5- and 10-year follow-up evaluations compared with 63% for knees that were corrected to 5° or less of valgus angulation. In another study, of 314 patients who were followed for 10 to 19 years, 54 of 170 patients who had undercorrection subsequently required revision surgery because of clinical deterioration compared with 8 of 144 patients with normalized or overcorrected alignment.[51] On the basis of this long-term experience, those authors suggested that the longevity of a knee with a properly performed high tibial osteotomy rivaled that of current prosthetic replacements.

The simultaneous performance of arthrotomy and joint débridement with osteotomy, although controversial, has been reported to enhance the final result.[52] Extrapolation of this experience would lead one to believe that some patients might benefit from arthroscopic débridement in conjunction with corrective osteotomy. In one study, the results of osteotomy and arthroscopic abrasion arthroplasty were compared with those of osteotomy alone.[53] At the 12-month follow-up visit, arthroscopic evaluation revealed a significantly higher prevalence of repair of grade II cartilage in the group that had had both osteotomy and arthroplasty ($P < 0.01$); however, there was no difference in the clinical outcome between the two groups at 2 to 9 years of follow-up.

Proliferation of fibrocartilage and regeneration of articular cartilage following osteotomy have been documented by second-look arthroscopy.[54,55] Importantly, only overcorrected knees demonstrated cartilage regeneration, supporting the concept of mechanical realignment facilitating the reparative capacity of the knee joint after unloading. Another reason for considering arthroscopy is the desire to evaluate the stage of the arthritis in order to predict the efficacy of osteotomy; however, its prognostic value for this application has not been demonstrated.[56]

It is clear that the reported outcomes of high tibial osteotomy have been quite variable. Patient selection factors, good surgical technique, appropriate postoperative alignment, and the passage of time all affect the final clinical outcome. Many studies of high tibial osteotomy have revealed satisfactory clinical results after 5 to 7 years of follow-up, with the percentage of such results then diminishing substantially[44-46,48-50,57-59] (Table 2). It is often difficult to ascertain the effects of patient selection and technical error on the long-term outcome when evaluating many of these clinical series. As with high tibial osteotomy, the reported success rates with distal femoral osteotomy have been variable[60-70] (Table 3).

The technical difficulties and the potential severity of complications associated with realignment osteotomy have undoubtedly contributed toward the decline in the popularity of this surgical procedure. Complications have been divided into those related to evaluation and those related to technical error.[71] Neurologic injury following osteotomy ranks as one of the most adverse consequences of this procedure. Postoperative peroneal nerve palsy appears to be associated with the use of an external fixation device.[54,72] Many external fixation techniques include a proximal fibular osteotomy, which is another etiologic factor.[72] Compartment syndrome is a rare yet devastating complication following osteotomy. Deep infection is also rare following corrective osteotomy, but the risk is higher when an external fixation device is used.[54] The frequency of thromboembolic disease is lower after osteotomy than that after TKA, and the proper method of prophylaxis is controversial.

Joint stiffness has been reported rarely following high tibial osteotomy, whereas it has been reported frequently following supracondylar osteotomy.[47,63,66,68] Rigid fixation and an early range of motion minimize stiffness, but rapid healing of the osteotomy site and maintenance of postoperative alignment should take priority. The stiffness associated with supracondylar osteotomy makes surgical exposure for a subsequent knee arthroplasty more difficult in some patients.[73] An early range of motion also helps to avoid quadriceps atrophy and may aid in the prevention of patellar tendon-shortening following tibial osteotomy.[74] The scarring and shortening of the patellar tendon often prevent eversion of the patella, and surgical exposure during a subsequent TKA may require specialized techniques.[75] Difficulties with successful union are mentioned in essentially all reports on corrective osteotomy and are more common after supracondylar osteotomy than after high tibial osteotomy.

The expected result of TKA following osteotomy must also be considered. The literature describing poor results of arthroplasty following osteotomy clearly indicates that technical difficulties or complications associated with the osteotomy lead to worse results after subsequent arthroplasty.[73,75,76] The results of conversion of an osteotomy to a TKA compared with those of conversion of a unicompartmental knee arthroplasty to a TKA are discussed in the next section. The poorer long-term radiographic results of TKA following high tibial osteotomy occur in a specific subset of patients consisting of younger, heavier, more active males,[41] which suggests that "buying time" with an osteotomy to avoid prosthetic replacement for as long as possible is a wise decision for these individuals. Although the current indications for osteotomy are relatively limited, the surgeon should be confident about performing a corrective osteotomy when the appropriate criteria are met. Successful long-term results are linked to careful patient selection, accurate surgical technique, and appropriate postoperative alignment.

Table 3
Results of distal femoral osteotomy

Study	No. of Patients	Rate of Success (%)	Duration of Follow-up* (yrs.)
Beaver et al[60]	42	83	3.6 (2-11.5)
Cameron et al[61]	49	87	7†
Conrad et al[62]	16	62	6.5
Edgerton et al[63]	24	71 (86‡)	8.3 (5-11)
Finkelstein et al[64]	21	64	11 (8-20)
Healy et al[65]	23	83 (93§)	4 (2-9)
Johnson and Bodell[66]	53	70	3.6 (1-9.3)
McDermott et al[67]	24	92	4 (2-11.5)
Mathews et al[68]	21	57	3 (1-8)
Miniaci et al[69]	35	86 (100#)	5.4 (2-16.7)
Terry and Cimino[70]	35	60	5.4 (2-19)

*The values are given as the average, with the range in parentheses

†End point of survival analysis

‡Value for patients who had isolated compartment disease

§Value for patients who did not have rheumatoid arthritis

#Value for patients who had valgus deformity without arthrosis

Unicompartmental Knee Arthroplasty

Unicompartmental knee arthroplasty is a potentially attractive alternative to tibial osteotomy or TKA in selected osteoarthritic patients. Traditionally, unicompartmental knee arthroplasty has been reserved for patients with unicompartmental arthritis who have a sedentary lifestyle and are older than 60 years of age.[77-79] However, there has been recent interest in performing this procedure in patients younger than 60 years as an alternative to tibial osteotomy or TKA.[1,80,81]

The advantages of unicompartmental knee arthroplasty compared with osteotomy include higher rates of initial success and fewer early complications; also, when unicompartmental knee arthroplasty is performed bilaterally the two procedures can be done simultaneously, during the same anesthesia session, whereas when osteotomy is performed bilaterally the procedures are best spaced apart.[82,83] The advantages of unicompartmental knee arthroplasty compared with TKA include retention of both cruciate ligaments and preservation of bone stock in the opposite compartment and the patellofemoral joint. Patients who have unicompartmental knee arthroplasty have less perioperative morbidity and an increased range of motion compared with those who have TKA.[84-86] Manipulation, extensor mechanism complications, and deep periprosthetic infection are more common with TKA than they are with unicompartmental knee arthroplasty.[1,86] Despite these advantages, unicompartmental knee arthroplasty has remained controversial for more than 25 years, as some authors have reported good or excellent results in most patients whereas others have reported less favorable results.[41,87-91] The keys to a successful unicompartmental knee arthroplasty are stringent patient selection criteria, careful surgical technique, and a proven prosthetic design.[92,93]

As with the other alternatives, patient selection is of great importance. Contraindications to unicompartmental knee arthroplasty have included obesity, severe angular deformity, a valgus knee with medial laxity, absence of the ACL, generalized arthritis of the knee, and inflammatory synovitis.[93,94] Increased body weight has been associated with an increased rate of failure of unicompartmental knee arthroplasty.[95] Unicompartmental metallic hemiarthroplasty is a rare but viable alternative for the patient with contraindications to osteotomy who is thought to be too young, heavy, and active for a metal-to-plastic arthroplasty.[93] The ideal candidate for unicompartmental knee arthroplasty is a thin individual with localized pain attributable to unicompartmental arthritis who has only mild to moderate angular deformity and no ligamentous laxity of the knee joint.

Many reported failures of unicompartmental knee arthroplasty have been attributed to technical error.[94,96-98] Slight undercorrection of the deformity with insertion of an adequate thickness of polyethylene are important contributors to a successful outcome.[88] Progressive arthritis is generally caused by overcorrection of a varus deformity into valgus alignment.[88,91,99,100]

The prosthetic design has also been associated with the long-term success of unicompartmental knee arthroplasty. In particular, major polyethylene wear, often related to the specific prosthetic design, has been a common finding in some studies.[98,101,103] Other reasons that have been mentioned for accelerated polyethylene wear include inadequate thickness of the polyethylene insert, increased rotational freedom, reduced conformity of the articular surfaces, and metal backing on the tibial component.[1] Use of a constrained unicompartmental knee arthroplasty design has resulted in significantly more poor results than use of an unconstrained design (P = 0.0009).[103] A meniscal-bearing unicompartmental knee arthroplasty design has been used in an effort to reduce polyethylene wear; however, these implants have been associated with initially inferior results and with the unique complication of meniscal-bearing dislocation.[104,105] Other meniscal-bearing unicompartmental knee arthroplasty designs may prove to be more successful.[79] In addition, it has been noted that the current femoral component design has not been optimized and that the prevalence of femoral loosening may be reduced with design modifications.[81,97,106]

In general, the initially good outcomes of unicompartmental knee arthroplasty appear to be comparable with the results of TKA in the first decade after the arthroplasty. Marmor[94] reported the 10- to 13-year results of 60 unicompartmental knee arthroplasties. He found that 70% of the knees still had a satisfactory result and that 87% were free of major pain. Scott and associates[107] reported an 85% rate of survival at 10 years after 100 unicompartmental knee arthroplasties. Heck and associates,[95] in a study of 294 implants, reported a 91% rate of survival at 10 years. Cartier and associates[88] reported a 93% rate of survival at 10 to 12 years after sixty unicompartmental knee arthroplasties. The highest reported rate of survival at 10 years after unicompartmental knee arthroplasty is 98%, after 143 Oxford medial arthroplasties.[90] The longest duration of follow-up after unicompartmental knee arthroplasty (15 years) revealed an 87.5% rate of survival with use of revision surgery as the end point.[91] It should be noted that these are among the best results that have been reported, but they are somewhat inferior to most survival rates after similar time intervals following modern TKA. It must also be remembered that these studies included many elderly patients with limited activity requirements; therefore, extrapolation of these results to a young and active patient population should be done with caution.

An early series of unicompartmental knee arthroplasties in middle-aged patients included 28 patients younger than 60 years of age.[81] At the 2- to 6-year follow-up evaluation, 90% had a good or excellent result and knee flexion averaged 124°. Two revisions had been performed for femoral component loosening, and one tibial component was associated with asymptomatic progressive radiolucency. Both of these problems were believed to be caused by the conformity of the fixed-bearing articulation. Those authors concluded that the results of unicompartmental knee arthroplasty in this patient population were comparable with those of osteotomy at an average of 4 years but were inferior to those of TKA in terms of the reoperation rate.

Of 46 knees in patients between 40 and 60 years of age who had a unicompartmental knee arthroplasty, 13 had a revision at an average of 7.1 years.[1] These patients had an average weight of 191 lb (86.6 kg). A higher rate of failure due to polyethylene wear was observed in association with one of the prosthetic designs used in this study. If the 9 knees with this specific type of prosthesis are excluded from the analysis, the remaining 37 knees had a success rate of 86% at the time of final follow-up. Those authors concluded that, in younger, active patients, the 10-year survival rate should be 80%, provided that an adequate thickness of polyethylene and a proven prosthetic design are used.

Revision of an osteotomy to a TKA has been reported to be difficult because of wound problems associated with prior incisions, a distorted joint line, technical difficulties in obtaining adequate surgical exposure, and retained hardware. In contrast, it has been suggested that conversion of a unicompartmental knee arthroplasty to a TKA is associated with fewer problems related to the surgical exposure and fewer technical difficulties.[108-110] The primary difficulty with conversion of a unicompartmental knee arthroplasty to a TKA has been the management of bone deficiencies.[111,112] Bone grafting, use of cement with screw augmentation, use of a long-stemmed tibial component, or a combination of these techniques is required in roughly 50% of patients.[96] Several studies have directly compared the results of conversion of an osteotomy to a TKA with those of conversion of a unicompartmental knee arthroplasty to a TKA.[108,113] Although it is commonly believed that revision of a unicompartmental knee arthroplasty is easier than revision of a TKA, in one report of 21 revisions of unicompartmental knee arthroplasties it was concluded that these procedures were technically demanding and that 76% of patients had a major osseous defect at revision.[112] Revision of a TKA is typically associated with a more difficult exposure and with global bone deficiency, whereas revision of a unicompartmental knee arthroplasty is usually associated with bone deficiency of only the medial tibial plateau and the femoral condyles.[110]

One may ask whether unicompartmental knee arthroplasty ought to be considered at all for the middle-aged patient. It may find its role as a conservative initial arthroplasty for patients with unicompartmental disease who have relative contraindications to tibial osteotomy, those who wish to avoid secondary angular deformity caused by osteotomy, those with very early changes in the opposite compartment, and some patients with bilateral involvement. If early loosening of the femoral component could be eliminated by changes in prosthetic design, unicompartmental knee arthroplasty could become very attractive as a conservative initial arthroplasty in selected younger patients. Surgical techniques that use less invasive exposures and implants are currently being studied, and their use may further increase the appeal of this procedure by allowing a markedly shorter hospital stay and a rapid recovery.

Total Knee Arthroplasty

Total knee replacement has been shown to have durable and predictable results in elderly patients, providing pain relief, improving function, and correcting deformity.[114-118] The possibility of multiple revisions due to loosening or wear initially discouraged the widespread use of TKA in young patients with degenerative arthritis.[119] These concerns arose from the poor results observed in young patients who had had a THA.[120-122] However, the early results of TKA in young patients did not reflect the experience with total hip arthroplasty, and the initial reports often included many patients with rheumatoid arthritis or juvenile rheumatoid arthritis.[123-126] On the basis of this initial success, the indications for TKA eventually were expanded to younger patients with osteoarthritis.[127] As the indications continue to expand, the decision to proceed with TKA in young, active patients needs to be individualized after careful consideration of alternatives.

Stuart and Rand[126] reported 38 good and excellent results at an average of 5 years after 44 TKAs with cement in patients with rheumatoid arthritis who were younger than 40 years old. Dalury and associates[124] reported the results of 103 TKAs in patients younger than 45 years old, most (87%) of whom had had a diagnosis of rheumatoid arthritis. At an average of 7 years, there were two patellar fractures and one infection, but no knee had been revised because of component loosening. In another study, an average of 6 years after 90 TKAs in patients with rheumatoid arthritis and osteoarthritis who were younger than 55 years of age, the average Hospital for Special Surgery knee score was 87 points.[125] In a study of only osteoarthritic knees, followed for an average of 6 years, there were 55 excellent and 13 good results in patients who were 55 years of age or younger.[128]

These short- and intermediate-term results have withstood the test of time, even in more active patients with degenerative or posttraumatic arthritis. Duffy and associates[129] reported the results of 74 consecutive TKAs in 54 patients who were 55 years of age or younger (average age, 43 years) at the time of the index procedure. All patients were followed for a minimum of 10 years (average, 13 years; range, 10 to 17 years). The preoperative diagnosis was rheumatoid arthritis in 47 patients; osteoarthritis in 12; posttraumatic arthritis in 6; osteonecrosis in 3; hemophilia in 2; and pigmented villonodular synovitis, tuberculosis, systemic lupus erythematosus, and achondroplasia in 1 patient each. All knees had a cemented condylar prosthesis. The functional knee score was 60 points at the time of the latest follow-up. Two knees had a revision: one because of ligamentous laxity at 3 years, and the other because of aseptic loosening of the tibial component at 13 years. At the last follow-up, there were no loose components. Duffy and associates concluded that TKA with cement in young patients is a reliable procedure that yields excellent results at 13 years and has an estimated survival rate of 99% at 10 years.

Because most long-term studies have had a larger percentage of older patients with a variety of diagnoses, including rheumatoid arthritis and multiple joint involvement, it is important that these results are interpreted carefully and are not extrapolated directly to younger patients with osteoarthritis. The latter subgroup of patients tends to be more active and more frequently employed as manual laborers, with activity requirements and demands that put higher stresses on the prosthetic surface and fixation. Diduch and associates[130] specifically evaluated this subgroup in a study of 108 knees in 84 patients with a diagnosis of either osteoarthritis or posttraumatic arthritis. Fifty-eight percent had had prior knee surgery, and all but one patient had a cemented posterior stabilized prosthesis. One hundred and three unrevised knees were available for clinical evaluation at an average of 8 years (range, 3 to 18 years), and 36 knees were followed for more than 10 years. Postoperatively, the average Hospital for Special Surgery knee score was 92 points, the average Knee Society score was 94 points, and the average functional score was 89 points. All knees were rated as either good or excellent. The average Tegner activity score[131] improved from 1.3 points preoperatively to 3.5 points (range, 1 to 6 points) postoperatively. All but two patients had an improvement in their level of activity, while 24% had an activity score of greater than 5 points, indicating regular participation in activities such as tennis, skiing, bicycling, or strenuous farm or construction work. There were two revisions for late infection, one for polyethylene wear, and one for flexion instability. In all of these patients, the femoral and tibial components were well fixed. With failure defined as revision of either the femoral or the tibial component, the cumulative survival rate was 94% at 18 years. Three additional patients required revision of a loose patellar component.[130] These durable results support the use of a cemented posterior stabilized prosthesis for the treatment of osteoarthritic knees in young, active patients when less invasive measures have failed.

Despite the good results obtained by several skilled surgeons and demonstrated by the clinical studies, common sense suggests that total knee replacement should continue to be considered with caution for some young patients. Deferment of the definitive surgical procedure for as long as possible may be the best option until the symptoms warrant total knee replacement. If total knee replacement is performed, these young patients need to realize that activities that involve high-impact loads, such as running and jumping, should be avoided. Finally, it should be remembered that, although the emerging data for long-term results at up to 18 years in some patients are encouraging, these are incidental cases with specific implant designs.[130] The results should therefore be interpreted cautiously, as differences in prosthetic design and fixation variables may alter the outcomes in future long-term studies. Additional long-term information must be gathered before total knee replacement for the treatment of osteoarthritis in young, active patients is universally accepted.

References

1. Engh GA, McAuley JP: Unicondylar arthroplasty: An option for high-demand patients with gonarthrosis. *Instr Course Lect* 1999;48: 143-148.
2. Goldman RT, Scuderi GR, Kelly MA: Arthroscopic treatment of the degenerative knee in older athletes. *Clin Sports Med* 1997; 16:51-68.
3. Stuart MJ: Arthroscopic management for degenerative arthritis of the knee. *Instr Course Lect* 1999;48:135-141.
4. McGinley BJ, Cushner FD, Scott WN: Debridement arthroscopy: 10-year followup. *Clin Orthop* 1999;367:190-194.
5. Aichroth PM, Patel DV, Moyes ST: A prospective review of arthroscopic debridement for degenerative joint disease of the knee. *Int Orthop* 1991;15:351-355.
6. Anderson JK, Goldstein WM: Arthroscopy in patients over the age of 50 years. *Am J Arthrosc* 1991;1:15-18.
7. Ogilvie-Harris DJ, Fitsialos DP: Arthroscopic management of the degenerative knee. *Arthroscopy* 1991;7:151-157.
8. Cameron JC, Saha S: Meniscal allograft transplantation for unicompartmental arthritis of the knee. *Clin Orthop* 1997;337:164-171.
9. Johnson LL: Arthroscopic abrasion arthroplasty historical and pathologic perspective: Present status. *Arthroscopy* 1986;2:54-69.
10. Stuart MJ: Treatment of chronic chondral injuries. *Sports Med Arthrosc Rev* 1994;2:50-58.
11. Linschoten NJ, Johnson CA: Arthroscopic debridement of knee joint arthritis: Effect of advancing articular degeneration. *J South Orthop Assoc* 1997;6:25-36.
12. Salisbury RB, Nottage WM, Gardner V: The effect of alignment on results in arthroscopic debridement of the degenerative knee. *Clin Orthop* 1985;198:268-272.
13. Merchan EC, Galindo E: Arthroscope-guided surgery versus nonsurgical treatment for limited degenerative osteoarthritis of the femorotibial joint in patients over 50 years of age: A prospective comparative study. *Arthroscopy* 1993;9:663-667.
14. Harwin SF: Arthroscopic debridement for osteoarthritis of the knee: Predictors of patient satisfaction. *Arthroscopy* 1999;15:142-146.
15. McLaren AC, Blokker CP, Fowler PJ, Roth JN, Rock MG: Arthroscopic debridement of the knee for osteoarthrosis. *Can J Surg* 1991;34:595-598.
16. Sherman OH, Fox JM, Snyder SJ, et al: Arthroscopy: "No-problem surgery": An analysis of complications in two thousand six hundred and forty cases. *J Bone Joint Surg Am* 1986;68:256-265.
17. Rodeo SA, Forster RA, Weiland AJ: Neurological complications due to arthroscopy. *J Bone Joint Surg Am* 1993;75:917-926.
18. Gibson JN, White MD, Chapman VM, Strachan RK: Arthroscopic lavage and debridement for osteoarthritis of the knee. *J Bone Joint Surg Br* 1992;74:534-537.
19. Moseley JB Jr, Wray NP, Kuykendall D, Willis K, Landon G: Arthroscopic treatment of osteoarthritis of the knee: A prospective, randomized, placebo-controlled trial: Results of a pilot study. *Am J Sports Med* 1996;24:28-34.
20. Johnson DL, Bealle D: Meniscal allograft transplantation. *Clin Sports Med* 1999;18: 93-108.
21. McEldowney AJ, Weiker GG: Open-knee Magnuson debridement as conservative treatment for degenerative osteoarthrosis of the knee. *J Arthroplasty* 1995;10:805-809.
22. Bert JM, Maschka K: The arthroscopic treatment of unicompartmental gonarthrosis: A five-year follow-up study of abrasion arthroplasty plus arthroscopic debridement and arthroscopic debridement alone. *Arthroscopy* 1989;5:25-32.
23. Friedman MJ, Berasi CC, Fox JM, Del Pizzo W, Snyder SJ, Ferkel RD: Preliminary results with abrasion arthroplasty in the osteoarthritic knee. *Clin Orthop* 1984;182:200-205.
24. Rand JA: Role of arthroscopy in osteoarthritis of the knee. *Arthroscopy* 1991;7:358-363.
25. Neuschwander DC, Drez D Jr, Paine RM: Simultaneous high tibial osteotomy and ACL reconstruction for combined genu varum and symptomatic ACL tear. *Orthopedics* 1993;16:679-684.
26. Shelbourne KD, Wilckens JH: Intraarticular anterior cruciate ligament reconstruction in the symptomatic arthritic knee. *Am J Sports Med* 1993:21:685-689.
27. Shelbourne KD, Stube KC: Anterior cruciate ligament (ACL)-deficient knee with degenerative arthrosis: Treatment with an isolated autogenous patellar tendon ACL reconstruction. *Knee Surg Sports Traumatol Arthrosc* 1997;5: 150-156.

28. Noyes FR, Barber-Westin SD: Anterior cruciate ligament reconstruction with autogenous patellar tendon graft in patients with articular cartilage damage. *Am J Sports Med* 1997;25: 626-634.

29. Boss A, Stutz G, Oursin C, Gachter A: Anterior cruciate ligament reconstruction combined with valgus tibial osteotomy: Combined procedure. *Knee Surg Sports Traumatol Arthrosc* 1995;3:187-191.

30. Dejour H, Neyret P, Boileau P, Donell ST: Anterior cruciate reconstruction combined with valgus tibial osteotomy. *Clin Orthop* 1994;299:220-228.

31. Jakob RP, Murphy SB: Tibial osteotomy for varus gonarthrosis: Indication, planning, and operative technique. *Instr Course Lect* 1992;41:87-93.

32. Lattermann C, Jakob RP: High tibial osteotomy alone or combined with ligament reconstruction in anterior cruciate ligament-deficient knees. *Knee Surg Sports Traumatol Arthrosc* 1996;4:32-38.

33. Noyes FR, Barber-Westin SD: Arthroscopic-assisted allograft anterior cruciate ligament reconstruction in patients with symptomatic arthrosis. *Arthroscopy* 1997;13:24-32.

34. O'Neill DF, James SL: Valgus osteotomy with anterior cruciate ligament laxity. *Clin Orthop* 1992;278:153-159.

35. Miller MD, Fu FH: The role of osteotomy in the anterior cruciate ligament-deficient knee. *Clin Sports Med* 1993;12:697-708.

36. Coventry MB: Upper tibial osteotomy for gonarthrosis: The evolution of the operation in the last 18 years and long term results. *Orthop Clin North Am* 1979;10:191-210.

37. Holden DL, James SL, Larson RL, Slocum DB: Proximal tibial osteotomy in patients who are fifty years old or less: A long-term follow-up study. *J Bone Joint Surg Am* 1988;70:977-982.

38. Nagel A, Insall JN, Scuderi GR: Proximal tibial osteotomy: A subjective outcome study. *J Bone Joint Surg Am* 1996;78:1353-1358.

39. Odenbring S, Tjornstrand B, Egund N, Hagstedt B, Hovelius L, Lindstrand A, Luxhoj T, Svanstrom A: Function after tibial osteotomy for medial gonarthrosis below aged 50 years. *Acta Orthop Scand* 1989;60:527-531.

40. Insall JN, Joseph DM, Msika C: High tibial osteotomy for varus gonarthrosis: A long-term follow-up study. *J Bone Joint Surg Am* 1984;66:1040-1048.

41. Johnson BG, Hanssen AD, Morrey BF: Abstract: Long-term radiographic analysis of cemented condylar TKA in patients with osteoarthritis who have had a prior high tibial osteotomy. *62nd Annual Meeting Proceedings*. Rosemont, IL, American Academy of Orthopaedic Surgeons, 1995, p 328.

42. Morrey BF: Upper tibial osteotomy for secondary osteoarthritis of the knee. *J Bone Joint Surg Br* 1989;71:554-559.

43. Slawski DP: High tibial osteotomy in the treatment of adult osteochondritis dissecans. *Clin Orthop* 1997;341:155-161.

44. Coventry MB, Ilstrup DM, Wallrichs SL: Proximal tibial osteotomy: A critical long-term study of eighty-seven cases. *J Bone Joint Surg Am* 1993;75:196-201.

45. Matthews LS, Goldstein SA, Malvitz TA, Katz BP, Kaufer H: Proximal tibial osteotomy: Factors that influence the duration of satisfactory function. *Clin Orthop* 1988;229:193-200.

46. Berman AT, Bosacco SJ, Kirshner S, Avalio A Jr: Factors influencing long-term results in high tibial osteotomy. *Clin Orthop* 1991; 272:192-198.

47. Chillag KJ, Nicholls PJ: High tibial osteotomy: A retrospective analysis of 30 cases. *Orthopedics* 1984;7:1821-1822.

48. Hernigou P, Medevielle D, Debeyre J, Goutallier D: Proximal tibial osteotomy for osteoarthritis with varus deformity: A ten to thirteen-year follow-up study. *J Bone Joint Surg Am* 1987;69:332-354.

49. Cass JR, Bryan RS: High tibial osteotomy. *Clin Orthop* 1988;230:196-199.

50. Rudan JF, Simurda MA: Valgus high tibial osteotomy: A long-term follow-up study. *Clin Orthop* 1991;268:157-160.

51. Odenbring S, Egund N, Knutson K, Lindstrand A, Larsen ST: Revision after osteotomy for gonarthrosis: A 10-19-year follow-up of 314 cases. *Acta Orthop Scand* 1990; 61:128-130.

52. MacIntosh DL, Welsh RP: Joint debridement: A complement to high tibial osteotomy in the treatment of degenerative arthritis of the knee. *J Bone Joint Surg Am* 1977;59:1094-1097.

53. Akizuki S, Yasukawa Y, Takizawa T: Does arthroscopic abrasion arthroplasty promote cartilage regeneration in osteoarthritic knees with eburnation? A prospective study of high tibial osteotomy with abrasion arthroplasty versus high tibial osteotomy alone. *Arthroscopy* 1997;13:9-17.

54. Hsu RW: The study of Maquet dome high tibial osteotomy: Arthroscopic-assisted analysis. *Clin Orthop* 1989;243:280-285.

55. Odenbring S, Egund N, Lindstrand A, Lohmander LS, Willén H: Cartilage regeneration after proximal tibial osteotomy for medial gonarthrosis: An arthroscopic, roentgenographic, and histologic study. *Clin Orthop* 1992; 277:210-216.

56. Keene JS, Dyreby JR Jr: High tibial osteotomy in the treatment of osteoarthritis of the knee: The role of preoperative arthroscopy. *J Bone Joint Surg Am* 1983;65:36-42.

57. Healy WL, Riley LH Jr: High tibial valgus osteotomy: A clinical review. *Clin Orthop* 1986;209:227-233.

58. Ritter MA, Fechtman RA: Proximal tibial osteotomy: A survivorship analysis. *J Arthroplasty* 1988;3:309-311.

59. Yasuda K, Majima T, Tsuchida T, Kaneda K: A ten- to 15-year follow-up observation of high tibial osteotomy in medial compartment osteoarthrosis. *Clin Orthop* 1992;282:186-195.

60. Beaver RJ, Yu J, Sekyi-Otu A, Gross AE: Distal femoral varus osteotomy for genu valgum: A prospective review. *Am J Knee Surg* 1991;4:9-17.

61. Cameron HU, Botsford DJ, Park YS: Prognostic factors in the outcome of supracondylar femoral osteotomy for lateral compartment osteoarthritis of the knee. *Can J Surg* 1997;40:114-118.

62. Conrad EU, Soudry M, Insall JN: Supracondylar femoral osteotomy for valgus knee deformities. *Orthop Trans* 1985;9:25-26.

63. Edgerton BC, Mariani EM, Morrey BF: Distal femoral varus osteotomy for painful genu valgum: A five-to-11-year follow-up study. *Clin Orthop* 1993;288:263-269.

64. Finkelstein JA, Gross AE, Davis A: Varus osteotomy of the distal part of the femur: A survivorship analysis. *J Bone Joint Surg Am* 1996;78:1348-1352.

65. Healy WL, Anglen JO, Wasilewski SA, Krackow KA: Distal femoral varus osteotomy. *J Bone Joint Surg Am* 1988;70:102-109.

66. Johnson EW Jr, Bodell LS: Corrective supracondylar osteotomy for painful genu valgum. *Mayo Clin Proc* 1981;56:87-92.

67. McDermott AG, Finklestein JA, Farine I, Boynton EL, MacIntosh DL, Gross A: Distal femoral varus osteotomy for valgus deformity of the knee. *J Bone Joint Surg Am* 1988;70:110-116.

68. Mathews J, Cobb AG, Richardson S, Bentley G: Distal femoral osteotomy for lateral compartment osteoarthritis of the knee. *Orthopedics* 1998;21:437-440.

69. Miniaci A, Grossmann SP, Jakob RP: Supracondylar femoral varus osteotomy in the treatment of valgus knee deformity. *Am J Knee Surg* 1990;3:65-70.

70. Terry GC, Cimino PM: Distal femoral osteotomy for valgus deformity of the knee. *Orthopedics* 1992;15:1283-1290.

71. Kettelkamp DB, Leach RE Nasca R: Pitfalls of proximal tibial osteotomy. *Clin Orthop* 1975;106:232-241.

72. Maquet P: Valgus osteotomy for osteoarthritis of the knee. *Clin Orthop* 1976;120:143-148.

73. Beyer CA, Lewallen DG, Hanssen AD: Total knee arthroplasty following prior osteotomy of the distal femur. *Am J Knee Surg* 1994;7:25-30.

74. Westrich GH, Peters LE, Haas SB, Buly RL, Windsor RE: Patella height after high tibial osteotomy with internal fixation and early motion. *Clin Orthop* 1998;354:169-174.

75. Windsor RE, Insall JN, Vince KG: Technical considerations of total knee arthroplasty after proximal tibial osteotomy. *J Bone Joint Surg Am* 1988;70:547-555.

76. Katz MM, Hungerford DS, Krackow KA, Lennox DW: Results of total knee arthroplasty after failed proximal tibial osteotomy for osteoarthritis. *J Bone Joint Surg Am* 1987;69:225-233.

77. Ansari S, Newman JH, Ackroyd CE: St. Georg sledge for medial compartment knee replacement: 461 arthroplasties followed for 4 (1-17) years. *Acta Orthop Scand* 1997;68:430-434.

78. Berger RA, Nedeff DD, Barden RM, et al: Unicompartmental knee arthroplasty: Clinical experience at 6- to 10-year followup. *Clin Orthop* 1999;367:50-60.

79. Hasegawa Y, Ooishi Y, Shimizu T, et al: Unicompartmental knee arthroplasty for medial gonarthrosis: 5 to 9 years follow-up evaluation of 77 knees. *Arch Orthop Trauma Surg* 1998;117:183-187.

80. Barrett WP, Scott RD: Revision of failed unicondylar unicompartmental knee arthroplasty. *J Bone Joint Surg Am* 1987;69:1328-1335.

81. Schai PA, Suh JT, Thornhill TS, Scott RD: Unicompartmental knee arthroplasty in middle-aged patients: A 2- to 6-year follow-up evaluation. *J Arthroplasty* 1998;13:365-372.

82. Ivarsson I, Gillquist J: Rehabilitation after high tibial osteotomy and unicompartmental arthroplasty: A comparative study. *Clin Orthop* 1991;266:139-144.

83. Weale AE, Newman JH: Unicompartmental arthroplasty and high tibial osteotomy for osteoarthrosis of the knee: A comparative study with a 12- to 17-year follow-up period. *Clin Orthop* 1994;302:134-137.

84. Bernasek TL, Rand JA, Bryan RS: Unicompartmental porous coated anatomic TKA. *Clin Orthop* 1988;236:52-59.

85. Newman JH, Ackroyd CE, Shah NA: Unicompartmental or total knee replacement? Five-year results of a prospective, randomised trial of 102 osteoarthritic knees with unicompartmental arthritis. *J Bone Joint Surg Br* 1998;80:862-865.

86. Rougraff BT, Heck DA, Gibson AE: A comparison of tricompartmental and unicompartmental arthroplasty for the treatment of gonarthrosis. *Clin Orthop* 1991;273:157-164.

87. Broughton NS, Newman JH, Baily RA: Unicompartmental replacement and high tibial osteotomy for osteoarthritis of the knee: A comparative study after 5-10 years' follow-up. *J Bone Joint Surg Br* 1986;68:447-452.

88. Cartier P, Sanouiller JL, Grelsamer RP: Unicompartmental knee arthroplasty surgery: 10-year minimum follow-up period. *J Arthroplasty* 1996;11:782-788.

89. Kozinn SC, Marx C, Scott RD: Unicompartmental knee arthroplasty: A 4.5-6-year follow-up study with a metal-backed tibial component. *J Arthroplasty* 1989;4(suppl):S1-S10.

90. Murray DW, Goodfellow JW, O'Connor JJ: The Oxford medial unicompartmental arthroplasty: A ten-year survival study. *J Bone Joint Surg Br* 1998;80:983-989.

91. Squire MW, Callaghan JJ, Goetz DD, Sullivan PM, Johnston RC: Unicompartmental knee replacement: A minimum 15 year followup study. *Clin Orthop* 1999;367:61-72.

92. Capra SW Jr, Fehring TK: Unicondylar arthroplasty: A survivorship analysis. *J Arthroplasty* 1992;7:247-251.

93. Thornhill TS, Scott RD: Unicompartmental total knee arthroplasty. *Orthop Clin North Am* 1989;20:245-256.

94. Marmor L: Unicompartmental arthroplasty of the knee with a minimum ten-year follow-up period. *Clin Orthop* 1988;228:171-177.

95. Heck DA, Marmor L, Gibson A, Rougraff BT: Unicompartmental knee arthroplasty: A multicenter investigation with long-term follow-up evaluation. *Clin Orthop* 1993;286:154-159.

96. Barnes CL, Scott RD: Unicompartmental knee arthroplasty. *Instr Course Lect* 1993;42:309-314.

97. Klemme WR, Galvin EG, Petersen SA: Unicompartmental knee arthroplasty: Sequential radiographic and scintigraphic imaging with an average five-year follow-up. *Clin Orthop* 1994;301:233-238.

98. Swank M, Stulberg SD, Jiganti J, Machairas S: The natural history of unicompartmental arthroplasty: An eight-year follow-up study with survivorship analysis. *Clin Orthop* 1993;286:130-142.

99. Bert JM: 10-year survivorship of metal-backed, unicompartmental arthroplasty. *J Arthroplasty* 1998;13:901-905.

100. Lewold S, Robertsson O, Knutson K, Lidgren L: Revision of unicompartmental knee arthroplasty: Outcome in 1,135 cases from the Swedish Knee Arthroplasty study. *Acta Orthop Scand* 1998;69:469-474.

101. Lindstrand A, Stenstrom A: Polyethylene wear of the PCA unicompartmental knee: Prospective 5 (4-8) year study of 120 arthrosis knees. *Acta Orthop Scand* 1992;63:260-262.

102. McCallum JD III, Scott RD: Duplication of medial erosion in unicompartmental knee arthroplasties. *J Bone Joint Surg Br* 1995;77:726-728.

103. Hodge WA, Chandler HP: Unicompartmental knee replacement: A comparison of constrained and unconstrained designs. *J Bone Joint Surg Am* 1992;74:877-883.

104. Cohen M, Buechel F, Pappas MJ: Meniscal-bearing unicompartmental knee arthroplasty: An 11-year clinical study. *Orthop Rev* 1991;20:443-448.

105. Lewold S, Goodman S, Knutson K, Robertsson O, Lidgren L: Oxford meniscal bearing knee versus the Marmor knee in unicompartmental arthroplasty for arthrosis: A Swedish multicenter survival study. *J Arthroplasty* 1995;10:722-731.

106. Riebel GD, Werner FW, Ayers DC, Bromka J, Murray DG: Early failure of the femoral component in unicompartmental knee arthroplasty. *J Arthroplasty* 1995;10:615-621.

107. Scott RD, Cobb AG, McQueary FG, Thornhill TS: Unicompartmental knee arthroplasty: Eight- to 12-year follow-up evaluation with survivorship analysis. *Clin Orthop* 1991;271:96-100.

108. Jackson M, Sarangi PP, Newman JH: Revision total knee arthroplasty: Comparison of outcome following primary proximal tibial osteotomy or unicompartmental arthroplasty. *J Arthroplasty* 1994;9:539-542.

109. Lai CH, Rand JA: Revision of failed unicompartmental total knee arthroplasty. *Clin Orthop* 1993;287:193-201.

110. Levine WN, Ozuna RM, Scott RD, Thornhill TS: Conversion of failed modern unicompartmental arthroplasty to total knee arthroplasty. *J Arthroplasty* 1996;11:797-801.

111. Chakrabarty G, Newman JH, Ackroyd CE: Revision of unicompartmental arthroplasty of the knee: Clinical and technical considerations. *J Arthroplasty* 1998;13:191-196.

112. Padgett DE, Stern SH, Insall JN: Revision total knee arthroplasty for failed unicompartmental replacement. *J Bone Joint Surg Am* 1991;73:186-190.

113. Gill T, Schemitsch EH, Brick GW, Thornhill TS: Revision total knee arthroplasty after failed unicompartmental knee arthroplasty or high tibial osteotomy. *Clin Orthop* 1995;321:10-18.

114. Colizza WA, Insall JN, Scuderi GR: The posterior stabilized total knee prosthesis: Assessment of polyethylene damage and osteolysis after a ten-year minimum follow-up. *J Bone Joint Surg Am* 1995;77:1713-1720.

115. Ewald FC, Jacobs MA, Miegel RE, Walker PS, Poss R, Sledge CB: Kinematic total knee replacement. *J Bone Joint Surg Am* 1984;66:1032-1040.

116. Insall JN, Lachiewicz PF, Burstein AH: The posterior stabilized condylar prosthesis: A modification of the total condylar design: Two to four-year clinical experience. *J Bone Joint Surg Am* 1982;64:1317-1323.

117. Insall JN, Kelly M: The total condylar prosthesis. *Clin Orthop* 1986;205:43-48.

118. Vince KG, Insall JN, Kelly MA: The total condylar prosthesis: 10- to 12-year results of a cemented knee replacement. *J Bone Joint Surg Br* 1989;71:793-797.

119. Ewald F, Christie MJ: Results of cemented total knee replacement in young patients. *Orthop Trans* 1987;11:442.

120. Dorr LD, Kane TJ III, Conaty JP: Long-term results of cemented total hip arthroplasty in patients 45 years old or younger: A 16-year follow-up study. *J Arthroplasty* 1994;9:453-456.

121. Joshi AB, Porter ML, Trail IA, Hunt LP, Murphy JC, Hardinge K: Long-term results of Charnley low-friction arthroplasty in young patients. *J Bone Joint Surg Br* 1993;75:616-623.

122. Solomon MI, Dall DM, Learmonth ID, Davenport JM: Survivorship of cemented total hip arthroplasty in patients 50 years of age or younger. *J Arthroplasty* 1992;7(suppl):S347-S352.

123. Boublik M, Tsahakis PJ, Scott RD: Cementless TKA in juvenile onset rheumatoid arthritis. *Clin Orthop* 1993;286:88-93.

124. Dalury DF, Ewald FC, Christie MJ, Scott RD: TKA in a group of patients less than 45 years of age. *J Arthroplasty* 1995;10:598-602.

125. Ranawat CS, Padgett DE, Ohashi Y: Total knee arthroplasty for patients younger than 55 years. *Clin Orthop* 1989;248:27-33.

126. Stuart MJ, Rand JA: Total knee arthroplasty in young adults who have rheumatoid arthritis. *J Bone Joint Surg Am* 1988;70:84-87.

127. Hungerford DS, Krackow KA, Kenna RV: Cementless total knee replacement in patients 50 years old and under. *Orthop Clin North Am* 1989;20:131-145.

128. Stern SH, Bowen MK, Insall JN, Scuderi GR: Cemented total knee arthroplasty for gonarthrosis in patients 55 years old or younger. *Clin Orthop* 1990;260:124-129.

129. Duffy GP, Trousdale RT, Stuart MJ: TKA in patients 55 years old or younger: 10- to 17-year results. *Clin Orthop* 1998;356:22-27.

130. Diduch DR, Insall JN, Scott WN, Scuderi GR, Font-Rodriguez D: Total knee replacement in young, active patients: Long-term follow-up and functional outcome. *J Bone Joint Surg Am* 1997;79:575-582.

131. Tegner Y, Lysholm J: Rating systems in the evaluation of knee ligament injuries. *Clin Orthop* 1985;198:43-49.

SECTION

9

Foot and Ankle

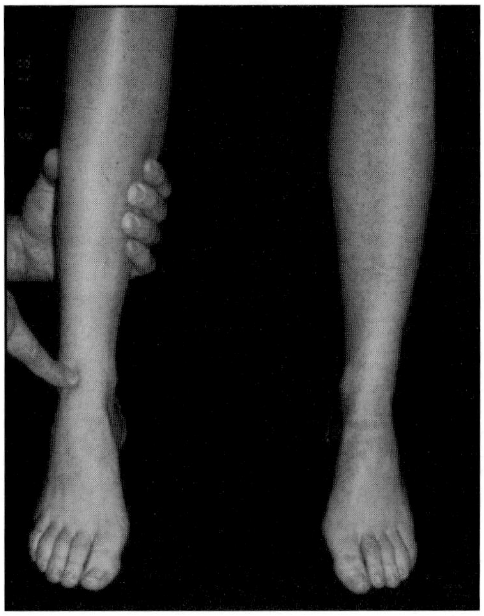

53 Ankle Sprains

54 Plantar Heel Pain

53

Ankle Sprains

Carol Frey, MD

Introduction

Inversion injuries to the ankle are one of the most common injuries seen in sports.[1] The incidence has been reported as high as one injury per 10,000 persons per day. The most common injury is to the anterior talofibular ligament followed by a combined injury to the anterior talofibular ligament and the calcaneofibular ligament. Although it has been noted that an isolated injury to the calcaneofibular ligament can exist, it is rarely seen. It is important for the orthopaedic surgeon to recognize that with a twisting injury to the foot and ankle, many structures are at risk for injury, including the peroneal tendons, syndesmosis, base of the fifth metatarsal, subtalar joint, lateral and anterior processes of the talus, Stieda process or the os trigonum, superficial peroneal and sural nerves, and the calcaneal-cuboid and Lisfranc joints. The complete differential diagnosis should be considered when evaluating the patient with an ankle sprain because a significant injury can be missed. Recent studies indicate that the subtalar joint may also be injured in the majority of grade II and III ankle sprains. In the case of an associated subtalar injury, the evaluating surgeon may note ecchymosis along the medial aspect of the heel, also known as the battle sign.

Lateral Collateral Ligament Injuries

Mechanism of Injury

Most injuries to the lateral collateral ligaments occur with a plantar flexion inversion injury to the ankle.[2-4] The lateral collateral ligaments are comprised of the anterior talofibular ligament, calcaneofibular ligament, and the posterior talofibular ligament. The anterior and posterior talofibular ligaments are capsular ligaments that represent discrete thickenings of the ankle joint capsule; the extracapsular calcaneofibular ligament is a distinct structure that is closely approximated to the inferior sheath of the peroneal tendons and is independent of the joint capsule. The anterior talofibular ligament is under maximum tension with the ankle in plantar flexion; in contrast, the calcaneofibular ligament is under most tension with the ankle in dorsiflexion.

Dynamic stabilization of the ankle is achieved with the help of the peroneal tendons, which protect the joint from the strong plantar flexion and inversion forces placed on it by the posterior tibial tendon. The nerves of proprioception that exist in the ankle joint and ligaments signal the peroneal tendons to contract when needed in order to stabilize the ankle joint.

Other biomechanical factors such as tight Achilles tendons, a varus hindfoot, or limited motion in the subtalar joint (for example, tarsal coalition) will cause excessive forces to fall to the lateral side of the foot and ankle and can place the ankle at an increased risk for inversion sprains.

Classification and Evaluation

Ankle sprains are classified as grades I, II, or III. The differences between these grades are outlined in Table 1. Physical examination with stress tests, radiographic stress tests, MRI, arthrograms, and tenograms have been recommended to help grade or assess the severity of the injury.[5-7]

Arthrograms and tenograms are rarely used because their results are difficult to obtain and interpret. The tests lack specificity and must be performed within the first 72 hours of an injury before fibrous clots develop.

MRI is a valuable tool in the evaluation of the patient with chronic ankle pain but does not provide information about ligamentous laxity and is not recommended in the workup of a patient with an acute ankle sprain.

Radiographic stress tests can sometimes provide objective data as to the extent of ligament damage.[8-10] The radiographic anterior drawer test (Fig. 1) is an evaluation of anterior talofibular damage and should be performed in approximately 10° of plantar flexion, the position that places most stress on the anterior talofibular ligament. The tibia is stabilized and the talus is pushed anteriorly, noting any subluxation of the talus with respect to the tibia. Any anterior displacement greater than approximately 4 mm has been considered abnormal, but a comparison should always be made to the opposite ankle.

The radiographic talar tilt test (Fig. 2) is performed by placing the ankle in neutral position (the position that places more stress on the calcaneofibular ligament) or in slight plantar flexion. A comparison is

Table 1
Classification of Ankle Sprains

	Anatomic Injury*	Physical Examination	Radiographic Findings
Grade I	Partial Tear ATF or CF	Negative or 1+ Drawer	– Drawer – Talar tilt
Grade II	Torn ATF Intact CF	2+ Drawer	+ Drawer – Talar tilt
Grade III	Torn ATF Torn CF	3+ Drawer	+ Drawer + Talar tilt

*ATF=anterior talofibular ligament; CF=calcaneofibular ligament

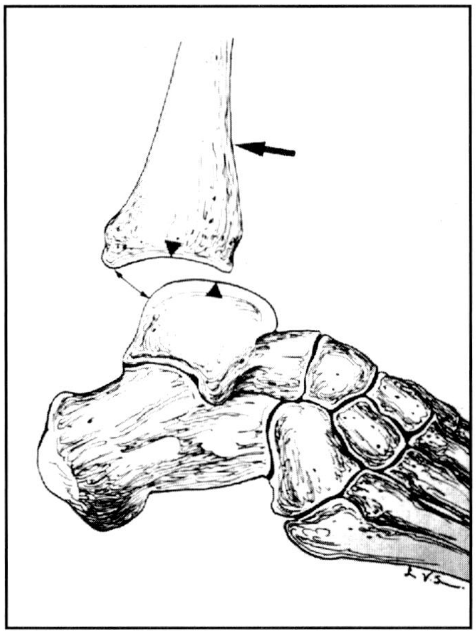

Fig. 1 Anterior instability demonstrated in a stress view. An anterior translation of more than 4.0 mm is usually considered abnormal. (Reproduced with permission from Pfeffer G, Frey C: Ankle instability, in *Current Practice in Foot and Ankle Surgery.* New York, NY, McGraw-Hill, 1993, pp 112-128.)

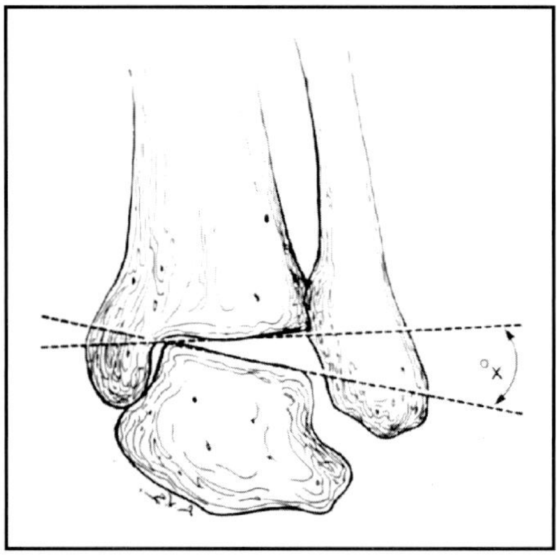

Fig. 2 Lateral instablility demonstrated on an inversion stress view. Using this measurement technique varies tilt. A value of 10° or a difference of more than 6° from the uninjured ankle is considered abnormal. (Reproduced with permission from Pfeffer G, Frey C: Ankle instability, in *Current Practice in Foot and Ankle Surgery.* New York, NY, McGraw-Hill, 1993, pp 112-128.)

always made to the opposite ankle. The tibia and the hindfoot are stabilized, and a varus stress is applied. The talar tilt is measured by drawing a line tangential to the distal aspect of the tibia and a line tangential to the proximal aspect of the talus. The angle where these two lines meet is the talar tilt angle. On average, a difference between the injured and the uninjured ankle of greater than 6° denotes a positive test.

Radiographic stress tests are considered by many to be unreliable because the results may vary depending on whether a machine or manual testing was performed; the position of the ankle; amount of relaxation, pain, or swelling; and amount or duration of load applied. Furthermore, normal values have been reported to range from 5° to 23° for the talar tilt test and 2 mm to 9 mm for the anterior drawer test. Although useful in evaluating chronic ankle instability, radiographic stress tests are not indicated in the workup of a patient with an acute lateral collateral ligament sprain.

The physical examination of the acute lateral ankle sprain should include an assessment of ligamentous laxity. If the patient's level of pain prevents a thorough evaluation, a local anesthetic may be used to block the injured ligaments. The anterior drawer test is performed as described for the radiographic stress tests.

The varus stress test is performed on both ankles for comparison. The ankle should be placed in neutral position to place more stress on the calcaneofibular ligament. The tibia is stabilized in one hand and the hindfoot in the other, making sure that varus stress is being applied through the ankle joint alone. The differences in the two ankles should be noted.

Treatment

Most authors agree that grade I and II ankle sprains should be treated conservatively. Phase 1 of treatment includes rest, ice, compression, elevation, and anti-inflammatory medications. Phase 2 includes range-of-motion stretching, particularly of the Achilles tendon, and strengthening, particularly of the peroneal tendons. Plantar flexion is deemphasized during this phase because this is the position that allows the most stress on the anterior talofibular ligament. Once the patient has full range of motion and has regained strength in the peroneal tendons, Phase 3 of treatment is instituted, which includes assessment of proprioception and agility, and a return to sports participation. A brace is recommended for grade II sprains through all phases of treatment and for sports participation until the end of the season or for a 3-month period, whichever is longer. It usually takes ankles with grade II sprains 2 to 4 weeks to regain full function.

There is some controversy with respect to the appropriate treatment of grade III ankle sprains.[11,12] Primary surgical treatment, cast immobilization, and early mobilization have been advocated.

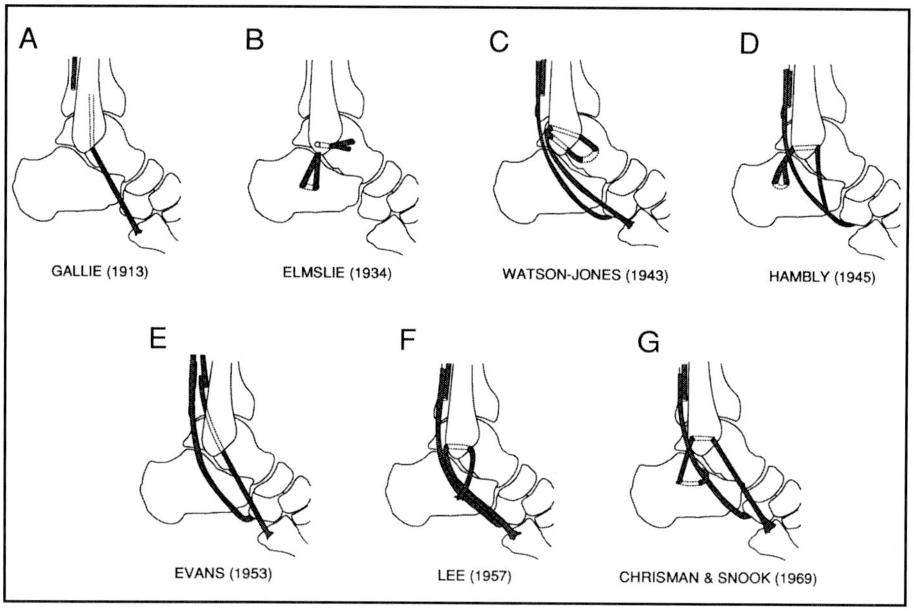

Fig. 3 Several techniques for reconstruction of the lateral collateral ligaments of the ankle are shown. (Reproduced with permission from Pfeffer G, Frey C: Ankle instability, in *Current Practice in Foot and Ankle Surgery.* New York, NY, McGraw-Hill, 1993, pp 112-128.)

In a review of all randomized prospective studies that compare primary surgical treatment versus the nonsurgical treatment of grade III ankle sprains, not one study shows the surgically treated patients to have better outcomes. Exceptions may be ballet dancers and other elite-level performers and athletes, although no randomized prospective study exists to support surgery in this group, either. Furthermore, even though acute repair may result in less talar tilt, patients may take a longer time to become symptom-free and at 1 year, a greater number of patients treated surgically have residual symptoms. In addition, there are more complications reported with acute surgical repair.

Generally, the same treatment protocol is used with grade III injuries as for grade I and II injuries. Grade III injuries progress more slowly through the phases of treatment. During phase 1 of treatment, grade III injuries require an ankle brace with a hindfoot lock or a short leg walking cast.

If a cast is elected, it should be a dorsiflexion walking cast that should not be used for more than 2 weeks. At 2 weeks, the repair process has commenced with the anterior talofibular ligament in apposition, and significant contracture formation has not begun. After this period, the patient progresses through phases 2 and 3 of treatment.

The patient with the grade III injury should wear a brace and/or have the injury taped for 3 months or until the end of the season, whichever is longer. A strength and balance program should continue through this period, especially for athletes and dancers. Bracing and tape can be used to stabilize the ankle by increasing mechanical stability and decreasing the range of ankle motion (particularly plantar flexion), and by amplifying and transferring the proprioception signals from the ankle. However, it should be kept in mind that tape is expensive to apply and can loosen after 20 to 30 minutes of play.

Proprioception

Freeman[13] introduced the concept of functional instability to describe the patient's subjective complaints of giving way. Functional ankle instability may be caused by damage to the proprioception fibers in the ankle ligaments and capsule or by peroneal weakness. Studies have indicated that balance exercises and a peroneal muscle strengthening program can restore functional stability to even a mechanically unstable ankle.[13,14] Exercise can increase the dynamic reaction time and ankle protection provided by the peroneal muscles. Failure to properly rehabilitate the peroneal muscles and proprioceptors is a major cause of chronic ankle instability.

Chronic Ankle Instability

A significant percentage of athletes will develop chronic instability of the ankle that will require further treatment. Chronic ankle instability may be documented by physical findings and radiographic stress tests. Prior to surgical intervention, the patient should complete an ankle rehabilitation program that includes peroneal muscle strengthening, proprioception training, and Achilles tendon stretching. If functional instability still exists after completion of this program, reconstruction of the ligaments is indicated. More than 50 procedures have been described to reconstruct the lateral collateral ligaments of the ankle. Many of these procedures use a portion or all of the peroneus brevis tendon to reconstruct the lateral ligaments. The most common are the Chrisman-Snook and the Evans procedures (Fig. 3). Most of these procedures have resulted in good outcomes.[15]

Anatomic repair of the ligaments, such as a direct ligament repair, will help preserve maximum ankle function[16] (Fig 4). In some cases this repair has been augmented with the inferior extensor retinaculum. Because the inferior extensor retinaculum has deep fibers that insert on the floor of the sinus tarsi, augmentation with the inferior extensor retinaculum is indicated in patients who have combined subtalar and ankle instability. The direct ligament repair has the advantages of preserving the peroneal tendons, creating minimal complications, and

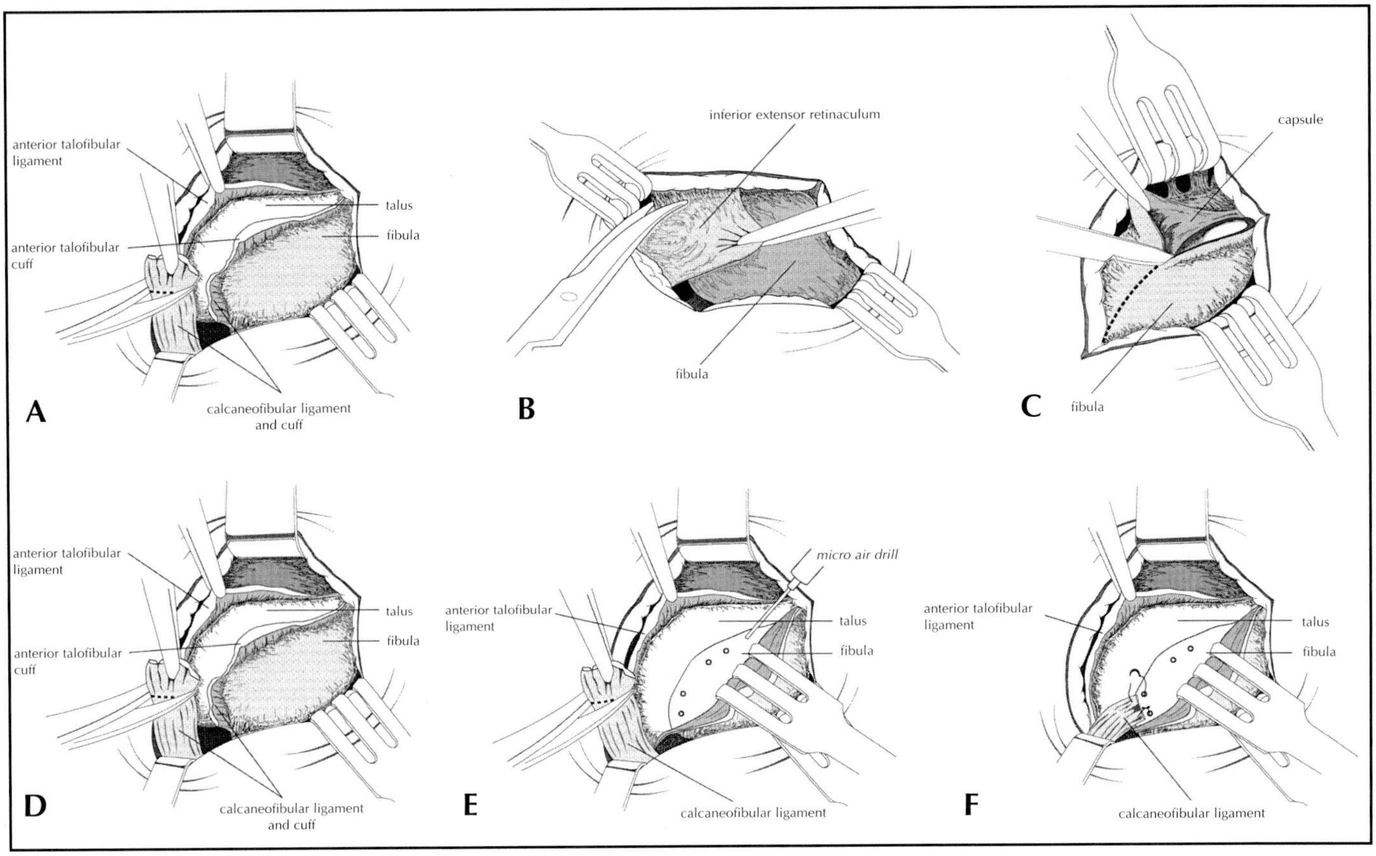

Fig. 4 The modified Brostrum procedure. The patient should be placed supine with a bolster under the ipsilateral hip. **A,** A small, curved incision at the tip of the lateral malleolus can be used. The inferior extensor retinaculum, peroneal tendons, and the lateral collateral ligaments are identified. **B,** The inferior extensor retinaculum is identified and freed to be used later for reinforcing the direct ligament repair. **C,** The capsule is opened in the region of the anterior talofibular ligament. **D,** The lax ligaments are transected, retaining approximately one third of the ligament attached to the distal fibula. **E,** The fibula is roughened with a burr inferior to the original ligaments' attachment. **F,** The distal stump of the anterior talofibular ligament and the calcaneofibular ligament is reattached to the fibula through drill holes, using a nonabsorbable braided suture. The ankle is placed in slight dorsiflexion and maximal eversion, and the sutures are tied. (Reproduced with permission from Pfeffer G, Frey C: Ankle instability, in *Current Practice in Foot and Ankle Surgery.* New York, NY, McGraw-Hill, 1993, pp 112-128.)

allowing retention of greater ankle and subtalar range of motion. Good long-term results have been reported using the direct ligament repair in high-performance athletes.

Exogenous ligament substitutes such as carbon fibers and bovine xenografts have been used more recently, but long-term results have not been reported.

Arthroscopic repair of the lateral collateral ligaments has been reported using suture anchors, staples, and capsular shrinkage (Figs. 5 through 8). Functional stability has been reported following these procedures but no long-term results have been reported.

Whatever the surgical technique selected, the athlete with a varus hindfoot places an added stress on the surgical repair and is at greater risk for reinjury. When extreme varus of the heel is present, a calcaneal osteotomy may be indicated.

Syndesmosis Injuries

Anatomy and Mechanism of Injury

The three ligaments that unite the distal fibula with the distal tibia are the anterior tibiofibular ligament, posterior tibiofibular ligament, and interosseous ligament. The lower aspect of the interosseous membrane also participates in stabilizing the distal fibula. When the ankle moves from full plantar flexion to full dorsiflexion, the fibula moves laterally 1.5 mm and takes a 2.5° lateral turn on its long axis.

Biomechanical tests have indicated that the anterior inferior tibiofibular ligament provides 35% of the strength of the syndesmosis, the interosseous ligament, 22%, and the posterior inferior tibiofibular ligament, 33%. The interosseous membrane does not add to the resistance to diastasis.

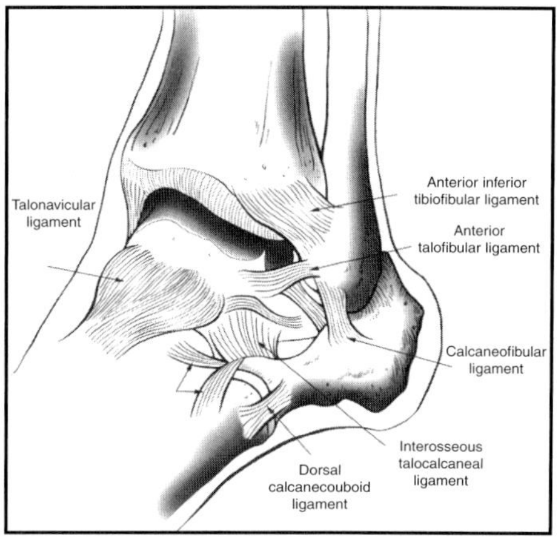

Fig. 5 The ligaments of the lateral side of the ankle.

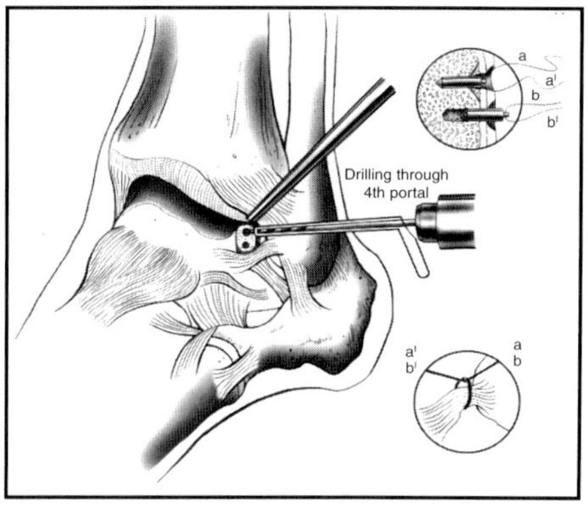

Fig. 6 A suture anchor technique to stabilize the ankle is shown.

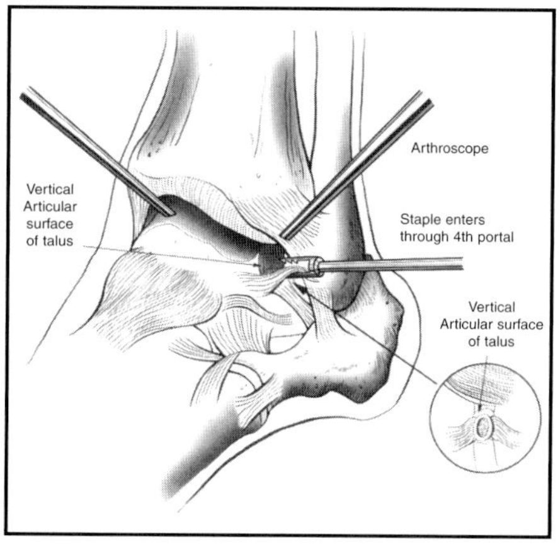

Fig. 7 A staple technique to stabilize the ankle is shown.

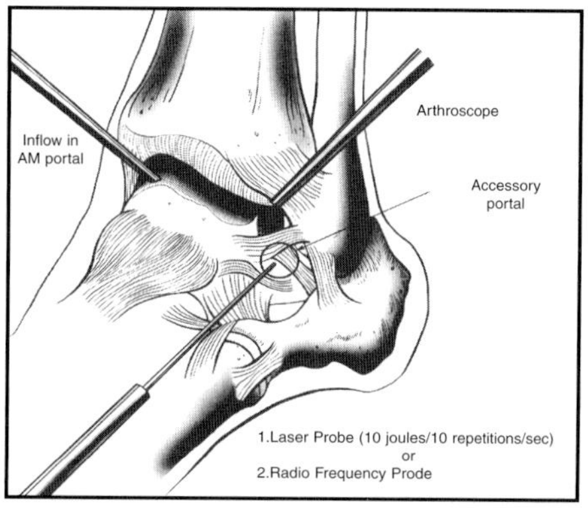

Fig. 8 Laser capsular shrinkage technique to stabilize the ankle.

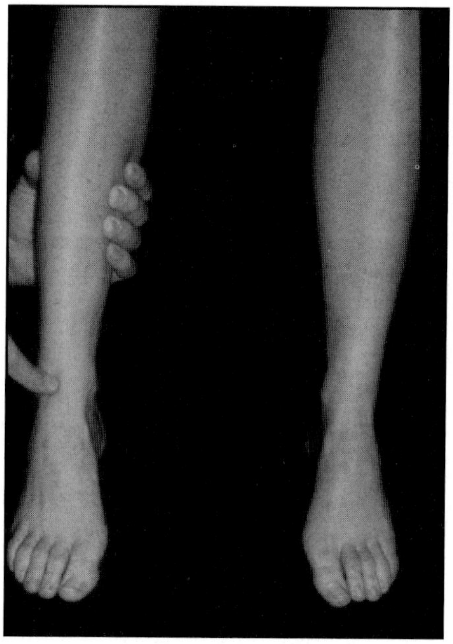

Fig. 9 The squeeze test demonstrates injury to the syndesmosis.

Injuries and sprains to the syndesmosis occur with much less frequency than do those to the lateral collateral ligament. They have been reported to represent approximately 11% of all ankle sprains. Disruption of the syndesmosis has been well described as occurring with or without fractures of the fibula. The mechanism of injury to the syndesmosis is primarily through external rotation or hyperdorsiflexion. This injury is commonly seen in skiers and football players.

Diagnosis

The patient's ankle is typically tender over the anterior syndesmosis, on the anterior lateral aspect of the ankle joint just proximal to the joint line. This may or may not be associated with swelling or tenderness over the deltoid ligament. The squeeze test may be performed by squeezing the fibula and the tibia at the midcalf area (Fig. 9). If the test is positive, it will elicit pain over the anterior syndesmosis. If there is an associated Maisonneuve fracture, the maximum tenderness will be felt in the area of the fracture. The syndesmosis may also be tested by performing the external rotation stress test. When performing this test, the foot is externally rotated on a stabilized leg with the knee flexed at a right angle. The external rotation stress test will create pain at the site of the syndesmosis if it is injured. These two tests should be included in any evaluation of an injured athlete after an ankle sprain. Syndesmosis injuries often have a longer rehabilitation time, requiring more long-term disability than injuries to the lateral collateral ligaments of the ankle.

Radiographs of the ankle are required in the evaluation of the athlete with a possible syndesmosis injury. In up to 50% of these cases, there may be a bone avulsion fracture from the anterior or posterior tubercle of the tibia. It is also important to evaluate the syndesmotic space. The tibiofibular clear space, measured 1 cm up from the joint line on the anteroposterior (AP) and mortise views, should be less than 6 mm. This is considered to be the most reliable criteria for detecting widening of the syndesmosis. The tibiofibular overlap on the AP view should be greater than 6 mm. The tibiofibular overlap on the mortise view should be greater than 1 mm. If there is any question as to widening of the syndesmosis, comparison views can be made of the opposite, uninjured ankle or external rotation stress views can be taken. Stress tests have been reported as difficult to obtain in many cases and occasionally other tests such as bone scans, CT, MRI, and arthrograms have been recommended. A positive bone scan will show increased uptake at the talofibular joint.

Treatment

There is universal agreement that sprains of the syndesmosis take considerably longer to heal than sprains to the lateral collateral ligaments of the ankle. It has also been noted that approximately one third of patients with syndesmotic ankle sprains have chronic mild to moderate pain with activity after recovery.

A partial injury to the syndesmosis should be treated in a walking cast for 2 to 4 weeks followed by an ankle rehabilitation program and tape/brace for 3 months or until the end of the season, whichever is longer. If syndesmosis widening is noted on plain or stress radiographs, then surgical repair is recommended. Surgery should include direct surgical repair of the torn anterior tibiofibular ligaments or repair of an avulsion fracture if present. Furthermore, the distal tibiofibular syndesmosis should be transfixed with a syndesmosis screw placed 1 to 2 cm proximal to the distal tibiofibular articulation, with the ankle held in maximum dorsiflexion. Postoperatively, the patient is treated in a non–weight-bearing short leg cast for 4 weeks, followed by 4 more weeks in a weight-bearing cast. The syndesmosis screw should be removed in approximately 12 weeks. It is not uncommon for heterotopic bone to form in the area of the syndesmosis injury, regardless of the treatment program. Unless there is frank synostosis that affects the normal motion of rotation and distal migration of the fibula with respect to the tibia, the results are not affected by heterotopic bone formation.

If a synostosis does occur, the athlete will particularly note pain during push-off and forced dorsiflexion. Dorsiflexion is limited. If symptoms cannot be managed with conservative treatment, including physical therapy, anti-inflammatory agents, and a cushioned heel lift, surgery to remove the synostosis is indicated when the heterotopic bone has matured. The recurrence rate is high with this type of surgery.

References

1. Holmer P, Sondergaard L, Konradsen L, Nielsen PT, Jorgensen LN: Epidemiology of sprains in the lateral ankle and foot. *Foot Ankle Int* 1994;15:72-74.
2. Kannus P, Renstrom P: Treatment for acute tears of the lateral ligaments of the ankle: Operation, cast, or early controlled mobilization. *J Bone Joint Surg Am* 1991; 73: 305-312.
3. Burks RT, Morgan J: Anatomy of the lateral ankle ligaments. *Am J Sports Med* 1994;22:72-77.
4. Colville MR, Marder RA, Zarins B: Reconstruction of the lateral ankle ligaments: A biomechanical analysis. *Am J Sports Med* 1992;20:594-600.
5. Johnson EE, Markolf KL: The contribution of the anterior talofibular ligament to ankle laxity. *J Bone Joint Surg Am* 1983;65:81-88.
6. Colville MR, Marder RA, Boyle JJ, Zarins B: Strain measurement in lateral ankle ligaments. *Am J Sports Med* 1990;18:196-200.
7. Rasmussen O: Stability of the ankle joint: Analysis of the function and traumatology of the ankle ligaments. *Acta Orthop Scand* 1985;211(suppl):1-75.
8. Ahovuo J, Kaartinen E, Slatis P: Diagnostic value of stress radiography in lesions of the lateral ligaments of the ankle. *Acta Radiol* 1988;29:711-714.
9. Louwerens JW, Ginai AZ, van Linge B, Snijders CJ: Stress radiography of the talocrural and subtalar joints. *Foot Ankle Int* 1995;16: 148-155.
10. Ishii T, Miyagawa S, Fukubayashi T, Hayashi K: Subtalar stress radiography using forced dorsiflexion and supination. *J Bone Joint Surg Br* 1996;78:56-60.
11. Thermann H, Zwipp H, Tscherne H: Treatment algorithm of chronic ankle and subtalar instability. *Foot Ankle Int* 1997;18:163-169.
12. Black HM, Brand RL, Eichelberger MR: An improved technique for the evaluation of ligamentous injury in severe ankle sprains. *Am J Sports Med* 1978;6:276-282.
13. Freeman MAR: Instability of the foot after injuries to the lateral ligaments of the ankle. *J Bone Joint Surg Br* 1965;47:669-677.
14. Mascaro TB, Swanson LE: Rehabilitation of the foot and ankle. *Orthop Clin North Am* 1994;25:147-160.
15. Colville MR, Grondel RJ: Anatomic reconstruction of the lateral ankle ligaments using a split peroneus brevis tendon graft. *Am J Sports Med* 1995;23:210-213.
16. Gould N, Seligson D, Gassman J: Early and late repair of lateral ligaments of the ankle. *Foot Ankle* 1980;1:84-89.

54

Plantar Heel Pain

Glenn B. Pfeffer, MD

Introduction

Plantar heel pain is one of the most common problems treated in orthopaedic practice.[1] Despite its frequency, little is known about the pathophysiology of this condition. Patients and physicians are often frustrated by symptoms refractory to varied and prolonged treatment modalities. The ability to effect a cure correlates with the precision of the diagnosis and is dependent on an understanding of both the complex anatomy of the heel and the multiple causes of plantar heel pain.

Diagnosis

The differential diagnosis of plantar heel pain includes atrophy of the fat pad; stress fracture of the calcaneus; rupture of the plantar fascia; proximal (and distal) plantar fasciitis; plantar fibromatosis; tendinitis of the flexor hallucis longus; tumor of the calcaneus; and nerve injury such as that to the first branch of the lateral plantar nerve, tarsal tunnel syndrome, and postoperative neuroma of the medial calcaneal sensory nerve.

In differentiating these varied diagnoses, a comprehensive medical history is essential. The history should include the patient's general medical condition, any substantial change in weight, the exact location and duration of pain and whether it radiates, and the relationship of pain to athletic activities, particularly those requiring running and jumping. The time of day that maximal pain occurs should be noted. Patients with proximal plantar fasciitis will frequently complain of disabling pain with the first few steps out of bed in the morning. Chronic pain at rest may be caused by a tumor of the calcaneus. Radiculopathy in the L5-S1 distribution should be considered in the patient with low back pain and, particularly when the heel pain is bilateral, a systemic process should be excluded. Pain at the sites of tendinous insertions (enthesiopathy) is often a prominent feature in patients with a seronegative spondyloarthropathy.[2,3] Ankylosing spondylitis, psoriatic arthritis, Reiter's syndrome, intestinal arthropathies, and Behçet's syndrome must be excluded in the patient with heel pain that occurs in conjunction with skin lesions, conjunctivitis, arthritis, back pain, or abdominal complaints. An HLA/B27 test and erythrocyte sedimentation rate are useful screening methods for these diagnoses. Gout, Paget's disease, or sarcoidosis are rare with isolated painful inflammation in the plantar heel. The ischemic changes of peripheral vascular disease are also an unusual cause of plantar heel pain.

The key to the examination of plantar heel pain is to determine the specific focal area of maximal tenderness (Fig. 1). Each diagnosis has a maximally tender spot. The medial calcaneal tuberosity, lateral calcaneal tuberosity, proximal plantar fascia, distal plantar fascia, proximal abductor (overlying the first branch of the lateral plantar nerve), tarsal tunnel, flexor hallucis longus at the knot of Henry, the fat pad, and any scar from a previous surgery should be percussed and compressed to determine tenderness and the reproduction of a patient's

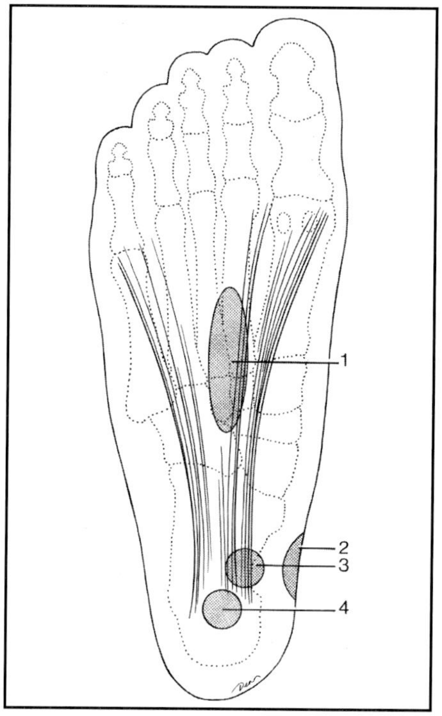

Fig. 1 Areas of maximal focal tenderness: 1 = midfoot plantar fasciitis, 2 = compression of first branch lateral plantar nerve, 3 = proximal plantar fasciitis, 4 = fat pat atrophy. (Reproduced with permission from Pfeffer GB, Baxter DE: Surgery of the adult heel, in Jahss MH (ed): *Disorders of the Foot and Ankle*, ed 2. Philadelphia, PA, WB Saunders, 1991, pp 1396-1416.)

symptoms. Deep pressure may often have to be applied. The windlass mechanism puts tension on the plantar fascia and may cause an increase in the patient's pain[4,5] (Fig. 2). When the fascia is taut, the plantar fascia should be palpated for defects proximally (rupture) or masses distally (plantar fibromatosis).

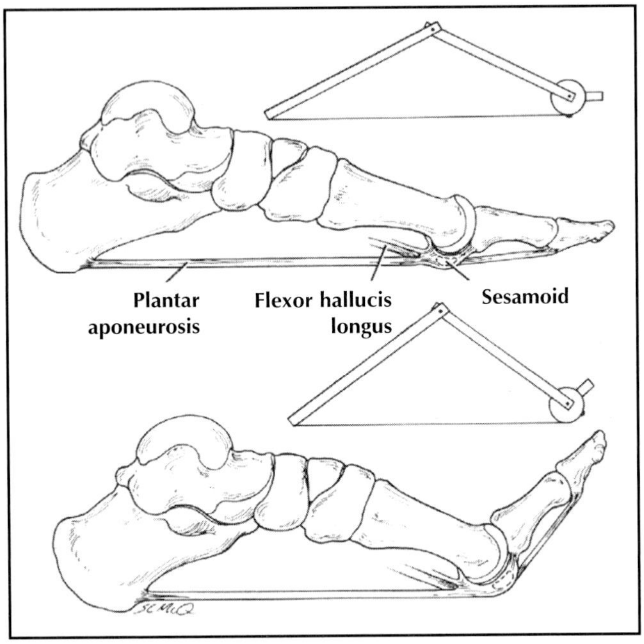

Fig. 2 The windlass mechanism. (Reproduced with permission from Richardson EG: The foot in adolescents and adults, in Crenshaw AH (ed): *Campbell's Operative Orthopaedics,* ed 7. St. Louis, MO, CV Mosby, 1987.)

The presence of a neuroma in a previous surgical scar will have a positive percussion sign directly over the cut nerve. Achilles tendon tightness is often associated with various causes of plantar heel pain (proximal plantar fasciitis and distal plantar fasciitis) and is tested by holding the foot in a neutral position and passive dorsiflexion of the ankle.

A patient's weight should also be documented on the physical examination. Increased body weight is associated with proximal plantar fasciitis.[6] It is often impossible, however, for a patient to achieve weight loss while a painful heel causes limitation of activity.

Anatomy of the Fat Pad

The fat pad cushions the foot with each heel strike.[7] A healthy middle-aged man has a gait velocity of approximately 82 m/min and a cadence of 116. This rate results in 58 heel strikes/min with a force of 110% of body weight. A middle- or long-distance runner generates a force of 200% of body weight. Considering timing, impact forces, and an average heel area of 23 cm^2, the loading pressure of a 70-kg man is approximately 9.3 kg/cm^2 when running.

Anatomic studies of the human heel pad have identified structural specialization that is capable of meeting these high impacts.[8,9] The anatomy of the heel pad was first described by Teitze in 1921. He emphasized the specialized anatomy of the heel pad, with elastic adipose tissue organized as spiral fibrous tissue septa anchored to one another, the calcaneus, and the skin. Designed to resist compressive loads, the tissue septa are U-shaped or comma-shaped, fat-filled columns.[10] The septa are reinforced internally with elastic transverse and diagonal fibers that connect the thicker walls and separate the fat into compartments.[11] The thickness of the heel pad is the most important factor in determining the stresses seen in the tissue beneath it. After age 40 years, the adipose tissue begins to deteriorate, with the insidious loss of collagen, elastic tissue, water, and overall thickness of the heel pad. These changes result in softening and thinning in the heel pad, loss of shock absorbency, and decreased protection of the underlying calcaneal tuberosity.

Causes of Chronic Heel Pain

The Fat Pad

Advanced atrophy of the plantar heel is an unusual problem and almost always occurs in the elderly patient. Heel pad atrophy can also occur in patients with rheumatoid arthritis.[12] A patient with calcaneodynia secondary to fat pad atrophy complains of plantar heel pain aggravated by hard-soled shoes and walking on nonresilient surfaces.[10,13] By clinical examination, the patient has soft, flattened heel pads, with prominence of the underlying calcaneal tubercles. Compression of this area by the examiner duplicates the symptoms, with pain maximal over the central weight-bearing portion of the heel pad. There is no radiation of the pain and the plantar fascia is not tender distally. The overlying plantar skin almost always demonstrates inflammation, from underlying bony irritation. This is not seen in any other cause of plantar heel pain. There is no reliable surgical treatment for this problem. A steroid solution should never be injected into the fat pad because it will promote further atrophy. The patient's symptoms are best treated with soft-soled shoes and a heel cup. A plastic heel cup that elevates the painful area and centralizes the fat pad under the prominent tuberosity is often the treatment of choice. A shock-absorbing insert, such as a cellular rubber gel or silicone pad, may also be beneficial. In addition, a slight heel elevation can be useful by shifting some of the weight bearing more anteriorly.

A rare cause of heel pain related to the fat pad is piezogenic ("piezo" meaning pressure) papules.[11] The normal fat chambers coalesce with degenerative changes in the dermis, creating piezogenic papules on the heel that appear with weight bearing. Multiple small papules are a common occurrence. Large, painful papules can form occasionally. It is not well understood why these larger papules are painful. Herniation of subcutaneous fat through defects in the dermis with subsequent local ischemia may be the cause. Heel cups may be sufficient treatment, but a custom orthosis molded to take pressure off of the painful papules is often required. In the absence of any papules, pinpoint tenderness on the heel can be caused by a glomus tumor, which is exquisitely tender to local pressure and changes in temperature. Surgical excision of the glomus tumor is curative.[14]

Another unusual cause of fat pad pain is separation of the fat pad from its anchor on the plantar aspect of the calcaneus. The heel pad becomes painful and freely mobile. The likely etiology for this separation is the presence of a fluid-filled cyst between the calcaneus and the fat pad, usually following direct trauma to the heel. MRI of the heel can confirm the diagnosis. Aspiration of the cyst and immobilization in a non-weight-bearing cast may permanently close the dead space. Surgical treatment consists of excision of the cyst through either a medial or lateral incision and removal of several millimeters of the plantar calcaneus. A compression dressing and adequate closed drainage should be used. The goal is for the heel pad to re-adhere to the underlying calcaneus.

Stress Fracture of the Calcaneus

Diffuse pain over the fat pad can occasionally be caused by an underlying stress fracture of the calcaneus.[15] Stress fractures of the calcaneus are uncommon and only occur in patients who place a significant stress on their heels. Military recruits who trained for more than 16 hours per day were found to be at particular risk for a calcaneal stress fracture. The stress fracture appears on the lateral radiographs as a vertical sclerotic band running from the posterior superior plateau into the cancellous region of the calcaneus. The trabecular pattern of bone is perpendicular to the line of the stress fracture. Often the stress fracture does not appear on initial radiographs and a technetium-99m bone scan may be required to detect early cases. The bone scan will demonstrate significant increased uptake on delayed images of the calcaneus. Although rare, a tumor of the calcaneus should be considered in the differential diagnosis of an abnormal bone scan.[16,17] Careful examination of the radiographs is essential. The sclerotic band of the stress fracture usually becomes evident on radiographs by 3 to 4 weeks after the onset of symptoms. On occasion, MRI may be required to evaluate the problem. Patients with proximal plantar fasciitis or heel pain syndrome will often have a hot bone scan directly over the medial calcaneal tuberosity related to inflammation of the periosteum. This finding is in clear distinction from a true stress fracture of the body of the calcaneus.

Clinically, a stress fracture of the calcaneus presents with diffuse pain about the entire heel. The patient has a history of progressive calcaneal pain almost always associated with a period of prolonged, intense activity. Mild erythema and swelling may be present. The hallmark of this condition is significant tenderness with simultaneous medial and lateral compression of the calcaneus. The pain is not localized to the plantar aspect of the heel alone. Casting is not required and symptoms usually resolve over 6 to 8 weeks. Weight bearing is allowed as tolerated with crutches. A removable cast may facilitate ambulation. Nonsteroidal anti-inflammatory agents, contrast baths, and a shock-absorbent heel insert may all be beneficial. Activity modification is essential to avoid recurrent injury.

Acute Rupture of the Plantar Fascia

If an active patient experiences the acute onset of proximal heel pain, rupture of the plantar fascia should be considered. Rupture is much less common than chronic proximal plantar fasciitis and can be easily differentiated on the basis of physical examination and history. A palpable defect in the proximal plantar fascia is present just distal to the medial calcaneal tuberosity. Ecchymosis and local hemorrhage occur with significant tenderness over the proximal plantar fascia. An athletic patient will often relate acute hyperextension of the midfoot that occurred while jamming the foot into a small pothole during running. There is often a history of proximal plantar fasciitis that has been treated with a steroid injection.[18-20] A short leg cast is helpful in a patient who needs to bear weight. Otherwise, crutches with weight bearing as tolerated is an appropriate treatment. Exercises directed at stretching the plantar fascia should be started when the acute inflammation lessens after several weeks.

Patients with a history of plantar fasciitis who rupture their plantar fascia often experience relief of their chronic plantar pain. However, they often develop a variety of new foot problems, including dorsal and lateral midfoot pain, midfoot swelling, metatarsalgia, and decreased toe-off strength.[21] These symptoms are best treated with supportive shoes, a medial longitudinal arch support, and, in refractory cases, prolonged casting for 8 weeks.

Proximal Plantar Fasciitis

Proximal plantar fasciitis is the most common cause of plantar heel pain, accounting for approximately 80% of patients with plantar symptoms. The average age of a patient with proximal plantar fasciitis is 45 years. The condition is twice as common in women as in men. There may be a history of increased stress on the foot from prolonged standing or athletic activity. There may be a history of recent weight gain. Symptoms are usually insidious in onset and often worse with the first few steps upon awakening. During sleep, the foot is in a plantar-flexed position, which allows the proximal plantar fascia to contract. The stretch placed on the plantar fascia by standing produces significant symptoms. The pain often resolves during the day, exacerbated by prolonged standing or athletic activity.[1,22-29]

Patients with proximal plantar fasciitis experience pain where the plantar fascia arises from the medial calcaneal tuberosity. A patient presents with maximal tenderness over the medial calcaneal tuberosity that may be associated with discomfort over the plantar fascia distally for 1 to 2 cm. The examiner frequently has to apply a considerable amount of pressure to localize this painful area. Radiation of pain is unusual. Contrary to many reports, the patient almost never has increased pain or duplication of symptoms with passive dorsiflexion of the toes, which causes traction on the plantar fascia by the windlass mechanism. Patients with proximal plantar fasciitis often have tightness of the Achilles tendon.[30,31] Achilles tendon tightness should be evaluated with the foot held in neutral position. In addition, there is a possible loss of dorsiflexion when compared to the contralateral, asymptomatic leg. A correlation has been postulated between proximal plantar fasciitis, pes planus, and pes cavus, although this relationship has never been clearly documented.

The diagnosis of proximal plantar fasciitis should be differentiated from other sources of plantar heel pain, especially distal plantar fasciitis and entrapment of the first branch of the lateral plantar nerve. Conservative and surgical treatments of these diagnoses are different. Proximal plantar fasciitis is a condition of chronic tears and inflammation in the origin of the plantar fascia where it arises from the medial calcaneal tuberosity. During gait, the plantar fascia places a repetitive traction stress on this area. The mechanism for this probably lies in the particular anatomic relationship of the plantar fascia to the calcaneus.[32]

The plantar fascia is a multilayered fibrous aponeurosis.[8] It arises predominantly from the medial calcaneal tuberosity and inserts distally through several slips into the plantar plates of the metatarsophalangeal joints, the flexor tendon sheaths, and the bases of the proximal phalanges of the digits. When the metatarsophalangeal joints are dorsiflexed during gait, the windlass of the plantar fascia tightens and raises the longitudinal arch.[5] A secondary effect is traction on the calcaneus by the inelastic plantar fascia fibers.[4]

Over time with repetitive stress, microtears can occur in the origin of the plantar fascia. Along with continued traumatic fatigue in the fascia, a reparative inflammatory response develops. As documented by MRI, the inflamed proximal plantar fascia becomes thickened, increasing from a mean thickness of 3 mm in a normal heel to a mean thickness of 7.4 mm in patients with chronic heel pain.[10] Surgical biopsy specimens of the origins of the plantar fascia in patients with proximal plantar fasciitis reveal collagen necrosis, angiofibroblastic hyperplasia, chondroid metaplasia, and matrix calcification. A similar process in all likelihood develops in the flexor brevis muscle directly deep to the plantar fascia, which accounts for the plantar spur that develops in the origin of that muscle in approximately 50% of patients with proximal plantar fasciitis. Nirschl and Pettrone[33] describe similar pathologic changes to the proximal planter fascia occurring in the extensor carpi radialis brevis origin in patients with tennis elbow. The striking similarity of these two conditions has in the past led clinicians to refer to chronic proximal plantar fasciitis as "tennis heel."

The diagnosis of proximal plantar fasciitis is largely a subjective one, based on tenderness and a reproduction of a patient's symptoms with pressure over the medial calcaneal tuberosity and proximal plantar fascia. Multiple tests have been suggested for the evaluation of this condition, including three-phase bone scan, ultrasound, CT scan, MRI, and sonography.[34-36]

It has also been suggested that oblique radiographs of the heel can reveal a fatigue fracture in the area of the medial calcaneal tuberosity. Ultrasound, sonography, and MRI are all able to demonstrate a thickening of the proximal plantar fascia consistent with chronic inflammatory changes.[37-39] All of these studies rarely contribute to the diagnosis and treatment of proximal plantar fasciitis, however, and should be reserved for the patient who presents a diagnostic challenge. Even the commonly obtained standing lateral radiograph of the painful heel is not required for the initial evaluation and treatment of a patient who presents with a classic history and examination for proximal plantar fasciitis.

A periosteitis of the medial calcaneal tuberosity frequently occurs in conjunction with the degenerative changes of the proximal plantar fascia. The majority of painful heels, in fact, have a positive delayed technetium-99m bone scan. The focal uptake in the medial calcaneal tuberosity is in clear distinction to the intense diffuse uptake on bone scan of a calcaneal stress fracture.

Conservative Treatment More than 90% of patients with proximal plantar fasciitis are cured with conservative care.[1,24,25,40,41] Nonsurgical treatment modalities include activity modification, shoe alteration, prefabricated inserts, custom-fabricated orthoses, stretching exercises, physical therapy, nonsteroidal anti-inflammatory agents, ultrasound, cortisone injections, night splints, casting, and recently, shock wave therapy.[42] The appropriate sequence of these treatments or which are most efficacious and cost-effective is not known. A large, prospective, randomized study of 236 patients demonstrated that an 8-week treatment course of Achilles tendon and plantar fascia stretching improved 72% of patients with proximal plantar fasciitis.[27] Stretching in addition to the use of a silicone or rubber heel cup yielded improvement in 95% and 88% of patients, respectively. The addition of a custom-made polypropylene orthotic device added no benefit to stretching alone. A reasonable conclusion, therefore, is that an 8-week program of stretching and the use of a prefabricated cushioned heel cup is a reasonable cost-effective first line of treatment for proximal plantar fasciitis.[43] Contrast baths, ice, massage, and anti-inflammatory agents may be of some additional benefit. Achilles tendon and plantar fascia stretching should be performed frequently during the day. If a patient is unable to master these techniques through a home program, a short formal consultation with a physical therapist may be helpful.

In the athletic patient, modification in training is essential. Mileage reduction, alternating activities, work reduction, and shortened workouts should be considered. Low-resistance cycling and running in the swimming pool are effective cardiovascular activities that are usually not stressful to the heel. A motion-control running shoe in the patient with pes planus or a cushioned shoe in the patient with pes cavus should also be prescribed.

If significant symptoms persist after 8 weeks of initial conservative care, a steroid injection is often beneficial. If a radiograph has not already been taken, it should be obtained prior to injecting the steroid. Care should be taken to inject deep to the plantar fascia so as not to cause atrophy of the fat pad.[21] A medial approach is easy to use and allows the steroid to spread along the broad origin of the plantar fascia[44] (Fig. 3). The needle is walked across the anterior border of the calcaneus just deep to the plantar fascia, thereby avoiding the plantar nerves. Multiple steroid injections may predispose a patient to plantar fascia rupture. Ninety-five percent of patients should expect improvement in their symptoms within the first few days after the injection. The maximum benefit of the injection, however, generally only lasts 6 to 8 weeks, with significant long-term benefits in less than 50% of patients.[21]

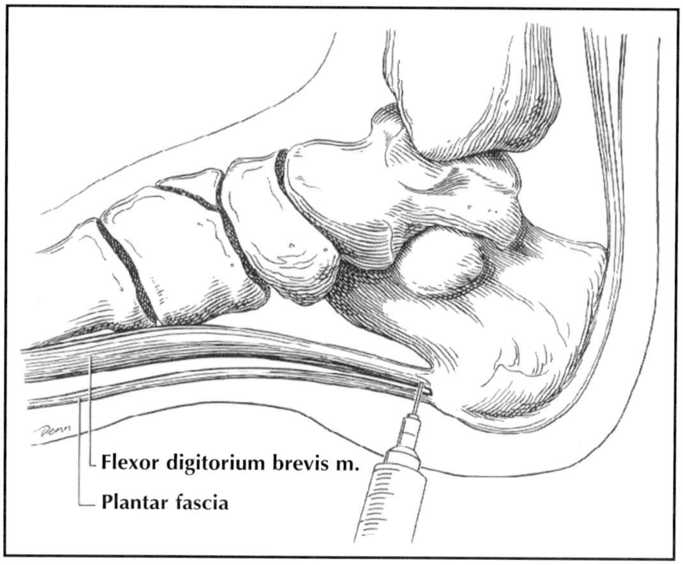

Fig. 3 Injection for proximal plantar fasciitis. (Reproduced with permission from Pfeffer GB, Baxter DE: Surgery of the adult heel, in Jahss MH (ed): *Disorders of the Foot and Ankle,* ed 2. Philadelphia, PA, WB Saunders, 1991, pp 1396-1416.)

Iontophoresis of dexamethasone is another popular treatment for a patient with persistent symptoms. A recent randomized double-blind placebo-controlled study, however, demonstrated that the iontophoresis provided no long-lasting benefit at only 1 month after treatment.[45] Patients who underwent iontophoresis did experience greater immediate relief of symptoms than those treated with traditional modalities alone. In the rare patient who requires immediate reduction of symptoms, such as the elite athlete, the modality of iontophoresis should be considered.

In patients who remain refractory to these initial conservative measures, other options include a custom orthotic device, a short-leg walking cast for 6 weeks, shoe modification with a rocker bottom and steel shank, and a dorsiflexion night splint.[46-48] The night splint has recently gained widespread acceptance with significant improvement in symptoms demonstrated in multiple studies.[49] A commercially available night splint provides a dorsiflexion stretch to the plantar fascia and metatarsophalangeal joints. Using this technique, a recent study by Powell and associates,[47] demonstrated that 88% of patients with refractory symptoms improved after only 1 month of treatment. Given the success of this device in patients with refractory symptoms, it should be considered as an addition to the initial treatment protocol.

Historically, the presence of a calcaneal spur was of great importance in the treatment of proximal plantar fasciitis.[50] In 1963, however, Tanz[51] demonstrated that only 50% of patients with plantar heel pain had a heel spur and that 16% with nonpainful heels also had a heel spur. Rubin and Witton[52] determined that same year that only 10% of patients with heel spurs were symptomatic. Multiple authors have since demonstrated that the successful treatment of proximal plantar fasciitis is not contingent on the surgical removal of a heel spur. This is not surprising, given that the spur arises deep to the plantar fascia in the non-weight-bearing substance of the flexor brevis muscle.

Surgical Treatment The majority of patients with proximal plantar fasciitis can be treated conservatively. A few patients will have symptoms that extend beyond several months. For patients with significant disability and more than 6 months of persistent pain, surgical intervention should be considered.[6,18,24,53,54] There are several options for the surgical treatment

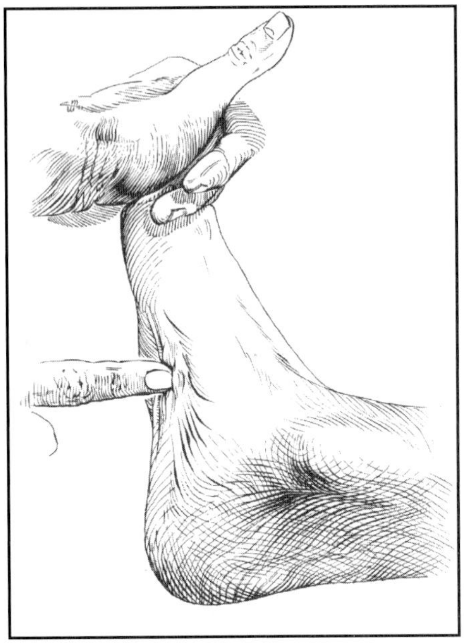

Fig. 4 Maximal tenderness exacerbated by the windlass mechanism in patient with midfoot plantar fasciitis. (Reproduced with permission from Campbell JW, Inman VT: Treatment of plantar fasciitis and calcaneal spurs with the UCBL shoe insert. *Clin Orthop* 1974;103:57.)

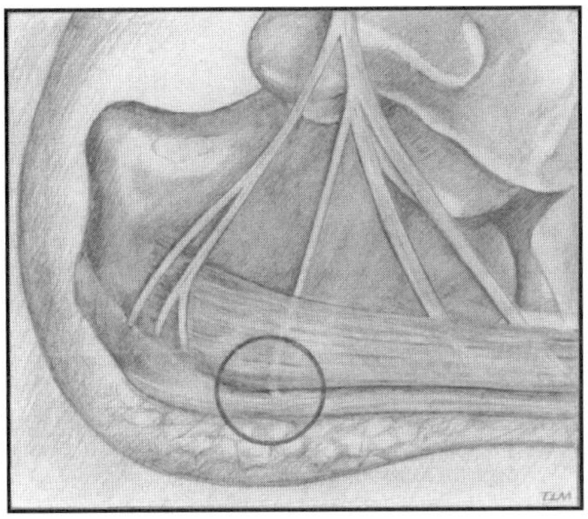

Fig. 5 Entrapment of the first branch of the lateral plantar nerve. (Reproduced with permission from Pfeffer GB, Baxter DE: Surgery of the adult heel, in Jahss MH (ed): *Disorders of the Foot and Ankle,* ed 2. Philadelphia, PA, WB Saunders, 1991, pp 1396-1416.)

of a patient with refractory proximal plantar fasciitis. All surgical treatments, however, have in common a partial, not complete, release of the plantar fascia where it arises from the medial calcaneal tubercle.

The plantar fascia plays a critical role in the static and dynamic stabilization of the longitudinal arch.[55] Nonsurgical, spontaneous rupture of the plantar fascia leads to some degree of a flatfoot deformity in patients and a complete surgical release produces a similar result. Several recent studies demonstrate the deleterious effect of a complete surgical plantar fascia release in that patients walk less energetically on the side treated surgically, place less force on the heel, and demonstrate a decrease in arch stability by 25%, creating a less rigid and more deformable arch.[56-59] Even a partial plantar fasciotomy decreases the arch-supporting function of the plantar fascia, but to a less significant degree than a complete release.[60] The average width of the entire plantar fascia, including the medial, central, and lateral bands, is approximately 3 cm. When the medial plantar fascial fibers are divided at surgery, an attempt should be made to preserve at least 50% of the lateral fibers.

The two most common surgical options for proximal plantar fasciitis are open and endoscopic partial plantar fascia release. An open release provides direct visualization of the plantar fascia, allowing the surgeon to divide only the thickened portion that is involved in the inflammatory process.[61-66] The endoscopic approach provides less morbidity and a more rapid return to function postoperatively.[67] Partial plantar fascia release is usually performed under regional anesthesia with intravenous sedation and standby general anesthesia. An ankle block is very useful, using a 1:1 solution of 0.25% bupivacaine hydrochloride (Marcaine) and 1% lidocaine, both without epinephrine. A well-padded ankle tourniquet set at 250 mm Hg is beneficial, although not required.

Distal Plantar Fasciitis and Tendinitis of the Flexor Hallucis Longus

An unusual but quite disabling cause of chronic heel pain is distal plantar fasciitis. The patient has tenderness over the midportion of the plantar fascia. As opposed to proximal plantar fasciitis, dorsiflexion of the toes almost always exacerbates the patient's symptoms by the windlass mechanism stretching the midfascial fibers. There is usually only minimal tenderness over the most proximal fascial fibers (Fig. 4). Distal plantar fasciitis is most frequently seen in sprinters and middle-distance runners who run on their toes. Significant pes cavus or pes planus may also predispose to this condition by placing increased stress on the midportion of the plantar fascia.

Tendinitis of the flexor hallucis longus tendon can be characterized by pain in the plantar medial midfoot. This condition can easily be distinguished from distal plantar fasciitis. Passive dorsiflexion of the great toe aggravates both plantar fasciitis and flexor hallucis longus tendinitis, but resisted flexion of the toe is painful only with involvement of the tendon. Careful palpation with motion of the tendon is usually sufficient to confirm the diagnosis. A painful plantar fibromatosis involving the midplantar fascia can also be detected by careful examination.

A medial longitudinal arch support is often not tolerated in a patient with distal plantar fasciitis because it pushes up on the inflamed plantar fascia and increases tension on its fibers. Circumferential taping of the foot with 1-in adhesive tape applied over a nonadhesive elastic wrap is usually most beneficial. Rest, alteration of training, nonsteroidal anti-inflammatory agents, ice, massage, contrast baths, and stretching exercises that emphasize plantar fascia and Achilles tendon stretching are also helpful. A 1/8-in medial heel wedge may take tension off the plantar fascia. If these modalities fail, a successful treatment option is the University of California Biomechanical Laboratory (UCBL) orthosis.[68] The theory of the UCBL orthosis is to hold the foot in supination and thereby decrease tension on the plantar fascia. The UCBL insert is usually not helpful in patients with proximal plantar fasciitis, as the rigid material used in construction of the insert often aggravates the inflamed heel. It is extremely unusual to operate on a patient for distal plantar fasciitis. If prolonged conservative treatment of more than 6 months fails, however, a partial plantar fascia release may help reduce symptoms.

Nerve Injury

Entrapment of the First Branch of the Lateral Plantar Nerve One of the most commonly overlooked causes of chronic plantar heel pain is entrapment of the first branch of the lateral plantar nerve.[69] Entrapment of the nerve accounts for approximately 15% of chronic plantar heel pain.[70] The first branch innervates the periosteum of the medial calcaneal tuberosity, the long plantar ligament, the abductor digiti quinti, and flexor brevis muscles. Entrapment occurs as the nerve changes from a vertical to a horizontal direction around the medial plantar aspect of the heel.[71-73] The exact site of compression is between the heavy deep fascia of the abductor hallucis muscle and the medial caudal margin of the medial head of the quadratus plantae muscle (Fig. 5). Athletes who spend a significant amount of time on their toes, such as sprinters, ballet dancers, and figure skaters, are prone to entrapment of the first branch of the lateral plantar nerve by the well-developed abductor hallucis. The medial calcaneal branches that innervate the plantar and medial aspects of the heel pass superficial to the abductor hallucis muscle and are not involved with the entrapment of the first branch.

Another potential site of entrapment of the first branch is where the nerve passes just distal to the medial calcaneal tuberosity. Inflammation and spur formation in the origin of the flexor brevis muscle can produce sufficient swelling to cause compression of the nerve against the long plantar ligament. The inflammatory changes of proximal plantar fasciitis can therefore predispose to chronic entrapment of the nerve, with both conditions often occurring simultaneously.

The diagnosis of entrapment of the first branch of the lateral plantar nerve is a clinical one. It is therefore incumbent on the examiner to differentiate entrapment of the first branch from other more common causes of heel pain. Early morning pain is not common with isolated nerve entrapment, which tends to cause more pain at the end of the day or after prolonged activity. The pathognomonic sign of entrapment of the first branch of the lateral plantar nerve is maximal tenderness where the nerve is compressed between the deep, taut fascia of the abductor hallucis muscle and the medial caudal margin of the quadratus plantae muscle. If simultaneous inflammation of the fascia occurs, the patient may have associated tenderness over the proximal plantar fascia and medial calcaneal tuberosity. Without maximal tenderness over the course of the nerve on the plantar medial aspect of the foot, the diagnosis of entrapment should not be made. Some patients may have paresthesias elicited with pressure over the nerve at the entrapment site, although this is not a common occurence. Entrapment of the isolated medial plantar nerve ("jogger's foot") occurs more distally at the level of the navicular tuberosity and should not be confused with entrapment of the first branch of the lateral plantar nerve more proximally.[74]

Motor weakness in the abductor digiti quinti may be detected, although no cutaneous sensory deficit occurs. Electromyography and nerve conduction studies are not consistent in the diagnosis entrapment of the first branch of the lateral plantar nerve.[75] Measurement of nerve conduction slowing across the site of entrapment is technically demanding, and denervation potentials in the intrinsic foot muscles may only rarely occur because of the possible dynamic nature of this particular compression neuropathy. A comparison may be drawn to the diagnosis of a posterior interosseous nerve entrapment in the upper extremity.

Treatment for athletes with entrapment of the first branch of the lateral plantar nerve is similar to that for proximal plantar fasciitis. Conservative care consists of rest, activity modification, nonsteroidal anti-inflammatory agents, contrast baths, ice, massage, stretching exercises, and the injection of a cortisone preparation. The addition of a prefabricated shock-absorbent heel insert will also help decrease inflammation in the area. In athletes with excessive pronation, especially long-distance runners, a nonrigid medial longitudinal arch support can decrease compression of the nerve.

The vast majority of patients can be cured with conservative care. As with the treatment of proximal plantar fasciitis, in a patient with persistent disabling symptoms of more than 6 months, surgical intervention should be considered. Eighty-five percent of patients can be expected to have a good or excellent result from surgical decompression of the nerve. Decompression of the first branch of the lateral plantar nerve requires an open procedure.[69] Adequate decompression of the nerve cannot be performed endoscopically. The endoscope is reserved for patients who have isolated proximal plantar fasciitis without evidence of nerve entrapment. The mean recovery time to resumption of everyday activity is 3 months.

Tarsal Tunnel Syndrome In making the diagnosis of entrapment of the first branch of the lateral plantar nerve, it is important not to miss a more extensive nerve entrapment consistent with a tarsal tunnel syndrome.[76] Posttraumatic adhesions, bony spurs from the medial

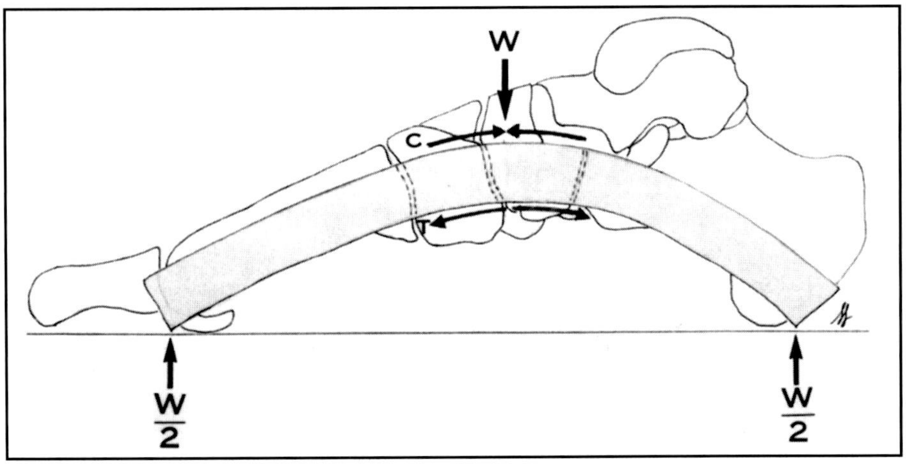

Fig. 6 Truss effect of plantar aponeurosis. (Reproduced with permission from Sarrafian FK: Functional characteristics of the foot and plantar aponeurosis under tibiotalar loading. *Foot Ankle* 1987;8:4-18.)

calcaneus or talus, chronic inflammation, benign tumors, and varicosities can all cause compression of the posterior tibial nerve within the tarsal tunnel. Excessive pronation has been postulated, but has never proven, to predispose to tarsal tunnel syndrome by placing repeated stress on the structures within the tarsal tunnel.

In general, the plantar heel pain produced by tarsal tunnel syndrome is more diffuse and less focal than that of either proximal plantar fasciitis or entrapment of the first branch of the lateral plantar nerve. A careful clinical examination should easily distinguish among these three entities. The salient clinical feature of tarsal tunnel syndrome is direct focal tenderness over the nerve as it passes beneath the flexor retinaculum. Percussion of the nerve in this area will reproduce the patient's symptoms, which can include pain, burning, or tingling on the plantar aspect of the foot. Subjective numbness of the toes may occur, although objective decreased sensibility is rarely demonstrated. Some patients may complain of proximal radiation of their symptoms. Electromyography and nerve conduction studies can be helpful in making a diagnosis. A normal study, however, does not exclude the diagnosis of tarsal tunnel syndrome. Entrapment of the first branch of the lateral plantar nerve with an associated chronic proximal plantar fasciitis may occur rarely in conjunction with a tarsal tunnel syndrome.

A medial heel wedge can decrease tension on the posterior tibial nerve and its branches. A steroid injection into the tarsal tunnel can also be beneficial, but usually produces only transient relief of symptoms. Surgical release of the flexor retinaculum and exploration of the tarsal tunnel can be expected to provide relief in a majority of patients, especially when the symptoms are unilateral and easily reproducible on preoperative examination. Internal neurolysis of the nerve is rarely indicated.

Complications of Heel Surgery

The most common problem encountered after plantar heel surgery is persistent pain. It is essential to determine if the pain is similar to or different from the patient's preoperative symptoms. Causes of similar continued heel pain include incorrect preoperative diagnosis, insufficient release of the plantar fascia, inadequate release of a nerve entrapment, and inadequate recovery time. The most common causes for postoperative pain that is different from preoperative symptoms are: incisional neuromas and biomechanical imbalance of the foot.

In the patient with persistent postoperative heel pain that has not changed in nature, it is essential to make sure that the initial diagnosis was correct. The plantar fascia may have been adequately treated, but the source of persistent symptoms may be tarsal tunnel sundrome that was overlooked. A partial release of the plantar fascia may have been performed for the diagnosis of proximal plantar fasciitis, without addressing the simultaneous occurrence of an entrapment of the first branch of the lateral plantar nerve. Careful postoperative examination of the patient to document areas of maximal tenderness can distinguish these diagnoses.

Persistent pain consistent with proximal plantar fasciitis is often a result of inadequate release of the plantar fascia. This problem most commonly occurs after minimal-incision heel surgery. Performed through a 1-cm incision, an attempt is made to divide the plantar fascia blindly just distal to the medial calcaneal tuberosity. Using this approach, it is possible to completely miss the plantar fascia, performing no release at all. A similar inadequate release can occur with endoscopic plantar fascia release. There is a clear learning curve using endoscopic technique and, unless the plantar fascia fibers are clearly visualized, it is easy to miss them entirely.

If the correct diagnosis has been made and the appropriate treatment carried out, a patient may have persistent heel pain simply on the basis of inadequate recovery time. The mean time to recovery after release of the first branch of the lateral plantar nerve is approximately 3.5 months, with some patients requiring up to 9 months. There is a similar range of recovery time after a partial release of the plantar fascia for proximal plantar fasciitis. In order to reduce the recovery period, an attempt should be made to minimize edema and decrease inflammation in the immediate postoperative period. Full weight bearing should be discouraged for at least 2 weeks after surgery, and the use of nonsteroidal anti-inflammatory agents and contrast baths can be helpful during the first 6 weeks of recovery. An injection of a steroid preparation may also be considered if some symptoms persist 4 months postoperatively. Continued plantar fascia stretching exercises can also be beneficial, especially in the patient recovering from a partial division of the plantar fascia.

Postoperative pain that is dissimilar to the patient's preoperative symptoms is most likely iatrogenic. An incisional neuroma is the most common significant complication of this type. Once a painful neuroma develops postoperatively, the results can be disastrous. Anything that touches the medial or lateral scar causes extreme pain and shoe wear is often impossible. A positive percussion/Tinel sign is present over the incision line, causing dysesthesias in the nerve distribution. Distal to the incision, there is a decrease in sensibility. While division of the superficial medial calcaneal sensory nerve is possible in an open procedure, nerve injury has increased because of the popularity of the endoscopic technique and inadequate visualization of the superficial sensory nerves.

Initial treatment should include a course of systematic desensitization performed by an experienced therapist. One injection of a steroid preparation into the painful area is also reasonable. More than one injection over a short period of time is unlikely to be beneficial and causes atrophy of the subcutaneous tissue. A transcutaneous electrical nerve stimulator may be helpful in some patients, as may modalities to decrease local edema and inflammation. A postoperative neuroma may serve as a trigger for a complex regional pain syndrome that may require sympathetic blocks and medical management.

If a patient is unable to tolerate the neuroma symptoms, surgical intervention should be considered. Repair of the nerve is usually impossible at this level because of the small size of the distal fibers and the difficulty in mobilizing the nerve. Excision of the neuroma with resection of the proximal nerve to a level within the tarsal tunnel above the shoe line is recommended. Rather than resecting the entire superficial medial or lateral sensory nerve, which would leave a significant area of numbness on the heel, only the branch involving the neuroma should be resected. This can be accomplished by intrafascicular dissection of the nerve branch under loupe magnification. The tourniquet should be deflated before closing the wound to obtain hemostasis and to prevent a hematoma postoperatively. No subcutaneous sutures should be used and a 3-0 nonabsorbable nylon skin suture will help minimize postoperative inflammation.

The first branch of the lateral plantar nerve can be cut inadvertently during surgery or significant postoperative adhesions can develop. Because this nerve runs deep to the abductor fascia, however, if a neuroma forms it is often asymptomatic. If chronic pain is present, the proximal fibers of the first branch of the lateral plantar nerve should be resected back to within the tarsal tunnel. If the patient complains of any symptoms referable to the posterior tibial nerve or its branches, a wide tarsal tunnel release should be performed simultaneously.

In some cases of persistent postoperative heel pain, a specific etiology cannot be determined. Previous surgery may obscure a definitive diagnosis. In these patients, there is often diffuse tenderness over the tarsal tunnel, the first branch of the lateral nerve, and the proximal plantar fascia. Salvage surgery consists of a release of the tarsal tunnel, decompression of entrapment of the first branch of the lateral plantar nerve, and complete division of the plantar fascia from its insertion on the calcaneal tuberosity. If at the original surgery the posterior tibial nerve and its branches have already been released in an adequate manner (proximal to the medial malleolus and distal beneath the abductor hallucis muscle), there is unlikely to be a benefit reexploration and neurolysis of the posterior tibial nerve is unlikely to be beneficial.

Perhaps the most difficult complication that can develop following surgery for proximal plantar fasciitis is a biomechanical imbalance of the foot. Patients have surgery to treat plantar heel pain, only to develop metatarsalgia or pain in the dorsal midfoot or calcaneocuboid joints. This clinical condition is referred to as lateral column syndrome. A truss mechanism exists in the foot through the plantar fascia as demonstrated by the windlass mechanism (Fig. 6). If the plantar fascia is divided surgically, either partially or completely, there are increased compressive forces transmitted to the dorsal and lateral aspect of the midfoot, and decreased flexion forces on the metatarsophalangeal joint complex.[31,58] These changes often produce pain with weight bearing.

As originally described, the endoscopic technique often involved complete release of the plantar fascia, and many patients developed lateral column symptoms. Complete plantar fascia release by either endoscopic or open techniques is no longer recommended, although inadvertent complete division of the plantar fascia may still cause similar symptoms. Treatment consists of either a custom-fabricated orthotic device or a short-leg walking cast. Metatarsalgia can often be treated with a custom-made orthotic device. Dorsal and lateral foot symptoms usually require a short-leg walking cast. Up to 12 weeks of casting may be needed before symptoms begin to abate. The lateral plantar heel pain that occasionally occurs following a partial plantar fascia release results from increased stress on the lateral calcaneal tuberosity from the remaining plantar fascia fibers. This condition usually resolves spontaneously without the need for an orthotic device or cast.

References

1. Gill LH: Plantar fasciitis: Diagnosis and conservative management. *J Am Acad Orthop Surg* 1997;5:109-117.
2. Gerster JC: Plantar fasciitis and Achilles tendinitis among 150 cases of seronegative spondarthritis. *Rheumatol Rehabil* 1980;19:218-222.
3. Gerster JC, Piccinin P: Enthesopathy of the heels in juvenile onset seronegative B-27 positive spondyloarthropathy. *J Rheumatol* 1985;12:310-314.
4. Hedrick MR: The plantar aponeurosis. *Foot Ankle Int* 1996;17:646-649.
5. Hicks JH: The mechanics of the foot. Part II: The plantar aponeurosis and the arch. *J Anat* 1954;88:25-30.
6. Hill JJ Jr, Cutting PJ: Heel pain and body weight. *Foot Ankle* 1989;9:254-256.
7. Miller WE: The heel pad. *Am J Sports Med* 1982;10:19-21.
8. Sarrafian SK (ed): *Anatomy of the Foot and Ankle: Descriptive, Topographic, Functional*, ed 2. Philadelphia, PA, JB Lippincott, 1993.
9. Jahss MH, Michelson JD, Desai P, et al: Investigations into the fat pads of the sole of the foot: Anatomy and histology. *Foot Ankle* 1992;13:233-242.
10. Prichasuk S: The heel pad in plantar heel pain. *J Bone Joint Surg Br* 1994;76:140-142.
11. Lin E, Ronen M, Stampler D, Suster S: Painful piezogenic heel papules: A case report. *J Bone Joint Surg Am* 1985;67:640-641.
12. Resnick RB, Hudgins LC, Buschmann WR, Kummer FJ, Jahss MH: Analysis of the heel pad fat in rheumatoid arthritis. *Foot Ankle Int* 1999;20:481-484.
13. Jorgensen U: Achillodynia and loss of heel pad shock absorbency. *Am J Sports Med* 1985;13:128-132.
14. Quigley JT: A glomus tumor of the heel pad: A case report. *J Bone Joint Surg Am* 1979;61: 443-444.
15. Protzman RR, Griffis CG: Stress fractures in men and women undergoing military training. *J Bone Joint Surg Am* 1977;59:825.
16. Hertzanu Y, Mendelsohn DB, Gottschalk F: Aneurysmal bone cyst of the calcaneus. *Radiology* 1984;151:51-52.
17. Khermosh O, Schujman E: Benign osteoblastoma of the calcaneous. *Clin Orthop* 1977;127:197-199.
18. Anderson RB, Foster MD: Operative treatment of subcalcaneal pain. *Foot Ankle* 1989;9:317-323.
19. Leach R, Jones R, Silva T: Rupture of the plantar fascia in athletes. *J Bone Joint Surg Am* 1978;60:537-539.
20. Sellman JR: Plantar fascia rupture associated with corticosteroid injection. *Foot Ankle Int* 1994;15:376-381.
21. Bordelon RL: Subcalcaneal pain: A method of evaluation and plan for treatment. *Clin Orthop* 1983;177:49-53.
22. Karr SD: Subcalcaneal heel pain. *Orthop Clin North Am* 1994; 25:161-175.
23. Furey JG: Plantar fasciitis: The painful heel syndrome. *J Bone Joint Surg Am* 1975;57: 672-673.
24. Gill LH, Kiebzak GM: Outcome of nonsurgical treatment for plantar fasciitis. *Foot Ankle Int* 1996;17:527-532.
25. Lapidus PW, Guidotti FP: Painful heel: Report of 323 patients with 364 painful heels. *Clin Orthop* 1965;39:178-186.
26. Pfeffer G, Bacchetti P, Deland J, et al: Comparison of custom and prefabricated orthoses in the initial treatment of proximal plantar fasciitis. *Foot Ankle Int* 1999;20:214-221.
27. Snook GA, Chrisman OD: The management of subcalcaneal pain. *Clin Orthop* 1972;82: 163-168.
28. Wolgin M, Cook C, Graham C; Mauldin D: Conservative treatment of plantar heel pain: Long-term follow-up. *Foot Ankle Int* 1994; 15:97-102.
29. Kibler WB, Goldberg C, Chandler TJ: Functional biomechanical deficits in running athletes with plantar fasciitis. *Am J Sports Med* 1991;19:66-71.
30. Carlson RE, Fleming LL, Hutton WC: The biomechanical relationship between the tendoachilles, plantar fascia, and metatarsophalangeal joint dorsiflexion angle. *Foot Ankle Int* 2000;21:18-25.
31. Sarrafian SK: Functional characteristics of the foot and plantar aponeurosis under tibiotalar loading. *Foot Ankle* 1987;8:4-18.
32. Cardinal E, Chhem RK, Beauregard CG, Aubin B, Pelletier M: Plantar fasciitis: Sonographic evaluation. *Radiology* 1996;201: 257-259.
33. Nirschl RP, Pettrone FA: Tennis elbow. *J Bone Joint Surg Am* 1979;61:832-839.
34. Wall JR, Harkness MA, Crawford A: Ultrasound diagnosis of plantar fasciitis. *Foot Ankle* 1993;14:465-470.
35. Williams PL, Smibert JG, Cox R, Mitchell R, Klenerman L: Imaging study of the painful heel syndrome. *Foot Ankle* 1987;7:345-349.
36. Berkowitz JF, Kier R, Rudicel S: Plantar fasciitis: MR imaging. *Radiology* 1991;179:665-667.
37. Sewell JR, Black CM, Chapman AH, Statham J, Hughes GR, Lavender JP: Quantitative scintigraphy in diagnosis and management of plantar fasciitis (calcaneal periostitis): Concise communication. *J Nucl Med* 1980;21:633-636.
38. Vasavada PJ, DeVries DF, Nishiyama H: Plantar fasciitis: Early blood pool images in diagnosis of inflammatory process. *Foot Ankle* 1984;5:74-76.
39. Davis PF, Severud E, Baxter DE: Painful heel syndrome: Results of nonoperative treatment. *Foot Ankle Int* 1994;15:531-535.
40. Lutter LD: Surgical decisions in athletes' subcalcaneal pain. *Am J Sports Med* 1986;14: 481-485.
41. Spiegl PV, Johnson KA: Heel pain syndrome: Which treatments to choose? *J Musculoskel Med* 1984;66-71.
42. Knuttgen HG: Ossatron: New treatment for sports injuries? *Georgia Tech Sports Medicine and Performance Newsletter* 1999;1:1.
43. Miller RA, Torres J, McGuire M: Efficacy of first-time steroid injection for painful heel syndrome. *Foot Ankle Int* 1995;16:610-612.
44. Dasgupta B, Bowles J: Scintigraphic localisation of steroid injection site in plantar fasciitis. *Lancet* 1995;346:1400-1401.
45. Gudeman SD, Eisele SA, Heidt RS, et al: Treatment of plantar fasciitis by iontophoresis of 0.4% dexamethasone: A randomized, double-blind, placebo-controlled study. *Am J Sports Med* 1997;25:312-316.
46. Mizel MS, Marymont JV, Trepman E: Treatment of plantar fasciitis with a night splint and shoe modification consisting of a steel shank and anterior rocker bottom. *Foot Ankle Int* 1996;17:732-735.
47. Powell M, Post WR, Keener J, Wearden S: Effective treatment of chronic plantar fasciitis with dorsiflexion night splints: A crossover prospective randomized outcome study. *Foot Ankle Int* 1998;19:10-18.
48. Tisdel CL, Harper MC: Chronic plantar heel pain: Treatment with a short leg walking cast. *Foot Ankle Int* 1996;17:41-42.
49. Wapner KL, Sharkey PF: The use of night splints for treatment of recalcitrant plantar fasciitis. *Foot Ankle Int* 1991;12:135-137.
50. DuVries HL: Heel spur (calcaneal spur). *Arch Surg* 1957;74:536-542.
51. Tanz SS: Heel pain. *Clin Orthop* 1963;28: 169-177.
52. Rubin G, Witten M: Plantar calcaneal spurs. *Am J Orthop* 1963;5:38-41; 53-55.
53. Lester DK, Buchanan JR: Surgical treatment of plantar fasciitis. *Clin Orthop* 1984;186:202-204.
54. Davies MS, Weiss GA, Saxby TS: Plantar fasciitis: How successful is surgical intervention? *Foot Ankle Int* 1999;20:803-807.
55. Daly PJ, Kitaoka HB, Chao EY: Plantar fasciotomy for intractable plantar fasciitis: Clinical results and biomechanical evaluation. *Foot Ankle* 1992;13:188-195.
56. Arangio GA, Chen C, Kim W: Effect of cutting the plantar fascia on mechanical properties of the foot. *Clin Orthop* 1997;339:227-231.

57. Huang CK, Kitaoka HB, An KN, Chao EY: Biomechanical evaluation of longitudinal arch stability. *Foot Ankle* 1993;14:353-357.

58. Katoh Y, Chao EY, Laughman RK Schneider E Morrey BF: Biomechanical analysis of foot function during gait and clinical applications. *Clin Orthop* 1983;177:23-33.

59. Kitaoka HB, Luo ZP, An KN: Mechanical behavior of the foot and ankle after plantar fascia release in the unstable foot. *Foot Ankle Int* 1997;18:8-15.

60. Thordarson DB, Kumar PJ, Hedman TP, Ebramzadeh E: The effect of partial versus complete plantar fasciotomy on the windlass mechanism. *Foot Ankle Int* 1997;18:16-20.

61. Kahn C, Bishop JO, Tullos HS: Plantar fascia release and heel spur excision via plantar route. *Orthop Rev* 1985;14:222-225.

62. Kinley S, Frascone S, Calderone D, Wertheimer SJ, Squire MA, Wiseman FA: Endoscopic plantar fasciotomy versus traditional heel spur surgery: A prospective study. *J Foot Ankle Surg* 1993;32:595-603.

63. Ward WG, Clippinger FW: Proximal medial longitudinal arch incision for plantar fascia release. *Foot Ankle* 1987;8:152-155.

64. Sammarco GJ, Helfrey RB: Surgical treatment of recalcitrant plantar fasciitis. *Foot Ankle Int* 1996;17:520-526.

65. Barrett SL, Day SV: Endoscopic plantar fasciotomy for chronic plantar fasciitis/heel spur syndrome: Surgical technique: Early clinical results. *J Foot Surg* 1991;30:568-570.

66. Barrett SL, Day SV, Pignetti TT, Robinson LB: Endoscopic plantar fasciotomy: A multi-surgeon prospective analysis of 652 cases. *J Foot Ankle Surg* 1995;34:400-406.

67. Palumbo R, Kudros SA, Baxter DE: Endoscopic plantar fasciotomy: Indications, techniques, and complications. *Sports Med Arthrosc Rev* 1994;2:317-322.

68. Baxter DE, Pfeffer GB: Treatment of chronic heel pain by surgical release of the first branch of the lateral plantar nerve. *Clin Orthop* 1992;279:229-236.

69. Baxter DE, Thigpen CM: Heel pain: Operative results. *Foot Ankle* 1984;5:16-25.

70. Przylucki H, Jones CL: Entrapment neuropathy of muscle branch of lateral plantar nerve: A cause of heel pain. *J Am Podiatry Assoc* 1981; 71:119-124.

71. Rondhuis JJ, Huson A: The first branch of the lateral plantar nerve and heel pain. *Acta Morphol Neerl Scand* 1986;24:269-279.

72. Rask MR: Medial plantar neurapraxia (jogger's foot): Report of 3 cases. *Clin Orthop* 1978;134:193-195.

73. Schon LC, Glennon TP, Baxter DE: Heel pain syndrome: Electrodiagnostic support for nerve entrapment. *Foot Ankle* 1993;14:129-135.

74. Radin EL: Tarsal tunnel syndrome. *Clin Orthop* 1983;181:167-170.

75. Clancy WG: Tendinitis and plantar fasciitis in runners. *Orthopedics* 1983;6:217-233.

76. Campbell JW, Inman VT: Treatment of plantar fasciitis and calcaneal spurs with the UC-BL shoe insert. *Clin Orthop* 1974;103:57-62.

SECTION

10

Pediatric Orthopaedics

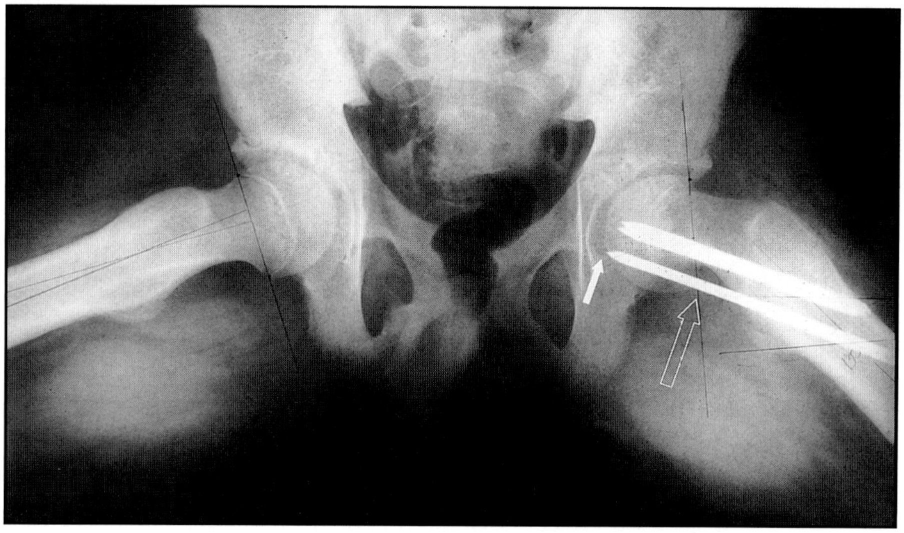

55 Developmental Dysplasia of the Hip: Etiology, Pathogenesis, and Examination and Physical Findings in the Newborn **(with video clip on enclosed CD)**

56 Developmental Dysplasia of the Hip: Assessment and Treatment Before Walking Age

57 Developmental Hip Dysplasia and Dislocation: Management of the Older Child

58 Slipped Capital Femoral Epiphysis

59 Natural History and Long-Term Outcomes of Slipped Capital Femoral Epiphysis **(with video clip on enclosed CD)**

55

Developmental Dysplasia of the Hip: Etiology, Pathogenesis, and Examination and Physical Findings in the Newborn

Richard J. Haynes, MD

Introduction

Edward S. Curtis included "Apache Babe in Carrier" in his written and photographic record *The North American Indian*[1] (Fig. 1). The cradle board depicted in his famous photograph has been a significant postnatal extrauterine risk factor for developmental dysplasia of the hip (DDH).

Until the last decade, the dislocation of the hip often seen in newborns was referred to as congenital dislocation of the hip. Confusion in the nomenclature involved the descriptors congenital versus developmental and dislocation versus dysplasia. The literature describes instability, dysplasia, subluxation, and dislocation. The Webster[2] definition of congenital is existing at birth but not hereditary; developmental is the act of developing or state of being developed; dysplasia is the abnormal development of tissues, organs, or cells; dislocation is displacement from the usual relationship with adjoining parts; subluxation is incomplete dislocation of a bone in a joint; and instability is the lack of resistance to sudden change. Developmental dysplasia has been described as a subluxated or dislocated hip. Weinstein[3] has included reducible dislocation.

Developmental dislocation has been described as a complete dislocation or a complete unreducible dislocation. Teratologic dislocation of the hip occurs prior to birth, is congenital, and is considered by most authors not to be representative of developmental dysplasia of the hip. According to Coleman,[4] "The hip joint at birth is seldom truly dislocated; rather it is merely unstable." Many authors believe that most irreducible dislocations at birth are teratogenic.

The current term, DDH, is accepted by the American Academy of Orthopaedic Surgeons,[5] the American Academy of Pediatrics, and *The Journal of Bone and Joint Surgery*. The term congenital dysplasia of the hip continues to be used by the International Classification of Diseases (ICD).[6] Because the ICD is the basis for documentation of all dysplastic or dislocated hips, the term congenital dysplasia hip continues to be present. It is clear to all authors that not all instances of DDH are either present or identifiable at birth. To avoid the implication that it should have been identified at birth was the prime motivating factor in changing the term from congenital dislocation to developmental dislocation. Missed or late dislocations have been discussed in the orthopaedic literature on numerous occasions. Ilfeld and associates[7] discussed initial normal examinations that subsequently became abnormal. The incidence is clearly significant. Bjerkreim and Arseth[8] in their review of 799 patients who had late diagnosis of DDH noted that 77% had had hip examinations when newborn.

All pediatric orthopaedic lower extremity examinations carry an implied guarantee in regard to the presence or absence of developmental dysplasia of the hip. It must be considered during the evaluation for metatarsus adductus, toeing-in, and so forth. It is important to tell the parents that the hip is being examined because they may not clearly understand the examination. **(CD-55.1)**

Epidemiology

Positive family history, gender, intrauterine position, and increased birth weight have been noted as being important epidemiologic factors.[9] The geographic incidence was presented by Stanisavljevic.[10] The incidence per 1,000 was noted to be 188 in Canadian Indians, 75 in Yugoslavia, 20 in Navajo Indians, 10 in Detroit, 0 in Hong Kong, and 0 in Africa. Wynne-Davies[11] discussed the familial incidence of DDH and documented the risks to subsequent children as 6% when there is one affected child, 12% with one affected parent, and 36% with one affected child and one affected parent. Twin concordance was documented in monozygotic twins as 43% and in dizygotic twins as 3%. The incidence in girls was noted to be five times higher than that in boys.

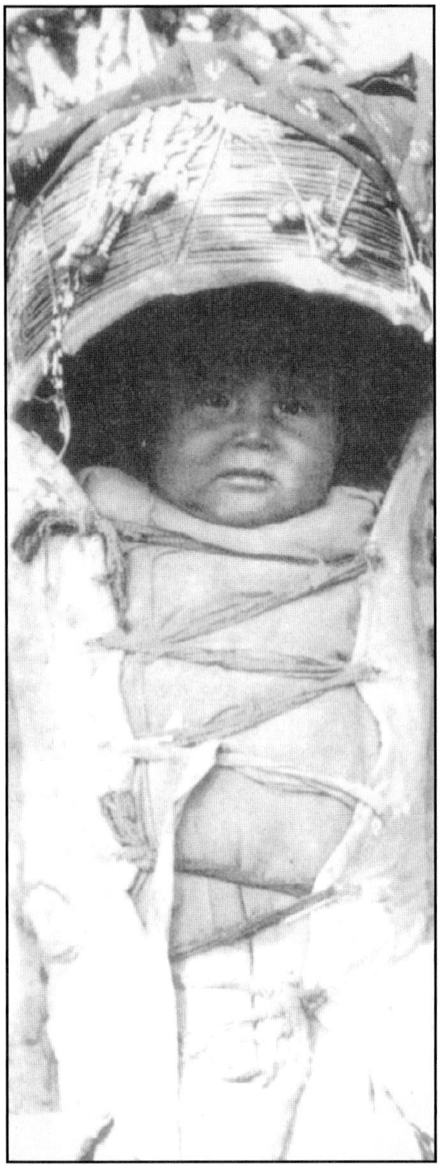

Fig. 1 "Apache Babe in Carrier," Edward S. Curtis, 1907. (Reproduced with permission from Curtis ES (ed): Apache babe in carrier, in *The North American Indian: List of Large Plates Supplementing v. 1-20.* Cambridge, MA, University Press, 1907,vol I, plate 17.)

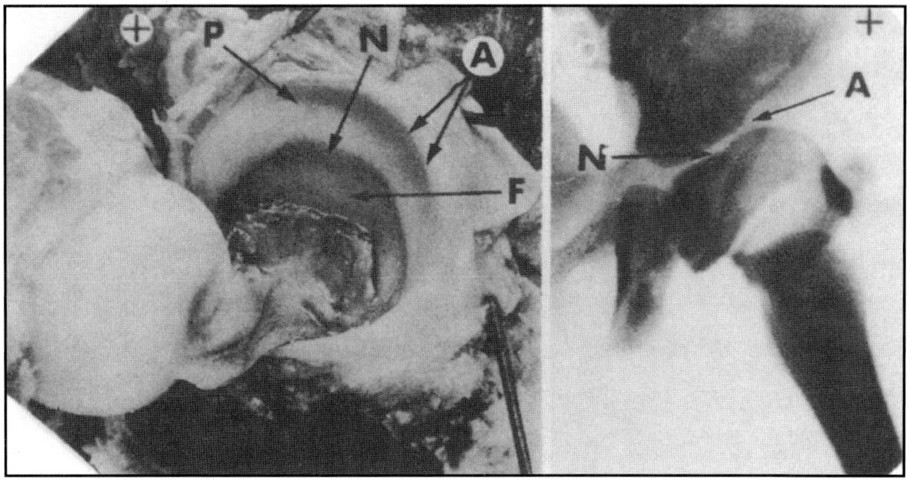

Fig. 2 The neolimbus. A = real limbus, N = neolimbus, F = real acetabulum, P = false acetabulum. (Reproduced with permission from Ortolani M: The classic: Congenital hip dysplasia in the light of early and very early diagnosis. *Clin Orthop* 1976;119:6-10.)

Wynne-Davies[11] described joint laxity using examination of the elbow, thumb, joints of the hand, ankle joint, and knee as evidence of joint laxity. When three of the five demonstrated increased mobility, joint laxity was considered to be present. It was documented that no children had joint laxity in the first week of life. Children were documented to have the most joint laxity at age 2 years. The age of the child at examination dramatically affects the incidence of the diagnosis of DDH. Examination at birth has an incidence of 17 per 1,000, examination at 1 week of 7 per 1,000, and examination at 2 months of 2 per 1,000. The true incidence was documented by Barlow[12] as being 1.55 per 1,000.

Caucasian first-born children have been documented as having increased risk of DDH, with associated torticollis and metatarsus adductus, because of limited fetal mobility (crowding phenomenon). Oligohydramnios increases the risk of developmental dysplasia of the hip. The left hip is affected more often than the right. Breech presentation and oligohydramnios are considered to be mechanical factors. Breech presentation occurs in 2% to 4% of vaginal deliveries, with a much higher incidence in developmental dysplasia of the hip. Carter and Wilkinson[13] document an incidence of 17% and Salter[14] an incidence of 23%. Twice as many girls are born with a breech presentation, 59% of breech patients are first born, and 7% of female breech patients have hip instability.

Dunn[15] evaluated 30 patients with Potter's syndrome (absence of fetal urination) and documented this as evidence for oligohydramnios being an etiologic factor. It was documented that 63% of these patients (19) had developmental dysplasia of the hip. Extrauterine environmental risk factors include swaddling cloths and cradle boards, which keep the hips in an extended position in the face of newborn hip flexion and hamstring contractures.

Growth and Development

Ponseti[16,17] best described growth and development of the acetabulum in the normal child and in the child with developmental dislocation of the hip. He notes that the hip joint, acetabulum, and femoral head develop from the same primitive mesenchymal cells, with the cleft developing at 7 weeks gestation. The hip joint is fully formed at 11 weeks gestation. There is continued development of the labrum. The femoral head is deeply seated in the acetabulum and held by the surface tension of the synovial fluid. Developmental dislocation of the hip is not merely capsular laxity, it is documented to be a pathologic entity.

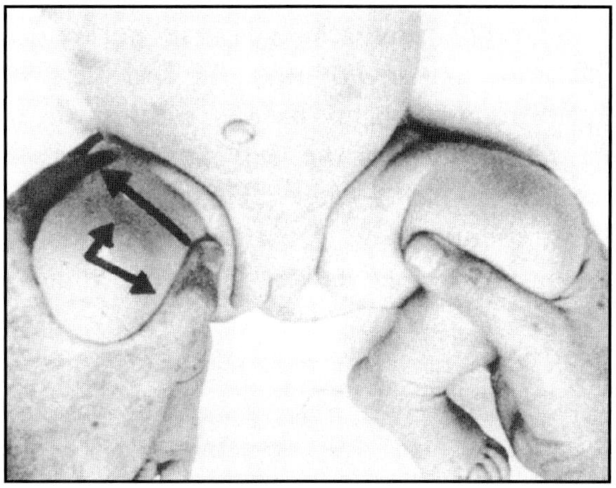

Fig. 3 Ortolani "click" sign with femoral head dislocating and click sign heard. (Reproduced with permission from Ortolani M: The classic: Congenital hip dysplasia in the light of early and very early diagnosis. *Clin Orthop* 1976;119:6-10.)

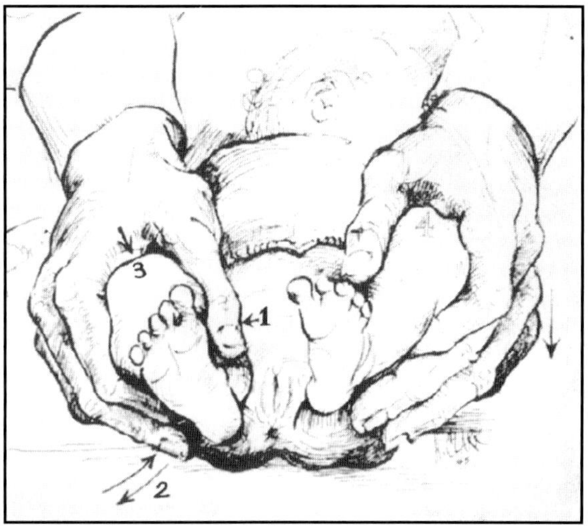

Fig. 4 Coleman jerk of exit sign with (1) thumb over the medial thigh, (2) fingers over the greater trochanter, (3) posterior lateral force resulting in an attempt to displace the femoral head. (Reproduced with permission from Schmidt H, Freyschmidt J, Holthusen W (eds): Acetabulum and anterior inferior spinous process of the ilium, in *Borderlands of Normal and Early Pathologic Findings in Skeletal Radiography/Köhler/Zimmer,* ed 4. Stuttgard, Germany, Thieme Medical Publishers, 1993, pp 649-665.

The acetabular cartilage complex has a cellular hyaline cartilage the lateral portion of which is homologous with other epiphyseal cartilages. Interstitial growth within the triradiate cartilage of the acetabulum causes the hip joint to expand in diameter. Because of this interstitial growth, innominate osteotomies affecting the triradiate cartilage may jeopardize further acetabular growth. The acetabular cartilage (triradiate) has a triphalangeal orientation in the horizonal, vertical, and anterior directions. There is a fibrocartilaginous labrum at the margin of the acetabular rim with a joint capsule inserting just above the rim.

Ortolani[18] described the neolimbus as a hypertrophied ridge of acetabular cartilage (Fig. 2). Its development was noted to be a reversible change in 95% of children and typical in 98% of those with developmental dysplasia of the hip.

The proximal femur is entirely cartilaginous in the infant.[16,17] The proximal femoral ossification center appears at 4 to 7 months of age with three main growth areas: the physeal plate, the growth plate of the greater trochanter, and the isthmus of the femoral neck. The cartilaginous isthmus of the femoral neck connects the femoral neck and trochanteric growth plates. It reflects the previous common origin and contributes to the lateral width of the femoral neck. The cartilaginous isthmus remains active until maturity. The proximal femoral physeal plate contributes 30% of the growth of the femur. Varus deformity may result from disruption of the blood supply or damage to the proximal physeal plate with continued growth of the trochanter or the isthmus of the femoral neck. The greater trochanter is a traction epiphysis with appositional growth stimulated by traction of the abductors. Secondary centers of ossification, the acetabulum (pubic epiphysis), acetabular epiphysis (iliac epiphysis), and ischial epiphysis, are commonly present in older children with DDH.

Avisse and associates[19] described the fetal acetabulum as always being deformable. The oval shaped cartilaginous cavity develops with an inverted labrum deformation preceding gliding of the femoral head in the acetabulum. Deformation in the neonate is entirely reversible. The cavity developed transforms into a bony cup by 3 months of age. No deformity of the acetabulum can be produced in older children. Later degenerative changes affect the central area.

Dysplasia appears to be the result rather than cause of dislocation. Therefore, screening tests need to be in the first weeks of life for diagnosis and reversal of the cartilaginous deformation.

Teratogenetic (antenatal) dislocations are present in 2% of patients with dysplasia of the hip. All of these patients demonstrate irreversible pathologic findings at birth.

Examination and Physical Findings

According to Ortolani, the ideal time for treatment of a congenital hip problem is the first day of life.[20] Ortolani[18] also described the pathology of the click sign, which occurs as the femoral head is dislocated from the acetabulum, or reduced into the acetabulum. This sign indicates a defect in the superior aspect of the

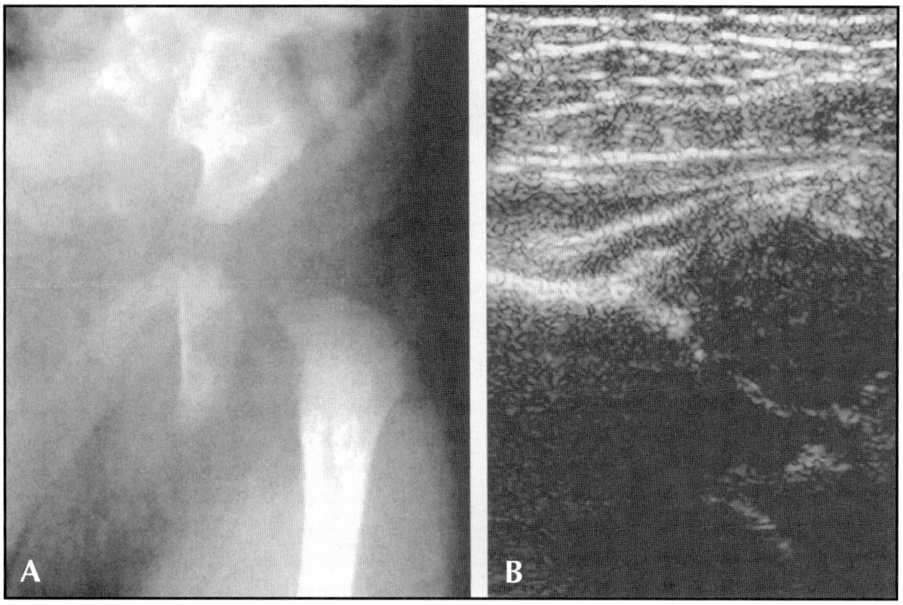
Fig. 5 AP radiograph of the hip (A) and coronal ultrasound (B).

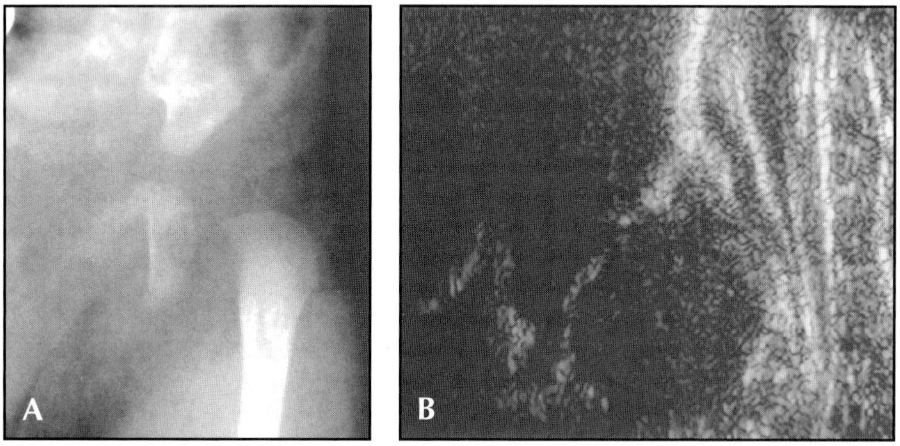
Fig. 6 AP radiograph of the hip (A) and coronal ultrasound rotated with ilium superior and abductor musculature lateral similar to the radiograph (B).

acetabulum (Fig. 3). The neolimbus subsequently forms if treatment was not initiated at birth.

Coleman[4] described the jerk of exit (Fig. 4). At birth, the joint is rarely truly dislocated; it is merely unstable. The jerk of exit was present in 27 of 3,500 children examined over a 10-month period. Coleman[4] has also stated that every newborn should receive a thorough orthopaedic examination. In his study, the hip in the newborn was documented as having abduction easily beyond 80°. He has stated that all of the examinations are tests for instability in newborns and neonates, and that it is difficult to always discern whether the instability is in-out or out-in.

Subsequent to Ortolani's and Coleman's presentations of instability, Barlow[12] in 1962 presented similar findings with the femoral head slipping forward into the acetabulum or the femoral head slipping out over the posterior lip of the acetabulum. He described this as the hip being unstable.

It is clear that Ortolani, Coleman, and Barlow are describing the identical test for instability. Because most hips are not dislocated at birth, it is clear that the click described by Ortolani is a test for instability. The click test, the jerk test of Coleman, and the femoral head slipping out over the posterior lip of the acetabulum by Barlow are all identical and represent the basis for instability testing. The proper terminology for the test should be instability.

Radiographic Findings

Radiographs of the newborn may be misleading and deceptive; they do not rule out the presence of dislocation. The femoral head is not ossified in the newborn and the bony landmarks are not distinct. Attempts to identify a frog-leg lateral view may reduce the dislocation. The normal flexion contracture of the newborn hip must be addressed. When a radiograph of a newborn is taken, it should consist of a single AP view with the hips held in 20° to 30° of flexion to accommodate the normal newborn hip deformity. Hilgenreiner's line and the acetabular index are often problematic. Hilgenreiner's line can be drawn as a horizonal line through the top of the clear area at the depths of the acetabulum. Perkins line can be drawn as a downward line from the most lateral ossified margin of the roof of the acetabulum and perpendicular to Hilgenreiner's line. When the medial margin of the ossified metaphysis of the femur was lateral to Perkins line, 58% of the hips were described as dislocatable by Coleman.[4]

The acetabular index is the angle formed between Hilgenreiner's line and a line from the depth of the acetabular socket to the most lateral ossified margin of the roof of the acetabulum. This index is helpful in measuring the development of the osseous roof of the acetabulum. In the newborn the acetabular index must be over 40° to be significantly abnormal.[4]

Other lines that had been referred to are Shenton's line,[21] which is from the medial border of the femoral neck to the superior border of the obturator foramen; in patients with no problem, the line is a continuous contour. It is interesting to note that the figures from Wenger's[21] chapter were of mature adolescent patients rather than of newborns. The teardrop shadow of Köhler describes three lines: the external semicircular line or the wall of the acetabulum, the long medial line or wall of the lesser pelvis, and the connecting line or semicylindrical cortex of the acetabular notch.[22] This teardrop shadow is not visible in the newborn and does not develop until the first few months of age.

Many observers believe that a radiograph should be taken of the newborn hip to document the absence of significant congenital abnormalities such as congenital coxa vera, proximal femoral focal deficiency, congenital short femur, and sacral agenesis.

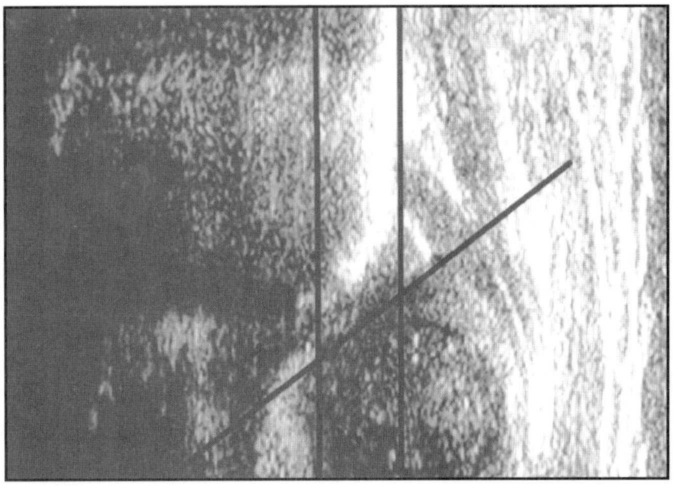

Fig. 7 Coronal ultrasound with 50% coverage of the femoral head and indicated alpha angle.

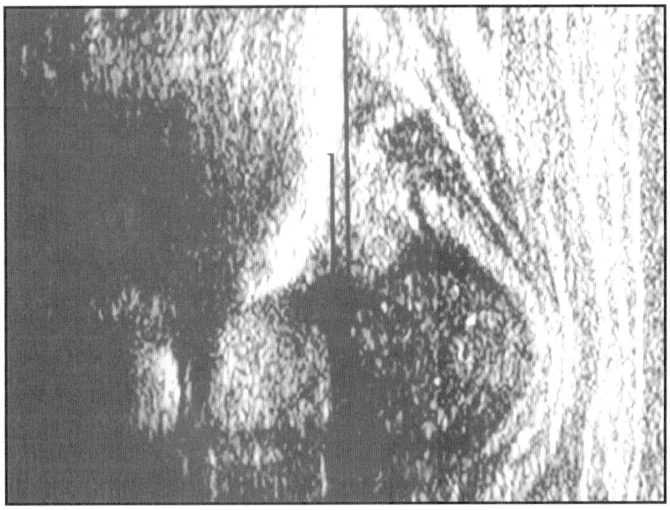

Fig. 8 Coronal ultrasound with 95% subluxation.

Ultrasound of the Newborn Hip

Graf and associates[23,24] described ultrasound of the newborn hip as being useful with static technique and Harcke and Grissom[25] describe it as useful with a dynamic technique. Graf and associates[23,24] describe static hip ultrasound as a single coronal image while the hip is held in a lateral decubitus position and the hips flexed 30° to 45° with two anatomic bony landmarks being identified. The configuration of the ossified ilium is a straight linear white line and the roof of the acetabulum is the ossified medial wall of the acetabulum and the labrum. An alpha line is described as the angle formed by the ossified lateral wall of the ilium and the bony roof line. The beta angle is described as the angle formed by the ossified lateral wall of the ilium and the cartilaginous roof line.[21,23] The Harcke dynamic technique describes axial and coronal images with real time stress of the femoral head similar to the Ortolani or the Barlow maneuver.[25] Four to 6 mm of laxity is normal in the first days of life. This is an operator-dependent study.

The American College of Radiology standards for ultrasound examination of the infant hip[26] includes five views: coronal neutral, coronal flexion mid acetabulum, coronal flexion posterior acetabulum, transverse flexion, and transverse neutral.

To more easily understand the ultrasound of the newborn, it is helpful to evaluate the ultrasound in the same way as a hip radiograph of a newborn. The AP view of the hip is similar to the coronal ultrasound. The ilium seen on the radiograph is similar to the lateral ilium seen on the ultrasound. The ischium seen on the radiograph is similar to the medial acetabulum on the ultrasound. The femoral metaphysis is identified on the radiograph; it is possible to identify the femoral head on the ultrasound. It is recommended to consider the coronal view only and to rotate it to view it as an AP radiograph (Figs. 5 and 6). Identification of the abductor muscles and the lateral wall of the ilium is completed first. The percentage of subluxation of the femoral head from this lateral wall line is then measured (Figs. 7 and 8). The alpha angle can be measured if desired, and the beta angle has not been shown to be helpful.

Early failure of the Pavlik harness treatment for DDH has been predicted when there is low percentage coverage of the femoral head (Lerman JA, Kasser JR, Emans JB, et al, unpublished data, 2000). A low alpha angle has not been shown to be a predictor.

Ultrasound of the newborn has led to an overdiagnosis of DDH. Moreover, it has been documented that high-risk screening with ultrasound does not reduce the prevalence of late diagnosed cases of DDH.[27] The ideal indication for the use of the ultrasound is for the guided reduction of the dislocated hip in the infant, that is, monitoring the hip in traction or evaluating closed reductions. Hip ultrasound of a newborn allows for anatomic evaluation of cartilaginous structures.

Clinical Screening

The incidence of the first surgical procedure has not changed since the introduction of screening.[27] It is clear that clinical screening in the newborn nursery still leads to many misdiagnoses of developmental dysplasia of the hip. Garvey and associates[28] have shown that at risk children with stable hips often had abnormal radiographs at 4 months. Of 375 children with abnormal radiographs at 4 months, 46 had continued abnormal radiographs at 15 months. No child with normal radiographs at 4 months had abnormal radiographs at 15 months.

Because there is no evidence that a child with a normal radiograph with an ossified femoral head at 4 months of age had an abnormal radiograph or development of dysplasia of the hip at 15 months, it is strongly recommended that all patients seen for DDH have a subsequent examination at 4 to 6 months to verify the presence of a normal radiograph. This is recommended because all examinations have an implied guarantee concerning the absence of DDH.

References

1. Curtis ES (ed): Apache babe in carrier, in *The North American Indian: List of Large Plates Supplementing v. 1-20.* Cambridge, MA, University Press, 1907.
2. *Webster's II New College Dictionary*. Boston, MA, Houghton Mifflin Company, 1995.
3. Weinstein SL: Development hip dysplasia and dislocation, in Morrissy RT, Weinstein SL (eds): *Lovell and Winter's Pediatric Orthopaedics,* ed 4. Philadelphia, PA, Lippincott-Raven, 1996, pp 903-950.
4. Coleman SS: Diagnosis of congenital dysplasia of the hip in the newborn infant. *JAMA* 1956:162;548-554.
5. American Academy of Orthopaedic Surgeons Advisory Statement: "CDH" should be "DDH". Park Ridge, IL, American Academy of Orthopaedic Surgeons, 1991.
6. Hart AC, Schmidt KM, Aaron WS (eds): *St. Anthony's ICD-9-CM Code Book.* Reston, VA, St. Anthony's Publishing, 1998.
7. Ilfeld FW, Westin GW, Makin M: Missed or developmental dislocation of the hip. *Clin Orthop* 1986;203:276-281.
8. Bjerkreim I, Arseth PH: Congenital dislocation of the hip in Norway: Late diagnosis CDH in the years 1970 to 1974. *Acta Paediatr Scand* 1978;67:329-332.
9. Beaty JH (ed): *Orthopaedic Knowledge Update 6.* Rosemont, IL, American Academy of Orthopaedic Surgeons, 1999.
10. Stanisavljevic S (ed): *Diagnosis and Treatment of Congenital Hip Pathology in the Newborn.* Baltimore, MD, Williams & Wilkins, 1964.
11. Wynne-Davies R: Acetabular dysplasia and familial joint laxity: Two etiological factors in congenital dislocation of the hip. A review of 589 patients and their families. *J Bone Joint Surg Br* 1970;52:704-716.
12. Barlow TG: Early diagnosis and treatment of congenital dislocation of the hip. *J Bone Joint Surg Br* 1962;44:292-301.
13. Carter CO, Wilkinson JA: Genetic and environmental factors in the etiology of congenital dislocation of the hip. *Clin Orthop* 1964;33:119-128.
14. Salter RB: Etiology, pathogenesis and possible prevention of congenital dislocation of the hip. *Can Med Assoc J* 1968;98:933-945.
15. Dunn PM: Perinatal observations on the etiology of congenital dislocation of the hip. *Clin Orthop* 1976;119:11-22.
16. Ponseti IV: Growth and development of the acetabulum in the normal child: Anatomical, histological, and roentgenographic studies. *J Bone Joint Surg Am* 1978;60:575-585.
17. Ponseti IV: Morphology of the acetabulum in congenital dislocation of the hip: Gross, histological, and roentgenographic studies. *J Bone Joint Surg Am* 1978;60:586-599.
18. Ortolani M: The classic: Congenital hip dysplasia in the light of early and very early diagnosis. *Clin Orthop* 1976;119:6-10.
19. Avisse C, Gomes H, Delvinquiere V, et al: Anatomic study of the pre- and neonatal hip: Physiopathologic considerations on dysplasia and congenital dislocation of the hip. *Surg Radiol Anat* 1997;19:155-159.
20. Stanisavljevic S: Tribute to Marino Ortolani. *Clin Orthop* 1976;119:4-5.
21. Wenger DR: Edward Warren Hine Shenton 1872-1955, in Wenger DR, Rang M (eds): *The Art and Practice of Children's Orthopaedics.* New York, NY, Raven Press 1993, p 269.
22. Schmidt H, Freyschmidt J, Holthusen W (eds): *Borderlands of Normal and Early Pathologic Findings in Skeletal Radiography/Köhler/Zimmer,* ed 4. Stuttgard, Germany, Thieme Medical Publishers,1993, pp 649-665.
23. Graf R: New possibilities for the diagnosis of congenital hip joint dislocation by ultrasonography. *J Pediatr Orthop* 1983,3:354-359.
24. Graf R, Scott S, Farkas P, Lercher K, Tschauner C, Benaroya A: Ultrasonography in the diagnosis and management of infant hip dysplasia, in *Manual for Hip Sonography.* Allgemeines u. orthopädisches Landeskrankenhaus Stolzalpe, Austria, 1999.
25. Harcke HT, Grissom LE: Performing dynamic sonography of the infant hip. *AJR Am J Roentgenol* 1990;155:837-844.
26. American College of Radiology Standards for the Performance of the Ultrasound Examination for Detection of Developmental Dysplasia of the Hip. American College of Radiology, Revised May 25, 1999.
27. Godward S, Dezateux C: Surgery for congenital dislocation of the hip in the UK as a measure of outcome of screening: MRC Working Party on Congenital Dislocation of the Hip: Medical Research Council. *Lancet* 1998;351:1149-1152.
28. Garvey M, Donoghue VB, Gorman WA, O'Brien N, Murphy JF: Radiographic screening at four months of infants at risk for congenital hip dislocation. *J Bone Joint Surg Br* 1992;74:704-707.

Reference to Video

Haynes R: *Dislocation of the Femoral Head in Infants.* Houston, TX.

56

Developmental Dysplasia of the Hip: Assessment and Treatment Before Walking Age

R. Baxter Willis, MD

Developmental dysplasia of the hip (DDH) is a term used to describe the condition formerly known as congenital dislocation of the hip. Its etiology and pathoanatomy are well understood but the management of this condition can be challenging in patients of any age.

Terminology

Many terms that are used interchangeably to describe this condition need clarification. Dislocation of the hip implies lack of contact between the femoral head and the acetabulum. A dislocatable hip dislocates with a provocative maneuver (Barlow maneuver) and relocates with flexion and abduction (Ortolani maneuver). Subluxation of the hip implies that the femoral head does not articulate with the true acetabulum. In the newborn, the experienced clinician may note a feeling of hip instability while performing the Barlow maneuver. The diagnosis may be confirmed with imaging modalities such as ultrasound, arthrogram, or plain radiographs.

Dysplasia is defined as an abnormality in development. Hip dysplasia is an all-encompassing term for the entire spectrum of congenital hip abnormalities from subluxation to dislocation.

Acetabular dysplasia implies abnormal development of the acetabulum; the acetabulum is shallow and more vertical than normal. Acetabular dysplasia can be primary or secondary to subluxation or dislocation of the hip.

A teratologic dislocation of the hip is one that occurs before birth.[1,2] It is synonymous with antenatal or intrauterine dislocation. This rare form of dislocation is associated with other conditions such as arthrogryposis, spina bifida, and Larsen's syndrome. This form of hip dislocation should be considered if the hip is irreducible at birth or the femoral head extremely high riding.

Incidence

The incidence of DDH varies widely depending on the definition of terms and geographic location. In North America, two large screening programs have reported their results. Gross and associates[3] screened 10,170 newborns and found an incidence of three to four dislocatable hips per 1,000 babies. Tredwell and Bell[4] reported an incidence of 9.8 dislocatable hips per 1,000 babies after screening 32,480 newborns. It appears from these and other studies that neonatal screening programs are effective for neonatal hip instability but not sensitive enough to discern acetabular dysplasia.

Physical Examination

The physical examination of the newborn is performed with the child quiet, warm, and on a relatively firm surface. The Ortolani maneuver is performed by gently flexing the hips to 90° and gently abducting the hips with forward and upward pressure on the greater trochanter. Dislocatability is produced by gently adducting the hip to the midline, using the thumb to exert firm posterior and outward pressure on the lesser trochanter. The Barlow maneuver confirms hip instability. It cannot be overemphasized that these tests should be performed gently and without force.

With time, the soft tissues about the hip will become contracted and prevent reduction of the femoral head into the acetabulum (the Ortolani maneuver is negative). As a consequence, limitation of abduction in the older child becomes the critical positive physical finding. In addition, apparent shortening of the femur (Galeazzi's sign) and asymmetric skin folds of the thigh should raise suspicions of the diagnosis.

Ultrasonography

Ultrasonography can be of significant value in imaging of the hip prior to ossification of the capital femoral epiphysis (up to 6 or 8 months of age).[5-9] It is superior to plain radiographs in evaluating DDH in infants because the cartilage and associated soft tissues of the hip can be seen.

Hip ultrasound has been used in some parts of Europe as a screening tool but is not a practical recommendation in North America because of the cost, both in manpower and in equipment, as well as the cost of interpretation. However, there are indications when ultrasound is of definite value. Absolute

Table 1
Ultrasonographic classification of hip dysplasia in the neonatal period

Type I	Normal	α angle > 60°
Type II	Normal-Dysplastic	α angle 44° to 60°
Type III	Dislocated	α angle < 43°
Type IV	Dislocated	α angle not measurable

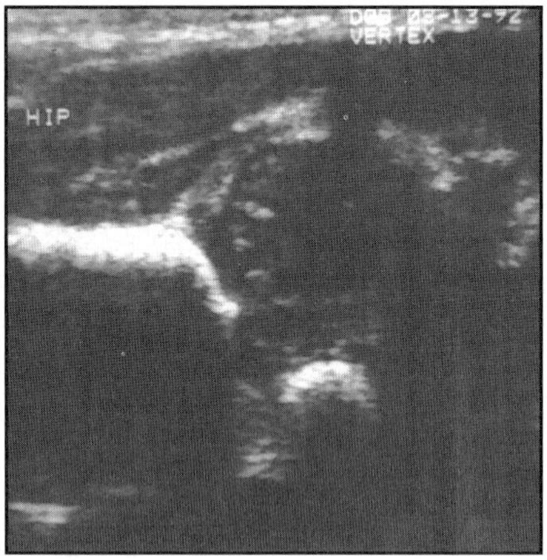

Fig. 1 Ultrasonographic image, coronal view, of a normal left hip. Dense white line represents bony ilium, which changes to become bony acetabulum. Cartilaginous labrum and capsule form other limb of a "V" with the femoral head in the joint.

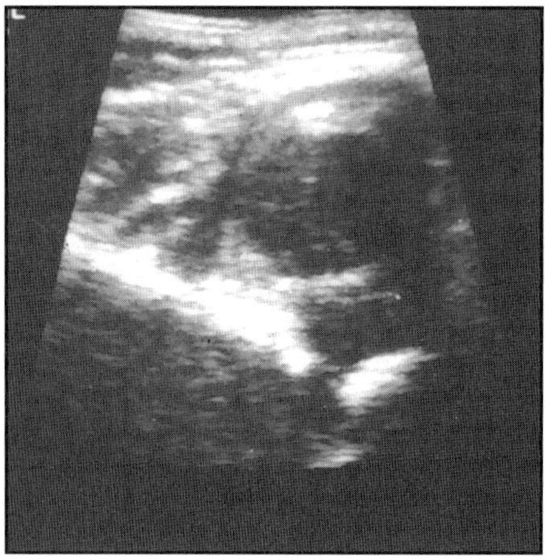

Fig. 2 Ultrasonographic image, coronal view, of a dislocated hip. The femoral head is displaced superiorly and laterally to the ilium.

indications include a positive or abnormal physical examination. Strong relative indications include high-risk infants—those with breech presentation, strong family history of DDH, or history of oligohydramnios and congenital torticollis.[5,6,8,9]

Static Technique

In the static technique popularized by Graf,[7] a coronal image of the hip is obtained with the transducer positioned lateral to the extended femur. An image of the hip joint is created that includes the bony ilium, bony acetabulum, triradiate cartilage, and cartilaginous labrum as well as the cartilaginous femoral head (Fig. 1). Two angles and a ratio are created that are consistently reproducible. Graf has classified four basic hip types depending on the measurement of the α angle (Table 1). The α angle assesses the inclination of the superior osseous acetabulum with respect to the lateral margin of the iliac bone.

Dynamic Technique

In North America, the dynamic technique has replaced the static technique as the most common.[6,8,10] The child is placed in the supine position and images of the hip are obtained with the hip extended. The hip is then flexed 90° and the thigh pistoned with direct posterior pressure while the hip is alternately adducted and abducted. Images are obtained in both the transverse and coronal planes.

In a normal hip up to 6 mm of femoral head translation or motion can be see in the newborn.[6,8,9] In the coronal view, 50% of the femoral head should be medial to a line drawn along the longitudinal axis of the ilium.[7-9]

In a dislocated hip, the femoral head is usually displaced posteriorly, laterally or superiorly. The acetabulum often appears shallow (dysplastic) and the labrum may be inverted (Fig. 2).

Sonography after treatment in a Pavlik harness should show the femoral head in a concentric reduced position.[6,7]

Management

The most important concept in the management of DDH at any age is the reduction of the femoral head into the true acetabulum by closed or open methods. In the child younger than 18 months, there is more potential for remodeling and correction of the concomitant dysplasia of the acetabulum. In the child older than 18 months, correction of the dysplasia of the acetabulum and upper femur often demands concomitant reconstructive osteotomies in addition to the open reduction. As a general rule, all unstable hips demand treatment. From natural history studies, treatment is more successful performed earlier than later with a lower incidence of residual acetabular dysplasia.

Closed Reduction: Newborn to Age 6 Months

In newborns and patients up to age 6 months, closed reduction and immobilization in a Pavlik harness is the treatment of choice. The hips should be flexed more than 90° and a sufficient amount of abduction used. The hip is stabilized and gently abducted until the hip is located to determine the safe zone. Forced abduction of greater than 60° is associated with osteonecrosis and should be avoided. A hip abduction orthosis, most commonly a Pavlik harness is used to maintain stability (Fig. 3). The brace is not removed until the hip is stable and imaging tests are normal, usually 2 to 3 months in a newborn.[11] The reduction of the hip should be confirmed by ultrasound. Once the hip is stable, the harness may be removed once or twice weekly for bathing.

Pitfalls If hip reduction is not achieved in approximately 3 weeks, the Pavlik harness should be discontinued and an alternative treatment selected. Options include a period of 2 weeks of home traction followed by closed reduction, or closed reduction alone under general anesthesia, or even open reduction.[11] It is critical to continue treatment for a long enough period of time. This usually means at least 6 weeks in the newborn or up to 3 or 4 months in the older child (up to 3 to 4 months of age). The endpoint of treatment is a stable hip and a normal imaging study (ultrasound or plain radiographs). Frequent follow-up and adjustment of the Pavlik harness is necessary because of growth of the child. Flexion of 100° should be maintained but flexion greater than this is associated with femoral nerve palsy and inferior hip dislocation.

Results of Pavlik Harness Treatment For acetabular dysplasia and subluxation, the long-term results of Pavlik harness treatment show a 95% success rate.[12] This success rate falls to 80% for frank dislocation of the hip. In a multicenter study from Europe, 30% of hips were reduced on the first day, 65% on the second day, and 85% by the end of the first week.[12] The rate of osteonecrosis was only 2.38%, but residual acetabular dysplasia was present at late follow-up in 20% of patients, this dysplasia was sometimes not present or identified until years later. Therefore, long-term follow-up is mandatory with radiographs every 1 to 2 years until skeletal maturity to ensure normal hip development.[10,13-17]

Closed Reduction: Age 6 Months to 1 Year

At age 6 months, treatment in a Pavlik harness is no longer effective.[11,12] The child becomes too strong and redislocation is common. Closed reduction under

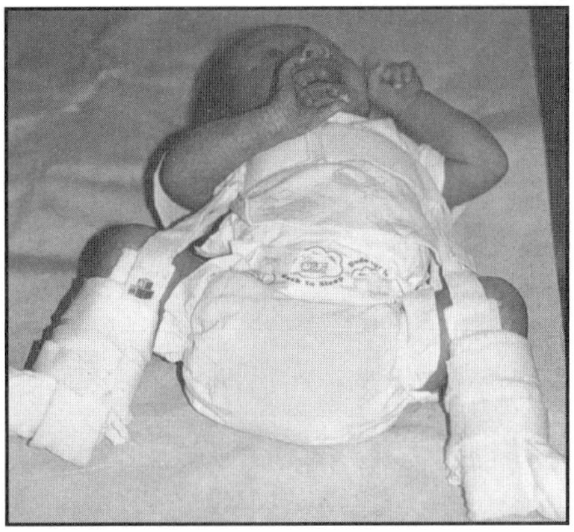

Fig. 3 Infant in a Pavlik harness. Note that flexion of the hips is greater than 90° and abduction is 60°.

general anesthesia and application of double hip spica cast is the treatment of choice. Preliminary traction has been favored historically to aid in the ease of reduction by stret ching out the soft tissues around the hip and lessening the incidence of osteonecrosis.[2,18] Home traction is usually used with the hips flexed 45° to 90° and abducted about 20° to 30°. Two weeks of traction is usually sufficient and is followed by a gentle closed reduction under general anesthesia.[18] The hips are flexed to about 100° and abducted about 40° to 60° in the so-called safe zone.[2,19,20] This position has been termed the human position by Salter because it avoids wide abduction, which is a potential cause of osteonecrosis[19-21] (Fig. 4). A percutaneous adductor longus tenotomy is almost always done to widen the safe zone and increase stability.[20]

An arthrogram should be performed at the time of the closed reduction.[15] It can be performed by a number of different approaches, but the medial approach is simple and effective. A 20- or 22-gauge spinal needle is introduced medially just anterior to the adductor longus. The needle, under fluoroscopic control, is aimed toward the ipsilateral shoulder and should enter the hip joint on the medial and inferior aspect of the femoral neck. Dye is instilled and the

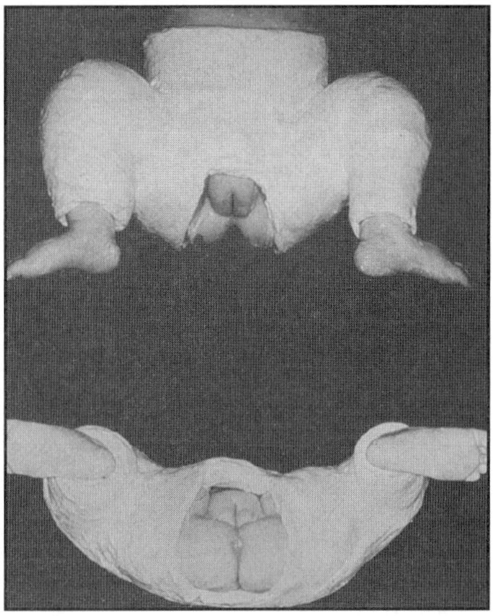

Fig. 4 Infant in a hip spica cast after closed reduction for developmental dislocation of the left hip. Note the "human" position of comfortable abduction (approximately 60°).

arthrogram performed. Up to 5 mm of medial dye pooling is acceptable with a 90% satisfactory outcome. If there is more than 7 mm of medial dye pooling, a poor result can be expected in 70% of cases.[14,17] A double hip spica cast is applied and a postoperative CT scan performed to confirm the concentric reduction of the femoral head in the acetabulum (Fig. 5). The hip spica is changed every 6 weeks and repeat arthrograms may be performed to assess stability and the development of the cartilaginous labrum. In the child up to 12 months of age, 12 or 18 weeks of immobilization in a hip spica cast is usually sufficient. If the hip is stable but there is persistent dysplasia on arthrogram or plain radiographs, a hip abduction splint should be used until the hip becomes normal.

Coleman[22] and Weinstein[17] have both documented no increase in the rate of osteonecrosis with gentle closed reduction alone without preliminary traction in this age group. From a personal standpoint, preoperative traction is not used unless the hip is particularly high riding.

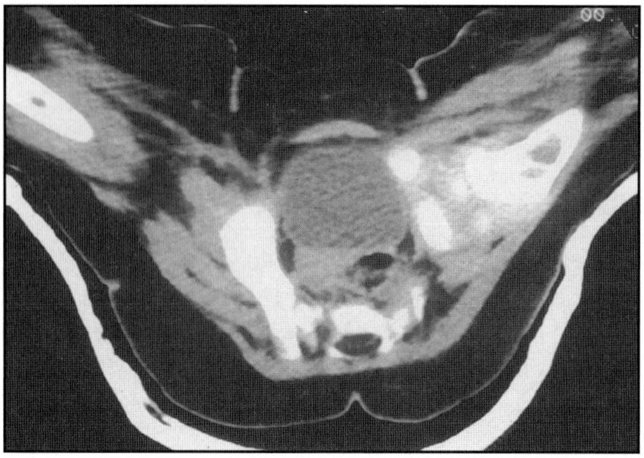

Fig. 5 CT scan of the pelvis after closed reduction for DDH. The child is placed in a hip spica cast and the scan confirms the reduction of the femoral head.

Open Reduction

If the hip is irreducible by closed methods or a concentric reduction is not achieved, an open reduction should be performed. There are three surgical approaches commonly used for an open reduction of DDH.[1,10,22-25] The medial or Ludloff approach is the most direct surgical approach to the obstacles to reduction.[2] Through this approach, the tendons of the adductor longus and iliopsoas can be lengthened and the hourglass constriction of the capsule addressed. In addition, the ligamentum teres and transverse acetabular ligament may be divided if necessary. However, this is a small and difficult anatomic area for most surgeons to navigate, especially if they are unfamiliar with the anatomy. The medial femoral circumflex vessels cross the field and must be protected. With this approach it is impossible to perform a capsulorrhaphy or capsular plication and reduction is dependent on the effectiveness of the postoperative immobilization.

Weinstein[25] has modified this approach by developing the interval between the pectineus and adductor brevis (the anteromedial approach). He has performed open reductions on 93 hips in 76 children with a mean patient age of 14.7 months. Osteonecrosis occurred in 13 patients (14%), 9 of whom had no previous treatment. There was no relationship between the rate of osteonecrosis and injury to the medial circumflex femoral vessels. In addition, preoperative traction did not affect the incidence of osteonecrosis.[25]

The anterolateral approach has been the most popular because it enables the surgeon to deal with the obstacles to reduction as well as allowing enough exposure for a capsular plication.[2,10,14,22-24] The upper portion of the Smith-Petersen anterior approach is used with development of the interval between the sartorius and tensor fascia lata. The iliac apophysis is split and the periosteum medially and laterally is reflected back to the sciatic notch. Recession of the illopsoas is almost always performed with resection of the redundant anterolateral capsule or a pants-over-vest repair to decrease the capsular volume. Immobilization is carried out in the most concentric position of reduction, usually 30° to 40° of flexion, abduction, and slight internal rotation. A hip spica cast is kept in place for 6 to 8 weeks followed by abduction casts for an additional 4 weeks.

An open reduction by any approach is a challenging procedure for even the most experienced surgeon. The results of repeat operations after failed open reductions are poor, with only one third of the hips having an acceptable result and an osteonecrosis rate approaching 50%.[10,17] This is not an operation for the inexperienced surgeon.

Recent work by Segal and associates[21,26] has suggested a protective effect from osteonecrosis once the ossific nucleus is visualized. Their work suggested no difference in osteonecrosis rates whether the reduction was performed open or closed but a significant decrease in osteonecrosis rates after appearance of the ossific nucleus.

A similar study (GS Bassett, MD, Alberta, Canada, unpublished data, 1997) has refuted these findings with no difference in osteonecrosis rates whether the ossific nucleus was present or not at the time of initial treatment. Therefore, it is safe to carry out appropriate treatment at the time of diagnosis of dislocated hips.

References

1. Gruel CR, Birch JG, Roach JW, Herring JA: Teratologic dislocation of the hip. *J Pediatr Orthop* 1986;6:693-702.
2. Herring JA: Congenital dislocation of the hip, in Morrissy RT (ed): *Lovell and Winter's Pediatric Orthopaedics,* ed 3. Philadelphia, PA, JB Lippincott, 1990, vol 2, pp 815-850.
3. Gross RH, Wisnefske M, Howard TC III, Hitch M: Infant hip screening. *Hip* 1982; 50-67.
4. Tredwell SJ, Bell HM: Efficacy of neonatal hip examination. *J Pediatr Orthop* 1981;1:61-65.
5. Berman L, Klenerman L: Ultrasound screening for hip abnormalities: Preliminary findings in 1001 neonates. *Br Med J* 1986;293:719-722.
6. Boal DK, Schwenkter EP: The infant hip: Assessment with real-time US. *Radiology* 1985;157:667-672.
7. Graf R: Classification of hip joint dysplasia by means of sonography. *Arch Orthop Trauma Surg* 1984;102:248-255.
8. Harcke HT, Clarke NM, Lee MS, Borns PF, MacEwen GD: Examination of the infant hip with real-time ultrasonography. *J Ultrasound Med* 1984;3:131-137.
9. Siegel MJ, McAlister WH: Musculoskeletal system and spine, in Siegel MJ (ed): *Pediatric Sonography,* ed 2. New York, NY, Raven Press, 1995, pp 513-551.
10. Tönnis D, Legal H, Graf R (eds): *Congenital Dysplasia and Dislocation of the Hip in Children and Adults.* Berlin, Germany, Springer-Verlag, 1987.

11. Mubarak S, Garfin S, Vance R, McKinnon B, Sutherland D: Pitfalls in the use of the Pavlik harness for treatment of congenital dysplasia, subluxation, and dislocation of the hip. *J Bone Joint Surg Am* 1981;63:1239-1248.

12. Grill F, Bensahel H, Canadell J, Dungl P, Matasovic T, Vizkelety T: The Pavlik harness in the treatment of congenital dislocating hip: Report on a multicenter study of the European Paediatric Orthopaedic Society. *J Pediatr Orthop* 1988;8:1-8.

13. Cooperman DR, Wallensten R, Stulberg SD: Acetabular dysplasia in the adult. *Clin Orthop* 1983;175:79-85.

14. Lindstrom JR, Ponseti IV, Wenger DR: Acetabular development after reduction in congenital dislocation of the hip. *J Bone Joint Surg Am* 1979;61:112-118.

15. Renshaw TS: Inadequate reduction of congenital dislocation of the hip. *J Bone Joint Surg Am* 1981;63:1114-1121.

16. Severin E: Contribution to the knowledge of congenital dislocation of the hip joint: Late results of closed reduction and arthrographic studies of recent cases. *Acta Chir Scand* 1941;84(suppl 63):1-142.

17. Weinstein SL: Natural history of congenital hip dislocation (CDH) and hip dysplasia. *Clin Orthop* 1987;225:62-76.

18. Joseph K, MacEwen GD, Boos ML: Home traction in the management of congenital dislocation of the hip. *Clin Orthop* 1982;165: 83-90.

19. Gage JR, Winter RB: Avascular necrosis of the capital femoral epiphysis as a complication of closed reduction of congenital dislocation of the hip: A critical review of twenty years'experience at Gillette Children's Hospital. *J Bone Joint Surg Am* 1972;54:373-388.

20. Ramsey PL, Lasser S, MacEwen GD: Congenital dislocation of the hip: Use of the Pavlik harness in the child during the first six months of life. *J Bone Joint Surg Am* 1976;58:1000-1004.

21. Segal LS, Boal DK, Borthwick L, Schwentker EP, Clark MW: Avascular necrosis following treatment of DDH: The protective influence of the ossific nucleus. *Orthop Trans* 1996-1997;20:297-298.

22. Coleman SS: Operative management of congenital dislocation of the hip. *Curr Orthop* 1987;1:275.

23. Powell EN, Gerratana FJ, Gage JR: Open reduction for congenital hip dislocation: The risk of avascular necrosis with three different approaches. *J Pediatr Orthop* 1986;6:127-132.

24. Ross ERS, Ford DJ, Evans GA: Abstract: Factors influencing the incidence of avascular necrosis in anterior open reduction for the congenitally dislocated hip. *J Bone Joint Surg Br* 1988;70:680.

25. Weinstein SL: Anteromedial approach to reduction for congenital hip dysplasia. *Strategies Orthop Surg* 1987;6:2.

26. Segal LS, Schneider DJ, Berlin JM, Bruno A, Davis BR, Jacobs CR: The contribution of the ossific nucleus to the structural stiffness of the capital femoral epiphysis: A porcine model for DDH. *J Pediatr Orthop* 1999;19:433-437.

57

Developmental Hip Dysplasia and Dislocation: Management of the Older Child

Colin F. Moseley, MD, BSc, CM

Management of Dislocation After 18 Months of Age

New Difficulties

As the child gets older and the femoral head has spent more time outside the acetabulum, developmental abnormalities become more severe. They become important factors in treatment, and require different management strategies than in a younger child. Whereas it may be possible to achieve a closed reduction of the dislocated hip in the older child, accepting a closed reduction alone may not lead to the best possible outcome.

It is worthwhile to review those aspects of the dysplasia that are factors in treatment.[1] The transverse acetabular ligament crosses the inferior portion of the fovea of the acetabulum. It can be thought of as completing the circle of the labrum. This circle of labrum and transverse ligament normally forms the margin of the acetabulum, but in the absence of a located head, gets drawn into the acetabulum and narrows its opening. This circle may be too small to accept the femoral head; therefore, a closed reduction may not be as deep as possible and may not exert pressure on the acetabular floor.

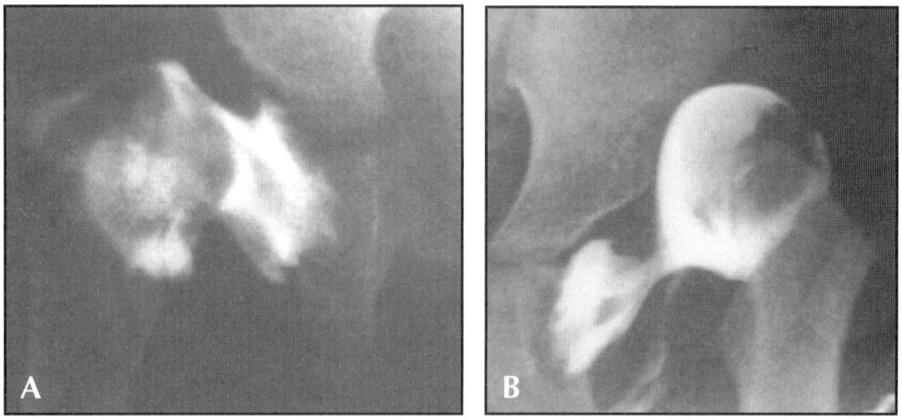

Fig. 1 A, Arthrogram showing the abnormal shape of the labrum with its medial border, sulcus beneath its inner edge, and broad attachment to acetabular subchondral bone. **B,** Arthrogram showing severe indentation of the capsule by the iliopsoas muscle and extreme narrowing of the capsule into the hourglass shape.

The labrum not only changes its location, but also becomes significantly deformed. It is unfortunate that the word infolded has achieved such wide usage because it implies that the labrum can simply be folded back out by the surgeon. The labrum undergoes a marked change in its shape and a marked widening and shifting of its attachment to the underlying bone. It is not simply folded in and cannot be folded out. The labrum is a thickened structure, which is located within the diameter of the rim of the acetabulum and has the effect of diminishing the size of the opening into the acetabulum.

The ligamentum teres is variable. It may be completely absent or may be considerably elongated and hypertrophied. Even if a closed reduction can be achieved, the ligamentum teres may serve as an obstruction to a deep reduction and may thereby impair future development.

The capsule may become hourglass shaped, with a severe narrowing between the femoral head and the acetabulum (Fig. 1). This narrowing occurs partly because there is nothing within that part of the capsule and partly because the iliopsoas tendon is tented across the inferior part of the capsule. If the femoral head cannot pass through this narrowed portion then it is impossible to obtain a deep closed reduction.

There is also significant deformity in the shapes of both the head and acetabulum. The degree of deformity of the head is extremely variable and may be severe in the very young child and, conversely, minimal in the occasional older child. All sorts of abnormal shapes may be encountered. The shape of the femoral head is impossible to determine from plain radiographs in the young child because most of the head is cartilage The acetabular dysplasia is evident as a decreased acetabular index and a teardrop shaped like a wedge rather than a teardrop. The combined effect of the dysplasias of the femoral head and acetabulum may result in a less than satisfactory fit after either closed or open reduction.

All of these components of the deformity decrease the possibility that a closed reduction will be successful or definitive in the management of the dislocated hip in the older child.

Principles of Treatment

The principle of treatment of the dislocated hip in the older child is the same as that in the younger child: obtain a deep reduction and maintain that reduction. The methodology of accomplishing that principle, however, is different as a result of the factors listed above. Because these obstructions must be dealt with, an open reduction is usually the best approach after the age of 18 months. At open reduction the surgeon can deal with the soft-tissue obstructions and with certain components of the bony dysplasia. It is worth noting that the surgeon cannot produce a normal hip, but can only set up the situation so that further development can gradually normalize the hip. At the time of open reduction, the surgeon can determine the position of the leg that produces the best fit and the best stability of the head in the acetabulum, and can decide whether derotation osteotomy of the femur or pelvic osteotomy is indicated.

At open reduction the surgeon must evaluate the tension that is produced by the reduction of the hip. It is widely believed that too much tension can produce osteonecrosis of the femoral head, but it is likely that too little tension can lead to instability and a failure to adequately stimulate normal acetabular modeling. The surgeon must therefore determine whether femoral shortening is necessary and, if it is, taking into account the tensioning effect of a possible Salter osteotomy, how much the femur should be shortened. If a femoral shortening is required, then the surgeon must decide whether or not a derotation component should be included. This question will be dealt with in detail.

Many patients with dislocation of the hip will require a pelvic osteotomy, such as a Salter osteotomy,[2,3] to improve the orientation and mechanics of the hip joint and to provide a beneficial stimulus to remodeling. Whether this should be done routinely at the time of open reduction or should be done at a later stage for hips that are not doing well is a matter of some controversy and will be dealt with in the next section.

Following open reduction the patient is immobilized in a cast to allow soft-tissue healing and a start to the remodeling process. During the time of immobilization the changes in pressure distribution on the femoral head can alter the process of ossification, and changes in pressure on the labrum can influence it to remodel into a more normal shape and position. The time of immobilization following open reduction varies, but is usually at least 3 months.

Controversial Aspects of Treatment

There are two areas in the surgical treatment of the dislocated hip that lack universal consensus. One is the benefit of routinely performing a pelvic osteotomy at the time of open reduction, and the other is the benefit and risk of performing a derotation femoral osteotomy.

It seems reasonable to believe, as Salter has taught, that it is beneficial to perform a pelvic osteotomy to redirect the acetabulum and provide more superior and lateral coverage. Providing more lateral coverage allows the resultant force across the hip to become more medially directed, thereby encouraging the acetabulum to deepen and improving the remodeling process.

Some argue that this operation is a purely geometric one and that the effect is the same at 4 years of age as it is at 2 years of age. This possibility has been investigated in the assessment of a fairly large cohort of patients who had or did not have a pelvic osteotomy at the time of open reduction. The group with the pelvic osteotomy fares better in the long run with respect to both acetabular index and center edge angle. It is also interesting to note that the patients who had the Salter osteotomy done later never caught up to the group that had it done early with respect to either of these parameters. This suggests that the Salter osteotomy is more than a geometric operation, that it does indeed have a beneficial effect on remodeling, and that it is best to do it at the earliest age possible. A Salter osteotomy performed rountinely at the time of open reduction adds minimally to the duration of surgery and does not add substantially to morbidity or risk.

Some surgeons, at the time of performing an open reduction, routinely derotate the proximal femur. It is their belief that the femur is always anteverted and that correction of anteversion is always indicated. There is no escaping the fact, however, that some patients are later found to be retroverted, and it thus seems clear that femoral derotation should not be performed in every patient.

I have performed very few femoral derotations at the time of open reduction, even in patients who have had femoral shortening. There is no indication that these patients have intoed significantly thereafter or that the development of the hip has been impaired.

The degree of anteversion in previously untreated children with dislocated hips was studied, and anteversion varied from 20° to 100°, with most being in the 40° to 60° range. It is extremely difficult for the surgeon to assess the degree of anteversion at the time of open reduction. The surgeon sees only the anterior part of a very deformed femoral head, has difficulty determining the location of its center, and can estimate the position of the greater trochanter only by palpation. Because anteversion can only be roughly estimated at the time of surgery, femoral derotation should be considered only in patients with obvious and severe anteversion and the degree of correction should be moderate.

Postoperative Management

The patient should be immobilized in a 1/2 hip spica cast for at least 3 months. It should be noted that the position of immobilization following open reduction surgery is very different from the position following a close reduction. Following a closed reduction, the most stable position is usually achieved with more than 90° of flexion and moderate abduction. Postoperative patients should not be immobilized in this position because it leads to extreme contractures of the anterior structures around the hip joint. When the cast is removed, the tightness of these structures can produce a tethering effect, and this effect can result in dislocation of the hip when the child attempts to extend the hip to stand or walk. It is preferable to immobilize the hip in 30° of abduction, 30° of flexion, and 30° of internal rotation. This position usually achieves satisfactory stability, particularly if a Salter osteotomy has been performed. In this position the leg is very close to the position of walking and the chance of dislocation after removal of the cast may be decreased.

The handling of the patient may be important during the postoperative period in the cast. It is possible that positioning the child in the upright position or in the prone position could lead to dislocation of the hip. In the upright position the patient's body weight is transmitted through the femurs to the cast. This has the effect of pushing the femurs upwards while the weight of the trunk is pushing downwards and could lead to dislocation. A similar effect happens when the patient is positioned prone. It may be advisable to have the parents control the child' s position by never putting the child upright or prone during the period of immobilization.

Upper Age Limits

The success of open reduction depends on the ability of a child's femoral head and acetabulum to remodel to spherical shapes with adequate coverage. The results of surgery are therefore much better in younger children than in older children, and older children have a much higher incidence of dysplasia and recurrent problems after open reduction. The surgeon who is about to perform an open reduction must keep in mind the natural history of the dislocated hip. Patients with long-standing untreated dislocated hips actually live good and productive lives. They walk with a noticeably asymmetric gait but can walk long distances with only minimal discomfort and fatigue. They generally are able to participate in almost all activities and can marry, have children of their own, and take care of their families for a long time.

Conversely, dysplastic hips have a much more difficult outcome, going on to degenerative arthritis, pain, stiffness, and disability. The surgeon, therefore, will be conferring a significant disadvantage by converting a dislocated hip to a dysplastic one. Performing an open reduction is only a reasonable strategy if there is a high likelihood of achieving a normal or near normal hip. Although it is technically possible to reduce the hip at almost any age, I believe that open reductions of unilateral dislocations should be avoided in children after their eighth birthday.

Special consideration must be given to children with bilateral dislocations. These children are symmetric in their gait and deformity, and for them to benefit from treatment, a surgeon must achieve excellent results with two hips, not just one. A patient who ends up with one excellent hip and one dysplastic arthritic hip will have significant pain and disability, and the excellent result in the good hip will be for naught. This fact means that the upper age limit for performing open reduction is younger in bilateral dislocations than in unilateral ones, and bilateral open reductions should be avoided after the fifth birthday. Such patients are better off with no treatment at all.

Management of Dysplasia in the Older Child

Pediatric orthopaedic surgeons are frequently faced with adolescent patients with dysplasia of the acetabulum. Sometimes they are patients who have been treated previously for developmental dysplasia of the hip, sometimes they have just begun to have pain, and sometimes the dysplasia is noticed as an incidental finding of a known problem in the contralateral hip. In any case, the pediatric orthopaedic surgeon must adopt a working approach that includes both a threshold for performing surgery, and an algorithm for selecting the best surgical procedure.

Classification of Acetabular Osteotomies

Many different procedures have been described to deal with dysplasia of the hip joint. Their goals are to prevent or delay degeneration of the hip joint and the associated loss of comfort and function. They do this by increasing the load-bearing area of the joint, or by increasing coverage as defined by the center-edge angle. Increasing the load-bearing area of the joint reduces the pressure born by the articular cartilage, and increasing coverage reduces the tendency for subluxation by increasing the medial component of the joint reaction force.

The various procedures fall into three groups, not only by their principles, but by the way they fit into the selection algorithm. The classification is seen in Table 1.

Redirectional Osteotomies

Redirectional osteotomies improve the orientation of the existing acetabulum.

Table 1
Classification of acetabular osteotomies

Redirectional Osteotomies	Reshaping Osteotomies	Augmentation Osteotomies
Salter	Pemberton	Chiari
Sutherland	Albee	Shelf (Staheli)
Steel	Dega	
Tonnis		
Ganz		
Wagner		
Eppright		

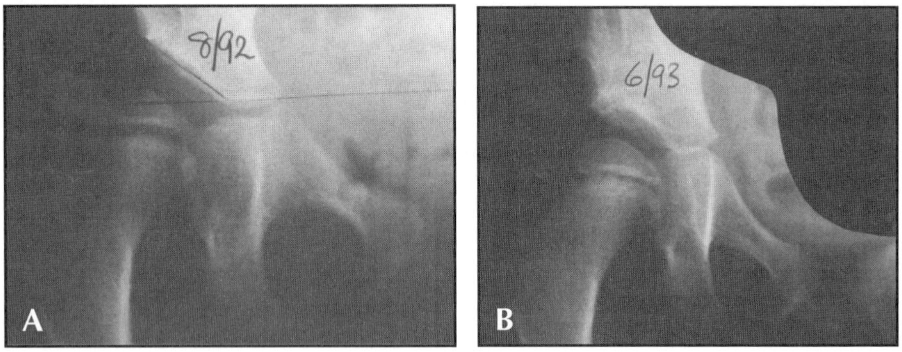

Fig. 2 A, Moderate dysplasia of the hip with a femoral head that is fairly round but has migrated somewhat superiorly and laterally. The acetabulum is shallow but the head is fairly concentric with its upper part. **B,** Five months after a Salter osteotomy, coverage has improved and the acetabular rim is sharp, indicating that remodeling is progressing well.

They share the prerequisite that acetabular size and shape are adequate; specifically, that the joint must be spherical and congruent, especially in this age group in which little benefit can be expected from remodeling. They move the acetabulum so that lateral and anterior coverage are increased, and posterior and inferior coverage are reduced.

The order in which these procedures are listed in Table 1 is not random. The Salter procedure, listed first, is the simplest and least technically demanding of the procedures in this category. Proceeding down the list, the procedures become technically more demanding until they become almost impossible. Why, then, do orthopaedic surgeons not simply do the Salter procedure in every case?

The answer is that the more technically demanding procedures lower on the list are more effective. They allow greater degrees of redirection and place more control over the final orientation in the hands of the surgeon. The pediatric orthopaedic surgeon, therefore, needs to have in his or her arsenal procedures from both ends of the list.

The Salter procedure involves a single cut through the pelvis just above the acetabulum.[2,3] The inferior segment is then rotated about an axis that passes through the posterior end of the cut in the sciatic notch and the symphysis pubis. This axis is defined by the anatomy of the pelvis and not by the surgeon who is limited with respect to both the direction and amount of redirection. The axis can be optimized by drawing the inferior segment anteriorly during the rotation, but the redirection depends mostly on the starting point of the cut and the size of the wedge inserted (Fig. 2).

Sutherland and Moore[4] described a variant of the Salter procedure in which a second cut is made adjacent to the symphysis pubis to facilitate rotation in older patients. Salter has shown, however, by performing the simpler procedure in patients of all ages, that this variation is unnecessary.

Rab[5] constructed a computerized geometric model of the pelvis and performed simulated Salter osteotomies. He found that coverage, as expressed by the center-edge angle, is increased by only 13° with a 30° wedge. This may be sufficient for some patients, particularly young ones who need only a catalyst for improved remodeling, but patients who need more coverage than that will require some other procedure. Although the Salter osteotomy appears to stimulate remodeling in younger patients, that potential is limited in adolescents.

The Steel triple osteotomy[6] permits greater redirection than the Salter procedure and gives the surgeon greater control over the direction of the redirection. It is, however, a bigger operation and more technically demanding because it requires a separate approach to the ischial tuberosity and an additional osteotomy of the pubic ramus. Although greater correction is possible the freedom of movement of the acetabular segment is still somewhat limited by the relatively long ischial tuberosity, which is tethered by ligaments and muscles.

In general, the closer the osteotomy cuts are to the acetabulum the greater the magnitude and versatility of the correction. Several procedures have been described that take advantage of this principle. Tonnis and associates[7] and Carlioz and associates[8] described variations of the Steel triple pelvic osteotomy in which the ischial cut is made higher on the ischial ramus and closer to the acetabulum, ideally above the sacrospinous ligament. The Tonnis procedure is preferred for patients in whom the correction offered by the Salter osteotomy would not be sufficient (Fig. 3).

Ganz and associates[9] have described a pelvic osteotomy that involves a difficult geometric cut around the acetabulum. This procedure is more demanding technically than Tonnis's

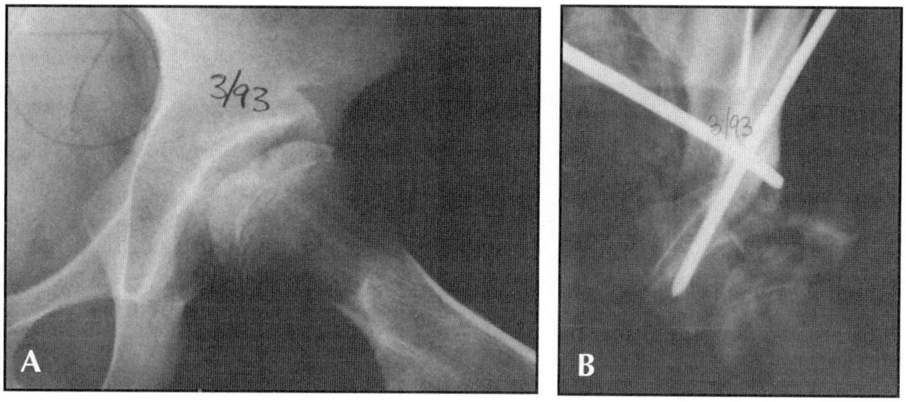

Fig. 3 A, Severe dysplasia of the hip in an adolescent. The femoral head is slightly flattened and enlarged but is relatively well concentric with the acetabulum. **B,** A Tonnis osteotomy has redirected the acetabulum approximately 40° providing excellent coverage and a much improved weight-bearing surface. This radiograph illustrates the extreme redirection that can be achieved when the osteotomies are close to the acetabulum.

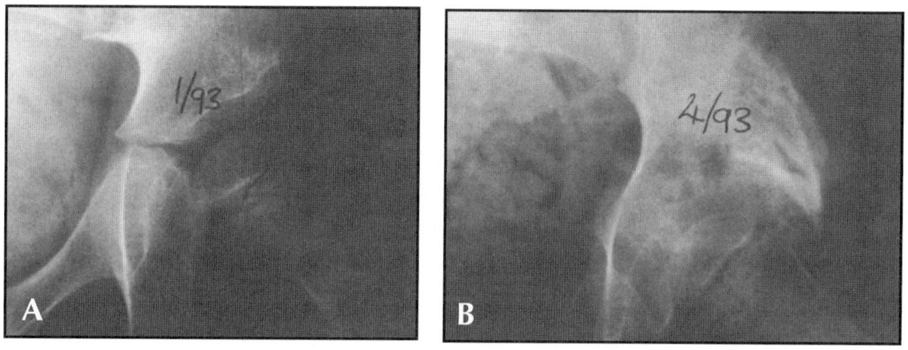

Fig. 4 A, Moderate dysplasia in an adolescent with cerebral palsy. The femoral head was egg-shaped and the acetabulum quite shallow. **B,** A large shelf was constructed using Staheli's technique and 3 months later a radiograph showed excellent coverage and stability.

osteotomy but can accomplish the same degree of redirection.

Wagner[10] and Eppright[11] described dial osteotomies that involved spherical and cylindrical cuts around the acetabulum, respectively. They are, however, of mainly historic interest. The Wagner osteotomy requires spherical osteotomes that are not readily available. It involves making a blind cut around the acetabulum passing in the floor of the acetabulum without invading either the inner table of the pelvis or the acetabulum. This is a very small target and it is impossible to make the cut consistently in just the right location.

Reshaping Osteotomies

Osteotomies in this group change the shape of the acetabulum and therefore share the obvious prerequisite that the shape of the acetabulum is not spherical or congruent to begin with. All three procedures in this group fold down the superior surface of the acetabulum and are intended to be used in patients whose femoral heads are fairly spherical but are articulating in an acetabulum that is much larger and has an upward sloping lip.

The Pemberton osteotomy[12] involves a periacetabular cut to the triradiate cartilage and a hinging down of the acetabular roof at the triradiate cartilage. In the Albee and Dega osteotomies the cut does not go as far.[13] Because they produce an acetabulum with a fold in its superomedial surface they are best reserved for patients with significant remodeling potential who can convert this shape to a spherical one. Because of this, the osteotomies in this group are not generally applicable to dysplastic hips in adolescent patients.

Augmentation Osteotomies

These procedures enlarge the articular surface of the acetabulum by adding bone superiorly and laterally and by depending on the capsule to act as weight-bearing articular tissue. The Chiari osteotomy[14] adds bone by shifting the cut surface of the osteotomy over the hip, and the shelf procedures do so by constructing a bony prominence over the capsule from pelvic bone graft.

The Chiari procedure[14] has the advantage that it provides immediate stability and a weight-bearing surface that can begin to bear weight immediately. It has the disadvantage that it is impossible to give the weight-bearing surface a spherical shape to match the head. Also the extent of additional weight-bearing surface is limited by the thickness of the pelvis at the level of the osteotomy, and, in dysplastic hips that have drifted somewhat superiorly, the pelvis can be quite thin (Fig. 4).

The shelf procedure[15] has the advantage that the added weight-bearing surface can be made as large or as small as necessary, and can be shaped to conform to the spherical shape of the femoral head in both the sagittal and coronal planes. It produces bony stability only after the bone graft has had time to heal, and therefore can be used only with femoral heads that are stable in the desired location or that can be made so by positioning the leg intraoperatively and postoperatively (Fig. 5).

Decision Parameters

The selection of an osteotomy will depend on the assessment of the patient and the

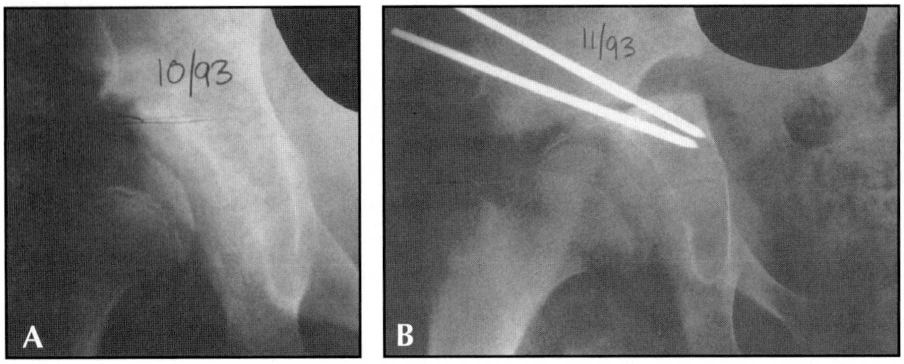

Fig. 5 A, Severe dysplasia in an adolescent. The acetabulum is very shallow with a blunt lateral rim, and the joint is not congruent. The femoral head wandered into the acetabulum with movement. **B,** A Chiari osteotomy provided good coverage and an immediately stable weight-bearing surface.

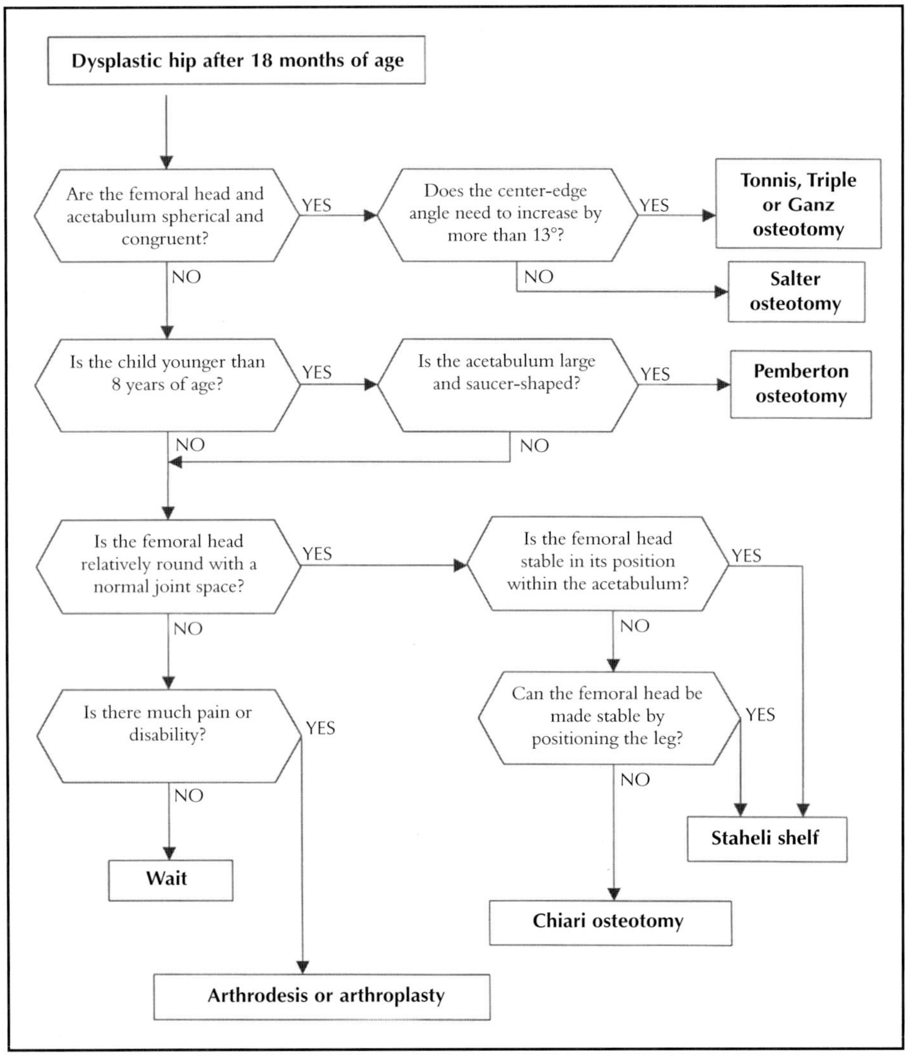

Fig. 6 Decision-making algorithm for dysplasia.

current state of the hip. Certain specific factors require assessment so that they can be used in the selection algorithm. These factors have been alluded to above and include the sphericity of the femoral head and acetabulum, the age of the patient, the diameter and capacity of the acetabulum, the area of the weight-bearing surface, and the existing coverage.

An algorithm can be devised that simulates the thought process of the pediatric orthopaedic surgeon who is selecting a pelvic osteotomy to treat an adolescent patient with developmental dysplasia of the hip. It uses the above parameters to travel down a decision tree leading to the most appropriate procedure. Such an algorithm is shown in Figure 6. The algorithm is not foolproof, and there are many times when other considerations are important. Indeed, the sequence in which the factors are taken into account is somewhat arbitrary. It does, however, bring together the concepts discussed above and may be illustrative to the pediatric orthopaedic surgeon who has not developed a working approach to this problem.

Conclusion

The treatment of the dislocated hip after walking age, and the management of dysplasia in the older child are challenging problems that demand that the surgeon master not only a variety of surgical techniques, but also the means of arriving at the correct treatment strategy. These situations are not forgiving of poor results, and the first operation, chosen correctly and performed well, offers the best chance for success.

References

1. Dunn PM: The anatony and pathology of congenital dislocation of the hip. *Clin Orthop* 1976:23-27.
2. Salter RB: Role of innominate osteotomy in the treatment of congenital dislocation and subluxation of the hip in the older child. *J Bone Joint Surg Am* 1966;48:1413-1439.

3. Salter RB, Best T: Abstract: Pathogenesis and prevention of valgus deformity following fractures of the proximal metaphysial region of the tibia in children. *J Bone Joint Surg Br* 1972;54:767.

4. Sutherland DH, Moore M: Clinical and radiographic outcome of patients treated with double innominate osteotomy for congenital hip dysplasia. *J Pediatr Orthop* 1991; 11: 143-148.

5. Rab GT: Biomechanical aspects of Salter osteotomy. *Clin Orthop* 1978;132:82-87.

6. Steel HH: Triple osteotomy of the innominate bone. *J Bone Joint Surg Am* 1973;55:343-350.

7. Tonnis D, Behrens K, Tscharani F: A modified technique of the triple pelvic osteotomy: Early results. *J Pediatr Orthop 1981*;1:241-249.

8. Carlioz H, Khouri N, Hulin P: Triple juxtacotyloid osteotomy [French]. *Rev Chir Orthop Reparatrice Appar Mot* 1982;68:497-501.

9. Ganz R, Klaue K, Vinh TS, Mast JW: A new periacetabular osteotomy for the treatment of hip dysplasias: Technique and preliminary results. *Clin Orthop* 1988;232:26-36.

10. Wagner H: Osteotomies for congenital hip dislocation, in Evarts CM (ed): *The Hip: Proceedings of the Fourth Open Scientific Meeting of the Hip Society, 1976*. St Louis, MO, CV Mosby, 1976, pp 45-66.

11. Eppright RH: Abstract: Dial osteotomy of the acetabulum in the treatment of dysplasia of the hip. *J Bone Joint Surg Am* 1976;58:726.

12. Pemberton PA: Pericapsular osteotomy of the ilium for treatment of congenital subluxation and dislocation of the hip. *J Bone Joint Surg Am* 1965;47:65-86.

13. Albee, FH: The bone graft wedge: Its use in the treatment of relapsing, acquired, and congenital dislocation of the hip. *NY Med J* 1915;102:433.

14. Chiari K: Medial displacement osteotomy of the pelvis. *Clin Orthop* 1974;98:55-71.

15. Staheli LT, Chew DE: Slotted acetabular augmentation in childhood and adolescence. *J Pediatr Orthop* 1992;12:569-580.

58

Slipped Capital Femoral Epiphysis

Randall T. Loder, MD
David D. Aronsson, MD
Matthew B. Dobbs, MD
Stuart L. Weinstein, MD

Slipped capital femoral epiphysis (SCFE) is a well-known disorder of the hip in adolescents that is characterized by displacement of the capital femoral epiphysis from the metaphysis through the physis. The term SCFE is a misnomer because the epiphysis is held in the acetabulum by the ligamentum teres, and thus it is actually the metaphysis that moves upward and outward while the epiphysis remains in the acetabulum. In most patients, there is an apparent varus relationship between the head and the neck, but occasionally the slip is into a valgus position, with the epiphysis displaced superiorly in relation to the neck.[1,2] In the vast majority of cases, the etiology is unknown. Although the condition may be associated with a known endocrine disorder,[3-5] with renal failure osteodystrophy,[6] or with previous radiation therapy,[4,7] this chapter deals only with idiopathic SCFE.

Etiology

Multiple theories have been proposed for the etiology of idiopathic SCFE, and it is likely a result of both biomechanical and biochemical factors.[8] The combination of these factors results in a weakened physis with subsequent failure.

Mechanical factors[9] associated with the disorder are obesity,[10,11] increased femoral retroversion,[9,12,13] and increased physeal obliquity.[14] The vast majority of children with an SCFE are obese, which increases the shear stress across the physis. Obesity is also associated with femoral retroversion, with anteversion averaging 10.6° in adolescents with normal weight but only 0.40° in obese adolescents.[12] This femoral retroversion increases the stress across the physis.[9] Children with an SCFE also have a more vertical proximal femoral physis (an increase of 8° to 11° compared with that in children without the disorder) even in the contralateral, normal hip. The combination of mechanical forces resulting from femoral retroversion and increased physeal slope is enough to cause an SCFE.[9] The mean shear load to failure of the proximal femoral physis in adolescents of normal weight is 4.0 times body weight; the mean shear load to failure in adolescents who are running, who are obese, or who have neutral version (or 10° of relative retroversion) is 5.1 times body weight. Finally, recent data[15] have shown that children with the disorder have deeper acetabula (a mean center-edge angle of Wiberg[16] of 37° compared with a mean of 33° in control subjects). Greater coverage of the femoral head yields more shear stress across the physis.

Biochemical factors are also likely involved. SCFE is a disease of puberty,[17] when many hormonal changes occur;[18] this raises the possibility of an association between the disorder and endocrine function. The increased prevalence of SCFE in children who have hypothyroidism, who are receiving growth hormone supplementation, or who have hypogonadism also suggests an association between the disorder and endocrine dysfunction. Rapid longitudinal growth occurs during puberty in response to growth hormone. This is due to the increased physiologic activity of the physis and is associated with widening of the physis. Decreased physeal strength occurs at puberty;[18] the cause is not clear, but it may be because of the increased cartilage width of the hypertrophic zones and to provisional calcification.[19]

The effects of the gonadotropins on the physis may explain the male predominance of SCFE; estrogen reduces physeal width and increases physeal strength,[20] whereas testosterone reduces physeal strength.[18] This probably also accounts for the fact that the disorder is extremely rare in girls after menarche.[21] Although most children with an SCFE do not have a demonstrable endocrine disorder,[22-26] a subtle but as yet undiagnosable endocrinopathy may be present. In some children, there is a delay in bone age compared with chronological age,[18-21] which further supports this concept.

SCFE does not appear to be a heritable disorder. Rennie[27] discovered that the risk of an SCFE in a second family member was 7.1% and that 14.5% of patients with an SCFE had a close relative who also had the disorder. A few families with the disorder may have an autosomal dominant inheritance with incomplete penetrance.[27] The findings of HLA-typing in children with an SCFE have varied.[28,29]

Routine histologic evaluation and electron microscopy studies of SCFE demonstrate a deficiency and abnormality in the supporting collagenous and proteoglycan framework of the physis. Both the hypertrophic and the proliferative zones are abnormal. Whether these abnormalities represent the cause or the effect of the SCFE is not known. Chondrocyte clustering and disarray occur in a thickened hypertrophic zone,[30,31] and ultrastructural studies have demonstrated defective collagen fibrils and defects in collagen banding in this zone.[32] The proliferative zone demonstrates changes in proteoglycan and glycoprotein concentrations, with increased glycoprotein staining in the territorial matrix and increased proteoglycan staining in the extraterritorial matrix.

Epidemiology and Demographics

The prevalence of SCFE is not completely known. The prevalence has been reported as 0.2 per 100,000 in eastern Japan,[33] as 2.13 per 100,000 in the southwestern United States, and as high as 10.08 per 100,000 in the northeastern United States.[34] Most series have demonstrated a male predominance. Early in the 20th century, 90% of the children with the disorder were boys, but more recently male predominance has decreased to 60%.[35] The mean duration of symptoms before the diagnosis of chronic SCFE is 5 months, with no difference noted with respect to gender. The mean age at diagnosis is 13.5 years for boys and 12.0 years for girls, with a typical age range of 9 to 16 years.[11] The majority of the children are obese; at least 50% of the children with the disorder are over the 95th percentile for weight according to age.[10,11] The age at onset decreases with increasing obesity.[11] The mean age at onset for children over the 95th percentile for weight according to age is 12.4 years; the mean age for children under the 10th percentile for weight according to age is 14.3 years. Although the chronologic age at the onset of SCFE varies, the physiologic age range appears to be smaller, with a "narrow window" of time during which it can occur.[36] In latitudes north of 40°, the onset of SCFE occurs more frequently in the summer and autumn months.[18,37-40]

The reported prevalence of bilaterality varies and depends on the study, the method of radiographic measurement, race, and possibly the type of treatment. In most series, a prevalence of 18% to 50% has been reported;[11] however, recent studies with follow-up into adulthood have demonstrated a prevalence of bilaterality as high as 63%.[39,41,42] The percentage of bilaterality has been found to be higher in black children (34%) than in Hispanic children (17%), white children (17%), and Asian children (18%), according to a study of 1,630 children.[11] Treatment may affect the prevalence of bilaterality. In one study,[43] the prevalence was 36% in 169 patients treated with in situ pinning and 7% in 30 treated with a spica cast. Therefore, it is mandatory that close attention be paid to the contralateral, normal hip in children who have a unilateral SCFE treated with in situ pinning.

Between 50% and 60% of patients with bilateral involvement have it when they are first seen.[11] Eighty-two percent of second cases of SCFE that develop in patients who initially presented with unilateral involvement are seen within 18 months after the first presentation.[11,21,39,44-46] In addition, children who are seen first with unilateral involvement and in whom bilateral SCFE later develops have a younger age at presentation than do children in whom the disorder does not develop bilaterally.[11,44,45,47,48] This difference is seen in both the chronologic age (12 compared with 13 years) and the pelvic bone age. Of those with unilateral involvement, 60% have an SCFE in the left hip.[11]

The predilection for SCFE varies by race. The relative racial frequency of SCFE is 1.0 for whites, 4.5 for Pacific Islanders, 2.2 for blacks, 1.05 for Amerindian peoples (Native Americans and Hispanics), 0.5 for Indonesian-Malay peoples (Chinese, Japanese, Thai, Vietnamese, and so on), and 0.1 for Indo-Mediterranean peoples (those of Near East, North African, or Indian subcontinent ancestry).[11] There are at least two possible explanations for these racial differences. One is that they reflect the mean body weight for each racial group, which further supports the theory that obesity is a major factor in the cause of the disorder.[11] The second explanation is that there is a racial variability in acetabular depth and femoral head coverage; the acetabula in adolescent black children are deeper than those in white children.[15]

Classification

SCFE is classified according to both the clinical nature and the magnitude of the disorder. The traditional clinical categories are preslip, acute, chronic, and acute-on-chronic.[49-53] Classification into these four categories depends on the patient's history, physical examination, and radiographs.

In the preslip stage, patients usually complain of weakness in the leg, limping, or pain in the groin or the knee on exertion. Prolonged standing or walking may produce these symptoms. On physical examination, the most consistent positive finding is lack of internal rotation. On radiographs, there may be generalized osteopenia of the hemipelvis and the proximal part of the femur in patients who limp or who have limited their activity. There may be widening and irregularity of the physis.[54]

An acute SCFE is an abrupt displacement through the proximal physis in which there was a preexisting epiphysiolysis.[52] Ten percent to 15% of

SCFEs have been acute in most large series.[45,51] The clinical criteria for an acute SCFE include a duration of symptoms of less than 3 weeks and demonstration of an external rotation deformity, shortening, and marked limitation of motion secondary to pain on physical examination. In general, the greater the amount of slip, the more the motion is restricted. However, 67% of patients with an acute SCFE have a 1- to 3-month history of mild prodromal symptoms before the acute episode, indicating that there was a preslip or a mild SCFE prior to the acute episode.[1,49,51,52,55] The traumatic episode may be as trivial as turning over in bed. The pain is usually severe enough to prevent weight bearing.

Chronic SCFEs are by far the most common and account for 85% of all slips.[45] Patients with a chronic SCFE have pain in the groin, thigh, and knee that varies in duration, often ranging from months to years. They may have a history of exacerbations and remissions of the pain and limp. Physical examination demonstrates an antalgic gait, with loss of internal rotation, abduction, and flexion of the hip.[56] In more severe cases, patients have a limb-length discrepancy and a natural positioning of the lower extremity in external rotation. As the hip is flexed, the lower extremity spontaneously moves into a position of increased external rotation. Importantly, 46% of the patients have pain in the knee or the distal part of the thigh as the initial symptom, emphasizing the importance of a hip examination in a child who complains of knee pain.[57,58]

An acute-on-chronic SCFE is one associated with chronic symptoms initially and with subsequent development of acute symptoms as well as a sudden increase in the degree of slip.

The traditional classification depends on the memory of the child or parent, or both, and may be inaccurate; it also does not give a prognosis with regard to the potential for osteonecrosis. Two newer and more clinically useful classifications, one clinical and one radiographic, depend on physeal stability. The clinical classification depends on the ability of the child to walk.[59] The SCFE is considered stable when the child is able to walk with or without crutches, and it is considered unstable when the child cannot walk with or without crutches. The radiographic classification depends on the presence or absence of a hip effusion on ultrasonography.[60,61] If the ultrasound demonstrates the absence of metaphyseal remodeling and the presence of an effusion, an acute event is likely to have occurred and the SCFE is considered unstable. If the ultrasound demonstrates metaphyseal remodeling and the absence of an effusion, an acute event has not occurred and the SCFE is considered stable.

This classification is important because it is predictive of the prognosis. The traditional classification of slips as acute or chronic is misleading because it does not consider the stability of the hip, which is highly predictive of the development of osteonecrosis. Unstable SCFEs have a much higher prevalence of osteonecrosis (up to 50% in some series) compared with stable SCFEs (nearly 0%).[59] The high rates of complications with unstable slips are most likely secondary to vascular injury caused at the time of the initial displacement.[59,62] The development of osteonecrosis is associated with the findings on bone scans made before treatment. A cold bone scan (demonstrating an absence of vascularity) essentially is seen only in unstable cases. When a patient has such a bone scan, the risk of subsequent development of osteonecrosis is 80% to 100%.[63] The symptoms of a child with an unstable SCFE mimic those of a child with a hip fracture, and indeed the SCFE may be considered a type of Salter-Harris type I fracture.[64] The child has severe pain and resists any passive or active attempt to move the lower extremity. The extremity is held in a flexed and externally rotated position.

Radiographs demonstrate an inferior and posterior slip of the proximal femoral epiphysis relative to the metaphysis. In a gradual slip, there are radiographic signs of superior and anterior remodeling on the femoral metaphysis and of periosteal new bone formation at the epiphyseal-metaphyseal junction posteriorly and inferiorly. In an early slip, the changes can be subtle, and both AP and lateral radiographs must be made. The epiphysis typically slips posteriorly[56] and as such is often seen only on a lateral radiograph in the earlier stages. Other helpful radiographic signs are the metaphyseal blanch sign of Steel[65] and Klein's line[66] (Fig. 1). The metaphyseal blanch sign of Steel is a double density seen at the level of the metaphysis on an AP radiograph; the double density reflects the posterior cortical lip of the epiphysis as it is beginning to slip posteriorly and is radiographically superimposed on the metaphyseal density. Klein's line is drawn on a radiograph along the anterior or superior aspect of the femoral neck; the epiphysis should normally intersect this line. In an early SCFE, the epiphysis is flush with or even below this line.

Other imaging methods may be needed in the evaluation of a child with an SCFE. A bone scan[63] and an MRI scan allow earlier diagnosis of osteonecrosis and chondrolysis. Advances in ultrasonography have allowed visualization of an effusion in the hip (a sign of an unstable SCFE) and remodeling of the femoral neck (a sign of a stable SCFE). CT scanning provides three-dimensional imaging of an SCFE, creating an awareness that the epiphysis remains in the acetabulum while the femoral neck displaces anteriorly. This process results in a retroversion deformity of the proximal part of the femur.

The severity of an SCFE is commonly assessed by two different methods. The first is evaluation of the amount of displacement of the epiphysis on the

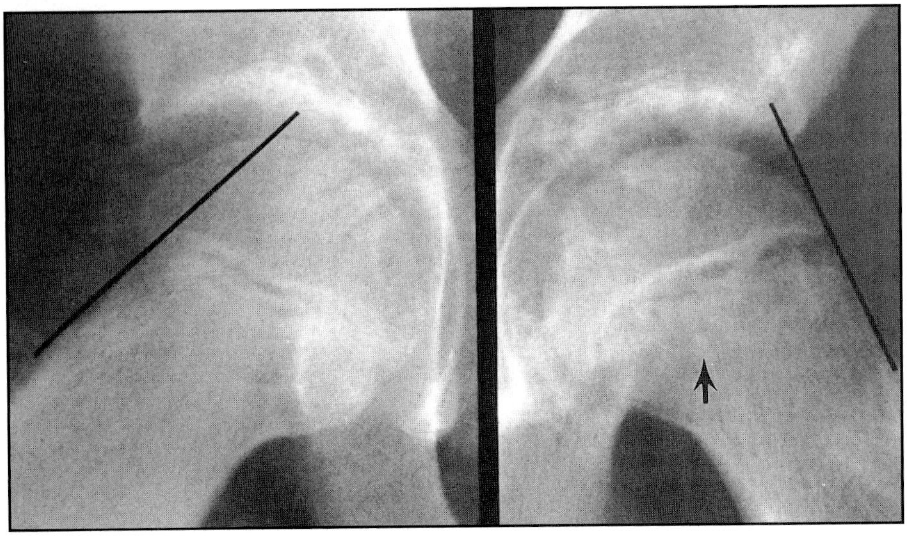

Fig. 1 AP radiographs showing the metaphyseal blanch sign and Klein's line. The metaphyseal blanch sign is a radiographic double density seen at the level of the metaphysis (*arrow*); this double density reflects the posterior cortical lip of the epiphysis as it is beginning to slip posteriorly and is radiographically superimposed on the metaphyseal density. Klein's line is drawn along the anterior or superior aspect of the femoral neck; the epiphysis should normally intersect this line (*left*). In an early SCFE, the epiphysis is flush with or even below this line (*right*).

metaphysis. The disorder is considered mild when the epiphyseal-metaphyseal displacement is less than one third of the width of the femoral neck, moderate when the displacement is one third to one half of the width of the femoral neck, and severe when the displacement is greater than one half of the width of the femoral neck.[58] However, because of the remodeling associated with a gradual slip,[67] this method is less accurate than the angular measurement method, which typically involves measurement of the epiphyseal shaft angle on the frog-leg lateral radiograph as described by Southwick.[68] The angle of slip can also be categorized into groups. Slip angles of less than 30° are considered mild; those of 30° to 50°, moderate; and those of more than 50°, severe.[51] This classification is probably most important with regard to long-term prognosis. Mild and moderate slips have an excellent long-term prognosis with regard to the Iowa hip score when treated with in situ pinning, whereas severe slips are associated with a more rapid decline in Iowa hip scores over time.[57,69]

Treatment

The most important priority in the management of a patient with an SCFE is primum non nocere (first, do no harm).[70] Most investigators agree that once an SCFE has been diagnosed, treatment is indicated to prevent progression of the slip. The goal of treatment is to prevent additional slippage while avoiding the complications of osteonecrosis and chondrolysis. Chondrolysis is defined as narrowing of the joint space to at least one half of that in the contralateral hip in unilateral cases and as narrowing of the joint space to less than 3 mm in bilateral cases.[58,71,72] There are several treatment methods, and each has its own advantages and disadvantages.

The treatment of a patient with an SCFE has changed because of improved imaging techniques. Twenty-five years ago, radiographs were the only imaging technique used to evaluate a patient with the disorder. Patients were often treated with in situ fixation with multiple pins, and intraoperative spot radiographs were used to control pin placement. Pin placement was not always ideal with this technique, and malpositioned pins were associated with complications, including additional slippage, chondrolysis, and osteonecrosis in 20% to 40% of patients.[70,73] The high rate of complications associated with in situ fixation with multiple pins led others to try treatment with a hip spica cast, open epiphysiodesis, or femoral osteotomy. The development of intraoperative fluoroscopy to assist in the placement of internal fixation devices has markedly lowered the complication rate associated with internal fixation.

Stable Slipped Capital Femoral Epiphysis

The current treatment methods for a patient with a stable (chronic) SCFE include (1) immobilization in a hip spica cast,[74] (2) in situ stabilization with single or multiple pins or screws,[50,53,70,75] (3) open epiphysiodesis with iliac crest[76,77] or allogeneic[78] bone graft, (4) open reduction with a corrective osteotomy through the physis and internal fixation with use of multiple pins,[79,80] (5) compensating base-of-neck osteotomy with in situ stabilization of the SCFE with use of multiple-pin fixation,[81,82] and (6) intertrochanteric osteotomy with internal fixation.[68] The advantages and disadvantages of each method are discussed below.

Hip Spica Cast Immobilization in a bilateral hip spica cast avoids the complications associated with a surgical procedure. The prevalence of bilateral SCFE is approximately 20% to 40%,[11,39,41,42] and a hip spica cast also provides prophylactic treatment of the contralateral hip. Hurley and associates[43] compared the results of in situ pinning in 169 patients with those of immobilization in a hip spica cast in 30 patients. After a mean follow-up of 2.8 years, SCFE had developed in

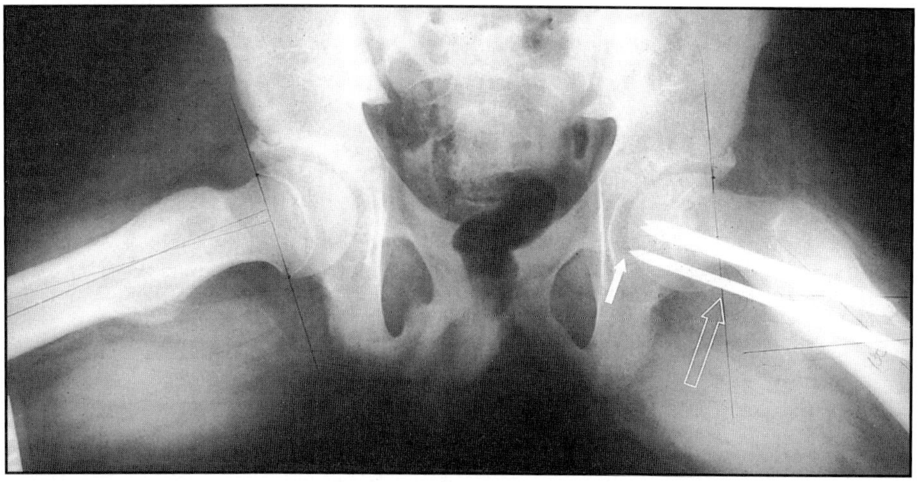

Fig. 2 Radiograph showing a pin (*open arrow*) exiting the posterior part of the femoral neck and entering the posterior aspect of the epiphysis. The pin also penetrates the femoral head and protrudes into the hip joint (*solid arrow*).

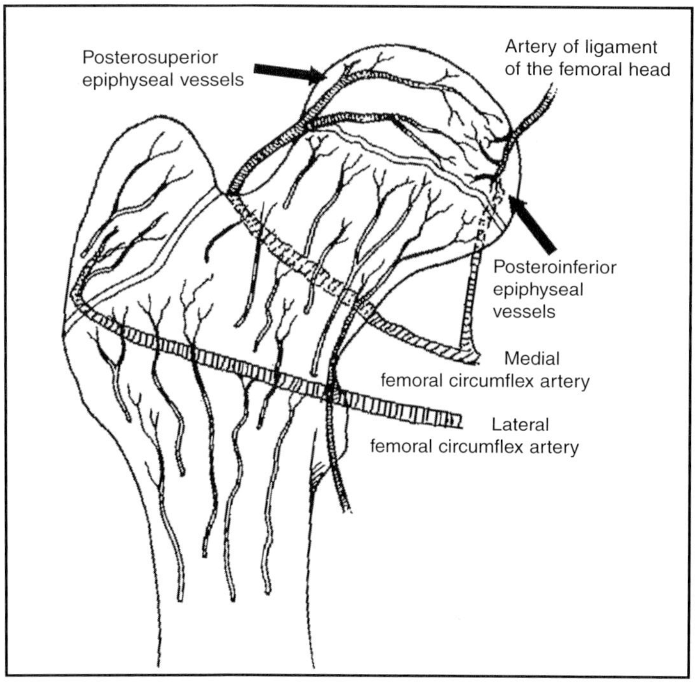

Fig. 3 Drawing showing the blood supply to the femoral head. The most important contribution to this blood supply is from the posterosuperior epiphyseal vessels that originate from the medial femoral circumflex artery.

the contralateral hip of 61 patients (36%) treated with in situ pinning. After a mean follow-up of 3.6 years, SCFE had developed in the contralateral hip of two patients (7%) treated with a hip spica cast. Betz and associates[74] evaluated 32 patients (37 hips) treated with a hip spica cast. A reduction was not attempted, and the cast was worn until the metaphyseal lucency adjacent to the physis was no longer visible on radiographs. The duration of immobilization in the cast averaged 12 weeks. Osteonecrosis did not develop in any hip, but the slip progressed in two hips (5%) and chondrolysis developed in seven (19%). Meier and associates[83] evaluated 13 patients (17 hips) who were treated with a hip spica cast for a mean of 12 weeks. The slip progressed in three hips, chondrolysis developed in nine, and full-thickness cast pressure sores developed in two. In total, complications occurred in 14 of the 17 hips, which led those authors to abandon the hip spica cast as a treatment for SCFE. In addition to the high rate of complications, the hip spica cast is awkward and cumbersome for the family, particularly if the patient is obese. The hip spica cast does not stabilize the SCFE, and most investigators have reported progression of the slip in 5% to 10% of patients, despite immobilization in the cast.[74,83] For all of these reasons, a hip spica cast for treatment of SCFE is not recommended.

In Situ Stabilization With Use of Single or Multiple Pins or Screws Since O'Brien and Fahey[84] reported on the remodeling potential of the proximal part of the femur in patients with an SCFE, in situ fixation with multiple pins has been the most popular treatment method. Long-term follow-up studies of in situ fixation have shown that postoperative remodeling occurs and that the loss of internal rotation of the hip in most patients is not clinically relevant.[85,86] In the past, the three-dimensional anatomy of SCFE was not well understood and reliable intraoperative imaging techniques were not available. As a result, insertion of the pins often was started on the lateral aspect of the femoral shaft, a technique similar to that used in treating a hip fracture in an adult. Because the proximal part of the femur is retroverted in a patient with an SCFE, the pins were often placed in the anterosuperior aspect of the epiphysis, achieving suboptimal fixation. To improve fixation, clinicians angled the pins more posteriorly. The pins often exited the posterior aspect of the femoral neck and entered the epiphysis in the posterosuperior quadrant, which jeopardized the blood supply to the femoral head (Fig. 2).

The most important contribution to the blood supply to the femoral head is from the lateral epiphyseal vessels.[87]

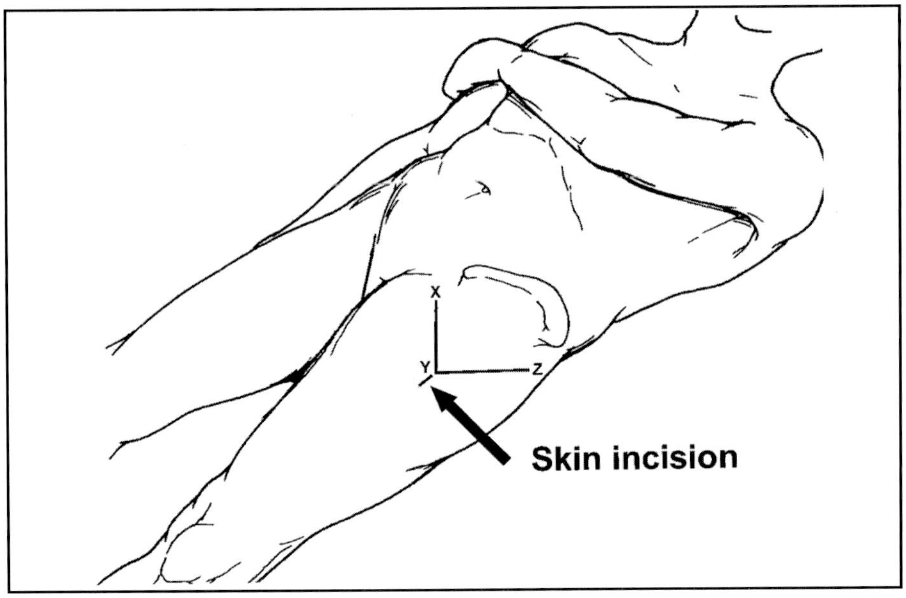

Fig. 4 Drawing showing the technique used for positioning the skin incision. The line X-Y represents a line overlying the center of the femoral head and perpendicular to the physis on the AP fluoroscopic image. The line Y-Z represents a line overlying the center of the femoral head and perpendicular to the physis on the lateral fluoroscopic image. The skin incision is made at the intersection of these lines.

Brodetti[88] demonstrated that the lateral epiphyseal vessels enter the femoral head in the posterosuperior quadrant and anastomose with the vessels from the round ligament at the junction of the medial and central thirds of the femoral head (Fig. 3). The ideal position for a screw, therefore, is in the central area or neutral zone of the femoral head. If a pin is placed in the posterosuperior quadrant, the risk of damage to the epiphyseal blood supply is increased. This risk is minimized by placement of a single screw in the center of the epiphysis, perpendicular to the physis.[50] A comparison of single-screw fixation and double-screw fixation in a calf model demonstrated only a slight increase in stiffness with two screws, which does not justify the increased risk of complications associated with the use of two screws.[89]

Another reason to use as few pins or screws as possible is that, even with the use of AP and true lateral radiographs, there is an area (the "blind spot") that cannot be seen.[73] This blind spot is often the site of unrecognized pin protrusion. Pin protrusion can be associated with the development of chondrolysis and subchondral bone changes. With multiple pins, the possibility that one or more will protrude into the joint is increased; this risk is lowered when a single screw is used.[53,90,91] The advantages of single-screw fixation in a patient with a stable SCFE include a high rate of success and a low prevalence of additional slippage and of complications.[50,92,93] It is presently the most common treatment for SCFE in North America.

Surgical Technique The technique for percutaneous insertion of a single screw has been described.[50,91] The patient is positioned on a fracture table or radiolucent table in the supine position to allow simultaneous biplane AP and lateral fluoroscopic imaging. It is important to emphasize that the technique is image-dependent, so excellent observation of the femoral head and neck is required before the procedure is begun. Because the procedure is performed percutaneously through a small skin incision with use of a cannulated screw, it is important to locate the proper starting position for the guide pin. To determine the starting point, a guide pin is placed on the skin overlying the proximal part of the femur and, under AP fluoroscopic guidance, the pin is positioned such that it projects over the center of the femoral neck and head, crossing the physis in a perpendicular fashion. Once this pin position has been obtained, a marking pen is used to draw a line on the skin reflecting the pin position on the AP image. The same procedure is used for the lateral fluoroscopic image, and a 1-cm skin incision is made at the intersection of the two lines (Fig. 4). The guide pin is advanced freehand through the soft tissues to engage the anterolateral femoral cortex. The position and angulation of the guide pin are adjusted, with fluoroscopic guidance, to obtain the proper alignment before the guide pin is drilled into the bone. It is ideal to advance the guide pin into the center of the femoral head, perpendicular to the physis, as seen on both the AP and the lateral fluoroscopic images on the first attempt, since multiple drill-holes can weaken the bone, causing a fracture through an unused hole.[94] After the appropriate screw length has been determined, a 7.3-mm stainless-steel cannulated screw is placed over the guide pin and is advanced until five threads engage the epiphysis (Fig. 5). The screw should not be left protruding beyond the lateral aspect of the femoral shaft, where it can be toggled by the soft tissues, leading to screw loosening.[95] After surgery, the patient begins partial weight bearing with use of crutches and gradually advances to full weight bearing as tolerated. Most patients can walk without crutches within 2 to 4 days.

The results of single-screw fixation in patients with SCFE have been gratifying. Aronson and Carlson[50] reported excellent or good results in 36 (95%) of

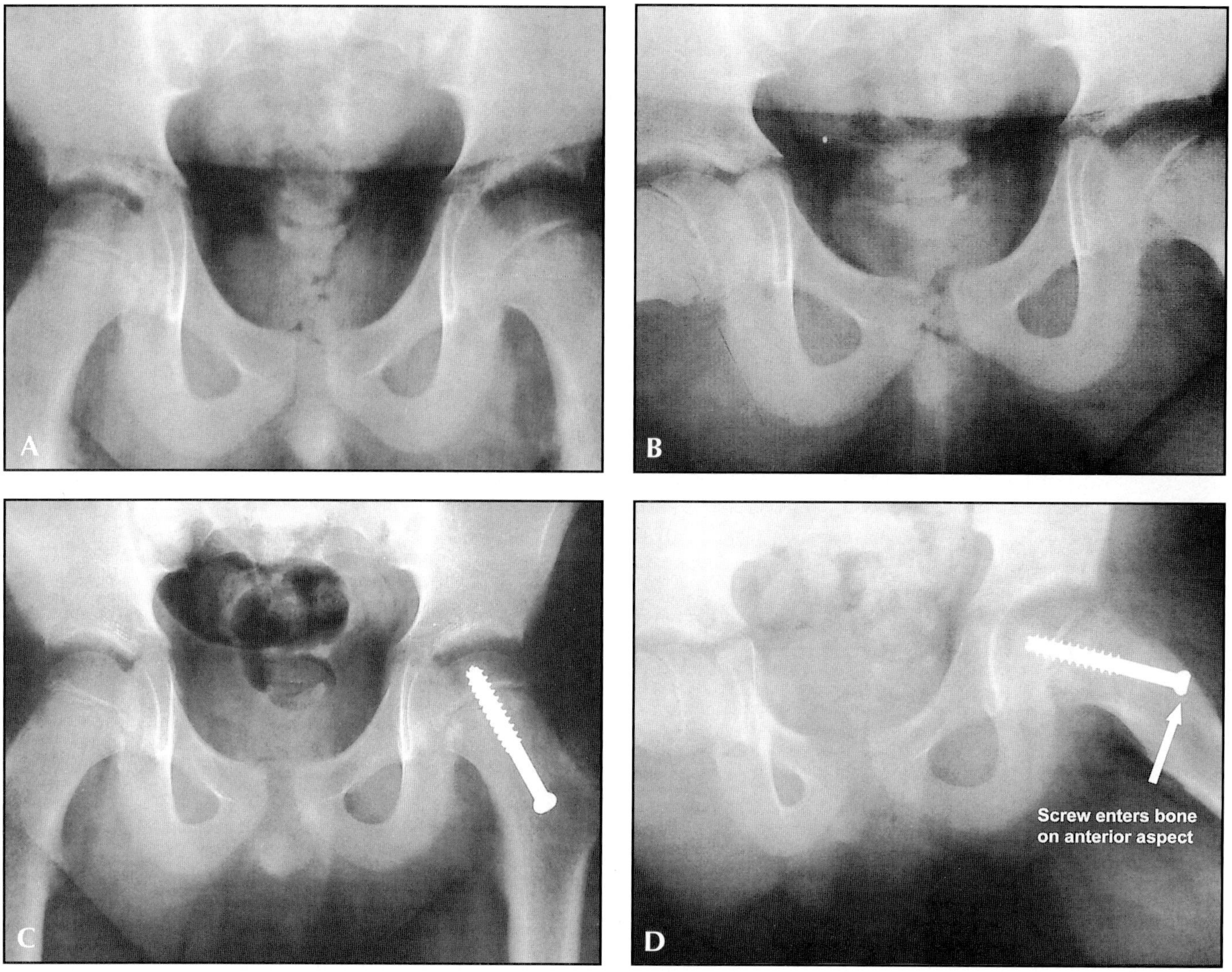

Fig. 5 A 10-year-old boy with a stable (chronic) mild SCFE involving the left hip. **A,** Preoperative AP pelvic radiograph. **B,** Preoperative frog-leg lateral pelvic radiograph. **C,** Postoperative AP radiograph. **D,** Pelvic radiograph showing placement of the screw perpendicular to the physis.

38 mild slips, 10 of 11 moderate slips, and 8 of 9 severe slips. Osteonecrosis developed in only one patient (2%), with an unstable SCFE, and chondrolysis developed in none. Ward and associates[53] reported on 42 patients (53 hips) with an SCFE treated with single-screw fixation. After a mean follow-up of 32 months, 92% of the patients demonstrated physeal fusion and were able to participate in full activities. Neither chondrolysis nor osteonecrosis developed in any patient. Samuelson and Olney,[96] using a similar percutaneous technique, reported excellent results in seven patients treated with two Knowles pins and in 17 patients treated with a single Knowles pin.

Open Epiphysiodesis With Iliac Crest or Allogeneic Bone Graft Open epiphysiodesis with iliac crest bone graft to stabilize the SCFE was first reported by Ferguson and Howorth[38] in 1931. This procedure avoids the complications associated with internal fixation, including unrecognized pin protrusion, damage to the lateral epiphyseal vessels, and hardware failure. The surgical technique involves an anterior iliofemoral exposure of the hip joint. A rectangular window of bone is removed from the anterior aspect of the femoral neck. A hollow mill is used to create a cylindrical tunnel across the physis, and multiple corticocancellous strips of iliac crest bone graft are driven into the tunnel as bone pegs across the proximal femoral physis (Fig. 6). Weiner and associates[77] reported on their 30-year experience with this technique, which they used to treat 159

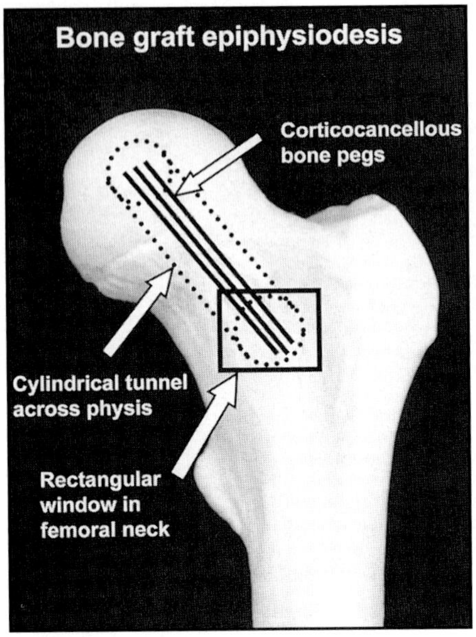

Fig. 6 Illustration showing the technique for performing an open epiphysiodesis. A rectangular window of bone is removed from the anterior aspect of the femoral neck, and a cylindrical tunnel is created across the physis. Multiple strips of corticocancellous bone from the iliac crest are then driven into the tunnel as bone pegs across the physis.

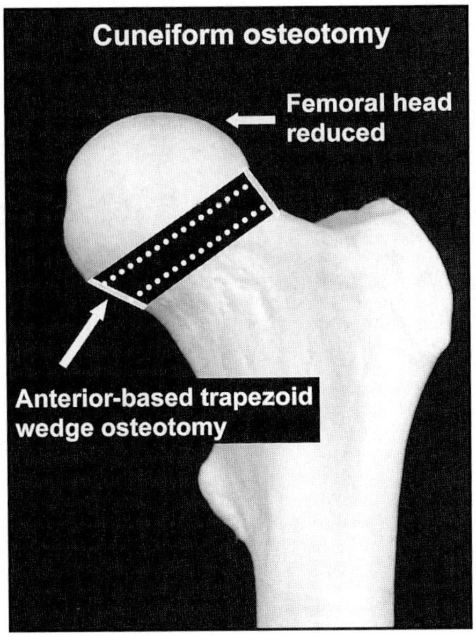

Fig. 7 Illustration showing the location of the anterior-based trapezoid wedge of bone that is removed from the metaphysis of the femoral neck during the cuneiform osteotomy. The epiphysis is then gently reduced and internally fixed with three pins.

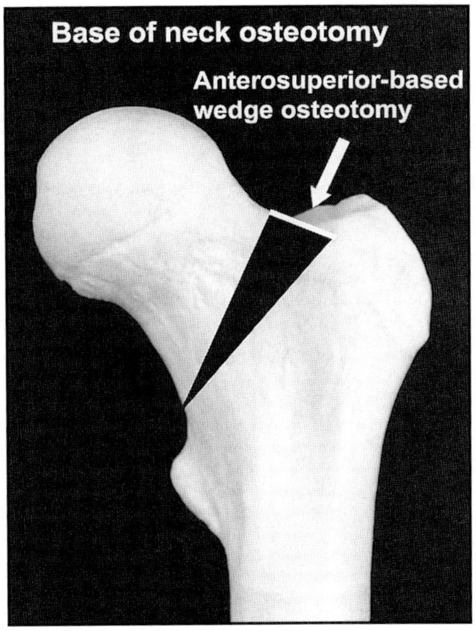

Fig. 8 Illustration showing the location of the anterosuperior-based wedge of bone that is removed during the compensating base-of-neck osteotomy. The osteotomy site is internally fixed with multiple pins.

patients (185 hips) who had an SCFE. Additional slipping developed in four hips (2%); osteonecrosis, in one (1%); and chondrolysis, in none.

An advantage of open epiphysiodesis with iliac crest bone graft is that the graft is inserted at the correct angle in the center of the femoral head, minimizing the risk of damage to the blood supply of the femoral head. The graft is not inserted as deeply as is recommended for internal fixation, so there is less risk of graft protrusion into the hip joint. However, the fixation provided by the iliac crest bone graft is not as secure as that achieved by internal fixation. Rao and associates[76] evaluated 43 patients (64 hips) treated by open bone-peg epiphysiodesis. At the time of healing, 27 hips (42%) had had additional slipping. Osteonecrosis developed in four hips (6%); chondrolysis, in three (5%); and additional complications, in 14 (22%). Other disadvantages of open bone-peg epiphysiodesis include increased blood loss, a longer duration of anesthesia, and a larger scar. As a result of these complications, Rao and associates[76] stated that they no longer recommend open bone-peg epiphysiodesis as the initial treatment for SCFE.

Schmidt and associates[78] developed a technique to percutaneously place a freeze-dried, irradiated cortical strut allograft across the physis. The technique is similar to that used for the percutaneous insertion of a single screw but, instead of a screw, a 10-mm cannulated reamer is placed over the guide pin to ream a channel to within 2 mm of the subchondral bone. A cortical strut allograft then is passed into the channel and is advanced until at least 1 cm is across the physis. Schmidt and associates[78] evaluated 31 patients (38 hips) who had a mean follow-up of 3 years and 6 months and reported that the Harris hip rating was excellent for 35 hips, good for one, and fair for two. Six patients (19%) had a major complication, including osteonecrosis, chondrolysis, femoral neck fracture, subtrochanteric hip fracture, bilateral coxa vara deformity, and unilateral coxa vara deformity in one patient each. Despite these complications, those authors still recommended this technique, particularly for a patient with a severe SCFE.

Open Reduction With Corrective Osteotomy Through the Physis and Internal Fixation With Use of Multiple Pins A cuneiform osteotomy through the physis is the ideal method with which to correct the retroversion deformity of the femoral neck, but is it safe? The surgical technique involves an anterior Smith-Petersen[79] or anterolateral[80] exposure of the hip. A wedge of bone is removed from the metaphysis of the femoral neck. This allows the epiphysis to be anatomically repositioned on the metaphysis without creating tension on the epiphyseal vasculature (Fig. 7). The osteotomy is created with use of osteotomes, rongeurs, curets, and a Kerrison punch (Codman, Raynham, MA). After the femoral neck is sufficiently shortened, the epiphysis is reduced and internally fixed with the use of three pins. Fish[97] performed the cuneiform osteotomy in 61 patients (66 hips) and reported that 55 hips (83%) had an excellent result; six (9%), a good result; two (3%), a fair result; and three (5%), a poor result. DeRosa and associates[79] evaluated 23 patients (27 hips) with a severe SCFE treated by cuneiform osteotomy. After a mean follow-up of 8 years and 5 months, no hip had an excellent result; 19 hips (70%) had a good result; four (15%), a fair result; and four, a poor result. Osteonecrosis developed in four hips (15%) and chondrolysis, in eight (30%). In addition, two patients (7%) lost fixation and required additional surgery, a skin erosion developed over one of the pins and required pin removal, and a buttock pressure sore developed in another patient. Despite the 15% rate of osteonecrosis in their study, DeRosa and associates[79] stated that they would still recommend the cuneiform osteotomy for patients with a severe SCFE.

Velasco and associates[80] evaluated 65 patients (66 hips) treated with open reduction of an SCFE. In 60 hips, the open reduction of the slip was combined with a cuneiform subcapital wedge resection of the femoral neck according to the technique described by Dunn and Angel.[98] At a mean of 16 years, chondrolysis had developed in eight hips (12%) and osteonecrosis, in seven (11%). Of the 48 hips that had been followed for a minimum of 10 years (mean, 20.6 years), 22 (46%) had a good result; 16 (33%), a moderate result; and 10 (21%), a poor result. Degenerative arthritis was seen in 19 (40%) of the 48 hips. Because of the high risk of osteonecrosis and subsequent poor results in most series, a physeal cuneiform osteotomy as the initial treatment of SCFE is not recommended.

Compensating Base-of-Neck Osteotomy With In Situ Stabilization of the SCFE With Use of Multiple-Pin Fixation Kramer and associates[82] described an anterosuperior-based wedge osteotomy of the femoral neck. They stabilized both the osteotomy site and the SCFE with multiple pins (Fig. 8). They reported on 55 patients (56 hips) who all had had a positive preoperative Trendelenburg test and had walked with a lurching gait. After the osteotomy, 48 patients (87%) had a negative Trendelenburg test. Nine hips (16%) had a poor result because of pain, a limp, or a decreased range of motion. Osteonecrosis developed in two patients (4%) and chondrolysis, in one (2%). Barmada and associates[81] described an extracapsular basilar neck osteotomy that was performed in an attempt to repair an SCFE while avoiding the risk of osteonecrosis. The prevalence of osteonecrosis associated with basilar neck osteotomy is less than that associated with cuneiform osteotomy. However, only 35° to 55° of correction is possible with this technique.[99] One benefit of the basilar neck osteotomy is improvement in hip motion. A disadvantage is that it shortens the femoral neck, which may result in impingement of the greater trochanter against the lateral aspect of the acetabulum during hip abduction. If there is premature closure of the proximal femoral physis, as is often seen in patients with an SCFE, shortening of the femoral neck may aggravate a limb-length discrepancy.

Intertrochanteric Osteotomy With Internal Fixation Southwick[68] described an intertrochanteric osteotomy through the lesser trochanter. This osteotomy improves hip motion and is not associated with osteonecrosis. The technique advocated by Crawford[100] involves an intertrochanteric osteotomy with flexion, abduction, and internal rotation of the distal fragment (Fig. 9). The osteotomy site is fixed with a compression hip screw, and the SCFE, if it is unstable, is fixed with a percutaneous cannulated screw. The intertrochanteric osteotomy is also a compensating osteotomy with correction limited to 45° on the AP radiograph and to 60° on the lateral radiograph as measured by the Southwick method.[101] An anterolateral wedge of bone is removed, so this osteotomy is also a shortening procedure. There is a risk that a limb-length discrepancy will be created if considerable correction is achieved. Schai and associates[102] evaluated 51 patients who had an SCFE of 30° to 60° that was treated with an intertrochanteric osteotomy and followed for a mean of 24 years. Moderate osteoarthritis developed in 14 patients (27%) and severe osteoarthritis, in nine (18%). Thirty-five patients (69%) had a shorter limb on the affected side, and two patients (4%) had a limb-length equalization procedure. Osteonecrosis developed in only one patient (2%). A summation of the results of these series indicates that intertrochanteric osteotomy with use of the Southwick technique is not the ideal initial treatment for an SCFE because the outcome of the procedure is relatively

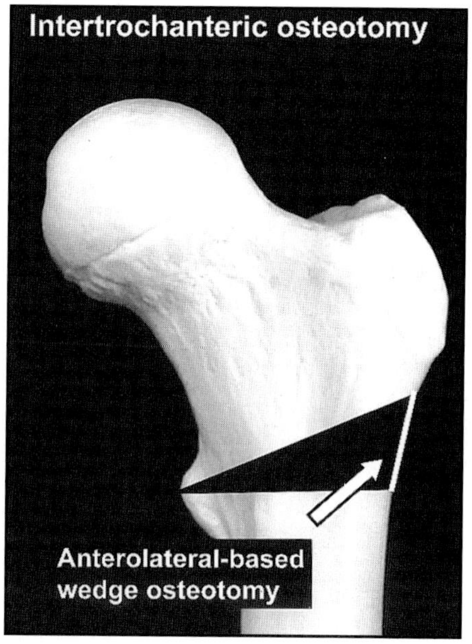

Fig. 9 Illustration showing the location of the anterolateral-based wedge of bone that is removed during the intertrochanteric osteotomy. This osteotomy includes flexion, abduction, and internal rotation of the distal fragment. The osteotomy site is internally fixed with a compression hip screw.

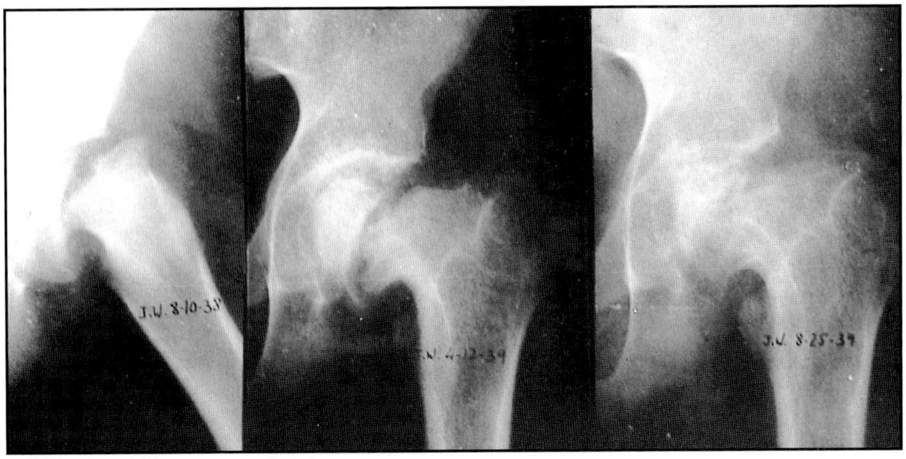

Fig. 10 Radiographs of the left hip of a 14-year-old boy who had immediate severe hip pain following acute trauma, without prior hip symptoms. The radiograph on the left was made at presentation. Those in the middle and on the right were made during a 1-year follow-up period and show the rapid development of osteonecrosis and severe degenerative changes.

poor compared with that of current techniques of in situ single-screw fixation.

Jerre and associates[103] evaluated the results of different realignment procedures in 36 patients (37 hips) after a mean follow-up of 33.8 years (range, 26 to 42 years). Serious short-term complications developed in seven (32%) of the 22 hips treated with subcapital osteotomy, 3 of the 11 hips treated with intertrochanteric osteotomy, and 3 of the 4 hips treated with manipulative reduction. Jerre and associates[103] reported that 41% of the hips treated with subcapital osteotomy, four of those treated with intertrochanteric osteotomy, and none of those treated with manipulative reduction had an excellent or good result.

Unstable Slipped Capital Femoral Epiphysis

The treatment of an unstable SCFE (acute or acute-on-chronic) is similar to that of a stable SCFE but is considerably more controversial. The role of immediate reduction compared with delayed reduction is controversial, as is the role of preoperative traction. Loder and associates[59] compared the results of treatment in 25 hips (24 patients) that had a stable SCFE with those in 30 hips (30 patients) that had an unstable SCFE. The result was satisfactory in 96% of the 25 hips that had a stable SCFE and in 47% of the 30 hips that had an unstable SCFE. Osteonecrosis developed in none of the hips in the former group and in 14 hips (47%) in the latter group. de Sanctis and associates[104] evaluated 70 patients (81 hips) who had an unstable SCFE (acute or acute-on-chronic) that was treated with a gentle closed reduction and fixation with use of one or two screws or pins. A complication developed in eight hips: three (4%) had chondrolysis, three had a wound infection, and two (2%) had osteonecrosis. de Sanctis and associates[104] concluded that a gentle reduction with percutaneous single-screw fixation is a stable, safe, and reliable method for treating patients who have an unstable SCFE.

Herman and associates[105] evaluated the cases of 21 patients (21 hips) with a severe SCFE (a displacement of more than 50%) after a mean follow-up of 2.8 years. Fifteen patients had an unstable SCFE; nine of them were treated with a gentle closed reduction and internal fixation with use of either one or two screws. Five of the nine hips had a complete reduction of the SCFE, and osteonecrosis developed in three of them. Four hips had an incomplete reduction, and none had osteonecrosis. The authors hypothesized that injury to the epiphyseal vasculature occurs at the time of the acute SCFE.

Peterson and associates[106] evaluated 91 patients (91 hips) with an unstable SCFE after a mean of 44 months. Forty-two hips had a closed reduction performed less than 24 hours after presentation, and osteonecrosis developed in three (7%). Forty-nine hips had a closed reduction performed more than 24 hours after presentation, and osteonecrosis developed in 10 (20%). The authors hypothesized that the acute displacement of the femoral head may kink the posterior blood vessels, compromising the blood flow to the epiphysis. In this situation, a timely reduction of the SCFE may restore blood flow to the epiphysis. In contrast, Loder and associates[59] assigned patients who had an acute slip into two groups on the basis of the time interval between the onset of symptoms and the surgical stabilization. Osteonecrosis developed in seven of eight hips that had surgical stabilization less than 48 hours after the onset of symptoms and in seven (32%) of 22 hips that had surgical stabilization more than 48 hours after the onset of symptoms. However, the present data cannot be used to develop guidelines with regard to the exact timing of surgical stabilization because the cause-and-effect relationship between the timing of surgical stabilization and the development of osteonecrosis cannot be determined. It is not known whether a hip with a more severe unstable SCFE, which would likely be associated with a higher risk of osteonecrosis, was stabilized sooner in an effort to reduce the child's discomfort as quickly as possible, or whether a hip with a less severe unstable SCFE, which theoretically might be associated with a lower risk of osteonecrosis, was stabilized later because the child may have been more comfortable.

Complications

Osteonecrosis

Osteonecrosis is the most devastating complication of SCFE (Fig. 10). The factors responsible for the development of osteonecrosis are an acute unstable SCFE, overreduction of an acute SCFE, attempts at reduction of the chronic component of an acute-on-chronic SCFE, placement of pins in the superolateral quadrant of the femoral head, and femoral neck osteotomy.[57,59,87,88,107,108] The frequency of osteonecrosis is increased if a cuneiform or basilar neck osteotomy is performed prior to physeal closure. The complication of osteonecrosis is rare in patients with a stable SCFE, but it occurs frequently in patients with an unstable SCFE.[59] A patient with osteonecrosis typically complains of pain in the groin or knee. On physical examination, there is a loss of motion of the hip, particularly internal rotation, and the hip is irritable on passive internal and external rotation. Plain radiographs are unremarkable early in the course of the disorder, but changes diagnostic of osteonecrosis (collapse of the femoral head with cyst formation and sclerosis) develop after a few months. All cases of osteonecrosis after SCFE are radiographically apparent within 1 year. An early bone scan[109] or MRI often shows asymmetry between the femoral heads, predicting the eventual development of osteonecrosis.

The treatment of osteonecrosis is not particularly rewarding for the patient or the clinician. Non–weight-bearing walking with crutches, range-of-motion exercises, and anti-inflammatory medication may help to minimize symptoms and epiphyseal collapse. An internal fixation device that protrudes into the hip joint should be backed out of the joint or removed, if the physis is closed, to reduce additional damage to the hip. In severe cases, a hip arthrodesis or joint arthroplasty may be needed.

Chondrolysis

The etiology of chondrolysis in SCFE is unknown. The possible role of an autoimmune phenomenon or some factor interfering with cartilage nutrition is yet to be defined. Risk factors leading to chondrolysis include immobilization in a cast, unrecognized permanent pin penetration, severe SCFE, and prolonged symptoms before treatment.

The prevalence of chondrolysis in patients with an SCFE is 5% to 7%.[110,111] A patient typically complains of pain in the groin or knee, and physical examination demonstrates a loss of hip motion, particularly internal rotation. The diagnosis is confirmed by radiographs that demonstrate a decrease in the width of the joint space of greater than 50% compared with the uninvolved side or, in patients who have bilateral involvement, a joint space of less than 3 mm. Hips that demonstrate increased uptake with premature closure of the greater trochanter on an early bone scan have been associated with an increased risk for the development of chondrolysis.[111] The prevalance of chondrolysis increases with the increasing severity of the SCFE, but it is not increased in the black population,[112-115] as previously reported.[110,116,117] The frequency of chondrolysis can be reduced with use of single-screw fixation rather than fixation with multiple screws or pins. With multiple pins or screws, the possibility that one or more may protrude into the joint is increased, and pin protrusion has been associated with an increased risk of chondrolysis.[118] The frequency of chondrolysis can also be reduced by not using a hip spica cast[83] and by waiting until physeal closure prior to performing a subtrochanteric osteotomy.[119]

As is the case with osteonecrosis, the treatment of chondrolysis is not particularly rewarding for the patient or the clinician. Non–weight-bearing walking with crutches, range-of-motion exercises, and anti-inflammatory medication may help to alleviate the symptoms. If there is pin protrusion, backing the pin out of the joint or removing it, if the physis is closed, helps to minimize damage to the hip. Some have recommended lengthening of the contracted muscle or muscles if a hip contracture develops. Arthrodesis may also be necessary in severe cases.

Internal Fixation Devices

The frequency of problems related to internal fixation devices (slip progression, pin breakage, and joint penetration by the pins) is decreasing with the use of fluoroscopic guidance and cannulated single-screw fixation. The risk of fracture through an unused pinhole can be avoided with use of fluoroscopy to position the guide pin correctly on the first attempt and by entering the bone proximal to the lesser trochanter.

Natural History Without Treatment

Two major issues arise when SCFE is untreated: the risk of additional progression and the risk of degenerative joint disease in adult life. Unfortunately, there are few long-term studies of patients with an SCFE and even fewer that have included untreated patients.[51,54,57,69,120-122]

Risk of Progression

The natural history of SCFE is unpredictable, and the risk of additional progression is difficult to ascertain. Ordeberg and associates[123] studied a series of patients 20 to 60 years after diagnosis of SCFE without primary treatment. Few patients had restrictions in working capacity or social life. However, there was a risk of slip progression as long as the physis remained open.[124] Carney and associates[57] reported on 36 cases of SCFE that were initially observed. Additional displacement occurred in six hips (17%) after the initial diagnosis; the SCFE became severe in five of them. Of these six hips, two were untreated and the other four were stabilized surgically. Eleven of the original 36 patients had an acute episode superimposed on the chronic SCFE. All 11 slips progressed to severe displacement and required surgical stabilization.

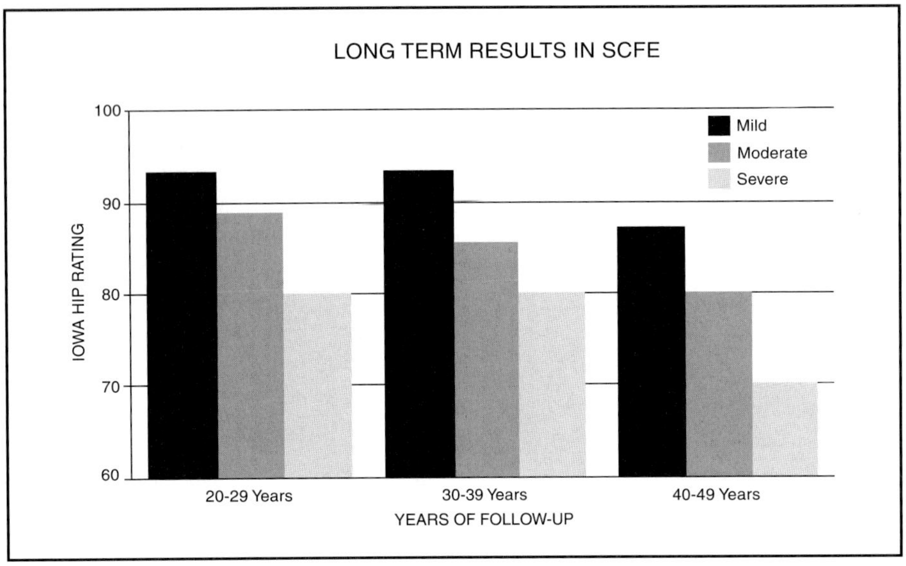

Fig. 11 Graph showing the worsening mean scores on the Iowa hip-rating scale for a group of 124 patients (155 hips) with an SCFE.[19]

Risk of Degenerative Joint Disease

Little is known about the risk of degenerative joint disease. Howorth[125] stated that SCFE is likely the most frequent cause of degenerative joint disease of the hip in middle-aged patients, and it is a common source of pain and disability. However, this theory is not necessarily supported by other studies. In reviews of a large series of patients with degenerative joint disease, the numbers of patients who were known to have an SCFE have been small, averaging approximately 5%.[126-128] Murray,[127] however, reported an association with SCFE in 40% of his 200 patients who were thought to have primary degenerative joint disease. He described a tilt deformity caused by bone resorption laterally with new bone formation medially, which he thought was compatible with an old SCFE. Stulberg and associates[129] described a similar deformity, the pistol-grip deformity, in 40% of patients without known prior hip disease who had total hip arthroplasty. This deformity was also thought to be compatible with an old SCFE. Resnick,[130] however, refuted this theory in a pathologic study of 48 femoral heads from patients with evidence of a tilt deformity on radiographs. The specimens suggested that the deformity was solely related to the remodeling changes of osteoarthritis. In summary, whether subclinical forms of SCFE lead to early osteoarthritis remains uncertain because of the controversy over the prevalence of the disorder.

What is known is that the severity of the untreated SCFE correlates with the long-term prognosis with regard to degenerative joint disease.[57,69,102,121,131,132] Oram[121] reported on 22 hips with an untreated SCFE, 11 of which were observed for more than 15 years. The hips with a moderate SCFE retained good function for years, whereas degenerative joint disease with resultant poor function developed within 15 years in the hips with a severe SCFE. Jerre[131,132] and Ross and associates[122] reported increasingly poor results with longer follow-up. In those studies, many patients did well early on, but symptoms increased and function decreased with increasing age. Carney and Weinstein[69] also studied the natural history of untreated, chronic SCFE. They evaluated 31 hips in 28 patients who had a mean age of 54 years and had been followed for a mean of 41 years. The mean Iowa hip rating score was 89 points for the entire group, 92 points for the 17 hips in which the SCFE was mild, 87 points for the 11 hips in which it was moderate, and 75 points for the three hips in which it was severe. There were four complications: displacement to a severe degree in two hips, and chondrolysis and osteonecrosis in one hip each. The chondrolysis developed in a hip in which the SCFE was mild and the osteonecrosis, in a hip in which it was severe. Although patients with a mild SCFE appear to have a favorable prognosis, patients in whom the disorder is moderate or severe have a high prevalence of degenerative joint disease. At a mean of 41 years after the diagnosis, all hips with a mild SCFE had an Iowa hip rating score of more than 80 points, whereas only 64% of the hips with a moderate or severe disorder had similar ratings. Thirty-six percent of the hips in which the disorder was mild had no degenerative changes; however, all of the hips in which the SCFE was moderate or severe had evidence of degenerative joint disease. Poor results, however, can occasionally be seen even with a minimal SCFE.[51,57,69,122] In summary, the natural history of chronic (stable) SCFE is favorable provided that displacement is mild and remains so.

Few data are available on the natural history of untreated acute SCFE. The acute episode is followed by a 2- to 3-week period of intolerance to weight bearing. As the pain and spasm subside, some motion returns, although the hip remains moderately painful in a position of external rotation. Degenerative changes (joint-space narrowing, subchondral bone cysts, and epiphyseal collapse) develop within a few months, and the patient is left with residual flexion, adduction, and external rotation contractures[54] (Fig. 10).

Long-Term Results of Treatment

Wilson and associates[46] reviewed the results in 300 hips in 240 patients treated between 1936 and 1960; 187 were treated with in situ pinning, with good clinical results in 81% and good radiographic results in 77%. Seventy-six hips in which correction of the deformity had been attempted had poorer results (60% had good clinical results, and 55% had good radiographic results). Hall,[120] in a study of 138 patients, reported that the best results were obtained with the use of multiple pins; 16 (80%) of 20 patients had an excellent result. The worst results were seen after realignment had been attempted with manipulation or osteotomy. Osteotomy of the femoral neck led to a poor result in 36% of the hips and to osteonecrosis in 38%.

Patients with an SCFE in southern Sweden were followed for more than 30 years.[35] Symptomatic treatment or in situ pinning resulted in high clinical ratings and few radiographic changes, with a secondary reconstructive procedure needed in only 2% of the hips. When closed reduction and a spica cast were used, the combined rate of osteonecrosis and chondrolysis was 16%, and a reconstructive procedure was needed in 35% of the hips. When femoral neck osteotomy was performed, the combined rate of osteonecrosis and chondrolysis was 30%, and a reconstructive procedure was necessary in 15% of 33 hips.

Carney and associates[57] reported on 155 hips in 124 patients who were followed for a mean of 41 years and were assessed with use of the Iowa hip rating system and a radiographic classification of degenerative joint disease, with grade 0 indicating no degenerative disease and grade 3 indicating severe degenerative disease. The SCFE was classified as acute, chronic, or acute-on-chronic. According to the head-shaft angle,[68] the degree of the slip was mild in 42%, moderate in 32%, and severe in 26%. Twenty-five percent of the hips that had a chronic SCFE received symptomatic treatment only; 30% were managed with a spica cast; 24%, with in situ pinning; and 20%, with osteotomy. The results worsened as the severity of the slip increased and when realignment had been performed (Fig. 11). Osteonecrosis, which developed in 12% of the hips, and chondrolysis, which developed in 16%, were more common with increasing severity of the slip. Reduction was performed in 39 hips and realignment, in 65 hips. For the 116 hips that had not been reduced, the mean Iowa hip rating was 85 points and the mean radiographic grade was 1.7. Osteonecrosis developed in seven (6%) of those hips, and chondrolysis, in 14 (12%). For the 39 hips with an SCFE that had been reduced, the mean Iowa hip rating score was 72 points and the mean radiographic grade was 2.4. Osteonecrosis developed in 12 of those hips (31%) and chondrolysis, in 11 (28%). Twenty-seven hips with a chronic SCFE that had in situ pinning demonstrated a mean Iowa hip rating score of 90 points and a mean radiographic grade of 1.5. Osteonecrosis developed in one of those hips and chondrolysis, in none. The long-term results of that study support the use of in situ pinning as the treatment of choice for SCFE. Realignment was associated with appreciable complications and had an adverse effect on the outcome. Regardless of the severity of the slip, in situ pinning provided the best long-term function and the longest delay of degenerative arthritis with the lowest risk of complications. Although limb-length discrepancy and motion in abduction and internal rotation were affected by the severity of the slip, function was not significantly impaired.

In conclusion, these series demonstrate that, regardless of the severity of the slip, in situ pinning provides the best long-term function, the lowest risk of complications, and the most effective delay of degenerative arthritis. Many patients with an SCFE respond well to this treatment, as seen at the time of long-term follow-up, if the SCFE is mild or moderate in severity, good congruity is maintained between the femoral head and the acetabulum, and osteonecrosis and chondrolysis do not develop. Hips with a severe SCFE and those with osteonecrosis or chondrolysis undergo more rapid deterioration with degenerative changes. SCFE differs from other pediatric disorders of the hip, such as Legg-Calvé-Perthes disease and developmental hip dysplasia, in that SCFE occurs at an age when the majority of acetabular development is completed and acetabular adaptation to a deformity of the femoral head cannot occur.

References

1. Schein AJ: Acute severe slipped capital femoral epiphysis. *Clin Orthop* 1967;51:151-166.
2. Segal LS, Weitzel PP, Davidson RS: Valgus slipped capital femoral epiphysis: Fact or fiction? *Clin Orthop* 1996;322:91-98.
3. Loder RT, Wittenberg B, DeSilva G: Slipped capital femoral epiphysis associated with endocrine disorders. *J Pediatr Orthop Am* 1995;15:349-356.
4. McAfee PC, Cady RB: Endocrinologic and metabolic factors in atypical presentations of slipped capital femoral epiphysis: Report of four cases and review of the literature. *Clin Orthop* 1983;180:188-197.
5. Wells D, King JD, Roe TF, Kaufman FR: Review of slipped capital femoral epiphysis associated with endocrine disease. *J Pediatr Orthop Am* 1993;13:610-614.
6. Loder RT, Hensinger RN: Slipped capital femoral epiphysis associated with renal failure osteodystrophy. *J Pediatr Orthop Am* 1997;17;205-211.
7. Loder RT, Hensinger RN, Alburger PD, et al: Slipped capital femoral epiphysis associated with radiation therapy. *J Pediatr Orthop Am* 1998;18:630-636.
8. Weiner D: Pathogenesis of slipped capital femoral epiphysis: Current concepts. *J Pediatr Orthop Br* 1996;5:67-73.
9. Pritchett JW, Perdue KD: Mechanical factors in slipped capital femoral epiphysis. *J Pediatr Orthop Am* 1988;8:385-388.
10. Kelsey JL, Acheson RM, Keggi KJ: The body build of patients with slipped capital femoral epiphysis. *Am J Dis Child* 1972;124:276-281.
11. Loder RT: The demographics of slipped capital femoral epiphysis: An international multicenter study. *Clin Orthop* 1996;322:8-27.
12. Galbraith RT, Gelberman RH, Hajek PC, et al: Obesity and decreased femoral anteversion in adolescence. *J Orthop Res* 1987;5:523-528.

13. Gelberman RH, Cohen MS, Shaw BA, Kasser JR, Griffin PP, Wilkinson RH: The association of femoral retroversion with slipped capital femoral epiphysis. *J Bone Joint Surg Am* 1986;68:1000-1007.

14. Mirkopulos N, Weiner DS, Askew M: The evolving slope of the proximal femoral growth plate relationship to slipped capital femoral epiphysis. *J Pediatr Orthop Am* 1988;8:268-273.

15. Kitadai HK, Milani C, Nery CA, Filho JL: Wiberg's center-edge angle in patients with slipped capital femoral epiphysis. *J Pediatr Orthop Am* 1999;19:97-105.

16. Wiberg G: Studies on dysplastic acetabula and congenital subluxation of the hip joint: With special reference to the complication of osteoarthrosis. *Acta Chir Scand* 1939; 58(suppl):7.

17. Exner GU: Growth and pubertal development in slipped capital femoral epiphysis: A longitudinal study. *J Pediatr Orthop Am* 1986;6:403-409.

18. Morscher E: Strength and morphology of growth cartilage under hormonal influence of puberty: Animal experiments and clinical study on the etiology of local growth disorders during puberty. *Reconstr Surg Traumatol* 1968;10: 3-104.

19. Speer DP: Experimental epiphysiolysis: Etiologic models of slipped capital femoral epiphysis, in Nelson JP (ed): *The Hip: Proceedings of the Tenth Open Scientific Meeting of the Hip Society*. St. Louis, MO, CV Mosby, 1982, pp 68-88.

20. Harris WR: The endocrine basis for slipping of the upper femoral epiphysis: An experimental study. *J Bone Joint Surg Br* 1950;32:5-11.

21. Sørensen KH: Slipped upper femoral epiphysis: Clinical study on aetiology. *Acta Orthop Scand* 1968;39:499-517.

22. Brenkel IJ, Dias JJ, Iqbal SJ, Gregg PJ: Thyroid hormone levels in patients with slipped capital femoral epiphysis. *J Pediatr Orthop Am* 1988;8:22-25.

23. Eisenstein A, Rothschild S: Biochemical abnormalities in patients with slipped capital femoral epiphysis and chondrolysis. *J Bone Joint Surg Am* 1976;58:459-467.

24. Mann DC, Weddington J, Richton S: Hormonal studies in patients with slipped capital femoral epiphysis without evidence of endocrinopathy. *J Pediatr Orthop Am* 1988;8:543-545.

25. Razzano CD, Nelson C, Eversman J: Growth hormone levels in slipped capital femoral epiphysis. *J Bone Joint Surg Am* 1972;54:1224-1226.

26. Wilcox PG, Weiner DS, Leighley B: Maturation factors in slipped capital femoral epiphysis. *J Pediatr Orthop Am* 1988;8:196-200.

27. Rennie AM: The inheritance of slipped upper femoral epiphysis. *J Bone Joint Surg Br* 1982;64:180-184.

28. Bednarz PA, Stanitski CL: Slipped capital femoral epiphysis in identical twins: HLA predisposition. *Orthopedics* 1998;21:1291-1293.

29. Günal I, Ates E: The HLA phenotype in slipped capital femoral epiphysis. *J Pediatr Orthop Am* 1997;17:655-656.

30. Agamanolis DP, Weiner DS, Lloyd JK: Slipped capital femoral epiphysis: A pathological study. I: A light microscopic and histochemical study of 21 cases. *J Pediatr Orthop Am* 1985;5:40-46.

31. Ponseti IV, McClintock R: The pathology of slipping of the upper femoral epiphysis. *J Bone Joint Surg Am* 1956;38:71-83.

32. Agamanolis DP, Weiner DS, Lloyd JK: Slipped capital femoral epiphysis: A pathological study. II: An ultrastructural study of 23 cases. *J Pediatr Orthop Am* 1985;5:47-58.

33. Ninomiya S, Nagasaka Y, Tagawa H: Slipped capital femoral epiphysis. A study of 68 cases in the eastern half area of Japan. *Clin Orthop* 1976;119:172-176.

34. Kelsey JL, Keggi KJ, Southwick WO: The incidence and distribution of slipped capital femoral epiphysis in Connecticut and southwestern United States. *J Bone Joint Surg Am* 1970;52:1203-1216.

35. Hansson LI, Hägglund G, Ordeberg G: Slipped capital femoral epiphysis in southern Sweden 1910-1982. *Acta Orthop Scand* 1987; 226(suppl):1-67.

36. Loder RT, Farley FA, Herzenberg JE, Hensinger RN, Kuhn JL: Narrow window of bone age in children with slipped capital femoral epiphyses. *J Pediatr Orthop Am* 1993;13:290-293.

37. Andrén L, Borgström K-E: Seasonal variation of epiphysiolysis of the hip and possibility of causal factor. *Acta Orthop Scand* 1958;28:22-26.

38. Ferguson AB, Howorth MB: Slipping of the upper femoral epiphysis: A study of 70 cases. *JAMA* 1931;97:1867-1872.

39. Hägglund G, Hansson LI, Ordeberg G: Epidemiology of slipped capital femoral epiphysis in southern Sweden. *Clin Orthop* 1984;191:82-94.

40. Loder RT: A worldwide study on the seasonal variation of slipped capital femoral epiphysis. *Clin Orthop* 1996;322:28-36.

41. Jerre R, Billing L, Hansson G, Wallin J: The contralateral hip in patients primarily treated for unilateral slipped upper femoral epiphysis: Long-term follow-up of 61 hips. *J Bone Joint Surg Br* 1994;76:563-567.

42. Jerre R, Billing L, Hansson G, Karlsson J, Wallin J: Bilaterality in slipped capital femoral epiphysis: Importance of a reliable radiographic method. *J Pediatr Orthop Br* 1996;5:80-84.

43. Hurley JM, Betz RR, Loder RT, Davidson RS, Alburger PD, Steel HH: Slipped capital femoral epiphysis: The prevalence of late contralateral slip. *J Bone Joint Surg Am* 1996;78: 226-230.

44. Dreghorn CR, Knight D, Mainds CC, Blockey NJ: Slipped upper femoral epiphysis: A review of 12 years of experience in Glasgow (1972-1983). *J Pediatr Orthop Am* 1987;7:283-287.

45. Loder RT, Aronson DD, Greenfield ML: The epidemiology of bilateral slipped capital femoral epiphysis: A study of children in Michigan. *J Bone Joint Surg Am* 1993;75:1141-1147.

46. Wilson PD, Jacobs B, Schecter L: Slipped capital femoral epiphysis: An end-result study. *J Bone Joint Surg Am* 1965;47:1128-1145.

47. Segal LS, Davidson RS, Robertson WW Jr, Drummond DS: Growth disturbances of the proximal femur after pinning of juvenile slipped capital femoral epiphysis. *J Pediatr Orthop Am* 1991;11:631-637.

48. Stasikelis PJ, Sullivan CM, Phillips WA, Polard JA: Slipped capital femoral epiphysis: Prediction of contralateral involvement. *J Bone Joint Surg Am* 1996;78:1149-1155.

49. Aadalen RJ, Weiner DS, Hoyt W, Herndon CH: Acute slipped capital femoral epiphysis. *J Bone Joint Surg Am* 1974;56:1473-1487.

50. Aronson DD, Carlson WE: Slipped capital femoral epiphysis: A prospective study of fixation with a single screw. *J Bone Joint Surg Am* 1992;74:810-819.

51. Boyer DW, Mickelson MR, Ponseti IV: Slipped capital femoral epiphysis: Long-term follow-up of one hundred and twenty-one patients. *J Bone Joint Surg Am* 1981;63:85-95.

52. Fahey JJ, O'Brien ET: Acute slipped capital femoral epiphysis: Review of the literature and report of ten cases. *J Bone Joint Surg Am* 1965;47:1105-1127.

53. Ward WT, Stefko J, Wood KB, Stanitski CL: Fixation with a single screw for slipped capital femoral epiphysis. *J Bone Joint Surg Am* 1992;74:799-809.

54. Ponseti I, Barta CK: Evaluation of treatment of slipping of the capital femoral epiphysis. *Surg Gynecol Obstet* 1948;86:87-97.

55. Casey BH, Hamilton HW, Bobechko WP: Reduction of acutely slipped upper femoral epiphysis. *J Bone Joint Surg Br* 1972;54:607-614.

56. Rab GT: The geometry of slipped capital femoral epiphysis: Implications for movement, impingement, and corrective osteotomy. *J Pediatr Orthop Am* 1999;19:419-424.

57. Carney BT, Weinstein SL, Noble J: Long-term follow-up of slipped capital femoral epiphysis. *J Bone Joint Surg Am* 1991;73:667-674.

58. Jacobs B: Diagnosis and natural history of slipped femoral capital epiphysis. *Instr Course Lect* 1972;21:167-173.

59. Loder RT, Richards BS, Shapiro PS, Reznick LR, Aronson DD: Acute slipped capital femoral epiphysis: The importance of physeal stability. *J Bone Joint Surg Am* 1993;75: 1134-1140.

60. Kallio PE, Paterson DC, Foster BK, Lequesne GW: Classification in slipped capital femoral epiphysis: Sonographic assessment of stability and remodeling. *Clin Orthop* 1993;294:196-203.

61. Kallio PE, Mah ET, Foster BK, Paterson DC, LeQuesne GW: Slipped capital femoral epiphysis: Incidence and clinical assessment of physeal instability. *J Bone Joint Surg Br* 1995;77:752-755.

62. Aronsson DD, Loder RT: Treatment of the unstable (acute) slipped capital femoral epiphysis. *Clin Orthop* 1996;322:99-110.

63. Rhoad RC, Davidson RS, Heyman S, Dormans JP, Drummond DS: Pretreatment bone scan in SCFE: A predictor of ischemia and avascular necrosis. *J Pediatr Orthop Am* 1999;19:164-168.

64. Salter RB, Harris WR: Injuries involving the epiphyseal plate. *J Bone Joint Surg Am* 1963;45:587-622.

65. Steel HH: The metaphyseal blanch sign of slipped capital femoral epiphysis. *J Bone Joint Surg Am* 1986;68:920-922.

66. Klein A, Joplin RJ, Reidy JA, Hanelin J: Slipped capital femoral epiphysis: Early diagnosis and treatment facilitated by "normal" roentgenograms. *J Bone Joint Surg Am* 1952;34:233-239.

67. Loder RT, Blakemore LC, Farley FA, Laidlaw AT: Measurement variability of slipped capital femoral epiphysis. *J Orthop Surg* 2000;7:33-42.

68. Southwick WO: Osteotomy through the lesser trochanter for slipped capital femoral epiphysis. *J Bone Joint Surg Am* 1967;49:807-835.

69. Carney BT, Weinstein SL: Natural history of untreated chronic slipped capital femoral epiphysis. *Clin Orthop* 1996;322:43-47.

70. Aronson DD, Peterson DA, Miller DV: Slipped capital femoral epiphysis: The case for internal fixation in situ. *Clin Orthop* 1992;281:115-122.

71. Maurer RC, Larsen IJ: Acute necrosis of cartilage in slipped capital femoral epiphysis. *J Bone Joint Surg Am* 1970;52:39-50.

72. Vrettos BC, Hoffman EB: Chondrolysis in slipped upper femoral epiphysis: Long-term study of the aetiology and natural history. *J Bone Joint Surg Br* 1993;75:956-961.

73. Walters R, Simon SR: Joint destruction: A sequel of unrecognized pin penetration in patients with slipped capital femoral epiphyses, in Riley LH Jr (ed): *The Hip: Proceedings of the Eighth Open Scientific Meeting of the Hip Society*. St. Louis, MO, CV Mosby, 1980, pp 145-164.

74. Betz RR, Steel HH, Emper WD, Huss GK, Clancy M: Treatment of slipped capital femoral epiphysis: Spica-cast immobilization. *J Bone Joint Surg Am* 1990;72:587-600.

75. Strong M, Lejman T, Michno P, Sulko J: Fixation of slipped capital femoral epiphyses with unthreaded 2-mm wires. *J Pediatr Orthop Am* 1996;16:53-55.

76. Rao SB, Crawford AH, Burger RR, Roy DR: Open bone peg epiphysiodesis for slipped capital femoral epiphysis. *J Pediatr Orthop Am* 1996;16:37-48.

77. Weiner DS, Weiner S, Melby A, Hoyt WA Jr: A 30-year experience with bone graft epiphysiodesis in the treatment of slipped capital femoral epiphysis. *J Pediatr Orthop Am* 1984;4:145-152.

78. Schmidt TL, Cimino WG, Seidel FG: Allograft epiphysiodesis for slipped capital femoral epiphysis. *Clin Orthop* 1996;322:61-76.

79. DeRosa GP, Mullins RC, Kling TF Jr: Cuneiform osteotomy of the femoral neck in severe slipped capital femoral epiphysis. *Clin Orthop* 1996;322:48-60.

80. Velasco R, Schai PA, Exner GU: Slipped capital femoral epiphysis: A long-term follow-up study after open reduction of the femoral head combined with subcapital wedge resection. *J Pediatr Orthop Br* 1998; 7:43-52.

81. Barmada R, Bruch RF, Gimbel JS, Ray RD: Base of the neck extracapsular osteotomy for correction of deformity in slipped capital femoral epiphysis. *Clin Orthop* 1978;132:98-101.

82. Kramer WG, Craig WA, Noel S: Compensating osteotomy at the base of the femoral neck for slipped capital femoral epiphysis. *J Bone Joint Surg Am* 1976;58:796-800.

83. Meier MC, Meyer LC, Ferguson RL: Treatment of slipped capital femoral epiphysis with a spica cast. *J Bone Joint Surg Am* 1992;74:1522-1529.

84. O'Brien ET, Fahey JJ: Remodeling of the femoral neck after in-situ pinning for slipped capital femoral epiphysis. *J Bone Joint Surg Am* 1977;59:62-68.

85. Bellemans J, Fabry G, Molenaers G, Lammens J, Moens P: Slipped capital femoral epiphysis: A long-term follow-up, with special emphasis on the capacities for remodeling. *J Pediatr Orthop Br* 1996;5:151-157.

86. Jerre R, Billing L, Karlsson J: Loss of hip motion in slipped capital femoral epiphysis: A calculation from the slipping angle and the slope. *J Pediatr Orthop Br* 1996;5:144-150.

87. Claffey TJ: Avascular necrosis of the femoral head: An anatomical study. *J Bone Joint Surg Br* 1960;42:802-809.

88. Brodetti A: The blood supply of the femoral neck and head in relation to the damaging effects of nails and screws. *J Bone Joint Surg Br* 1960;42:794-801.

89. Karol LA, Doane RM, Cornicelli SF, Zak PA, Haut RC, Manoli A II: Single versus double screw fixation for treatment of slipped capital femoral epiphysis: A biomechanical analysis. *J Pediatr Orthop Am* 1992;12:741-745.

90. Blanco JS, Taylor B, Johnston CE II: Comparison of single pin versus multiple pin fixation in treatment of slipped capital femoral epiphysis. *J Pediatr Orthop Am* 1992;12:384-389.

91. Morrissy RT: Slipped capital femoral epiphysis: Technique of percutaneous in situ fixation. *J Pediatr Orthop Am* 1990;10:347-350.

92. Goodman WW, Johnson JT, Robertson WW Jr: Single screw fixation for acute and acute-on-chronic slipped capital femoral epiphysis. *Clin Orthop* 1996;322:86-90.

93. Stevens DB, Short BA, Burch JM: In situ fixation of the slipped capital femoral epiphysis with a single screw. *J Pediatr Orthop Br* 1996;5:85-89.

94. Canale ST, Azar F, Young J, Beaty JH, Warner WC, Whitmer G: Subtrochanteric fracture after fixation of slipped capital femoral epiphysis: A complication of unused drill holes. *J Pediatr Orthop Am* 1994;14:623-626.

95. Maletis GB, Bassett GS: Windshield-wiper loosening: A complication of in situ screw fixation of slipped capital femoral epiphysis. *J Pediatr Orthop Am* 1993;13:607-609.

96. Samuelson T, Olney B: Percutaneous pin fixation of chronic slipped capital femoral epiphysis. *Clin Orthop* 1996;326:225-228.

97. Fish JB: Cuneiform osteotomy of the femoral neck in the treatment of slipped capital femoral epiphysis: A follow-up note. *J Bone Joint Surg Am* 1994;76:46-59.

98. Dunn DM, Angel JC: Replacement of the femoral head by open operation in severe adolescent slipping of the upper femoral epiphysis. *J Bone Joint Surg Br* 1978;60:394-403.

99. Crawford AH: Role of osteotomy in the treatment of slipped capital femoral epiphysis. *J Pediatr Orthop Br* 1996;5:102-109.

100. Crawford AH: Osteotomies in the treatment of slipped capital femoral epiphysis. *Instr Course Lect* 1984;33:327-349.

101. Southwick WO: Compression fixation after biplane intertrochanteric osteotomy for slipped capital femoral epiphysis: A technical improvement. *J Bone Joint Surg Am* 1973;55:1218-1224.

102. Schai PA, Exner GU, Hansch O: Prevention of secondary coxarthrosis in slipped capital femoral epiphysis: A long-term follow-up study after corrective intertrochanteric osteotomy. *J Pediatr Orthop Br* 1996;5:135-143.

103. Jerre R, Hansson G, Wallin J, Karlsson J: Long-term results after realignment operations for slipped upper femoral epiphysis. *J Bone Joint Surg Br* 1996;78:745-750.

104. de Sanctis N, Di Gennaro G, Pempinello C, Corte SD, Carannante G: Is gentle manipulative reduction and percutaneous fixation with a single screw the best management of acute and acute-on-chronic slipped capital femoral epiphysis? A report of 70 patients. *J Pediatr Orthop Br* 1996;5:90-95.

105. Herman MJ, Dormans JP, Davidson RS, Drummond DS, Gregg JR: Screw fixation of Grade III slipped capital femoral epiphysis. *Clin Orthop* 1996;322:77-85.

106. Peterson MD, Weiner DS, Green NE, Terry CL: Acute slipped capital femoral epiphysis: The value and safety of urgent manipulative reduction. *J Pediatr Orthop Am* 1997;17:648-654.

107. Dietz FR: Traction reduction of acute and acute-on-chronic slipped capital femoral epiphysis. *Clin Orthop* 1994;302:101-110.

108. Krahn TH, Canale ST, Beaty JH, Warner WC, Lourenco P: Long-term follow-up of patients with avascular necrosis after treatment of slipped capital femoral epiphysis. *J Pediatr Orthop Am* 1993;13:154-158.

109. Strange-Vognsen H, Wagner A, Dirksen K, et al: The value of scintigraphy in hips with slipped capital femoral epiphysis and the value of radiography and MRI after 10 years. *Acta Orthop Belg* 1999;65:33-38.

110. Ingram AJ, Clarke MS, Clark CS Jr, Marshall WR: Chondrolysis complicating slipped capital femoral epiphysis. *Clin Orthop* 1982;165: 99-109.

111. Mandell GA, Keret D, Harcke HT, Bowen JR: Chondrolysis: Detection by bone scintigraphy. *J Pediatr Orthop Am* 1992;12:80-85.

112. Aronson DD, Loder RT: Slipped capital femoral epiphysis in black children. *J Pediatr Orthop Am* 1992;12:74-79.

113. Bishop JO, Oley TJ, Stephenson CT, Tullos HS: Slipped capital femoral epiphysis: A study of 50 cases in black children. *Clin Orthop* 1978:135:93-96.

114. Kennedy JP, Weiner DS: Results of slipped capital femoral epiphysis in the black population. *J Pediatr Orthop Am* 1990;10:224-227.

115. Spero CR, Masciale JP, Tornetta P III; Star MJ, Tucci JJ: Slipped capital femoral epiphysis in black children: Incidence of chondrolysis. *J Pediatr Orthop Am* 1992;12:444-448.

116. Orofino C, Innis JJ, Lowrey CW: Slipped capital femoral epiphysis in Negroes: A study of ninety-five cases. *J Bone Joint Surg Am* 1960;42:1079-1083.

117. Tillema DA, Golding JSR: Chondrolysis following slipped capital femoral epiphysis in Jamaica. *J Bone Joint Surg Am* 1971;53:1528-1540.

118. Gonzalez-Moran G, Carsi B, Abril JC, Albinana J: Results after preoperative traction and pinning in slipped capital femoral epiphysis: K wires versus cannulated screws. *J Pediatr Orthop Br* 1998;7:53-58.

119. Frymoyer JW: Chondrolysis of the hip following Southwick osteotomy for severe slipped capital femoral epiphysis. *Clin Orthop* 1974;99:120-124.

120. Hall JE: The results of treatment of slipped femoral epiphysis. *J Bone Joint Surg Br* 1957;39:659-673.

121. Oram V: Epiphysiolysis of the head of the femur: A follow-up examination with special reference to end results and the social prognosis. *Acta Orthop Scand* 1953;23:100-120.

122. Ross PM, Lyne ED, Morawa LG: Slipped capital femoral epiphysis: Long-term results after 10-38 years. *Clin Orthop* 1979;141:176-180.

123. Ordeberg G, Hansson LI, Sandström S: Slipped capital femoral epiphysis in southern Sweden: Long-term result with no treatment or symptomatic primary treatment. *Clin Orthop* 1984;191:95-104.

124. Jerre R, Karlsson J, Romanus B, Wallin J: Does a single device prevent further slipping of the epiphysis in children with slipped capital femoral epiphysis? *Arch Orthop Trauma Surg* 1997;116:348-351.

125. Howorth B: Slipping of the capital femoral epiphysis: History. *Clin Orthop* 1966;48:11-32.

126. Johnston RC, Larson CB: Results of treatment of hip disorders with cup arthroplasty. *J Bone Joint Surg Am* 1969;51:1461-1479.

127. Murray RO: The aetiology of primary osteoarthritis of the hip. *Br J Radiol* 1965;38:810-824.

128. Solomon L: Patterns of osteoarthritis of the hip. *J Bone Joint Surg Br* 1976;58:176-183.

129. Stulberg SD, Cordell LD, Harris WH: Unrecognized childhood hip disease: A major cause of idiopathic osteonecrosis of the hip, in *The Hip: Proceedings of the Third Open Scientific Meeting of the Hip Society*. St Louis, MO, CV Mosby, 1975, pp 212-230.

130. Resnick D: The "tilt deformity" of the femoral head in osteoarthritis of the hip: A poor indicator of previous epiphysiolysis. *Clin Radiol* 1976;27:355-363.

131. Jerre T: A study in slipped upper femoral epiphysis: With special reference to the late functional and roentgenological results and to the value of closed reduction. *Acta Orthop Scand* 1950;6(suppl):5-157.

132. Jerre T: Early complications after osteosynthesis with a three flanged nail in situ for slipped epiphysis. *Acta Orthop Scand* 1958;27:126-134.

59

Natural History and Long-Term Outcomes of Slipped Capital Femoral Epiphysis

Matthew B. Dobbs, MD
Stuart L. Weinstein, MD

Introduction

Slipped capital femoral epiphysis (SCFE) is a disorder in which there is a displacement of the capital femoral epiphysis from the metaphysis through the physeal plate. The term slipped capital femoral epiphysis is actually a misnomer, because the head of the femur is held in the acetabulum by the ligamentum teres, and thus it is actually the neck that comes upward and outward while the head remains in the acetabulum. In the majority of cases, there is a varus relationship between the head and neck, but occasionally the slip is into a valgus position, with displacement superiorly and posteriorly in relation to the neck.[1,2]

Classification

Traditionally, on the basis of the patient's history, physical examination, and radiographs, SCFE can be classified into four clinical categories: preslip, acute, acute on chronic, and chronic.

In the preslip stage, patients usually have a limp, complain of weakness in the leg, or have exertional pain in the groin or knee with prolonged standing or walking. On physical examination, the most consistent positive finding is lack of medial rotation. Radiographs reveal generalized bone atrophy of the hemipelvis and upper femur only in those patients who limped or limited their activity. There may be some widening and irregularity of the physeal plate region.[3]

An acute slip is an abrupt displacement through the proximal physeal cartilaginous plate in which there was a preexisting epiphyseolysis.[4] Acute slips account for only 10% to 15% of the slips in most large reported series.[5,6] The clinical criteria for having an acute slip include the onset of symptoms for less than 2 weeks. Physical examination demonstrates an external rotation deformity, shortening, and marked limitation of motion secondary to pain. In general, the greater the amount of slip, the greater the motion restriction. However, 67% of patients with acute slips give a history of mild prodromal symptoms for 1 to 3 months before their acute episode, indicating that they probably had a preslip or mild slip preceding their acute episode.[1,4,5,7,8] The traumatic episode may be as trivial as turning over in bed. The pain is usually severe enough to prevent weight bearing. Slips in those patients with a history of mild prodromal symptoms may be better classified as acute-on-chronic slips.

An acute-on-chronic SCFE is one associated with chronic symptoms initially and with subsequent development of acute symptoms as well as a sudden increase in the degree of slip.

Chronic slips are by far the most common type, accounting for 85.5% of all slips.[6] Patients with chronic SCFE generally have a history of groin or medial thigh pain for months to years. They may have a history of exacerbations and remissions of the pain and limp. Importantly, 46% will have knee or lower thigh pain as their initial symptom, emphasizing the importance of a hip examination in any child complaining of knee pain.[9,10] All of these patients demonstrate limited motion, particularly medial rotation.

A newer and more clinically useful classification of slips is stable versus unstable.[6,11,12] Unstable slips are those in which weight bearing is not possible, with or without crutches, and stable slips are those in which weight bearing is possible, with or without crutches. The reason this classification is important is that in a large series of patients with acute symptomatology classified as stable versus unstable (all treated with pinning in situ), the incidence of aseptic necrosis in the unstable slip was significantly greater than in those patients with stable slips. The traditional classification of acute versus chronic is considered to be misleading because it does not consider hip stability. The high complication rates in the unstable slip are most likely secondary to vascular injury caused at the time of the initial displacement.[6,11]

Slips can also be classified radiographically by the amount of displacement anteriorly, posteriorly, or laterally.[13] The minimal slip is classified as one with maximal displacement of less than one third of the diameter of the neck. Moderate slip is greater than 1 cm of displacement but less

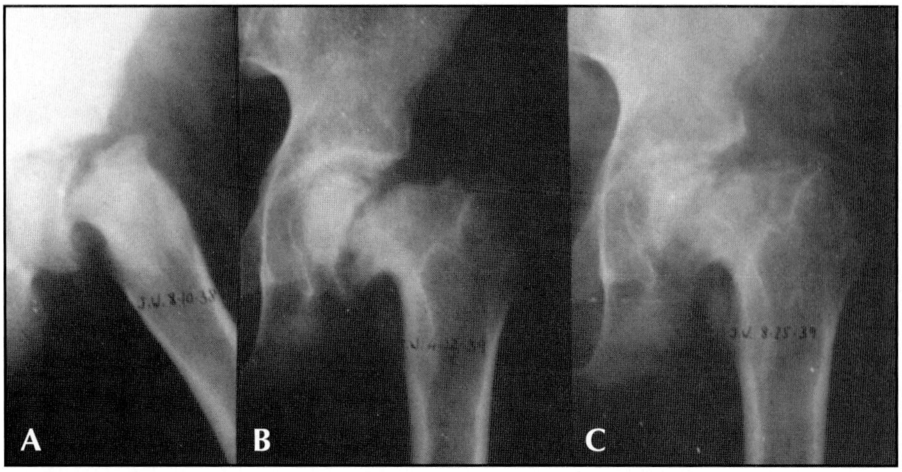

Fig. 1 A, Radiograph of the left hip in a 14-year-old boy with immediate severe hip pain following acute trauma, without prior hip symptoms. **B** and **C,** Follow-up radiographs over a 1-year period showing the rapid development of severe degenerative changes.

than one half the diameter of the neck, and a severe slip is displacement greater than half the diameter of the neck. This classification is probably most important when considering long-term prognosis, because mild and moderate slips have an excellent long-term prognosis when treated by pinning in situ, whereas severe slips tend to deteriorate with time.[9,14]

Natural History

Howarth[15] stated that SCFE is probably the most frequent cause of degenerative joint disease of the hip in middle-aged patients and is a common source of pain and disability, but there are few long-term studies of patients with slipped capital femoral epiphysis, and included in these are few untreated patients.[3,5,9,14,16-18] However, there are some data on the natural history of true acute slips. The acute episode is followed by a 2- to 3-week period of intolerance to weight bearing. As the pain and spasm subside, some motion returns, though the hip remains moderately painful in external rotation. Degenerative changes develop within only a few months and the patient is left with residual flexion, adduction, and external rotation contractures[3] (Fig. 1).

In reviewing a large series of patients with degenerative joint disease, the number of patients with known SCFE is small, averaging around 5%.[19-21] Murray,[20] however, reported an association with SCFE in 40% of 200 patients thought to have primary degenerative joint disease. He described a tilt deformity caused by bone resorption laterally with new bone formation medially and thought this to be compatible with old SCFE. Stulberg and associates[22] also described a similar deformity, the pistol grip deformity, in 40% of patients without known prior hip disease undergoing total hip arthroplasty. This deformity was also thought to be compatible with old SCFE. Resnick,[23] however, refuted this theory in a pathologic study of 48 femoral heads of patients with a tilt deformity on radiographs. The specimens suggested that the deformity was solely related to the remodeling changes of osteoarthritis. In summary, whether subclinical forms of SCFE lead to early osteoarthritis remains uncertain because of the controversy over its incidence.

The severity of deformity does correlate with the overall long-term prognosis with regard to the development of degenerative joint disease and function.[9,14,17,18,24,25] Oram[17] reported results of 22 untreated slips, 11 of which were observed for more than 15 years. Patients with moderate slips retained good function for years, whereas those with severe slips developed early degenerative joint disease with resultant poor function. Poor results are occasionally seen even with minimal slips.[5,9,14,18]

Carney and Weinstein[14] reported results in 31 hips in 28 patients with SCFE observed without surgical intervention. The mean duration of patient follow-up from the onset of symptoms was 41 years. The mean patient age was 54 years at review. Complications occurred in four slips: displacement to a severe degree occurred in two hips; chondrolysis and aseptic necrosis in one hip each. In this natural history group, chondrolysis, defined as early loss of width of the joint space, was seen in one mild slip, and osteonecrosis, defined as collapse of some portion of the femoral head, was seen in one severe slip. The mean Iowa Hip Rating (100-point scale) for the entire group was 89 points. The mild slips had a mean rating of 87 points and the severe slips had a mean Iowa Hip Rating of 75. At the 41-year follow-up, all mild slips had an Iowa Hip Rating of more than 80 points, whereas only 64% of moderate and severe slips had similar ratings. Mild slips had good long-term results regarding Iowa Hip Rating and degenerative disease rating. There were no degenerative changes in 36% of the mild slips; however, all moderate and severe slips had evidence of degenerative joint disease.

In an earlier study, Carney and associates[9] reported on 35 slips that were observed initially. After the time of initial diagnosis, additional displacement occurred in six (17%), five of which became severe. Two of these six were untreated. The other four slips were stabilized surgically and excluded from the natural history study. Eleven of the original 35 patients had an acute episode superimposed on the chronic slip. These 11 slips all progressed to severe displacement and were stabilized surgically and also were excluded from the natural history study.[9]

Ordeberg and associates[26] studied a series of patients with slipped capital femoral epiphyses without primary treatment, from 20 to 40 years after diagnosis. Few patients had restrictions in working capacity or social life.

In summary, the natural history of chronic SCFE is favorable provided that displacement is mild and remains so. Jerre[24,25] and Ross and associates[18] reported a decline in favorable results with older age at follow-up. Both groups reported many patients doing well early on but having increasing symptoms and decreasing function with increasing age.

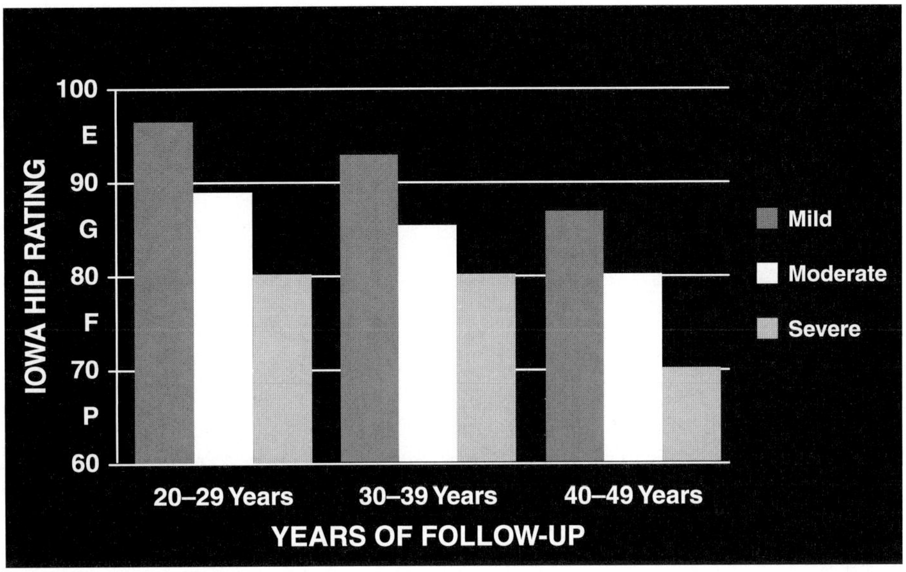

Fig. 2 Bar graph depicting worsening scores on the Iowa Hip Rating when following a group of patients long term with SCFE. Deterioration over time was most marked with increasing severity of the slip. (Adapted with permission from Carney BT, Weinstein SL, Noble J: Long-term follow-up of slipped capital femoral epiphysis. *J Bone Joint Surg* 1991;73: 667-674.)

Long-Term Results

Carney and associates[9] reported long-term results for 155 hips in 124 patients who were reviewed at a mean follow-up of 41 years after the onset of symptoms.[5] The slips were classified by duration of symptoms as acute, chronic, or acute on chronic. As determined by the head shaft angle,[27] 42% of slips were mild, 32% were moderate, and 26% were severe. Reduction was performed on 39 hips and realignment in 65 hips. Treatment of chronic slips included symptomatic treatment only in 25% of the hips, spica cast in 30%, pinning in situ in 24%, and osteotomy in 20%. The Iowa Hip Rating and radiographic classification of degenerative joint disease were determined at follow-up and both worsened with increasing severity of the slip and where reduction or realignment had been done (Fig. 2). Osteonecrosis (12%) and chondrolysis (16%) were also more common with increasing severity of the slip. Poor results were common when either reduction or realignment had been performed. Deterioration over time was most marked with increasing severity of the slip. The authors reported that the long-term natural history of malunited slips is mild deterioration related to the severity of the slip and complications.

Realignment techniques are associated with risk of appreciable complications and adversely affect the natural history of the disease. Regardless of the severity of the slip, pinning in situ provided the best long-term function and delay of degenerative arthritis with a low risk of complications. Although limb-length discrepancy and motion in abduction and internal rotation were affected by the severity of the slip, function was not significantly impaired.

Wilson and associates[28] reviewed the results of 300 hips in 240 patients who had been seen for SCFE at the Hospital for Special Surgery between 1936 and 1960. Of these hips, 187 had been treated by pinning in situ, with good clinical results in 81% and good radiographic results in 77%. The results were worse (60% good clinical results and 55% good radiographic results) for the 76 hips in which correction of the deformity had been attempted. Hall[16] reported on 100 patients from a study of the British Orthopaedic Association as well as an additional 38 patients in regard to the results of various types of treatment. The best results were obtained with the use of multiple pins: 16 of 20 patients (80%) had excellent results. The worst results were seen after realignment had been attempted with manipulation or osteotomy. Osteotomy of the femoral neck was followed by a poor result in 36% of the hips and osteonecrosis in 38%.

Patients with SCFE in southern Sweden were observed for more than 30 years.[9,26,29] Symptomatic treatment or pinning in situ resulted in high clinical ratings and few radiographic changes, with only 2% of the hips requiring a secondary reconstructive procedure. When closed reduction and spica cast were used, the combined rate of osteonecrosis and chondrolysis was 13% and reconstructive procedures were needed in 35% of the hips. Osteotomy through the femoral neck was followed by a combined rate of osteonecrosis and chondrolysis of 30%, and reconstructive procedures were necessary in 15% of the hips.

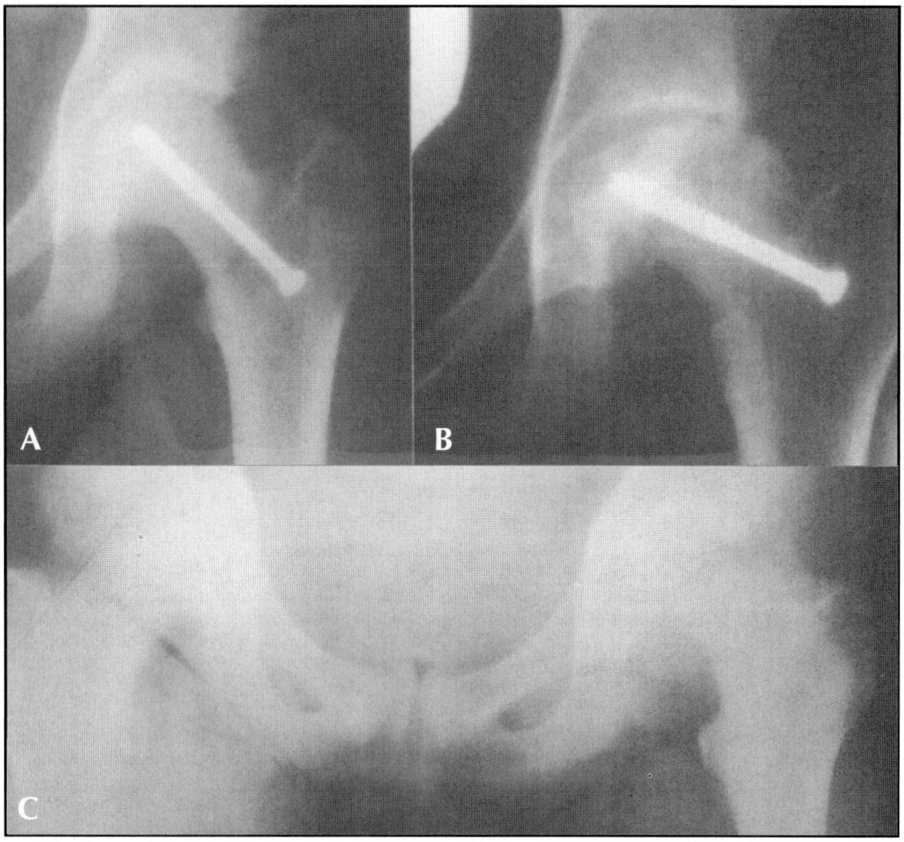

Fig. 3 A and **B,** Radiographs of the the left hip of a 13-year-old girl with immediate severe hip pain after running sprints, without prior hip symptoms. Patient was thought to have an acute slip and was therefore placed on the fracture table and in situ pinning was performed in the operating room. **C,** Follow-up radiograph demonstrates aseptic necrosis with collapse of the femoral head.

In several series, the use of multiple pins in situ resulted in good or excellent results in more than 90% of the hips. The high percentage of good results has been attributed to remodeling of the femoral neck. However, difficulty with pin removal and a relatively high incidence of unrecognized penetration of the joint space by pins have also been reported. Because of the significant prevalence of early osteoarthritis, reduction by closed or open means currently is not advocated.[4,9,30]

Carney and associates[9] reported on a series of 39 slips that had been reduced. Their mean Iowa Hip Rating was 72 points, and the mean radiographic degenerative score was 2.4 of 3 (0 = no degenerative disease, 3 = severe degenerative disease). Osteonecrosis developed in 12 of the hips (31%) and chondrolysis in 11 (28%). For the 116 hips that had not been reduced, the mean Iowa Hip Rating was 85 points and the mean radiographic grade was 1.7 of 3. Osteonecrosis developed in 7 hips (6%) and chondrolysis in 14 (12%). Results of this long-term study support the use of pinning in situ as the treatment of choice for SCFE. Twenty-seven hips in which the slip was chronic were so treated, and at the most recent follow-up the mean Iowa Hip Rating was 90 points and the mean radiographic degenerative score was 1.5 of 3. Osteonecrosis developed in one of these hips and chondrolysis did not develop in any.

The natural history of a malunited slip is one of mild deterioration that is related to the severity of the slip and the complications of treatment. Realignment is associated with the risk of substantial complications and adversely affects the natural course of disease. Regardless of the severity of the slip, pinning in situ provides the best long-term function with a low risk of complications and most effectively delays the development of degenerative arthritis. Remodeling of the metaphyseal prominence is seen in many radiographs during the course of time.

The development of aseptic necrosis is the most devastating complication of SCFE (Fig. 3). The factors noted to be responsible for the development of aseptic necrosis are acute slips, unstable slips, overreduction of acute slips, attempts at reduction of the chronic component of an acute-on-chronic slip, placement of pins in the superolateral quadrant of the femoral head, or osteotomies of the femoral neck.[9,12,31-34]

The etiology of chondrolysis in the treatment of SCFE is unknown. Clinically, chondrolysis presents with loss of range of motion, pain, limp, and joint contracture. The question of whether it is an autoimmune phenomenon or has some factors interfering with cartilage nutrition is yet to be defined. Risk factors leading to chondrolysis include cast immobilization, unrecognized pin penetration (only if the pin is left in the joint), severe slips, and long duration of symptoms before treatment. The treatment of chondrolysis is difficult, with most patients requiring anti-inflammatory agents and bed rest with skeletal traction to relieve their contractures. Rarely, patients may require surgical capsulectomy and continuous passive motion.[9,11,35-37]

The treatment of SCFE is somewhat controversial, but most authors now agree that pinning in situ offers the best long-term results, with secondary corrective osteotomies as necessary to relieve mechanical symptoms or pain once the physis is closed. In general, patients with the condition do well over the long term if the slip is of mild or moderate degree and good congruity between the femoral head and the acetabulum remains. It is only in the severe slips that the deterioration occurs with degenerative changes over time. **(CD-59.1)**

SCFE differs from other pediatric hip disorders such as Legg-Calvé-Perthes disease and developmental dysplasia of the hip in that slips occur at an age when the majority of acetabular development is completed. Because of the maturity of the acetabulum, no adaptation to head deformity can occur. Mild and most moderate slips may cause some incongruity and eventually lead to degenerative disease. Aseptic necrosis and chondrolysis, which may also compromise outcome, are associated with a high incidence of degenerative disease.

References

1. Schein AJ: Acute severe slipped capital femoral epiphysis. *Clin Orthop* 1967;51:151-166.
2. Segal LS, Weitzel PP, Davidson RS: Valgus slipped capital femoral epiphysis: Fact or fiction? *Clin Orthop* 1996;322:91-98.
3. Ponseti I, Barta CK: Evaluation of treatment of slipping of the capital femoral epiphysis. *Surg Gynecol Obstet* 1948;86:87-97.
4. Fahey JJ, O'Brien ET: Acute slipped capital femoral epiphysis: Review of the literature and report of ten cases. *J Bone Joint Surg Am* 1965;47:1105-1127.
5. Boyer DW, Mickelson MR, Ponseti IV: Slipped capital femoral epiphysis: Long-term follow-up and study of one hundred and twenty-one patients. *J Bone Joint Surg Am* 1981;63:85-95.
6. Loder RT, Aronson DD, Greenfield ML: The epidemiology of bilateral slipped capital femoral epiphysis: A study of children in Michigan. *J Bone Joint Surg Am* 1993;75:1141-1147.
7. Aadalen RJ, Weiner DS, Hoyt W, Herndon CH: Acute slipped capital femoral epiphysis. *J Bone Joint Surg Am* 1974;56:1473-1487.
8. Casey BH, Hamilton HW, Bobechko WP: Reduction of acutely slipped upper femoral epiphysis. *J Bone Joint Surg* Br 1972;54:607-614.
9. Carney BT, Weinstein SL, Noble J: Long-term follow-up of slipped capital femoral epiphysis. *J Bone Joint Surg Am* 1991;73:667-674.
10. Jacobs B: Diagnosis and natural history of slipped femoral capital epiphysis. *Instr Course Lect* 1972;21:167-173.
11. Aronsson DD, Loder RT: Treatment of the unstable (acute) slipped capital femoral epiphysis. *Clin Orthop* 1996;322:99-110.
12. Loder RT, Richards BS, Shapiro PS, Reznick LR, Aronson DD: Acute slipped capital femoral epiphysis: The importance of physeal stability. *J Bone Joint Surg Am* 1993;75:1134-1140.
13. Wedge JH, Wasylenko MJ: The natural history of congenital dislocation of the hip: A critical review. *Clin Orthop* 1978;137:154-162.
14. Carney BT, Weinstein SL: Natural history of untreated chronic slipped capital femoral epiphysis. *Clin Orthop* 1996;322:43-47.
15. Howorth B: Slipping of the capital femoral epiphysis: History. *Clin Orthop* 1966;48:11-32.
16. Hall JE: The results of treatment of slipped femoral epiphysis. *J Bone Joint Surg Br* 1957;39:659-673.
17. Oram V: Epiphysiolysis of the head of the femur: A follow-up examination with special reference to end results and the social prognosis. *Acta Orthop Scand* 1953;23:100-120.
18. Ross PM, Lyne ED, Morawa LG: Slipped capital femoral epiphysis: Long-term results after 10-38 years. *Clin Orthop* 1979;141:176-180.
19. Johnston RC, Larson CB: Results of treatment of hip disorders with cup arthroplasty. *J Bone Joint Surg Am* 1969;51:1461-1479.
20. Murray RO: The aetiology of primary osteoarthritis of the hip. *Br J Radiol* 1965;38: 810-824.
21. Solomon L: Patterns of osteoarthritis of the hip. *J Bone Joint Surg Br* 1976;58:176-183.
22. Stulberg SD, Cordell LD, Harris WH: Unrecognized Childhood Hip Disease: A Major Cause of Idiopathic Osteoarthritis of the Hip, in *The Hip: Proceedings of the Third Open Scientific Meeting of the Hip Society.* St. Louis, MO, CV Mosby 1975, pp 212-230.
23. Resnick D: The 'tilt deformity' of the femoral head in osteoarthritis of the hip: A poor indicator of previous epiphysiolysis. *Clin Radiol* 1976;27:355-363.
24. Jerre T: A study in slipped upper femoral epiphysis: With special reference to the late functional and roentgenological results and the value of closed reduction. *Acta Orthop Scand* 1950;6(suppl):5-157.
25. Jerre T: Early complications after osteosynthesis with a three flanged nail in situ for slipped epiphysis. *Acta Orthop Scand* 1958;27:126-134.
26. Ordeberg G, Hansson LI, Sandstrom S: Slipped capital femoral epiphysis in southern Sweden: Long-term result with no treatment or symptomatic primary treatment. *Clin Orthop* 1984;191:95-104.
27. Southwick WO: Osteotomy through the lesser trochanter for slipped capital femoral epiphysis. *J Bone Joint Surg Am* 1967;49:807-835.
28. Wilson PD, Jacobs B, Schecter L: Slipped capital femoral epiphysis: An end-result study. *J Bone Joint Surg Am* 1965;47:1128-1145.
29. Mickelson MR, Ponseti IV, Cooper RR, Maynard JA: The ultrastructure of the growth plate in slipped capital femoral epiphysis. *J Bone Joint Surg Am* 1977;59:1076-1081.
30. Billing L, Severin E: Slipping epiphysis of the hip: A roentgenological and clinical study based on a new roentgen technique. *Acta Radiol* 1959;174(suppl):5-76.
31. Brodetti A: The blood supply of the femoral neck and head in relation to the damaging effects of nails and screws. *J Bone Joint Surg Br* 1960;42:794-801.
32. Claffey TJ: Avascular necrosis of the femoral head: An anatomical study. *J Bone Joint Surg Br* 1960;42:802-809.
33. Dietz FR: Traction reduction of acute and acute-on-chronic slipped capital femoral epiphysis. *Clin Orthop* 1994;302:101-110.
34. Krahn TH, Canale ST, Beaty JH, Warner WC, Lourenco P: Long-term follow-up of patients with avascular necrosis after treatment of slipped capital femoral epiphysis. *J Pediatr Orthop* 1993;13:154-158.
35. Frymoyer JW: Chondrolysis of the hip following Southwick osteotomy for severe slipped capital femoral epiphysis. *Clin Orthop* 1974;99:120-124.
36. Ingram AJ, Clarke MS, Clarke CS Jr, Marshall WR: Chondrolysis complicating slipped capital femoral epiphysis. *Clin Orthop* 1982;165: 99-109.
37. O'Brien ET, Fahey JJ: Remodeling of the femoral neck after in situ pinning for slipped capital femoral epiphysis. *J Bone Joint Surg Am* 1977;59:62-68.

Reference to Video

Moseley C, Canale ST, Morrissy R: Pediatric: At issue in orthopaedics. *Slipped Capital Femoral Epiphysis (SCFE): Diagnosis, Treatment, and Postoperative Care.* Rosemont, IL, American Academy of Orthopaedic Surgeons, 1994.

VOLUME 50 2001

Cumulative Index 1997-2001

Please note: Page numbers in bold refer to information in this volume, ICL Volume 50, published in 2001. All other page numbers refer to Volumes 46, 47, 48, and 49 published in 1997, 1998, 1999, and 2000. Page numbers in italic/bold italic refer to figures or figure legends.

A

Abduction orthosis
- prescription of, 48: 24
- and rehabilitation, for acetabular transplants, 48: 73
- use of, 49: 126

Abduction pillow, 47: 62, 83
Abductor digiti quinti, weakness, **50: 527**
Abductor hallucis muscle, 47: 426-427
Ablation, glenohumeral capsules, **50: 31**
Abrasion, wear particles, **50: 186**
Abrasion arthroplasty
- arthroscopic, 48: 139
- treatment of chondral injuries, 48: 634-635

Abrasion arthroscopy, knee joint, **50: 501-502**
Abscesses. *see also* Infections
- drainage of, 49: 589-590
- and early osteomyelitis, *49: 588*
- prevalence in diabetic foot, 48: 298

Accreditation, and performance measurement, 48: 677-678
Accreditation Council for Graduate Medical Education, clinical ethics requirement, 49: 639
Acetabular components, constrained, **50: 281-287, 283-284**
Acetabular cups
- cavitary defects, 48: *59*
  - and bone loss, 48: *51, 52*
  - outcomes of treatment, 48: 63
  - treatment of, 48: 57-65
- centralization, **50: 311-312, 314**
- difficult sockets, 49: 57-61
- fixation, **50: *283***
- migration, **50: 216**
- modular bilobed, **50: *344***
- oblong, **50: 314**
- placement and coverage, **50: 309**
- polyethylene, **50: *165***
- porous spread-press-fit, migration of, **50: 285**
- stability after reconstruction, **50: 227, 212-213**
- UHMWPE, **50: 169-170**

Acetabular dysplasia
- pathomechanism, **50: 229**
- septic arthritis, **50: 318**

Acetabular fractures, 48: 481-494
- anterior column, 48: 488
- anterior wall, 48: 488
- associated anterior column and posterior hemitransverse, 48: 489
- associated both-column, 48: 489
- associated transverse and posterior wall, 48: 489
- complications to surgical treatment, 48: 490-491
- contraindications to surgery, 48: 485
- failure of fixation, **50: *345***
- heterotopic ossification, 48: 491-492, **50: 346-348**
- insertion of femoral stems, **50: 343-344**
- nonunion, **50: 342-343**
- open reduction and internal fixation, 48: 485-489
- osteonecrosis, **50: 348-349**
- periprosthetic, 47: *231-232,* 231-235, *234,* 252
- posterior column, 48: 488
- posterior wall, 48: 487-488, **50: *342, 343***
- primary THA after, **50: 335-354**
- radiographic assessment, 48: 482-483, **50: 336**
- salvage of late cases, **50: 349**
- surgical outcomes, 48: 489-490
- T-type, 48: 489, **50: *338, 340, 341***
- THR after, 48: 494
- timing of THA, **50: 338**
- transverse, 48: 488-489
- types of, 48: *486, 487*

Acetabular osteotomy, classification of, **50: 549, *550***
Acetabular revision arthroplasty
- clinical results of, 47: 271-273
- instrumentation used for, 47: *268*
- morcellized allografting for, 47: 265-273
- surgical technique, 47: *268*-269

Acetabular rim liners
- components, **50: *282***
- dissociation, **50: *284***
- elevated, **50: 268**
- types of, **50: *277***

Acetabular screws, four-quadrant system for safe placement of, 47: *280*-281
Acetabulum
- allografts of, 48: 67-75
- anterior-posterior view landmarks, 48: *482*-483
- AP view, *49: 7*
- assessment of components, 48: *30*
- augmentation, 49: 30-31, **50: 551**
- biomechanics, 48: 483-484
- bone grafts, motion in sheep model, 49: *108*
- bone loss
  - evaluation of, 48: 45-47
  - and preoperative planning, 48: 50-55
  - and revision hip arthroplasty, 48: 57-65
  - views of, 48: *53*
- capsular healing, **50: 291**

capsular insufficiency, **50: 291**
class III metastatic defect, 49: *469*
classification of deficiencies, 48: 67-68, *68,* **50: *337***
radiographic criteria, 48: 68-69
classification of periacetabular lesions, 49: 467
component failure, 48: 43
computed tomography of fractures, 48: 483
constrained implants, **50: 272**
contained defects, **50: 340**
coverage of, 49: 29, **50: *233***
CT, 48: 47
defects of, radiographs, 48: *81*
development and growth, **50: 537**
dysplasia, **50: 255, 541**
fixation of, 46: 543
and perioperative acetabular fractures, 47: 252
iliac oblique view, 48: *483*
imaging of defects, **50: *337***
impaction grafting
four-month biopsy, 49: *106*
goat model, 49: *104*
histologic analysis, 48: 84-86, *85*
new bone formation in, 48: *86*
impaction instruments, 48: *82*
intrinsic defects, surgical strategies, **50: *341***
metal backing of components, 49: 77
obturator oblique view, 48: *483*
osteolysis, 49: *71*
classification system for, 48: 37-42
type I, 48: 38-39
type II, 48: 39-40, *40*
type III, 48: 40
position, Ranawat's method of determination, 48: 46
preoperative and postoperative coverage, **50: *258***
radiographs
anteroposterior view, 48: *47*
iliac oblique view, 48: *47*
obturator oblique view, 48: *47*
reaming of, **50: *303***
reconstruction, 48: *83,* 49: 28-32, *58,* **50: *226***
clinical results, **50: 224-226**
with impaction bone graft, **50: 221-228**
late, **50: *339***
outcomes, 48: 73-74
postoperative care, 48: 73, **50: 224**
preoperative planning, 48: 68-70
preparation for, **50: *339-343***
surgical technique, 48: 70-73
technique, **50: 223-224**
redirectional osteotomies, **50: 549-551**
replacement, **50: *223***
reshaping osteotomies, **50: 551**
revision surgery technique, **50: 222**
revisions, long-term follow-up of, 48: 87, *88*
roof arc measurement, 48: *484, 485*
small components, 49: 29
templating, 49: 7-9
type IIA defects, 48: *61*
type IIB defects, 48: *62*
type IIIB defects, 48: *69*
uncontained defects, **50: 340-342**
use of fracture table, 48: 485-487
vascular structures adjacent to, 47: *280*-281
vascularity, **50: *235***
Acetaminophen, pain management, 49: 515
Achilles/patellar tendon, allografts, 48: 520
Achilles tendon
ACL reconstruction graft, **50: 469**
acute ruptures of, 48: 219-220
anatomy, 48: 211-212
biomechanics of, 47: 405
chronic rupture, 48: 224-229
Haglund's deformity, 48: 215-217
heel pain, 47: 425-427
nerve entrapment syndromes, 47: 426-427
plantar fasciitis, 47: 405, 425-426
posterior, 47: 421-422
incidence of, 46: 577, 47: 419
insertion disorders, 48: 211-218
insertional tendinitis, 47: 424-*425*
nodular deformity, 47: *421*
peritendinitis, 47: *420*-421
and posterior heel pain, 48: 213
problems in athletes, 47: 419-427
retrocalcaneal bursitis, 47: 422-424, 48: 217-218
rupture of
chronic, 48: 224-229
complications after repair, 48: 223-224
diagnosis, 48: 220
nonsurgical treatment of, 48: 220-222
rehabilitation after surgery, 48: 223
surgical treatment of, 48: 222-224
stretching, **50: 516, 526**
tendinitis, 46: 577-580, 48: 211-218
insertional, 48: 213-215
noninsertional, 48: 212-213
Achondroplasia, cause of, 46: 477, 47: 466, 471
ACL. *See* Anterior cruciate ligament
Acquired flatfoot deformity, 46: 393-404
anatomy and pathophysiology, 46: 393-394
diagnosis of, 46: 394-395
etiology of, 46: 394
treatment of
arthrodesis, 46: 400-404
calcaneal osteotomy, 46: 397-*398*
flexor tendon transfer, 46: 398-*400,* 401
nonsurgical, 46: 395-396
surgical, 46: 396-397
tenosynovectomy, 46: 397
Acromed system, 48: 440
Acromioclavicular joints (AC)
classification injuries, 49: 407
complete dislocations, complications of treatment, 49: 404-412
evaluation of, 46: 43-*45,* 47: 29-30
and failed rotator cuff repair, 47: 80-81
osteoarthritis, 47: *36*
rheumatoid arthritis, 47: 36-37
Acromion
assessing shape of, 47: *6*-7, 23, 30
postoperative fractures of, 47: *89*
three types of, 47: 22, *30*
Acromioplasty
advantages of, 47: 21-22, 27
arthroscopic, 47: 21-27
conservative, **50: *46***
technique, 47: 24-26, 88-90
Active range of motion, postoperative protocols for anterior instability, **50: 14**
Activities of daily living (ADLs)
in the elderly, 46: 410-411
Japanese Orthopaedic Association Score, 48: 420

Acupuncture
autonomic effects, 49: 560-561
bioelectrical properties, 49: 561-562
humeral mechanisms, 49: 560
local effects, 49: 561
middle effects, 49: 562
pain management, 49: 559-562
pathways, 49: 559-560
scientific basis, 49: 559
treatment of CRPS, 49: 554
trigger points, 49: 562
Acute brachial neuritis. *See* Parsonage-Turner syndrome
Acute normovolemic hemodilution (ANH), use in the orthopaedic setting, 48: 658
Adductor releases, and hip contractures, 48: 97
Adhesive capsulitis, diabetic, 49: 283-293
Adhesive wear, occurrence, **50: 165**
Administrative responsibility, and medical malpractice, 48: 701
Adolescents, dynamic scapholunate instability, **50: 129-130**
Adrenocorticoid deficiency, consideration in preoperative planning, 48: 98
Adson test, 47: 87
older nerve compression, 49: 307
Advance directives, teaching of ethics, 49: 640
Aeonian process, polyethylene cross-linking, **50: 173**
Age
arthroplasty results, **50: 83**
DDH open reduction, **50: 549**
and disk constituents, **50: 146**
dynamic scapholunate instability, **50: 129-130**
education selection, **50: 502**
and glenohumeral instability, **50: 23**
and infection rates, 49: 36
OA of the knee, **50: 499-511**
plantar fasciitis, **50: 523**
proximal femoral megaprostheses, 49: *142*
scaphoid fractures, **50: 105**
surgery for obstetrical brachial plexus palsy, 49: *319*
symptoms of spinal stenosis, **50: 150**
volumetric wear rates, THA, 49: 74
Aggrecans, 47: 480-*481*
in the meniscus, 49: 208
in osteoarthritis, 49: 486
Agility ankle, outcomes, 48: 264-265, 264-*265*
Aging
ankle osteoarthritis, 48: 233
articular cartilage, 46: 461-463, 47: 489, 48: 235
tensile fracture stress, 48: *236*
of cartilage, compared to osteoarthritis, 49: *484*
cervical spine, 49: 339
chondrocytes, 46: 461-462
distribution of bone lesions, 48: *610*
evaluation of bone tumors, 48: 609
infection at arthroplasty sites, 48: 112
intervertebral disks, 46: 463-464
musculoskeletal system function, 46: 459-460
and pharmacology, 46: 415
population trends, 49: 569
and skeletal muscle, 46: 460-461
and soft tissues, 46: 460-465
theories of, 46: 410
total joint arthroplasty, 46: 418-420
total knee arthroplasty, 46: 421-422
Agonist/antagonist activity, 46: 40
AIDS. *See* HIV/AIDS
Akin procedure, 46: 366-*367, 368*
Albee osteotomies, **50: 551**
Albumin, decision making in foot amputations, 48: 323
Alcohol, allograft sterilization, 49: 617
Alcoholism
in the elderly, 46: 413-*414*
and osteonecrosis of the humeral head, 48: 350
total contact casting and lesions due to, 48: 305
Algorithms
for anterior knee pain, 47: 339-343
elbow dislocations and fractures, **50: *100***
failed lateral epicondylitis surgery, 47: *171*
femoral osteolysis, **50: *199, 203***
femoral reconstruction, 49: *117*
infection after TKA, **50: *374, 409***
malunited proximal humerus fractures, 47: 140
osteolysis after total hip arthroplasty, 47: *322, 323, 325*
osteolysis treatment, 48: *38*
osteonecrosis treatment, 49: 181
periprosthetic patellar fractures, 47: *457*
posterior cruciate ligament (PCL) injuries, 48: *204*
primary treatment of chondral injuries, 48: *630-631*
prostatic hip infections, **50: *328***
RSD management, 49: *555*-556
supracondylar femoral fracture, **50: *384***
supracondylar periprosthetic fractures, 47: *452*
treatment for dysplasia, **50: *552***
Alignment
limb, and periarticular osteotomies, 48: 279-285
using intramedullary instruments, 48: *180*
Alkaline phosphatase, serum, laboratory investigations of bone tumors, 48: 608
Allen classification, of cervical trauma, 48: 438
Allen test, ulnar nerve compression, 49: 315
Allergies, local anesthetics, 49: 527
Allografts, 47: 526-527
acetabular, 48: 67-75
acetabular augmentation, 49: 31-32
acetabular revision arthroplasty, 47: 265-273
clinical results of, 47: 271-273
surgical technique, 47: *268*-269
ACL revision, **50: *455***
articular cartilage restoration, 48: 624
bone, 48: 58, 648-650
acceptance of, 48: 70
advantages of, 48: 67
defined, 46: 230-231
and disease transmission, 48: 64-65
immunogenicity, 49: 97-98
inflammatory responses, 49: 98
preparation of, 48: 60
use in hip revision surgery, 48: 645
circumferential replacement, revision THA, 49: 147-159
composite, 46: *233,* 234
corticocancellous bone, immunogenicity, 49: 97
defined, 48: 79
extensor mechanism, **50: *405***
immunology of, 48: 650-651
impaction grafts
biomechanics, 49: 107
complications, 49: 114-117
femoral fractures, 49: 114-115
femoral revision, 49: *116*
THA outcomes, 49: *112-113*
THA revisions, 49: 103-110
interface with prosthesis, 49: 152
junction with host bone, 49: 152
for knee ligaments and meniscal reconstruction, 47: 379-394

ACL reconstruction, 47: 385-388
LCL reconstruction, 47: 389-391
meniscal allografts, 47: 392-393
PCL reconstruction, 47: 388-389
management of type 3 defects, 48: 171-173
meniscal, 49: *196*
morcellized bone, 48: 79-88
impacted
and cement, 48: 79-88
mechanical stability of reconstructions, 48: 83
musculoskeletal, screening, 49: 615-618
onlay, 49: 97-101
osteochondral, **50: 484**
osteochondral allografts for the knee, 47: 500, 517-*521*
results of, 47: 512
screening for donors, 47: 517-518
surgical procedure, 47: *518-521*
periprosthetic femoral fracture treatment, 47: 257-*263*
advantages and disadvantages of, 47: 262
technique, 47: 257-259
planning revision TKA, 48: 164
reconstruction, and medial epicondylar osteotomy, 48: 155-156
revascularization, **50: 216-217**
in revision knee arthroplasty, 46: 231-234
selection of preparation, 49: 151-152
sterilization of, 47: 380-385
and disease transmission, 47: 385, 527
structural
considerations, 49: 148-149
femoral, 49: *156*
preparation of, 49: *154*
strut, reinforcement of femoral allografts, 49: *155*
tendon, **50: 63**
TKA, **50: 397**
in total knee arthroplasty, 46: 234-236
treatment of malignant bone tumors, 48: 599-600
treatment of osteonecrosis, **50: 492**
use after infection, **50: 330**
viral transmission, **50: 469**
Allogrip, 46: 233
Alumina ceramics
physical properties of, **50: *167***
retrieval analysis, 49: 75
in THA, 49: 43
Alumina-on-alumina bearings, **50: 167**
Alzheimer's disease, 46: 423
American Academy of Orthopaedic Surgeons (AAOS)
acetabular defects due to metastatic disease, 49: 467
bone loss classification, 49: *91,* 92-93, 148
classification of acetabular deficiencies, 48: 47-48, *48*
classification of osteolysis, **50: 202**
Guide to the Ethical Practice of Orthopaedic Surgery, 49: 633
HIV serosurvey, 49: 621-622
land mine initiatives, 49: 433
outcomes assessment questionnaires, 48: 679-683
principles of involvement in the Third World, 49: 580-583
services in the developing world, 49: 572
and the SF-36, 48: 420
traveling faculty program, 49: *572*
Web site, 49: 573
American Association of Tissue Banks (AATB), 47: 385, 527
donor screening, 49: 617
guidelines for graft selection, 48: 70
American College of Radiology, diagnostic criteria for osteoarthritis, 49: *483*
American Joint Committee on Cancer
soft-tissue sarcomas staging, 49: *445*
staging system for soft-tissue tumors, 49: *444*-446
American Medical Association (AMA)
Guides to the Evaluation of Permanent Impairment, 4th edition, 48: 451-461
landmine initiatives, 49: 433
American Public Health Association (APHA), land mine initiatives, 49: 433
American Shoulder and Elbow Surgeons (ASES) Assessment, thermal capsulorrhaphy, **50: 26-27**
American Spinal Injury Association (ASIA)
impairment scale, 46: 117
and neurological status, 48: 438
E-Aminocaproic acid, use in the orthopaedic setting, 48: 656
Aminoglycosides, treatment of diabetic foot infection, 48: 319
Amitriptyline, and aging, 46: 415
Amoxicillin-clavulanic acid, treatment of diabetic foot infection, 48: 319
Amoxicillin-sulbactam acid, treatment of diabetic foot infection, 48: 319
Amputation surgery
below the knee, 48: *328*
comparison with reconstruction, for Charcot arthropathy, 48: 276-277
cost compared with nonsurgical treatment, 48: 313
diabetic foot, 48: 322-323
digits, 49: *384*
following infected TKA, **50: 411**
foot and ankle, 48: 687-689
for infected knee arthroplasty, 46: 217
infected knees, **50: 370**
injuries to the upper extremities, 49: 379
land mine injuries, 49: 432
versus limb salvage, 46: 511-517
cost of, 46: 517
factors affecting outcome, 46: 513-517
factors affecting salvage, 46: 511-512
scoring systems, 46: 512-513
which injuries, 46: 511
lower extremities, frequency, 48: *321*
partial, diabetic foot, 48: 321-329
in peripheral vascular disease, 46: 501-508, 48: 687-691
cognitive and psychological requirements for walking in amputees, 46: 502
functional levels, 46: 505-508
joints as energy couples, 46: *501*-502
load transfer, 46: *502-503*
rehabilitation, 46: 508
selection of level, 46: 504-505
wound healing, 46: 503-*504*
reasons for, 48: 321-322
risk in diabetes, 48: 317
through knee, 48: 689
transfemoral, 48: 689-*690*
transmetatarsal, 48: *688*
transtibial, 48: *688, 689*
treatment of malignant bone tumors, 48: 599-600
treatment of RSD, 49: 555
Anabolic steroids, and collagen dysplasia, 48: 219-220
Analgesia
drug groups, 49: 514
postoperative, total hip arthroplasty, 48: 35
in treating loxoscelism, 46: 71
use in cervical degenerative disease, 48: 434
Anaphylaxis, defined, 48: 548-549
Anconeus compartment syndrome, 47: 170
Anderson Orthopaedic Research Institute (AORI), bone defect classification, 46: 229-230, 48: *168*-169

Anemia
consideration in preoperative planning, 48: 97
normocytic normochromic, 49: 458
and wound healing, **50: 359-360**
Anesthesia
arthroscopic shoulder surgery, **50: 56**
arthroscopy of the elbow, 49: 239
continuous epidural, postoperative, 49: 219-220
invasive techniques, 49: 519
laryngeal general masked, **50: 56**
pain in orthopaedic surgery, 49: 523-537
total shoulder arthroplasty, **50: 79**
Anesthetics
history of, 49: 523-524
local
complications, 49: 527-533
molecular structure, 49: *525*
perineural dosage, 49: *527*
pharmacology of, 49: 524-525
Aneurysmal bone cysts
and pediatric back pain, 48: 538-539
treatment of, 48: 593-594, *595*
Angiofibroblastic hyperplasia, 46: 572
Angiography
of bone tumors, 48: 611
of iliac vessels, 48: 54
of left external iliac artery, 48: *34*
preoperative investigations, 48: 31, *31*
soft-tissue tumors, 48: 618, 49: 439, 448-449
Angiolipomas, description, 49: 438
Ankle
amputation, 48: 687-689
anatomic dissection, 49: *262*
anatomy, 48: *234*-235, 49: 262
arthritis, 48: *281*
arthrodesis, 46: 348-351, 48: 255-261, 49: 259-279
chronic instability, **50: 517-518**
débridement, 49: *269*
débridement and fusion, 48: 243-247
diastasis, 49: *266*
dynamic stabilization, **50: 515**
fusion with bone loss, 46: 354
guide pin placement, 49: *269*
imaging of, 46: 524-526
instrumentation for débridement, 49: *268*
inversion injuries, 49: 261-263
lateral distraction instrumentation, 49: *268*
lateral instability, **50: *516***
measurement of intra-articular pressure, 48: *251*
medial distraction instrumentation, 49: *268*
motion of, 48: 234
osteoarthritis, 48: 233-240
joint distraction as treatment for, 48: 249-254
posterior capsular disruption, 49: *263*
postreduction fusion position, 49: *269*
prevalence of joint degeneration, 48: *237*
prioritization of reconstructive surgeries, 48: 94-95
protection of the talar body, 48: *543*
solid fusion, 49: *269*
sprains, **50: 515-520**
classification of, **50: 515-516, *516***
treatment, **50: 516-517**
stabilization techniques, **50: *519***
surgical treatment for neuropathic arthropathy, 48: 269-277
syndesmosis injuries, 49: 263-266, **50: 518-520**
valgus and myelomeningocele, 48: 545
Ankle arthroplasty, state of the art, 48: 263-268
Ankle-brachial index (ABI), 48: 296
Ankle/brachial pressure index, 46: 183
Ankle disarticulation, 46: 506
Syme's, 48: 688-689
Ankle equinus, polio-related deformities, 49: 597-*598*
Ankle-foot orthoses (AFOs)
bivalved, 48: 308, 312
calf-lacer, 48: *276*
in myelomeningocele patients, 48: 546-547
polypropylene clamshell-type, 48: *276*
use of, 49: 277
Ankle fractures, 46: 311-318. *see also* Fractures
anatomy and biomechanics, 46: 311-*312*
association of tibial shaft fractures with ipsilateral, 46: 276-277
classification of, 46: 312-315
current issues in, 46: 315
deltoid ligament injuries, 46: 315-316
isolated lateral malleolar, 46: 315
posterior malleolar, 46: 316
postoperative and postinjury management, 46: 318
radiographic evaluation, 46: 312, *313*
syndesmotic injuries, 46: 316-318
Ankle-pressure index (API), 48: 296
Ankylosing spondylitis, 46: 394
arthroplasty procedure, 49: 65
cementless fixation, 49: *66*
etiology, 48: 102
evaluation in preoperative planning, 48: 97
and fusion in the spine, 48: *97*
total hip arthroplasty in, 48: 104
use of femoral allograft, 48: *646*
Ankylosis, evaluation of, **50: 300**
Anterior cervical diskectomy, Robinson-type, 48: 423
Anterior cruciate ligament (ACL)
with focal chondral damage, 48: 641
injuries
and knee envelope of function, 48: *195*
knee function after, 48: 185-196
treatment factors, 48: 195
injuries in skeletally immature patients, 47: 351-358
diagnosis, 47: 351
tibial eminence fractures, 47: 352-*354*
treatment for, 47: 354-358
interference screws, **50: *453***
LCL deficiency, **50: 451**
load transference, 48: 187
loss of motion following surgery on, 46: *251-259,* 47: 361
literature review, 46: 252-256
and meniscal repair, 49: 195-196
protocols, 49: 208
relationship to meniscus, 49: 189
revision, 47: 361-366
rupture
assessment of trauma, 48: *194*
and envelope of function of a knee, 48: *189*
Anterior cruciate ligament (ACL) reconstruction
and aged patients, **50: 502**
allograft, 47: 385-388, **50: 454-455**
autograft revision, **50: *457***
bioresorbable implants, 46: *541-542*
classification of failure, **50: 463-464**
graft failure rates, **50: 458**
graft selection, **50: 468-470**
graft tensioning, **50: 453-454**
notchplasty revision, **50: 453**

outcomes, **50: *454***
placement of graft, 49: *212*
preoperative evaluation, **50: 467-468**
pseudolaxity, 48: *204*
recurrent instability, **50: 463-474**
revision, **50: 451-461**
revision outcomes, **50: *456***
secondary stabilizers, **50: 466**
Anterior cruciate ligament transection (ACLT), and induction of osteoarthritis, 48: 253
Anterior-inferior subluxation, complication in humeral head replacement, 46: 19
Anterior inferior tibiofibular (AITF) ligament, 49: 263-264
Anterior instability, after TSA, **50: 84**
Anterior labrum, heat probes application, **50: *33***
Anterior-posterior translation, mobile-bearing TKR, **50: 434-435, *435-436***
Anterior release for spinal deformity, 46: 135
Anterior talofibular ligaments (ATFL), anatomy, 49: 262
Anterior tibial talar spurs, arthroscopic approach, 48: 245
Anterolateral approaches
THA revisions, 49: 86
THAs, 49: 15-16
Anterolisthesis, spinal, **50: *143***
Anteromedial approaches, in knee arthroplasty, 48: 165
Anteromedial bone grafting for tibial shaft fractures, 46: 283
Anteroposterior technetium scintiscan, of the knees, in osseous homeostasis, 48: *192*
Antiadhesion membrane, 46: 543-544
Antiarrhythmics, pain management, 49: 519
Antibiotics. *see also* Infections
acute osteomyelitis, 49: 589
arthroplasty site infection, 48: 115-117
cement impregnated with, **50: *323*, 329-330, *412***
deep periprosthetic joint infection, 46: 557-558
diabetic foot infections, 48: 318, 319
elution from bone cement, 48: 117
impregnated beads, **50: 329-330**
infected arthroplasties, **50: 369**
infected hip arthroplasty, 47: 300
antibiotic-loaded cement, 47: 303-304
infected knee arthroplasty, 46: 217
intravenous administration of, in tibial shaft fractures, 46: 293-294
local delivery systems, 48: 117
perioperative, bone graft management, 49: 153
periprostatic infections, **50: 410**
prophylactic, 49: 611-612
after acetabular transplantation, 48: 73
after total hip arthroplasty, 48: 105
and bone grafts, 49: 152
and infection at arthroplasty sites, 48: 113
wound complication management in THA, 46: 167-168
Antibodies, polyclonal, indium labeled, **50: 321**
Anticholinergic drugs and aging, 46: 415
Anticoagulants, contraindication for chondroitin sulfate, 49: 492
Anticonvulsants, pain management, 49: 519
Antidepressants
and aging, 46: 415
pain management, 49: 519
use in cervical degenerative disease, 48: 434
Antifibrinolytics, use in the orthopaedic setting, 48: 656
Antigen-presenting cells (APCs), immune response to allografts, 49: 150
Antihistamines, and aging, 46: 415
Antimalarials, treating rheumatoid arthritis, 46: 78
Antimetabolic agents, consideration in preoperative planning, 48: 98
Antineoplastic agents, consideration in preoperative planning, 48: 98
Antiprotrusio cage, and acetabular defect reconstruction, 48: 68, *69*
Antiprotrusio rings, use of, 49: 8
Antipruritics, in treating loxoscelism, 46: 71
Antipyretics, in treating loxoscelism, 46: 71
Anxiety, and pain, 49: 541
AO/ASIF classification for soft-tissue injuries, 46: 294
AO classification system
for ankle injury, 46: 313, 315
intra-articular fracture of the radius, 48: 469-*470*
AO dynamic compression plate, 49: *327*
AO/Orthopaedic Trauma Association classification, of pilonfractures, 46: 318-319
AO plates
femoral fractures and children, 49: 419
internal fixation in children, 49: 418
Apert syndrome, 46: 477
Apprehension sign, 46: 571, 47: 347
Aprotinin, use in the orthopaedic setting, 48: 656
Arcade of Frohse, PIN compression, 49: *298*
Arcade of Struthers, and the ulnar nerve, 49: 305
Arcs of motion, in modular femoral heads with flanges, 49: 78
Armed conflicts, children at risk, 49: 569-570
Arteriography
decision making in foot amputations, 48: 323
as preoperative evaluation, 46: 183
vascular evaluation using, 48: 297
Arteriosclerosis, and Achilles tendon rupture, 48: 220
Arthritis. *see also* Osteoarthritis
ankle
classification of, 48: *281*
treatment of, 48: 255-256
degenerative, 49: 247-248, 256
of the knee, 48: 135-140
elbow, arthroscopic treatment, 49: 247-252
facet joints, **50: 146-147**
following instability repairs, **50: 83**
following scaphoid nonunion, **50: 118-119**
in geriatric population, 46: 409
glenohumeral joint, **50: *76***
gouty, 46: 75
inflammatory
difficult femurs, 49: 64-65
of the elbow, 49: 247
laboratory tests in diagnosis, 48: 255
surgical management of, 48: 93-106
juvenile, effects on bone quality, 48: 97
juvenile rheumatoid, total knee arthroplasty, **50: 507**
lateral compartmental, after Girdlestone arthroplasty, 48: 161
monoarticular, 46: 78
sternoclavicular joint, 49: 404
and osteonecrosis, 49: 173
palindromic, 46: 78
polyarticular inflammatory, occupational therapy evaluation, 48: 94
postoperative, acromioclavicular joint, 49: 412
posttraumatic, 49: *267*
acromioclavicular joint, 49: 408-409
with offset of tibial metaphysis, 48: *162*
prevalence rates, 49: *431*
progressive, after unicondylar knee arthroplasty (UKA), 48: 143
rheumatoid
elbow, 49: 256
glenohumeral joint, **50: 73-77**
sternoclavicular joint, 49: 404
total knee arthroplasty, **50: 507**
and wound healing, **50: 359**
scapholunate advanced collapsed, **50: 130-131**
septic, 46: 78
femoral head, **50: *327***

spontaneous fusion, **50: *323***
sternoclavicular joint, 49: 404
shoulder arthroplasty for, 47: 128-129
tibiotalar, arthroscopic ankle fusion, 49: 266-267
tubercular, after arthroplasty, **50: *326***
Arthritis Impact Measurement Scale (AIMS), 46: 441
Arthrodesis. *See also* Fusion
and acquired flatfoot deformity, 46: 400-404
in active infection, **50: 321-322**
ankle, 46: 348-351, 48: 255-261, 49: 266-270
arthroscopic, 48: 243-247
arthroscopic technique, 48: 245-*247, 246-247*
arthroscopic treatment, 49: 259-279
complications and failures, 48: 257-258
methods for, 48: 256-257
ankle arthroplasty, outcomes, 48: 263-267
Blair-type, 46: 333, *336, 350*-351
conversion of, 49: 6, 8, 60
conversion technique, **50: 301-302**
conversion to THA, **50: 297-305**
failure, and biomechanical forces, 48: *556*
first metatarsophalangeal joint, 46: 380-382
hip joint pain after, **50: *297***
outcomes, **50: 297-298, 302-304**
salvage procedures for rheumatoid arthritis, 48: 100-101
indications for conversion of, **50: 298**
infected knees, **50: 370**
infected TKA, **50: 410-411**
intercalary allograft, 48: *600*
joints injuries, 49: 385-386
lumbar spinal stenosis, 49: 368
malrotation of, complications of shoulder surgery, 48: 368-369
metatarsocuneiform joint (modified Lapidus procedure), 46: 378-380
with osteotomy, 46: 343-344
pantalar, 46: *353,* 354-355
paralytic poliomyelitis, 49: 599
preoperative assessment, **50: 298-299**
reconstruction of neuropathic deformities, 48: 273-275
scapholunate, 47: 226, 227
shoulder, 49: *327*
for complications of surgery, 48: 368-369
unreconstructible, 47: 147-148
subtalar, 46: 343, 351
treatment of malignant bone tumors, 48: 599-600
triple, 46: 351-354, 400
osteotomy through, 46: *355,* 356
triscaphoid, 47: 226-227
in vertebral corpectomies, 48: 424
without osteotomy, 46: 344-345
Arthrofibrosis, 46: 216
defined, 46: 254, 255
of the knee, operative treatment, 49: 211-220
loss of motion secondary to, 46: 251
management of, 46: 256-259
pathophysiology, 49: 214-215
symptoms, 49: 212
treatment of, 49: 215-219
Arthrography
for carpal instability, 47: 223
DDH, **50: *547***
diagnosis of ankle sprains, **50: 515**
midcarpal, **50: *126***
periprostatic femoral osteolysis, **50: 201**
Arthroplasties. *See also* Hip arthroplasty; Shoulder arthroplasty; Total knee arthroplasty
abrasion, shoulder joint, **50: 75**
ankle, state of the art, 48: 263-268
diagnosis of infection, 48: 114-115
first metatarsophalangeal joint, 48: 336-338
imaging of infected, 46: 527
shoulder
counterindications, **50: 77-78**
indications, **50: 77**
young patients, **50: 73-88**
soft-tissue, injured upper extremities, 49: 385-386
total shoulder, complications following, 48: 364-367
treatment of malignant bone tumors, 48: 599-600
Arthroscopes, wrist arthroscopy, 49: 226
Arthroscopic acromioplasty, 47: 21-27. *See also* Rotator cuff repair
advantages of, 47: 21-22, 27
technique, 47: 24-26
errors in, 47: 88-90
Arthroscopic microdiskectomy (AMD) procedures, 46: 147-148
Arthroscopic test, joint openings, **50: *452***
Arthroscopy
abrasion, **50: 501**
ankle
arthrodesis, 49: 259-279
in chronic instability, 49: 262-263
débridement and fusion, 48: 243-247
fusion outcomes, 49: 269-270
general technique principles, 48: 243
débridement of disk-space infection, 46: 156
diabetic frozen shoulder, 49: 287
diagnostic, and PCL damage, 48: 201-*203*
distal clavicle resection, 47: 35-41
advantages of, 47: 37, 41
direct approach, 47: *38*-39
indirect approach, 47: 39-41
elbow, 49: 239-246
complications of, 49: 252, 255-257
treatment of arthritis, 49: 247-252
elbow instability, **50: 98-99**
for epicondylitis, 48: 380
fractures of the proximal tibia, 48: 502-505
indications, metatarsophalangeal (MTP) joint, 48: 344-345
knee
arthrofibrosis, 49: 214-215
complications of, 48: *140*
management of degenerative arthritis, 48: 135-140
lateral collateral ligament repair, **50: 518**
and ligament reconstruction, TKA, **50: 500-502**
lumbar spine, 46: 148-155
instruments, 46: *151-152*
intervertebral disk, 46: 150-*151*
intradiskal approach, 46: 152-*155*
myoligamentous structures, 46: 149
neurovascular structures, 46: *150*
posterolateral approach to lower thoracic and lumbar spine, 46: 145-148
technique for posterolateral intradiskal and extra-annular access to spinal canal, 46: 151
triangular working zone, 46: *149-150*
meniscal repair, outside-in technique, 49: 195-206
midcarpal, 47: 223-224
PCL reconstruction, 48: 205
portals, metatarsophalangeal (MTP) joint, first, 48: 343, *344*
postoperative care and rehabilitation, metatarsophalangeal (MTP) joint, first, 48: 345-346
rotator cuff repair, 47: 59-65 (*See also* Rotator cuff repair)
combined with open treatment, 47: 51-57

shoulder, **50: 56-58**
acromioplasty, 47: 21-27
complications of, 48: 369-372
distal clavicle resection, 47: 35-41
rotator cuff repair, 46: 572, 47: 59-65 (*See also* Rotator cuff repair)
for stiffness after rotator cuff repair, 47: 69-*72*
subacromial decompression, 47: 25-26, 29-33
subacromial decompression, 47: 25-26
avoidance of complications, 47: 29-33
subtalar arthrodesis, 49: 275-279
syndesmosis injuries, 49: 263-266
thermal capsulorrhaphy, **50: *25-26*, 29-30**
glenohumeral joint, **50: 13-15**
treatment of chondral injuries symptoms, 48: 632-633
treatment of osteonecrosis, **50: 484**
treatment of posterior elbow impingement, 48: 399-404
wrist, 49: 225-235, **50: 126**
Arthrosis
after shoulder instability surgery, 47: *123-124*
glenohumeral joint, **50: *75***
Arthrotomy, total knee arthroplasty, **50: 362**
Articular cartilage. *See also* Cartilage; Hyaline cartilage
after acute trauma, 48: *194*
and aging, 46: 461-463, 47: 489
chondrocytes, 47: 469-470, *478*-479
chondrocyte-matrix interactions, 47: 483-484
collagen in, 47: 469
composition, 47: 478-481
chondrocytes, 47: *478*-479
extracellular matrix, 47: 479-481
degeneration
age-related, 46: 461-463, 47: 489
and growth factors, 47: 472-473
joint use and joint degeneration, 47: 491-492
and osteoarthritis, 47: 487-491
development, 47: 461-466
limb buds in embryos, 47: *462*-463
lesions in young individuals, 47: 505-*513*
diagnostic tests for, 47: 505-506
grading systems for defects, 47: *506*-508
treatment for, 47: 509-*513*
in osteoarthritis, 49: 486-487
osteochondral allografts for articular defects of the knee, 47: 500, 517-*521*
results of, 47: 512
surgical procedure, 47: 518-*521*
properties of, 48: 235
regulation of cartilage proliferation, 47: 464-466, 469-473
bone morphogenetic proteins, 47: 471-472
fibroblast growth factor, 47: 465, 471
insulin-like growth factors, 47: 465, 470
parathyroid hormone related protein (PTHrP), 47: 465, 466, 472
transforming growth factor-ß, 47: 465, 470-471
repair and regeneration, 47: 492-501
artificial matrices, 47: 499-500
cell transplantation, 47: 497-*498*
decreased joint loading combined with joint motion, 47: 496-497
growth factors, 47: 498-*499*
osteochondral allografts, 47: 500, 517-521
osteotomy, 47: 495-496
penetration of subchondral bone, 47: 492-*495*
soft-tissue grafts, 47: 497
tensile fracture stress, and age, 48: *236*
zones, 47: *477-478*
calcified cartilage zone, 47: 483
middle zone, 47: 483
superficial zone, 47: 482
transitional zone, 47: 482-483
Articular disks, wrist, torn, 49: *230, 231*
Articular interfaces
biologic restoration of surfaces, 48: 623-626
between radius, ulna and carpus, 48: 465-466
reduction in treatment of fractures, 48: 510
Articular tissues, effects of hyaluronate, 49: *496*
Artzal (hyaluronic acid), use of, 49: 497-498
Aseptic loosening. *See also* Osteolysis
after unicondylar knee arthroplasty (UKA), 48: 143
compared to osteolysis, 47: 307
definition, **50: 197**
diagnosis of, 47: 309-*310*
and failed total hip arthroplasties, 47: 265, 272-273
of prosthesis, 49: 78
recommendations, **50: 226-228**
tibial component, 48: *173*
Aspiration biopsies
and diagnosis of active infection, 48: 114-115, **50: 321, 369**
hip joint, 47: 289-291, *293*
periprosthetic femoral osteolysis, **50: 201**
Aspirin. *See also* Nonsteroidal anti-inflammatory drugs
consideration in preoperative planning, 48: 98
for juvenile rheumatoid arthritis, 46: 78
prevention of DVT, **50: 417**
for rheumatoid arthritis, 46: 78
Assistive devices
consideration in planning surgery, 48: 97
ordering of, 48: 94
Atherosclerosis, spinal arteries, 49: 341
Atherosclerotic plaques, fractures of, in hip arthroplasty, 48: 29
Athletes
Achilles tendon problems in runners, 47: 419-427
biomechanics of, 47: 405
heel pain, 47: 425-427
incidence of, 46: 577, 47: 419
insertional Achilles tendinitis, 47: 424-*425*
nodular deformity, 47: *421*
peritendinitis, 47: *420*-421
retrocalcaneal bursitis, 47: 422-424
tendinitis, 46: 577-580
ACL reconstruction failure, **50: 466-467**
elbow, medial collateral ligament and ulnar neuritis in, 48: 383-391
epicondylitis in, 48: 375-381
hand injuries
fractures, 47: 187-190
soft-tissue, 47: 181-185
lateral plantar nerve entrapments, **50: 527**
osteochondritis dissecans of the elbow, 48: 393-398
patellar instability in school-age athletes, 47: 345-349
imaging for, 47: 347-348
physical examination for, 47: 347
plantar fasciitis, **50: 525**
tendon problems in, 46: 569-581
Achilles, 46: 577-580, 47: 419-427
elbow, 46: 572-573
hand, 47: 181-184
hip, 46: 573-574
jumper's knee, 46: 574-575, 47: 404, 411-412
pathophysiology, 46: 569-570
posterior tibial, 46: 575-577
rotator cuff, 46: 570-572
throwing, 46: 570, 47: 26-27
anterior microinstability, **50: *35***
internal impingement, **50: 34**

shoulder injuries, **50: 17-21**
shoulder instability, **50: 29**
subacromial impingement, **50: 19**
Atlanto-occipital joint, inflammatory arthritis in, 48: 94
Atlantoaxial joint, inflammatory arthritis in, 48: 94
Atropine, affect on acupuncture analgesia, 49: 560
Attorneys, role in medical malpractice, 48: 699-703
Aufranc test
evaluation of component version, 48: 23
version of components, 49: 125
Augmentation osteotomies, **50: 551**
Austin-Moore prostheses, failure rates, 49: 179
Autografts
ACL revision reconstruction, **50: 455-458**
articular cartilage restoration, 48: 624
bone, 46: 230, 47: 525-526, 48: 58
advantages of, 48: 67
choice of, **50: 468**
defined, 48: 79
immunogenicity, 49: 97
tunnels, **50: 453**
Autologous chondrocyte transplantation (ACT)
categories, 48: 636-637
complications, 48: 638
failures, 48: 638
location of defects treated with, 48: *636*
magnetic resonance imaging of knee after, 48: *640*
treatment of chondral injuries, 48: 635-638
Autologous tissue-derived cell therapies, treatment of chondral injuries, 48: 635-638
Automated percutaneous nucleotomy, 46: 144
Autonomic neuropathy
and diabetic foot, 48: 291
in the diabetic foot, 48: 317
effect on skin, 48: 301
Autophor implants, critical results, 49: 46
Avascular necrosis, 46: 173
Axial compression test
disc herniation, 49: *337*
radicular symptoms, 49: *342*
Axial pain, cervical spondylosis, 49: 335
Axillary nerves
complications of thermal capsulorrhaphy, **50: 32, 40**
and proximal humeral fractures, 46: 31
in rotator cuff repair, 47: 72, 79, 90
subscapularis tendon repair, **50: 67**
and tendon transfers, 49: 325-326
total shoulder arthroplasty, **50: 79**
Axonotmesis, 47: 276
Azathioprine, immunosuppression, 49: 151

B
Back pain
following hip arthrodesis, **50: 297, 302-303**
pediatric, 48: 525-539
history, 48: 525-526
imaging studies, 48: 526-527
incidence, 48: 525
laboratory examinations, 48: 527
physical examination, 48: 526
Scheuermann's disorder, 48: 527-528
spinal stenosis, **50: 137-144**
Baclofen, children with multiple injuries, 49: 428
Bacteremia, potential sites, **50: 84**
Bacterial pyoderma, 46: 72
Bactericidal titer testing, serum, 48: 116
Bacteroides, infection in the diabetic foot, 48: 318
Bailey-Bradgley graft, 49: *348*
Balkan beams, simple construction, 49: 594-*595*
Bankart lesions
arthroscopic repair, **50: 33**
arthroscopic view, **50: *39***
defined, 47: 13
incomplete correction of, 47: 113, *114*
and multidirectional instability, 47: 101
thermal capsulorrhaphy, **50: 37**
and treatment for recurrent instability, 47: 116
Barlow maneuver, hip dislocation, **50: 541**
Base-of-neck osteotomy, **50: *562*, 563**
Baseball players
external rotation of the arm, **50: *17***
thermal capsulorrhaphy, **50: 27**
Basement membranes, thickening in diabetes, 48: 292
Basic fibroblast growth factor (bFGF). *See also* Fibroblast growth factors
and cartilage repair, 46: 489-490
for fracture healing, 47: 530
Battered root syndrome, 46: 143
Bauer and Jackson classification of cartilage injury patterns, 47: *506*-507
Beach-chair position, 47: 24
Bearing surfaces
finish and stem migration, 49: 108-109
total hip arthroplasty, 49: 41-54
Behavioral therapies, pain management, 49: 520
Benzocaine
molecular structure, 49: *526*
use of, 49: 525-526
Benzodiazepines
management of subcortical seizures, 49: 527-528
sympathetically maintained pain, 46: 265
Bernese periacetabular osteotomy (PAO), **50: 230-231**
approach, **50: 234-235**
clinical results, **50: 240-242**
complications, **50: 242**
experience with, **50: 239-245**
indications, **50: 233-234**
outcomes, **50: 239-240**
perioperative care, **50: 237**
radiographic analysis, **50: 253-261**
subsequent surgeries, **50: *243***
technique, **50: 235-237**
Beta-lactam antibiotics, resistance of enterococci, 49: 607-608
Betadine, allografts preparation, 49: 152
Biceps tendons
electromyography of long head of, 46: 59-60
injury to, 48: 405-410
complications of treatment, 48: 407-409
etiology, 48: 405
incidence, 48: 405
mechanism of, 48: 405
outcomes, 48: 407
postoperative care, 48: 407
presentation, 48: 405-406
surgical technique, 48: *408*
treatment of, 48: 406-407
partial distal rupture, 48: 409-410
surgical technique, 48: *409*
Bicondylar disease, and outcome of arthroscopic debridement, 48: 136
Bier blocks, treatment of CRPS, 49: 554
Biglycan, 47: 480
Bilateral intradiskal access, 46: 154

Bimalleolar fracture, malunited, 48: *281*
Biomaterials, with impaction grafting, **50: 214**
Biomechanics
acetabulum, 48: 483-484
center of hip rotation, 49: 30
first metatarsophalangeal (MTP) joints, 48: 343
of forward human locomotion, 47: 397-402
gait cycle, 47: 398, *399*
kinematics, 47: 398-399, *401*
kinetics, 47: 399-402
and hip and spine fractures in osteoporotic bone, 46: 431-437
hip fracture prevention, 46: 434-435
vertebral fracture prevention, 46: 436
knee, 47: 370-371
imaging of biomechanical patella disorders, 46: 526-*527*
of radial head and forearm stability, 47: 173-174
of rotator cuff repair, 47: 43-50
bone tunnels vs suture anchors, 47: 43-44
suture anchors, 47: 45-49
and running injuries, 47: 397-406
forward human locomotion, 47: 397-402
injury mechanisms, 47: 402-*403*
soft-tissue stresses, 47: 403-405
of throwing, 48: 383-384
wrist, 47: 220-221
Biopsies
aspiration
diagnosis of active infection, **50: 321, 369**
hip joint, 47: 289-291, *293*
joint, and diagnosis of infection, 48: 114-115
periprosthetic femoral osteolysis, **50: 201**
core needle, 48: 590
decision-making, 49: 439-440
defined, 48: 587
examination of soft-tissue tumors, 48: 619
excisional, soft-tissue tumors, 49: 440
fine needle aspiration, 48: 589-590
metastatic bone disease, 49: 456
metastatic disease of the spine, 49: 474
principles and techniques, 48: 587-590
and seeding of neoplasms, 48: 588
types of, 49: 440
vertebral bodies in lumbar and lower thoracic spine, 46: 158
Bioresorbable implants
applications in orthopaedic surgery
in adults, 46: 538-*539*
advantages and disadvantages, 46: 536-538
in anterior cruciate ligament reconstruction, 46: *541-542*
biodegradation of, 46: 535-536
in children, 46: 539-*540*
future of, 46: 542-545
historic overview, 46: *531-532*
manufacturing methods, 46: 533-535
mechanical properties of materials, 46: 535
properties and characteristics, 46: 532-533
for rotator cuff fixation, 47: 47
suture anchors, 47: 47
sterilization of, 46: 535
Bioresorbable polymers
processing of, 46: 533-534
production of, 46: 533
Bipolar cautery devices, 46: 133
Biportal technique, 46: 144
Bisphosphonates
effect on particulate-induced bone resorption, **50: 192**
metastatic bone disease, 49: 461
for osteoporosis, 46: 453
use of, 49: 4
Blair arthrodesis, 46: 333, *336, 350*-351
Blast injuries
pattern 1, 49: *432*
pattern 2, 49: *432*
Blastomycosis, 46: 72
Blood coagulation, 47: 331
Blood management
anticipation of losses, **50: 347**
autologous donation, **50: 154**
current options, 48: *656*
hip arthroplasty, 49: 4
investigational options, 48: *659*
options in orthopaedic settings, 48: *662*
during orthopaedic surgery, 48: 655-662
salvage techniques, 48: 655, 657
Blood pressure, control during shoulder surgery, **50: 57**
Blood supply
autonomic neuropathy and diabetic foot, 48: 291
in diabetics, 48: 292
effect of nerve compression, 49: 364
femoral head, **50: *559***
maintenance of, injured upper extremities, 49: 381
and osteonecrosis, 49: 170-171
osteonecrosis and, **50: 478**
and partial foot amputations, 48: 322
patellar, **50: *386***
skin incisions, **50: 360**
and steroids, **50: 489**
Blood transfusions, allogeneic
and infection rates, 48: 655
and length of stay, 48: 655
prevalence in orthopaedic patients, 48: *662*
Blood vessels. *See also* Vascularization
consequences of injury, during total hip arthroplasty, 48: 30
in inner aspect of pelvis, 48: *27*
reconstruction of, upper extremities, 49: 386
revascularization of grafts, 48: 80
supply of the humeral head, 48: *350*
Blunt trauma, effect of, on cartilage, 46: 488
Body weight
failure of unicompartmental knee arthroplasty, **50: 506**
force at osteotomy interface, **50: *249***
plantar fasciitis, **50: 522**
SCFE, **50: 555**
treatment of spinal stenosis, **50: 153**
Böhler-Braun frame, use in the developing world, 49: *586*
Bone. *See also* Articular cartilage
chronic infections, least developed countries, 49: 580
defects
Anderson Orthopaedic Research Institute (AORI), classification, 48: *168*-169
classification of, 48: 59-60
selection of management method, 48: 167-168
deficits
acetabular, 48: 47-50
ankle arthrodesis in, 48: 259
clinical results of revision arthroplasty, 48: 173-175
and planning revision surgery, 48: 163-164
radiographic assessment, 48: 46-47
development, 47: 461-466
cascade theory of, 46: 497
growth plate development, 47: *464*
limb buds in embryos, 47: *462*-463
regulatory control of, 46: 495-497, 47: 464-465

diagnosis of destructive lesions, 49: *453*
evaluation in preoperative planning, 48: 97
formation of, in acetabular impaction grafting, 48: *86*
freeze-dried, and disease transmission, 48: 64-65
frequency of defects, 48: 167
function of, 46: 445
heterotopic formation, and range of motion, 48: 44
impacted morcellized allografts, mechanical stability of reconstructions, 48: 83
induction, by allografts, 48: 65
management of type 1 defects, 48: 169
management of type 2 defects, 48: 169-171
management of type 3 defects, 48: 171-173
measurement of turnover, 48: 102
metabolism in osteoporosis, 46: 445-447
metabolism of, 49: 78-79
morcellized
  reconstruction of type I acetabular defects, 48: 60-61
  use in hip arthroplasty, 48: 645
osteoclastic resorption, 48: 37-38
pathophysiology of metastatic disease, 49: 453-*454*
quality of
  effect of arthritis on, 48: 97
  in elderly, 46: 424
resection in total knee replacement, 46: 192
resorption, 46: 445
  impaction morcellized graft, **50: *218***
  particulate-induced, **50: 192**
  response to particulate debris, **50: 189**
sclerotic
  removal of, **50: 222**
  and revisions, **50: 393**
structural grafts, 48: 57-65
  failure rates, 48: 58
subchondral, changes in osteoarthritis, 49: 487
types of healing, 49: 97
Bone cement
  antibiotic-impregnated, 48: 115-116, 117
    timing of reconstruction and use, 48: 117-118, *119*
  and impaction morcellized allografting, 48: 79-88
  removal from femoral canal, 48: 9-11
  removal from femur, 48: 15
  thermal injury from curing of, in hip arthroplasty, 48: 29
  total hip arthroplasty, assessment of, 48: *30*
Bone chips, stability of cemented impaction grafting, 49: 109
Bone cysts
  aneurysmal, treatment of, 48: 593-594
  unicameral, treatment of, 48: 593-594
Bone density, following morcellized bone graft, **50: 215**
Bone grafts, 47: 525-532. *See also* Bone remodeling
  acetabular augmentation, outcomes, 49: 31-32
  acetabular reconstructions, **50: 221-228**
  ACL reconstruction, **50: 464-466**
  allogeneic
    advantages of, 48: 67
    reconstruction of type IIA acetabular defects, 48: 61-62
  allografts, 47: 526-527, 48: 648-650
    for acetabular revision arthroplasty, 47: 265-273
    for the knee, 47: 500, 517-*521*
    in periprosthetic femoral fracture treatment, 47: 257-*263*
    in revision knee arthroplasty, 46: 231-236
    sterilization of, 47: 380-385, 527
  autogenous, 47: 525-526, 48: 647-648
    advantages of, 48: 67
    femoral heads, 49: 176-178
  biology of, 48: 645-651, 646-647
  biosynthetic graft materials, 47: 528-532
    ceramics, 47: 528-530, 532
    in composite grafts, 47: 530, 532
    osteoinductive growth factors, 47: 530-532
  with bone marrow, 47: 527-528
  cancellous, femoral neck or head, 49: 177
  conversion to TKA, **50: 507**
  cortical, femoral neck or head, 49: 177
  "Crawford Campbell," 46: 354
  with demineralized bone matrix, 47: 527, 532
  femoral, **50: 213-214**
  femoral head, trapdoor procedure, 49: *176, 177*
  flying buttress, 49: *59*
  freeze-dried, 49: 150, **50: 214**
  fresh allografts, immune responses, 49: 150
  guidelines for selection, 48: 70
  hip arthroplasty, 49: 8
  history of, 47: 265, 48: 79-80
  impaction, **50: 211-219**
    acetabular cup migration, **50: 216**
    acetabular reconstructions, **50: 221-228**
    alternative materials, **50: 214**
    revision THA, 49: 103-110
  and infection of arthroplasty sites, 48: 119-120
  morcellized, **50: 211-212**
  nonvascularized, treatment of precollapse osteonecrosis, 48: 100
  onlay allografts, 49: 97-101
  osteochondral
    femoral head, 49: 177
    isolated articular cartilage defects, 47: *511-513*
  overview of types, 48: *80*
  perioperative antibiotics, 49: 153
  preparation of, 49: 152-153, **50: 222-223, 227**
  prophylactic antibiotics, 49: 152
  resorption, **50: 215**
  revitalization of, 48: 80
  scaphoid, **50: 113-117**
    preoperative planning, **50: 113-114**
  SCFE, **50: 561-562**
  selection of preparation, 49: 151-152
  shear-strain-relieved, 46: 350, 351, 354
  structural, 49: 148-149, 176-177
  structural femoral autograft, **50: 314-315**
  substitutes, 46: 543
  for tibial shaft fractures, 46: 283, 285, 299
  use after infection, **50: 330**
  vascularized, 49: 177-178
    treatment of precollapse osteonecrosis, 48: 100
  vascularized medical, **50: 105**
Bone loss. *see also* Osteolysis
  AAOS classification system, 49: *91,* 92-93
  acetabular
    evaluation of, 48: 45-47
    and preoperative planning, 48: 50-55
    and revision hip arthroplasty, 48: 57-65
  bone preparation techniques, 48: 178-179
  Chandler and Penenberg classification system, 49: *88*-89
  classification systems, 49: *91, 49: 92-93,* 49: 147-148
  etiology, 49: 83-84
  with failed cemented component, 48: *180*
  femoral, 49: 83-95
    distal bypass fixation, 49: 119-129
    fixation with modular stem, 49: 131-138
    in revision hip replacement, 49: 147-159
    tibia and patella, 48: *177*
    treatment options, 49: 148-149

grade III, 49: *94*
with implant loosening, 46: 228
level of, 49: 93
preoperative planning, 49: *83*
radiographic assessments, 49: 85
with revision total knee arthroplasty, 48: 167-175
segmental defects, 49: *93*
surgical revision techniques, 48: 80-83
Bone marrow, 47: 527-528
pressures, **50: 489**
Bone marrow edema syndrome (BMES), and osteonecrosis, 49: 171
Bone mineral density, measurement of, 46: 450
Bone morphogenetic proteins (BMPs)
articular cartilage restoration, 48: 624
in autocrine regulation of articular cartilage, 47: 471-472
and bone formation, 46: 496
in bone grafting, 47: 525, 530-532
and bone grafts, 48: 647
for fracture healing, 46: 484, 47: 530
in limb buds, 47: 51
as a therapeutic agent, 47: 498
as therapeutic agents, 46: 473-474
Bone remodeling. *see also* Bone grafts
after morcellized bone graft, **50: 216-219**
of cancellous grafts, 48: 648
histology of biopsy specimens, 48: *181*
prosthetic-induced, 46: 227
Bone scans
3-phase diagnosis of RSD, 49: 551
carpal instability, **50: 125**
diagnosis of arthroplasty site infection, 48: 114
diagnosis of osteonecrosis, **50: 496**
in evaluation of diabetic foot, 48: 298
examination of bone tumors, 48: 609-610
periprosthetic femoral osteolysis, **50: 201**
and posterior cruciate ligament damage, 48: 201
technetium, 49: 471-472
diagnosis of active infection, **50: 320**
exclusion of active infection, **50: 320**
follow-up for orthopaedic oncology patients, 48: 604-605
infected bones, **50: 369**
metastatic bone disease, 49: 455
scaphoid fractures, **50: 106**
soft-tissue tumors, 49: 439
tibial osteonecrosis, **50: 478**
Bone scans, technetium
for infection following total hip arthroplasty, 47: 288-289
for reflex sympathetic dystrophy, 46: 264
Bone stock deficiencies, 46: 418
Bone tumors
benign, treatment of, 48: 591-596
clinical presentation, 48: 607-608
common sites of, 48: *609*
diagnostic by plain film alone, 48: *611*
juxtacortical, differential diagnosis of, 48: *610*
laboratory investigations, 48: 608
malignant, treatment of, 48: 598-600
multiple lesions, differential diagnosis of, 48: 611
pathologist's role in diagnosis of, 48: 613-616
physical examination, 48: 608
presentation and evaluation of, 48: 607-611
radiographic examination, 48: 608-609
Bone tunnels
autografts, **50: 453**
femoral, **50: 470-471**
femoral placement, **50: *465***
femur, improper tunnel placement, **50: 464-465**
inappropriate positioning, **50: 464-465**
in rotator cuff repair, 47: *43*-44, 63
sutures, ulnar osseous tunnels, **50: *99***
technique, **50: *470*-471**
tendon graft passage, 48: *387*
tibial, **50: 464-*465*, *468*, 471**
ulnar osseous, **50: *99***
Bostrum procedure, modified, **50: *518***
Bourne-Rorabeck classification, femoral bone deficiency, **50: *203***
Boutonnière deformity, 47: 181-*182*
pseudo-, 47: 182, *183*
Boxer's knuckle, 47: 182-183
Braces, simple construction, in developing countries, 49: 593-*594*
Brachalgia cord syndrome, 49: 341
Brachial plexuses blocks, 49: 528-529
Brachioradialis tendons
electromyographic analysis of, 46: 59-60
tapping, 49: *344*
Bracing
and arthrodesis for neuropathic deformities, 48: 275
management of chronic Achilles tendon rupture, 48: 225
nonsurgical treatment of epicondylitis, 48: 377
pediatric thoracic myelomeningocele, 48: 564-566
postoperative
dynamic hip abduction brace, **50: *292***
following THA, **50: 268**
soft-tissue imbalances, **50: 289**
static hip abduction brace, **50: *291***
unstable THA, **50: 289-293**
treatment for kyphosis, 48: 528
treatment of lumbar and thoracic fractures, 48: 413
Brain injuries, risk of CRPS, 49: 550
Breast cancers
metastatic bone disease, hypercalcemia, 49: 458
metastatic disease, 49: *454*
Bristow procedure, 47: 118, 120, *124*
loss of motion after, 47: 119
Brittain procedure, **50: 301, *302***
Broca-Perthes-Bankart lesion, 47: 105-106
Brown recluse spider, bites of, 46: 70-71, 72
Brown-Séquard syndrome, cord compression, 49: 341
Brucella, and infection at arthroplasty sites, 48: 113
Büchler and Hastings classification, traumatic injuries, 49: 379
Buck's traction, use for femoral fractures, developing world, 49: 587
Buechel-Pappas Ultra Total Ankle Replacement, outcomes, 48: 266-267
Bunions, 46: 357, 362
with normal hallux valgus angle, 48: 333
Bupivacaine (Marcaine, Sensorcaine)
diagnostic nerve blocks, 49: 535
molecular structure, 49: *526*
postoperative infiltration, 49: 533
preoperative analgesia, 49: 533-534
Burns, fractures complicated by, in children, 49: 425-430
Bursal resection, subacromial, **50: 46**
Bursectomy, subacromial, **50: 57**
Bursitis
calcific, 47: 18
differential diagnosis, **50: 477, 491**
pes anserine, 47: 412-413
retrocalcaneal, 47: 422-*424*
superficial peritendinous Achilles, 47: 425
Vochel's, 47: 412-413

C

C-reactive protein (CRP)
  diagnosis of arthroplasty site infection, 48: 114
  for diagnosis of infection following THA, 47: 286-287, 292-*293*
  exclusion of active infection, **50: 319**
  infected knees, **50: 368-369**
  laboratory investigations of bone tumors, 48: 608
  levels, 47: 287
  periprosthetic femoral osteolysis, **50: 200-201**
  in preoperative assessments, 48: 45
Cages
  acetabular, **50: *343***
  acetabular fracture, **50: 340**
Caisson disease, and osteonecrosis, 49: 171
Calandruccio triangular external fixation device, and ankle arthrodesis, 48: 257
Calcaneal osteotomy, 46: 397-*398*
Calcaneal tubercles, prominence of, **50: 522**
Calcanectomy, partial, in diabetic feet, 48: 326-327
Calcaneofibular ligament (CFL), anatomy, 49: 262
Calcaneus, posterior facets, 49: *274*
Calcaneus fractures
  bony changes, 46: 339-341
  initial management, 46: 339
  salvage procedures for, 46: 339-345
  stress, **50: 523**
  treatment of, 46: 341-345
Calcar deficiencies, after THA, 49: 88-89
Calcific tendinitis, acute, 46: *69*-70
Calcitonin
  nasal, treatment of spinal stenosis, **50: 153**
  for osteoporosis, 46: 447, 452-453
  treatment of RSD, 49: 554
  use of, 49: 4
Calcitropic hormones, in osteoporosis, 46: 446-447
Calcium
  absorption of, in treating acute calcific tendinitis, 46: 70
  cytosolic, response to cellular deformation, 48: 193
  in osteoporosis, 46: 445-446, 451
  serum, laboratory investigations of bone tumors, 48: 608
Calcium channel blockers
  in treating spinal cord injuries, 46: 119
  treatment of CRPS, 49: 553
Calcium pyrophosphate (CPP) crystals, intrasynovial deposition of, 46: 76-77
Calcium pyrophosphate deposition disease, 46: 76-77
Calluses, sanding down of, 48: 301
Campomelic dysplasia, 47: 466
Canal of Guyon, anatomy, 49: 314-315
Cancellization, cortical onlay allografts, 49: 101
Cancellous bone grafting, 47: 526. *See also* Bone grafts
  versus ceramics, 47: 528
  versus composite grafts, 47: 530
  for tibial shaft fractures, 46: 283
Cancellous bones, impaction revision, 49: *105*
Cancellous screws, placement, hip arthroplasty, 48: 72
Cancellous trabeculae, photomicrograph, 48: 351
Cancer, management of chronic pain, 49: 513-520
Candida, infected hip arthroplasties, **50: 318**
Capillary permeability, in diabetes, 48: 292
Capillary refill, in diagnosis of diabetic foot, 48: 295
Capitellar osteophytes, arthroscopic view, 49: *248*
Capitellum
  arthroscopic view of osteochondritis dissecans of, 48: 397
  osteochondritis dissecans of, 48: 395
Capsaicin, pain management, 49: 520
Capsular fibrosis, and medial epicondylar osteotomy, 48: 155
Capsular laxity, visualization, **50: 30**
Capsular ligaments, sternoclavicular joint, 49: 397
Capsular release, glenohumeral joint, efficacy of, **50: 75**
Capsular releases
  arthroscopic technique, diabetic frozen shoulder, 49: 287-289
  forceps, 49: *288*
  LBO, 49: 256-257
Capsular repair, for patellofemoral instability, 46: 172
Capsulectomies
  anterolateral approach, 49: 15
  total shoulder arthroplasty, **50: 80**
Capsules, joint, type 1 collagen, **50: 3-4**
Capsulodesis for scapholunate instability, 47: 225, 226
Capsuloligamentous structures
  anatomy, 47: *98,* 99-100
  nontraumatic instability of, 46: 3
Capsulorrhaphy. *See also* Thermal capsulorrhaphy
  arthropathy, 47: 132
  Putti-Platt, **50: 75**
Capsulotomies, anterolateral approach, 49: 15
Cardiopulmonary disease in elderly, 46: 423
Cardiotoxicity, local anesthetics, 49: 528
CARE, disaster relief, 49: 576
Carpal instability. *See* Wrist, instability
Carpal tunnel release, area specific annual rates of, 48: 667
Carpal tunnel syndrome (CTS)
  literature reviews of, 48: 693
  symptoms, 48: 694
Carpus. *See also* Wrist
  adaptive instability, **50: 131-132**
  bony anatomy, **50: 105-106**
  dynamic instability, **50: 130**
  instability, **50: 123-134**
  mechanisms of injury, **50: 125**
  midcarpal arthrograms, **50: *126***
  terminology, **50: 124-125**
Cartilage
  age-related changes in collagens, 46: 462-463
  articular
    repair of, 48: 623-626
    strategies for biological restoration of, 48: 624
  defined of repair, 48: 624
  degeneration, **50: 147**
  erosion and septic arthritis, **50: 317**
  hyaline, 46: 487
    composition of, 48: 623
    durability of, 48: 140
    hypocellular, in an enchondroma, 48: *613*
    repair of, 48: 135
  injuries to, 48: 623-624
  meniscus, response to injury, 49: 189-192
  prevalence of fibrillation in, 48: 235-237
  repair
    effect of growth factors, 46: 487-488
    effect of growth factors on, 46: 488-490, 47: 498-*499*
    effect of growth factors on carriers, 46: 491-492
    growth factors as agents of healing, 46: 490-491
    inflammatory disease, 46: 488
    techniques, 48: 629-642
Cartilage matrix, repair, and joint distraction, 48: 251-254
Cascade theory of bone formation, 46: 497
Casts
  acute scaphoid fractures, **50: *111***
  DDH, older children, **50: 549**
  hip pantaloon, **50: 291-292**
  immobilization following THA, **50: 268**

plantar fasciitis, **50: 525**
proposed mechanism of action, 48: 306-307
spica cast, **50: *290***
supracondylar femoral fracture, **50: 380-381**
walking, syndesmosis injuries, **50: 520**
Catecholamines, role in acupuncture analgesia, 49: 560
Cathepsin G, response to particulate debris, **50: 191**
Cauda equina
anatomy, 49: 361-362
spinal compression, **50: 147**
Causalgia, 46: 261. *See also* complex regional pain syndrome
after hip arthroplasty, 47: 278
minor, 46: 263
risk of, 49: 550
Cautery, rotator cuff repair, **50: 57**
Cavitary defects
contained, acetabulum, 48: 59
femoral, definition, 49: 92
Cavus, in patients with myelomeningocele, 48: 545-546
CD44 receptors, and hyaluronic acid, 49: 496
Cefazolin
open fractures, pediatric use, 49: 416
wound infections, 49: 426
Ceftzidime, wound infections, 49: 426
Ceiling effect
of generic-based outcome study, 48: 419
and opioids use, 49: 516
Ceiling traction, 47: *271*
Cell death
response to particulate debris, **50: 188**
and steroids, **50: 489**
Cell membranes, deformation of, 48: 193-195
Cellulitis
in the diabetic foot, 48: 318
prevalence in diabetic foot, 48: 298
Cement. *See also* Bone cement; Polymethylmethacrylate (PMMA)
acetabular augmentation, 49: 30
acetabular component, **50: 282**
antibiotic-loaded, 47: 303-304, **50: 327, 329-330**
THA revision, **50: *323***
in TKA, **50: 412**
femoral stems, **50: 213**
fixation without, issues in revision total knee arthroplasty, 48: 177-182
removal, infected knees, **50: 371-373**
removal from femur, 49: 86-87
spacers, **50: 372**
thermal damage, **50: 372**
Cement disease, 49: 71
Cement mantle, cold flow, 49: 111
Cemented stem, loosening of, 48: *25*
Cementless components, **50: 392-393**
Cementless sockets
extended proximal femoral osteotomies for, 48: *22*
with osteolysis, classification system for, 48: 38
Center edge angle (CEA), measurement of, **50: 254-*257***
Center of rotation and angulation (CORA), planning periarticular osteotomies, 48: 282
Centers for Disease Control and Prevention (CDC), isolation precautions, 49: 608-611
Central deficiency, longitudinal failure of upper-limb formation in hand, 46: 97-*104*
Central sacral line (CSL), and spinal alignment, 48: *554*
Centralia, scaphoid osteogenesis, **50: 105**
Cephalic vein, total shoulder arthroplasty, **50: 79**
Cephalosporins, treatment of diabetic foot infection, 48: 319
Ceramic-on-ceramic implants, total hip replacements, **50: 167-168**
Ceramic-on-polyethylene bearings, **50: 168-169**
Ceramics, 47: 528-529
alumina
physical properties of, **50: *167***
retrieval analysis, 49: 75
in THA, 49: 43
biologic response to, **50: 188**
implant fracture, 49: 44-45
and osteolysis, 49: 46
on polyethylene, 49: 43-44
replamineform, 47: 528-529
THA implants, 49: 75
in total hip arthroplasty, 49: 43-47
used with polyethylene, **50: 168-169**
zirconia
surface of, 49: 75
in THA, 49: 43
Cerclage wires
placement, 48: *24*
strut-grafting with, 47: *248*
for treatment of periprosthetic fractures, 47: 244-*245,* 251-252
Cerebral palsy
management of spinal deformity, 48: 556-557
THA in, 49: 163-165
Cerebrospinal fluid (CSF), spinal stenosis, **50: 148**
Cervical corpectomy
lateral decompression, 49: *349*
and struct graft fusion, 49: 349-352
Cervical degenerative disease, nonsurgical treatment of, 48: 433-435
Cervical diskectomy, anterior
with fusion, 49: 346-348
without fusion, 49: 348-349
Cervical disorders, outcomes instruments for, 48: 419-421
Cervical facet dislocations, closed cervical reduction for, 46: 121-122
Cervical lordosis, age-related changes, 49: 345
Cervical myelopathy
advantages of anterior and posterior approaches, 48: *425*
laminectomy, 48: 425
laminoplasty, 48: 425
measuring outcomes of, 48: 417-421
surgical management of, 48: 423-426
Cervical nerves, level of roots, 49: *342*
Cervical radiculopathies, differential diagnosis, 49: 297, 301, *343*
Cervical soft-disk herniation, outcomes, 48: 417
Cervical spine
canal stenosis, 49: 340
changes in sagittal alignment, 49: *340*
degenerative disorders, 49: 335-337
evaluation in preoperative planning, 48: 96
instability, prioritizing surgical treatment, 48: 94
metastatic disease
MRI, 49: *475*
surgical treatment, 49: 474
motion segments, 49: *339*
range-of-motion model, 48: *458*
spondylitic myelopathy and radiculopathy, 49: 339-357
Cervical spondylitis, radiologic evaluation, 49: 344-345
Cervical spondylosis, definition, 49: 335
Cervical spondylotic myelopathy, after corpectomy and fibular strut, 48: *424*
Cervicothoracic area, spinal impairment, *Guides to the Evaluation of Permanent Impairment,* 4th edition, 48: 456
Chain scission, 46: 207
Chandler and Penenberg bone loss classification, 49: *88,* 88-89, 147-148
of acetabular deficiencies, 48: 48-*49*
Charcot arthropathy. *see also* Neuropathic arthropathy
reconstruction compared with amputation, 48: 276-277

Charcot joints, 46: 356
pain at presentation, 48: 292-293
results of reconstruction, 48: 275-276
Charcot-Marie-Tooth disease, total contact casting and, 48: 305
Charcot restraint orthotic walker (CROW), use of, 48: 308, 312
Charnley acetabular cementing technique, 48: 46
Charnley arthroplasty, outcomes, 49: 29, 30
Charnley cup, outcomes, 49: 49
Charnley hips, revision rates, 49: 73-74
Charnley osteotomy, biomechanics, **50: 247-252**
Charnley prosthesis, **50: 166**
Charnley total hip replacements, outcomes, **50: 314**
Cheiralgia paresthetica, SRN entrapment, 49: 302-303
Cheirarthropathy, in diabetes, 49: 283-284, 290
Chemical sympathectomy, treatment of RSD, 49: 552-553
Chemokines, response to particulate debris, **50: 191**
Chemoprophylaxis, impact of, on thromboembolic disease, 46: 186-187
Chemotaxis, of polymorphonuclear leukocytes, impairment by polymethylmethacrylate, 48: 114
Chemotherapy
consideration in preoperative planning, 48: 98
and high-grade bone sarcomas, 48: 601-602
metastatic disease of the spine, 49: 473
and osteonecrosis, 49: 170
pain reduction, 49: 514
Chevron osteotomy, 46: 370-*372, 373*
malunion after, 48: 334-335
Chiari malformation, 46: 120
association of SCIWORA with, 46: 120
Chiari osteotomy, **50: 230, 551**
outcomes, 49: 26
Child abuse, and pediatric spinal fractures, 48: 536-537
Children, with multiple injuries, treatment of fractures, 49: 415-423
Chlorazepate, and aging, 46: 415
Chlordiazepoxide, and aging, 46: 415
Chondral injuries
algorithm for primary treatment of, 48: *630-631*
evaluation of, 48: 632
and osteoarthritis, 48: 629-632
symptom management, 48: 632
Chondroblastoma, treatment of, 48: 592-593
Chondrocalcinosis, and outcome of arthroscopic débridement, 48: 136
Chondrocyte transplantation, treatment of chondral injuries, 48: 632
Chondrocytes
age changes in, 46: 461-462
articular, 47: 469-473, *478*-479
in articular cartilage, 48: 623
growth factors, and articular cartilage restoration, 48: 624
in limb development, 47: 463-464
transplantation of, 47: *510,* 511-512
Chondrodysplasias, 47: 465-466
Chondroitin sulfate
identification in menisci, 49: 191
treatment of osteoarthritis, 49: 491-493
Chondrolysis, complication of SCFE, **50: 565, 574-575**
Chondroma, differentiation from chondrosarcoma, 48: 613-615
Chondromalacia, imaging of, 46: 528
Chondroprotective agents, nutritional supplementation, 49: 491-493
Chondrosarcomas
clinicopathologic features of, 48: *614*
differential diagnosis of, 48: 613-615
pelvic, 48: *585*
radiograph, 48: *581*
Chordomas, and low back pain, 48: 586
Chow technique, triangular fibrocartilage complex repair, 49: 232
Christianson hip, 49: 41
Chromium, serum levels, 49: 49
Chromium phosphate, corrosion, **50: 186**
Cicatrix formation, shoulders stabilization, **50: 8**
Cimetadine, and aging, 46: 415
Cincinnati knee scores, results of autologous chondrocyte transplantation (ACT), 48: 637-*638*
Circumflex vessels, subscapularis tendon repair, **50: 67**
Claudication, neurogenic, spinal degeneration, **50: *139***
Claudication, spinal stenosis, **50: 142-143**
Clavicles
ligamentous supports, 49: 397-398
ossification pattern, 49: 398
osteolysis, 49: 408, 411-412
Clawtoe deformities, in the diabetic foot, 48: 293, 317
Cleft hand, 46: 97
classification of, 46: 98-100
surgical treatment of, 46: 100-104
Clindamycin
fluocinolone with, treatment of diabetic foot infection, 48: 319
treatment of diabetic foot infection, 48: 319
Clinodactyly, in fingers, 49: *286*
Clogs, simple construction, in developing countries, 49: 593-*594*
Clonidine, treatment of RSD, 49: 553
Closed cervical reduction, for cervical facet dislocations, 46: 121-122
Clostridium perfringens, tibial shaft fractures infection, 46: 293-294
Cloward graft, 49: *348*
Coactivation, 46: 40
Coagulation factors, and osteonecrosis, **50: 490**
Cobalt, serum levels, 49: 49, 75
Cobalt-chromium (Co-Cr) alloy
femoral head, **50: *186***
immune responses to, **50: 193**
implant elasticity, 49: 75
macrophage response, 49: 72
Cobb elevators, 46: 133
Cobra head plate, **50: 297**
Cocaine
as anesthetic, 49: 523-524
molecular structure, 49: *525*
Cognition, in elderly, 46: 410
Cognitive therapies, pain management, 49: 520
Colchicine
for gout, 46: *76*
for pseudogout, 46: 77
Coleman jerk of exit sign, **50: *537*, 538**
Colitis, and arthritis, 48: 97
Collaborative care tracks. *See* critical pathways
Collagen
as articular cartilage structural macromolecules, 47: 479-480
capsular healing, **50: 291**
and chondrodysplasias, 47: 465
denaturation, **50: 3, 31**
diabetic frozen shoulder, 49: *284*
fibers, thermal modification, **50: 7**
glycosylation of, 48: 293
in growth plate development, 47: 464
inconsistent shrinkage, **50: 30-31**
mechanism of shrinkage, **50: *4***
meniscus implants, 49: 196-197
meniscus microanatomy, 49: 190-191
necrosis and corticosteroids, 48: 219
nonenzymatic glycosylation in diabetes, 48: 307
renaturation, **50: 5**
spinal degeneration, 49: 362
thermal shrinkage, **50: 13**
type I, thermal shrinkage, **50: 3-4**

type II, 47: 465, 469, 480
in hyaline cartilage, 48: 623
in osteoarthritis, 49: 486
type IX, in osteoarthritis, 49: 486
type XI, and osteoarthritis, 49: 486
Collagen fibrils, 47: *480*
analysis of, quantitative ultrastructural, 46: 242
population, normal and ultrastructure, 46: 242-245
Collagen genes, particulate-induced bone resorption, **50: 192**
Collagenases
production of, 49: 72
response to particulate debris, **50: 189**
Collarless Polished Tapered (CPT) stem, use of, 49: 111-113, *116*
Colles' fractures, risk of CRPS I, 49: 550
Columnar carpus, **50: *124***
kinematics, **50: 124**
Coma, general anesthesia for children, 49: 415
Committee for Development Planning of the United Nations, 49: 567
Common peroneal nerve block, 49: 531
Communications, ethical pitfalls, 49: 635-636
Community-acquired infections, antibiotic-resistant organisms, 49: 605
Comorbidities, in outcomes measurement, 48: 419
Compartment syndrome
associated with tibial fracture, 46: 303-308
children with multiple injuries, 49: 427
Competency, ethical issues, 49: 634-635
Complex regional pain syndrome (CRPS). *See also* reflex sympathetic dystrophy
pain management, 49: 549-556
Complications. *See* specific procedures/treatments
Components. *See also* Implants; Prostheses
cemented, osteolysis, 50: 393
computer-generated models, 50: 277
positioning of, 50: 285
treatment of dysplastic hips, 50: 310
Composite grafts, 47: 530
Compound muscle action potentials to (CMAP), ulnar nerve compression, 49: 308
Comprehensive Classification of Fractures, 47: 193-*194*
Comprehensive Omnibus Budget Reconciliation Act (COBRA), and medical malpractice, 48: 701-702
Compression plating, for tibial shaft fractures, 46: 288-289
Computed tomography (CT), **50: *299***
acetabular dysplasia, **50: 256-258**
acetabular fractures, 48: 483
carpal instability, **50: 125**
cervical radiculopathy or myelopathy, 49: 345
evaluation of bone stock, 49: 85
examination of bone tumors, 48: 610-611
examination of soft-tissue tumors, 48: 618
follow-up for orthopaedic oncology patients, 48: 604-606
osteochondral lesion of the talar dome, 49: *259*
preoperative investigations, total hip arthroplasty, 48: 31-32
scaphoid fractures, **50: 106**
soft-tissue tumors, 49: 439, 447, 448
in spinal cord injury, 46: 119-121
spinal stenosis, 49: 366-367, **50: 138-141**
spondylitic myelopathy, 49: 337
sternoclavicular joint injuries, 49: 399
and thoracolumbar trauma, 48: 429-430
three-dimensional scans, **50: 256-258**
Computer-assisted surgery, acetabular osteotomies, **50: 259**
Computer technology for orthopaedic presentations, 46: 595-610
basic hardware guidelines, 46: 597
digital graphic images, 46: 600-601
general design guidelines, 46: 597-600
multimedia, 46: 604-610
poster exhibits, 46: *601*-603
slides, 46: *603*-604
Concavity-compression effect, 46: 39
Confidentiality
ethical pitfalls, 49: 636
MODEMS program, 48: 681-682
teaching of ethics, 49: 640
Conflicts of interest, teaching of ethical issues, 49: 640
Confusion assessment method, 46: 410, 411
Congenital convex pes valgus foot deformity, in patients with myelomeningocele, 48: 544
Congenital dislocation of the hip (CDH)
femoral implants, 49: 64
total hip arthroplasty, 49: 20-21
Congenital hip dysplasia, 47: 277
difficult femur, 49: 63-64
Congenital vertical talus, in patients with myelomeningocele, 48: 544
Connective tissues, thermal modification, **50: 3-11**
Constipation, side effect of opioids use, 49: 516
Contact stress, and development of osteoarthritis, 48: 238-239
Continuous passive motion (CPM)
and atrophy, 48: 510
devices, 46: 185-186, 191
knee rehabilitation, 49: 219
postarthroscopic drilling, 48: 137-138
prevention of DVT, **50: 416**
treatment of chondral injuries, 48: 634-635
Continuous postoperative anesthesia, use of, 49: 534-535
Contractures
consideration in preoperative planning, 48: 97
Dupuytren's, 49: 290
flexion
in myelomeningocele patients, 48: 564, 565
pediatric thoracic myelomeningocele, 48: 566
lower limb, correction of, 49*: 598*
motor neuropathy and diabetic foot, 48: 291-292
and partial foot amputations, 48: 322
polio-related, correction of, 4
soft-tissue, and medial epicondylar osteotomy, 48: 153-156
Controlled cortical perforation, removal of cement, 49: 87
Coracoacromial arch
defined, 47: 5
insufficiency, 47: 90, *91*
Coracoacromial ligament
in rotator cuff repair, 47: 82-*83*
and subacromial impingement, **50: 45**
and unstable shoulder arthroplasty, 47: 146-*147*
Coracoclavicular ossification, acromioclavicular joint, 49: 411
Coralline hydroxyapatite, 47: 528
Cord compression, and Steinberg Staging System, 49: *180*
Core decompression
knees, 48: 101
for osteonecrosis, 49: 174, 175, **50: 483-484, 492**
for precollapse osteonecrosis, 48: 99
tibial osteonecrosis, **50: *486***
in treatment of humeral head osteonecrosis, 48: 354-355
Core needle biopsy, 48: 590
examination of soft-tissue tumors, 48: 619
Coronal plane malunion, and total knee arthroplasty, 48: 161
Coronal ultrasound
newborn femoral head, **50: *539***
newborn hip, **50: *538***
Coronoid process
and elbow stability, 47: 158
fractures, 47: 162-164

fractures of, **50: 92-93**
internal fixation, **50: *93***
Corpectomy, 46: 130
cervical spondylotic myelopathy after, 48: *424*
for excision of tumor or fracture, 46: 135
L3, 48: *444*
Corrosion
metal implants, 49: 75
modularity and, 49: 76
process of, **50: 186**
Cortical bridge, 48: *154*
Cortical onlay strut allografts
canine model, 49: 99, *49: 99-100*
human retrievals, *49: 100-101*
Cortical perforation, fail to THA, 49: 89
Cortical strut grafts, incorporation, 49: 128
Corticocancellous bone, autogenous wafers of, in hip arthroplasty revision, 48: 81
Corticosteroids
and collagen necrosis, 48: 219
osteonecrosis, **50: 489-493**
osteonecrosis of the humeral head, 48: 349
pain management, 49: 519-520
and posterior heel pain, 48: 213
for rheumatoid arthritis, 46: 78
for sympathetically maintained pain, 46: 265
treatment of RSD, 49: 553
and wound healing, **50: 359**
Cost management
and blood management in orthopaedic surgery, 48: 655
revision total knee replacement, 46: 237-240
Costoclavicular ligaments, sternoclavicular joints, 49: 397
Cotyloides, terminology, **50: 105**
Cotyloplasty
centralization of socket, 49: 60
outcomes, 49: 29-30
Council of Musculoskeletal Specialty Societies (COMSS), outcomes assessment questionnaires, 48: 679-683
Council of Spine Societies (COSS), MODEMS development, 48: 681
Counterforce brace, 47: *166*
Coventry staples, 47: 433
Coxa valga, choice of implant, 49: 64
Coxa vara, neck cut, 49: 10
Craig biopsy cannula, 46: 144
Crawfish claw, 46: 97
"Crawford Campbell" bone graft, 46: 354
Creep-test loading apparatus, **50: *212***
Cricoarytenoid cartilage, rheumatoid arthritis in, 48: 97
Critical pathways
barriers to development, 49: 644-646
implementation of, 49: 647
need for, 49: 644
orthopaedic, development of, 49: 643-649
types of, 49: 644
Cross-arm adduction test, 47: *35*
Cross-linking
polyethylene, optimum methods, **50: 174-175**
UHMWPEs, **50: *170*-174**
Crossfire process, polyethylene cross-linking, **50: 173, 183**
Crouzon's syndrome, 46: 477, 496
Crowe classification system, hip dislocation, **50: 307**
Cruess classification, osteonecrosis of the humeral head, 48: *353*
Crutches, simple construction, 49: 594-*595*
Cuff tuberosity failure, and shoulder fracture management, 48: 368
Cultures
intraoperative, **50: 374**
periprosthetic femoral osteolysis, **50: 201**
Cuneiform, osteotomy of first, 46: 386
Cuniform osteotomy, **50: *562***
Cycle of disablement, 46: 417
Cyclic adenosine monophosphate agonists, effect on particulate-induced bone resorption, **50: 192**
Cyclooxygenase (COX), inhibitors, 49: 515
Cyclooxygenase-II (COX-II)
inhibitors, 49: 515
production of, 49: 79
treatment of spinal stenosis, **50: 153**
Cyclops lesion, 46: 257
Cyclosporine, and immunology of allografts, 48: 651
Cysts
aneurysmal, bone, 48: 538-539, 593-594, *595*
around hips, **50: 236**
dorsal ganglion, 49: *235*
extracapsular, **50: 391**
ganglion, 47: *12*
unicameral, bone, 48: 593-594
Cytokines
and bone resorption, 49: 72
and osteoarthritis, 49: 486
production of, 49: 78
Cytotoxic agents, treating rheumatoid arthritis, 46: 78

D

D'Antonio classification system, acetabular deficiencies, **50: *337***
Dantrolene, malignant hyperthermia treatment, 48: 560
Darrach procedure, 47: 211
Data management
Musculoskeletal Outcomes Data Evaluation and Management System (MODEMS), 48: 680-683
and outcomes research, 48: 667-683
Davis technique, **50: *300***
Deadman angle, 47: 45-*47*, 63
Deaths, leading causes of, 49: 567, *568*
Débridement
adequacy of, 49: 380
arthroscopic
of the ankle, 48: 243-247
in degenerative arthritis of the knee, 48: 136-137
for infected hip arthroplasty, 47: 300-301
for open tibial fracture, 46: 294-295
for osteoarthritis of the knee, 47: 429
periprostatic infections, **50: 410**
for rotator cuff repair, 47: 59
for stiff total knee replacement, 46: 194
treatment of chondral injuries symptoms, 48: 633
treatment of diabetic foot infection, 48: 319-320
treatment of osteonecrosis, **50: 492**
Debris-generated osteolytic defects, 46: 227-228
Decision making
at the end of life, 49: 640
orthopaedic critical pathways, 49: 643
Decompression. *See also* Core decompression
spinal stenosis, **50: 154-155**
subacromial
avoidance of complications, 47: 29-33
technique, 47: 25-26
subacromial impingement, **50: 45**
Deconditioning, geriatric patients, 46: 414

Decorin, 47: 480
Deep periprosthetic joint infection
prevention of, 46: 555-565
operating room environment, 46: 558-562
postoperative period, 46: 562-564
preoperative period, 46: 555-557
prophylactic antibiotics, 46: 557-558
Deep peroneal nerve, blocks, 49: 532
Deep vein thrombosis (DVT)
after hip arthroplasty, 47: 331-335
incidence of, 47: 331
prevention of, 47: 332-333
after knee arthroplasty, 46: 185-188
current prophylaxis, 46: 187-188
epidemiology, 46: 185-186
impact of chemoprophylaxis, 46: 186-187
treatment of, 46: 188
duration of prophylaxis/surveillance, **50: 418**
following TKA, **50: 415**
minimizing risk of, **50: 416-418**
prevention of, **50: 293**
risk of, 49: 4
Deformities
clinical presentation of bone tumors, 48: 607
as indication for surgery, 48: 93-94
and partial foot amputations, 48: 322
Dega osteotomies, **50: 551**
Degenerative arthritis, complication in humeral head replacement, 46: 19
Degenerative disk disease, 46: 129, 144
Dehydration, laser heating, **50: 5**
Delayed union, definition, 46: 281
Delirium, in geriatric patients, 46: 414
Deltoid ligament, injuries, 46: 315-316
following rotator cuff repair, 47: *78*-80, 89-*90*
with shoulder stiffness, 47: 73-74
Deltoid muscles
lateral head, rotator cuff reconstruction, **50: 66**
reattachment, **50: 49-50**
transfer of, 49: 325-326
Deltopectoral interval, identification of, 46: 8
Demineralized bone matrix, 47: 527
Demographics, reasons for changes in, 46: *409*
Denis classification system
stability of spinal tumors, *49: 473*-474
thoracolumbar fractures, 48: 437
Depo-Medrol, treatment of spinal stenosis, **50: 153**
Depositions, by expert witnesses, 48: 702-702
Depression
effect on musculoskeletal function, 46: 418
in elderly, 46: *413*
multiple-injury patients, 49: 394-395
and pain, 49: 541
Depth-ischemia classification, diabetic foot lesions, 48: *297,* 298-*299, 307*
de Quervain's disease, overdiagnosis of, 48: 694
de Quervain's extensor tenosynovitis, differential diagnosis, 49: 302
Dermatan sulfate, identification in menisci, 49: 191
Desmopressin, use in the orthopaedic setting, 48: 656-657
Developing countries
AAOS principles of involvement, 49: 580-583
appliances and surgery for poliomyelitis, 49: 593-600
burden of disease, 49: 570
common orthopaedic diseases, 49: 571
correction of lower limbs deformities, 49: 594-598
epidemiologic profiles, 49: 569
orthopaedic surgery in, 49: 567-573
selected orthopaedic conditions common in, 49: 585-591
United Nations classification, 49: *568*
volunteer opportunities for orthopaedists, 49: 575-577
Developmental dysplasia of the hip (DDH)
closed reduction
newborn to 6 months, **50: 542-543**
6 months to 1 year, **50: 543-544**
congenital, **50: *536***
hip arthroplasty, 49: 6
incidence, **50: 541**
newborns, **50: 535-540**
older children, **50: 547-553**
treatment, **50: 548-549**
open reduction, **50: 544**
physical examination, **50: 541**
planning hip arthroplasty, 49: 3
Salter osteotomy, **50: *550***
templating, 49: *9*
Dexamethasone, iontophoresis of, **50: 525**
Dextran, 47: 332
prevention of DVT, **50: 417**
Dextrose, generalized inflammatory reaction, **50: 8**
Diabetes mellitus
and infection at arthroplasty sites, 48: 111
management of stiff shoulder, 49: 283-293
and neuropathic osteoarthropathy, 48: 269-270
prevalence of, 48: 289
type 1, 49: 284
type 2, 49: 284
wound healing, **50: 359**
Diabetic foot
classification of ulcerations, 48: 305-306
considerations in healing, 48: *323*
depth-ischemia classification of lesions, 48: *297, 307*
diagnosis, 48: 294-298
financial impact, 48: 290
impact of infections, 48: 317
infections of, 48: 317-320
outpatient diagnosis and management, 48: 289-302
outpatient treatments, 48: 299-302
pathophysiology, 48: 290-294
risk of amputation, 48: 317
total contact casting and, 48: 305
Diagnosis-related estimates (DREs), evaluation of the spine, 48: 451
Diagnostic fixation of lumbar motion segments, 46: 157-158
Diagnostic thoracoscopy, 46: 144-145
Diastrophic dwarfism, 47: 466
Diazepam and aging, 46: 415
Dicloxacillin, treatment of diabetic foot infection, 48: 319
Die-punch fracture, scaphoid facet, 48: *467, 468*
Diet, postoperative, total hip arthroplasty, 48: 35
Differential spinal blockade, 46: 264
Digital Encryption Standard (DES), and MODEMS data, 48: 681-682
Digital flexor tendon, entrapment, 48: 694
Digital nerves, block, 49: 530-531
Digits, transmetacarpal amputation, 49: *384*
1,25-Dihydroxyvitamin D_3, effect on particulate-induced bone resorption, **50: 192**
Dilator knots, meniscus repair, 49: *199*
N,N-Dimethylparatoluidine, sensitivity to, 49: 79
Dimethylsulfoxide (DMSO), in treating spinal cord injuries, 46: 119
Diphenhydramine and aging, 46: 415
Direct lateral approach, hip arthroplasty, 49: 16-17, *16-17*
Directional osteotomies, **50: 549-551**
Disability of the Arm, Shoulder and Hand (DASH), MODEMS program, 48: 680
Disability prevention strategies, 46: 417-418

Disaster relief
management of, 49: 575
volunteering, 49: 576
Disclosure, respect for autonomy, 49: 635-636
Disease burden, disability-adjusted life years, 49: 569, *570*
Disease-specific outcome assessment instruments, use after fractures in elderly, 46: 441
Diseases, new, emergence of, 49: 569
DISI (dorsal intercalated segment instability) deformity
and analysis of wrist instability, 47: 203-205
defined, 47: 222
Disk excision, failures following
identification, 46: 143
natural causes, 46: 144
technique, 46: 143-144
Disk herniations
classification, 46: *148*
foraminal and extraforaminal, 46: 143
infraforaminal herniation, 49: 339
L5-S1, 48: *529*
pediatric, 48: 535-536
test for, 49: *337*
Diskitis
bone scan of, 48: *531*
and pediatric back pain, 48: 530-531
Diskogenic pain, anatomy of, 46: 145
Diskography
evaluation of cervical degenerative disk disease, 49: 337
spinal cord compression, 49: 341
Dislocations. *See also* Developmental dysplasia of the hip
acute, elbow, **50: 91-92**
after total hip arthroplasty, **50: 265**
chronology of, **50: 265-266**
developmental, **50: 535**
elbow, **50: 89-90**
hinged external fixation, **50: 96-98**
hip
abductor muscle deficiencies, **50: 270**
classifications, **50: 307**
differential diagnosis, **50: *269***
risk of, 49: 4
THR for, **50: 307-316**
and implant choice, **50: 267**
implants locations, **50: 266-267**
implants orientation, **50: 266**
of the knee, 48: 515-521
mobile-bearing knee prostheses, **50: 433-434**
postoperative rate of, revision total hip arthroplasty, 48: 24
prevention of, **50: 266-267**
recurrent, and revision total hip arthroplasty, 48: 53
risk factors, **50: 265**
THA, classification of, **50: 289-290**
total congenital hip, 49: 20-21
treatment of, **50: 267-273**
use of constrained acetabular component, **50: 281-287**
use of megaprostheses, 49: 145
Disodium pamidronate, effect on particulate-induced bone resorption, **50: 192**
Distal amputation surgery, 46: 508
Distal bypass fixation
femoral defects, 49: 120-121
treatment of femoral bone loss, 49: 119-129
Distal clavicle resection, arthroscopic, 47: 35-41
advantages of, 47: 37, 41
direct approach, 47: *38*-39
indirect approach, 47: 39-41
Distal femoral osteotomy, outcomes, **50: *505***
Distal femoral varus osteotomy, 47: 430, 434
Distal metatarsal articular angle (DMAA), 46: 362
Distal metatarsal osteotomy (Mitchell or Wilson osteotomy), 46: 372-*375,* 385-386
Distal phalanx fractures, 47: 187
Distal radial tilt, radiographic measurement, 48: *465*
Distal radioulnar joint (DRUJ)
anatomy, 47: 191, 209
disorders after radial fracture, 47: 199-200
exposure of, 47: 200-201
imaging of, 47: 209
instability, 47: 209-213
acute, 47: 210
chronic, 47: 210-213
Distal radius fractures, 47: 191-201
classification of, 47: *192*-195
radiography of, 47: *195*
treatment
of compression fractures, 47: 197-*199*
of shearing fractures, 47: 195-*197*
Distal soft-tissue reconstruction
for correction of hallux valgus deformity, 46: 367-370
with osteotomy of first metatarsal, 46: 374-378
Distal tibiofibular synostosis, 48: 328
Distraction
ankle
and cartilage matrix repair, 48: 251-254
technique of, 48: 250-251
in dog knee joint, 48: *254*
joint, and formation of articular surfaces, 48: 239-240
osteogenesis, 49: 503-509
and reframing, pain management, 49: 520
Distraction osteogenesis, 46: 284, 547
preoperative planning, 48: 282
Do-not-resuscitate (DNR) orders, teaching of ethics, 49: 640
Donors, screening of, infection control, 49: 617-618
Doppler. *See* Ultrasonography
Dorsal angulation, 46: 372-374
Dorsal carpal ganglia, wrist, removal of, 49: 234-235
Dorsal ganglion cysts, removal of, 49: *235*
Dorsal intercalated segment instability (DISI) deformity, 47: 203-205
Dorsal intercarpal ligaments, **50: *123***
Dorsal radiocarpal ligaments, **50: 123**
Dorsal radioulnar ligament, **50: *123***
Dorsal root ganglia, pain transmission, 49: 513
Dorsal root ganglia (DRG), and spinal stenosis, **50: 145**
Dorsal wrist ganglia, **50: 130**
Down syndrome, THA in, 49: 163
Doxepin and aging, 46: 415
Drapes
and infection at arthroplasty sites, 48: 113
infection control, 49: 612
Drawer test
posterior, for posterior cruciate ligament damage, 48: 200
posterolateral, for posterior cruciate ligament damage, 48: 200
prone, for posterior cruciate ligament damage, 48: 200
Drilling
sanding down calluses, 48: *301*
treatment of chondral injuries, 48: 633-635
Drop sign, positive, rotator cuff tear, **50: 43**
Drug abuse, and recurrent sepsis, **50: 318**
Duchenne muscular dystrophy, neuromuscular scoliosis in, 48: *557,* 559-560
Dupuytren's contractures, 49: 290
of palmar fascia, 46: 246, *248*
Durasul process, polyethylene cross-linking, **50: 173, 183**

Dwarfism
diastrophic, 47: 466
and fibroblast growth factors, 46: 481, 47: 466
Dwyer-type osteotomy, 46: 343
Dynamic hip abduction brace, **50: *292***
Dynamic Joint Distractor, 47: *161,* 163-164
Dynamic posterior shift test, for posterior cruciate ligament damage, 48: 200
Dynamic scapholunate instability, **50: 129-130**
Dynamic splinting, 46: 547-*548*
Dysbaric exposure, and osteonecrosis, 49: 171-172
Dysplasia
definition, **50: 541**
hip, classifications, 49: 24-26, *25*
older children management of, **50: 549**

E
Early active-assisted joint motion, use in the developing world, 49: *588*
Economic aspects of medical care, teaching of ethics, 49: 640
Economic impacts, synovial joint degeneration, 49: 481-482
Education, ethics, 49: 634-635
case-based curriculum, 49: 640-641
Effusion, joints, **50: 391**
Effusions, knee joint, 49: 220
Eichenholtz classification system, for neuropathic arthropathy, 48: *269*
Elastase, response to particulate debris, **50: 191**
Elastic stockings, prevention of DVT, 47: 332, **50: 416**
Elastic wraps, tendinitis, **50: 526**
Elasticity, cobalt-chromium implants, 49: 75
Elbow. *See also* Olecranon
acute dislocations, **50: 91-92, 100-101**
acute fracture-dislocations, **50: 92**
algorithm for dislocations, **50: *100***
anatomy, 49: 255-256
anterolateral portal, 49: 242, *243*
arthritis
arthroscopic treatment, 49: 247-252
radiograph, 49: *248*
arthroscopy, 49: 239-246
complication risk by procedure, 49: *257*
complications, 49: 245, 252, 255-257, *257*
contraindications, 49: 249
patient position, 49: 239-240
technique, 49: 249-251
classification of instability, **50: 90-91**
constraints to instability, **50: 90, *91***
dislocation, **50: 89-90, *95***
extensor mechanism, 47: *151-152*
hinged external fixation, **50: 96-98**
imaging of, 46: 522-523
instability, 47: 157-164
contributions to normal stability, 47: 157-159
fractures of proximal ulna, olecranon or coronoid, 47: *161*-164
laxity, 47: *102*
radial head fracture with dislocation of elbow, 47: 160-*161*
radial head fracture with MCL tear, 47: 159-*160*
recurrent, **50: 98-100**
lateral pivot-shift test, **50: *91***
loose bodies, 49: 248-249
medial instability
diagnosis of, 48: 384
nonsurgical treatment of, 48: 384-385
outcomes, 48: 387-388
rehabilitation, 48: 387
surgical treatment of, 48: 385-387
midlateral portal, 49: *242,* 242-243
nerve distances, 49: *255*
options for tendon transfers, 49: *319*
osteochondritis dissecans of, 48: 393-398
portal placement, 49: 240-244
posterior impingement
arthroscopic treatment of, 48: 399-404
nonsurgical management, 48: 402
patient evaluation, 48: 400-402
postoperative rehabilitation, 48: 403
results, 48: 403-404
surgical technique, 48: 402-403
posterior view, after ulnohumeral arthroplasty, 49: *251*
posterolateral portal, 49: 243-*244*
posttraumatic, 49: 256
proximal lateral portal, *49: 241*-242
proximal medial portal, 49: *240*
risk of complication, by diagnosis, 49: *256*
surgical management of extensor mechanism, 47: 151-156
excision of olecranon, 47: 153-155
for triceps avulsion injuries, 47: 152-153
for triceps tendinitis, 47: 152, 170
tendon transfers, 49: 328-331
tennis, 47: 165-171
anconeus compartment syndrome, 47: 170
lateral epicondylitis, 46: 572-573, 47: 165-167
medial epicondylitis, 46: 573, 47: 168-170
triceps tendinitis, 47: 152, 170
terrible-triad injury, **50: 92-94**
treatment of radial head fractures, **50: 94-95**
ulnar nerve compression, 49: 305
unstable, **50: 89-102**
valgus-stress testing, **50: 92**
varus-stress testing, **50: 92**
work related illnesses, 48: 694
Elderly. *See also* Aging
activities of daily living (ADL) in, 46: 410-411
alcoholism in, 46: 413-*414*
Alzheimer's disease in, 46: 423
cardiopulmonary disease in, 46: 423
outcome assessment after fracture in, 46: 439-443
quality of bone in, 46: 424
Electrical stimulation, and osteonecrosis, 49: 174-175
Electroacupuncture, treatment of CRPS, 49: 554-555
Electrodiagnostic studies
cervical reticulopathy myelopathy, 49: 345
high radial nerve palsy, 49: 297
PIN palsy, 49: 299
usefulness of, 49: 308-309
Electromagnetic energy, pain management, 49: 545-546
Electromagnetic medicine, safety issues, 49: 546
Electromyography (EMG)
axonal degeneration, 49: 309
high medial nerve palsy, 49: 297
PIN palsy, 49: 299
shoulder, 46: 53-64
analysis of long head of biceps tendon, 46: 59-60
analysis of manual muscle testing for rotator cuff strength, 46: 57-58
of aquatic physical therapy, 46: *60*-62
of dynamic shoulder motion during therapeutic rotator cuff, exercise, 46: 62-64
electrode placement, 46: 53-55
normalization of EMG signal, 46: 55-57
ulnar nerve compression, 49: 308
Electrophysiology, effect of nerve compression, 49: 364

Embryology, limb development, 47: *462*-463
Emergency medical services (EMS), management of acute spinal trauma, 46: 113-114
Emergency Medical Technicians-Basic (EMT-B) management of acute spinal trauma, 46: 114
Emergency medicine
 children with multiple injuries, 49: 416
 multiply-injured patients, 49: 377-379
Emergency rooms
 airway, breathing, and circulation management in, 46: 114-115
 evaluation of spinal cord injury in, 46: 116-117
 infection control precautions, 49: 605-613
 treatment of tibial shaft fractures in, 46: 293-300
Emotions, and pain, 49: 541
Employers
 choice of health plan, 48: *677*
 and the cost of health care, 48: 673-674
 health insurance spending, 48: *675*
EMT-P (paramedic) in acute spinal trauma management, 46: 114
Enchondroma
 clinicopathologic features of, 48: *614*
 differentiation from chondrosarcoma, 48: 613-615
 hypocellular hyaline cartilage in, 48: *613*
 treatment of, 48: 592
Endo-Klinik bone loss classification, 49: 89, *89*
Endocrinologic problems, in the elderly, 46: 423
Endorphins, and acupuncture, 49: 559-560
Endoscopic clip appliers, 46: 132
Endoscopic retractors, 46: 132
Endoscopic scissors, 46: 132
Endoscopic surgery
 development of, 46: 127
 introduction, history, and benefits, 46: 127
Energy/fatigue measurement, outcomes instrument for, 48: 420-421
Engh and Glassman classification
 of acetabular deficiencies, 48: 48, *48*
 bone loss, 49: *89,* 89-90
Enterobacter cloacae, in factitious disease of the hand, 46: 74
Enterococcus
 antibiotic resistance, 49: 607-608
 glycopeptide resistance, 49: *608*
 infection in the diabetic foot, 48: 318
 vancomycin resistance (VRE), 49: 606
Enterococcus casseliflavus, vancomycin resistance, 49: 607
Enterococcus faecalis, prevalence of, 49: 607
Enterococcus faecium, prevalence of, 49: 607
Enterococcus gallinarum, vancomycin resistance, 49: 607
Envelope of function
 concept of, 48: 187-188
 dynamic changes in, 48: *190*
 knee
  and anterior cruciate ligament injury, 48: *195*
  loading examples, 48: *188*
Eosinophilic granuloma, and pediatric back pain, 48: 538-539
Epicondyle, osteotomized, 48: *154*
Epicondylitis. *See also* Tennis elbow
 arthroscopy for, 48: 380
 in the athlete, 48: 375-381
 diagnosis, 48: 376
 etiology, 48: 375
 lateral, surgical treatment, 48: *379*
 medial, surgical treatment, 48: *380*
 nonsurgical treatment, 48: 376-378
 pathophysiology, 48: 375-376
 postoperative care, 48: 379
 surgical outcomes, 48: 379-380
 surgical treatment, 48: 378-380
Epidural sympathetic blockade, 46: 264
Epinephrine
 use with bupivacaine, 49: 527
 use with lidocaine, 49: 526
Epiphyseodesis, open, **50: *562***
Epoetin alfa
 efficacy in major orthopaedic surgery, 48: *661*
 physiologic effects of, 48: *660*
 use in the orthopaedic setting, 48: *660*-662
Equinovarus deformity, management of, 48: 543-*544*
Equinus contracture, and plantar metatarsal ulcerations, 48: 293
Equinus deformity, in patients with myelomeningocele, 48: 545
Equipment, maintenance in the Third World, 49: 582
Ertl procedure, 48: 328
Erythema, periprosthetic femoral osteolysis, **50: 200**
Erythema multiforme, 46: 72
Erythrocyte sedimentation rate (ESR)
 in arthritis, 48: 97
 defined, 47: 286
 diagnosis of arthroplasty site infection, 48: 114
 diagnosis of infection following arthroplasty, 47: 286-287, 292-*293*
 exclusion of active infection, **50: 319**
 infected knees, **50: 368-369**
 laboratory investigations of bone tumors, 48: 608
 periprosthetic femoral osteolysis, **50: 200-201**
 in preoperative assessments, 48: 45
Erythromycin, antibiotic-loaded cement, **50: 327**
Escharotomy, children with multiple injuries, 49: 425
Escherichia coli
 in factitious disease of the hand, 46: 74
 infection in the diabetic foot, 48: 318
 penicillin resistance, 49: 606
Essex-Lopresti lesion, 47: 173
Estrogens
 for osteoporosis, 46: 447, 452
 SCFE, **50: 555**
Ethical dilemmas, 46: 415
Ethics, clinical, residency training, 49: 634-635, 639-642
Ethylene oxide, 47: 380, 527
 UHMWPE sterilization, 49: 74
Ewing's sarcoma
 extraosseous soft-tissue, 48: *580*
 knee radiographs, 48: *578*
 nuclear features, 49: 437
 treatment of, 48: 598-600
Examination under anesthesia (EUA), of knee dislocation, 48: 517
Excessive Lateral Pressure Syndrome (ELPS), 46: 527
Excisional biopsies, soft tissue tumors, 49: 440
Exeter stems, use of, 49: 111
Exopolysaccharide-glycocalyx slime. *see* Glycocalyx slime
Expenditures, for national health care, 48: 673
Expert witnesses, and malpractice actions, 48: 702-702
Extensor carpi radialis brevis (ECRB), anatomy, 49: 295
Extensor carpi radialis longus (ECRL), anatomy, 49: 295
Extensor compartment artery, **50: *115*, 115-117**
Extensor hallucis longus, 46: 358
 with arthrodesis, 48: 340
Extensor mechanism
 function of, 49: 386-387
 and implant failures, 48: 163
 lag, 48: 158-159
 patellar clunk syndrome, 46: 177
 patellar fractures, 46: 173-174
 rupture, **50: 405**

Extensor pollicis longus, ruptured, differential diagnosis, 49: 299
External rotation recurvatum test, for PCL damage, 48: 200
External-rotation stress test, syndesmosis instability, 46: 317
Extra-abdominal desmoid, treatment of, 48: 597-598
Extra-annular arthroscopic approach, 46: 155
Extracellular matrix (ECM)
articular cartilage, 47: 479-*481*
chondrocyte remodeling of, 48: 193
collagens, 47: 479-480
proteoglycans, 47: 480-*481*
tissue fluid, 47: 479

F

FABER test, 49: 366
Facet arthrosis, **50: *142***
Facet joints
degeneration of, 49: 363
removal of, spinal stenosis, 49: 369
Facet tropism, **50: *141***
Factitious diseases of hand, 46: 74-*75*
Falls
distinct phases of, 46: *432*
in geriatric patients, 46: 414-415
and hip fractures, 46: 449-450
Familial hyperlipidemia, and posterior heel pain, 48: 213
Fascia lata, autograft, latissimus dorsi transfer, **50: *69***
Fasciitis, plantar, **50: 521**
Fasciocutaneous flaps, **50: 361**
Fasciotomy
children with multiple injuries, 49: 425
surgical technique for, 46: 305-*307*
Fat emboli, and osteonecrosis, 49: 171
Fat embolism during hip arthroplasty, 47: 275-*276*
Fat pads
atrophy, **50: *521***
chronic heel pain, **50: 522-523**
foot, anatomy of, **50: 522**
heel, separation, **50: 523**
infrapatellar, 49: *214*
Fatigue, polyethylene wear, **50: 165**
Fear, and pain, 49: 541
Federation of the Red Cross (FRC), disaster relief, 49: 575
Femoral artery, occlusion, 48: 157-158
Femoral canal
exposure of, 49: *14*
vascularized scaphoid window for access to, revision total hip arthroplasty, 48: 9-11
Femoral components
anterior stem location and stability, 48: *170*
catch-coated, **50: 202**
classification of fixation, 49: 128
constrained system, **50: 282-283**
fixation of, total knee arthroplasty, 48: *179*
loosening, extended proximal femoral osteotomy, 48: 19
mobile-bearing TKA, **50: *435***
New Jersey LCS, **50: *443***
porous-coated, outcomes, 49: 127-129
revision, 49: 86-87
Femoral condyle, spontaneous osteonecrosis, **50: 483-486**
Femoral condyles, allograft for defects of, 47: 518-*520*
Femoral defects
classification, 49: 121-122, **50: 203-206**
cortical, bridging of, **50: *214***
focal, loading of, 48: *633*
type 1, **50: 202-*204***
type 2, **50: 203-*204***
type 3, **50: *204-206***
type 4, **50: *206***
type I, 49: *121*
type II, 49: *121, 127*
type IIIA, 49: *122, 127*
type IIIB, 49: *122*
type IV, 49: *122*
Femoral discontinuity, definition, 49: 93
Femoral fractures
children with multiple injuries, 49: 418-419
in the developing world, 49: 585-587
pathologic
intertrochanteric, 49: 463-465
subtrochanteric, 49: 465-467
periprosthetic
after total hip arthroplasty, 47: 237-241
classification of, 47: 253
intraoperative, 47: 237-238, 251-252
postoperative, 47: 238-241, 243-248
prevalence of, 47: 243-244
treatment and results, 47: 244-248
after total knee arthroplasty, 46: 197-202, 47: 437-448
incidence of, 46: 197, 47: 253-254
internal fixation for supracondylar fractures, 46: 199-*201,* 47:439-442, 452-*453*
intraoperative, 47: *437*-438, 449-*450*
and notching of the femur, 46: 197, 47: 253-254
postoperative, 46: 197-202, 47: 439-445, 451-*453*
and revision total knee replacement, 46: 201, 47: 444-445
treatment, 46: 197-*199,* 47: 439-445
treatment algorithm for supracondylar fractures, 47: *452*
treatment results, 46: 201-202, 47: 439-445
allografts in treatment of, 47: 257-*263*
advantages and disadvantages of, 47: 262
technique, 47: 257-259
proximal replacement prosthesis, 49: 466-467
subtrochanteric, nonunion, 49: *142*
supracondylar, **50: 379-384**
classifications, **50: 379**
displaced, **50: *381, 383***
risk factors, **50: 379**
treatment options, **50: 379-384**
Femoral grafts
impaction allografting, 49: 111-117
stem migration, 49: 108-109
Femoral head
allograft reconstruction, 46: 232-234
blood supply, **50: *559***
cancellous grafts, 49: 177
classification of osteonecrosis, 49: *172*
conversion to bipolar, **50: 270-271**
corrosion, **50: *186***
cortical grafts, 49: 177
displacement of, **50: 255**
limited endoprosthesis for osteonecrosis, 48: 100
osteochondral grafts, 49: 177
osteonecrosis, 49: 169-181
osteonecrosis in SLE, 48: 98-99
pathologic fractures, surgical treatment, 49: 463
protrusion of prostheses, **50: *225***
resurfacing, 48: 100
septic arthritis, **50: *327***
subluxation, **50: *276***

trapdoor procedure, nonvascularized bone grafting, 49: *176, 177*
vascularized fibular graft, 49: *177*
Femoral neck
anteversion, **50: 254**
development and growth, **50: 537**
osteotomies, **50: *562***
pathologic fractures, surgical treatment, 49: 463
Femoral nerves
block, 49: 531
Halsey, Pavlik harness, **50: 543**
Femoral osteolysis, 47: 321-324
algorithm for treatment of, 47: *323*
classification, 47: 321-322
epidemiology, 47: 316-317
Femoral osteotomy, correctional, 49: *67*
Femoral peel, in knee arthroplasty, 48: 165-166
Femoral resurfacing, and the Steinberg Staging System, 49: *181*
Femoral S-ROM stems, Solution, 49: *1126*
Femoral shafts, retraction of, 49: *18*
Femoral stems
calcar replacement, pathologic intertrochanteric fractures, 49: 464-465
insertion of, **50: 343-344**
migration with impaction morcellized bone graft, **50: 216**
modularity, 49: 76
porous-coated, failure rates, 49: *120*
precoated, collared, 49: 114, *115*
in situ prosthesis removal, 49: 124
subsidence, 49: 111-112
Femoral stenosis, definition, 49: 92-93
Femur
angular deformities, 49: 67-68
bone loss, 48: *177,* 49: 83-95
distal bypass fixation, 49: 119-129
treatment options, 49: 148-149
bone preparation techniques, 48: 178
canal distortion, and arthroplasty, 49: 68
canal preparation, for proximal femoral osteotomy, 48: 22-23
cementless revisions, outcomes, 49: 120-121
choice of components, 49: 34
classification of osteolysis, **50: 202**
controlled perforations, 48: *15*
cortical allograft repair, 49: 98-99
creation of controlled windows, 48: 9
deficient, longitudinal split, 48: 77, *78*
deficient proximal, transfemoral approach, 48: 77-79
diagnosis of osteolysis, **50: 199-200**
difficult, in THA, 49: 63-68
distal, quadriceps myocutaneous composite flap for exposure of, 48: 157-159
distal, spontaneous osteonecrosis, **50: 495**
distortion, 49: 63
dysplastic hips, 49: *24*
failure of prosthesis components, 48: 43
gunshot wound, 49: *585*
hemiresurfacing, 49: 178-179
impaction grafting, biomechanics, 49: 105-110
improper tunnel placement, **50: 464-465, *465***
level to bone loss, 49: *92*
loading schedule of intramedullary grafts, 48: *84*
loose long-stem prosthesis, 49: *143*
maximal subsidence and graft stability, 48: *84*
medial condyle, articular lesion, **50: *501***
modular fixated stem, 49: *66*
osteolysis of, **50: 197-209**
preparation of structural allografts, 49: *154*
proximal
development and growth, **50: 537**
metastatic disease, surgical treatment, 49: 461-469
replacement implants, 49: *144*
replacement with megaprosthesis, 49: 141-146
varus remodeling, 48: *20*
radiographic anatomy, **50: 255-256**
reconstruction algorithm, 49: *117*
reconstruction of, 49: 32-34
restoration of bone stock, 49: 97-101
revision with structural allografts, complications, 49: 156-159, *157*
right distal, surgical schematic, 48: *126*
shortening, **50: 308-309**
slipped capital epiphysis, **50: 555-570**
stability after impaction graphing, **50: 213-214**
structural allografts, 49: *156*
reinforcement, 49: *155*
templating, 49: 9-10
tunnel formation, **50: 470-471**
type 1 defect, 48: *169*
type 2 defects, 48: *170*
type 3 defects, 48: *171*
use of vastus slide for access to, 48: 13-17
Fernandez classification of distal radius fractures, 47: *192*-193
Fibrin clots
arthroscopic image, 49: *196*
in healing menisci, 49: 208
meniscal repair, 49: 201
meniscal tear, 49: *201*
Fibroblast growth factors. *See also* Basic fibroblast growth factor
and achondroplasia, 46: 481, 47: 466, 471
articular cartilage restoration, 48: 624
and bone formation, 46: 496
for fracture healing, 46: 484
as regulator of articular cartilage, 47: 465, 471
as therapeutic agents, 46: 473
Fibroblastic responses, after hip arthroplasty, 48: 97
Fibroblasts
and metal implants, 49: 75
response to particulate debris, **50: 189**
Fibrocartilage
proliferation, **50: 504**
reparative, and arthroscopic drilling, 48: 137-139
and retrocalcaneal bursitis, 48: 211
Fibrocartilaginous anlage, resection of, 46: 107
Fibrocytes, diabetic frozen shoulder, 49: *284*
Fibromatosis, 48: *598*
MRI, 49: *448*
treatment of, 48: 597
Fibromodulin, 47: 480
Fibronectin, in osteoarthritis, 49: 486
Fibroproliferative scar nodule, 46: 257
Fibrous dysplasia
correction, 49: *507*
differentiation from parosteal osteosarcoma, 48: 615-*616*
treatment of, 48: 594-*595*
Fibrous histiocytoma
malignant, 48: 601
MRI of, 48: *579*
Fibrous hyperplasia, and arthrofibrosis, 49: 212
Fibrous tissues, age-related changes in dense, 46: 464-465
Fibula transfer, tibial stabilization, 49: *591*
Fibular fracture, malunited, 48: *280*
Ficat and Arlet system, classification of osteonecrosis, 49: *172-173*
Fine needle aspiration biopsy (FNAB), 48: 589-590
Fine needle aspiration (FNA), examination of soft-tissue tumors, 48: 619

Finger escape sign, 49: *343*
tests for myelopathy, 49: *337*
Fingers. *See also* Digits
clinodactyly, 49: *286*
Finkelstein's test, de Quervain's extensor tenosynovitis, 49: 302
"Fish hook" osteophyte, in insertional Achilles tendinitis, 47: 424-*425*
Fixation
and allograft healing, 48: 182
cementless, issues in revision total knee arthroplasty, 48: 177-182
children with multiple injuries, 49: 429-430
circular, limb lengthening, 49: 506-507
external
for tibial shaft fractures, 46: 284, 296-297
use in the developing world, 49: 587
long-stem, total knee arthroplasty, 48: 179
Flail shoulder, polio-related, 49: 599
Flaps
risk of necrosis, 48: 157-158
soft-tissue management, injured upper extremities, 49: 389-390
Flexible intramedullary rods, internal fixation in children, 49: 417
Flexible nails, use in children, 49: 430
Flexor carpi ulnaris tendon, acute calcific tendinitis in, 46: *69*
Flexor hallucis longus (FHL), 46: 358-359
tendinitis, **50: 526-527**
and walking, 48: 220
Flexor-pronator mass, reattachment of, 48: *390*
Flexor-protonator muscles
exposure of origin, 48: *386*
proximal transfer, 49: 328
Flexor retinaculum, 46: 393
Flexor system, function of, 49: 386-387
Flexor tendon transfer
for Achilles tendon reconstruction, 46: 579-*580*
for posterior tibial tendon dysfunction, 46: 398-*400, 401*
Floating joints, children with multiple injuries, 49: 420
Fluid extravasation, and complications of shoulder arthroscopy, 48: 369-370
Fluocinolone, with clindamycin, treatment of diabetic foot infection, 48: 319
Fluoride, for osteoporosis, 46: 453-454
Fluoroquinolones, 47: 300
and collagen dysplasia, 48: 219-220
oral, and posterior heel pain, 48: 213
Fluoroscopy
mobile-bearing TKR, **50: 434-437**
for wrist instability, 47: 205, 208, 223
Flurazepam and aging, 46: 415
Flying buttress graft, **50: *312***
Foam models, preoperative, use of, 48: 47
Foil templates, use in distal femoral varus osteotomy, 48: 126, 128
Follow-up regimens
frequency of examinations, 48: *605*
orthopaedic oncology patients, 48: 603-606
Foot
acquired flatfoot deformity, 46: 393-404
anatomy and pathophysiology, 46: 393-394
diagnosis of, 46: 394-395
surgical treatment for, 46: 396-404
amputation of, 48: 687-689
anatomy, 46: *358*-364
hindfoot, 47: 421-422
arch support, **50: 526**
calcaneus fractures, salvage procedures for, 46: 339-345
bony changes, 46: 339-*341*
initial management, 46: 339
treatment of, 46: 341-*345*
deformities, and myelomeningocele, 48: 543-546
hallux valgus, 46: 357-388
history and physical examination, 46: 364-365
radiography for, 46: 365
surgical correction, 46: 365-*387*
heel pain, 47: 425-427
nerve entrapment syndromes, 47: 426-427
plantar fasciitis, 47: 405, 425-426
hypersensitivity, spinal stenosis, **50: 149**
imaging of, 46: 524-526
partial amputation, in the diabetic, 48: 321-329
pathophysiology of ulceration, 48: 305
planovalgus deformity, relation of valgus knee arthritis with, 48: 94
prioritization of reconstructive surgeries, 48: 94-95
surgical treatment for neuropathic arthropathy, 48: 269-277
talus fractures, 46: *323-337*
outcome of, 46: *335, 337*
talar body fractures, 46: 332-*333*
talar neck fractures, 46: *326-332*
windlass mechanism, **50: *522***
Foraminotomy
lumbar spinal stenosis, 49: 367
posteroanterior view, **50: *156***
Forced vital capacity (FVC), and pulmonary distress, 48: 552, 559
Forearm
gunshot wound, 49: *387*
skeletal reconstruction, 49: 333-384
soft-tissue sarcomas, 49: *446*
Forefoot, prioritizing surgeries, 48: 94
Foreign body giant cells, bone-cement interface, 49: 72
Foreign-body reaction in hand, 46: 74
Format selection, of outcomes assessment instruments, 48: 668
Foundation for Accountability (FACCT), and performance measurement, 48: 677, 679
Fractures
acetabular (*See* Acetabular fractures)
ankle, 46: 311-318
associated with neuropathic arthropathy, 48: *271*-272
calcaneus, 46: 339-345
of cementless components, **50: 392-393**
in children, complicated by burns or head injuries, 49: 425-430
children with multiple injuries, 49: 426-429
classification of, 49: 416, 418-419
clinical presentation of bone tumors, 48: 607
coronoid process, 47: 162-164, **50: 92-93**
distal aspect of the radius, 49: 233-234
in the elderly, outcome assessment, 46: 439-443
external fixation, children with multiple injuries, 49: 419-420
femoral (*See* Femoral fractures)
femoral components, 49: 89
fixation, children with multiple injuries, 49: 417-419
growth factor treatment of, 46: 483-486, 47: 530-532
hand, 47: 187-190
hip, in rheumatoid arthritis, 48: 102
humeral impression, 47: *106,* 109-110
iatrogenic intraoperative, THA, 48: 24
implant, 49: 44-45
intertrochanteric, metastatic bone disease, 49: 463-465
intra-articular, distal aspect of the radius, **48: 465-479**
intraoperative, TSA, **50: 84-85**
lumbar spine, frequency, **48: 429**
malunited, 48: *280*
neuroarthropathic, use of total contact casting, 48: 307-308
nonunion, upper extremities, 49: 382-383
olecranon, 46: *539,* 47: *162*
open
and ankle dislocation, 48: *284*
sepsis rate for HIV-positive patients, 49: 627-628

upper extremities, 49: 382
osteoporotic, 46: 7
patellar, following TKA, **50: 385-387, 403-404**
pathologic, 48: 581-583
metastatic bone disease, 49: 457
risk scoring, 49: *462*
spinal, probability of, 49: *474*
pelvic, children with multiple injuries, 49: 420-423
periprosthetic, 47: 251-254
acetabular, 47: 231-235
after total shoulder arthroplasty, 48: 365-366
femoral, 47: 237-241, 243-254, 257-*263*
following TKA, **50: 379-389**
patellar, 46: 173-*174,* 47: 254, 438, 445-448, 450-451, 455-*457*
tibial, **50: *385***
proximal humeral (*See* Proximal humeral fractures)
radial head (*See* Radial head fractures)
scaphoid (*See* Scaphoid fractures)
shoulder (*See* Shoulder joint fractures)
spine (*See* Spinal fractures)
stabilization burn injuries, 49: 426
stress, 48: *583,* **50: 523**
structural femoral allografts, 49: 158
supracondylar femoral, **50: 379-384**
talus (*See* Talar fractures)
thoracolumbar, 48: 427-428, 437-441, 443-449, 448-449
tibia (*See* Tibial fractures)
timing of surgery, children with multiple injuries, 49: 427
ulnar styloid process, 48: 475-476
worldwide prevalence, 49: 571
Free microvascular bone transfer, for tibial shaft fractures, 46: 284
Free radicals
in polyethylene, 49: 52
and UHMWPEs, **50: 169-170**
Freeze drying
allograft bone, 49: 97-98
and immunology of allografts, 48: 650-651
Freezing, allograft bone, 49: 97-98
Frictional force, at osteotomy interface, **50: 250**
Friedreich's ataxia, neuromuscular scoliosis in, 48: 560
Froment's sign, ulnar nerve compression, 49: 308
Frozen sections, intraoperative, **50: 373-374**
Frozen shoulder
after rotator cuff repair, 47: 78, 91
after shoulder surgery, 48: 369
and proximal humeral fractures, 46: 32-33
Frykman classification, intra-articular fracture of the radius, 48: *468*
Full-thickness soft-tissue necrosis, total knee arthroplasty, 46: 167
Functional assessment, in the elderly, 46: 410-*412*
Functional Recovery Score (FRS), for elderly hip fracture patients, 46: 442-443
Fungi
bone and joint infections, **50: 318**
and infection at arthroplasty sites, 48: 113
Fusion. *see* Arthrodesis
Fusion levels, in neuromuscular scoliosis, 48: 555

G

Gait analysis
abnormalities in diabetic neuropathy, 48: 294
high knee adduction, **50: 451**
limp following arthrodesis, **50: 303**
pelvic osteotomies, **50: 231-232**
plantar heel pain, **50: 522**
Gait cycle, 47: 398, *399*
Gait training, pediatric thoracic myelomeningocele, 48: 564-566
Gallium citrate scanning, 47: 288
diagnosis of active infection, **50: 320**
infected bones, **50: 369**
Galveston technique, segmental spinal fusion, 48: 556, *558*
Gamekeeper's thumb, 47: 184-*185*
Gamma irradiation, 47: 380, 382-385
sterilization of polyethylene, 49: 42
Ganglia
around hips, **50: 236**
distinguished from sarcoma, 48: 584
dorsal wrist, **50: 130**
palpitation, 49: 438
Ganglion cysts, denervation caused by, 47: *12*
Gangrene, wet, 48: *687*
Gastrocnemius muscle
anatomy, 47: 419
transfer of medial head, for reconstruction of posterior cruciate ligament, 48: 205
Gastronemius-soleus, strength of complex, 48: 225
Gate Control Theory of pain, 49: 541
Gaucher's disease
and osteonecrosis, 49: 171
osteonecrosis of the humeral head, 48: 350
Gender
and spinal stenosis, **50: 145**
symptoms of spinal stenosis, **50: 150**
General Accounting Office (GAO), on health insurance premiums, 48: 674
General health assessment instruments, use after fractures in elderly, 46: 441-442
Gentamicin
antibiotic-impregnated cement, 48: 117
antibiotic-loaded cement, **50: 327**
in cement spacers, **50: 372**
resistant organisms, **50: 329**
Gentamicin-impregnated beads, and serum bactericidal titer testing, 48: 116
Gerber retractors, 47: 81, **50: 46**
Gerber test for subscapularis function, 46: *58,* 47: 137, 144
Gerdy's tubercle, 47: *373, 374*
in iliotibial band syndrome, 47: 413
Geriatrics for orthopaedists, 46: 409-416
changes in focus of medical care, 46: 410-414
ethical dilemmas, 46: 415
iatrogenic conditions, 46: 415
medical conditions, 46: 414-415
pharmacology and aging, 46: 415
reasons for change in demographics, 46: *409*
theories of aging, 46: 410
Geyser sign, 47: 79
Giant cell tumors
differentiation from metaphyseal fibrous defect, 48: *615*
treatment of, 48: 595-596
Girdlestone arthroplasty, 47: 301
in active infection, **50: 321**
conversion of, 49: 68
septic arthritis, **50: *326***
and total knee arthroplasty, 48: 161
Glenohumeral capsules
ablation, **50: 31**
RF heating, **50: 5**
thermal capsulorrhaphy, **50: 29-36**
Glenohumeral joint
anterior, thermal modification, **50: 13-15**
arthroscopy, 47: 59 (*See also* Shoulder arthroscopy)
arthrosis, **50: *75***

capsular nerves, **50: 32**
evaluation of, 46: 44
instability, 47: 97-110
and age, **50: 23**
biomechanical considerations, 47: 98-101
failed repairs for, 113-125
multidirectional, 47: 101-109
and posterior capsular contracture, 46: 571
reconstruction for severe glenoid loss, 47: 109-110
thermal modification, **50: 37**
loss of motion with arthrosis, after surgery for shoulder instability, 48: 360
osteoarthritis, 47: 129, *130*
postoperative protocols, **50: 13-14**
radiograph, arthritis, **50: *76***
rheumatoid arthritis, **50: 73-77**
septic arthritis of, 46: *33*
surgical stabilization, **50: 24-25**
Glenohumeral ligaments
release, **50: 48**
rotator capsular closure, **50: *35***
Glenohumeral ligaments/labrum, imaging of, 46: 521-522
Glenohumeral proprioceptive neuromuscular facilitation patterns, 46: 47
Glenohumeral stability
and arthrodesis, 49: 327
estimation of, 46: 44
provocative tests for, 46: 44
Glenoid arthritis, complication in humeral head replacement, 46: 20
Glenoid bone
indications for replacement, **50: 78**
loosening, 48: 364
loss of, 47: *108,* 110
resurfacing, **50: 78**
Glenoid labrum, function of, 47: 97, *98*
Gloves, perforations of, and infection at arthroplasty sites, 48: 113
Glucocorticoids in osteoporosis, 46: 447
Glucosamine
pain management, 49: 520
side effects, 49: *493*
treatment of osteoarthritis, 49: 491-493
versus ibuprofen, osteoarthritis, 49: 492
Glutei, forces at osteotomy interface, **50: *249-251***
Gluteus medius tubercle, **50: *235***
Glycocalyx slime
and antibiotics, 48: 116
and infection at arthroplasty sites, 48: 114
Glycosaminoglycans (GAG), 47: 480
chain size, in osteoarthritis, 49: 486
identification in menisci, 49: 191
and meniscus immobilization, 49: 208
and nutritional supplements, 49: 491
GM-1 gangliosides in treating spinal cord injuries, 46: 118
Gold compounds in treating rheumatoid arthritis, 46: 78
Gonadotropins, SCFE, **50: 555**
Gonarthrosis
unicompartmental, arthroscopic treatment of, 48: 139
unicondylar knee arthroplasty for, 48: 143-148
Gore-Tex grafts, 47: 365
Gout, 46: 75-76
and Achilles tendon rupture, 48: 220
arthritis, 46: 75
and posterior heel pain, 48: 213
Gracilis muscle, free microneurovascular transfer, 49: 330-331
Grafts. *See also* Allografts; Autografts; Bone grafts; Xenografts
ACL reconstruction, causes of failure, **50: 463-465**
bone
biology of, 48: 645-651
classification of, 48: 58
donors of, 48: 58
dynamic bone turnover in, 48: 84-85
history of, 48: 79-80
incorporation of, 48: 86-87
and infection of arthroplasty sites, 48: 119-120
principles of, 48: 58-59
revitalization of, 48: 80
surgical technique, 48: 70-73
and bone loss, total knee arthroplasty, 48: 179
impaction, histologic analysis, 48: 84-86
ligament, selection of, 48: 520
morcellized bone, 48: 58-59
nerves, 49: 388
preparation and placement, total knee arthroplasty, 48: 180-181
soft-tissue management, injured upper extremities, 49: 388-390
Gram stain, 47: 291
Gram stains, intraoperative, **50: 374**
Granulation tissue, and osteonecrosis, **50: 490**
Graspers, 46: 131-132, 135
Greater trochanter
deficiency, 49: 89
development and growth, **50: 537**
fractures of, 47: 252
free-body diagram, **50: *248***
longitudinal split, 48: 77
reapproximation, 49: *20*
reattachment, 49: *19*
slide, 49: *19*
Greater tuberosity nonunions, 46: 26
Groin flap, pedicled, 49: 389-390
Gross bone loss classification, 49: 91, *91,* 148
acetabular deficiencies, 48: 50, *50,* **50: *337***
Gross domestic profit, health care percentage, 48: *674*
Ground reaction force (GRF), 47: 399, *401*
Growth factor receptors, 46: 474-475
Growth factors
articular cartilage restoration, 48: 624
effect on cartilage repair, 46: 488-490
acute mechanical damage, 46: 487-488
as agents of healing, 46: 490-491
carriers, 46: 491-492
inflammatory disease, 46: 488
and repair capacity, 47: 498-*499*
for fracture healing, 46: 483-486, 47: 530-532
bone morphogenetic proteins, 46: 484, 47: 530-531
fibroblast growth factors, 46: 484, 47: 530
insulin-like growth factors, 46: 485
platelet-derived growth factor, 46: 485, 47: 531-532
transforming growth factor-ß, 46: 483-484, 47: 531
and joint degeneration, 47: 472-473
and regulation of cartilage proliferation,
47: 464-466, 469-473
bone morphogenetic proteins, 47: 471-472
fibroblast growth factor, 47: 465, 471
insulin-like growth factors, 47: 465, 470
parathyroid hormone related protein (PTHrP), 47: 465
transforming growth factor-ß, 47: 465, 470-471
as therapeutic agents, 46: 473-474
challenges to clinical application, 46: 475-476
in osteoporosis, 46: 495-497
receptors, 46: 27-28, 474-475
in treating skeletal disorders, 46: 477-481
ethics of intervention, 46: 481
growth hormone-IGF-I axis, 46: 477, 47: *478*
growth hormone resistance, 46: 477-481

Growth hormone, 47:465, 465
  resistance, 46: 477-481
  SCFE, **50: 555**
Growth plates
  development, 47: *464*
  zones, 47: 464
Guanethidine
  Bier block, 49: 554
  treatment of RSD, 49: 553
Guepar prosthesis, 46: 215
Guide to the Ethical Practice of Orthopaedic Surgery, 49: 640
Guides to the Evaluation of Permanent Impairment, 4th edition, AMA
  philosophy, 48: 452-455
  spine evaluation, 48: 451-461
Guillain-Barré Syndrome, 46: 118
Gunshot wounds
  elbow injury, 49: *588*
  femoral, 49: 585
  forearm, 49: *387*
Gustilo's classification, injuries, 49: 379
Gustilo and Pasternak bone loss classification, 49: *91,* 91-92

H

Haemophilus influenzae, septic arthritis, **50: 317**
Haglund's deformity, treatment of, 48: 215-217
Hair growth, in diagnosis of diabetic foot, 48: 295
Hallux valgus, 46: 357-388
  anatomy of, 46: 358-364
  bilateral, 48: *333*
  clinical considerations in treatment of, 48: *332*
  complications after surgery for, 48: 331-341
  with cross-over deformity of second toe, 48: *333*
  deformity following second toe amputation, 48: *324*
  history and physical examination, 46: 364-365
  pain in, 48: 294
  radiographic evaluation
    nonweightbearing medial oblique view, 48: 332
    weightbearing anteroposterior view, 48: 331
    weightbearing lateral view, 48: 331-332
    weightbearing sosamoid view, 48: 332, *334*
  radiographic examination, 46: 365
  recurrent deformity, 48: 335-336
  recurrent valgus deformity after surgery for, 48: 333-334
  surgical correction, 46: 365-366
    arthrodesis of first metatarsophalangeal joint, 46: 380-382
    arthrodesis of metatarsocuneiform joint, 46: 378-380
    chevron osteotomy, 46: 370-372, *373*
    distal metatarsal osteotomy, 46: 372-*375*
    distal soft-tissue reconstruction, 46: 367-370
    distal soft-tissue reconstruction with osteotomy of first metatarsal, 46: 374-378
    excisional arthroplasty, 46: 382-384
    multiple osteotomies, 46: 385-387
    proximal phalangeal osteotomy, 46: 366-*367, 368*
Hallux varus
  acquired, 48: 337
  after basilar metatarsal osteotomy, 48: *336*
  after failed McBride bunionectomy, 48: *332*
  after replacement arthroplasty, 48: *337*
  dynamic, 48: 340-341
  static (uniplanar), 48: 337-340
Halo vest immobilization in acute spinal trauma, 46: 122-124
Hammertoes, and diabetic foot, 48: 293, 294
Hamstrings
  ACL reconstruction graft, **50: 469**
  peak torque, 48: 191
Hand
  crush injury, 49: *390*
  fractures in athletes, 47: 187-190
    metacarpal, 47: 188-190
    on-the-field examination of, 47: 187
  imaging of, 46: 523-524, *525*
  index finger amputation, 49: *393*
  lateral arm flap, 49: *392*
  longitudinal failure of upper-limb formation, 46: 83-*108*
    central deficiency, 46: 83, 97-*104*
    radial deficiency, 46: 83-97
    ulnar deficiency, 46: 83, 104-*108*
  postoperative pain, 49: 541-542
  punch-press injuries, 49: *394*
  simulators of infection in, 46: 69-79
    acute calcific tendinitis, 46: *69*-70
    bites of brown recluse spider, 46: 70-71
    factitious diseases, 46: 74-75
    foreign-body reaction, 46: 74
    gout, 46: 75-76
    metastatic lesions, 46: 73-74
    pyoderma gangrenosum, 46: 72-73
    pyrogenic granuloma, 46: 71-72
    rheumatoid arthritis, 46: 77-79
  soft-tissue injuries in athletes
    dislocation of carpometacarpal joint of thumb, 47: *185*
    dislocation-subluxation of extensor tendons at metacarpophalangeal joint, 47: 183-184
    tendon injuries, 47: 181-183
  work-related illnesses, 48: 694
Handicap International (HI), land mine initiatives, 49: 433
Hands/forearm antisepsis, surgical personnel, 49: 611
Hansen's disease
  in developing nations, 49: 571
  total contact casting and, 48: 305
Harcke dynamic technique, **50: 539**
Hardinge approach, compared to vastus slide, 48: 17
Hardware complications of internal fixation of proximal humeral fractures, 46: 28-30
Hardware failures, acromioclavicular joint, 49: 410-411
Harrington instrumentation, outcomes analysis in neuromuscular scoliosis treatment, 48: 552
Harrington rod fixation, 48: 440
Harris Hip Scores (HHS), 46: 419, 420
  Metasul articulation, 49: 47, *48*
  and outcome of hip arthroplasties, 48: 87
Hartofilakidis classification system, hip dislocation, **50: *307-308***
Hassan technique, 46: 136
Hawkins classification of talar neck injuries, 46: *326*-327
Hawkins sign, 46: *330,* 331, 47: 23
Head injuries
  children with multiple injuries, 49: 415
  and fractures, children with multiple injuries, 49: 427-430
  fractures complicated by, in children, 49: 425-430
Head size, femoral components, 49: 126
Health, defined of, 48: 418
Health assessment questionnaire, 46: 441
Health care, value in, 48: *676*-677
Health-care workers (HCWs), and occupational risk of HIV/AIDS infection, 49: 621-624
Health insurance premiums, General Accounting Office (GAO)report, 48: 674
Health law, recent developments, 48: 701-702

Health Maintenance Organizations (HMOs)
evaluation of, 48: *677*
premium growth rates, 48: 674
and reporting of work-related disorders, 48: 696
Health Outcomes Institute, 48: 679
Health Plan Employer Data and Information Set (HEDIS)
and performance measurement, 48: 677-678
use of data, 48: 677
Health-Related Quality-of-Life (HRQL)
instruments and scoring resources, 48: *671*
steps in development of instruments, 48: 668-670
Health status instruments
generic *versus* disease-specific, 48: 418-419
measurement of, 48: 418
Health Status Scores, diabetics, 49: 290
Health Volunteers Overseas (HVO)
services in the developing world, 49: 572
volunteer teachers, 49: 576
Web site, 49: 573
Heat, as therapeutic modality, **50: 3-11**
Heat probes. *See also* Thermal modification
application in anterior stabilization, **50: *33***
thermal capsulorrhaphy, **50: 29-32**
Heel
complications of surgery, **50: 528-530**
pad pain, 46: 339, 47: 427
pain, 47: 425-427, 48: 213-214
nerve entrapment syndromes, 47: 426-427
plantar fasciitis, 47: 405, 425-426
plantar pain, **50: 521-531**
spurs, **50: 525**
Heelcord lengthening, 46: 349, 354
Helmet aspirator suits, and infection at arthroplasty sites, 48: 112-113
Hemangiomas
imaging of, 48: 618
intramuscular, 48: 598
Hematologic testing, diagnosis of arthroplasty site infection, 48: 114
Hematomas
misdiagnosis of, 48: 579
postoperative, **50: 529**
Hematopoiesis
evaluation in preoperative planning, 48: 97
metastatic bone disease, 49: 458
Hemiarthroplasty, resurfacing, radiograph, 49: *178*
Hemiarthrosis, incidence of, chondral injuries and, 48: 629
Hemilaminotomy, oblique view, **50: *157***
Hemiplegia, plastic, THA in, 49: *165*
Hemiresurfacing, femoral, 49: 178-179
Hemoglobin-based oxygen carriers, use in the orthopaedic setting, 48: 658
Hemoglobinopathy, bone and joint infections, **50: 318**
Hemophiliac patients, HIV-positive, infection complications, 49: 628
Hemorrhages
intramedullary, and osteonecrosis, 49: 171
intraoperative, Paget's disease, 49: 66
Henry approach, vastus slide technique, 48: *16*
Heparin
prevention of DVT, **50: 417-418**
for thromboembolic disease, 46: 186-187, 188, 47: 333
Hepatitis, transmission through grafts, 49: 149
Hepatitis B
allograft transmission, 49: 616
laboratory screening, 49: 618
transmission through allografts, 48: 64
Hepatitis C
and allograft sterilization, 47: 385
allograft transmission, 49: 616
laboratory screening, 49: 618
transmission through allografts, 48: 64
Herbert scaphoid fracture classification, **50: *108***
Herniated disks, C5-C6, 49: *386*
Herniated nucleus pulposus (HNP), 46: 145
Heterotopic ossification (HO)
acetabular fractures, 48: 491-492
after rotator cuff repair, 47: *91, 92*
in ankylosing spondylitis, 48: 97
as complication of internal fixation of proximal humeral fractures, 46: *34*
patellar tendon, 46: 272
Hexosaminidase, response to titanium, **50: 189**
High-density polyethylene (HDPE), 46: 206
High hip centers, **50: 309**
use of, **50: 313**
High proximal tibial osteotomy, **50: 484-485**
High tibial osteotomy (HTO)
correcting lower limb malalignment, **50: 451**
survival rates, **50: *504***
Hilgenreiner's line, newborn hip, **50: 538**
Hill-Sachs deformity
defined, 47: 13
and reconstruction for anterior dislocation, 47: *108,* 109
Hindfoot
amputations, 46: 506, 48: 325-*326,* 688
anatomy, 47: 421-422
arthrodesis, 46: 347-356
ankle, 46: 348-351
basic principles, 46: 347-348
special circumstances, 46: 354-356
triple, 46: 351-354
prioritizing surgeries, 48: 94
pronation of, 46: 357
valgus, in patients with myelomeningocele, 48: 544
Hinged external fixation, elbow, surgical technique, **50: 97-98**
Hip
abductor muscle deficiencies, **50: *270***
anterolateral approach, 49: 15-16
arthrodesis, conversion to THA, **50: 297-305**
bilateral dysplasia, **50: *241, 307***
biomechanical considerations of fractures, in osteoporotic bone, 46: 431-437
biomechanics, **50: 240-241**
center of rotation, 49: 30
childhood problems, 49: 3-4
classification of dislocations, **50: 307**
developmental dysplasia, **50: 535-540**
differential diagnosis of dislocation, **50: *269***
dislocations, THR for, **50: 307-316**
dysplastic
anatomy, 49: 23-24
classifications, 49: 24-26
computed tomography, **50: 256-258**
primary total replacement, 49: 23-36
radiographic analysis, **50: 253-255**
flexion deformities, polio-related, 49: *597*
fractures in rheumatoid arthritis, 48: 102
high center, socket placement, 49: 60
hip joint aspiration, 47: 289-291, *293*
imaging of, 46: 527-*528*
insufficient acetabular coverage, **50: *233***
moderate dysplasia, **50: *551***
multifactorial instability, **50: 270**
natural history of problems, in myelomeningocele patients, 48: 564
newborns, **50: *538***

osteoarthritis, 46: 418
  radiograph, 49: *482*
osteoarthrosis, **50: 229**
physical examination, **50: 231-232**
posterior surgical approach, 49: 13-15
prioritization of reconstructive surgeries, 48: 94
problems in myelomeningocele patients, 48: 563-573
pseudarthrosis, **50: *298***
recurrent instability, **50: *271***
rheumatoid arthritis in
  clinical manifestations of, 48: 102-103
  treatment of, 48: 103-105
salvage procedures, in rheumatoid arthritis, 48: 100-101
severe dysplasia, **50: *551, 552***
soft-tissue abnormalities, 49: *35*
spica cast, **50: *290***
stiff, 49: 5
  trochanteric slide, 49: 86
surgical management of inflammatory arthritis, 48: 93-106
tendinosis about, 46: 573-574
teratologic dislocation, **50: 541**
total congenital dislocation, 49: 20-21

Hip arthroplasty. *See also* Total hip arthroplasty
acetabular revision
  clinical results of, 47: 271-273
  instrumentation used for, 47: *268*
  morcellized allografting for, 47: 265-273
  surgical technique, 47: 268-269
bacteriology of infections, 49: *606*
bipolar, 49: 179-180
diagnosis of site infection, 48: 114-115
direct lateral approach, 49: 16-17
effect of previous surgeries, 49: 26-27
femoral canal distortion, 49: 68
Harris Hip Scores (HHS) and outcome of, 48: 87
infection following THA
  diagnosis, 47: 285-293
  treatment, 47: 297-304
neurovascular injury after, 47: 275-281
  neurologic sequelae of fat embolism, 47: 275-*276*
  peripheral nerve complications, 47: 276-279
  vascular complications, 47: 279-281
options for revision, 49: 131-132
and osteonecrosis, 49: 169-170
periprosthetic acetabular fractures after THA, 47: 231-235
  intraoperative, 47: 232-233, *234,* 252
  postoperative, 47: 233-234
  in vitro studies, 47: 231-232
periprosthetic femoral fractures after THA, 47: 237-241
  classification of, 47: 253
  intraoperative, 47: 237-238, 251-252
  postoperative, 47: 238-241, 243-248
postoperative management, 48: 24-25
preoperative planning, 48: 19-20
primary total
  difficult, surgical exposures, 49: 13-21
  planning, 49: 3-10
  preoperative planning, 49: 26-27
resection, 49: *132*
revision
  and acetabular bone loss, 48: 57-65
  femoral bone loss, 49: 147-159
  impaction allografting, 49: 103-110
  instances of vascular injuries, 48: *28*
  preoperative planning, 49: *83*
  proximal femoral replacement with megaprosthesis, 49: 141-146
  retroperitoneal exposure, 48: 27-35
  and risk of vascular injury, 48: 30-31
  surgical approaches, 48: 3-8
  two-stage implantation, 49: 67
  use of a vastus slide, 48: 13-17
  use of an extended proximal femoral osteotomy, 48: 19-26
  vascular injuries, 48: 27-35
  vascularized scaphoid window for femoral canal access, 48: 9-11
subtrochanteric osteotomy, 49: 20-*21*
surgical approaches, 49: 28
surgical technique, 48: 32-35
timing of surgery, 48: 32
total
  bearing surfaces, 49: 41-54
  the difficult femur, 49: 63-68
  fixation with modular system, outcomes, 49: 136-137
  and neuromuscular disease, 49: 163-168
  and osteolysis, 49: 71-80
  patient with osteonecrosis, 49: *169*
  revision, fixation with modular stem, 49: 131-138
transtrochanteric osteotomy, 49: 17-20
treatment of femoral bone loss, 49: 119-129
treatment of site infection, 48: 115-117
uncemented, outcomes, 48: 104
venous thromboembolic complications, 47: 331-335
  diagnosis of, 47: 333-334
  prevention of, 47: 332-333
  treatment for, 47: 335

Hip aspirations, periprosthetic femoral osteolysis, **50: 201**

Hip dysplasia
complications following total hip arthroplasty, 49: 35-36
pediatric lumbar myelomeningocele patients, 48: 566, 569-571

Hip fusion, conversion of, 49: *61*

Hip-knee-ankle-foot orthoses (HKAFOs), in myelomeningocele patients, 48: 547

Hip pantaloon cast, **50: 291-292**

Hippocrates, shoulder stabilization, **50: 8**

Histiocytosis, and pediatric back pain, 48: 538-539

HIV/AIDS
allograft transmission, 49: 616
blood transmission of, 48: 665
infection in the orthopedic setting, 49: 621-624
laboratory screening, 49: 618
postexposure prophylaxis of, 49: 623
risk of HCW-to-patient transmission, 49: 623-*624*
seroprevalence in groups of patients, 49: *622*
seroprevalence in HCW, 49: *622*
skeletal tuberculosis, **50: 318**
surgical risks for patients with, 49: 627-628
transmission
  and allograft sterilization, 47: 380, 385, 527
  and osteochondral allografts, 47: 517-518
transmission and allograft sterilization, 47: 380, 385, 527
transmission and osteochondral allografts, 47: 517-518
transmission through allografts, 48: 64
transmission through grafts, 49: 149

HLA/B27 test, plantar heel pain, **50: 521**

Hoffman's reflex, tests for myelopathy, 49: *337*

Hoffman's test, radicular symptoms, 49: *344*

Holmium:YAG laser
adsorption of, **50: 6**
thermal capsulorrhaphy, **50: 13**

Homeobox genes, 47: 461, 463

Homeostasis
osseous, technetium scintiscan of the knees, 48: *192*

tissue
and the envelope of function, 48: 187-188
imaging of, 48: 192-195
zone of, and loading, 48: *188*
Hopf's double osteotomy, **50: 231**
Horii circle, definition, **50: 89, *90***
Hospital Infection Control Practices Advisory Committee (HICPAC), isolation precautions, 49: 608-611
Hospital law, recent developments, 48: 701-702
Howmedica ankle, outcomes, 48: 265
Human leukocyte antigen (HLA)
and immunology of allografts, 48: 651
matching in bone grafts, 49: 151
Humeral component loosening, in humeral head replacement, 46: 21, 380-382
Humeral head
blood supply, 48: *350*
circular defect, 49: *287*
exposure of, **50: *80***
osteonecrosis of, 48: 349-356
etiology, 48: 349-350
pathology, 48: 350-352
progressive degeneration of, 48: *355*
replacement for proximal humeral fractures, 46: 15-23
indications for acute fractures, 46: 7
indications for malunited fractures, 47: 138
literature, 46: 15-16
Mayo Clinic experience, 46: 16-21
preventive measures, 46: 21-22, 374-378
prosthetic arthroplasty for malunion, 47: 135-140
clinical evaluation, 47: *137*
imaging studies, 47: 137-*138*
review of literature, 47: 135-136
treatment algorithm, 47: 140
surgical technique for acute 4-part fracture, 46: 7-14
humeral shaft preparation, 46: 9-*10*
positioning, 46: *8*
surgical approach, 46: 8-*9*
tuberosity fixation, 46: 10-*13*
treatment options, 46: 22-23
resection, **50: 76**
Humeral head replacement (HHR), **50: 77**
indications, **50: 77**
Humeral impression fractures, 47: *106,* 109-110
bone grafting for, 47: *107,* 110
and recurrent instability, 47: 114
Humerus
fractures, children with multiple injuries, 49: 418
skeletal reconstruction, 49: 383
total shoulder arthroplasty, **50: 78-79**
Hyalgan (hyaluronan), use of, 49: 497-498
Hyaline cartilage, 46: 487
composition of, 48: 623
durability of, 48: 140
hypocellular, in an enchondroma, 48: *613*
in osteoarthritis, 49: 491
repair of, 48: 135
Hyaluronan (Hyalgan), use of, 49: 497-498
Hyaluronic acid (HA), 47: 480-481
adverse reactions, 49: 499
derivatives, and articular cartilage restoration, 48: 625
identification in menisci
inter-articular injection, 49: 485-496
for osteoarthritis, 49: 495-501
postsurgical adhesion formation, 49: 499
structure of, 49: *495*
Hydrothermal heating, in vitro studies, **50: 5**
Hydroxyapatite (HA)
femoral stems, **50: 213**
with impaction graphing, **50: 214**
on implants, 49: 75-76
Hylamer, performance of, 49: 50-51
Hylan G-F 20 (Synvisc), use of, 49: 497
Hyperbaric oxygen, and wound healing, 48: 300
Hypercalcemia, metastatic bone disease, 49: 458
Hyperextension test, radicular symptoms, 49: 342-343
Hyperglycemia, and diabetic neuropathy, 48: 293
Hyperkyphosis
inflexible thoracic, in Scheuermann's disorder, 48: *527*
lateral radiograph of, 48: *528*
Hyperlipidemia, and osteonecrosis, 49: 171
Hyperlordosis, 46: 136-137
Hyperostosis, sternoclavicular, 49: 404-405
Hyperplasia, thermal modification, **50: 5, 7**
Hyperreflexia, systemic causes, 49: 344
Hypersensitivity, osteolysis, **50: 192-193**
Hyperthyroidism, and Achilles tendon rupture, 48: 220
Hypnosis
medical, and pain management, 49: 541-543
pain management, 49: 520
Hypofibrinolysis, and osteonecrosis, **50: 490**
Hypoplastic thumb, 46: 89
classification of, 46: 89-*91*
pollicization for, 46: 94-97
reconstructive procedures for, 46: 91-*94*
Hypothyroidism in geriatric patients, 46: 414
Hypovascularity
and Achilles tendon degeneration, 48: 219
and Achilles tendon rupture, 48: 211, 220
Hypovolemia, impact on wound healing, 46: 166-167

I

Iatrogenesis, and reporting of work-related disorders, 48: 696
Iatrogenic damage, implant removal, 48: 167
Iatrogenic sciatic nerve injury, acetabular fractures, 48: 492-493
Ibuprofen
consideration in preoperative planning, 48: 98
versus glucosamine sulfate, osteoarthritis, 49: 492
Idiopathic peripheral neuropathy, total contact casting and, 48: 305
Idiopathic tibial rotation deformity, assessment of, 48: *283*
Ileitis, and arthritis, 48: 97
Ileum, soft-tissue releases, 49: 28
Iliac artery, left external, angiography, 48: *34*
Iliofemoral approach, arthroplasty, 49: 28
Iliofemoral distraction, outcomes, 49: 34
Iliopsoas, and hip contractures, 48: 97
Iliotibial band syndrome
biomechanics of, 47: 404-405
corticosteroid injections for, 47: 416
diagnosis and treatment of, 47: 413-414
Ober's test for, 46: 574, *575,* 47: 414
Ilizarov technique
for ankle distraction, 48: *250*-251
tibial shaft fractures, 46: 284
use in the developing world, 49: 587
Imaging studies, diagnostic evaluation of diabetic foot, 48: 297-298
Imipenem-cilastatin, treatment of diabetic foot infection, 48: 319
Immobilization
casts, scaphoid fractures, **50: 110-111**
control of range of motion, **50: 293**

following thermal capsulorrhaphy, glenohumeral joint, **50: 13-15**
of knee joints, 49: 212
long-term, and arthrodesis for neuropathic deformities, 48: 275
meniscus, effect on glycosaminoglycans, 49: 208
shoulder capsulorrhaphy, **50: 25-26**
spinal, after anterior decompression and fusion, 48: 424
in spinal injury, 48: 413
thermal capsulorrhaphy, **50: 31-32**
treatment for Achilles tendon rupture, 48: 221
treatment of Charcot deformities, 48: 270
wrist sprains, 49: 225
Immune system
effect of methotrexate, 48: 97
evaluation in preoperative planning, 48: 97
Immunity, cell-mediated, bone grafts, 49: 97
Immunization, polio, global coverage, 49: *571*
Immunocompatibility, and allograft healing, 48: 182
Immunocompetence, decision making in foot amputations, 48: 323
Immunocompromise, and infection at arthroplasty sites, 48: 111
Immunodeficiency syndromes. *See also* HIV/AIDS
and effect on joint replacement, 46: 555
HIV transmission and allograft sterilization, 47: 380, 385
Immunogenicity, bone grafts, 49: 149-150
Immunoglobulin G, radiolabeled, diagnosis of infection, **50: 369**
Immunologic factors, role of, in allograft incorporation, 46: 231-234
Immunology, of allografts, 48: 650-651
Immunosuppression
azothioprine, 49: 97
and immunology of allografts, 48: 651
incorporation of bone grafts, 49: 151
Impaction grafting
acetabular cup, **50: 212-213**
acetabular fractures, **50: 346**
clinical results, 49: 111-114
goat model, 49: *104*
prosthesis motion, 49: *107*
histology, **50: *218***
with morcellized bone, 48: 645
in revision hip surgery, 49: 103-110
Impairment categories, spine, *Guides to the Evaluation of Permanent Impairment,* 4th edition, 48: *453*
Impairment percents, whole-person, *Guides to the Evaluation of Permanent Impairment,* 4th edition, 48: *454*
Impingement
after fixation of proximal humeral fractures, 46: 32, *33*
assessment of, in management of instability, 48: 23
clinical evaluation for, 47: 22-23
defined, 47: 21
and dislocation, **50: 269-270**
effect of component design, **50: 275-279**
glenohumeral joint, **50: 17-18**
magnetic resonance imaging of, 47: 4-7
management of instability, 49: 125-126
persistent, 47: 80
soft tissue, following TKA, **50: 405-406**
Impingement test, 47: 23, **50: *232***
Implantation, revision prosthesis, 48: *24*
Implants. *See also* Components
bone preparation techniques, 48: 178-179
choice of, **50: 267**
complications in neuromuscular scoliosis, 48: 552
constrained, **50: 271-273**
cost of, 49: 44
custom components, 48: 174
design and failure, 48: 162
femoral, cost of, 49: 116-117
hinged components, 48: 174
infection seeded from foot wounds, 48: 289
knee, size selection, 48: 164
loosening, and polyethylene wear, 48: 162
loosening of, **50: 198-199**
malpositioning, and extensor mechanisms, 48: 163
migration, acromioclavicular joint, 49: 410-411
migration of, **50: 201**
orientation, and dislocation risk, **50: 266**
porous-coated, 49: 119
removal
knee arthroplasty, 48: 166
minimalization of bone loss, 49: 88
removal and iatrogenic damage, 48: 167
selection of, total knee arthroplasty, 48: 167
stemmed, 48: 174-175
type 3 bone defects, 48: 175
subsidence, and type 2 bone defects, 48: 169
In-field responder in acute spinal trauma management, 46: 114
In vivo degradation, ultra-high molecular weight polyethylene in, 46: 207
Incidental findings, clinical presentation of bone tumors, 48: 607-608
Incisions
postoperative care, 49: 612
SCFE, **50: *560***
sham, **50: 360-361**
vascular anatomy, **50: 360**
Indium-labeled polyclonal antibodies, diagnosis of active infection, **50: 321**
Indium-labeled WBC scans
diagnosis of active infection, **50: 320-321, 369**
Indomethacin
effect on particulate-induced bone resorption, **50: 192**
elbow dislocations, **50: 96**
for gout, 46: 76
for pseudogout, 46: 77
Infections. *See also* Abscesses
after acetabular transplant, 48: 74
after Achilles tendon rupture repair, 48: 224
after rotator cuff surgery, 48: 363
after surgery for acetabular fractures, 48: 493-494
after total shoulder arthroplasty, 48: 366
after TSA, **50: 84**
antibiotic-resistant organisms, 49: 605
at arthroplasty sites, 48: 111-120
diagnosis of, 48: 114-115
etiology, 48: 111-115
bacterial, allograft transmission, 49: 615-616
classification of, 48: 318, **50: 367-368**
complication of humeral head replacement, 46: 18
complication of internal fixation of proximal humeral fractures, 46: 33-34
contact precautions, 49: *610*
contraindication in total joint replacement, 46: 419
débridement, **50: 370, 410**
deep periprosthetic joint, 46: 557-565
and operating-room environment, 46: 558-562
during postoperative period, 46: 562-564
prevention with antibiotics, 46: 557-558
diabetic foot, 48: 298, 317-320
diagnosis of, **50: 367-368**
exclusion of, **50: 319-321**
and failure of knee arthroplasty, 48: 163
following THA, 46: 215-218
diagnosis, 46: 216, 47: 285-*293*
management, 46: 216-218
prevalence of deep sepsis, 46: 215-216
treatment, 47: 287-304

following TKA, **50: 409-414**
hip treatment algorithm, **50: *328***
imaging of infected arthroplasty, 46: 528
imaging of infected hip arthroplasty
radiography, 47: 287-288
radionuclide imaging, 47: 288-289
implants, seeded from foot wounds, 48: 289
intraoperative investigation, **50: 373-374**
joint, treatment of antibiotic-resistant bacteria, 49: *613*
management of, **50: 369-375**
occult
after acetabular open reduction, **50: 348**
preoperative investigations for, 48: 44-45
organisms and eradication rates, **50: 330**
predictive value of investigations, **50: *320***
preoperative assessments, 49: 84-85
primary THA after, **50: 317-333**
pyrogenic, outcome of THA after, **50: 322-324**
rates and age, 49: 36
recurrent, **50: *322***
reinfecting organisms, **50: 323**
revision TKA, **50: 367-377**
risk for HIV-positive patients, 49: 627-628
screening of musculoskeletal allografts, 49: 615-618
seeding of implants, from bowel infection, 48: 97
simulators of infection in the hand, 46: *69*-79, 472
standard precautions, 49: *609*
structural femoral allografts, 49: 157
surgeon's "gut feeling," **50: 374**
surgical site, recommendations for prevention, 49: *609*
surgical technique, **50: 330-331**
treatment for painful hip degeneration, **50: 321-322**
use of allografts after, **50: 330**
and vascular injury in THA, 48: 31
Infectious diseases, blood transmission of, 48: 665
Infectious spondylitis, and pediatric back pain, 48: 529-530
Inferior capsular sling, idiopathic frozen shoulder, 49: *284*
Inferior glenohumeral ligament complex
anatomy, 47: *99*
function, 47: 97
Inferior subluxation
as complication in humeral head replacement, 46: 19
as complication of internal fixation of proximal humeral fractures, 46: 34
Inferior vena cava filters, prevention of embolism, **50: 418**
Inflammatory disease
cartilage destruction, 46: 488
relief in nonsurgical treatment of epicondylitis, 48: 377
Informed consent, teaching of ethics, 49: 640
Infraspinatus muscles
amplitude, **50: 66**
magnetic resonance imaging of, 47: *12*
substitution of teres major, **50: 63**
tendon transfers, 49: 323-327
Infraspinatus tendon
tear of, **50: 43**
transfer of, 49: 321-323
undersurface tear, **50: *18***
Infraspinatus/teres minor weakness, 46: 5
Insall-Salvati ratio, 47: 342
Insertional Achilles tendinitis, 47: 424-*425*
Insertional enthesopathy, and posterior heel pain, 48: 213
Insomnia, and pain, 49: 542
Instability
after acetabular transplant, 48: 74
after shoulder arthroplasty, 47: 141-148, 48: 364-365
etiology, 47: 142-*143*
management of, 47: 144-148
preoperative evaluation of, 47: 143-144
after total hip arthroplasty, **50: 265-274**
ankle, **50: *516***
anterior cursive ligament reconstruction, **50: 463-474**
biomechanical considerations, 47: 98-101
carpal, **50: 123-134**
cervical spine, prioritizing surgical treatment, 48: 94
classification scheme for, 47: 203-204
distal radioulnar joint instability, 47: 199-201, 209-213
acute, 47: 210
chronic, 47: 210-213
dynamic scapholunate, **50: 129-130**
elbow, **50: 91, 96-98**
arthroscopic test, 48: *401*
and posterior impingement, 48: 399, *400*
recurrent, **50: 98-100**
failed repairs for, 47: 113-125
arthrosis after instability surgery, 47: 123-*124*
etiology of recurrence, 47: 113-*115*
revision surgical treatment, 47: 115-117
stiffness after instability surgery, 47: 117-123
and head size, in revision total hip arthroplasty, 48: 23-24
ligamentous, in TKA, **50: 399-401**
management of, in revision total hip arthroplasty, 48: 23-24
medial collateral ligament, in the athlete's elbow, 48: 383-391
midcarpal (MCI), 47: 204-208
diagnosis of, 47: 204-205
Lichtman's classification for, 47: 205-206
multidirectional, 47: 101-109
of the shoulder, failed surgery for, 48: 362
patellofemoral, and implant failures, 48: 163
radial-sided, 47: 219-227
diagnosis of, 47: 221-222
imaging for, 47: 222-224
treatment for scapholunate instability, 47: 224-227
reconstruction for severe glenoid loss, 47: 109-110
shoulder, 47: 97-110
and arthritis, **50: 75**
complications of arthroscopic surgery for, 48: 371-372
complications of surgery for, 48: 359-362
thermal capsulorrhaphy, **50: 29-36**
total hip arthroplasty, **50: 289-291**
ulnar-sided, 47: 215-218
wrist, 47: 203-208
Instruments
in outcomes research, 48: 668-683
used for acetabular impaction, 48: *82*
Insulin-dependent growth factor I, in osteoarthritis, 49: 486
Insulin-like growth factor binding protein-3 (IGFBP-3), 46: 480
Insulin-like growth factor binding proteins (IGFBPs), 46: 477
Insulin-like growth factor-I (IGF-I)
and bone formation, 46: 496-497
and cartilage regulation, 47: 465, 470
and cartilage repair, 46: 489
complications of therapy, 46: 480
direct action of, 46: 480-481
effects in humans, 46: 479-480
in fracture repair, 46: 485
growth hormone-IGF-I axis, 46: 477, *478*
as a therapeutic agent, 46: 473, 475-476
two classes of, 46: 473
Insulin-like growth factors, articular cartilage restoration, 48: 624
Insurance
factors contributing to premium increases, 48: *676*
and national health expenditures, 48: *675*

role in medical malpractice, 48: 699-703
Intercarpal ligaments, categorization of injuries, 48: 476
Interclavicular ligament, sternoclavicular joint, 49: 397
Intercompartmental supraretinacular artery, **50: *115*-117**
Interleukin-1 (IL-1), 46: 205
in osteoarthritis, 49: 486
and osteoclasts, 49: 78
production of, effect of intermittent fluid pressure on, 48: 252
and proteoglycan synthesis, 48: 235
response to particulate debris, **50: 190-191**
Interleukin-6 (IL-6), 46: 205
and osteoclasts, 49: 78
response to particulate debris, **50: 188-190**
simulation of osteoclasts by, 48: 37
Interleukin-1α (IL-1α)
response to particulate debris, **50: 188-189**
simulation of osteoclasts by, 48: 37
Interleukin-1β (IL-1β), response to particulate debris, **50: 188-189**
Interlocking tibial nailing in treating tibial shaft fractures, 46: 297-298
Intermittent pneumatic compression, prevention of DVT, **50: 416**
Internal fixation
complications of
frozen shoulder, 46: 32-33
hardware, 46: 28-30
heterotopic ossification, 46: *34*
iatrogenic fracture displacement, 46: 34
infection, 46: 33-34
inferior subluxation, 46: 34
malunion, 46: 27-28, 29
neurovascular injury, 46: 31-32
nonunion, 46: 25-27
osteonecrosis, 46: 30-31
in proximal humeral fractures, 46: 25-35
subacromial impingement, 46: 32
of supracondylar periprosthetic fractures, 46: 199-*201,* 47: 452-453
plate-and-screw fixation, 47: 440-442
Rush rods and Zickel supracondylar rods, 47: 439-440
techniques of, 46: 25
Internal impingement
heat probes used, **50: 34**
throwing athletes, **50: 29**
International Association for the Study of Pain, 49: 513
International Campaign to Ban Land Mines (ICBL), 49: 433
International Center for Orthopaedic Education (ICOE), services in the developing world, 49: 573
International Committee of the Red Cross (ICRC)
land mine initiatives, 49: 433
relief programs, 49: 575
International Medical Core (IMC), international relief, 49: 576
International Rescue Committee (IRC), refugee relief, 49: 576
International Standards for Neurological and Functional Classification of Spinal Cord Injury, 48: 438
Interosseous edema, and osteonecrosis, 49: 171
Interosseous ligaments
ankle, disruption of, 49: *265*
of the forearm, 47: 175-176
tears, 49: 227-229
wrist, chronic tears, 49: 229-230
Interosseous talocalcaneal ligaments, 49: *274*
Interscaphoid angles, measurement of, **50: *110***
Interstitial fibrosis, 46: 129
Intertrochanteric osteotomy, **50: *563*-564**
Interventional study designs, clinical trials in outcome assessment of fractures in elderly, 46: 440-441
Intervertebral disks, 49: *339*
age-related changes, 50: 145-146, **50: 145-146**
and aging, 46: 463-464
arthroscopic visualization of, 46: 150-151
biochemical constituents, **50: 146**
bulging of, **50: *144***
degeneration, segmental instability, **50: 138**
degeneration of, 49: 335-337
degenerative process, 49: 362-363
displacements, 49: *340*
excision, spinal stenosis, 49: 369
Intervertebral fusion cages, 46: 133
Intestines, evaluation in preoperative planning, 48: 97
Intra-articular disks, sternoclavicular joints, 49: 397
Intra-articular disorders, 46: 572
Intra-articular fractures, in the elderly, 46: 425
Intra-articular pressure, measurement in ankle joint, 48: *251*
Intracapsular pressure, septic arthritis, **50: 317-318**
Intracompartmental pressure, measurement of, in evaluation of compartment syndrome, 46: 304
Intradiskal approach, 46: 152-155
Intramedullary hip-screw, pathologic intertrochanter fractures of the femur, 49: 464
Intramedullary nailing
children with multiple injuries, 49: 430
femoral, in children, 49: 419
for knee arthrodesis, 46: 217
for tibial shaft fractures, 46: 284-285
Intraosseous pressure, release of, **50: 483-484**
Intraosseous tibial exposure, 46: 224
Intrathecal pressure, spinal stenosis, **50: 147-148**
Intrinsic minus hallux, after failed metatarsal osteotomy, 48: *332*
Intubation, difficulties, rheumatoid arthritis and, 48: 97
Inverted radial reflex
radicular symptoms, 49: *344*
test for myelopathy, 49: *337*
Involucrum, formation of, 49: *589-590*
IPOS postoperative shoe, use of, 48: 312
Ipsilateral ankle and foot injuries and amputation, 46: 516
Irrigation, injured upper extremities, 49: 380
Ischemia, and pain, 48: 293
Ischemia, septic arthritis, **50: 318**
Isolation precautions, for resistant bacteria, 49: 608-611
Isometric exercises, rotator cuff rehabilitation, **50: 50**
Item development, of outcomes assessment instruments, 48: 668
Item reduction, of outcomes assessment instruments, 48: 668

J

Jackson-Weiss syndrome, 46: 477
Japanese Investigation Committee on Osteonecrosis, 49: 173
Japanese Orthopaedic Association Score, outcomes instrument for myelopathy, 48: 420
Japanese Orthopedic Association Traveling Fellowship, 49: 572
Jeanne's sign, ulnar nerve compression, 49: 308
Jersey finger, 47: 183-184
Job dissatisfaction, and reporting of work-related disorders, 48: 696
Johansson classification for periprosthetic fractures, 47: 253
Joint Commission on Accreditation of Healthcare Organizations (JCAHO), accreditation by, 48: 677, 679
Joint degeneration
age-related, 46: 461-463, 47: 489
and growth factors, 47: 472-473
and joint use, 47: 491-492
and osteoarthritis, 47: 487-491
repair and regeneration for, 47: 492-501
artificial matrices, 47: 499-500

cell transplantation, 47: 497-*498*
decreased joint loading combined with joint motion, 47: 496-497
growth factors, 47: 498-*499*
osteochondral allografts, 47: 500, 517-521
osteotomy, 47: 495-496
penetration of subchondral bone, 47: 492-*495*
soft-tissue grafts, 47: 497
Joint distraction
and formation or articular surfaces, 48: 239-240
as treatment for ankle osteoarthritis, 48: 249-254
Joint effusion, **50: 391**
Joint function
concept of, 48: 186-187
contributing factors, 48: 188-195
Joint injuries, skeletal reconstruction, 49: 385-386
Joint laxity, thermal modification, **50: 7-8**
Joint line elevation, 46: 229
Joint replacement, critical pathways for, 49: 646-*647*
Joint space, and outcome of arthroscopic debridement, 48: 136
Joint transfer, injured upper extremities, 49: 385-386
Joints. *See also* Specific joints
contracture, and range of motion, 48: 44
deformity, as indication for surgery, 48: 93-94
degenerative disease, arthroscopic ankle débridement, 48: 243-245
effective hyaluronic articular tissue, 49: *496*
functional disturbance, as indication for surgery, 48: 93
infections, treatment of antibiotic-resistant bacteria, 49: *613*
injury and osteoarthritis, 48: 237-239
pain in, as indication for surgery, 48: 93
process of degeneration, 49: *485*
Journal of the American Medical Association (JAMA), volunteer opportunities, 49: 575
Jumper's knee
biomechanics of, 47: 404
diagnosis and treatment of, 47: 411-412
brace for, 46: 575, *576*
surgical treatment for, 46: 575, *576,* 47: 412
Jupiter and Fernandez classification, intra-articular fracture of the radius, 48: 468-469
Juvenile rheumatoid arthritis (JRA), 46: 78
hip arthroplasty, 48: 102
joint destruction, 49: 64
total knee arthroplasty, **50: 507**

K

Keller excisional arthroplasty, 46: 382-384
Kenny Howard sling, problematic use, 49: *408*
Keratan sulfate, identification in menisci, 49: 191
Kerrison rongeurs, 46: 133
Kinematic rotating hinge prosthesis, 46: 172
Kinematics, 47: 398-399, *401*
mobile-bearing TKR, **50: 434-437**
Kinetics, 47: 399-402
Kirschner wires, internal fixation in children, 49: 417
Kitners, 46: 136
Klein's line, **50: *558***
Knee. *See also* Meniscus; Total knee arthroplasty
adult, surgical management of inflammatory arthritis, 48: 93-106
algorithm for anterior knee pain, 47: 339-343
clinical tests recommended in, 47: 339, 342
allografts for ligament and meniscal reconstruction, 47: 379-394
ACL reconstruction, 47: 385-388
LCL reconstruction, 47: 389-391
meniscal allografts, 47: 392-393
PCL reconstruction, 47: 388-389
anatomy, 46: *165,* 47: 345-*346,* 370
anterior cruciate ligament
injuries in skeletally immature patients, 47: 351-358
loss of motion following ACL surgery, 46: 251-259
revision ACL reconstruction, 47: 361-366
arthritic, arthroscopic photograph, 48: *138*
arthrodeses, polio-related deformities, 49: 596-597
arthrodesis, intramedullary nailing for, 46: 217
arthrofibrosis, lateral view, 49: *217*
arthroscopic gap test, **50: *452***
arthroscopy, complications of, 48: *140*
biomechanics of anterior knee pain, 47: *404*
capsular thickening, 49: *213*
congenital hyperextension, in myelomeningocele patients, 48: 572
degeneration after reconstruction, 48: 186
degenerative arthritis of, arthroscopic management, 48: 135-140
disarticulation, 46: *507,* 48: *670,* 689, 49: *189*
dislocations, 48: 515-521
anterior external fixation, 48: *519*
classification, 48: 515-516, 517
and medial epicondylar osteotomy, 48: 156
paramedian approach for access to, 48: *520*
physical examination, 48: 516-517
posterolateral approach for access to, 48: *521*
radiographic evaluation, 48: 517
sequence of injury, 48: 515
surgical management, 48: 519-521
and tibial avulsion, 48: *518*
with torn popliteal artery, 48: *516*
treatment, 48: 517-521
energy absorbed, 48: 187
envelope of function, and anterior cruciate ligament injury, 48: *195*
flexion deformities, polio-related, 49: *597*
function, after anterior cruciate ligament injury, 48: 185-196
fusions, and medial epicondylar osteotomy, 48: 156
loss of motion, arthrofibrosis, 49: 213-214
medial peripatellar incision, 49: *218*
metaphyseal region, 48: *169*
mobile-bearing prostheses, **50: 431-449**
normal, lateral view, 49: *217*
normal motion, 49: 211
operative treatment of arthrofibrosis, 49: 211-220
osteoarthritis, 47: 429-434
pathophysiology, 47: 429-430
radiographs, 49: *482*
surgical options, **50: 499-511**
treatment for, 47: 430-434
osteochondral allografts for articular defects, 47: 500, 517-*521*
screening for donors, 47: 517-518
surgical procedure, 47: *518-521*
osteonecrosis, **50: 483-488**
patella infera syndrome, 46: 241-249, 251-259
collagen fibril population of patellar tendon, 46: 242-245
quantitative ultrastructural collagen fibril analysis, 46: 242
patellar instability in school age athletes, 47: 345-349
imaging for, 47: 347-348
physical examination for, 47: 347
posterior capsular release, 49: 218
posterolateral rotatory instability (PLRI), 47: 369-378
physical examination for, 47: 371-372
surgical technique for, 47: 373-377
prioritization of reconstructive surgeries, 48: 94
problems in myelomeningocele patients, 48: 571-573
proximal valgus tibial osteotomy, 48: 131-133
pseudogout in, 46: 77

quadriceps myocutaneous composite flap for exposure of, 48: 157-159
realignment osteotomies, **50: 502-505**
reflex sympathetic dystrophy, 46: 251
in algorithm for anterior knee pain, 47: *340,* 342
and pain dysfunction in lower extremity, 46: 261-267
salvage procedures, in rheumatoid arthritis, 48: 100-101
total replacement, rheumatoid arthritis patients, 48: 105-106
types of bearing configurations, **50: *443***
valgus arthritis, relation to planovalgus foot deformity, 48: 94
vascular anatomy, 46: *165*
villonodular synovitis, 49: *448*
Knee arthroplasty. *See also* Total knee arthroplasty
bone defects in revision cases, 46: 227-236
causes of, 46: 227-228
classification for, 46: 228-230
clinical results of allografts in, 46: 234-236
options for reconstruction of major bone deficiencies, 46: 230-231
techniques for allograft reconstruction in, 46: 231-234
cost effectiveness of revision total knee replacement, 46: 237-240
diagnosis of site infection, 48: 114-115
extensor mechanism problems in, 46: 171-177
patellar clunk syndrome, 46: 176, *177*
patellar component failure, 46: *175*-176
patellar component loosening, 46: 174-175
patellar fractures, 46: 173-*174,* 47: 254
patellofemoral instability, 46: 171-173
surgical technique, 46: 176-177
tendon rupture, 46: 176
implant removal, 48: 166
infected, 46: 215-218
diagnosis, 46: 216
management, 46: 216-218
prevalence of deep sepsis, 46: 215-216
medial epicondylar osteotomy, 48: 153-156
neurovascular complications following, 46: 181-184
direct injury to vascular structures around knee, 46: 183-184
peroneal nerve palsy, 46: 181
wound-healing problems, 46: 181-183
for osteoarthritis, 47: 429
periprosthetic fractures in TKA
incidence of, 47: 253-254
intraoperative, 47: 437-439, 449-451
postoperative, 47: 439-448, 451-*457*
polyethylene wear and osteolysis following, 46: *205*-212, 47: 254
incidence of, 46: 205-206
pathophysiology of osteolysis, 46: 211
prevalence of osteolysis following, 46: 210-211
prevention of osteolysis, 46: 212
structure of polyethylene, 46: *206-207*
treatment of osteolysis, 46: 211-*212*
UHMWPE damage following, 46: 208-210
UHMWPE in vivo degradation, 46: *207*
UHMWPE quality, 46: 207
UHMWPE sterilization, 46: 207
UHMWPE thickness, 46: *208*
revision total
bone loss with, 48: 167-175
goals of, 48: 167
stiff total knee replacement, 46: 191-195
causes of, 46: 192-193
diagnostic considerations, 46: 193
prevention of, 46: 194-195
treatment alternatives, 46: 193-194
supracondylar fracture of distal femur proximal to total knee replacement
incidence, 46: 197-202
revision, 46: 201
surgical technique, 46: 199-201
treatment, 46: 197-199
treatment results, 46: 201-202
surgical exposure in revision total knee arthroplasty, 46: 221-225
closure, 46: 225
exposure of posterior recess, 46: 224
intraosseous exposure, 46: 224
quadriceps transection exposure, 46: 221-222
tibial tubercle osteotomy, 46: 222-224
thromboembolic disease following, 46: 185-188
current prophylaxis, 46: 187-188
epidemiologic considerations, 46: 185-186
impact of chemoprophylaxis, 46: 186-187
treatment of, 46: 188
wound complications in, 46: 165-168
choice of skin incision, 46: 165-166
management, 46: 167-168
patient risk factors, 46: 166-167
technical factors, 46: 166
vascular anatomy, 46: 165
Knee prostheses
LCS mobile-bearing, **50: 443-445**
mobile-bearing, design features, **50: 433-434**
New Jersey LCS, **50: *444***
Oxford Unicompartmental replacement, **50: 437-440**
Knee Society Scores (KSS), results of autologous chondrocyte transplantation (ACT), 48: 637, *639*
Kummel's disease, **50: *139***
Kyphosis, 46: 43
brace treatment for, 48: 528
spinal stenosis, 49: 368

L

Laboratory investigations. *See also* Specific tests
diagnosis of infection, **50: 319-321, 367-369**
preoperative assessment, **50: 298-299**
Labral lesions, Bernese periacetabular osteotomy, **50: 242**
Labral reattachment, laxity, **50: 29**
Labral tears
attritional, 46: 3
detection of, 47: 13-*16*
Labrum, developmental changes, **50: 547**
Lacerations, from acetabular screws, in hip arthroplasty, 48: 29
Lachman tests, 47: 381, *382*
posterior, for PCL damage, 48: 200
and restoration of knee function, 48: 195
shoulder, **50: 18**
Lamina splendens, 46: 487
Laminar airflow, and infection at arthroplasty sites, 48: 113
Laminectomies
complications, 49: 356
decompression, lumbar spinal stenosis, 49: 367
multiple-level, 49: 353-357
outcomes, **50: 156**
posterior cervical spine prepared for, 49: *354*
spinal stenosis, **50: *155*-156**
Laminoforaminotomies (LF), nerve root decompression, 49: 352-353
Laminoplasty
canal-expansive, 49: 354-356
trap-door technique, 48: *425*
Laminotomies, with foraminotomy, 49: 352-353
Land mines
epidemic of, 49: 431-433
history, 49: 431-432

number of unexploded, 49: 580
patterns of injury, 49: 432
types of, 49: *431*
Lap belt injury, spinal imaging following, 46: 119
Laparoscopic approach to lumbar spine, 46: 135-137
Laparoscopic lumbar diskectomy, 46: 144
Laron dwarfism, 46: 477
Laryngeal masked anesthesia (LMA), shoulder surgery, **50: 56**
Laser energy
delivery of, **50: 6**
generators, **50: 7**
thermal capsulorrhaphy, **50: 23**
Laser heating, in vitro experiments, **50: 5**
Lateral antebrachial cutaneous (LABC) nerve, symptoms from, 49: 303
Lateral collateral ligament (LCL)
classification of sprains, **50: 515-516**
deficiency, **50: 451**
mechanisms of injury, **50: 515**
reconstruction, **50: *517***
Lateral complex of ankle, 46: 311
Lateral cruciate ligament, allograft reconstruction of, 47: 389-391
Lateral distal tibial angle (LDTA)
assessment of limb alignment using, 48: 281
use in preoperative planning, 48: 283
variation in measurement of, 48: *282*
Lateral epicondylitis, 46: 572-573, 47: 165-167
Lateral epicondylitis, differential diagnosis, 49: 301
Lateral femoral cutaneous nerve block, 49: 531
Lateral plantar nerve
complications of surgery, **50: 529**
entrapments, **50: *526*-528**
Lateral pivot-shift test, **50: *91*, 92**
Lateral recess stenosis, 46: 143, 156
Lateral runner's knee, 46: 574
biomechanics of, 47: 404-405
corticosteroid injections for, 47: 416
diagnosis and treatment of, 47: 413-414
Ober's test for, 46: 574, *575,* 47: 414
Lateralvolar vessel, **50: 105**
Latex allergies
preoperative prophylaxis, in myelomeningocele patients, 48: 549-550
reaction types, in myelomeningocele patients, 48: 548-549
Latissimus dorsi muscles
amplitude, **50: 66**
bipolar flexorplasty, 49: *330*
bipolar transfer, 49: 326, 329-330
bipolar tricepsplasty, 49: 331
Latissimus dorsi tendons
rotator cuff reconstruction, **50: 68-70**
transfer, 49: 323-324, **50: 63, *68***
Lauge-Hansen classification system for ankle injury, 46: 313
Lavage for treatment of articular cartilage defects, 47: 509
Laxity
generalized ligamentous, 47: *102*
knee
and response to reconstruction, 48: 186
and restoration of function, 48: 195
posterior, for posterior cruciate ligament damage, 48: 200
shoulder, 47: 100
thermal modification, **50: 7-8**
Least developed countries (LDCs)
definition, 49: 567
transfer of appropriate technology, 49: 579-583
Leg pain, spinal stenosis, **50: 150**
Leprosy. *See* Hansen's disease
Lesser toes, amputation of, 46: 505-508
Leukemia, and knee pain, 48: *580*
Leukotrienes, effects of, 49: 79
L'Hermitte's sign
radicular symptoms, 49: 343
test for myelopathy, 49: *337*
Liability, physicians, and medical malpractice, 48: 699-703
Lichtleiter, 46: 127
Lidocaine (xylocaine)
diagnostic nerve blocks, 49: 535
molecular structure, 49: *526*
preoperative analgesia, 49: 533-534
use of, 49: 526
Life expectancies, 46: 409
trends, 49: 567
Lifestyle, in cervical degenerative disease, 48: 435
Lift-off test, Gerber's, 46: *58,* 47: 137, 144
Ligamentous lumbosacral dislocations, 48: 414
Ligaments
age-related changes in, 46: 465
augmentation, 46: 544
imbalance, in inflammatory arthritis, 48: 105
instability in TKA, **50: 399-401**
knee, reconstruction, 47: 379-392
ACL allograft reconstruction, 47: 385-388
LCL allograft reconstruction, 47: 389-391
PCL allograft reconstruction, 47: 388-389
and movement of joints, 48: 190
reconstruction, and formation or articular surfaces, 48: 240
sprains, **50: 515**
type 1 collagen, **50: 3-4**
wrist, **50: 123**
Ligamentum teres, development, **50: 547**
Light touch, testing of, 49: 307
Likert scale, outcomes instrument for cervical disorders, 48: 420-421
Limb alignment
assessment of, 48: 218-282
and periarticular osteotomies, 48: 279-285
Limb development, 47: 461-466
cartilage proliferation, 47: 464-465
embryology, 47: *462*-463
growth hormones in, 47: 465
growth plate development, 47: 464
limb buds, 47: *462*-463
Limb Instrument, MODEMS program, 48: 680
Limb-length discrepancies
after arthrodesis, **50: 303**
and THR, **50: 307-309**
Limb lengths
and acetabular bone loss, 48: 44
compensation for discrepancies, total hip arthroplasties, 48: 58-59
femoral reconstruction, 49: 33-34
finding before the correction, 49: 503-509
inequalities of, revision total hip arthroplasty, 48: 23
leg, templating, 49: 7
and neural injury during hip arthroplasty, 47: 277, 278
patient management during, 46: *547-554*
ambulation, 46: *549*-550
in external fixation, 46: *550-554*
functional use, 46: 549
joint mobility, 46: 549
night positioning, 46: *548*
splinting, 46: *547-548*
stretching, 46: 548-549
preoperative assessments, 49: 87-88
preoperative discussions, 49: 126

and trochanter slides, 48: 78
true, 49: 5
Limb salvage
versus amputation, 46: 511-517
cost of, 46: 517
factors affecting outcome, 46: 513-517
factors affecting salvage, 46: 511-512
scoring systems, 46: 512-513
which injuries, 46: 511
treatment of malignant bone tumors, 48: 599
Limb salvage index (LSI), 46: 512, 513
Limited joint mobility syndrome, in diabetics, 48: 293
Limited to joint motion syndrome, in diabetes, 49: 283-284
Lincomycin, deactivation by bone cement, 48: 117
Lipomas
deep, imaging of, 48: 618
treatment of, 48: 596-597
Liposarcoma, anterior groin, 48: *580*
Litigation, trauma of, 48: 699
Load and shift test, 46: 571
Load testing, alumina ceramics and, 49: 44
Load transfer
in amputees, 46: 502-503
and the envelope of function, 48: 187-188
Loading
of femoral intramedullary grafts, 48: *84*
impact on bone graft incorporation, **50: 215**
and ligament imbalance, in inflammatory arthritis, 48: 105
MTS testing, **50: 212**
response of articular cartilage, 48: 193
subphysiologic, and healing, **50: 5-6**
trochanteric slide, **50: 250-251**
Lobster claw, 46: 97
Locked intramedullary rods, 46: 200-*201, 202*
Loge de Guyon. *See* canal of Guyon
Long bones
fractures, children with multiple injuries, 49: 415-423
risk of pathologic fracture, 49: *462*
Long radiolunate ligaments, **50: *123***
Longevity process, polyethylene cross-linking, **50: 173, 183**
Loose bodies
arthroscopic removal from ankles, 48: 244
elbow, 49: 248-249, 256
arthroscopic view, 49: *248*
glenohumeral joint, **50: 75**
MRI scan, medial talar dome, 49: *260*
osteochondral, 49: 483
Lordosis, spinal stenosis, **50: 147**
Loss of motion
after rotator cuff surgery, 48: 363
with glenohumeral arthrosis, after surgery for shoulder instability, 48: 360
without arthrosis, after surgery for shoulder instability, 48: 359-360
Loss of motion segment integrity, spine, 48: *452*
Loss of reduction, acromioclavicular joint, 49: 410
Low back pain
and chordomas, 48: 586
spinal stenosis, 49: 364-365
Lower limbs. *See also* Specific limbs
surgical correction of deformities, developing countries, 49: 594-598
Loxoscelism, 46: *70*-71
Ludloff approach, DDH, **50: 544**
Lumbar corset, treatment of spinal stenosis, **50: 153**
Lumbar diskectomy
laparoscopic, 46: 144
and posterior fragmentectomy, 46: 155-156
Lumbar flexibility, 46: 43
Lumbar fractures, nonsurgical treatment of, 48: 413-416
Lumbar lordosis, 46: 43
Lumbar myelomeningocele
and bilateral dislocation of the hip, 48: *571*
at fourth lumbar level, 48: *569*
in pediatric patients, 48: 566-569, *568*
and sublaxation of the hip, 48: *571*
Lumbar spine
adolescent back pain, 48: *537*
metastatic disease, surgical treatment, 49: 474-475
range-of-motion model, 48: *460*
Lumbar sympathectomy, 46: 265-267
Lumbar sympathetic blocks, 49: 537
treatment of CRPS, 49: 553
Lumbosacral spine, impairment
due to abnormal motion, 48: *461*
Guides to the Evaluation of Permanent Impairment, 4th edition, 48: 455-456
Lunate
acute perilunate dissociation, **50: 127-129**
perilunate instability, **50: 129**
Lung carcinomas
acral metastases, 49: 453
metastatic bone disease, 49: 462
Lungs
evaluation in preoperative planning, 48: 97
follow-up for orthopaedic oncology patients, 48: 605
Lunotriquetral interosseous ligaments, **50: *123***
Lunotriquetral ligaments
acute tears, 49: 228-229
appearance of, 49: *228*
instability, 49: 225, 229
tear, **50: *126***
Luque-Galveston technique, segmental spinal fusion, 48: 556
Luque rod and wire stabilization, 48: 440
Lymph nodes, follow-up for orthopaedic oncology patients, 48: 605-606

M

Macrophages
bone-cement interface, 49: 71-72
bone debris, 49: *79*
cell death, 49: 79
response to particulate debris, **50: 188-190**
Macrotrauma, acute, 46: 3
Magnetic coils, stimulation of human nervous system, 49: 546
Magnetic resonance arthrography, pelvic, **50: 232-233**
Magnetic resonance imaging (MRI)
acetabular dysplasia, **50: 258-259**
of Achilles tendon, 47: *421*
assessment of cement, 49: 85
carpal instability, **50: 125-126**
cervical radiculopathy or myelopathy, 49: 345
diagnosis of ankle sprains, **50: 515**
diagnosis of osteonecrosis, **50: 496**
in elbow imaging, 46: 522-523
examination of bone tumors, 48: 611
examination of soft-tissue tumors, 48: 618
exclusion of active infection, **50: 320**
follow-up for orthopaedic oncology patients, 48: 605-606
in foot and ankle imaging, 46: 524-526
gadolinium-enhanced, shoulder injuries, **50: 19**
for knee pain, 47: 342
metastatic bone disease, 49: 455
metastatic disease of the spine, 49: 472
osteonecrosis of the femoral condyle, **50: *497***

ostial contributions of the talar dome, 49: 259
and posterior cruciate ligament damage, 48: 201
preoperative investigations, total hip arthroplasty, 48: 32
and restoration of knee function, 48: 195
rotator cuff tears, **50: 43, *44*, *65***
scaphoid fractures, **50: 106**
of shoulder, 47: 3-18
instability, 46: 521-522, 47: 13-*16*
muscle injury, 47: 11-13
rotator cuff, 46: 521, 47: 4-11, 92, *93*
soft-tissue sarcomas, 49: 447-448
of soft-tissue sarcomas, 48: 583-584
soft-tissue tumors, 49: 439
in spinal cord injury, 46: 119-121
spinal stenosis, 49: 366, **50: 138-141**
spondylitic myelopathy, 49: 336
sternoclavicular joint injuries, 49: 399
and thoracolumbar trauma, 48: 430
tibial osteonecrosis, **50: 479-480**
Magnetic resonance spectroscopy, soft-tissue tumors, 49: 249-450
Magnuson-Stack procedure, 47: 118, 120
loss of motion after, 47: 119
Maisonneuve fracture, 46: 317, **50: 519**
Major histocompatibility complexes (MHCs), and immunology of allografts, 48: 651
Malalignment
femoral deficiencies, 49: 92
and outcome of arthroscopic débridement, 48: 136
Malignant hyperthermia, neuromuscular scoliosis in, 48: 560
Malleolus
fracture of posterior, 46: 316
isolated fractures of lateral, 46: 315
Mallet finger, 47: 181
Mallory bone loss classification, 49: *90,* 90-91
Malnutrition, seroconversion of vaccinations, 49: 580
Malpositioning, and polyethylene wear, **50: 422**
Malunion. *See also* Nonunion
in ankle necrosis, 48: 257-258, 259-260
of proximal humeral fractures
as complication of internal fixation, 46: 27-*29*
prosthetic arthroplasty for, 47: 135-140
radial head fractures, **50: 96**
radius, **50: *132***
scaphoid, **50: 112-113, 118-120**
of tibial shaft fracture, defined, 46: 281
Managed care. *See also* Health Maintenance Organizations (HMOs)
and the cost of health care, 48: 674-675
and physician liability, 48: 701
premium increases, 48: 674-675
Mangled extremities severity score (MESS), 49: 381
Mangled extremity severity index (MESI), 46: 512-513
Manipulation for stiff total knee replacement, 46: 194
Mantoux test, diagnosis of active infection, **50: 321**
Manual muscle testing for rotator cuff strength, 46: 57-58
Maquet osteotomies of tibial tubercle, 46: 246
Marathon process
cross-linked polyethylene, **50: 182-183**
polyethylene cross-linking, **50: 172-173**
Marcaine (bupivacaine)
postarthroscopic releases, 49: 219
use of, 49: 526-547
Margin convergence, in rotator cuff repair, 47: 44-*46*
Marginal wound necrosis, 46: 182-183
Marrow stem cells, pluripotential, treatment of chondral injuries, 48: 633-635
Marrow stimulation techniques, treatment of chondral injuries, 48: 633-635
Mason classification for radial head fractures, 47: 160-*161,* 174-175
Masses
clinical presentation of bone tumors, 48: 607
misdiagnosis of, 48: 578-579
Mast cells
bone debris, 49: *79*
phagocytosis by, 49: 72
Matrix metalloproteinase-8 (MMP-8). *See also* Neutrophil collagenase
in knee articular cartilage chondrocytes, 48: 235
Matrix metalloproteinases (MMPs)
and osteoarthritis, 49: 78
in osteoarthritis, 49: 486
response to particulate debris, **50: 191**
Maximal treadmill stress (MTS), loading, **50: 212**
Maximal voluntary contraction, 46: 55-57
Mayo classification system
intra-articular fracture of the radius, 48: 468, *469*
periprosthetic tibial fractures, **50: *385***
McAfee classification, thoracolumbar fractures, 48: 438, 441
McConnell arm-holder, 47: 53
McConnell headrest, **50: 44**
McKee-Farrar hips, **50: 166**
McLee-Farrar articulation, outcomes, 49: 49
McMurray's test, 47: 412
Meary's line, 46: 343
Mechanical axes, preoperative planning, 49: 504-505
Media, orthopaedic care in least developed countries, 49: 579-580
Media/legal system, and reporting of work-related disorders, 48: 697
Medial collateral ligament (MCL)
deficiency, **50: 451**
iatrogenic injury, **50: 399**
instability of, in the athlete's elbow, 48: 383-391
Medial complex of ankle, 46: 311
Medial cutaneous nerve blocks, 49: 529
Medial eminence, 46: 362
Medial epicondylar osteotomy
in knee arthroplasty, 48: 153-156
rehabilitation following, 48: 155
repair of, 48: 154-155
Medial epicondylectomy
surgical technique, 49: 313
ulnar nerve compression, 49: 311
Medial epicondylitis, 46: 573, 47: 168-170
Medial malleolar fracture, malunited, 48: *280*
Medial wedge osteotomies, technique, 48: 283-285
Median hand, ulnar nerve compression, 49: 308
Median nerves
blocks, 49: 530
capsular release, 49: 256
Medical malpractice, defenses, 48: 699-703
Medical Outcomes Trust, 48: 679
Medicalization, and reporting of work-related disorders, 48: 696
Medications, evaluation in preoperative planning, 48: 98
Medicin Sans Frontiere (MSF), disaster relief, 49: 576
Megaprosthesis
proximal femoral replacement with, 49: 141-146
reconstruction of proximal femur, 48: *601*
Melanoma, differentiation of pyogenic granuloma from, 46: 71
Melone classification, intra-articular fracture of the radius, 48: 468, *469*
Meniscal allografts, 47: 392-393
transplantation treatment of chondral injuries, 48: 640-641
Meniscal lesions in runners, 47: 412
Meniscus. *See also* Knee
arthroscopic repair, outside-in technique, 49: 195-206
blood supply, 49: 207-208
degenerative tears, 49: 192, *192*

gross anatomy, 49: 189-190
indications for repair, 49: 195-196
lateral, repair technique, 49: 200-201
medial, repair technique, 49: 197-200
microanatomy, 49: 190-191
outside-in repairs, outcomes, 49: 204-205
pain following hip arthrodesis, **50: 297**
postoperative rehabilitation, 49: 202-203
rehabilitation after repair, 49: 207-209
repairs during ACL revision, **50: 459**
response to injury, 49: 189-192
sutures for repair, 49: 201-202
tears, differential diagnosis, **50: 491**
unstable tears, 48: 136
Wrisberg-type discoid, 49: 197
Mental status exam, mini-, 46: 410, *411*
Meperidine, toxicity of, 49: 517
Mesenchymal stem cells, 46: 466-467, 487
and articular cartilage repair, 48: *626*
Metacarpal fractures, 47: 188-*189*
of thumb, 47: 189-*190*
Metacarpals, skeletal reconstruction, 49: 384
Metal ions, release from bearing surface, 49: 50
Metal-on-metal bearings, total hip replacements, **50: 166-167**
Metal-on-polyethylene bearings, **50: 168**
Metals, THA implants, 49: 75
Metaphyseal blanch sign, ***50: 558***
Metaphyseal bone, strength of, 46: 227
Metaphyseal fibrous defect, differentiation from giant cell tumor, 48: *615*
Metaphyseal region, of the knee, 48: *169*
Metaphyses, circumferential deficiency, 49: 89
Metastatic bone disease, 49: 453-459
classification of periacetabular lesions, 49: 467
features, treatment, and management, 49: 453-459
guidelines for prophylactic fixation, 49: *458*
pathophysiology, 49: 453-*454*
pelvis and proximal femur, surgical treatment, 49: 461-469
presentation, 49: 454-455
radiation therapy, 49: 459
spine, 49: 471-476
Metastatic disease
intramuscular, 49: 438
orthopaedic neoplasms, 48: 605-606
Metastatic lesions of hand, 46: *73*-74
Metasul articulations, outcomes, 49: 47-50
Metatarsalgia, **50: 529**
Metatarsocuneiform (MC) joint, 46: 364
arthrodesis of, 46: 378-380
Metatarsophalangeal (MTP) joints
arthrodesis of first, 46: 380-382
first
arthroscopy of, 48: 343, *346*
gross anatomy and biomechanics, 48: 343
resection and replacement arthroplasty, 48: 336-338
hyperextention, and diabetic foot, 48: *292*
Metatarsus primus varus, 46: 357
Methicillin, organisms resistant to, 49: 605
Methicillin-resistant *Staphylococcus aureus* (MRSA), isolation precautions, 49: 608-609
Methotrexate, consideration in preoperative planning, 48: 98
N-Methyl-d-aspartate receptor agonists, pain management, 49: 520
Methylmethacrylate, inhibition of white cell function, 48: 97
Microfractures
arthroscopic photograph, 48: *138*
technique for articular cartilage defects, 46: 510-511, 47: *508*
treatment of chondral injuries, 48: 634-635
in treatment of degenerative arthritis, 48: 137-139
Microinstability, thermal capsulorrhaphy, **50: 32**
Microorganisms. *See also* Specific organisms
and infection at arthroplasty sites, 48: 113
Microtrauma, repetitive, 46: 3
and Achilles tendon degeneration, 48: 219
and MDI, **50: 24**
and posterior subluxation, **50: 24**
Microvasculature, and steroids, **50: 489-490**
Midcarpal instability (MCI), 47: 204-208
diagnosis of, 47: 204-205
Lichtman's classification of, 47: 205-206
Middle finger test, radial tunnel syndrome, 49: 301
Middle phalangeal fractures, 47: 187
Midfoot
amputations, 46: *504,* 506
diabetic feet, 48: 325, *326*
focal tenderness, ***50: 521***
Military AntiShock Trousers (MAST), 46: 115
Mimo-causalgia, 46: 261
Mini Mental Status Exam, 46: 410, *411*
Minor causalgia, 46: 263
Misoprostol, effect on particulate-induced bone resorption, **50: 192**
Mobility
in elderly, 46: 412
maintaining and restoring, in middle and old age, 46: 459-467
Mobilization, prevention of DVT, **50: 416**
Modular components, revision arthroplasty, 49: 133-135
Modular implants, 46: 230
Molecular analysis, 47: 292
Monarthritis, 46: 78
Monoarticular arthritis, 46: 78
sternoclavicular joint, 49: 404
Monteggia fractures, PIN palsy, 49: 298
Morcellized cancellous bone
and allograft healing, 48: 182
impaction grafting, 49: 106
Morel-Lavelle's lesion, 48: 481
Morphine, anesthetic action, 49: 523
Morton neuroma, 46: 264
Motion segment unit (MSU), 46: 145
Motor conduction velocities, ulnar nerve compression, 49: 308
Motor neuropathy
and diabetic foot, 48: 291-292
in the diabetic foot, 48: 317
Motor ulnar nerve symptoms, 48: 386
Motor vehicle accident, patient extrication from, 46: 115
Mulberry knots
meniscal terror reduction, 49: 200
meniscus surface, 49: *198*
outside-in meniscus repair, 49: 197
Multitasking, 46: 544
Multidirectional instability (MDI)
diagnosis, **50: 23-24**
heat probes used, **50: 34**
joint capsule volume, **50: 23**
shoulder, 47: 101-109
approach for inferior capsular shift, 47: 104-108
clinical presentation, 47: 101-*103*
nonsurgical treatment for, 47: 102, 104
surgical technique, 47: 104-108
thermal capsulorrhaphy, **50: *26*, 37-38**
Multidisciplinary committees, critical pathways development, 49: 645
Multiple joint disease, arthrodesis in, 48: 260
Multiple osteotomies, 46: 385-387

Muscle flaps, **50: 361**
Muscle hypertrophy, misdiagnosis of, 48: 579-580
Muscle relaxants
treatment of spinal stenosis, **50: 153**
use in cervical degenerative disease, 48: 434
Muscles, pulled, misdiagnosis of, 48: 579
Musculocutaneous nerves
block, 49: 529
obstetrical brachial plexus palsy, 49: 328
Musculoskeletal function
age-related changes in, 46: 459-460
disorders in elderly populations, 46: 417
effect of depression on, 46: 418
Musculoskeletal Functional Assessment (MFA) Index
development of, 48: 670-671
use in orthopaedic practice, 48: 668
Musculoskeletal Outcomes Data Evaluation and Management System (MODEMS), 48: 680-683
communication with, 48: 683
Musculoskeletal tissues, homeostasis in, 48: 187
Musculoskeletal Tumor Society (MSTS), staging system, 49: 438-439, 444
Mycobacteria, and infection at arthroplasty sites, 48: 113
Mycobacterium tuberculosis, and spinal osteomyelitis, 48: 532
Myelography, spinal stenosis, **50: 141-142**
Myelomeningoceles
current concepts, 48: 543-550
THA in, 49: 163
treatment of hip and knee problems in, 48: 563-573
Myelopathies
cervical spondylitic, 49: 339-357
cervical spondylosis, 49: 335
differential diagnosis, 49: *344*
spinal cord involvement, 49: *341*
stability, diagnosis of, 49: 336
tests suggesting, 49: *337*
Myelopathy hand, description of, 49: 343
Myocardial infarction in geriatric patients, 46: 414
Myoligamentous structures, arthroscopic visualization of, 46: 149
Myositis ossificans
imaging of, 48: 618
radiographs, 48: *583*

N
Nail care instruments, for the clinic, 48: *300*
Nail splitter, 48: *302*
Nailing
in surgical stabilization of tibia, 46: 271
tibial
and compartment syndrome, 46: 304-305
interlocking, 46: 297-298
Nails, outpatient care, for diabetic foot, 48: 300
Naloxone
administration of, 49: 517
affection acupuncture, 49: 560
in treating spinal cord injuries, 46: 118
Narcotics in treating sympathetically maintained pain, 46: 265
National Acute Spinal Cord Injury Study (NASCIS), 46: 118
National Committee for Quality Assurance (NCQA), and performance measurement, 48: 677-678, 679
National health care
expenditures for, 48: 673
percapita expenditures, 48: *674*
projected national expenditures, 48: *674*
projected procapita expenditures, 48: *675*
total national expenditures, 48: *674*
National Institute of Occupational Safety and Health (NIOSH)
criteria for work relatedness, 48: 694
illness and work activities, 48: 693
National Institutes of Health/National Institute of Child Health and Human Development (NIH/NICHHD), development of the Musculoskeletal Functional Assessment (MFA), 48: 670-671
National Nosocomial Surveillance System, surgical site pathogens, 49: *605*
National Union Against Cancer, TNM system for staging, 49: 445
Nausea, and opioids use, 49: 516
Navicular, terminology, **50: 105**
Neck
evaluation in preoperative planning, 48: 97
work related illnesses, 48: 694
Neck Disability Index (NDI), 48: 419
outcomes instrument for cervical disorders, 48: 419
Neck pain
and cervical degenerative disease, 48: 433-435
cervical degenerative disorders, 49: 335-337
outcome prediction, 48: 417-418
Necrobiosis lipoidica diabeticorum, 46: 72
Necrosis
full-thickness soft-tissue, in total knee arthroplasty, 46: 167
marginal wound, 46: 182-183
superficial soft tissue, in total knee arthroplasty, 46: 167
Necrotizing vasculitis, 46: 72
Needle biopsies, soft-tissue tumors, 49: 440-441
Needs assessments, critical pathways, 49: 645
Neer classification, rotator cuff tears, 47: 52
Neer test, 46: 571
Neoplasms. *See also* Oncology; Tumors
biopsies and seeding of, 48: 588
musculoskeletal
staging, 48: 591
treatment options for, 48: 591-602
and pediatric back pain, 48: 537-539
Neovascularization. *See also* Vascularization
in drilled channels, 48: 99
thermal modification, **50: 5**
Nerve blocks
diagnostic, 49: 519
intravenous regional, 49: 532-533
regional, 49: 528-533
Nerve conduction studies (NCS)
high medial nerve palsy, 49: 297
PIN palsy, 49: 299
Nerve injuries, complication of local anesthetics, 49: 528
Nerve palsies, after total hip arthroplasty, 49: 35-36
Nerve roots, spinal stenosis, **50: 145**
Nerves
conduction block, 49: 524
reconstruction, upper extremities, 49: 388
Neural axis, MRI study, 48: *527*
Neurapraxia, 47: 276-277
Neurilemoma, treatment of, 48: *597*
Neuritis, ulnar, in the athlete's elbow, 48: 383-391
Neuroarthropathic fractures, use of total contact casting, 48: 307-308
Neurofibromas, treatment of, 48: 597
Neurologic injury, after total shoulder arthroplasty, 48: 366-367
Neurologic problems in elderly, 46: 423
Neurological level, defined, 48: *563*
Neuromas, postoperative, **50: 529**
Neuromuscular diseases. *See also* Specific diseases
THA in, 49: 163-168

Neuromuscular scoliosis
in Duchenne muscular dystrophy, 48: *557*
instrumentation, 48: 556
outcomes analysis, 48: 551-553
in patient with spastic quadriplegia, 48: *559*
spinal alignment, 48: 553-554
treatment goals, 48: 553
treatment of, 48: 551-560
Neuropathic ankle, arthrodesis in, 48: 260
Neuropathic arthropathy. *See also* Charcot arthropathy
Eichenholtz classification system, 48: *269*
of the foot and ankle, surgical treatment for, 48: 269-277
shoulder, **50: 77-78**
Neuropathic deformities, reconstructive procedures for, 48: 272-275
Neuropathic joints, radiographic staging and treatment, 48: 308
Neuropathic osteoarthropathy, natural history and clinical presentation, 48: 269-270
Neuropathies
compressive, ulnar nerve, 49: 305-316
and diabetic foot, 48: 290
radial nerves, 49: 295-303
Neurotmesis, 47: 276-277
Neurotoxicity, local anesthetics, 49: 528
Neurotransmitters, effective acupuncture, 49: 559
Neurovascular injuries
acromioclavicular joint instability, 49: 409
after surgery for shoulder instability, 48: 361
avoidance of, in hip arthroplasty, 48: 13
following hip arthroplasty, 47: 275-281
neurologic sequelae of fat embolism, 47: 275-*276*
peripheral-nerve complications, 47: 276-279
vascular complications, 47: 279-281
following internal fixation of proximal humeral fractures, 46: 31-32
following total knee replacement, 46: 181-184
direct injury to vascular structures around knee, 46: 183-184
peroneal nerve palsy, 46: 181
wound-healing problems, 46: 181-183
and shoulder fracture management, 48: 367
Neurovascular status
documentation of, in preoperative assessment, 48: 44
preoperative planning, 49: 84
Neurovascular structures, arthroscopic visualization of, 46: 150
Neutrophil collagenase. *See also* Matrix metalloproteinase-8 (MMP-8)
in knee articular cartilage chondrocytes, 48: 235
Newborns, DDH, **50: 535-540**
Nifedipine, treatment of the CRPS, 49: 553
Night pain, osteolysis, **50: 198**
Nijmegen technique
for acetabular reconstruction, 47: 266-269, 273
rationale for, 48: 80-82
Nitrous oxide synthase (NOS)
inducible, production of, 49: 79
response to particulate debris, **50: 191**
Nocebo, and reporting of work-related disorders, 48: 696
Nociception, definition, 49: 513
Noncircumferential splinting, children with multiple injuries, 49: 428
Nongovernmental organizations (NGOs), health programs, 49: 575
Nonossifying fibroma, differentiation from giant cell tumor, 48: 615
Nonsteroidal anti-inflammatory drugs (NSAIDs). *See also* Aspirin; Ibuprofen
consideration in preoperative planning, 48: 98
glenohumeral arthritis, **50: 74**
for gout, 46: 76
for juvenile rheumatoid arthritis, 46: 78
in osteoarthritis, 49: 497
pain management, 49: 515
for pseudogout, 46: 77
for rheumatoid arthritis, 46: 78
treatment of CRPS, 49: 553
treatment of spinal stenosis, **50: 153**
use in cervical degenerative disease, 48: 434
Nonunion. *See also* Malunion
acetabular fracture, **50: 342-343**
after nailing without reaming for tibial shaft fractures, 46: 285-287
in ankle arthrodesis, 48: 257-258
as complication of internal fixation of proximal humeral fractures, 46: 25-27
defined of, 46: 281
radial head fractures, **50: 96**
rate of, revision total hip arthroplasty, using extended proximal femoral osteotomies, 48: 24
risk of, 49: 6
scaphoid, **50: 112-113**
structural femoral allografts, 49: 157-158
Norepinephrine, and naloxone, 49: 560
North American Indians, Apache baby carrier, ***50: 536***
Nosocomial infections
antibiotic-resistant organisms, 49: 605
ICU patients, resistant organisms, 49: *606*
Notch technique, 46: 347
Nottingham Health Profile (NHP), 48: 419
validity of, 48: 669
Novocaine. *See* procaine
Nuclear factor-κB, response to particulate debris, **50: 189**
Nudge test, 46: 412
Nurick Criteria, outcomes instrument for cervical disorders, 48: 420
Nutraceuticals, osteoarthritis, 49: 491-493
Nutritional status
decision making in foot amputations, 48: 323
in diabetics, 48: 294
evaluation in preoperative planning, 48: 98
and infection at arthroplasty sites, 48: 111-112
wound healing, **50: 359**
Nutritional supplementation, chondroprotective agents, 49: 491-493

O

Ober test, 46: 574, *575,* 47: 414
Obesity
and infection at arthroplasty sites, 48: 112
and knee osteotomy, 47: 496
and revision total knee arthroplasty, 46: 221
SCFE, **50: 555**
Oblique dorsal artery, of the distal ulna, **50: *115*-117**
Observational study designs, outcome assessment of fractures in elderly, 46: 439-440
Obstetrical brachial plexus palsy
tendon transfers, 49: 319-332
timing of operative procedures, 49: 319
Obstructive pulmonary disease, 46: 129
Obturator nerves, block, 49: 531
Occult fractures, imaging of, 46: 526
Occupational therapy
evaluations, polyarticular inflammatory arthritis, 48: 94
glenohumeral arthritis, **50: 74**
pain of, 49: 542
treatment of RSD, 49: 552
Odom Criteria, outcomes instrument for cervical disorders, 48: 419-420
Oh-Harris rings, class to acetabular defects, 49: 467
Olecranon. *See also* Elbow
after fenestration for posterior impingement, 48: *403*
after spur excision, 48: *403*

central spurring of, 48: *399*
fractures, 47: *162,* **50: 93**
bioresorbable implants for, 46: *539*
osteotomy, 47: 155
spurring of, 49: *250*
spurs, 47: 152-*153,* 170
Oncology. *See also* Neoplasms; Tumors; Specific cancers
follow-up regimens for orthopaedic patients, 48: 603-606
orthopaedic
index of suspicion, 48: 577-578
introduction and common errors, 48: 577-586
Oncology patients, orthopaedic, follow-up regimens, 48: 603-606
Onlay allografts, basics of, 49: 97-101
Open biopsies, soft-tissue tumors, 49: 440-441
Opening wedge osteotomy, preoperative planning, 48: 282
Operating rooms
environment, and infection at arthroplasty sites, 48: 112-113
infection control precautions, 49: 605-613
Opioids
common side effects, 49: *516*-517
duration of action, 49: *518*
hypersensitivity, 49: 517
pain management, 49: 515
pharmacology, 49: 515-516
routes of administration, 49: 517-518
time to peak effect, 49: *518*
toxicity of, 49: 517
use with peripheral nerve blocks, 49: 535
Oral contraceptives, and deep vein thrombosis, **50: 415**
Orthopaedic assistants, training, developing countries, 49: 593, 600
Orthopaedic care
issues related to delivery, 49: 571-572
lack in developing nations, 49: 571
needs for, 49: 570-571
technology for less-developed countries, 49: 579-583
training resources, 49: 572
Orthopaedic challenges, in aging population, 46: 417-422
total joint arthroplasty, 46: 418-420
total knee arthroplasty, 46: 421-422
trauma treatment and related clinical issues, 46: 423-429
anesthesia considerations, 46: 427
bone quality, 46: 424
fixation enhancement, 46: 427-428
impact choice, 46: 427
metastatic disease, 46: 426
open fractures, 46: 424
Paget's disease, 46: 426, *427*
patient factors in, 46: 423-424
periarticular fractures, 46: 424-425
periprosthetic fractures, 46: 425-426
polytrauma, 46: 424
postoperative management, 46: 428-429
soft-tissue quality, 46: 424
surgical indications, 46: 426
timing of surgery, 46: 426-427
Orthopaedic oncology
index of suspicion, 48: 577-578
introduction and common errors, 48: 577-586
misdiagnoses
of hematomas, 48: 579
of masses, 48: 578-579
of pulled muscles, 48: 579
Orthopaedic surgery
bioresorbable implants in
in adults, 46: 538-539
advantages and disadvantages, 46: 536-538
in anterior cruciate ligament reconstruction, 46: 541-542
biodegradation of, 46: 535-536
in children, 46: 539-540
future of, 46: 542-545
historic overview, 46: 531-532
manufacturing methods, 46: 533-535
mechanical properties of materials, 46: 535
properties and characteristics, 46: 532-533
blood management during, 48: 655-662
in the developing world's, 49: 567-573
ethical considerations, 49: 633-636
hand, post operative pain, 49: 541-542
Lowe technology, developing world, 49: 587-588
management of pain, 49: 523-537
and prevention of deep periprosthetic joint infection, 46: 555-565
prevention of infections, 49: 611-612
risk on HIV-infected patients, 49: 627-628
teaching ethics to residents, 49: 639-642
Orthopaedic Trauma Association, trauma registries and outcomes research, 48: 672
Orthopaedics
advanced imaging in, 46: 521
elbow, 46: 522-523
foot and ankle, 46: 524-526
hip, 46: 527-528
knee, 46: 526-527
shoulder, 46: 521-522
wrist and hand, 46: 523-524
clinical teaching of, 46: 583-593
in clinic and conference, 46: 592-593
by lecture, 46: 590-592
in operating room, 46: 587-590
computer technology in improving presentations, 46: 595-610
basic hardware guidelines, 46: 597
digital graphic images, 46: 600-601
general design guidelines, 46: 597-600
multimedia, 46: 604-610
poster exhibits, 46: *601*-603
slides, 46: *603*-604
Orthopaedics Overseas (OO)
goals of, 49: 577
land mine initiatives, 49: 433
services in the developing world, 49: 572
volunteer orthopedic surgeons, 49: 600
Orthopaedists
geriatrics for, 46: 409-416
changes in focus of medical care, 46: 410-414
ethical dilemmas, 46: 415
iatrogenic conditions, 46: 415
medical conditions, 46: 414-415
pharmacology and aging, 46: 415
reasons for change in demographics, 46: 409
theories of aging, 46: 410
need in Africa, 49: 579
Orthotic devices for running injuries, 47: 415-416
Orthotics, lower extremity, in patients with myelomeningocele, 48: 546-548
Ortolani "click" sign, **50: *537*-538**
Os acromiale, 47: 7, 88
Os trigonum, 46: 324
Osgood-Schlatter's syndrome, 47: 339, *341*
Osmotic diuretics in treating spinal cord injuries, 46: 119
Osseointegrated stems, removal of, 49: 87
Osseous homeostasis, anteroposterior technetium scintiscan, of the knees, 48: *192*

Osseous tumor, 46: 572
Ossification
of allograft segments, 48: 179
ectopic, after biceps tendon injury, 48: *408*
heterotropic
acetabular fractures, **50: 346-348**
after hip arthroplasty, 48: *105*
in ankylosing spondylitis after THA, 48: 104
newborn hip, **50: 538-539**
Ossification of the posterior longitudinal ligament (OPLL), occurrence of, 48: 423
Ostectomy
reconstruction of neuropathic deformities, 48: 272-273
simple, 46: 341-343
Osteoarthritis (OA)
acromioclavicular joint, 47: *36*
animal models, effect of hyaluronic acid, 49: 496-497
ankle
joint distraction as treatment for, 48: 249-254
pathogenesis, 48: 237-239
posttraumatic, stages in development, 48: *238*
prevalence of, 48: 235-237
of the ankle, 48: 233-240
etiology and epidemiology, 48: 233-234
Bernese periacetabular osteotomy, **50: 240-245**
chondral injuries and, 48: 629-632
compared to aging of cartilage, 49: *484*
distal femoral osteotomy knees, **50: 504-505**
early detection of, 46: 417-418
etiology, 49: 484-485
etiology of, 48: 279
experimental induction of, 48: 253
glenohumeral, 47: 129, *130*
high tibial osteotomy, **50: 505**
hip, 46: 418
hyaluronic acid therapy, 49: 495-501
joint degeneration, 49: *485*
and joint degeneration, 47: 487-491
knee, 46: 418, 47: 429-434
osteotomy for, 47: 430-434
pathophysiology, 47: 429-430
proximal valgus tibial osteotomy, 48: 131-133
knees, middle-aged patients, **50: 499-511**
longitudinal studies, 49: 487-488
medial compartment, 48: *284*
oral glucosamine and chondroitin sulfate, 49: 491-493
radiographic changes, 49: *482*
radiographic science, **50: 73**
realignment osteotomies, **50: 502-505**
in runners, 47: 413
secondary
causes of, 49: *483*
hip, 49: 23
selection of surgical procedures, **50: *499***
shoulder joint, **50: 73-77**
staging of, 48: 279-281
sternoclavicular joint, 49: 403-404
subtalar fusion, 49: *278*
synovial joint degeneration, 49: 481-488
in talar body fractures, 46: 333
treatment of spurs, 49: 249
trials of hyaluronate, 49: *500*
unicompartmental knee arthroplasty, **50: 505-507**
and unstable shoulder arthroplasty, 47: 142-*143*
worldwide prevalence, 49: 571
Osteoarthrosis
and hardware complications, after surgery for shoulder instability, 48: 360-361
of the hip, **50: 229**
and infection at arthroplasty sites, 48: 111
posttraumatic, 46: 320
shoulder, 47: 17, 73
Osteoarticular allograft reconstruction, distal femoral, 48: *600*
Osteoblastomas
and pediatric back pain, 48: 537-538
treatment of, 48: 591-592
Osteoblasts
in bone grafts, 48: *85*
inhibition by metal, 49: 75
Osteocartilaginous plugs, harvesting of, 48: 245
Osteochondral allografts for the knee, 47: 500, 517-521
results of, 47: 512, 521
surgical procedure, 47: 512, *513, 518*-521
for defects of femoral condyles, 47: 518-*520*
for malunion after tibial plateau fracture, 47: *518*
for replacement of patella facet, 47: 520, *521*
Osteochondral defects, 47: 512
ankles, 48: 244-245
Osteochondral grafts, for isolated articular cartilage defects, 47: *511-513*
Osteochondral lesions
débridement, 49: 260-261
medial talar dome, after débridement, 49: *260*
talar dome, drilling of intact lesions, 49: 261
Osteochondral progenitor cells, and articular cartilage restoration, 48: 625
Osteochondral transplantation
fresh and cryopreserved, treatment of chondral injuries, 48: 640
treatment of chondral injuries, 48: 639-640
Osteochondritis dissecans, 46: 572
computed tomography of lesion, 48: *244*
of the elbow, 48: 393-398
clinical presentation, 48: 394
diagnosis, 48: 394-395
etiology, 48: 393-394
histopathology, 48: 393-394
outcomes, 48: 396-397
treatment, 48: 395-396
Osteochondroma, treatment of, 48: 593
Osteoclastic resorption, and bone grafts, 48: 646-647
Osteoclasts
in bone grafts, 48: *85*
control of, 49: 78
Osteogenesis
and bone grafts, 48: 646-647
distraction, 46: 284
Osteogenesis imperfecta, arthroplasty procedure, 49: 65-66
Osteoid osteoma
and pediatric back pain, 48: 537-538, *539*
treatment of, 48: 591-592
Osteoinducive properties, of bone grafts, 48: 647
Osteoinductive growth factors, 47: 530-532
Osteolysis, 47: 307-317. *See also* Aseptic loosening; Bone loss
acetabular, 49: *71*
after total hip arthroplasty, classification system for, 48: 37-42
classification system for, 48: *39*
and particle generators, 48: 40-42
and aseptic loosening, 47: 307, 309-*310*
cemented hip arthroplasty, 49: *73*
cemented total hip replacement, **50: *185***
with cementless components, **50: 392**
cementless sockets with, classification system for, 48: 38
ceramics and, 49: 46

clinical presentation, **50: 391**
cracks in cement mantle, 49: 76
critical presentation, **50: 198-199**
definition, **50: 197**
design of prosthesis, 49: 76-78
diagnosis of, 47: 309-310
differential diagnosis, **50: 199-200**
direction of, influences on, 48: 46
epidemiology
after total hip arthroplasty, 47: 314-317
after total knee replacement, 46: 210-*211*
etiology, prosthetic factors, and pathogenesis, 49: 71-80
femoral
classification of, **50: 202**
clinical management, **50: 201-202**
preoperative planning, **50: 202-203**
principles of management, **50: 197-209**
femoral component, **50: *395***
and fractures, 47: 239, 254
intraoperative inspection, **50: 394**
management options, **50: 394-397**
materials used, 49: 74-76
minimization in THA, 49: 50
pathology of, **50: 428**
pathophysiology, **50: 197-198**
pathophysiology of, 46: 211, 47: 307-309, 48: 37-38
patterns of, **50: 392-393**
periprosthetic, 48: *52,* **50: 181-182**
after total hip arthroplasty, 48: 37-42
basic science of, **50: 185-195**
with TKA, **50: 391-398**
periprosthetic femoral, clinical investigations, **50: 200-201**
polyethylene promotion of, 49: 52-53
and polyethylene wear, 48: 162
preoperative investigations, **50: 368-369**
prevention of, 46: 212
and proinflammatory cytokines, **50: 190-191**
radiographic appearance of, 47: 310-314
and resorbable implants, 46: 537
revision arthroplasty, 49: 119
risk factors for, 47: 317
surgical approaches, 49: 86-87
surgical factors, 49: 76-78
treatment, 46: 211-*212,* 47: 321-328
for acetabular defects, 47: 324-328
for femoral defects, 47: 321-324
treatment algorithm, 48: *38*
in weight lifters, 47: 37
Osteolytic defects, debris-generated, 46: 227-228
Osteomyelitis
in the diabetic foot, 48: 318
hematogenous, in the developing world, 49: 588-590
imaging of, 46: 525-526
vertebral
and pediatric back pain, 48: 531-532
secondary to atypical mycobacterium, 48: *532*
Osteomyelitis
incidence, **50: 317**
neonatal, **50: 317**
Osteonecrosis (ON)
acetabular, **50: *349***
of the acetabulum, **50: 348-349**
after distal metatarsal osteotomy, 48: *335*
classification of lesions, **50: 480**
as complication of internal fixation of proximal humeral fractures, 46: 30-31
complication of SCFE, **50: 564-565, 574-575**
as complication of talar injuries, 46: 324
corticosteroid-induced, 48: *354*
differential diagnosis, **50: 491**
evaluation, 48: 353
femoral condyle, **50: *496***
femoral head, classification of, 49: *172*
of the femoral head to, 49: 169-181
following surgery, **50: 490**
hip-preserving surgical approaches, 48: 98-99
humeral head, 48: *356*
of the humeral head, 48: 349-356
Cruess classification, 48: *353*
of the knee, **50: 483-488**
large lesions, 49: 178
magnetic resonance imaging of, 47: 16-*17*
medial femoral condyle, **50: *485***
natural history of, 48: 352-353
path of physiology, 49: 170-172
pathology, **50: 490, 496-497**
Pavlik harness, **50: 543**
postcollapse disease, 48: 100
precollapse disease, 48: 99-100
prostatic replacement, **50: 485-486**
radial head fractures, **50: 96**
radiograph and computed tomography scan, 48: *352*
radiographic staging of progression, 48: 351-352
septic arthritis, **50: 318**
shoulder arthroplasty for, 47: 132
and shoulder fracture management, 48: 367-368
spontaneous
of the distal femur, **50: 495-498**
prognosis, **50: 497-498**
stages of, **50: 491-*492*, 495-496**
steroid-associated, **50: 487, 489-493**
in talar body, 46: 337, 350
in talar neck fractures, 46: 328-329, 331-332
tibial, **50: 477-481**
etiology, **50: 477-478**
pathology of, **50: 478**
treatment of, **50: 486-487**
treatment, 48: 353-356
treatment algorithms, 49: 181
treatment methods, 49: 174-181
vascularized bone grafts, 49: 177-178
Osteopenia
condylar fragment, distal fixation, **50: *382***
diabetic frozen shoulder, 49: *285*
in elderly, 46: 424
in rheumatoid arthritis of the hip, 48: 102
supracondylar femoral fracture, **50: *380***
Osteophytes, 47: 491
nerve root compression, 49: 340
osteoarthritis, 49: 483
removal of, 49: 256
Osteoporosis
bone biomechanics, 46: 447
physical activity, 46: 448
bone metabolism in, 46: 445
calcitropic hormones, 46: *446*-447
calcium, 46: 445-446
cause of death, 49: 571
in elderly, 46: 424
evaluation of, 46: *448-449*
bone histomorphometry, 46: 451
history, 46: 449-450

imaging studies and measurement of bone mineral density, 46: 450
laboratory studies, 46: 450-451
growth factors as potential therapeutic agents in, 46: 495-497
insufficiency fractures, **50: 477**
treatment of, pharmacologic therapy, 46: 451-454
Osteoporotic bone, hip and spine fractures in, 46: 431-437
Osteoporotic fractures, 46: 7
Osteosarcomas
knee radiographs, 48: *578*
pain and diagnosis of, 48: 580
telangiectatic extraosseous, 48: *584*
treatment of, 48: 598-600
treatment using limb salvage techniques, 48: *646*
Osteosynthesis, 46: 544
Osteotomies. *See also* Specific techniques
affect on later hip arthroplasty, 49: 26-27
arthrodesis with, 46: 343-344
arthrodesis without, 46: 344-345
and articular cartilage regeneration, 47: 495-496
bilateral varus, 49: 175
calcaneal, 46: 397-*398*
chevron, 46: 370-*372, 373*
choice of type, revision total hip arthroplasty, 48: 3
corrective, of radius, 46: 107
distal femoral varus, 47: 434, 48: 125-129
distal metatarsal, 46: 372-*375,* 385-386
Dwyer-type, 46: 343
effective angles, **50: 249-250**
extended conventional, revision total hip arthroplasty, 48: 3, 6-7, *8*
extended femoral, 48: 9-10
extended proximal femoral
for cementless implants, 48: *22*
for hip arthroplasty, 48: 19-26
length of procedure, 48: 24
outcomes, 48: 24-25
surgical technique, 48: *21*
femoral, 49: 123-124
fibular, 47: 433
of first cuneiform, 46: 386
of first metatarsal, distal soft-tissue reconstruction of, 46: 374-378
forces that interface, **50: *251***
and formation of articular surfaces, 48: 240
frictional force, **50: 250**
glenohumeral arthritis, **50: 76**
greater trochanter, 49: *18*
hip, salvage procedures for rheumatoid arthritis, 48: 100-101
intertrochanteric, **50: 242**
of the knee, 47: 429-434
and articular cartilage regeneration, 47: 496
indications for, 47: 430-431
patient assessment, 47: 431-432
knees, results in rheumatoid arthritis, 48: 101
medial epicondylar, 48: 153-156
medial transfer of tibial tubercle by, 46: 172-173
multiple, 46: 385-387
multiple drill holes, 49: *124*
olecranon, 47: 155
for osteonecrosis, 49: 175-176
pediatric, 46: 540
pelvic, **50: 229-230**
reorientation, **50: *230***
periacetabular, **50: 229-245**
periarticular, importance of limb alignment, 48: 279-285
proximal phalangeal, 46: 366-367
radiographic analysis, **50: 253-261**
realignment, **50: 502-505**
revision total hip arthroplasty, 48: *4*
rotational, of first metacarpal, 46: 108
scaphoid malunion, **50: 118**
simple, 46: 343
through previous ankle fusion, 46: 356
through triple arthrodesis, 46: 356
tibial
proximal tibial osteotomies, 47: 432-434
tubercle, 46: 222-*224,* 246
treatment of precollapse osteonecrosis, 48: 99-100
trochanteric, in total hip arthroplasty, 48: 54
trochanteric slide, **50: 247-252**
valgus-extension, 49: 176
Osteotomy slide, 48: *10*
Oswestry Disability Index, 48: 419
Oswestry Low Back Disability Index, outcomes instrument for cervical disorders, 48: 419
Outcomes assessments
importance of, 48: 418
instrument for cervical disorders, 48: 419-421
instruments, data collection and utilization of data, 48: 667-683
recommendations for, 48: 671-672
selection of instruments, 48: 419
steps in development of instruments, 48: 668-670
Outcomes management, 49: 643-648. *See also* Critical pathways
Outcomes research
defined, 48: 667
recommendations for, 48: 671-672
Outerbridge-Kashiwagi procedure, 49: 251
Outside-in technique
arthroscopic meniscal repair, 49: 195-206
triangular fibrocartilage complex repair, 49: 231
Oxford Unicompartmental knee replacement, **50: 437-440, *438, 440***
Oxidative degradation of ultra-high molecular weight polyethylene, 46: 207
Oxygen carriers, use in the orthopaedic setting, 48: 658
Oxygen free radical scavengers, treating spinal cord injuries, 46: 118
Oxygenated blood, and wound healing, 46: 503-504

P

Paget's disease
arthroplasty procedure, 49: 66
and hip arthroplasty, 49: 4
pathologic fractures in, 46: 426, *427*
Pain
adjunctive psychological treatment, 49: 542
algorithm, 47: *340-341*
anterior knee, 47: 339-343
chronic, management for cancer patients, 49: 513-520
classification of, 49: 541
clinical presentation of bone tumors, 48: 607
components of, 49: 541
definition of, 49: 513
degenerative arthritis, outcome of arthroscopic surgery, 48: 137
diagnosis of osteoarthritis, 49: 482-484
electromagnetic medicine, 49: 545-546
invasive therapies, 49: 519-520
joints, as indication for surgery, 48: 93
metastatic disease of the spine, 49: 471
misdiagnosis of, 48: 580-581
neuropathic, 49: 514
nociceptive, 49: 514
pelvic, and the risk of vascular injury, in total hip arthroplasty, 48: 31
phantom limb, 48: 690-691
physiology of, 49: 513-514

and posterior subluxation, **50: 24**
relief in chondral injuries, 48: 632
relief in nonsurgical treatment of epicondylitis, 48: 376-377
rotator cuff tear, **50: 43**
soft-tissue tumors, 49: 438
upper extremity, 48: 695
and vascular disease, 48: 292
weight bearing, metastatic bone disease, 49: 454-455
on weight bearing, 48: 581
Pain dysfunction syndrome
defined of, 46: 262
primary components of, 46: 262
secondary components of, 46: 262
Pain management
acupuncture, 49: 559-562
modalities for RSD, 49: 549-556
through hypnosis, 49: 541-543
Pain teams, multidisciplinary approach, 49: 555-556
Palindromic arthritis, 46: 78
Palmar tilt, radiographic measurement, 48: *465*
Palmaris lingus tendon, harvesting of, 48: *386*
Pantalar arthrodesis, 46: *353,* 354-355, 48: 260
Paprosky classification
of acetabular deficiencies, for total hip arthroplasty, 48: *49*-50
bone loss, 49: 90, *90*
Parameniscal synovial abrasion, 49: 201
Paraplegia, defined, 48: 438
Parapodium, pediatric thoracic myelomeningocele, 48: 564-566
Paratendinitis, Achilles, 48: 212
Parathyroid hormone, laboratory investigations of bone tumors, 48: 608
Parathyroid hormone in osteoporosis, 46: 446
Parathyroid hormone-related protein (PTHrP)
as autocrine/paracrine growth factor in cartilage, 47: 465, 472
and Jansen-type chondrometaphyseal dysplasia, 47: 466
Paravertebral blockade, 46: 264
Parkinson's disease, 46: 423
THA in, 49: 165-168, *167*
Parosteal osteosarcomas, differentiation from fibrous dysplasia, 48: 615-*616*
Parsonage-Turner syndrome, differential diagnosis, 49: 296-297, 299, 301
Particle generators, and osteolysis, 48: 37-38, 40-42
Particulate debris
biologic response to, **50: 187-188**
and osteolysis, **50: 197-198**
polyethylene wear, **50: 424-426**
sources of, **50: *198***
Passive range of motion, postoperative protocols for anterior instability, **50: 13-14**
Patella facet, allograft replacement of, 47: 520, *521*
Patella infera syndrome, 46: 241-249, 251-259
normal and ultrastructure collagen fibril population of patellar tendon, 46: 242-245
quantitative ultrastructural collagen fibril analysis, 46: 242
Patellae
blood supply, **50: *386*, 403**
dislocating, **50: *404***
fractures, **50: *404***
following TKA, **50: 385-387**
fractures following TKA, **50: 403-404**
metal-backed, and type 1 bone defects, 48: 169
Patellar bone, loss of, 48: 164
Patellar clunk syndrome, 46: 176, *177*
Patellar component failure, 46: *175*-176
Patellar component loosening, 46: 174-175
Patellar component revision, 46: 177
Patellar fractures, periprosthetic
etiologies and risk factors for, 46: 173-*174*
incidence of, 47: 254
intraoperative, 47: 438, 450-451
postoperative, 47: 445-448, 455-*457*
Patellar instability
following total knee arthroplasty, 46: 171-*173*
in runners, 47: 410-411
in school-age athletes, 47: 345-349
imaging for, 47: 347-348
physical examination for, 47: 347
Patellar ligament, histology of, 48: *191*
Patellar osteotomy, 48: *158*
Patellar pain, algorithm for, 47: 339-343
Patellar resection, 46: 173, 176
Patellar tendinosis, 46: 574, 47: 411-412
Patellar tendon
autografts using, 48: 520
normal and ultrastructure collagen fibril population of, 46: 242-245
normal rabbit, **50: *8***
rabbit, thermal shrinkage, **50: *4***
read harvesting, **50: 468-469**
reharvesting, **50: 459**
rupture, and extensor mechanism evaluation, 48: 163
rupture of, **50: *404***
ruptures, 46: 176
Patellar tilt in runners, 47: 410
Patellar turndown, revision total knee arthroplasty, 48: 149-152, *151*
Patellar vascularity, efforts to preserve, 46: 177
Patellofemoral instability, following TKA, **50: 404**
Patient compliance, and dislocated THA, **50: 285**
Patient-controlled analgesia (PCA), pain management, 49: 518
Patient education
and cervical degenerative disease, 48: 433
instructions on total contact casts, 48: *314*
Patient education, and dislocated THA, **50: 285**
Patient extrication, from motor vehicle accident, 46: 115
Patient history, periprosthetic femoral osteolysis, **50: 200**
Patient immobilization in acute spinal trauma management, 46: 115
Patient positioning
rotator cuff surgery, **50: 44-45**
shoulder surgery, **50: 56-57**
surgical management of spinal stenosis, **50: *154***
Patient satisfaction, cervical myelopathy and radiculopathy, 48: 417-421
Patient selection
realignment osteotomies, **50: 503-505**
for revision of total knee arthroplasty, 48: 161-162
Patient Self-Determination Act, teaching of ethical issues, 49: 640
Pavlik harness
DDH, **50: 542-543**
patient selection, **50: 540**
Pectoralis major muscles
bipolar flexorplasty, 49: *329*
bipolar transposition, 49: 329
Pectoralis major tendon
amplitude of, **50: 65**
clavicular head, **50: *67***
transfer, **50: *66*-68**
Pediatric Instrument, MODEMS program, 48: 680
Pediatrics
back pain, 48: 525-539
DDH, **50: 535-540**
and dislocation, **50: 547-553**
infants, **50: 541-545**
fractures in children with multiple injuries, 49: 425-430
hip development, **50: 536-537**
long bones fractures with multiple injuries, 49: 415-420
myelomeningocele, 48: 564-566

neonatal osteomyelitis, **50: 317**
SCFE, **50: 555-570**
septic arthritis, **50: 317-318**
Pelvic obliquity, in neuromuscular scoliosis, 48: 554, *555*
Pelvic osteotomy, DDH, **50: 540**
Pelvis
associated deformities of ring, **50: *341***
bilateral dysplasia, **50: *307*, 50: *310***
blood vessels in inner aspect of, 48: *27*
displaced iliac-wing, **50: *340***
dysplasia and OA, **50: *311***
dysplastic right hip, **50: *254***
fractures, children with multiple injuries, 49: 415-423, 424-423
hip dislocation, **50: *308***
metastatic disease, surgical treatment, 49: 461-469
osteolysis of, 48: *41*
preoperative radiographs, **50: 253-256**
reconstruction of table, **50: *346***
recurrent instability, **50: *271***
Pemberton osteotomies, **50: 551**
Penicillamine, consideration in preoperative planning, 48: 98
Penicillin, resistance to, 49: 606
Perceived Pain Affect (PPA), 49: 542
Perceived Pain Intensity (PPI), 49: 542
Percutaneous electrical nerve stimulation (PENS), pain management, 49: 520
Percutaneous screw fixation, scaphoid fractures, **50: 110-112**
Perfluorocarbons
oxygen-carrying capacity, 48: *659*
use in the orthopaedic setting, 48: 658-660
Performance measurement, and accreditation, 48: 677-678
Periacetabular lesions, metastatic bone disease, 49: 467-469
Periarticular osteotomies
importance of limb alignment, 48: 279-285
preoperative planning for, 48: 282-283
Periarticular tissues, changes in osteoarthritis, 49: 487
Perichondral grafts, articular cartilage restoration, 48: 624
Perichondrium, autologous, treatment of chondral injuries, 48: 635
Periodic perineural infusion, pain management, 49: 537
Perioperative morbidity, and unicondylar knee arthroplasty (UKA), 48: 144
Periosteal chondroma
clinicopathologic features of, 48: *614*
differentiation from chondrosarcoma, 48: 613-615
Periosteal grafts, articular cartilage restoration, 48: 624
Periosteal-perichondral grafts, 47: 511
Periosteal reactions, differential diagnosis of, 48: *610*
Peripheral nerves
blocks, 49: 536-537
stimulation to acupuncture, 49: 559
Peripheral neuropathy, spinal stenosis, **50: 150**
Peripheral vascular disease
amputation surgery in, 46: 501-508, 48: 687-691
cognitive and psychological requirements for walking in amputees, 46: 502
functional levels, 46: 505-508
joints as energy couples, 46: 501-502
load transfer, 46: 502-503
rehabilitation, 46: 508
selection of level, 46: 504-505
wound healing, 46: 503-504
and diabetic foot, 48: 292
Periprosthetic fractures
acetabular, 47: 231-235
intraoperative, 47: 232-233, *234*, 252
postoperative, 47: 233-234
in vitro studies, 47: 231-232
after and during total knee implants, 47: 437-448
decision making and principles of management, 47: 449-*457*
incidence of, 47: 253-254
intraoperative, 47: 437-439
postoperative, 47: 439-448
after total shoulder arthroplasty, 48: 365-366
in elderly, 46: *425*-426
epidemiology, 47: 251-254
femoral, 47: 237-241
allografts in treatment of, 47: 257-*263*
intraoperative, 47: 237-238, 251-252, 437-439
postoperative, 47: 238-241, 243-248, 439-445
Vancouver classification for, 47: 241, 247
Johansson classification for, 47: 253
Periradicular fibrosis, 46: 146
Perkins line newborn hip, **50: 538**
Perkins traction, use in the developing world, 49: *586*
Peroneal mononeuropathy, and diabetic foot, 48: 292
Peroneal muscles, and walking, 48: 220
Peroneal nerves
early treatment of injury, 46: 181
meniscal repair, 49: 196
palsy, 46: 181
Peroneal tendinitis, imaging of, 46: 525
Peroneal tendon, imaging of tears, 46: 525
Pes anserine bursitis, 47: 412-413
Pfeiffer syndrome, 46: 477
Phagocytosis
particulate debris, **50: 188**
by polymorphonuclear leukocytes, impairment by polymethylmethacrylate, 48: 114
Phalanges, skeletal reconstruction, 49: 384-385
Phalen's tests, 48: 694
Phantom limb pain, 48: 690-691
Phantom sensation, after amputation, 48: 328-329
Pharmacologic prophylaxis, for thromboembolic disease, 47: 332-333
Pharmacologic therapy, for osteoporosis, 46: 451-454
Pharmacology, and aging, 46: 415
Phenols, ablation of nail matrix with, 48: 302
Phenoxybenzamine, treatment of RSD, 49: 552-553
Phentolamine, treatment of RSD, 49: 553
Phosphorus, serum, laboratory investigations of bone tumors, 48: 608
Physeal arrest, correction, 49: 507-*508*
Physeal plates, development and growth, **50: 537**
Physical therapy
aquatic, electromyography, 46: *60*-62
arthritis of the shoulder, **50: 74**
casted patients, **50: 293**
and exercise in management of sympathetically maintained pain, 46: 267
following tibial shaft fractures, 46: 300
postoperative pain, **50: 529**
for stiff total knee replacement, 46: 193
treatment of RSD, 49: 552
treatment of spinal stenosis, **50: 153**
Physician-patient relationships, teaching of ethics, 49: 640
Physician support groups, and medical malpractice, 48: 699
Physicians for Human Rights (PHR), land mine initiatives, 49: 431
Piezogenic papules, heel pain, **50: 522-523**
Pilon fractures, 46: *314*
classification of, 46: 318-320
complications in, 46: 320
Pin-tract infections, associated with thermal necrosis of bone, 46: 296
Pins, placements, right distal femur, 48: *126*, 127-128
Piperacillin-tazobactam, treatment of diabetic foot infection, 48: 319
Pisohamate tunnel. *see* canal of Guyon
Pisotriquetral joint, 47: 218

Pivot-shift test, reversed, for posterior cruciate ligament damage, 48: 200-201
Pivoting sports, meniscus repair rehabilitation, 49: 208
Plane of deformity, definition, 49: *505*
Plantar aponeurosis, truss effect, **50: *528***
Plantar arch, ulceration of, 48: 294
Plantar fascia
  acute rupture, **50: 523**
  complications of surgery, **50: 528-530**
Plantar fasciitis, 47: 425-426, **50: 521**
  biomechanics of, 47: 405
  distal, **50: 526-527**
  injection for, **50: *525***
  proximal, **50: 523-526**
  treatment, **50: 524-525**
  treatment for, 47: 426
Plantar heel pain, **50: 521-531**
  focal tenderness, **50: *521***
Plantar pressure, measuring system, 48: 306
Plantar ulceration
  chronic recurrent, 48: *273*
  proposed mechanism of cast action, 48: 306-307
  total contact casting and, 48: 305
  treatment of, 48: 319
Plasma gas, UHMWPE sterilization, 49: 74
Plasminogen activator inhibitor-1 (PAI-1), in osteoarthritis, 49: 486
Plate-and-screw fixation, periprosthetic supracondylar fractures, 47: 440-442
Platelet-derived growth factor (PDGF), 46: 473, 485
  affect on osteoclasts, 49: 78
  and bone formation, 46: 496
Platelet-derived wound-healing factor (PDWHF), use of, 48: 314-315
Plethysmography, diagnosis of thromboemboli disease, **50: 416**
Plica, pathologic, 47: 412
Pneumatic AntiShock Garments (PASG), 46: 115
Pneumatic compression devices, 46: 186
Pneumatic tourniquet, effect of, 46: 185
Pneumonia and delirium in geriatric patients, 46: 414
Poliomyelitis
  appliances and surgery, developing countries, 49: 593-600
  contractures, 49: *595*
  in developing nations, 49: 571
  global immunization coverage, 49: *571*
  immunization can pain, 49: 580
  THA in, 49: 163
Pollicization, 46: 108
  for hypoplastic thumb, 46: 94-97
Poly-beta-hydroxybutyric acid (PHBA)
  biodegradation of, 46: 536
  in bioresorbable implants, 46: 533
Poly-p-dioxanone (PDS)
  biodegradation of, 46: 536
  in bioresorbable implants, 46: 533
Polyarticular inflammatory arthritis, bilateral surgery in, 48: 95
Polyarticular joint infections, 46: 78
Polydactyly
  classification of, 46: 98-100
  surgical treatment of, 46: 100-104
Polydioxanone, structure, 49: 198
Polyethylene. *See also* Ultra-high molecular weight polyethylene
  ceramics on, 49: 43-44
  ceramics used with, **50: 168-169**
  chemical structure, 49: *50*
  cross-linked, 49: 50-54, *51*
  cross-linking, **50: 170-175, 181-184**
  debris within cells, **50: *190***
  improvement of, **50: 169-170**
  metals used with, **50: 168**
  oxidation of, 49: *51*
  particles in tissues, **50: *187***
  remelted, **50: 172-173**
  thermally stabilized, **50: *172-175***
  thickness, **50: *424***
  tibial components, **50: *394***
  types of, 49: 42, *48*
Polyethylene, tibial components, aseptic loosening, 48: 143
Polyethylene wear
  acetabular cup, **50: *165***
  backside, **50: 395**
  compressive contacts stress, **50: *425***
  factors influencing, **50: 422-424**
  and impingements, **50: 275**
  implant design and failure, 48: 162
  knee replacement, **50: *423***
  mobile-bearing TKR, **50: 431-432**
  and osteolysis, 48: *163,* **50: 428**
  and osteolysis following total knee replacement, 46: 205-212
    incidence of, 46: 205-206
    pathophysiology of osteolysis, 46: 211
    prevalence of osteolysis following, 46: 210-211
    prevention of osteolysis, 46: 212
    structure of polyethylene, 46: 206-207
    treatment of osteolysis, 46: 211-212
    UHMWPE damage following, 46: 208-210
    UHMWPE in vivo degradation, 46: 207
    UHMWPE quality, 46: 207
    UHMWPE sterilization, 46: 207
    UHMWPE thickness, 46: 208
  treatment of, **50: 427-428**
  without osteolysis, and type 1 bone defects, 48: 169
Polyglycolic acid (PGA)
  biodegradation of, 46: 536
  in bioresorbable implants, 46: 533
Polyglyconate tack, 47: 47
Polyhydroxides, metabolic routes of biodegradation of, 46: 536
Polylactic acid (PLA)
  biodegradation of, 46: 536
  in bioresorbable implants, 46: 533
Polymerase chain reactions (PCR), 47: 292
  and diagnosis of arthroplasty site infection, 48: 115
  diagnosis of infection, **50: 374**
Polymethylmethacrylate (PMMA). *See also* Cement
  bone cement
    and morcellized bone grafts, 48: 79-88
    use of, 48: 596
  curing of, 49: 76
  hypersensitivity to, **50: 192-193**
  identification of, 49: 71-72
  and impaction graft, **50: 215**
  and infection at arthroplasty sites, 48: 114
  morcellized allografts used with, 47: 265-273
  reinforcement for nonunion of proximal humeral fractures, 46: 25
  screw-reinforced, 46: *230*
  toxicity of, **50: 188**
Polymorphonuclear leukocytes (PMNLs)
  altered chemotaxis in diabetes, 48: 294
  frozen sections, **50: 373-374**
  periprostatic femoral osteolysis, **50: 201**
Polymyxin-bacitracin cream, burn treatment, 49: 425, 426
Polypropylene ankle-foot orthosis (AFO), management of chronic Achilles tendon rupture, 48: 225
Polytomography, carpal instability, **50: 125**
Polytrauma, in elderly, 46: 424

Popliteal tenosynovitis, 47: 414
Popliteus dynamic transfer, for reconstruction of posterior cruciate ligament, 48: 205
Positron-emission tomography (PET) scans
follow-up for orthopaedic oncology patients, 48: 605
imaging of osseous homeostasis, 48: 193
and restoration of knee function, 48: 195
Posttraumatic osteoarthrosis, in pilon fractures, 46: 320
Posterior approaches, hip arthroplasty, 49: 13-15
Posterior cruciate ligament (PCL)
allograft reconstruction, 47: 388-389
clinical evaluation of injury, 48: 200-203
evaluation and treatment of injury, 48: 199-206
and flexion instability, **50: 400-401**
footprints of, 48: *199*
functional anatomy of, 48: 199-200
injuries to, treatment algorithms for, 48: *204*
instability following TKA, **50: 399**
mechanism of injury, 48: 200
natural history, 48: 200
preservation of, 48: 105-106
relation to meniscus, 49: 190
surgical indications of damage, 48: 203-205
surgical reconstruction techniques, 48: 205-206
tear, 48: *205*
Posterior inferior tibiofibular ligament (PITF) ligament, 49: 263-264
Posterior inlay procedures, posterior cruciate ligament reconstruction, 48: 205
Posterior instability
after TSA, **50: 84**
thermal capsulorrhaphy, **50: *25***
Posterior interosseous flap, management of, 49: 389
Posterior interosseous nerve (PIN)
anatomy, 49: 295, *295*
compression syndrome, 49: 298-301
palsy, 49: *299*
surgical approaches, 49: 299-301
syndromes associated with, 49: 297
Posterior longitudinal ligament (PLL), 46: 145
Posterior subluxation
complication in HHR, 46: 19
recurrent
arthroscopy, **50: *34***
stabilization of, **50: 33**
Posterior talofibular ligament (PTFL), anatomy, 49: 262
Posterior tibial muscles, and walking, 48: 220
Posterior tibial tendon, treatment of dysfunction of, 46: 393-403
anatomy and pathophysiology, 46: 393-394
diagnosis of, 46: 394-395
etiology of, 46: 394
treatment of, 46: 395-404
Posterolateral arthroscopic interbody fusion, 46: 156-*157*
Posterolateral bone grafting for tibial shaft fractures, 46: 283
Posterolateral ligament complex, 47: 176
Posterolateral rotatory instability (PLRI) of the knee, 47: 369-378
physical examination for, 47: 371-372
surgical technique for, 47: 373-377
Posteromedial capsule, 48: *154*
Postoperative care, patients with rheumatoid arthritis, 48: 105
Postoperative wound infections, staphylococcus, 49: 607
Posttraumatic arthritis, 46: 335
of distal radioulnar joint, 47: *211*
shoulder arthroplasty for, 47: 130
Potassium channels, blocking agents in treating spinal cord injuries, 46: 118
Power density, laser energy, **50: 6**
Practice guidelines, 49: 643-648. *See also* Critical pathways
Practice responsibility, and medical malpractice, 48: 701
Practice standards, for transfusions, 48: 655-656
Prayer sign, 49: *286,* 290
Prazepam and aging, 46: 415
Predictive salvage index (PSI), 46: 512, 513, 514
Prednisone
pyoderma gangrenosum, 46: 73
treatment of RSD, 49: 553
Preemptive analgesia, regional blocks, 49: *534*
Preferred provider organizations (PPO), premium growth rates, 48: 674
Prehospital care in spinal cord injury, 46: 113-116
Preoperative autologous blood donation (PAD)
and orthopaedic surgery, 48: 655
use in the orthopaedic setting, 48: 657-658
Preoperative investigations, total hip arthroplasty, 48: 19-20, 31-32
assessment of acetabular bone loss, 48: 43-55
Preoperative planning
for acetabular defect reconstruction, 48: 68-70
deformity correction, 49: 503-509
femoral, 49: *34*
fixation with modular system, 49: 132-133
hip arthroplasty, 49: 27-28
in inflammatory arthritis, 48: 95-98
for periarticular osteotomies, 48: 282-283
primary hip replacement, 49: 3-10
steps in, for acetabular revision, 48: *44*
templating, 49: 85-86
templating for DDH, 49: *9*
total shoulder arthroplasty, **50: 78-79**
Pressure devices, in vitro, 48: *253*
Pretesting, of outcomes assessment instruments, 48: 668
Prioritization, regional, in planning surgeries, 48: 94-95
Procainamide, acute calcific tendinitis, 46: 69-70
Procaine (novocaine)
anesthesia, 49: 524
molecular structure, 49: *525*
use of, 49: 525
Profilimetry, definition, 49: 77
Progressive intervertebral disk space, 46: 144
Proinflammatory cytokines, response to particulate debris, **50: 189**
Prolific enzymes, and metal particles, 49: 75
Prolotherapy, cicatrix formation, **50: 8**
Pronation-external rotation injury, 46: 313
Propranolol, treatment of CRPS, 49: 553
Proprioception, ankle instability, **50: 517**
Proprioceptive neuromuscular conditioning, importance of, 48: 191
Prostaglandin D_2 (PGD_2), effects of, 49: 79
Prostaglandin E_2 (PGE_2), 46: 205
affect on osteoclasts, 49: 78
production of, 49: 72
response to particulate debris, **50: 187-188, 190, 191**
stimulation of osteoclasts by, 48: 37
PROSTALAC components, **50: *324*, *325*, 372**
antibiotic-loaded cement, 47: 303-304
choice of, **50: 331**
Prostate cancer, 5-year survival, 49: 461
Prostate specific antigen (PSA), laboratory investigations of bone tumors, 48: 608
Prostheses
allograft composite reconstruction, 48: *601*
below-knee, land mine victims, 49: 433
femoral
extraction, 49: 123
removal of, 48: 9-11
hip, failure of components, 48: 43
implantation, total hip arthroplasty, 48: *24*
insertion without cement, 48: 119

interface with allografts, 49: 152
knee, mobile-bearing, **50: 432**
longevity, **50: 185**
medial protrusion, in total hip arthroplasty, 48: 31
megaprosthesis, 48: *601*
monopolar, fixed-head, 49: 179
proximal femoral replacement with, 49: *141*
reimplantation
antibiotic protocols, 48: 115-116
and site infections, 48: 115
in situ removal, 49: 124
total hip, migration of, 48: *30*
upper extremities, 49: 386
Prosthetic-induced bone remodeling, 46: 227
Prosthetic replacement in elderly, 46: 425
Protasul 21 WF, outcomes, 49: 47
Protein electrophoresis, serum, laboratory investigations of bone tumors, 48: 608
Proteoglycans, 47: 480-*481*
aggregation, in osteoarthritis, 49: 486
function of, **50: 146**
hyaluronic acid structure, 49: *495*
interleukin-1 and synthesis of, 48: 235
in intervertebral disks, 49: 362
Proteus, infection in the diabetic foot, 48: 318
Protrusio acetabuli, 47: 266-*267,* 49: 5
definition, 49: 8
radiographic follow-up, 48: 102
radiographs, 48: *81*
Proximal humeral fractures
complications of humeral head replacement for, 46: 15-23
literature, 46: 15-16
Mayo Clinic experience, 46: 16-21
preventive resources, 46: 21-22
treatment options, 46: 22-23
complications of internal fixation of, 46: 25-35
frozen shoulder, 46: 32-33
hardware, 46: 28-30
heterotopic ossification, 46: 34
iatrogenic fracture displacement, 46: 34
infection, 46: 33-34
inferior subluxation, 46: 34
malunion, 46: 27-28
neurovascular injury, 46: 31-32
nonunion, 46: 25-27
osteonecrosis, 46: 30-31
subacromial impingement, 46: 32
humeral head replacement for, 46: 7-14
humeral shaft preparation, 46: 9-10
positioning, 46: 8
postoperative rehabilitation, 46: 12-13
results, 46: 13-14
surgical approach, 46: 8-9
tuberosity fixation, 46: 10-12
malunion
clinical evaluation, 47: *137*
as complication of internal fixation, 46: 27-28
imaging studies, 47: *137-138*
prosthetic arthroplasty for, 47: 135-140
review of literature, 47: 135-136
treatment algorithm, 47: 140
Proximal phalangeal articular angle (PPAA), 46: 362
Proximal phalangeal osteotomy (Akin procedure), 46: 366-*367, 368*
Proximal phalanx fracture, 47: 187-*188*
Proximal tibial osteotomy, in osteonecrosis, **50: 484-485**
Proximal tibial varus osteotomy, 47: 434
Proximal valgus tibial osteotomy, 47: 430, 432-434
knee, surgical technique, 48: 132
Pseudo-Boutonnière deformity, 47: 182, *183*
Pseudoaneurysms, relation to trauma, 48: 617
Pseudarthrosis
negative aspiration of, 46: 218
occurrence in neuromuscular scoliosis fusion, 48: 552
Pseudarthrosis, hip, **50: *298***
Pseudocysts, osteolysis, **50: *391***
Pseudogout, 46: 76-77
Pseudomonas
infection in the diabetic foot, 48: 318
recurrent infections, **50: 330**
Psoriasis, 46: 394
evaluation in preoperative planning, 48: 95
Psychosocial status assessment of elderly, 46: 412-414
Pulmonary distress, and forced vital capacity (FVC), 48: 552
Pulmonary emboli, 47: 331-335
symptoms, **50: 416**
Pulse volume recordings (PVRs), 48: 297
Pulsed high peak power electromagnetic energy, biologic effects, 49: 545-546
Pulses, peripheral, spinal stenosis, **50: 150**
Pump bumps, 47: 425
Purchasers of health care, expectations of, 48: 572
Putti-Platt capsulorrhaphy, **50: 75**
Putti-Platt procedure, 47: *118*
loss of motion after, 47: *118,* 119, 120
Pyoderma gangrenosum, 46: 72-73
Pyogenic granuloma, 46: 71-72

Q

Q angle, 47: 339
in patellar instability, 47: 347, 410-411
in patellar tendinosis, 47: 411
QSART (quantitative pseudomotor axon reflex test), diagnosis of RSD, 49: 551
Quadriceps active test, for posterior cruciate ligament damage, 48: 200
Quadriceps deficiency, 46: 252
Quadriceps inhibition, acute knee injury, 49: 211
Quadriceps myocutaneous composite flap, exposure of distal femur and knee, 48: 157-159
Quadriceps rehabilitation, 46: 172
Quadriceps snip, 46: 221-222
exposure for revision total knee arthroplasty, 48: 149-152
revision total knee arthroplasty, 48: *150*
total knee arthroplasty, **50: 362, *362***
Quadriceps tendon
ACL reconstruction graft, **50: 469**
autografts using, 48: 520
ruptures, 46: 176
tendinosis, 47: 411-412
Quadriceps transection exposure, 46: 221-222
Quadriceps turndown, 48: *158*
Quadricepsplasty, VY curves, revision total knee arthroplasty, 48: *152*
Quadriplegic, polio-related, 49: *599*
Quality, and outcomes measurement, 48: 678
Quality Adjusted Life Years (QALYs), validity of, 48: 669-670
Quality improvement, orthopedic critical pathways, 49: 643-648
Quality of life, defined of, 48: 418
Quality-of-life scores, autologous chondrocyte transplantation, 48: 637
Quality of Well-Being (QWB) scale, 46: 442
validity of, 48: 669-670
Quantitative CT scanning, bone mineral density, 46: 450
Quebec Task Force on Spinal Disorders, **50: 153**

R

Race, DDH, **50: 535-536**
Racquet grip, and epicondylitis rehabilitation, 48: 377-378
Radial artery, vascular supplies for the scaphoid, **50: 105**
Radial clubhand
appearance of, 46: 83-*84*
classification of, 46: 83-84
function in, 46: 84-85
surgical treatment of, 46: 85-89
Radial fractures
adaptive instability, **50: 131-132**
fixation in children, 49: 417-418
intra-articular
AO type B, 48: 470
AO type C, 48: *471*
arthroscopically guided reduction, 48: 474-*475*
classification, 48: 467-471
combined volar and dorsal approach, 48: 473-474
complex, 48: 470-471
dorsal approach, 48: 471-*472*
effect of, 48: 466
limited dorsal approach, 48: 472-473
rehabilitation, 48: 478-479
surgical approaches, 48: *470*
volar radial approach, 48: *473*
volar ulnar approach, 48: 473
Radial head
anatomy and biomechanics, **50: 94**
degenerative, arthroscopic view, 49: *249*
and elbow stability, 47: 157-*158*
and forearm stability, 47: 173-174
fracture of, **50: 94-96, 100-101**
classification, **50: 94**
postoperative management, **50: 96**
PIN palsy, 49: 298
prosthetic replacement of, 47: 175-176
resection, AP radiograph, 49: 248
surgical fracture repair, **50: 95-96**
Radial head fractures
and coronoid fracture with dislocation, 47: 163-164
with dislocation of elbow, 47: 160-*161*
Mason classification for, 47: 160-*161,* 174-175
with MCL tear, 47: 159-*160*
treatment for, 47: 174-175
Radial nerves
anatomy, 49: 295-296, *298*
blocks, 49: 529-530
capsular release, 49: 256
compressive neuropathies, 49: 295-303
high nerve palsy, 49: 296-297
Radial tunnel syndrome, 46: 572, 49: 301-302
posterior interosseous nerves, 49: 297
Radiation
allograft preparation, 49: 151
allograft sterilization, 49: 617
of allografts
and bone induction, 48: 65
and disease transmission, 48: 64-65
effect on UHMWPEs, **50: *169*-170**
and immunology of allografts, 48: 650-651
of polyethylene, 49: 42
polyethylene cross-linking, **50: 172-173**
prevention of heterotropic ossification, 48: 104
UHMWPE sterilization, 49: 74
Radiation necrosis, and osteonecrosis, 49: 170
Radiation therapy
heterotopic ossification (HO) in acetabular fractures, 48: 492
heterotrophic ossification, **50: 348**
and high-grade bone sarcomas, 48: 602
metastatic bone disease, 49: 459, *462*
metastatic disease of the spine, 49: 473
for pain, 49: 514
Radicular compression, anatomy of, 46: 145-*146*
Radicular pain, cervical spondylosis, 49: 335
Radicular symptoms, metastatic disease of the spine, 49: 471
Radiculopathy
cervical spine, 49: 339-357
foraminal compression, 49: *340*
measuring outcomes of, 48: 417-421
Radioallergosorbent test (RAST), and latex allergy, 48: 550
Radiocapitellar osteoarthrosis, 46: 572
Radiocarpal capsule, arthrotomy, **50: *117***
Radiocarpal joint, arthroscopic image, 49: *227*
Radiofrequency (RF) energy
delivery of, **50: 6-7**
generators, **50: 7**
thermal capsulorrhaphy, **50: 23**
Radiofrequency (RF) heating
probes, **50: 6**
thermal capsulorrhaphy, **50: 14**
in vitro studies, **50: 5**
Radiographic analysis
acetabular fracture, **50: 336**
of the acetabulum, evaluation of bone loss, 48: 45-47
analysis of femoral impaction grafting, 49: 116
of ankle fracture, 46: 312
AP views, 49: 6-7
assessment bone loss, 49: 85
assessment of ankle and hindfoot disorders, 48: 255
in assessment of osteolysis, 48: 38
Bernese periacetabular osteotomy, **50: 240**
bilateral standing AP, 49: 503-509
bone tumors diagnostic by plain film, 48: *611*
carpal instability, **50: 125-126**
in cervical degenerative disease, 48: 433-434
chest films, and thoracolumbar trauma, 48: 429
classification of ankle arthritis from, 48: *281*
diagnosis of arthroplasty site infection, 48: 114
diagnosis of infection, **50: 368**
of distal radius fractures, 47: 195
dysplastic right hip, **50: *254***
elbow, **50: 98**
examination of bone tumors, 48: 608-609
examination of soft-tissue tumors, 48: 618
exclusion of active infection, **50: 319-320**
femoral osteolysis, **50: 199**
of gout, 46: *76*
hip arthrodesis, **50: 299-301**
for impingement syndrome, 47: 23
for infection following total hip arthroplasty, 47: 287-288
for knee pain, anterior, 47: 410
metastatic bone disease, 49: 455
metastatic disease of the spine, 49: 471-473
newborn hip, **50: *538*-539**
osteolysis, **50: 393**
osteonecrosis, **50: 490-491**
shoulder, **50: *74***
osteotomies around the hip, **50: 253-261**
pelvis, **50: 232**
periprosthetic femoral osteolysis, **50: 200**
in planning revision total knee arthroplasty, 48: 164

and posterior cruciate ligament damage, 48: 201
preoperative TSA planning, **50: 78-79**
rheumatoid arthritis, shoulder, **50: *74***
rotator cuff tear, **50: 43**
scaphoid fractures, **50: 106**
scaphoid imaging, **50: 106**
SCFE, **50: 557-558**
for shoulder pain, 47: 6-7
soft-tissue sarcomas, 49: 447
soft-tissue tumors, 49: 439
spinal stenosis, **50: 137-144**
spontaneous ON of the distal femur, **50: 495**
sternoclavicular joint, 49: 399
subluxation of femoral heads, **50: *276***
syndesmosis injuries, **50: 519-520**
templating, 49: 7-10
tibial osteonecrosis, **50: 478**
Torg ratios, 49: 336
for wrist instability, 47: 222-223
Radiolucent lines, and osteolysis, **50: 197**
Radiolunate ligaments, structure of, 49: 227
Radionuclide imaging, 47: 288-289
and posterior cruciate ligament damage, 48: 201
Radioscaphocapitate ligaments, **50: *123***
Radioscaphocapitate (RSC) ligaments, arthroscopic image, 49: *227*
Radioulnar synostosis, establishment of proximal, 46: 107
Radius
distal, fractures, 47: 191-201, 49: 233-234
classification of, 47: *192*-195
compression fractures, 47: 197-*199*
intra-articular, 48: 465-479, 49: *234*
radiography of, 47: *195*
of shearing fractures, 47: 195-*197*
distal articular surface, 48: *466*
malunion, **50: *132***
vascular supply, **50: *115*-117**
Range-of-motion (ROM)
assessment of, in planning revision of total hip arthroplasty, 48: 44
code of motion, **50: *278***
control by immobilization, **50: 293**
diabetic stiff shoulder, 49: *291*
effect of component design, **50: 275-279**
evaluation of the spine, 48: 451
measurement of, **50: 275-277**
postoperative bracing, **50: 290**
preoperative planning, 49: 84
resisted, postoperative protocols for anterior instability, **50: 14**
spinal impairment, *Guides to the Evaluation of Permanent Impairment,* 4th edition, 48: 457-461
Ray resection, 46: 506
Rays, amputation in diabetic feet, 48: *324*-325
Realignment, reconstruction of neuropathic deformities, 48: 273-275
Reamers, **50: *470***
Reaming
acetabula, **50: *303***
distal bypass fixation, 49: 125
femoral canal preparation, in hip arthroplasty, 48: 22-23
in surgical management of tibial fractures, 46: 273-276
for tibial shaft fractures, 46: 297
type IIIB acetabular defect, 48: *71*
Reciprocal-gait orthoses (RGOs), in myelomeningocele patients, 48: 547
Reconstruction. *See also* Specific anatomic area
acetabular
for contained defects, 48: 60-62
preoperative planning for, 48: 50
amputation surgery as, 46: 501
anterior cruciate ligament, knee function after, 48: 185-196
blood vessels, injured upper extremities, 49: 386
comparison with amputation, for Charcot arthropathy, 48: 276-277
delayed procedures, 48: 118-119
direct exchange procedures, 48: 118
distal femur and knee, quadriceps myocutaneous composite flap for exposure of, 48: 157-159
femoral algorithm, 49: *117*
imagination and innovation, 49: 392-393
with impacted morcellized allografts, mechanical stability of, 48: 83
injured upper extremities, 49: 381-390
timing of, 49: 390-392
nerves, upper extremities, 49: 388
of tendons, upper extremities, 49: 386-388
type, and infection at arthroplasty sites, 48: 112
use of antibiotic-impregnated cement, 48: 117-118, *119*
Reconstruction cages
hip salvage with, 48: *647*
surgical technique, 48: 72-73
Reconstruction nails. *See also* Specific nails
pathologic subtrochanteric fractures, 49: 465
Rectus femoris muscle, **50: *235***
Rectus snip, **50: 371**
in knee arthroplasty, 48: 165
Red blood cell substitutes, use in the orthopaedic setting, 48: 658
Reflex algodystrophy, 46: 261
Reflex dystrophy, in humeral head replacement, 46: 20
Reflex sympathetic dystrophy (RSD), 46: 216, 251-259. *See also* complex regional pain syndrome
after total knee arthroplasty, 48: 161
in algorithm for anterior knee pain, 47: *340,* 342
alternative modalities for management of pain, 49: 549-556
diagnosis, 49: 550-552
management of pain, 49: 535-536
and pain dysfunction in lower extremity, 46: 261-267
pathophysiology, 49: 552
treatment, 49: 552-553
upper-extremity, management algorithm, 49: *555*-556
Reflexes, spinal stenosis, **50: 150**
Regional pain syndrome, complex, use of sympathetic blocks, 49: 535-537
Rehabilitation
ACL reconstruction, **50: 452**
after posterior cruciate ligament reconstruction, 48: 205
after running injuries, 47: 416-417
developing countries, 49: 600
elbow, **50: 99**
to enhance cell-based therapies for chondral injury, 48: 638-*639*
following amputation surgery, 46: 508
following medial epicondylar osteotomy, 48: 155
following meniscal repair, 49: 202-203, 207-209
glenohumeral joint instability, **50: 13-15**
nonsurgical treatment of epicondylitis, 48: 377-378
pain of, 49: 542
and partial foot amputations, 48: 322
plantar fasciitis, **50: 525**
postoperative, revision total hip arthroplasty, 48: 7-8
rotator cuff repair, **50: 50**
syndesmosis injuries, **50: 520**
TACS, throwing athletes, **50: 20-21**
for tibial shaft fractures, 46: 299-300
upper extremities, 49: 393-395
Reinforcement rings, acetabular reinforcement, 49: 32
Reiter syndrome, 46: 394
Rejection, of allograft segments, 48: 179-180
Reliability, MODEMS program, 48: 681
Relocation test, 46: 571

Renal insufficiency, and Achilles tendon rupture, 48: 220
Reoperations, revision total hip arthroplasty, 48: 24
Repetitive stress, plantar fasciitis, **50: 524**
Replamineform ceramics, 47: 528-529
Reproducibility, of outcomes assessment instruments, 48: 668
Reshaping osteotomies, DDH, **50: 551**
Residency training
    clinical ethics, 49: 634-635
    teaching clinical ethics, 49: 639-642
Resorption, structural femoral allografts, 49: *158*-159
Resource utilization, critical pathways development, 49: 645
Respect for economy, clinical ethics, 49: 635-636
Respiratory depression, and opioids use, 49: 517
Responsiveness, of outcomes assessment instruments, 48: 668
Rest, treatment of spinal stenosis, **50: 153**
Resting sweat output test, diagnosis of RSD, 49: 551
Resuscitation
    children with multiple injuries, 49: 425
    head injuries, children with multiple injuries, 49: 427-428
Retractors
    endoscopic, 46: 132
    mechanism of vascular injury, 48: 29
Retrocalcaneal bursitis, 47: 422-*424*
    diagnosis of, 47: 422-*423*
    and fibrocartilages, 48: 211
    treatment for, 47: 423-*424*
    treatment of, 48: 217-218
Retrocalcaneal ostectomy, 47: 423-*424*
Rett syndrome, neuromuscular scoliosis in, 48: 560
Revascularization
    allografts, **50: 216-217**
    bone allografts, 49: 149
    bone graft, **50: 226**
    cortical allografts, 49: 98-99
Revo screw, 47: *60*-61
RF. *See* Radiofrequency
Rhabdomyosarcomas, nuclear features, 49: 437
Rheumatoid arthritis, 46: 77-79
    of acromioclavicular joint, 47: 36-*37*
    ankle arthrodesis in, 48: 258
    cementless stem fixation, 49: *65*
    elbow, 49: 256
    evaluation in preoperative planning, 48: 97
    glenohumeral joint, **50: 73-77**
    hip, clinical manifestations, 48: 102-103
    hip arthroplasty, 49: 64-65
    hip fractures in, 48: 102
    and infection at arthroplasty sites, 48: 111
    juvenile, loosening of cemented components, 48: 103
    postoperative care, 48: 105
    and primary cavitary defects, 48: 81
    salvage procedures, 48: 100-101
    shoulder arthroplasty for, 47: 130-*131*
    sternoclavicular joint, 49: 404
    steroid-dependent, effects on bone quality, 48: 97
    total knee arthroplasty, **50: 507**
    total knee replacement, 48: 105-106
    and unstable prosthetic shoulder arthroplasty, 47: 142-*143*
    and wound healing, **50: 359**
Rheumatoid disease, and infection in total knee replacement, 46: 215, 216
Rheumatoid factor, rheumatoid arthritis, 46: 78
Rheumatologists, collaboration with, 49: 65
Rhomboid ligaments, sternoclavicular joints, 49: 397
Rib head resection, 46: 137
Rickets, in developing nations, 49: 571
Rifampin, reaction with bone cement, 48: 117
Rings, acetabular fracture, **50: 340**
Risk-benefit analyses, THA revision, 49: 84
Roentgen stereogrammetric analysis (RSA), displacement
        measurement, 49: 106
Roland Disability Questionnaire, 48: 419
Rongeur, double-action, 48: *300*
Roo's test, older nerve compression, 49: 307
Rotation
    loss of, thermal capsulorrhaphy, **50: 32**
    preoperative planning, 49: 5
Rotational alignment, for bone grafting, total knee arthroplasty, 48: *179*
Rotationplasty, treatment of malignant bone tumors, 48: 599-600
Rotator cuff
    arthroscopic visualization, **50: *58***
    assessment of tears, **50: 46**
    complications of surgery for, 48: 362-364
    deficiencies, **50: 49**
    electromyography (EMG) of, 46: *62*-64
    function and shoulder stability, 47: 97, 100
    imaging of, 46: 521, 47: 4-11
    indications for tendon transfer, **50: 65**
    infection, 48: 363
    injury to, 46: 3, 5
    management of irreparable tears, **50: 63-72**
    manual muscle testing for strength in, 46: 57-58
    mobilization, **50: *46*-48**
    open repair, **50: 43-52**
    reconstruction, **50: 65-66**
        latissimus dorsi transfer, **50: 68-70**
        postoperative care, **50: 69-70**
    recurrent tear, after total shoulder arthroplasty, 48: 365
    tear arthropathy, 47: *131*-132
    tearing as complication in humeral head replacement, 46: 20
    tendinitis/tendinosis of, 46: 3, 50
    tendinosis of, 46: 570-572
Rotator cuff repair
    arthroscopic, 47: 59-65
        approach, 47: 48-*49*
        indications, 47: 59, 63
        results, 47: 62-63
        surgical technique, 47: 59-62
    biomechanics of, 47: 43-50
        bone tunnels vs suture anchors, 47: *43*-44
        suture anchors, 47: 45-49, 63
    closure, **50: 50**
    combined arthroscopic and open, 47: 51-57
        for complete tears, 47: 47: 55-56
        for partial-thickness tears, 47: 55-56
        rationale for, 47: 51-52
    comparison of techniques, **50: *55***
    complications, 47: 90-91
    deltoid reattachment, **50: 49-50**
    errors in surgical technique, 47: 88-*90*
    failed, 47: 77-84, 87-94, 48: 362-363
        causes of, 47: 87-94
        clinical presentation, 47: 77-*79*
        and large rotator cuff tears, 47: 81-*83*
        results of revision surgery for, 47: 84
        subacromial decompression for, 47: 80-81
    fundamentals of, **50: *53***
    historical considerations, **50: 53-54**
    interval slide technique in, 47: 82
    mini-open, **50: 53-61**
        approach, **50: *59***
        historical perspectives, **50: 53-54**
        indications for surgery, **50: 54-56**

outcomes, **50: 58-60**
surgical technique, **50: 56-58**
mini-open approach, 47: 48
minimally invasive, **50: *56***
mobilization, **50: 56-57**
and persistent rotator cuff defects, 47: 91-94
preparation of tendon bone, **50: 48**
rehabilitation, **50: 50**
rehabilitation after, 47: 54-55, 56-57, 83
shoulder stiffness after, 47: 67-*74*
etiology and clinical evaluation, 47: 67-69
treatment options for, 47: 69-74
and size of tear, 47: 81
sutures and anchors, **50: 48-49**
Rotator cuff tears
mass of the repairable, **50: 63-64**
massive
MRI, **50: *65***
pathoanatomy and mechanics, **50: 64-70**
preoperative evaluation, **50: 43**
radiographic evaluation, **50: 43**
surgical approach, **50: 44-45**
surgical technique, **50: 44-50**
throwing athletes, **50: 17-18**
Rotator interval, defined, 47: 105
Rotators, external, exposure of, 49: *13*
Rotatory malalignment in tibial shaft fracture, 46: 281
Running injuries, 47: *397*-406
and Achilles tendinitis, 48: 212
Achilles tendon problems, 47: 419-427
biomechanics of, 47: 405
heel pain, 47: 425-427
nerve entrapment syndromes, 47: 426-427
plantar fasciitis, 47: 405, 425-426
posterior, 47: 421-422
incidence of, 46: 577, 47: 419
insertional Achilles tendinitis, 47: 424-*425*
nodular deformity, 47: *421*
peritendinitis, 47: *420*-421
retrocalcaneal bursitis, 47: 422-424
tendinitis, 46: 577-*580*
biomechanical approach to, 47: 397-406
forward human locomotion, 47: 397-402
injury mechanisms, 47: 402-*403*
soft-tissue stresses, 47: 403-405
of the knee, 47: 407-417
anterior knee pain, 47: 410-412
iliotibial band friction syndrome, 46: 574, *575,* 47: 413-414
physical examination, 47: 409-410
Running shoes, 47: 415
Rush rods
femoral shaft fracture, developing world, 49: *587*
internal fixation in children, 49: 417
for periprosthetic femoral fractures, 47: 439-440
use the developing world, 49: 586-587
Russell-Taylor nails, pathologic subtrochanteric fractures, 49: 465-466
Russell traction, use for femoral fractures, developing world, 49: 587
Russe's scaphoid fracture classification, **50: *107***

S

S-ROM components
combinations available, 49: *134*
femoral reconstruction, 49: 33, 34
prostheses considerations, 49: 134-136
proximal femoral replacement, 49: *144*
Saddle prosthesis, metastatic acetabular defects, 49: 468
SADOA (slow-acting drugs for the treatment of osteoarthritis), 49: 491
"Sag" sign, for posterior cruciate ligament damage, 48: 200
Salmonella, bone and joint infections, **50: 318**
Salter osteotomy, DDH, **50: 540**
Saphenous nerves
blocks, 49: 531-532
injury to, 49: 196
Sarcoidosis, and posterior heel pain, 48: 213
Sarcomas
grading, 49: 437
MRI of, 48: *582*
soft-tissue, staging and imaging, 49: 443-450
Satisfaction, patient, and unicondylar knee arthroplasty (UKA), 48: 144
Scandinavian Total Ankle Replacement (STAR), outcomes, 48: *266,* 267
Scaphocapitate intercarpal arthrodesis, **50: 127**
Scaphoid
anterior interpositional wedge graft technique, **50: 113-115**
collapsed pattern arthritis, **50: *120***
dislocation, **50: 129**
dorsal capsulodesis, **50: *130***
dynamic scapholunate instability, **50: 129-130**
interscaphoid angles, **50: *110***
osteogenesis, **50: 105**
percutaneous screw fixation, **50: 110-112**
reconstruction, **50: *118***
reconstructive problems, **50: 105-122**
screw placement, **50: *114***
unstable nonunion, **50: *113***
vascular supply, **50: 105-106, *106***
Scaphoid facet, die-punch fracture, 48: *467*
Scaphoid fractures
classification of, **50: 106-107**
confirmation of healing, **50: *108***
malunion, **50: *119***
nonsurgical treatment, **50: 107-110**
occult, **50: *107***
stable, **50: *108, 109, 111***
surgical management, **50: 110-112**
unstable, **50: *109-111***
Scaphoid shift maneuver, **50: *130***
Scaphoid shift test, 47: 222
Scaphoideum, terminology, **50: 105**
Scapholunate advanced collapse, **50: 130-*131***
Scapholunate interosseous ligaments, **50: *123***
acute static dissociation, **50: 126-*127***
acute tears, 49: 228-229
appearance of, 49: *228*
chronic dissociation, **50: 127**
instability, 49: 225, 229
treatment for instability, 47: 224-227
Scaphotrapeziotrapezoid intercarpal arthrodesis, **50: 127**
Scapula, evaluation of, 46: 43
Scapular muscle failure, 46: 5
Scapular proprioceptive facilitation patterns, 46: 47
Scapular winging, 46: 571, 47: 101
Scapularis transfer, rotator cuff repair, **50: 48**
Scapulothoracic motion, 47: 100-101
Scarring
capsular, **50: 290**
collagen fibers, **50: *4***
hypertrophic, acromioclavicular joint, 49: 411
from prior surgery, 49: 6
thermal modification, **50: 5**

SCFE. *see* Slipped capital femoral epiphysis
Scheuermann's disorder, pediatric back pain, 48: 527-528
Schwannomas
imaging of, 48: 618
MRI, 49: *449*
treatment of, 48: 597
Schwartzman phenomena, and osteonecrosis, 49: 171-172
Sciatic nerves
block, 49: 531
iatrogenic injury, acetabular fractures, 48: 492-493
identification of, **50: 311**
injury, acetabular fracture, **50: 344-345**
injury after hip arthroplasty, 47: 277
and limb length changes, 49: 6
during limb lengthening, **50: 307-308**
palsy after revision total hip arthroplasty, 48: 44
Sciatica, 46: 143
Scintigraphy, 47: 288-289
exclusion of active infection, **50: 320-321**
infected joints, **50: 369**
soft-tissue tumors, 49: 449
Scissors, endoscopic, 46: 132
SCIWORA (spinal cord injury without radiographic abnormality), association with Chiari malformation, 46: 120
Scoliosis, 46: 43
frontal view of spine, 48: *555*
neuromuscular, treatment of, 48: 551-560
painful, in children and adolescents, 48: 528-529
paralytic, complication rates, 48: *551*
spinal fusion, **50: 147-158**
spinal stenosis, 49: 368, **50: 137-138**
Screening, preoperative, and complication rates, 48: 140
Screw fixation, potential pitfalls, **50: *112***
Sedative-hypnotics, and aging, 46: 415
Sedatives, treating loxoscelism, 46: 71
Segmental defects, femoral, definition, 49: 92
Segmental spinal instrumentation (SSI), failure, occurrence in neuromuscular scoliosis fusion, 48: 552
Seizures
children with multiple injuries, 49: 428
local anesthetics, 49: 527-528
Semimembranousus reconstruction, of posterior cruciate ligament, 48: 205
Semmes-Weinstein monofilaments
in diagnosis of diabetic foot, 48: *291,* 295
Sensorcaine (bupivacaine), use of, 49: 526-527
Sensory conduction velocities
ulnar nerve compression, 49: 308
use of, 49: 309
Sensory neuropathy, in the diabetic foot, 48: 290-291, 317
Sensory radial nerves (SRN)
anatomy, 49: 295, *296*
entrapment, 49: 302-303
Sensory receptors, shoulder joint, **50: 8-9**
Sensory testing, in diagnosis of diabetic foot, 48: 295
Separated bipolar electrode insertion technique, EMG study, 46: 54
Sepsis, ongoing, ankle arthrodesis in, 48: 258-259
Septic arthritis, 46: 78
of glenohumeral joint, 46: 33
incidence, **50: 317-318**
spontaneous fusion, **50: *323***
sternoclavicular joint, 49: 404
Serotonin, role in acupuncture analgesia, 49: 560
Serratus anterior tendons, transfer of, 49: 326-327
Sesamoidectomy, lateral, 46: 377
SF-36 Health Status Questionnaire, diabetic stiff shoulder, 49: *292*
Sham incisions, **50: 360-361**
Shaving, and infection at arthroplasty sites, 48: 113
Shear forces, and osteotomy ankle, **50: *249***
Shear-strain-relieved bone grafts, 46: 350, 351, 354
Sheet grafts, management of, 49: 389
Shelf autograft, **50: *312***
Shelf reconstructions
with grafts, 49: 59
outcomes, 49: 31-32
Shoes
running, 47: 415
shock absorbing inserts, **50: 522**
Short Form-36 (SF-36), 46: 442
AAOS approval of, 48: 679
domains of, 48: *420*
outcome measurement with, 48: 419
results of autologous chondrocyte transplantation (ACT), 48: *637*
validity of, 48: 669
Short Musculoskeletal Functional Assessment (SMFA), development of, 48: 671
Short radiolunate ligament, **50: *123***
Shoulder abduction relief sign, 49: *343*
disk herniation, 49: *337*
Shoulder arthroplasty
for capsulorrhaphy arthropathy, 47: 132
for glenohumeral osteoarthritis, 47: 129-*130*
history of, 47: 127-128
indications for, 47: 128-132
for osteonecrosis, 47: 132
for posttraumatic arthritis, 47: 130, *131*
for proximal humerus fractures, 47: *129*
humeral head replacement complications, 46: 15-23
humeral head replacement for acute fractures, 46: 7-14
and malunion, 47: 135-140
for rheumatoid arthritis, 47: 130-*131*
for rotator cuff arthropathy, 47: *131*-132
technique, 47: 128
unstable, 47: 141-148
etiology, 47: *142-143*
management of, 47: 144-148
preoperative evaluation of, 47: 143-*144*
Shoulder arthroscopy, 46: 572
acromioplasty, 47: 21-27
advantages of, 47: 21-22, 27
technique, 47: 24-26
distal clavicle resection, 47: 35-41
rotator cuff repair, 47: 59-65
for shoulder stiffness after rotator cuff repair, 47: 69-70
anterior capsular release, 47: *70*-71
arthroscopic release, 47: 70
posterior capsular release, 47: *71*
subacromial arthroscopy, 47: 71, *72*
subacromial decompression
avoidance of complications, 47: 29-33
technique, 47: 25-26
Shoulder fractures
complications of humeral head replacement for, 46: 15-23
literature, 46: 15-16
Mayo Clinic experience, 46: 16-21
preventive measures, 46: 21-22
treatment options, 46: 22-23
complications of internal fixation of, 46: 25-35
frozen shoulder, 46: 32-33
hardware, 46: 28-30
heterotopic ossification, 46: 34
iatrogenic fracture displacement, 46: 34
infection, 46: 33-34

inferior subluxation, 46: 34
malunion, 46: 27-28
neurovascular injury, 46: 31-32
nonunion, 46: 25-27
osteonecrosis, 46: 30-31
subacromial impingement, 46: 32
Shoulder girdle, work related illnesses, 48: 694
Shoulder joints
alternatives to arthroplasty, **50: 73-77**
anterior instability, thermal capsulorrhaphy, **50: *40***
anterior microinstability, **50: *35***
arthrodesis, 49: *327*
biomechanics, 49: 320-323
complications of surgery, 48: 359-372
electromyography
of aquatic physical therapy, 46: *60*-62
electrode placement, 46: 53-55
of long head of biceps tendon, 46: 59-60
of manual muscle testing for rotator cuff strength, 46: 57-58
normalization of EMG signal, 46: 55-57
during therapeutic rotator cuff exercise, 46: 62-64
following thermal capsular shrinkage, **50: *9***
history of stabilization, **50: 8**
idiopathic frozen, symptoms, 49: 289-290
impingement syndrome, 47: 21-27
clinical evaluation for, 47: 22-23
radiography for, 47: 23
surgical treatment for, 47: 24-27
indications for arthroplasty, **50: 77**
injuries in throwing athletes, **50: 17-21**
instability, 47: 97-110, **50: 23-24**
anatomic factors, 47: 97-100
biomechanical considerations, 47: 98-101
failed repairs for, 113-125
magnetic resonance imaging of, 47: 13-*16*
multidirectional, 47: 101-109
reconstruction for severe glenoid loss, 47: 109-110
internal impingement, **50: 34**
lateral view, 49: *325*
magnetic resonance imaging of, 47: 3-18
glenohumeral ligaments/labrum, 46: 521-*522,* 47: 13-*16*
muscle injury, 47: 11-13
rotator cuff, 46: 521-522, 47: 4-11
management of posterior instability, **50: 24**
multidirectional instability, **50: 34**
neuropathic arthropathy, **50: 77-78**
normal, MRI, **50: *9***
normal mechanics and function, 46: 39-41
constraint systems, 46: 39-41
implications for rehabilitation, 46: 41
mobility *versus* stability, 46: 39
options for tendon transfers, 49: *319*
overconstrained, **50: 31-32**
pathophysiologic alterations in injury to, 46: 3-6
ranges of motion, 49: *285*
recurrent posterior subluxation, **50: 33**
rehabilitation, 46: *43*-50
evaluation before, 46: *43*-44
phases of, 46: 44-*46*
postoperative, 46: *46*-50
rotator cuff repair
arthroscopic, 47: 59-65
biomechanics of, 47: 43-50
combined arthroscopic and open, 47: 51-57
failed, 47: 77-84, 87-94
shoulder stiffness after, 47: 67-*74*
stabilization, thermal modification, **50: 8**
stiff, in diabetes, 49: 283-293
tendon transfers, 49: 323-327
thermal capsulorrhaphy for instability, **50: 23-36**
total arthroplasty, young patients, **50: 73-88**
traumatic anterior instability, **50: 33**
Shoulder stiffness
after instability surgery, 47: 117-123
treatment for, 47: 121-123
after rotator cuff repair, 47: 67-74
etiology and clinical evaluation, 47: 67-69
treatment options for, 47: 69-74
Sickle-cell disease
bone and joint infections, **50: 318**
and osteonecrosis, 49: 171-172
osteonecrosis of the humeral head, 48: 349-350
Sickness Impact Profile (SIP), 46: 442, 48: 419
validity of, 48: 669
Sigmoid notch, 47: 191, 209
Silver nitrate in treating pyogenic granuloma, 46: 71
Silver-sulfurdiazine, burn treatment, 49: 425, 426
Simmons-Bhalla graft, 49: *348*
Simple Shoulder Test (SST), 49: 290
diabetic stiff shoulder, 49: 291-292, *292*
Sinding-Johansson-Larsen syndrome, 47: 339, *341*
Single-beam densitometry in measuring bone mineral density, 46: 450
Single photon emission computed tomography (SPECT), in pediatric back pain, 48: 526
Sinus formation and resorbable implants, 46: 537-538
Sinus tarsi, anatomy of, 49: 270
Sinuvertebral nerve, cross-sections of, 46: *145*
Skeletal dysfunction, metastatic bone disease, 49: 456-458
Skeletal growth
achondroplasia, cause of, 46: 477, 47: 466, 471
growth factor treatment of disorders of, 46: 477-481
ethics of intervention, 46: 481
growth hormone-IGF-I axis, 46: 477, *478*
growth hormone resistance, 46: 477-481
Skeletal hyperostosis, diffuse idiopathic, and posterior heel pain, 48: 213
Skeletal muscle and aging, 46: 460-461
Skeletal scintigraphy, examination of bone tumors, 48: 609-610
Skeletal stability, reconstruction, injured upper extremities, 49: 381-385
Skier's thumb, 47: 184
Skin
for diabetic foot, 48: 300
diagnosis of diabetic foot, 48: 295
effect of autonomic neuropathy, 48: 301
evaluation in preoperative planning, 48: 95-96
management of grafts, 49: 389
preservation of bridges, 49: 380
pressure lesions, 48: 552
substitutes, 48: 300
temperature, 48: 291
SLAC (scapholunate advanced collapse), 47: 224
SLAP lesions. *See* Superior labrum anterior and posterior lesions
Slipped capital femoral epiphysis (SCFE), **50: 555-570**
classification, **50: 556-558, 571-572**
demographics, **50: 556**
epidemiology, **50: 556**
etiology, **50: 555-556**
long-term outcomes, **50: *573*-575**
natural history, **50: 572-573**
prognosis, **50: 565-567**
radiographic analysis, **50: 557-558, 561**
remodeling, **50: 559-561**

treatment, **50: 558-564**
unstable, **50: 564**
Smith-Petersen approach
anterior, outcomes analysis, 49: 28
Bernese periacetabular osteotomy, **50: *234*-235**
DDH, **50: 544**
vastus slide technique, 48: *16*
Smoking
and osteonecrosis, 48: 350
and wound healing, **50: 359**
Snapping hip, 46: 573-574
Social supports for elderly, 46: 414
Sockets
centralization, 49: 60
difficult, 49: 57-61
Sodium channels, local anesthesia, 49: *524*
Sofamor-Danek Horizon system, 48: 440
Soft-tissue allografts
disease transmission and, 47: 385
sterilization for, 47: 380
Soft-tissue chondromas
clinicopathologic features of, 48: *614*
differentiation from chondrosarcomas, 48: 613-615
Soft-tissue deficiency, and planning revision surgery, 48: 163-164
Soft-tissue expansion, preoperative, total knee arthroplasty, 48: 164
Soft-tissue sarcomas
American Joint Committee on Cancer, staging, 49: *445*
development of staging systems, 49: 443-444
5-year survival by grade, 49: *445*
staging and imaging, 49: 443-450
Soft-tissue tumors
benign, 48: 596-598
classification and grading, 49: 437-438
diagnostic maneuvers, 49: 439-440
evaluation of, 48: 617-619
malignant, treatment of, 48: 600-602
presentation, 49: 438
Soft tissues
abnormalities with hip dislocation, 49: *35*
age-related changes in, 46: 460-465
causes of, 46: 465
biopsy of masses, 49: 437-442
chondrification, arthrofibrosis, 49: 212-213
damage and limb salvage, 46: 511-512
evaluation in preoperative planning, 48: 97
expansion techniques, 46: 166
flaps, **50: 361**
hand soft-tissue injuries, 47: 181-185
ileum releases, 49: 28
imbalance of the hip, **50: 289-290**
impingement following TKA, **50: 405-406**
injury, Horii circle, **50: *90***
insufficiency, **50: 260**
management of, injured upper extremities, 49: 388-390
quality in elderly, 46: 424
running injuries and stresses on, 47: 403-405
swelling, 49: 425
tissue expanders, **50: 361**
Software, Lightwave 3D, **50: 275-276**
Somatization, and reporting of work-related disorders, 48: 696
Southern approach. *See* Posterior approaches
Space available for the cord (SAC), spinal impingement, 49: 344-345
Spacer blocks, TKR, **50: *445***
Spasticity, children with multiple injuries, 49: 428
Spectron EF stem, use of, 49: 113-114
Speed test, 47: 88
Spica casts
children with multiple injuries, 49: 415
DDH, older children, **50: 549**
hip, **50: *290***
DDH, **50: 543-544**
SCFE, **50: 558-559**
Spina bifida
lumbar spine spondylolisthesis, 48: *533*
management of spinal deformity, 48: 557-559
Spinal canal
compromise of, 48: 415, 416
posterolateral intradiskal and extra-annular access to, 46: 151
Spinal cord
compression, and cervical myelopathy, 48: 423
impingement, 49: 344-345
involvement in myelopathy, 49: *341*
segmental instability, 49: 363
stenosis of, 49: 361-371
Spinal cord injury. *See also* Spinal fractures
bone remodeling, 48: 414
complete, definition of, 48: 438
hypotension in, 46: 116
magnetic resonance imaging and thoracolumbar trauma, 48: 430
with neurologic deficit, nonsurgical treatment of, 48: 414
pathophysiology of, 46: 117-118, 120
plan of treatment, 48: 414-415
without neurologic deficit, nonsurgical treatment of, 48: 414
without radiographic abnormalities (SCIWORA), 48: 536
Spinal deformity, anterior release for, 46: 135
Spinal fractures. *See also* Spinal cord injury
biomechanical considerations of, in osteoporotic bone, 46: 431-437
and deep venous thrombosis, 48: 416
L1 and L3 burst fracture, 48: *445*
L5 burst fracture, 48: *444*
L1 flexion-compression burst fracture, 48: *446*
multiple, 48: 415-416
pediatric, 48: 536-537
rotational fracture-dislocation, 48: *447*
surgical stabilization and pain, 48: 416
T3 burst fracture, 48: *444*
thoracic and lumbar fractures, nonsurgical treatment of, 48: 413-416
thoracolumbar fractures, 48: 437-441, 443-449
Spinal imaging, 46: 119-*121*
Spinal injuries
classification of, 48: 414
L1, L2 level distraction extension, 48: *448*
management of acute trauma
drug therapy, 46: 118-119
emergency room evaluation, 46: 116-117
medical therapy, 46: 119-124
pathophysiology of spinal cord injury, 46: 117-118
prehospital care, 46: 113-116
Spinal instrumentation, 49: 350-351
spinal stenosis, 49: 369-370
Spinal muscular atrophy, neuromuscular scoliosis in, 48: 559-560
Spinal nerves
root compression, 49: 363-364
unilateral root impairment, *Guides to the Evaluation of Permanent Impairment,* 4th edition, 48: *455*
Spinal paralysis poliomyelitis, developing countries, 49: 599
Spinal stenosis, 46: *147,* 49: 361-371, **50: 135-161, *141*, 145, *148***
acquired, **50: 145**
canal, **50: *142***
classification of, 49: *361*
critical presentation, **50: 149-150**
description of, **50: 145-152**

developmental, **50: 140**
diagnosis, **50: 142-144**
differential diagnosis, 49: *365*
fusion, **50: 156-158**
intrathecal pressure, **50: 147-148**
lumbar
postoperative care, **50: 158-159**
treatment of, 49: 367-370
treatment options, **50: 153-161**
outcomes of treatment, 49: 370-371
radiologic imaging, **50: 137-144**
recurrent, 49: 368-369
thecal sac compression, **50: *138***
treatment options, **50: 153-161**
Spinal surgery
endoscopic, 46: 127
minimally invasive arthroscopic, 46: 143-159
anatomy, surgical technique, and treatment of lumbar spine disorders, 46: 148-155
biopsy of vertebral bodies in lumbar and lower thoracic spine, 46: 158
failures following disk excision, 46: 143-144
posterolateral approach to lower thoracic and lumbar spine, 46: 145-148
posterolateral treatment of disorders of lumbar spine, 46: 155-158
technical developments, 46: 144-145
postoperative care, **50: 158**
preoperative planning, 48: 96
Spinal sympathetic blockade, methods for, 46: 264
Spinati muscles, atrophy of, **50: 43**
Spine, 46: 127
AMA *Guides to the Evaluation of Permanent Impairment,* 4th edition, 48: 451-461
compression, **50: 147**
cord compression, metastatic disease, 49: *476*
degenerative disease, **50: *139*-141**
facet joint, **50: *145***
fusion in ankylosing spondylitis, 48: *97*
herniated disks and vertebral apophysis, 48: 535-536
impairment categories, 48: *453*
L3 corpectomy and strut grafting, 48: *444*
metastatic disease, 49: 471-476
percentage of slip of L5 on S1, 48: *534*
sagittal section, **50: *146***
stenotic canal, **50: *147***
thoracic, metastatic disease, 49: *472*
video-assisted thoracic surgery (VATS)
advantages and disadvantages, 46: 127-128
indications and contraindications, 46: 128-130
Spine Instrument, MODEMS program, 48: 680
Splash basins, and infection at arthroplasty sites, 48: 113
Splinting
for distal radioulnar joint injury, 47: 201
dynamic, 46: 547-*548*
immobilization of the wrist, 49: 315
night splinting for plantar fasciitis, 47: 426
noncircumferential, children with multiple injuries, 49: 428
static, 46: 547
static progressive, of the forearm, 48: *478*
Split hand, 46: 97
Spondyloarthropathies
and posterior heel pain, 48: 213
seronegative, 48: 102
Spondylolisthesis
and back pain, **50: 137**
cephalocaudal stenosis, **50: *144***
definition, **50: 140**
degenerative, 49: 368
isthmic, **50: *149***
and pediatric back pain, 48: 532-535
spinal fusion, **50: 157-158**
and spinal stenosis, **50: 145**
Spondylosis
and back pain, **50: 137**
cervical, 49: 335-337
and pediatric back pain, 48: 532-535
of triple joint complex, 46: 144
in weightlifters, 48: *533*
Sprains
ankle, **50: 515-520**
classification of, 49: 261-262
sternoclavicular joint, 49: 399-400
Spurling's test, 47: 87
cervical radiculopathy, 49: *342*
disk herniation, 49: *337*
radicular symptoms, 49: 343
Spurs, olecranon, 47: *170*
Squeeze test
syndesmosis injuries, **50: *519***
syndesmosis instability, 46: 317
St. Georg Sledge, femoral component, 48: *145*
Standards of care
See also critical pathways, 49: 643-648
Standing-frame orthoses, in myelomeningocele patients, 48: 547
Staphylococcus aureus
as agent in infected knee arthroplasty, 46: 215
as agent in proximal humeral fracture infection, 46: 18
and diskitis, 48: 531
hematogenous osteomyelitis, 49: 588-590
and infection at arthroplasty sites, 48: 113-114
infection following TKA, **50: 410**
infection in neuromuscular scoliosis fusion, 48: 552
infection in the diabetic foot, 48: 318
intermediate resistance to vancomycin (VISA), 49: 606
methicillin resistance, 49: 606
methicillin-resistant, recurrent infection, **50: 330**
osteomyelitis, **50: 317**
penicillin resistance, 49: 606
postoperative wound infections, 49: 607
septic arthritis, **50: 317**
septic arthroplasties, **50: 367**
treatment in the diabetic foot, 48: 319
Staphylococcus epidermidis
in infected knee arthroplasty, 46: 215
and infection at arthroplasty sites, 48: 113-114
infection in the diabetic foot, 48: 318
osteomyelitis, **50: 317**
postoperative wound infections, 49: 607
in proximal humeral fracture infection, 46: 18
septic arthroplasties, **50: 367**
treatment in the diabetic foot, 48: 319
Staphylococcus hemolyticus, vancomycin resistance, 49: 606
State Anxiety (SANX), 49: 542
State-Trait Anxiety Inventory, 49: 542-543
Static hip abduction brace, **50: *291***
Static splinting, 46: 547
Stationary bicycle riding, treatment of spinal stenosis, **50: 153**
Steel triple pelvic osteotomy, **50: 550**
Steinberg staging system, and treatment of osteonecrosis, 49: *180-181*
Steinmann pins
internal fixation in children, 49: 417, 418
metastatic acetabular defects, 49: *468*

Stellate ganglion blocks, 49: 536
treatment of CRPS, 49: 553-554
Stem cells, mesenchymal, 46: 487
Stemless titanium surface hemiarthroplasty, results of, 48: 100
Stenosing tenosynovitis, imaging of, 46: 524-525
Stenosis, spinal, **50: 135-161**
Steri-strips, instead of sutures, 49: 277
Sterile strap distraction, non-invasive technique, 49: *260*
Sterilization
allografts, infection control, 49: 616-618
of bioresorbable implants, 46: 535
polyethylene, 49: 42
UHMWPE, 49: 74, **50: 169-172, 423**
Sternoclavicular joint (SCJ)
acute anterior dislocation, 49: 400-401
acute posterior dislocations, 49: 401-402
atraumatic posterior dislocation, 49: 403
atraumatic spontaneous anterior subluxation, 49: 403
biomechanics, 49: 398
chronic dislocation, 49: *402*-403
cross-sectional anatomy, 49: *399*
degenerative disorders, 49: 403-404
dislocations, 49: *398, 400*
gross anatomy, 49: *397*
injuries, 49: 398-404
injuries and disorders, 49: 397-405
intra-articular disk injury, 49: 403
medial clavicular physeal injury
sprained, 49: 399-400
Sternocleidomastoid muscle, transfer of, 49: *328*
Sternum, hyperossification, 49: 404
Steroids
ON associated with, **50: 489-493**
consideration in preoperative planning, 48: 98
epidural injections, treatment of spinal stenosis, **50: 153**
fat pat atrophy, **50: 522**
induction of osteonecrosis, **50: 487**
oral, and infection at arthroplasty sites, 48: 112
and osteonecrosis, 49: 171
plantar fasciitis, **50: 525**
for pyoderma gangrenosum, 46: 73
risk of infection, 49: 64
SCFE, **50: 555**
spinal cord edema, 49: 473
in spinal cord injury, 46: 118
use in cervical degenerative disease, 48: 434
Stickler syndrome, 47: 465
STIR (short tau inversion recovery), soft-tissue tumors of, 49: 447-448
Straight leg raising test, lumbar spinal stenosis, 49: 366
Strain
response of cytosolic calcium to, 48: 194-195
response of tenocytes to, 48: *194*
Streptococcus group B
infection in the diabetic foot, 48: 318
treatment in the diabetic foot, 48: 319
Stress
consideration in preoperative planning, 48: 98
contact, and development of osteoarthritis, 48: 238-239
Stress fractures
after total hip arthroplasty, 47: 252
calcaneus, **50: 523**
cortical allografts, 49: 99
differential diagnosis, **50: 477**
tibial, 47: 413, 48: *583*
Stress radiographs, **50: 526**
diagnosis of sprains, **50: 515**
and posterior cruciate ligament damage, 48: 201
Sunrise, and posterior cruciate ligament damage, 48: *203*
X-Stress, and posterior cruciate ligament damage, 48: *204*
Stress shielding
severe, 49: 128
use of megaprostheses, 49: 145
Stress tests, varus, **50: 516**
Stretching
and Achilles tendinitis, 48: 212
diabetic frozen shoulder, 49: 283, 286
Stroke
risk of CRPS, 49: 550
THA in, 49: 168
Stromelysin, response to particulate debris, **50: 189**
Strut grafts
final position, 49: *351*
seating holes, 49: *351*
Whitecloud and LaRocca, 49: *350*
Stryker views, shoulder injuries, **50: 19**
Suavé-Kapandji procedure, 47: 211-212
Subacromial bursa, resection, **50: 46**
Subacromial decompression (SAD), efficacy of, **50: 75**
Subacromial impingement
decompression, **50: 45-46**
and internal fixation of proximal humeral fractures, 46: 32
and subacromial decompression, 47: 80
throwing athletes, **50: 19**
Subacromial space procedures, complications of arthroscopy, 48: 370-371
Subaxial joints, inflammatory arthritis in, 48: 94
Subchondral drilling, in treatment of degenerative arthritis, 48: 137-139
Subcutaneous lipomas, palpitation, 49: 438
Subcutaneous tenotomy, Achilles tendon, polio-related deformities, 49: *598*
Subfascial dissection technique, 46: 221
Subligamentous approach to herniation, 46: 155
Subluxation
elbow, **50: 91**
femoral head, **50: *276***
Subluxation/dislocation/splits, imaging of, 46: 524
Subscapular nerves, tendon transfers, 49: 323, 326-327
Subscapularis
recession, 47: 145, *146*
release of, 49: 321, *322*
rupture, 47: *144*
rupture after surgery for shoulder instability, 48: 361-362
weakness, 46: 5
Subscapularis muscles
amplitude of, **50: 65**
humoral heads exposure, **50: *80***
Subscapularis tendon
irreparable tear, **50: 64**
tear, reconstruction, **50: 66-68**
Subscapularis tendon transfer, 47: 82
Subsidence, femoral stem, 49: 111-113, 115-116
Subtalar arthrodesis, 46: 351
Subtalar bone block distraction, 46: 344-345
Subtalar joints
anatomy, 49: *270,* 270-272
arthroscopic arthrodesis, 49: 275-279
arthroscopic technique, 49: 273-*274*
compartments, 49: *272*-273
letter of capsule, 49: *274*
outcome of arthroscopy, 49: 274-275
portal anatomy, 49: 270-272
portals for arthroscopy, 49: *271*
Subtalar valgus, in patients with myelomeningocele, 48: 544-545
Subtotal diskectomy, 46: 144

Subtrochanteric osteotomies, femoral shortening, **50: 308-*309***
Suction irrigation systems, 46: 132
Suction tips, and infection at arthroplasty sites, 48: 113
Sulcus sign, 46: 571, 47: 102-*103*
Sulfamylon (mafenide acetate), burn treatment, 49: 425
Sulfonamides, resistance to, 49: 606
Superficial perennial nerve blocks, 49: 532
Superficial soft-tissue necrosis, 46: 167
Superior labra
  detachment, **50: *18***
  tears, throwing athletes, **50: 29**
Superior labrum anterior and posterior (SLAP) lesions
  thermal capsulorrhaphy, **50: 37**
  throwing athletes, **50: 17-21**
Supination-external rotation injury, 46: 313
Support groups
  pain management, 49: 520
  physician, and medical malpractice, 48: 699
Supracondylar fracture, femur proximal to total knee replacement, 46: 197-202, 47: 439-445
  incidence, 46: 197
  revision, 46: 201
  surgical technique, 46: 199-*201*
  treatment, 46: 197-199, 47: 439-445
    for displaced supracondylar fractures, 47: 440-443
    results, 46: 201-202
    with revision of implant, 47: 443-445
    for undisplaced supracondylar fractures, 47: 439-440
Supracondylar intramedullary rods, 46: 200-*201,* 47: 442-*443*
Supracondylar osteotomy, femoral, polio-related deformities, 49: 595-*596*
Suprapatellar approach, scarring, 49: 219
Suprapatellar pouch, arthroscopic view, 49: *214*
Supraspinatus muscles, tendon transfers, 49: 323
Supraspinatus outlet
  defined, 47: 5
  radiograph, 47: 7, 23, 30, *31, 32*
Supraspinatus weakness, 46: 5
Sural nerve blocks, 49: 532
Surfaces, total hip replacements, **50: 165-179**
Surgical attire, infection control, 49: 612
Surgical history, and infection at arthroplasty sites, 48: 112
Surgical margins, treatment of malignant bone tumors, 48: 599
Surgical personnel, infection control, 49: 611
Surgical sites, preparation of, and infection at arthroplasty sites, 48: 113
Surgical stabilization, and pain, 48: 416
Suture anchors
  designs of, 48: *407*
  in rotator cuff repair
    versus bone tunnels, 47: *43*-44, 63
    how to insert, 47: 45-47
    ideal, 47: 47-48, 63-64
Sutures
  revision TKA, **50: 373**
  rotator cuff repair, **50: 48-49**
  ulnar osseous tunnels, **50: *99***
Sweating, autonomic neuropathy and diabetic foot, 48: 291
Sweet syndrome, 46: 72
Swimmers, loose shoulders in, 47: 100, 101
Swimmer's sign, 47: *35*
Symbrachydactyly-cleft hand deformity, treatment of, 46: 104
Syme's amputations, 48: 688-689
  in diabetic feet, 48: *32,* 327
Sympathectomy, surgical, 49: 554
Sympathetic blockade, 46: 264
  treatment of CRPS, 49: 553-554
Sympathetic nervous system, 46: 262
  dysfunction, 46: 261-262
Sympathetically maintained pain (SMP), 46: 261
  cause of, 46: 263
  description of, 49: 549
  diagnostic studies of, 46: 264
  history of, 46: 263
  pharmacologic therapy of, 46: 265-267
  physical therapy and exercise, 46: 267
  presentation of, 46: 263-264
  signs and symptoms of, 46: 263-264
  treatment of, 46: 264-265
Syndactylized fingers, release of, 46: 107
Syndactyly
  classification of, 46: 98-*100*
  surgical treatment of, 46: 100-104
Syndesmosis, injuries, **50: 518-520**
Syndesmotic complex of ankle, 46: 311
Syndesmotic ligaments, injuries, 46: 316-318, 49: 263-266
Synovectomy
  hip, salvage procedures for rheumatoid arthritis, 48: 100-101
  knees, results in rheumatoid arthritis, 48: 101
Synovectomy surgical, glenohumeral joint, **50: 75-76**
Synovial fluid
  analysis of
    in diagnosing gout, 46: 75-76
    in diagnosing pseudogout, 46: 77
  from degenerative joints, 49: 484
  hyaluronic acid in osteoarthritis, 49: 495
Synovial joints
  causes of degeneration, 49: *483*
  osteoarthritic degeneration, 49: 481-488
Synovial-lined pseudarthrosis, 46: 25-26
Synovial sarcomas
  imaging of, 48: 618
  malignant, 48: 601
  nuclear features, 49: 437
Synovitis
  with intra-articular use, 46: 538
  loss of flexion, **50: 391**
  rheumatoid, in hip joints, 48: 101
  villonodular, knee, 49: *448*
Synvisc (Hylan G-F 20), use of, 49: 497
Syringomyelia, total contact casting and, 48: 305
SYSADOA (symptomatic slow-acting drug for osteoarthritis), 49: 491
Systemic lupus erythematosus (SLE), hip-preserving surgical approaches, 48: 98-99

T

T-lymphocytes, in osteolysis, 49: 79
Tabes dorsales, total contact casting and, 48: 305
Tachycardia, and thromboemboli disease, **50: 416**
TACS. *See* Thermal-assisted capsular shrinkage
Talar body, Kirschner wire introduction, 48: *545*
Talar dome
  drilling of intact lesions, 49: 261
  osteochondral lesions, 49: 259-261
Talar fractures
  anatomy, 46: *323-324*
  circulation, 46: *324*-325
  head injuries, 46: *325*-327
  history of injuries, 46: 323
  neck
    classification of, 46: 327

complications, 46: 331
malalignments, 46: 327-328
osteonecrosis, 46: 331-332
treatment of, 46: 328-331
open, 46: 334-335
outcome of, 46: 335-337
salvage problems, 46: 333
talar body, 46: 332-333
Talar osteonecrosis, ankle arthrodesis in, 48: 259
Talar tilt tests, radiographic, **50: 515-516**
Talectomy, 46: 333
in patients with myelomeningocele, 48: 544
Talocalcaneal ligament, 46: 324
Talus
neuropathies and necrosis of, and development of osteoarthritis, 48: 238
posterior facets, 49: *274*
Tarsal canals
anatomy of, 49: 270
contents of, 49: *271*
Tarsal tunnel syndrome, 47: 426, **50: 527-528**
Television, worldwide exposure, 49: 580
Templating
acetabulum, 49: *8*
femoral, 49: *9*, 9-10, 122-*123*
planning reconstruction, 49: 85-86
preoperative, difficult femurs, 49: 63-64
and preoperative planning, in total hip arthroplasty, 48: 53
radiographic, 49: 7-10
total hip arthroplasty, **50: 266**
Temporomandibular joints, rheumatoid arthritis in, 48: 97
Tendinitis
Achilles, 46: 577-580
biomechanics of, 47: 405
Achilles tendon, 48: 212-215
flexor hallucis longus, **50: 526-527**
labeling, 48: 695
Tendinosis
cycle, 47: 402-*403*
of elbow, 46: 572-573
of hip, 46: 573
patellar, 46: 574-575, 576, 47: 404, 411-412
of rotator cuff, 46: 570-572
Tendon grafts
passage through bone tunnels, 48: *387*
suture fixation, 48: *387*
Tendon problems in athletic individuals, 46: 569-581
Achilles tendinopathy, 46: 577-580, 47: 405
jumper's knee, 46: 574-575, *576*, 47: 404, 411-412
pathophysiology, 46: 569-570
popliteal tenosynovitis, 47: 414
posterior tibial tendon dysfunction, 46: 575-577
tendinosis about hip, 46: 573-574
tendinosis of elbow, 46: 572-573
tendinosis of rotator cuff, 46: 570-572
Tendon rupture, 46: 176
Tendon transfers
indications for, **50: 65**
irreparable rotator cuff tears, **50: 63-72**
latissimus dorsi, **50: *68*-70**
pectoralis major, **50: *66***
shoulder and elbow, 49: 319-332
Tendons
age-related changes in, 46: 464-465
in diagnosis of diabetic foot, 48: 295
reconstruction of, 49: 386-388
response to loading, 48: 193-194
transfers, 49: 387-388
Tennis elbow, 47: 165-171. *See also* Epicondylitis; Radial tunnel syndrome
anconeus compartment syndrome, 47: 170
lateral epicondylitis, 46: 572-573, 47: 165-167
medial epicondylitis, 46: 573, 47: 168-170
triceps tendinitis, 47: 170
Tennis players, pain syndrome, **50: 35**
Tenocytes, response to strain, 48: *194*
Tenograms, diagnosis of ankle sprains, **50: 515**
Tenosynovectomy, 46: 397
Tenosynovitis, 46: 397
acute, 46: 577
Tenosynovium, 46: 569
Tenovagium, 46: 569
Tensile fracture stress, articular cartilage, and age, 48: *236*
Teratologic dislocation of the hip, **50: 541**
Teres major tendons
amplitude, **50: 66**
infraspinatus transfer to, 49: 321-323
tear of, **50: 43**
transfer of, 49: 324, **50: 63**
Testosterone, SCFE, **50: 555**
Tetracaine (pontocaine), use of, 49: 525
Tetracycline, deactivation by bone cement, 48: 117
Tetragonal zirconia polycrystals (TZP), **50: 167-168**
Tetraplegia, defined, 48: 438
THA. *see* Total hip arthroplasty
THARIES (Total Hip Articular Replacement with Internal Eccentric Shells), 49: 178-179
Thecal sac, neural organization, 49: *362*
Therabands, 46: 571
Thermal-assisted capsular shrinkage (TACS)
injuries in throwing athletes, **50: 17-21**
postoperative care, **50: 20-21**
Thermal capsulorrhaphy
complications, **50: 31-32, 37-41**
concurrent procedures, **50: 39**
contact sports participation, **50: 39**
failures in MDI group, **50: 39**
heat probes, **50: 29-36**
motion restriction, **50: 40**
multiple postoperative dislocations, **50: 39**
nerve injuries, **50: 40-41**
postoperative care, **50: 40**
postsurgical care, **50: 31-32**
risks of failure, **50: *38*-41**
shoulder
outcomes, **50: 26-27**
postoperative care, **50: 25-26**
for shoulder instability, **50: 23-28**
a thermal impingement with SLAP repair, **50: *20***
treatment of anterior instability, **50: *40***
Thermal energy. *See* Heat
Thermal injury
from curing of cement, in hip arthroplasty, 48: 29
and osteonecrosis, 49: 170
Thermal modification
ankle, **50: *519***
anterior glenohumeral instability, 50: 13-15, **50: 13-15**
connective tissues, **50: 3-11**
delivery of energy, **50: 6-7**
fibroblastic response, **50: *8***
glenohumeral instability, **50: 37-41**
in vitro studies, **50: 4-6**
Thermography, diagnosis of CRPS, 49: 551

Third party liability, and contracts, 48: 701
Thomas splint, use in the developing world, 49: 586
Thomas test, and flexion contractures, in myelomeningocele patients, 48: 564
Thompson test, and Achilles tendon rupture, 48: 220
Thoracic disk herniation, 46: 135, 138-*139*
Thoracic fractures, nonsurgical treatment of, 48: 413-416
Thoracic myelomeningocele, hip problems in pediatric patients, 48: 564-566
Thoracic outlet syndrome (TOS), 48: 694
differential diagnosis, 49: 297
ulnar nerve compression, 49: 307
Thoracic spine
metastatic disease
MRI, 49: *475*
surgical treatment, 49: 474-475
range-of-motion model, 48: *459*
Thoracolumbar area, spinal impairment, *AMA Guides to the Evaluation of Permanent Impairment,* 4th edition, 48: 456-457
Thoracolumbar fractures
classification of, 48: 437-441
combined anterior and posterior surgery for, 48: 443-449
introduction to, 48: 427-428
posterior instrumentation, 48: 440-441
prophylactic decompression, 48: 439
timing of surgery, 48: 438-439
treatment by type, 48: *438*
treatment of, 48: *440*
Thoracolumbar junction, injuries to, 48: 414
Thoracolumbar spine, evaluation in preoperative planning, 48: 96-97
Thoracolumbar trauma, imaging overview, 48: 429-430
Thoracoscopic procedures
anterior release for spinal deformity, 46: 135
corpectomy for excision of tumor or fracture, 46: 135
laparoscopic approach to lumbar spine, 46: 135-137
surgical technique, 46: 133-135
thoracic disk herniation, 46: 135, 138-*139*
Thoracoscopy, 46: 127, 128
diagnostic, 46: 144-145
indications and contraindications, 46: 129-130
indications for, 46: 129
video-assisted thoracic surgery, instruments used in, 46: 131-*133*
Thoracotomy, 46: 128
Thromboembolic disease
after hip arthroplasty, 47: 331-335
epidemiology, 47: 331
prevention of, 47: 332-333
treatment of, 47: 335
after knee arthroplasty, 46: 185-188
current prophylaxis, 46: 187-188
epidemiology, 46: 185-186
impact of chemoprophylaxis, 46: 186-187
treatment of, 46: 188
diagnosis of, **50: 415-416**
following TKA, **50: 415-419**
pathogenesis, **50: 415**
predisposing factors, **50: 415**
Thrombophilia, and osteonecrosis, **50: 490**
Thrombophlebitis, 46: 425
Thrombosis, deep vein, total hip arthroplasty, 48: 35
Thromboxane inhibitors in treating spinal cord injuries, 46: 118
Throwing athletes
anterior microinstability, **50: *35***
athlete's elbow, 48: 383-391
biomechanics of, 48: 383-384
internal impingement, **50: 34**
phases of, 48: *384*
shoulder instability, **50: 29**
subacromial impingement, **50: 19**
Thumb
acute rupture of ulnar collateral ligament of metacarpophalangeal joint of, 47: 184-*185*
dislocation of carpometacarpal joint of, 47: *185*
hypoplastic, 46: 89-97
classification for, 46: 89-*91*
pollicization for, 46: 94-*97*
reconstructive procedures for, 46: 91-*94*
laxity, 47: *102*
Thyroid hormone in osteoporosis, 46: 447
Thyroid-releasing hormone (TRH), spinal cord injuries, 46: 118
Tibia
bone graft stabilization, 49: *591*
bone preparation techniques, 48: 178-179
classification of ON lesions, **50: 480**
dislocation of cruciate-retaining component, 48: *155*
lateral plateau
after complete reduction, 48: *508*
fracture of, 48: *504, 506*
split depressed fracture of, 48: *508*
medial condyle, fracture of, 48: *499*
medial plateau, high energy fracture of, 48: *498*
osteonecrosis, **50: 477-481, *486*-487**
posterior displacement, 48: *202*
proximal
compression screws, 48: *511*
fracture-dislocation, 48: *509*
proximal valgus tibial osteotomy, 48: 131-133
stability of hybrid frame fixation of, 48: *507*
tunnel enlargement, **50: *468***
tunnel formation, **50: 471**
tunnel placement, **50: 464-*465***
type 1 defect, 48: *169*
type 2 defects, 48: *170*
type 3 defects, 48: *171*
valgus deformity, 48: *147*
Tibial components
aseptic loosening, 48: *173*
fixation of, 48: *180*
mobile-bearing TKR, **50: *435***
shifted, **50: *394***
thickness of polyethylene, **50: 424-426**
undersurface wear, **50: 427**
Tibial fractures
base plate, **50: *393***
children with multiple injuries, 49: 418
compartment syndrome associated with, 46: 303-308
clinical problem, 46: 303
diagnosis of, 46: 303-304
outcome of, 46: 307
surgical technique for fasciotomy, 46: 305-*307*
and tibial nailing, 46: 304-305
following TKA, **50: 384-387**
leg placement during surgery, 48: *505*
periprosthetic
intraoperative, 47: 438, 450
postoperative, 47: *445,* 453-455
placement of guide wire, 48: *507*
plateau
hybrid frame fixation of, 48: 505-511
postoperative treatment, 48: 511-512
proximal, 48: 497-512
arthroscopic management, 48: 502-505
diagnosis, 48: 499-500

management, 48: 500-501
with patellar dislocation, 48: *500*
shaft, 46: 293-*300*
bone grafting, 46: 299
classification of, 46: 294
delayed union and nonunion of, 46: 281-289
assessment of tibial nonunion, 46: 282
defect nonunion, 46: 283-284
goals of tibial nonunion treatment, 46: 282
incidence and etiology, 46: 281-282
treatment of tibial nonunion, 46: 282-283
treatment protocols for common tibial nonunions, 46: 284-289
initial surgical treatment, 46: 294-295
rehabilitation, 46: 299-300
stabilization of, 46: 295-298
treatment in emergency room, 46: 293-294
treatment of wound, 46: 298-299
stress fractures in runners, 47: 413
technical considerations in surgical management of, 46: *271*-279
combined injuries, 46: 276-278
portal placement, 46: 271-272
position, 46: *272*-273
proximal fractures, 46: *276, 278*-279
reaming, 46: 273-276
setup, 46: *271*
tibial plateau fractures, osteochondral allograft for, 47: *518*
tibial spine fractures, 47: 352-*354*
Tibial joint surface on the lateral view (TLS), use in preoperative planning, 48: 283
Tibial nerve, blocks, 49: 532
Tibial osteotomy
at 12 weeks, 48: *467*
for knee osteoarthritis, 47: 430-434
fixation methods for, 47: 433
indications for, 47: 430-431
patient assessment for, 47: 431-432
proximal tibial varus osteotomy, 47: 434
Tibial tendon, dysfunction of posterior, 46: 575-577
Tibial tubercle osteotomy, 46: 222-224, 224
in knee arthroplasty, 48: 165
total knee arthroplasty, **50: 363**
Tibiocalcaneal arthrodesis, 46: 333, 48: 260
Tibiofibular joint-external rotation, 49: *264*
Tibiofibular joint-internal rotation, 49: *264*
Tibiotalar angle, assessment of limb alignment using, 48: 281
Tibiotalar fusion
indications and contraindications, 49: *267*
surgical technique, 49: 267-269
Tibiotalar joints, fusion of, 49: 266-271
Tibiotalocalcaneal arthrodesis, 48: 260
reconstruction, 48: *275*
Ticarcillin-clavulanate, treatment of diabetic foot infection, 48: 319
Tinel's sign, 48: 694
radial nerve compression, 49: 296
SRN entrapment, 49: 302-303
ulnar nerve compression, 49: 307
Tissue cultures, for assessment of infection, 48: 45
Tissue engineering, 46: 544
and articular cartilage restoration, 48: 625-626
Tissue expanders, use of, **50: 361**
Tissue factors, local, in diabetics, 48: 294
Tissue homeostasis, and the envelope of function, 48: 187-188
Tissue inhibitor of metalloproteinase (TIMP), response to particulate debris, **50: 189**
Tissues
response, **50: 7**
thermal properties, **50: 3**
Titanium
femoral heads, 49: 42
phagocytosis of particles, 49: 72
response of hexosaminidase, **50: 189**
wear rates, 49: 75
Titanium-aluminum-vanadium (Ti6Al4V)
biologic response, **50: 187**
implant elasticity, 49: 75
macrophage response, 49: 72
Titanium monoblock femoral stems, removal of, 48: 40-41
Titanium nails, internal fixation in children, 49: 417
TNK ankle, outcomes, 48: 265-*266*
Tobramycin
antibiotic-impregnated cement, 48: 117
cement beads loaded with, **50: 330**
cement loaded with, **50: 329, 331**
in cement spacers, **50: 372**
Toenails
hypertrophic onychomycotic, 48: *301*
ingrown, and diabetic foot, 48: 293
Toes
amputation in diabetic feet, 48: 324
amputations, 48: 688
Tomography, elbow, **50: 94**
Tongue-type fracture, 46: 341
Tonnis osteotomy, **50: 550**
Torg ratio, spondylitic myelopathy, 49: 336
Total ankle arthroplasty, satisfaction rates after, 48: *263*
Total ankle replacements, radiographic loosening after, 48: *267*
Total articulating resurfacing arthroplasties, results of, 48: 100
Total contact casts, 48: 305-315
advantages of, 48: 306-307
alternatives to, 48: 311-312
application, 48: 309-*312*
and arthrodesis for neuropathic deformities, 48: 275
contraindications for, 48: 308-309
indications for, 48: 308
patient instructions, 48: *314*
postcasting care, 48: 310-311
treatment of plantar ulcers, 48: 319
Total hip arthroplasty (THA)
abductor muscle deficiencies, **50: 270**
with active sepsis, **50: 319**
after acetabular fracture, **50: 349-352**
allografts, 48: 67-75
in ankylosing spondylitis, 48: 104
approaches, **50: 266**
capsular defects, **50: *289***
cemented, outcomes, 48: 103-104
chronology of dislocation, **50: 265-266**
component design, **50: *279***
component malposition, **50: 268-269**
constrained acetabular opponents, **50: 281-287**
constrained implants, **50: 271-273**
conversion of arthrodesis to, **50: 297-305**
diagnosis of infection, **50: *320***
dislocation after, **50: 265, *281, 289***
effect of component design, **50: 275-279**
impingements, **50: 269-270**
incidence of dislocation, **50: 284**
infection at site of, 48: 111-120
infection following
diagnosis, 47: 285-293

treatment, 47: 297-304
multifactorial instability, **50: 270**
osteolysis, **50: 197**
periprosthetic acetabular fractures after 47: 231-235
intraoperative, 47: 232-233, *234,* 252
postoperative, 47: 233-234
in vitro studies, 47: 231-232
periprosthetic femoral fractures after, 47: 237-241
classification of, 47: 253
intraoperative, 47: 237-238, 251-252
postoperative, 47: 238-241, 243-248
periprosthetic osteolysis after, 48: 37-42
postoperative management, **50: 350**
preoperative investigations, 48: 31-32
preoperative planning, **50: 266**
prevention of dislocation, **50: 266-267**
primary
acetabular reconstruction, **50: 224**
after acetabular fracture, **50: 335-354**
after infection, **50: 317-333**
outcome after infection, **50: 322-325**
reconstruction after infection, **50: 325-331**
recurrent hip instability, **50: *271***
recurrent tuberculosis infection, **50: 324-325**
results in adult-onset rheumatoid arthritis, 48: 101-102
retroperitoneal exposure, 48: *33*
revision, acetabular reconstruction, **50: 224-226**
risk factors for revision, **50: 352**
soft-tissue tension insufficiency, **50: 269**
sources of infection, **50: 318-319**
surgical approaches, **50: *339***
timing of, **50: 338**
treatment of dislocation, **50: 267-273**
unstable
overview, **50: 265-274**
postoperative bracing, **50: 289-293**
use of allograft bone, 48: 645
Total hip replacement (THR)
after acetabular fractures, 48: 494
arthrodesis conversion to, outcomes, **50: 312-313**
bearing surfaces in replacements, **50: 165-179**
choices of bearings, **50: *174***
cross-linked polyethylene, **50: 181-184**
for dislocated hips, **50: 307-316**
failure of, **50: 182**
wear of materials, **50: 165**
Total joint arthroplasty, 46: 418-420
Total knee arthroplasty (TKA). *See also* Knee arthroplasty
allograft reconstruction, **50: 396-397**
anatomic considerations, **50: 360**
arthroscopic débridement, **50: 500**
bone defects in revision, 46: 227-236
causes of, 46: 227-228
classification for, 46: 228-230
clinical results of allografts in, 46: 234-236
options for reconstruction of major bone deficiencies, 46: 230-231
techniques for allograft reconstruction in, 46: 231-234
bone loss and grafting techniques, 48: 179
bone loss from femur, tibia and patella, 48: *177*
cementless fixation issues in revision, 48: 177-182
classification of instability, **50: *399***
cost effectiveness of revision, 46: 237-240
distal femoral varus osteotomy, 48: 125-129
durability of revisions, 48: 146-148
in the elderly, 46: 421-*422*
excisional, 46: 382-384
extensor mechanism problems in
patellar clunk syndrome, 46: 176, *177*
patellar component failure, 46: *175*-176
patellar component loosening, 46: 174-175
patellar fractures, 46: 173-*174*
patellofemoral instability, 46: 171-173
surgical technique, 46: 176-177
tendon rupture, 46: 176
extensor mechanism rupture, **50: 405**
flexion instability, **50: *400***
fractures of femur, tibia and patella after, 47: 449-*457*
intraoperative, 47: 437-439, 449-451
postoperative, 47: 439-448, 451-*457*
infected, 46: 215-218
diagnosis, 46: 216
management, 46: 216-218
prevalence of deep sepsis, 46: 215-216
infection after, **50: 404-414**
infection at site of, 48: 111-120
knees, results in rheumatoid arthritis, 48: 101
landmarks for resection, 48: *178*
ligament instability, **50: 399-401**
neurovascular complications following, 46: 181-184
direct injury to vascular structures around knee, 46: 183-184
peroneal nerve palsy, 46: 181
wound-healing problems, 46: 181-183
osteoarthritis, middle-aged patients, **50: 507-508, 599-511**
for osteonecrosis, **50: 485-486**
patellar component, **50: 405**
patellofemoral complications, **50: 403-407**
periprostatic patellar fractures, **50: 385-387**
and periprosthetic fractures, 47: 437-448
decision making and principles of management, 47: 449-457
incidence of, 47: 253-254
intraoperative, 47: 437-439, 449-451
postoperative, 47: 439-448, 451-457
periprosthetic fractures following, **50: 379-389**
periprosthetic osteolysis, **50: 391-398**
planning for revision, 48: 161-166
preoperative evaluation, **50: 359-361**
preoperative soft-tissue expansion, 48: 164
reimplantation following infection, **50: 411-412**
resection arthroplasty, **50: 410**
revision, **50: 359-365, 367-377**
principles of, **50: 357-358**
reimplantation after infection, **50: 370-373**
timing of, **50: 396**
revision of unicondylar implants, 48: 144-148
skin incisions, **50: 360-361**
stiff, 46: 191-195
causes of, 46: 192-193
diagnostic considerations, 46: 193
prevention of, 46: 194-195
treatment alternatives, 46: 193-194
supracondylar fracture of distal femur proximal to, 46: 197-202
incidence, 46: 197
revision, 46: 201
surgical technique, 46: 199-201
treatment, 46: 197-199
treatment results, 46: 201-202
supracondylar fractures, **50: 382**
surgical exposure, **50: 361-364**
surgical exposure for revision, 48: 149-152
surgical exposure in revision
closure, 46: 225
exposure of posterior recess, 46: 224

intraosseous exposure, 46: 224
quadriceps transection exposure, 46: 221-222
tibial tubercle osteotomy, 46: 222-224
thromboembolic disease, **50: 415-419**
thromboembolic disease following, 46: 185-188
tibial fractures, **50: 384-387**
treatment of osteonecrosis, **50: 492**
treatment regimens for infection of, 48: 177-178
wound complications in, 46: 165-168
choice of skin incision, 46: 165-166
management, 46: 167-168
patient risk factors, 46: 166-167
technical factors, 46: 166
vascular anatomy, 46: 165
Total knee replacement (TKR)
incidence of polyethylene wear, **50: 426-427**
mobile-bearing, **50: 431-449**
polyethylene damage, **50: 424-426**
range of motion, **50: *437***
results of mobile-bearing designs, **50: *446***
self-aligning, **50: 440-443**
spacer blocks, **50: *445***
Total shoulder arthroplasty
complications, **50: 83-86**
complications following, 48: 364-367
indications, **50: 78**
outcomes, **50: 82-83**
postoperative course, **50: 82**
preoperative planning, **50: 78-79**
technique, **50: 79-82**
Tourniquet-induced ischemia, pain relief, 49: 554
Tourniquets, and DVT, **50: 416**
Trabeculae, resorption of, 48: 627
Trabecular bone, in Paget's disease, 49: 66
Tracings, preoperative planning, 49: 503-509
Traction
Buck's apparatus, developing world, 49: 587
DDH, **50: 543-544**
Perkins apparatus, 49: *586*
Russell apparatus, 49: 587
use in cervical degenerative disease, 48: 434
in wrist arthroscopy, 49: 225-227
Training, and Achilles tendinitis, 48: 212
Tramadol, pain management, 49: 515
Tranexamic acid, use in the orthopaedic setting, 48: 656
Trans-syndesmotic fixation, 46: 317
Transcutaneous electrical nerve stimulation (TENS)
and phantom sensation, 48: 329
treatment of RSD, 49: 554
use in cervical degenerative disease, 48: 435
use of, 49: *394*
Transcutaneous oxygen tension ($TcPO_2$)
decision making in foot amputations, 48: 323
vascular studies using, 48: 296-297
Transfemoral amputation, 48: *689*-690
Transfemoral type of amputation, 46: 507-508
Transforming growth factor-ß
and bone formation, 46: 495-496
and cartilage regulation, 47: 465, 470-471
and cartilage repair, 46: 490, 47: 498-*499*
for fracture healing, 46: 483-484, 47: 531
as a therapeutic agent, 46: 473
Transforming growth factors, articular cartilage restoration, 48: 624
Transfusions
autologous donation, **50: 154**
practice standards, 48: 655-656
Transillumination
arthroscopy of meniscus, 49: 197
ganglia, 49: 438
Transpedicular approach to vertebral bodies, 46: 158
Transplants. *See* Allografts; Grafts
Transportation in acute spinal trauma management, 46: 115-116
Transposons, role in bacterial resistance, 49: 606
Transscaphoid perilunate dislocation, **50: 129**
Transthoracic diskectomy, 46: 138
Transtibial amputations, 46: 506
in diabetic feet, 48: 327-328
Transtrochanteric osteotomies, approach to hip, 49: 17-20
Trapezius muscle
rotator cuff reconstruction, **50: 66**
transfer of, *49: 325*-326
Trapezius tendon, transfer for rotator cuff tear, **50: 63**
Trauma
classification of injuries, 49: 378-379
cumulative disorders, 48: 695
land mine injuries, 49: 431-433
and osteonecrosis of the humeral head, 48: 350
relation with soft-tissue tumors, 48: 617
Trauma registries, and outcomes research, 48: 672
Trauma room, severely injured upper extremities, 49: 377-379
Traverse lesions syndrome, 49: *341*
Treadmill exercises, treatment of spinal stenosis, **50: 153**
Trendelenburg sign
hip dysplasia, 49: 26
periprosthetic femoral osteolysis, **50: 200**
preoperative planning, 49: 5
spinal stenosis, **50: 150**
Triscaphoid arthrodesis, 47: 226-227
Trial reductions
in revision total hip arthroplasty, 48: 23
THA, 49: 125
and use of reconstruction cages, 48: 73
Triangular fibrocartilage complex (TFCC), 46: 77, 47: 176
anatomy and function, 49: 230-233
categorization of injuries, 48: 476
and distal radioulnar joint instability, 47: 209-210
Triangular working zone (TWZ), 46: 144
anatomy of, 46: *147-148*
arthroscopic visualization of, 46: *149-150*
Tricalcium phosphate, 47: 528-529
Triceps tendinitis, 47: 152, 170
Triceps tendons, anterior transfer, 49: 328-329
Tricompartmental wrist arthrography, intra-articular abnormalities, 49: 225
Tricyclic antidepressants and aging, 46: 415
Trigger finger, 48: 694
Trigger point injection, use in cervical degenerative disease, 48: 434-435
Trihexyphenidyl and aging, 46: 415
Triple arthrodesis, 46: 351-354, 400
Trocar insertion techniques, 46: 134-135
Trocars, 46: 131, 136
Trochanteric osteotomies, 49: *60*
healing, 49: *133*
outcomes, 49: 34
revision THA, 49: 86
total hip replacements, **50: 310-311**
Trochanteric slide
anterior, revision total hip arthroplasty, 48: 3-6
with femoral bone loss, 49: 86
hip arthroplasty, 49: 28
osteotomy, **50: 247-252, *312***
THA revision, femoral bone loss, 49: 151
Tubercle sulcus angle (TSA), 47: 339

Tuberculosis, 47: 304
allograft transmission, 49: 616
diagnosis, **50: 319**
diagnosis of active infection, **50: 321**
recurrent infection, **50: 324-325**
skeletal, **50: 318**
Tuberculosus spondylitis, and pediatric back pain, 48: 532
Tuberosities, nonunions, 46: 26-27
Tuberosity fixation, 46: 10-12
Tuberosity malunion, in humeral head replacement, 46: 20
Tuberosity nonunion, in humeral head replacement, 46: 19-20
Tug test, 46: 9
Tumor necrosis factor-α receptors, response to particulate debris, **50: 192**
Tumor necrosis factor-α (TNF-α)
antibody, particulate-induced bone resorption, **50: 192**
effect of hyaluronic acid, 49: 496
in osteoarthritis, 49: 486
production of, effect of intermittent fluid pressure on, 48: 252
response to particulate debris, **50: 187-188, 190**
simulation of osteoclasts by, 48: 37
Tumor necrosis factors, 46: 205
and osteoclastic activity, 49: 79
and osteoclasts, 49: 78
Tumor resection, quadriceps myocutaneous composite flap for exposure of, 48: 157-159
Tumors. *See also* Neoplasms
benign, and pediatric back pain, 48: 537-539
bone, presentation and evaluation of, 48: 607-611
magnetic resonance imaging of shoulder, 47: 16-17
orthopaedic presentation, 48: *578*
soft tissue
evaluation of, 48: 617-619
and history of traumatic events, 48: 617
physical examination, 48: 617-618
radiographic examination, 48: 618
unexpected surgical encounters, 48: 584-585
Two-bundle procedures, posterior cruciate ligament reconstruction, 48: 205
Two-plane fluoroscopic imaging, 46: 137
Two-point discrimination, innovation density, 49: 307
Two-screw danger sign, **50: *300*, 301**

U

UHMWPE. *See* Ultra-high molecular weight polyethylene
Ulceration
evaluation in preoperative planning, 48: 95-96
foot, pathophysiology of, 48: 305
Ulcers. *See also* Diabetic foot
amputation compared with nonsurgical treatment, 48: 313
evaluation of, 48: *295*
foot
classification of, 48: 318
etiology of, 48: 317
healing of, 48: 313
of the plantar arch, 48: 294
propensity for, 48: 270
total contact casting and, 48: 305-315
and treatment of neuropathic deformity, 48: 271
use of platelet-derived wound-healing factor (PDWHF), 48: 314-315
Ulna
AO classification of the distal aspect of, 48: *476*
fractures, 49: 382
fixation in children, 49: 417-418
sutures through osseous tunnels, **50: *99***
vascular supply, **50: *115***
Ulnar artery flap, management of, 49: 389
Ulnar deficiency, longitudinal failure of upper-limb formation in hand, 46: 104-*108*
Ulnar hand, ulnar nerve compression, 49: 308
Ulnar nerves
anterior submuscular transposition, 48: *390*
blocks, 49: 530
classification of function, 49: 309
compression at the rest, 49: 314-316
compressive neuropathies, 49: 305-316
decompression, surgical techniques, 49: 312-314
decompression without transposition, 49: 310-312
irritation of, 48: 694
Ulnar neuritis
in the athlete's elbow, 48: 383-391
diagnosis, 48: 388-389
nonsurgical treatment, 48: 389
rehabilitation, 48: 391
surgical treatment and technique, 48: 389-391
Ulnar styloid process, fractures of, 48: 475-476
external fixation devices, 48: *477*-478
Ulnar tunnel. *See* canal of Guyon
Ulnar variance, radiographic measurement, 48: 465
Ulnolunate ligaments, **50: *123***
Ulnotriquetral ligaments, **50: *123***
Ultra-high molecular weight polyethylene (UHMWPE), 46: 206. *See also* Polyethylene
available resins, **50: *169***
cross-linking, **50: 170-174**
drainage following total knee replacement, 46: 208-210
fabrication, **50: 421-422**
features of, **50: 182-183**
improvement in, **50: 169-170**
induction of osteolysis by, 48: 37-38
maximum performance in TKR, **50: 421-429**
methods in making devices, 46: 206-207
molecular structure, **50: *421***
and osteolysis, 49: 74
quality, 46: 207
sterilization, 46: 207
thickness, 46: 208
use in arthroplasty, 49: 71
in vivo degradation, 46: 207
wear in metal-backed cups, 49: 77
Ultra Power Drill System, 46: 133
Ultrasonography
and Achilles tendon rupture, 48: 220
coronal, newborn femoral head, **50: *539***
DDH, **50: 541-*542***
decision making in foot amputations, 48: 323
Doppler arterial pulse-volume recording, 48: *296*-297
dynamic technique, hip joint, **50: 542**
newborn hip, **50: 539-540**
removal of cement, 49: 87
soft-tissue tumors, 49: 439, 449
static technique, hip joint, **50: 542**
Ultraviolet light, and infection at arthroplasty sites, 48: 113
Uncovertebral joints, 49: *339*
Underwriting results, Blue Cross/Blue Shield, 48: *676*
Unicompartmental knee arthroplasty, **50: 505-507**
Unicondylar arthroplasties, and type 1 bone defects, 48: 169
Unicondylar implants, revision of, 48: 144-146
Unicondylar knee arthroplasty (UKA)
for gonarthrosis, 48: 143-148

outcomes studies, 48: *143*
Unilateral biportal access, 46: 154-155
Uniportal intradiskal access, 46: 152-154
United Nations, health programs, 49: 575
United Nations High Commissioner for Refugees (UNHCR), relief for nation, 49: 575
United Nations International Children's Emergency Fund (UNICEF), health programs, 49: 575
University of Pennsylvania Staging System
classification of osteonecrosis, 49: 173-174
treatment plants for osteonecrosis, 49: *180*
Upper extremities
classification of injuries, 49: 379
severely injured, treatment of, 49: 377-395
work-related complaints, 48: 693-697
Upper limb deformities, polio-related, 49: 599
Urbanization, global shifts, 49: 569
Urinary dysfunction, and spinal stenosis, 49: 365
Urinary tract infections
and delirium in geriatric patients, 46: 414
and infection at arthroplasty sites, 48: 112
occurrence in neuromuscular scoliosis fusion, 48: 552

V

V-Y quadriceps turn-down, **50: 362-363**
V-Y quadricepsplasty, in knee arthroplasty, 48: 165
Valgus deformities
after Girdlestone arthroplasty, 48: 161
neuropathic arthropathy with, 48: *274*
prioritizing surgical treatment, 48: 94
severe, 48: *106*
of the tibia, 48: *147*
Validity, of outcomes assessment instruments, 48: 668-670
Valsalva maneuver, radicular symptoms, 49: 342
Value, defineds, 48: *676*
Vancomycin
antibiotic-impregnated cement, 48: 117
appropriate use, 49: *610*-611
cement loaded with, **50: 331**
in cement spacers, **50: 372**
combined with metronidazole and aztreonam, treatment of diabetic foot infection, 48: 319
resistance to, 49: 605
wound infections, 49: 426
Vancomycin intermediately-resistant *Staphylococcus aureus* (VISA)
isolation precautions, 49: 608-611
occurence, 49: 605
Vancomycin-resistant enterococci (VRE)
isolation precautions, 49: 608-611
prevalence of, 49: 605
Vancouver classification for periprosthetic femoral fractures, 47: 241, 247
Varus deformities
distal femoral osteotomy
indications, 48: 125-126
surgical technique, 48: 126-129
medial epicondylar osteotomy, 48: 153-156
and progressive arthritis, 48: 144
Varus remodeling
femoral, 49: *123*
of the proximal femur, 48: *20*
Varus stress tests, **50: 516**
Varus-valgus angulation in tibial shaft fracture, 46: 281
Vascular anatomy
knee, 46: *165*
pelvic, 47: 280
talus, 46: *324*-325
Vascular diseases
in the diabetic foot, 48: 317
peripheral, and diabetic foot, 48: 292
Vascular injury
after revision total hip arthroplasty, 48: 44
following hip arthroplasty, 47: 279-281
and limb salvage, 46: 511
in proximal humeral fractures, 46: 31-32
in total hip arthroplasty, 48: 27-35
Vascular insufficiency, in elderly, 46: 423
Vascular insults, elbow arthroscopy, 49: 257
Vascular invasion, and autogenous bone grafts, 48: 647-648
Vascular occlusive disease, comparison with diabetic vascular disease, 48: 292
Vascular studies, in diagnosis of diabetic foot, 48: 295-297
Vascularization. *See also* Neovascularization; Revascularization
of allograft segments, 48: 179
Vascularized fibular grafts
femoral head, 49: 177-178
and Steinberg Staging System, 49: *180*
Vasodilation, and acupuncture, 49: 561
Vastus intermedius, reflected, 48: *15*
Vastus lateralis
magnitude of pull, **50: 250**
pool at osteotomy interface, **50: *250***
reflected, 48: *15*
shear forces and osteotomy interface, **50: *249***
Vastus slides
approaches, 48: *16*
exposure, 48: *14*
use of, revision total hip arthroplasty, 48: 13-17
Vaughn-Jackson syndrome, differential diagnosis, 49: 299
Venography
diagnosis of DVT, **50: 416**
preoperative investigations, total hip arthroplasty, 48: 31
Venous thromboembolism complications
in hip arthroplasty, 47: 331-335
diagnosis of, 47: 333-334
prevention of, 47: 332-333
treatment for, 47: 335
in knee arthroplasty, 46: 185-188
Ventilation, intraoperative, infection control, 49: 612
Ventilation/perfusion scan, **50: 416**
Ventral inclination angle (VCA), measurement of, **50: 254-255**
Version
component, assessment of instability, 48: 23
management of instability, 49: 125
Vertebral apophysis, slipped, 48: 536
Vertebral bodies, arthroscopic biopsy of, in lumbar and lower thoracic spine, 46: 158
Vertebral corpectomies, technique of, 48: 423-424
Vertebral height, compression of, 48: 415
Vertebral osteomyelitis, and pediatric back pain, 48: 531-532
Vertebral vein plexus, 49: *454*
Vertebral vein system, role in bone metastases, 49: 453
Vertebrate development, 47: 461-462
cartilage proliferation, 47: 464-465
growth hormones in, 47: 465
growth plate development, 47: 464
limb buds, 47: *462*-463
limb development, 47: 463-464
Vesper's curse of LaBan, 46: 147
Vibratory sensation
spinal stenosis, 49: 365
ulnar nerve compression, 49: 307

Video-assisted thoracic surgery (VATS), 46: 144-145
advantages and disadvantages, 46: 127-128
cameramonitors, insufflator, and video recorder, 46: 131
indications and contraindications, 46: 128-130, 129
operating room setup personnel and basic equipment, 46: 130-*131*
thoracoscopic instruments, 46: 131-*133*
thoracoscopic procedures
anterior release for spinal deformity, 46: 135
corpectomy for excision of tumor or fracture, 46: 135
laparoscopic approach to lumbar spine, 46: 135-137
preliminary results, 46: 138-139
surgical technique, 46: 133-135
thoracic disk herniation, 46: 135
Video printer, documentation by, 49: 226
Villonodular synovitis, knee, 49: *448*
Viruses
allograft transmission, 49: 616
blood transmission of, 48: 665
graft transmission of, **50: 469**
transmission through grafts, 49: 149, 151
transmission via allografts, 48: 64
Viscosupplementation, intra-articular hyaluronic acid, 49: 497
VISI (volar intercalated segment instability) deformity, 47: 203-206
causes of, 47: 215
defined, 47: 222
midcarpal clunk test for, 47: *216-217*
and staging for ulnar-sided perilunate instability, 47: 215-216, 218
Vitallium mini-fragment screw-and-plate construct, 46: *382*
Vitamin A, 47: 464
Vitamin C, 47: 464
Vitamin D
in osteoporosis, 46: *446,* 451-452
in regulation of cartilage proliferation, 47: 464
Vochel's bursitis, 47: 412-413
Volunteers
orthopaedists, opportunities in the developing world, 49: 575-577
short-term service, developing countries, 49: 576
teaching, 49: 576-577

W

Wages, and health insurance spending, 48: *676*
Wagner classification, ulcerations of the diabetic foot, 48: *306*
Wagner end-bearing long stem prosthesis, use of, 49: 120
Wagner-Meggitt classification, in evaluation of diabetic foot, 48: 298
Wagner osteotomy, **50: 551**
Wake-up test, **50: 308**
sciatic nerve identification, **50: 312**
Walking
biomechanics of forward human locomotion, demarcation between walking and running, 47: 397-*398*
energy demands in amputees for, 46: *501*-502
gait cycle, 47: 398, *399*
potential and kinetic energy in, 47: 398, *400*
psychological requirements in amputees, 46: 502
Walking sticks, simple construction, 49: 594-*595*
Warfarin
prevention of DVT, **50: 417-418**
as prophylactic agent after total knee replacement, 46: 186
for thromboembolic disease, 46: 188, 47: 332-333
Wartenberg sign, ulnar nerve compression, 49: 307
Wartenberg's syndrome, SRN entrapment, 49: 302-303
Washington Business Group of Health (WBGH)-Watson Wyatt Worldwide, survey of employers, 48: 676-677
Water
and hyaline cartilage, 49: 491
interstitial flow, in menisci, 49: 191
Weakness, disuse, **50: 293**
Weaknesses, spinal stenosis, **50: 150**
Wear
adhesive, **50: 165**
on bearing surfaces, 49: *73*
debris and osteonecrosis, 49: 180
fatigue, **50: 165**
metal-metal hip prostheses, **50: *166***
morphology of particles, **50: 186**
periprosthetic, **50: 185-186**
polyethylene components, **50: 165-166**
volumetric rates, effect of age, 49: 74
Wear testing
ceramic implants, 49: 45-46
cross-linked polyethylene, 49: 52-53
Weather, arthritic pain, 49: 482
Weber classification system for ankle injury, 46: 313
Weight bearing
meniscus repair rehabilitation, 49: 208
protected, for osteonecrosis, 49: 174
Weightlifter's shoulder, 47: 37
Weight reaction line, and spinal alignment, 48: *554*
Werner syndrome, 46: 497
Wheelchairs, simple construction, developing countries, 49: *596*
White blood cell (WBC) counts
in diabetic infections, 48: 297
diagnosis of arthroplasty site infection, 48: 114
exclusion of active infection, **50: 321**
infected knees, **50: 368**
laboratory investigations of bone tumors, 48: 608
periprosthetic femoral osteolysis, **50: 200-201**
White cells, inhibition of function, by methylmethacrylate, 48: 97
Whitecloud and LaRocca strut graft, 49: *350*
Whole-person impairment percents, *AMA Guides to the Evaluation of Permanent Impairment,* 4th edition, 48: *454*
Windlass mechanism
foot, **50: *522***
maximal tenderness, **50: *526***
Wires
cerclage, placement, 48: *24*
placement of, revision total hip arthroplasty, 48: *7, 8*
Wiring, prophylactic, revision total hip arthroplasty, 48: 24
WOMAC scores, results of autologous chondrocyte transplantation (ACT), 48: *637*
Work, upper extremity complaints related to, 48: 693-697
Work-related disorders, upper extremities
epidemiology, 48: 695
factors influencing reporting of, 48: 695-697
Workers' compensation, and reporting of work-related disorders, 48: 696
World Food Program (WFP), food distribution, 49: 575
World Health Organization (WHO), health programs, 49: 575
World Orthopaedic Concern (WOC)
foundation of, 49: 599-600
services in the developing world, 49: 572
Web site, 49: 573
Wound care, outpatient, for diabetic foot, 48: 300
Wound classification, in evaluation of diabetic foot, 48: 298-299
Wound excision, severely injured upper extremities, 49: 379-381
Wound healing
amputation, 46: 503-*504*
assessment of, 48: 44
collagen synthesis and, **50: 291**
comorbidities and, **50: 359-360**

in diabetics, 48: 294
effect of chemotherapeutic agents, 48: 98
factors affecting, 48: 687
and infection at arthroplasty sites, 48: 111
postoperative, total hip arthroplasty, 48: 35
thermal modification, **50: 3-11**
Wound lavage, injured upper extremities, 49: 380
Wound treatment in tibial shaft fractures, 46: 298-299
Wright test, 47: 87
Wright's maneuver, Alder nerve compression, 49: 307
Wrist. *See also* Carpus
adaptive carpal instability, **50: 131-132**
anatomy, 47: 219-220
arthritis, **50: 130-131**
arthritis following scaphoid nonunion, **50: 118-119**
arthroscopic techniques, 49: 225-235
arthroscopy, **50: 126**
carpal instability, **50: 123-134**
classification of degenerative lesions, 49: *230*
classification of traumatic injuries, 49: *230*
coronal section, 49: *226*
dorsal carpal ganglia, removal of, 49: 234-235
dorsal ganglia, **50: 130**
imaging of, 46: 523-524
for carpal instability, 47: 222-224
instability, 47: 203-208, **50: *125***
arthroscopic treatment, 49: 227-230
classification of, 49: *228*
classification scheme for, 47: 203-204
distal radioulnar joint instability, 47: 199-201, 209-213
acute, 47: 210
chronic, 47: 210-213
midcarpal (MCI), 47: 204-208
diagnosis of, 47: 204-205
Lichtman's classification for, 47: 205-206
radial-sided, 47: 219-227
diagnosis of, 47: 221-222
imaging for, 47: 222-224
treatment for scapholunate instability, 47: 224-227
ulnar-sided, 47: 215-218
mechanics, 47: 220-221
midcarpal instability, **50: *132***
reconstructive procedures, **50: 105-122**
scaphoid problems, **50: 105-122**
ulnar nerve compression of, 49: 314-316
work related illnesses, 48: 694-695

X

X-Change Acetabular Revision Instrumentation System, 48: 82
Xenografts, defined, 48: 79
Xenografts, bovine, **50: 214**
Xenon 133 skin clearance, decision making in foot amputations, 48: 323
XLPE process, polyethylene cross-linking, **50: 173**
Xylocaine (lidocaine)
treatment of spinal stenosis, **50: 153**
use of, 49: 526

Y

Yergason test, 47: 88

Z

Zanca radiographic view of acromioclavicular joint, 47: 23, *36*
after failed rotator cuff repair, 47: 88
postoperative heterotopic ossification, 47: *92*
for weight lifter's shoulder, 47: 37
Zickel supracondylar rods, 47: 439-440
Zickel nails, pathologic subtrochanteric fractures, 49: 465
Zirconia, physical properties of, **50: *167***
Zirconia ceramics
surface of, 49: 75
in THA, 49: 43